MEDICAL MICROBIOLOGY

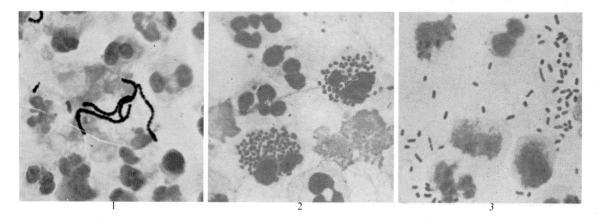

Plate 1   Gram-stained film of pus containing *Streptococcus pyogenes*. Streptococci can be seen in pairs and in chains of varying length; the chain length is no guide to the cultural type of streptococcus. × 1000. (From Gillies and Dodds *Bacteriology Illustrated*, 3rd edn. Churchill Livingstone, 1973.)

Plate 2   A Gram-stained film of the centrifuged deposit of cerebrospinal fluid from a case of acute meningitis. Two poly-morphonuclear leucocytes are crammed with Gram-negative diplococci; this intracellular appearance is typical of the patho-genic neisseriae. On cultivation a pure growth of oxidase-positive organisms proved on biochemical testing to be *N. meningitidis*. × 1000. (From Gillies and Dodds *Bacteriology Illustrated*, 3rd edn. Churchill Livingstone, 1973.)

Plate 3   Gram-stained film of urinary deposit showing Gram-negative bacilli and polymorphonuclear leucocytes; some of the latter are disintegrating. The bacilli, which are morphologically indistinguishable from other enterobacteria by Gram's method, were shown to belong to the genus *Klebsiella*. × 1000. (From Gillies and Dodds *Bacteriology Illustrated*, 3rd edn. Churchill Livingstone, 1967.)

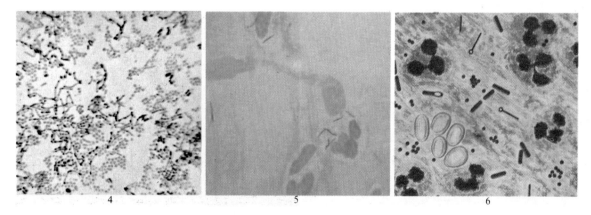

Plate 4   Film, stained by Albert's method, of material harvested from Loeffler's serum medium from a patient with sore throat and exudate. *C. diphtheriae* appear as slender straight or slightly curved bacilli coloured green with volutin granules stained black. The green-stained cocci were noted as *Strept. pyogenes* by parallel cultivation on blood agar. × 1000. (From Gillies and Dodds *Bacteriology Illustrated*, 3rd edn. Churchill Livingstone, 1973.)

Plate 5   Film of concentrated specimen of sputum stained by the Ziehl-Neelsen method. Acid- and alcohol-fast bacilli can be noted: saprophytic members of the genus are acid-fast only. × 1000. (From Gillies and Dodds *Bacteriology Illustrated*, 3rd edn. Churchill Livingstone, 1973.)

Plate 6   This Gram-stained film of material from a wound shows pus cells and clumps of Gram-positive cocci which on culture proved to be coagulase positive staphylococci. Two species of *Clostridia* were also isolated, *Cl. tetani* which is repre-sented by the slender Gram-positive rods and also rods with spherical, terminal and projecting spores (drumstick) which have stained Gram-negatively. The stouter Gram-positive bacilli, some of which bear oval, sub-terminal, projecting spores were identified as *Cl. oedematiens*. (From Gillies and Dodds *Bacteriology Illustrated*, 3rd edn. Churchill Livingstone, 1973.)

CHURCHILL LIVINGSTONE

Medical Division of Longman Group Limited

Represented in the United States of America by Longman Inc., New York, and by associated companies, branches and representatives throughout the world.

© **Longman Group Limited 1973**

First edition	1925
Second Edition	1928
Third Edition	1931
Fourth Edition	1934
Fifth Edition	1938
Sixth Edition	1942
Seventh Edition	1945
Reprinted	1946
Eighth Edition	1948
Reprinted	1949
Reprinted	1950
Ninth Edition	1953
Reprinted	1956
Reprinted	1959
Tenth Edition	1960
Reprinted	1962
Eleventh Edition	1965
Revised Reprint	1968
Reprinted	1969
Reprinted	1970
Reprinted	1972
E L B S Edition first published	1965
Reprinted	1968, 1969, 1970, 1972
Twelfth Edition, Vol. 1	1973
Reprinted	1975
E L B S Edition of Twelfth Edition Vol. 1	1974

ISBN 0 443 01099 4 (limp)

0 443 01202 4 (cased)

Library of Congress Catalog Card Number 73-86121

Printed in Great Britain

PREFACE

There are several good reasons for the publication
of a new edition of this textbook on Medical
Microbiology. The last (11th) edition was first
published in 1965; despite numerous reprintings,
there has been only one revised reprint, and in a
rapidly expanding specialty like microbiology,
textbooks soon become outdated. In the last
edition, a considerable expansion of the text had
given the book a middle-aged spread but a more
serious defect from the viewpoint of the medical
student and the young doctor was the large amount
of space allocated to laboratory procedures of
interest mainly to professional and technical staff
concerned with the isolation and identification of
pathogenic microbes. It may, however, be noted
that the English Language Book Society (E.L.B.S.)
paperback edition has become popular in many
Commonwealth and other English-speaking
countries, probably because of its comprehensive
coverage of the subject. The time seemed opportune
to separate the contents into two volumes—
Volume 1 aimed primarily at medical and science
students and doctors, and Volume 11 directed to
professional and technical laboratory staff—the
'bench book' which will be published within the
next few months.

Medical textbooks have not always been popular
with the undergraduate student, partly because
they tend to be overloaded with scientific and
technical details of interest mainly to the specialist.
In Volume 1 of this 12th edition of *Medical
Microbiology*, we have aimed to present a well-
illustrated text which the student would find to be
interesting as well as informative—and without too
much technical detail. At the same time, recent
outgrowths in the broad field of microbiology, e.g.,
microbial genetics and immunology, have been
given additional attention.

Volume 1 is divided into five parts: Part 1 deals
with microbial anatomy and physiology and the
basic principles of infection and immunity; Parts 2
and 3 are concerned with the common bacterial

and viral infections with emphasis on the pathogenesis of the infection. sources and modes of
spread of the pathogen in the community and
methods for the diagnosis, control and prevention
of the infection; Part 4 is devoted to (a) infections
by small microorganisms (chlamydia, rickettsia and
mycoplasma) formerly thought to bridge the gap
between bacteria and viruses, and (b) to the
common protozoal and fungal infections of man.
In Part 5, some of the more applied aspects in the
laboratory diagnosis and treatment of infective
syndromes and in the epidemiology and prevention
of community, including hospital, infections are
discussed.
Every chapter dealing with specific pathogens has
been re-written, a number of new chapters have
been added and new contributors co-opted. The
editorial staff has been augmented by the inclusion
of Professor B. P. Marmion. Although this textbook was born and nurtured in the Department of
Bacteriology, Edinburgh University, inevitably some
of the contributors have sought new pastures
whilst a satellite colony has been formed by
Professor J. P. Duguid and his colleagues in the
Bacteriology Department of Dundee University.
As in the assessment and preparation of previous
editions, we have had most valuable criticisms,
comments and constructive suggestions from
many colleagues, both in Britain and overseas.
To them and to our helpful and patient publishers,
we express our sincerest gratitude.

October, 1973.   The Editors.

LIST OF CONTRIBUTORS
and the topics and pathogens for which they have had sole or shared responsibility

JOYCE D. COGHLAN, B.Sc., Ph.D.
Brucella; pasteurella group; leptospira.

J. G. COLLEE, M.D., M.R.C.Path.
Bacterial morphology and classification; sterilization and disinfection; bacterial genetics; clostridia; bacteroides.

R. CRUICKSHANK, C.B.E., M.D., F.R.C.P., F.R.C.P.E., D.P.H., F.R.S.E., Hon.Ll.D.
Microbiology and medicine; bacterial pathogenicity; epidemiology of community infections; prophylactic immunization; streptococcus; pneumococcus; neisseria; bordetella; haemophilus; corynebacterium; erysipelothrix; listeria; mycobacterium; vibrio; spirillum; rabies virus.

J. P. DUGUID, M.D., B.Sc., F.R.C.Path.[1]
Bacterial morphology and classification; sterilization and disinfection; infection in the community; staphylococcus; lactobacillus; dental caries; pathogenic fungi.

A. G. FRASER, B.Sc., M.B., Ch.B.
Bacterial genetics.

R. R. GILLIES, M.D., F.R.C.P.E., M.R.C.Path., D.P.H.
Salmonella; shigella; escherichia; other enterobacteriaceae; proteus; pseudomonas; loefflerella; actinomyces; nocardia.

J. C. GOULD, B.Sc., M.D., F.R.C.P.E., F.R.C.Path., F.R.S.E.
Strategy of antimicrobial therapy; epidemiology of community infections.

D. M. GREEN, M.D., F.R.C.Path.[1]
Anthrax; picornaviruses; infective syndromes.

W. H. R. LUMSDEN, M.B., D.Sc., F.R.C.P.E., F.R.S.E.[3]
Arboviruses; protozoal infections.

---

[1] Department of Bacteriology, University of Dundee.
[2] Central Microbiological Laboratories, Edinburgh.
[3] Department of Medical Protozoology, London School of Hygiene and Tropical Medicine.

B. P. MARMION, M.D., D.Sc., F.R.C.Path., F.R.C.P.E., F.R.S.E.

Hepatitis viruses; chlamydia; rickettsia; mycoplasma.

J. M. K. MACKAY, M.R.C.V.S., Ph.D.

Slow and oncogenic viruses.

J. F. PEUTHERER, B.Sc., M.B., Ch.B.

Viruses; virus-cell interaction; virus genetics; antiviral agents; herpes viruses.

R. H. A. SWAIN, M.A., M.D., F.R.C.P.E., F.R.C.Path., F.R.S.E.

Viruses; virus infections; treponema; borrelia; poxviruses; adenoviruses; myxoviruses; paramyxoviruses; rubella; corona and arenaviruses.

A. T. WALLACE, M.D., F.R.C.Path., M.R.C.P.E., D.P.H.[4]

Atypical mycobacteria.

D. M. WEIR, M.D.

Immunological principles; natural and acquired immunity; hypersensitivity; autoimmunity.

J. F. WILKINSON, M.A., Ph.D.[5]

Bacterial growth and nutrition; action of antimicrobial drugs.

A. M. M. WILSON, B.A., B.M., B.Ch., F.R.C.Path., Dip.Bact.

Pathogenic fungi.

[4] Bacteriology Laboratory, City Hospital, Edinburgh.
[5] Department of Microbiology, School of Agriculture, University of Edinburgh.

CONTENTS

PART 3   PATHOGENIC VIRUSES AND ASSOCIATED DISEASES

**PART 4   OTHER PATHOGENIC MICROORGANISMS AND
            ASSOCIATED DISEASES**

Volume I: Part I
Microbial Biology: Infection and Immunity

1. Microbiology and Medicine

Microbiology is, as a biological science, just over a century old. Although its ancestry is rather nebulous, the first productive seed was implanted by a French chemist, Louis Pasteur, who a century ago was persuaded to turn his inquisitive mind from a study of tartrate crystals to the troubles that were affecting the wine industry in France. Pasteur, brooding over the age-old phenomenon of fermentation, which has given us both bread and wine, was not prepared to accept the pontifical pronouncements of the leading chemists of the day that this was a purely chemical reaction. Having satisfied himself that the souring of milk was due to the formation of lactic acid by multiplying bacteria, he proceeded to turn sugar into alcohol with only ammonia and some organic salts as a source of nutrient for the growing yeast cells. He concluded his paper in 1857 with these words: 'Alcoholic fermentation is an act correlated with the life and with the organization of these (yeast) globules, and not with their death or their putrefaction'.

In his early work in microbiology Pasteur also made the fundamental observation that certain bacteria (which he called *anaerobic*) would grow only in the absence of oxygen, a momentous discovery at a time when oxygen was still regarded as the essential elixir for all living creatures. A few years later, his monograph on 'The Study of Wines' and his demonstration of the value of differential heating—or *pasteurization* as we now call it—revolutionized the whole wine and beer industry of Europe and established the importance of microbiology in industry.

Joseph Lister (1867), an English surgeon working in Scotland, saw in Pasteur's work on fermentation a possible explanation of the tragic fate that befell so many of his patients who after compound fracture or amputation were dying in large numbers from hospital gangrene and 'blood poisoning'. By treating the wound with carbolic acid and covering it with a phenolic dressing, he prevented bacterial growth in the exudate and so satisfied himself that putrefaction or sepsis was caused, like fermentation, by these invisible but living microbes which Leeuwenhoek (1675), two centuries earlier, had called his 'little animals'. Some years before Lister's work, Semmelweis (1848), an obstetric surgeon in Vienna, proved in one of the first controlled trials that disinfection of the hands in chloride of lime by students and surgeons after examination of a patient or the performance of a necropsy reduced the case-fatality from puerperal sepsis from 8·3 to 2·3 per cent in the hospital teaching clinic, that is, to a rate equivalent to that in the midwife clinic or in private practice.

In an era dominated by the physical sciences it required great courage and pertinacity as well as ingenuity and technical skill for these pioneers in microbiology to persuade their fellows of the validity of the new gospel. However, they had strong support from one of the outstanding physicists of the day, John Tyndall (1877), who interested himself in the new biological science and gave us intermittent sterilization (or *tyndallization*) as a method for destroying sporing bacteria; he was, incidentally, one of the first observers to note the antibacterial properties of the mould penicillium. About this time (1876) Robert Koch, a country doctor in Germany, became acutely aware of the havoc which a disease called 'splenic fever', or anthrax, was causing among the sheep and cattle of the farming community. By most ingenious methods devised in a home-made laboratory, Koch was able to prove that a large square-ended sporing rod was constantly present in the blood of animals dying of anthrax, and that the bacilli or spores derived from them could reproduce septicaemic anthrax in mice. Later, after further experience with anthrax and tuberculosis, he formulated the well-known Koch's postulates (1884) which must be fulfilled before a specific microorganism was accepted as the cause of a specific disease. These required, in addition to the constant presence of the microorganism in the tissues of the naturally infected host, that it be grown artificially in *pure culture* (for this he devised boiled potato slices and nutrient gelatin as *solid media*) and after many subcultures should reproduce the specific disease when inoculated into a susceptible animal. And so, by the eighteen eighties, the new science of microbiology was firmly founded and its importance in the economy of men, animals and industry was beginning to be appreciated.

Pasteur was again a pioneer in two early offshoots of this science—immunology and virology. He was the first to extend Jenner's (1794) protective *vaccination* (vacca – cow), a word coined by Pasteur in honour of Jenner's work with cowpox, by the use of living attenuated cultures of pathogenic microbes against important infections like anthrax, swine erysipelas and chicken cholera. Today the *attenuated vaccine* is being used with outstanding success in such diverse diseases as tuberculosis, yellow fever, poliomyelitis, dog distemper and contagious abortion of cattle.

Pasteur's contribution to animal virology was equally fertile. From his boyhood days in the Jura hills, he had known of the horrible deaths that might follow the bite of a wolf or a mad dog, and in due course he turned his attention to the aetiology of rabies. After some false trails, his assistant Roux eventually injected some of the infective material from the brain of a fatal case into the brain of a dog, which fourteen days later developed rabies. Thus the use of selective living tissue for the growth of viruses—which today is practised on an enormous scale—was born in Pasteur's laboratory and this experimental work with rabies led on to the anti-rabies vaccine which was his last great effort in the field of immunology. Later, the demonstration of bacterial toxins by both French and German workers was the precursor of antitoxin therapy through the experimental studies of von Behring who showed that the serum of animals given inoculations of sublethal doses of diphtheria or tetanus toxin could specifically neutralize these toxins *in vitro* and *in vivo*.

Ehrlich who like von Behring was trained in Koch's laboratory later developed an analogous concept of chemotherapy whereby his 'magic bullets' would specifically attack the invading parasite. His success with Hata (1906) in the treatment of syphilis with an organic arsenical,

Salvarsan (or 606) was followed in time by the flowering of chemotherapy, pioneered by the discoveries of penicillin by Fleming, a Scot, in 1929 and of prontosil (the prototype of the sulphonamides) by Domagk, a German, in 1930.

This brief historical sketch illustrates the importance of microbiology as an applied science, particularly in fermentation processes and in infectious diseases. The term *microbiology*, 'biology of the small organisms', is preferred to *bacteriology* since it includes in the present context viruses, fungi and protozoa in addition to bacteria. Only a small proportion of the myriads of microorganisms that abound in nature are disease-producing or *pathogenic* for man. The majority of microorganisms are *free living* in soil, water and similar natural habitats, and are unable to invade the living human or animal body. Some free-living microorganisms obtain their energy from daylight or by oxidation of inorganic matter, but most feed on dead organic matter; these last microorganisms are termed *saprophytes* ('grow on dead matter'). In contrast, a *parasite* is defined as a microorganism or a larger species (e.g. helminth) that lives in or on, and obtains nourishment from, a living host. Parasitic microorganisms are either commensal or pathogenic. *Commensals* (table companions) constitute the normal flora of the healthy body. They live on the skin and on the mucous membranes of the upper respiratory tract, the intestinal and female genital canals, and obtain nourishment from the secretions and food residues. Since normally they do not invade the tissues, they are generally harmless, though under certain circumstances, usually when the body's defences are impaired, they may invade the tissues and cause disease, thus acting as *opportunistic pathogens*. True pathogens are the parasitic microorganisms that are adapted to overcoming the normal defences of the body and invading the tissues; their growth in the tissues, or their production of poisonous substances, or *toxins*, often causes damage to the tissues and thus the manifestations of disease.

MICROBIOLOGY AND THE PATIENT

Medical microbiology is concerned with the *aetiology* (causation), *pathogenesis* (mechanism of attack on tissues), laboratory diagnosis and treatment of infection in the individual and with the *epidemiology* (study of mass disease among the people) and control or prevention of infection in the community. It therefore has close links with several other disciplines into which the training of the doctor has been divided to form the medical curriculum, e.g. pathology, clinical medicine and surgery, pharmacology and therapeutics, and preventive medicine.

The changes that occur in the host's tissues as the result of infection are often recognized by the pathologist as specific or pathognomonic of a particular pathogenic microorganism, e.g. the circumscribed boil of the staphylococcus, the spreading cellulitis of the streptococcus, the red liver-like appearance (hepatization) of the lung in pneumococcal pneumonia, the tubercles and the subsequent necrotic changes (called caseation) of tuberculosis, the aortic disease and granulomata (gummata) of syphilis, and the typical intestinal ulcerations of typhoid fever and the dysenteries. But the prudent pathologist will usually seek to confirm his diagnosis of the cause of these macroscopic changes by taking smears and preparing cultures from the lesions to demonstrate the microscopic germ. The pathology of infection provides a fascinating but relatively unexplored field of study since it includes the affinity of pathogens for particular tissues and the initiation of infection as well as the characteristic tissue reactions.

Microbiology has a close link with curative medicine in regard to the precise diagnosis and the rational treatment of microbial diseases. The doctor engaged in the care of sick patients will often be able to identify the pathogenic microorganisms from the typical clinical features of an infection and will accordingly prescribe the appropriate treatment. Sometimes, however, the patient presents with a fever but no characteristic signs or symptoms that will allow the doctor to make a precise diagnosis; this pyrexia of unknown—or uncertain—origin (PUO) will require laboratory help to elucidate the cause of the fever. Even when the doctor identifies the disease from the patient's signs or symptoms— sore throat, acute diarrhoea, pneumonia, meningitis—he will still need laboratory help since many of these syndromes are caused by different kinds of microorganisms, e.g. acute diarrhoea

may be due to a wide range of pathogenic bacteria, protozoa and possibly viruses. Therefore with modern selective *chemotherapy* the effective treatment of the patient with a clinical infection requires the early isolation and identification of the infecting microorganisms and tests for its drug-sensitivities. In other words, the doctor has to identify and treat specific infections rather than clinical syndromes. When an infection is not amenable to chemotherapy as is the case with the toxic infections and most virus infections, *antisera* containing neutralizing antibodies against the pathogenic agent (either specially prepared in animals like the horse or derived from human blood containing the specific antibodies, called immunoglobulins), may be used either to treat the patient as in diphtheria or to give temporary (passive) protection to a person exposed to the risk of infection as in measles or tetanus.

MICROBIOLOGY AND THE COMMUNITY

Microbiology is closely concerned with the epidemiology and the control of infection in any community where the transmission and disease-producing capacity of the infecting microorganisms may be facilitated by environmental or host factors, e.g. overcrowding, contaminated food, drink or air, malnutrition, tissue damage. The term epidemiology has in the past been applied particularly to the study of the factors contributing to the endemic or epidemic prevalence of an infectious or communicable disease; but, as the name implies, it may be concerned with the distribution and determinants of any disease or disability in the community and in recent years epidemiological methods have been applied to many non-infective conditions. As a medical science, epidemiology is particularly concerned with aetiological factors and it has had remarkable successes in their elucidation among both infectious and noninfectious diseases. Thus, the evidence that cholera and typhoid fever were due to living agents spread by water was produced from epidemiological data collected respectively by John Snow, a London anaesthetist and William Budd, a West Country doctor, 30 to 40 years before the aetiological agents were identified. Pellagra was shown by Goldberger to be a deficiency disease long before vitamins were defined. While in our own time, heavy cigarette smoking has been proved to be causally related to lung cancer although the carcinogenic agent has not yet been identified.

Certain infections are not ordinarily transmissible from one person to another because they are due to opportunistic invasion of tissues by commensal microorganisms previously resident elsewhere in the body, e.g. urinary tract infections or subacute bacterial endocarditis, and for these the term *endogenous* (originating from within) infection may be used. Most of the common fevers—measles, whooping-cough, chickenpox, etc., are *infectious* or *communicable* diseases in the sense that they are transmissible from one person to another and are therefore called *exogenous* (originating from without) infections. Other infections that are transmissible from vertebrate animal hosts to man, called the *zoonoses*, are not ordinarily communicable from man to man, e.g. bubonic plague, brucellosis, rabies; the same is true of some infections derived from microbes in the soil, e.g. tetanus.

In the study of the sources and modes of spread of infectious diseases, the importance of *carriers* was first demonstrated when on Koch's recommendation 'bacteriological stations' were established around 1900 in typhoid-ridden parts of Germany. Combined bacteriological and epidemiological studies brought to light convalescent and more persistent stool excreters of typhoid bacilli, and these findings with other data confirmed Koch's hypothesis that in typhoid fever the acute or convalescent patient was a common source for further infection. Later it was shown that carriers, that is, individuals who while not showing any clinical symptoms of infection, carry and disperse a pathogenic microorganism, were important links in the chain of dissemination of various infections in a community. Again, tests for the presence of antibodies to specific pathogens or their toxins have shown that inapparent infections may play an important part in raising the resistance of a community to epidemic outbursts of disease. With a good knowledge of the epidemiology of a specific communicable disease, the Health Officer concerned with preventive medicine, knows what measures for its control are most likely to be effective and here again, in the field of prophylactic immunization, the microbiologist has been a most valuable partner.

Mortality and Morbidity Rates

In the economically more developed countries the past century has seen a phenomenal decrease in the death rate from infections. Some examples may be taken from Scotland, a small but representative country, where the population has increased from approximately 2·5 millions in 1865 to 5·0 millions in 1965. Deaths from the principal infectious diseases contributed, at a rate of 1 167 per 100 000 population, more than half the total deaths in the quinquennium to 1865 whereas in the corresponding five years to 1965 they were reduced to one tenth (111 per 100 000) of the earlier death rate, and constituted less than one tenth of the total deaths. The main causes of death among the infections a century ago were tuberculosis, pneumonia and bronchitis, diarrhoeal diseases (including typhoid fever) and scarlet fever whereas in the period 1961–65 only pneumonia and bronchitis took a heavy toll of life; the death rates from tuberculosis (8·2 per 100 000) and the diarrhoeal diseases (2·3 per 100 000) have fallen precipitously and scarlet fever has become a mild non-hospitalized infection although rheumatic heart

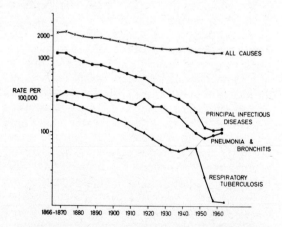

FIG. 1.1. Crude death rates in Scotland per 100 000 population for all causes, principal infectious diseases, pneumonia and bronchitis, and respiratory tuberculosis. Five year averages 1866–1965.

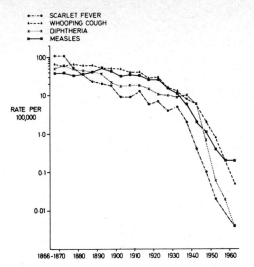

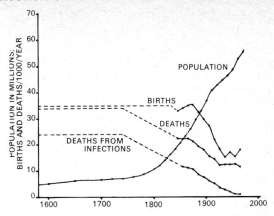

FIG. 1.4. Schematic representation of birth rates, death rates (total and for infectious diseases) and population growth in Britain from 1600 to 1965.

FIG. 1.2. Death rates from scarlet fever, whooping-cough, measles and diphtheria per 100 000 population in Scotland, five year averages 1866–1965.

disease, a sequela of streptococcal infection, still has a relatively high death-rate (14·2 per 100 000). The dramatic decline in the death rates in Scotland from most of the main infectious diseases during the past century is illustrated in Figs. 1.1, 1.2 and 1.3; this decline has been a major contributor to the so-called 'population explosion' since it was not accompanied by a sufficiently great decline in the birth rate as is illustrated in Fig. 1.4.

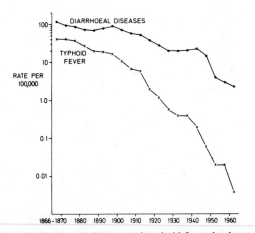

FIG. 1.3. Diarrhoeal diseases and typhoid fever death rates per 100 000 of population in Scotland. Five year averages, 1866–1965.

The extraordinary reduction in deaths from infection initiated by improvements in nutrition, environmental sanitation and living conditions, and accelerated in the past 30 years by the increasing range and use of antimicrobial drugs, has led to a widespread belief, particularly among hospital staff, that infection has ceased to be a major health problem. Unfortunately, the rapid decline in mortality rates has not been paralleled by a corresponding decline in morbidity rates in a wide range of infections. Indeed, infection is still the major cause of sickness in children as is illustrated by the data in the Newcastle thousand-families study (Miller *et al.*, 1960). There, in a large city, 847 children had 8 467 significant incidents of illness in the first five years of life: of these, 6 845 (80 per cent) were infections, half of them respiratory (colds, sore throat, febrile catarrh, bronchitis), rather more than one fifth were specific fevers (measles, whooping cough, chickenpox, mumps, etc.) and one tenth were diarrhoeal diseases; staphylococcal infections contributed 5 per cent and pyrexias of unknown origin (PUO) 3 per cent. In a comprehensive study of disease and disability in general practice during one year (1955–56), involving 171 doctors in 106 practices, the large part which infections played in doctors' consultations and time was again very manifest. The great mass of data has been analysed and published in three reports of which Volume III is a selectively narrative and epidemiological account of the main infections and other diseases seen in general practice; it deserves to be widely read by students and teachers of medicine (Report, 1962). Most of these illnesses do not require hospital care and are therefore seldom seen by students in training; yet the infections, if not treated promptly and effectively, may lead to impairment of physical or mental development or death. It has been estimated that more than 1 000 children between 3 months and 14 years of age die each year in Britain as a result of primary infection and in at least another 2 000, infection is a contributory cause; a high proportion of these deaths are preventable by early and accurate diagnosis (Selwyn and Bain, 1965). Laboratory services for general practitioners are therefore essential and are nowadays available in most areas; good liaison between the practitioner and the microbiologist will help to improve the quality of patient care in the community (see Chapter 30 and Thomson, 1971).

A community infection of a special kind still occurs among patients congregated in hospitals (nosocomial infections). Although the consequences of hospital cross-infection are much less serious than they were in Lister's day, we are reminded of the aphorisms of two great hospital reformers of the nineteenth century—Florence Nightingale's pungent comment that 'the first requirement of any hospital (is) that it do the sick no harm' and Sir James Y. Simpson's conclusions after a most remarkable epidemiological survey of deaths from infection following amputations that 'in treatment of the sick, there is ever danger in their aggregation and safety only in their segregation; and our hospitals should be constructed so as to avoid . . . the former and secure . . . the latter condition'. We are still far from achieving these worthy objectives.

Most of the major pestilences—typhus and typhoid fever, plague, cholera, smallpox and yellow fever—that used to decimate armies and beleaguered cities or spread like wild-fire round the world are now being controlled by good environmental sanitation, by the destruction of insect vectors such as louse, flea and mosquito, or by prophylactic vaccination. However, some of these great plagues, together with other global infections like malaria, tuberculosis and leprosy, the diarrhoeal diseases and the pneumonias, still take a heavy toll of life and health in most of the developing countries.

MICROBIOLOGY AND BASIC SCIENCES

Microbiology owed much of its early recognition to its usefulness in medicine, agriculture and industry. But it soon became obvious that the bacterial cell and its products had many attractions for the general biologist, the chemist, the physicist, the geneticist, the pharmacologist and other scientists as well as the bacteriologist, immunologist and pathologist. In its free living form, the bacterial cell with its simple food requirements, rapid growth and remarkable plasticity, and its great range of enzymes and diffusible products is very suitable for detailed study and, in the past few decades, bacterial physiology (sometimes called microbial chemistry) has made many contributions to advances in our knowledge of cellular and molecular biology. Together with bacteriophage (its own particular parasite) the bacterial cell has been specially useful in advancing the science of genetics while the biochemist interested in enzymology finds it a most valuable granary. Although many of the developments in general microbiology are not immediately relevant to medicine, it is essential that the medical student should have some understanding of the anatomy, physiology, genetic behaviour and interaction with host tissues of the microbial cell and these aspects of microbiology are discussed in the chapters that follow in Part I.

REFERENCES AND FURTHER READING

BROCK, T. D. (1961) *Milestones in Microbiology*. Translated by N. J. Englewood. London: Prentice Hall.

BULLOCH, W. (1960) *The History of Bacteriology*. London: Oxford University Press.

BURNET, F. M. (1962) *Natural History of Infectious Diseases*. 3rd edn. Cambridge University Press.

DUBOS, R. (1950) *Louis Pasteur, Free Lance of Science*. Boston: Little Brown.

FOSTER, W. D. (1970) *A History of Medical Bacteriology and Immunology*. London: Cox and Wyman, Ltd.

GODLEE, R. J. (1917) *Lord Lister*. London: Macmillan.

KRUIF, DE P. (1958) *Microbe Hunters*. London: Hutchinson.

LEDINGHAM, J. C. G. & ARKWRIGHT, J. A. (1912) *The Carrier Problem in Infectious Diseases*. London: Arnold.

MAUROIS, A. (1959) *The Life of Sir Alexander Fleming, Discoverer of Penicillin*. London: Cape.

MILLER, F. J. W., COURT, S. D. M., WALTON, W. S. & KNOX,

E. G. (1960) *Growing Up in Newcastle-upon-Tyne*. London: Oxford University Press.

REPORT (1962) *Studies on Medical and Population Subjects*: No. 14. Morbidity Statistics from General Practice. Volume III. (Disease in General Practice.) H.M.S.O. London.

SMITH, T. (1934) *Parasitism and Disease*. Princeton: University Press.

SELWYN, S. & BAIN, A. D. (1965) Deaths in childhood due to infection. *British Journal of Preventive and Social Medicine*, **19**, 123.

THOMSON, W. A. R. (1971) *Calling the Laboratory*, 3rd edn. Edinburgh and London: Churchill Livingstone.

WINSLOW, C. E. A. (1943) *The Conquest of Epidemic Disease: a Chapter in the History of Ideas*. Princeton: University Press.

ZINSSER, H. (1937) *Rats, Lice and History*. London: Routledge.

2. Morphology and Nature of Bacteria

Living material, or protoplasm, is organized in units known as *cells*. Each cell consists of a body of protoplasm, the *protoplast*, enclosed by a thin semipermeable membrane, the *cytoplasmic membrane* or *plasma membrane*, and also, in some cases, by an outer, relatively rigid *cell wall*. The protoplast is differentiated into a major part, the *cytoplasm*, and an inner body, the *nucleus*, which contains the hereditary determinants of character, the *genes*, borne on thread-like *chromosomes*.

Microorganisms are generally regarded as living forms that are microscopical in size and relatively simple, usually unicellular, in structure. The diameter of the smallest body that can be resolved and seen clearly with the naked eye is about 100 μm. All but a few of the microorganisms are smaller than this and a microscope is therefore necessary for their observation. However, when bacteria or fungi are allowed to grow on a relatively solid supporting medium, their numerous progeny accumulate locally to form *colonies* and these colonies are readily visible to the naked eye.

Biologists have found it useful to draw a clear distinction between relatively primitive (*prokaryotic*) cells and more advanced (*eukaryotic*) cells (Stanier and van Niel, 1962). The bacteria and related organisms (rickettsiae, chlamydiae and mycoplasmas—see Chapter 4) are prokaryotic cells whereas the cells of fungi, protozoa, plants and animals are eukaryotic. The main distinguishing features of the prokaryotic cell are as follows:

(1) Its nucleus appears as a simple, homogeneous body not possessing a nuclear membrane separating it from the cytoplasm, nor a nucleolus, nor a spindle, nor a number of separate non-identical chromosomes. (2) It lacks the internal membranes isolating the respiratory and photosynthetic enzyme systems in specific organelles, comparable with the membrane-bounded mitochondria and chloroplasts of eukaryotic cells. Thus, the respiratory enzymes in bacteria are located mainly in the peripheral cytoplasmic membrane and their effective functioning is dependent upon the integrity of the cell protoplast as a whole. (3) Its rigid cell wall contains as its main strengthening element a specific mucopeptide substance not found in eukaryotic organisms. This mucopeptide is the 'target' of the antibacterial actions of penicillin, D-cycloserine and lysozyme.

The bodies of higher plants and animals are multicellular, with interdependence and specialization of function amongst the cells, the different kinds of cells being segregated in separate tissues. Many microorganisms, on the other hand, are unicellular, existing as single cells, unattached to their fellows. Other microorganisms grow as aggregates of cells joined together by their cell walls in clusters, chains, rods, filaments (hyphae) or mycelia (i.e. meshworks of branching filaments). Generally, these morphologically multicellular microbes are physiologically unicellular, each cell being self-sufficient and, if isolated artificially, able to nourish itself, grow and reproduce the species. Some specialization of cell function, approaching that of true multicellular organisms, is encountered in colonies of moulds and filamentous 'higher' bacteria in which certain cells form an aerial mycelium and are specialized for the formation and dissemination of spores; these cells are dependent for their nutrition on the activities of other cells comprising a vegetative mycelium.

In summary, bacteria are small microorganisms with a prokaryotic form of cellular organization. They are generally unicellular, but the cells may grow attached to one another in clusters, chains, rods, filaments or, as in the 'higher bacteria' (*Actinomycetales*), a mycelium. Their cells are smaller (usually between 0·4 and 1·5 μm in short diameter) than those of fungi and protozoa (Chaps. 53 and 54), and in most cases they have relatively rigid cell walls that maintain their characteristic shape; this may be spherical (coccus), rod-shaped (bacillus), comma-shaped (vibrio), spiral (spirillum and spirochaete), or filamentous (Fig. 2.1). They

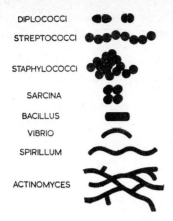

DIPLOCOCCI

STREPTOCOCCI

STAPHYLOCOCCI

SARCINA

BACILLUS

VIBRIO

SPIRILLUM

ACTINOMYCES

FIG. 2.1. The shapes and characteristic groupings of various bacterial cells.

show little structural differentiation when examined by ordinary microscopical methods.

ANATOMY OF THE BACTERIAL CELL

The principal structures of the bacterial cell are shown in Fig. 2.2. The *protoplast*, i.e. the whole body of living material (*protoplasm*), is bounded peripherally by a very thin, elastic and semi-permeable cytoplasmic membrane. Outside, and closely covering this, lies the rigid, supporting *cell wall*, which is porous and relatively permeable. Cell division occurs by the development, from the periphery inwards, of a transverse cytoplasmic membrane and a transverse cell wall, or *cross wall*.

The *cytoplasm*, or main part of the protoplasm, consists of a watery sap packed with large numbers of small granules called *ribosomes* and a few convoluted membranous bodies called *mesosomes* (see below). The nuclear material may be referred to as the *nuclear body* or *chromatin*; the word *nucleus* is now generally accepted—provided that it is borne in mind that the bacterial nucleus is not normally seen with the light microscope. Plate 2.1 is an electron-micrograph of a thin section of a dividing bacterial cell.

In addition to these essential structures, other intracellular and extracellular structures may be present in some species of bacteria; their occurrence sometimes depends upon particular conditions of growth. *Inclusion granules* of storage products such as volutin (polyphosphate), lipid (poly-β-hydroxybutyrate), glycogen or starch may occur in the cytoplasm. Outside the cell wall, there may be a protective gelatinous covering layer called a *capsule* or, when it is too

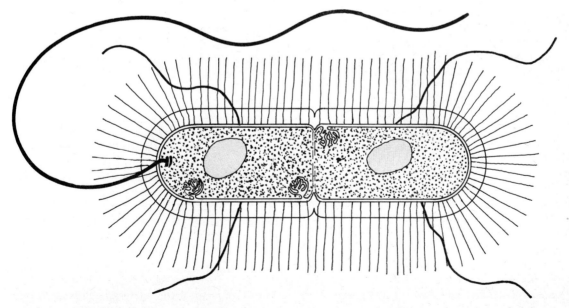

FIG. 2.2. A diagram of a dividing bacterial cell with a single flagellum, four sex fimbriae, numerous common fimbriae, a cell wall, a cytoplasmic membrane, two nuclear bodies, three mesosomes and numerous ribosomes.

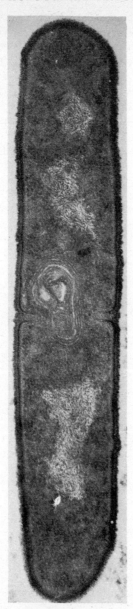

PLATE 2.1. A thin section of a dividing bacillus showing cell wall, cytoplasmic membrane, ribosomes, a developing cross-wall, and a mesosome. (By courtesy of Dr P. J. Highton and editors of *Journal of Ultrastructure Research.*) ×50 000.

the cell wall, one or both of two kinds of fila-mentous appendages, (1) *flagella*, which are organs of locomotion, and (2) *fimbriae* (syn. pili), which appear to be organs of adhesion. Because they are exposed to contact and inter-action with the cells and humoral substances of the body of the host, the surface structures of bacteria—the cell wall, capsule or microcapsule, flagella and fimbriae—are the structures most likely to have special roles in the processes of infection.

Bacterial Nucleus (DNA)

The genetic information of a bacterial cell is contained in a single long molecule of double-stranded deoxyribonucleic acid (DNA) which occurs in the form of a closed circle. It can be extracted in the form of a circular thread about 1 000 μm long, but it is coiled and tightly packed up in a bundle resembling a skein of woollen thread. Geneticists refer to it as the chromo-some. As it is not bound to proteins, it does not stain like a eukaryotic chromosome and in un-stained bacteria examined normally with the light microscope or in bacteria stained by the usual methods, there is no obvious differentia-tion into nucleus and cytoplasm. The appear-ance of the nuclear body in ultrathin sections examined with the electron microscope is com-patible with the bacterial chromosome occurring as a very long thin fibre folded backwards and forwards on itself. Only a single nuclear body is present in some cells, whilst in others, as a result of nuclear division preceding cell division, two, four or even more rounded, ovoid or irregularly shaped nuclear bodies may be present. These can be revealed by special staining procedures. Unlike the intracellular storage granules des-cribed below, they are constantly present in all cells and under all conditions of culture. The nuclear bodies replicate by growth and simple fission, and not by mitosis; they show no outer nuclear membrane separating them from the cytoplasm, and they have no nucleolus.

Cytoplasm of Bacteria

The cytoplasm of the bacterial cell is a viscous watery solution, or soft gel, containing a variety of organic and inorganic solutes, and numerous

thin to be resolved with the light microscope (<0·2 μm), a *microcapsule*. Soluble large-molecular material may be dispersed by the bacterium into the environment as *loose slime*. Some bacteria bear, protruding outwards from small granules called *ribosomes*. The cytoplasm of bacteria differs from that of the higher eukaryotic organisms in not containing an endoplasmic reticulum or membrane bearing microsomes, in not containing mitochondria and in not showing signs of internal mobility, e.g. cytoplasmic streaming, the formation, migration and disappearance of vacuoles, and amoeboid movement.

Ribosomes

Bacterial ribosomes are slightly smaller (10–20 nm) than those of eukaryotic cells and they have a sedimentation constant of 70S, being composed of a 30S and a 50S subunit (cf. 40S and 60S in the 80S eukaryotic counterparts). They may be seen with the electron microscope and number tens of thousands per cell. They are strung together on strands of mRNA to form *polysomes* and it is at this site that the code of the mRNA is translated into peptide sequences. Thus the ribosomal components link up and travel along the mRNA strand and here determine the sequence of amino acids brought to the site on tRNA molecules and built into specific polypeptides. Although there are many similarities between bacterial ribosomes and those of cellular tissues, there are some considerable differences. This fortunately allows us to use antibacterial agents such as streptomycin, which interfere with bacterial metabolism at the ribosomal level without unduly upsetting human ribosomal function.

Inclusion Granules

In many species of bacteria, round granules are observed in the cytoplasm. These are not permanent or essential structures, and may be absent under certain conditions of growth. They appear to be aggregates of substances concerned in cell metabolism, e.g. an excess metabolite stored as a nutrient reserve. Generally, they are present in largest amount when the bacteria have access to an abundance of energy-yielding nutrients, and diminish or disappear under conditions of energy-source starvation (Duguid and Wilkinson, 1961). They consist of volutin (polyphosphate), lipid, glycogen, starch or sulphur.

Volutin and lipid granules, $0 \cdot 1$–$1 \cdot 0$ μm in diameter, are seen in many parasitic and saprophytic bacteria, and their demonstration may assist in the identification of certain organisms; thus, the diphtheria bacillus may be distinguished from related bacilli found in the throat by its content of volutin granules.

Volutin granules (syn. metachromatic granules). These granules have an intense affinity for basic dyes. With toluidine blue or methylene blue, they stain metachromatically a red-violet colour, contrasting with the blue staining of the bacterial protoplasm. By special methods such as those of Neisser and Albert the granules can be demonstrated with even greater colour contrast. Their metachromatic staining is thought to be due to their large content of polymerized inorganic polyphosphate (Harold, 1966). This is an energy-rich compound that may act as a reserve of energy and phosphate for cell metabolism or it may be a by-product. Volutin granules are slightly acid-fast, resisting decolourization by 1 per cent sulphuric acid; they are more refractile than the protoplasm and are sometimes distinguishable in unstained wet films. By electron microscopy they appear as very opaque, clearly demarcated bodies.

Lipid granules. These granules have an affinity for fat-soluble dyes such as Sudan black; they are then coloured black in contrast to the remaining protoplasm, which can be counterstained pink with water-soluble basic fuchsin. The granules are spherical, of varying size and highly refractile, being easily seen in unstained preparations. They are slightly acid-fast and may be stained by the modified Ziehl-Neelsen method used for spores. They resist staining by basic dyes and appear as unstained spaces in bacteria treated with simple stains or by Gram's method. Lipid granules resemble endospores (see below) in their acid-fast staining and their resistance to simple stains, but are distinguished by their staining with Sudan black, their smaller size and their frequent occurrence in numbers of more than one per cell. In the bacteria so far subjected to chemical analysis, the granules appear to consist mainly of polymerized β-hydroxybutyric acid (or poly-β-hydroxybutyrate). The manner in which the lipid content of bacteria, e.g. in the *Bacillus* genus, varies with the conditions of culture suggests that this sub-

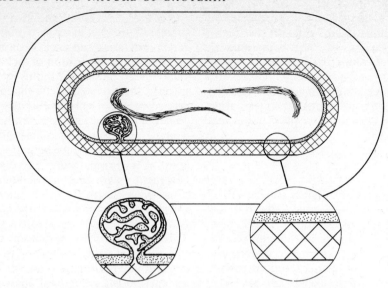

FIG. 2.3. A simplified diagram of a capsulate bacterium showing nuclear material, a mesosome and details of the relation of the cytoplasmic membrane to the cell wall.

stance may act as a carbon and energy storage product.

Polysaccharide granules of either glycogen (red-brown) or starch (blue) can be seen in the cytoplasm of certain bacteria when they are stained with iodine. Many other species, e.g. *Escherichia coli*, do not form granules visible with the light microscope but, when grown with abundant carbon and energy-yielding nutrients, show a diffuse staining of their cytoplasm with the periodic acid-Schiff stain for polysaccharides. In *Esch. coli* this cytoplasmic polysaccharide is

glycogen and it is present as minute granules visible as clear areas with the electron microscope.

Mesosomes

These are convoluted or multilaminated membranous bodies and they are visible with the electron microscope. They develop by complex invagination of the cytoplasmic membrane into the cytoplasm, sometimes in relation to the nuclear body and often from the sites of cross-

FIG. 2.4. A diagram of a unit membrane. A lipid bilayer with polar (hydrophilic) regions externally orientated towards a layer of protein at each surface has a characteristic appearance when stained and seen in cross-section in the electron-microscope.

wall formation in Gram-positive bacteria (Figs. 2.2 and 2.3). Similar structures have been noted in Gram-negative bacteria, but they are much less commonly observed in this group. Mesosomes are thought to be involved in mechanisms responsible for the compartmenting of DNA at cell division and at sporulation. They may also have a function analogous to the mitochondria of the eukaryotic cell—providing a membranous support for respiratory enzymes. Moreover, they may be involved in mechanisms of ejection or excretion of material from the cytoplasm to the exterior.

Cytoplasmic Membrane

The bacterial protoplast is limited externally by a thin, elastic cytoplasmic membrane, which is 5–10 nm thick, consists mainly of lipoprotein and is visible in some ultrathin sections examined with the electron microscope. *Membranes* are important features of prokaryotic and eukaryotic cells. In cross-section they generally appear in suitably stained electronmicroscope (EM) preparations as two dark lines about 2·5 nm wide separated by a lighter area of similar width. The classical model of a 'unit membrane' is illustrated in Fig. 2.4; lipid molecules are arrayed in a double layer with their hydrophilic polar regions externally aligned and in contact with a layer of protein at each surface. The functions of membranes differ widely in nature and it is clear that this simplified model cannot account for all of the variations of function that are already known. More complex membrane architecture is gradually being revealed by special EM techniques such as freeze etching which uses heavy-metal shadowing to reveal details of the faces of fractured frozen membranes imprinted on a carbon replica. In bacteria, the cytoplasmic membrane lacks cholesterol which is a normal constituent of animal cell membranes. The cytoplasmic membrane constitutes an osmotic barrier that is impermeable to many small molecular solutes and is responsible for maintaining the differences in solute content between the cytoplasm and the external environment. It permits the passive diffusion inwards and outwards of water and certain other small molecular substances, especially lipid-soluble ones, and it actively effects the selective transport of specific nutrient solutes into the cell and that of waste products out of it. In addition to the enzymes, or *permeases*, responsible for the active uptake of nutrients, the cytoplasmic membrane contains many other kinds of enzymes, notably respiratory enzymes and pigments (cytochrome system), certain enzymes of the tricarboxylic acid cycle and, probably, polymerizing enzymes that manufacture the substances of the cell wall and extracellular structures. It has little mechanical strength and is supported on the outside by the cell wall (Fig. 2.3).

Cell Wall

The cell wall encases the protoplast and lies immediately external to the cytoplasmic membrane (Salton, 1964; Rogers and Perkins, 1968; Sharon, 1969). It is 10–25 nm thick, strong and relatively rigid, though with some elasticity, and openly porous, being freely permeable to solute molecules smaller than 10 000 daltons and 1 nm in diameter. It supports the weak cytoplasmic membrane against the high internal osmotic pressure of the protoplasm (usually between 5 and 25 atmospheres) and maintains the characteristic shape of the bacterium in its coccal, bacillary, filamentous or spiral form. From a mechanical point of view the cell wall may be likened to the outer cover, and the plasma membrane to the inner tube of the pneumatic tyre of a motor car.

The integrity of the cell wall is essential to the viability of the bacterium. If the wall is weakened or ruptured, the protoplasm may swell from osmotic imbibition of water and burst the weak cytoplasmic membrane. This process of lethal disintegration and dissolution is termed *lysis*. When the rupture occurs locally in some part of the cell wall and a bubble of protoplasm is extruded there, the process is called *plasmoptysis*.

When intact bacteria, particularly Gram-negative bacteria, are placed in a solution of very high solute concentration and osmotic pressure, water may be withdrawn osmotically so that the protoplast shrinks, detaching and retracting the plasma membrane from the cell wall. This process is called *plasmolysis*. A similar process takes place when bacteria are dried, as in preparing a dry film on a microscope slide.

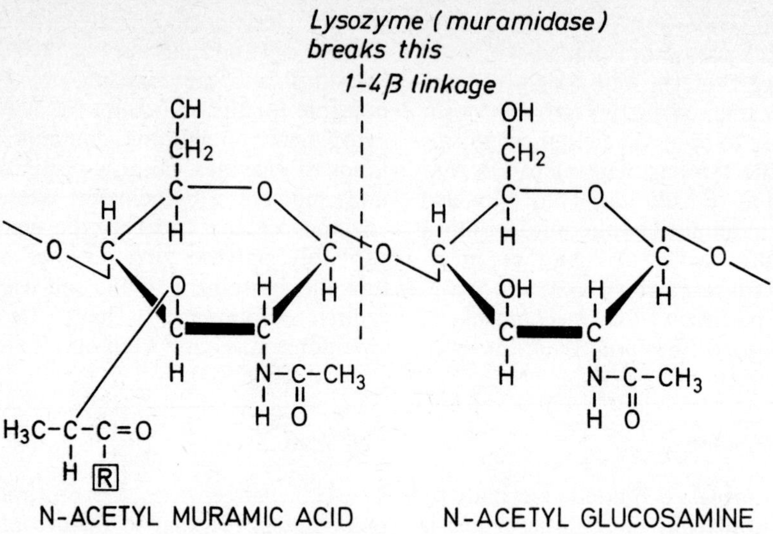

FIG. 2.5. The mucopeptide structure of the bacterial cell wall. Alternating molecules of *N*-acetyl muramic acid and *N*-acetyl glucosamine form chains that bear short peptide side chains (R) attached to each of the muramic acid units. These side chains are further cross-linked by peptide chains.

Plasmolysis may be reversible or it may be lethal.

The cell wall plays an important part in *cell division*. A transverse partition of cell wall material grows inwards, like a closing iris diaphragm, from the lateral wall at the equator of the cell and forms a complete *cross-wall* separating two daughter cells (Chap. 3). The cell wall is not seen in conventionally stained smears examined with the light microscope; it generally remains unstained and lies, invisible, outside the stained shrunken bacterial protoplast. It can be demonstrated by special staining methods but most readily and clearly by electron microscopy; it is seen both in ultrathin sections and, as an empty fold surrounding the shrunken protoplast, in whole-cell preparations shadow-cast with heavy metal.

The chemical composition of the cell wall differs considerably between different bacterial species, but in all species the main strengthening component (the 'basal structure') is a *mucopeptide* (glycopeptide) substance. The mucopeptide is composed of *N*-acetylglucosamine and *N*-acetylmuramic acid molecules linked alternately in a chain (Fig. 2.5), the *N*-acetylmuramic acid molecules each carrying a short tri-, tetra- or penta-peptide side-chain containing D- and L-alanine, D-glutamic acid and either L-lysine or diaminopimelic acid. These are further cross-linked by peptide chains (Fig. 2.6). The wall also contains some other components (collectively called the 'special structure') whose nature and amount vary with the species and whose role is unknown. In Gram-positive bacteria the special structure is generally simple and minor in amount; e.g. in *Staphylococcus aureus* it consists of teichoic acid (ribitol phosphate and *N*-acetylglucosamine polymer) and glycine, and makes up only about 20 per cent of the weight of the wall. In Gram-negative bacteria it is complex and large in amount; e.g. in *Escherichia coli* it comprises lipid, polysaccharide, protein and lipopolysaccharide (endotoxin) and makes up over 80 per cent of the wall weight. The special structure of the cell wall may have an important role in protecting the mucopeptide from attack by the body's lysozyme.

The presence of a muramic acid-containing mucopeptide has recently been demonstrated in rickettsiae and chlamydiae, and this is taken to indicate that these organisms are phylogenetically related to the bacteria rather than to the viruses, in which muramic acid has not been found.

The cell wall, and in particular its basal mucopeptide component, is the target of the action of

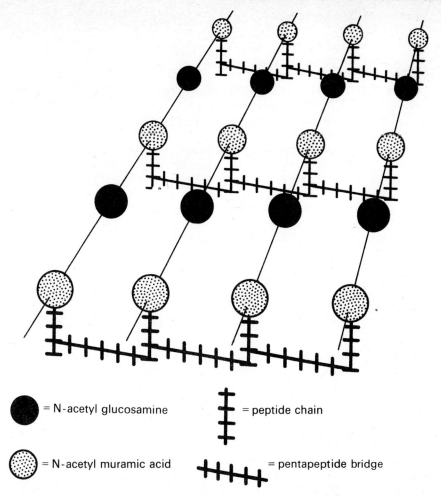

Fig. 2.6. The structure of cell-wall mucopeptide (after Sharon, N. (1969). The bacterial cell wall. *Scientific American*, **220**, 92).

a variety of antibiotics and other antibacterial agents (Chap. 6). Bacteria growing in the presence of one of these agents form defective cell walls (and cross-walls) and, as a result, undergo lysis and die. The body defence substance, lysozyme, which lyses bacteria of many species, dissolves the mucopeptide by cleaving the acetylglucosamine from the acetylmuramic acid molecules. Bacteriophages possess a lysozyme-like enzyme that allows their initial penetration into the bacterium and, after they have reproduced, causes lysis of the bacterium.

It should be noted, moreover, that bacteria themselves possess enzymes, called *autolysins*, able to hydrolyse their own cell-wall substances.

Under some unfavourable physiological conditions the autolysins may act to bring about massive lysis, but normally their action is kept in check and is probably confined to the minor removal of wall substances necessary for remodelling of the cell wall in the course of growth. These enzymes may also be important in bringing about the competence of organisms to take up DNA in the process of transformation (Chap. 7).

Weakening, removal or defective formation of the cell wall is involved in the production of the various abnormal forms called *spheroplasts*, *free protoplasts*, *pleomorphic involution forms*, and *L-forms* or *L-phase organisms* (see below).

Capsules, Microcapsules and Loose Slime

Many bacteria are surrounded by a discrete covering layer of a relatively firm gelatinous material that lies outside and immediately in contact with the cell wall. When this layer, in the wet state, is wide enough (0·2 μm or more) to be resolved with the light microscope, it is called a *capsule*. When it is narrower, and detectable only by indirect, serological means, or by electron microscopy, it may be termed a *microcapsule* (Wilkinson, 1958). The capsular gel consists largely of water and has only a small content (e.g. 2 per cent) of solids. In most species, the solid material is a complex polysaccharide, though in some species its main constituent is polypeptide or protein.

Loose slime, or *free slime*, is an amorphous, viscid colloidal material that is secreted extracellularly by some non-capsulate bacteria and also, outside their capsules, by many capsulate bacteria. In capsulate bacteria the slime is generally similar in chemical composition and antigenic character to the capsular substance. When slime-forming bacteria are grown on a solid culture medium, the slime remains around the bacteria as a matrix in which they are embedded and its presence confers on the growths a watery and sticky 'mucoid' character. The slime is freely soluble in water and, when the bacteria are grown or suspended in a liquid medium, it passes away from them and disperses through the medium.

Demonstration. Capsules and slime have little affinity for basic dyes and are usually invisible in films stained by ordinary methods, e.g. Gram and Leishman stains. Capsules are most likely to be visualized by these stains, as either clear or coloured haloes, when the bacteria are contained in blood, pus or serous fluid. Special methods are available for the 'positive' or 'negative' staining of capsules and loose slime, some being applied to dry, and some to wet films (Duguid, 1951). Since capsules consist largely of water, they shrink very greatly on drying. For this reason, dry-film methods of demonstrating capsules are unreliable; the capsules may shrink so much that they become invisible or, on the other hand, shrinkage artefacts may give the appearance of capsules on non-capsulate bacteria. The most reliable method of demonstration is by 'negative'

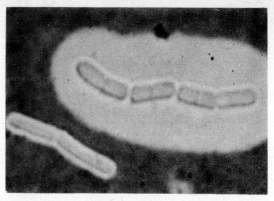

PLATE 2.2. *Bacillus megatherium.* Chain of bacilli with large capsule and pair with very small capsule in wet film with India ink. × 3 500.

staining in wet films with India ink; the carbon particles of the ink make a dark background in the film, but cannot penetrate the capsule, which thus appears as a clear halo around the bacterium (Plate 2.2). When bacteria that have been grown on solid medium are being examined for capsules, it is important that they should first be washed or suspended for a sufficient time in water to ensure the removal of any loose slime which can be observed when films are made directly from the solid medium.

Because of their low solid content and tendency to shrink greatly on drying, capsules and microcapsules are not easily demonstrated with the electron microscope. A large capsule is commonly seen only as an indefinite narrow zone of slight opacity that blurs the otherwise clear-cut edge of the cell wall. Microcapsules may not be seen at all and for this reason the presence of microcapsules has generally to be deduced from serological evidence that the cell-wall antigen (e.g. the O, or somatic antigen in Enterobacteriaceae) is masked by a covering layer (e.g. of K, or 'capsular' antigen).

In attempts to demonstrate capsules it should be remembered that their development is often dependent on the existence of favourable environmental conditions. Thus, their size may vary with the amount of carbohydrate in the culture medium available for nutrition of the bacteria. In the later stages of growth in artificial culture (e.g. 12–24 h) they may become reduced in size due to carbon and energy starvation or they may disappear due to the accumulation in

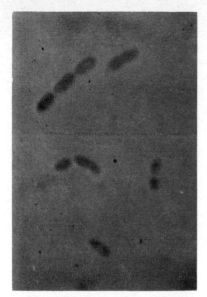

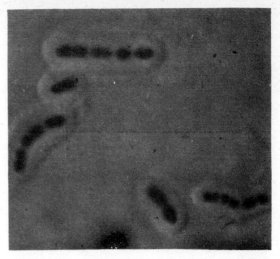

PLATE 2.4. **Pneumococcu**s type 19 showing 'capsule swelling' reaction in wet film with homologous (type-19) antiserum and methylene blue. × 3 750.

PLATE 2.3. Pneumococcus type 19 (from same culture as in Plate 2.4) showing absence of 'capsule swelling' reaction in wet film with heterologous (type-1) antiserum and methylene blue. × 3 750.

the medium of capsule-degrading enzymes (e.g. hyaluronidase in the case of *Streptococcus pyogenes*).

Function. It is not known with certainty what are the functions of capsules and microcapsules, but it is probable that their principal action is in protecting the cell wall against attack by various kinds of antibacterial agents, e.g. bacteriophages, colicines, complement, lysozyme and other lytic enzymes, that otherwise would more readily damage or destroy it. In the case of certain capsulate pathogenic organisms (e.g. pneumococcus, pyogenic streptococci, anthrax bacillus and plague bacillus) good evidence has been obtained to show that the capsule protects the bacteria against ingestion by the phagocytes of the host. The capsule is thus an important agent determining virulence, and non-capsulate mutants of these bacteria are found to be non-virulent. In some organisms the capsule contains more than one functional component. Thus, *Streptococcus pyogenes*, which under favourable conditions of growth may form an anti-phagocytic capsule composed of hyaluronic acid, also possesses a second surface substance, M protein, which inhibits either the ingestion or the intracellular digestion of the cocci by the

phagocytes; the M protein occurs in association with the hyaluronic acid capsule or, when the latter is absent, by itself in the form of a microcapsule. In *Bacillus anthracis* the capsule is a polymer of *D*-glutamic acid and protects the bacteria not only against phagocytosis but also, to some extent, against the action of a bactericidal basic polypeptide present in animal tissues.

The capsular substance is usually antigenic (see below) and the capsular antigens play a very important part in determining the antigenic specificity of bacteria (Chap. 17). When capsulate pneumococci are treated with type-specific antiserum, the sharpness of outline of the capsule is greatly enhanced. This is referred to as the 'capsule-swelling reaction' (see Plates 2.3 and 2.4).

Flagella and Motility

Motile strains of bacteria possess filamentous appendages known as *flagella*, which effect screw-like propulsive movements and act as organs of locomotion. The flagellum is a long, thin filament, twisted spirally in an open, regular wave-form. It is about 0·02 μm thick and is usually several times the length of the bacterial cell. It originates in the bacterial protoplasm and is extruded through the cell wall. According to the species, there may be one or several (e.g.

1–20) flagella per cell, and in elongated bacteria the arrangement of the flagella may be *peritrichous*, or *lateral*, when they originate from the sides of the cell, or *polar*, when they originate from one or both ends. Where several occur on a cell, they may function coiled together as a single 'tail'. Flagella consist largely or entirely of a protein, *flagellin*, belonging to the same chemical group as myosin, the contractile protein of muscle. They can be demonstrated easily and clearly with the electron microscope, particularly in metal-shadowed preparations or preparations 'negatively' stained with phosphotungstic acid (PTA), usually appearing as simple fibrils without internal differentiation. In some PTA preparations the flagellum appears as a hollow tube formed of helically twisted fibrils, and the flagella of some bacteria, e.g. vibrios, have an outer sheath; but bacterial flagella do not have the complex structure of the flagella and cilia of plants and animals, which in all cases consist of two central and nine peripheral fibrils contained in a tube-like sheath. They are invisible in ordinary preparations by the light microscope, but may be shown by the use of special staining methods that involve mordanting and deposition of stain, and in special circumstances by dark-ground illumination. Because of the difficulties of these methods, the presence of flagella is commonly inferred from the observation of motility.

Motility may be observed either microscopically or by noting the occurrence of spreading growth in semi-solid agar medium. On microscopic observation of wet films, motile bacteria are seen swimming in different directions across the field, with a darting, wriggling or tumbling movement. True motility must be distinguished from a drifting of the bacteria in a single direction due to a current in the liquid, and also from Brownian movement, which is a rapid oscillation of each bacterium within a very limited area due to bombardment by the water molecules.

Among the spirochaetes, motility appears to be a function of the cell body, since flagella do not occur. The most characteristic movement is a fast spiral rotation on the long axis with slow progression in the axial line; movements of flexion and lashing movements may be observed. Some spirochaetes possess an axial filament and others a band of fibrils wound around their surface from pole to pole. It has been suggested that these structures may contribute to motility, either through being themselves contractile or by acting as stiffeners for recoil against the contractile protoplast (Chap. 38).

Function. It is not known with certainty what advantage a bacterium derives from its ability to move actively. Motility may be beneficial in increasing the rate of uptake of nutrient solutes by continuously changing the environmental fluid in contact with the bacterial cell surface. Random movement and dispersion through the environment may be beneficial in ensuring that at least some cells of a strain reach every locality suitable for colonization. There is, moreover,

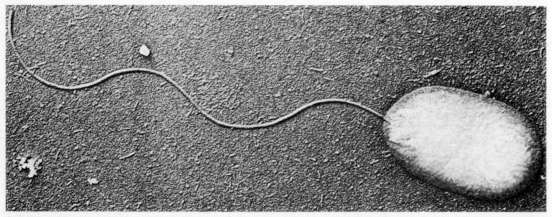

PLATE 2.5. *Pseudomonas aeruginosa* (*pyocyanea*). Bacillus with single polar flagellum. Whole bacillus dried and shadow-cast. Electron microscope ×38 000. (From Wilkinson, J. F. and Duguid, J. P. (1960). The influence of cultural conditions on bacterial cytology. *International Review of Cytology*, **9**, 1–76.)

good evidence that the movement of many bacteria is *directed* by responses of the organism towards localities favourable to growth and away from unfavourable regions. Thus, bacteria tend to migrate towards regions where there is a higher concentration of nutrient solutes and away from regions containing higher concentrations of disinfectant substances. Motile aerobic bacteria show positive aerotaxis and migrate towards regions where there is a higher concentration of dissolved oxygen; anaerobes migrate away from such regions.

It might be supposed that the power of active locomotion would assist pathogenic bacteria in penetrating through viscid mucous secretions and epithelial barriers, and in spreading throughout the body fluids and tissues, but it must be noted that many non-motile pathogens (e.g. brucellae and streptococci) are not any less invasive than motile ones.

Fimbriae

Certain Gram-negative bacilli, including saprophytic, intestinal commensal and pathogenic species in the family Enterobacteriaceae, possess filamentous appendages of a different kind from the flagella (Duguid *et al.*, 1955; Duguid, 1968). These are called *fimbriae* or *pili*, and they occur in some non-motile, as well as in some motile strains. They are far more numerous than flagella (e.g. 100–500 being borne peritrichously by each cell) and are much shorter and only about half as thick (e.g. varying from 0·1 to 1·5 μm in length and having a uniform width between 4 and 8 nm). They do not have the smoothly curved spiral form of flagella and are mostly more or less straight. They cannot be seen with the light microscope but are clearly seen with the electron microscope in preparations that have been metal-shadowed or negatively stained with phosphotungstic acid (see Plates 2.6 and 2.7).

Most potentially (i.e. genetically) fimbriate strains of bacteria readily undergo a reversible variation between a fimbriate phase and a non-fimbriate phase and this variation is affected by the conditions of growth. The fimbriate phase becomes predominant, and the majority of bacilli in the culture become fimbriate, as a result of prolonged culture or serial (48-hourly)

subculture, in static liquid medium incubated aerobically. The non-fimbriate phase predominates and cultures consist entirely or almost entirely of non-fimbriate bacilli when subcultures are made serially on a solid culture medium.

Function. There is evidence that fimbriae may function as organs of adhesion. The possession of fimbriae confers on bacilli the power of adhering firmly to solid surfaces of various kinds, including those of the cells of animals, plants and fungi. Comparable non-fimbriate bacilli do not adhere when they collide with such surfaces. The adhesive property may be of value to the

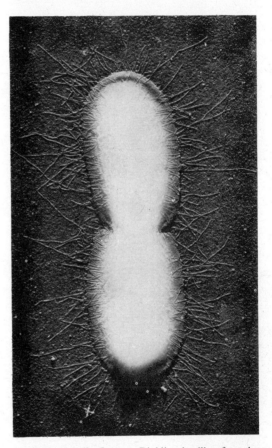

PLATE 2.6. *Shigella flexneri.* Dividing bacillus from log-phase culture bears numerous fimbriae on both daughter cells. Note dense (white) shrunken protoplast surrounded by empty fold of cell wall. Whole bacillus dried and shadow-cast. Electron microscope. × 24 000. (From Duguid, J. P. and Wilkinson, J. F. (1961) Environmentally induced changes in bacterial morphology. *Symposia of the Society of General Microbiology*, **11**, 69–99.)

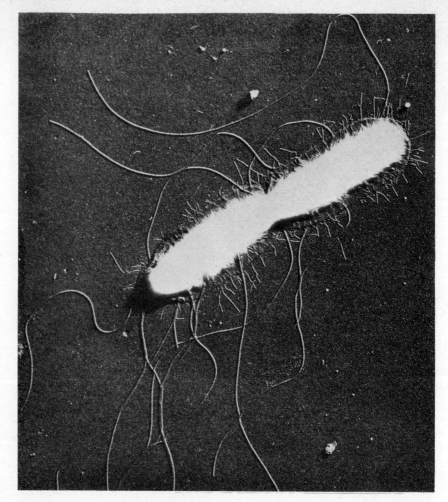

PLATE 2.7. *Salmonella typhi.* Dividing bacillus from log-phase culture bears about fifteen long wavy flagella and over a hundred short fimbriae. Note dense (white) shrunken protoplast surrounded by empty fold of cell wall. Whole bacillus dried and shadow-cast. Electron microscope. ×16 000. (From Duguid, J. P. and Wilkinson, J. F. (1961) Environmentally induced changes in bacterial morphology. *Symposia of the Society of General Microbiology*, **11**, 69–99.)

bacteria in holding them in nutritionally favourable micro-environments. Moreover, bacteria growing in stagnant liquid medium under air are assisted by the possession of fimbriae to grow attached together in the form of a *pellicle* that floats on the surface of the medium where the growth is greatly enhanced by the free supply of atmospheric oxygen.

Haemagglutination. The majority of fimbriate bacteria bear fimbriae of a type that enables them to adhere to, among other kinds of tissue cells, the red blood cells of many animal species (e.g. to guinea-pig, fowl, horse and pig red cells

very strongly, to human cells moderately strongly, to sheep cells weakly and to ox cells scarcely at all). If a drop of a concentrated suspension of fimbriate bacilli is mixed for a few minutes with a drop of a suspension of red cells, preferably guinea-pig red cells, the adhering bacilli bind the red cells together in clumps visible to the naked eye. A simple haemagglutination test can thus be used to determine whether a culture contains fimbriate bacilli.

There exist different types of fimbriae having different adhesive properties. The commonest kind type 1, which occurs in escherichia, klebsiella, serratia, salmonella and shigella organisms is about 8 nm in width, and it may be recognized by the observation that its adhesive and haemagglutinating actions are completely and specifically inhibited by the addition of a small amount (0·1–0·5 per cent) of *D*-mannose to the test mixture (i.e. its activities are mannose-sensitive). In addition to, or instead of type 1 fimbriae, some klebsiella and serratia organisms possess type 3 fimbriae, about 5 nm in width; these do not agglutinate red cells unless the cells are first heated or tanned, and their adhesive properties are unaffected by mannose. Proteus organisms possess a third kind of fimbriae (type 4), which have mannose-resistant haemagglutinating activity against untreated red cells of certain species. A few salmonella organisms (e.g. *S. gallinarum* and *S. pullorum*) possess a fourth kind of fimbriae (type 2), apparently devoid of all haemagglutinating and adhesive properties. It should be noted also that some bacteria, e.g. many strains of *Esch. coli*, possess haemagglutinating factors (mannose-resistant) that are not associated with fimbriae.

Sex fimbriae (*sex pili*). The fertility factors of enterobacteria, such as the F factor, which confer 'maleness', or conjugating and DNA-donor abilities on the bacteria in which they are present, determine the formation by the bacterium of a few exceptionally long, specialized fimbriae. These sex fimbriae appear to attach specifically to non-male bacteria and may play a part in the transfer of DNA (Chap. 7). They also act as receptor sites for certain bacteriophages described as being 'male-specific'.

BACTERIAL REPRODUCTION

Among the 'lower' or true bacteria, multiplication takes place by *simple binary fission* (Symposium, 1965). The cell grows in size, usually elongating to twice its original length, and the protoplasm becomes divided into two approximately equal parts by the ingrowth of a transverse septum from the plasma membrane and cell wall. In some species, the cell wall septum, or cross-wall, splits in two and the daughter cells separate almost immediately. In others, the cell walls of the daughter cells remain continuous for some time after cell division and the

organisms grow adhering in pairs, clusters, chains or filaments. If cross-wall splitting is thus delayed in an organism in which the cross-walls of successive cell divisions are all formed in parallel planes, the cells will be grouped in pairs, chains, rods or filaments. If it is delayed in an organism that forms successive cross-walls in different planes, e.g. ones at right angles to each other, the cells will be grouped in pairs and either cubical or irregular clusters. Under favourable conditions, growth and division are repeated with great rapidity, e.g. every half-hour or less, so that one individual cell may reproduce thousands of millions of new organisms in less than a day. A bacterium dividing every 20 min under suitable conditions in artificial culture medium multiplies about 1 000 000 000-fold in 10 h. Generation times of pathogens *in vivo* are much longer. Among the spirochaetes, transverse fission occurs as in other bacteria.

In the 'higher', or mycelial bacteria, growth takes place by extension of the vegetative filaments, and multiplication by transverse division of these into shorter forms, or by the liberation of numerous conidia (*vide supra*) which later germinate and give rise to fresh mycelia.

Some observers have described more complex processes of reproduction among bacteria and postulated life cycles comprising different morphological phases. In many cases, however, the forms presumed to be 'intermediate phases' have in fact been degenerate involution cells, and the evidence at present available does not warrant acceptance of such views. In some bacterial species there can be conjugation of two individual cells with genetic recombination.

Bacterial Spores

Some species, particularly those of the genera *Bacillus* and *Clostridium*, develop a highly resistant resting-phase or *endospore*, whereby the organism can survive in a dormant state through a long period of starvation or other adverse environmental condition (Gould and Hurst, 1969). The process does not involve multiplication: in *sporulation*, each vegetative cell forms only one spore, and in subsequent *germination* each spore gives rise to a single vegetative cell. Certain specific antigens develop in the spore that are not found in the vegetative cells.

Sporulation. Although it has been suggested that spores are formed spontaneously, as an intermediate stage in a bacterial life cycle, it seems more likely that sporulation occurs as a response to starvation or, at least, the exhaustion of a limiting substance. It does not take place as long as conditions continue to favour maximal vegetative growth, but occurs when multiplication is being arrested, as at the end of the log phase and in the early stationary phase of artificial culture. In certain species, sporulation may be induced by depletion of the supply of one of the nutrients necessary for vegetative growth, e.g. the carbon and energy source, the nitrogen source, sulphate, phosphate or iron salt; at the same time, the process requires a continued supply of other minerals (K, Mg, Mn and Ca salts), and favourable conditions of moisture, temperature, pH, oxygen tension, etc. The spore is formed inside the parent vegetative cell (hence the name 'endospore'). It develops from a portion of proto-plasm near one end of the cell (the 'forespore'), incorporates part of the nuclear material (equivalent to one genome) of the cell and acquires a thick covering layer, the 'cortex', and a thin, but tough, outer 'spore coat' consisting of several layers. Spores of some species have an additional, apparently rather loose covering known as the exosporium and this structure sometimes bears characteristic ridges and folds that can be visualized in the electron microscope (Plate 2.8). Mesosomes seem to play a part in the development of the endospore and may be involved in the compartmentation of the spore's share of the nuclear material. The appearance of the mature spore varies according to the species, being spherical, ovoid or elongated, occupying a terminal, subterminal or central position, and being narrower than the cell, or broader and bulging it (Fig. 2.7). Finally, the remainder of the parent cell disintegrates and the spore is freed. Fig. 2.8 shows a cross-section of a typical spore.

Viability. Spores are much more resistant than the vegetative forms to injurious chemical and physical influences, including exposure to disinfectants, drying and heating. Thus, their killing requires application of moist heat at 100°–120°C for a period (e.g. 10 min) although heating at 60°C suffices to kill the vegetative cells. Spores may remain viable for many years, either in the dry state or in moist conditions unfavourable to growth, as in absence of nutrients sufficient to maintain the minimal metabolism

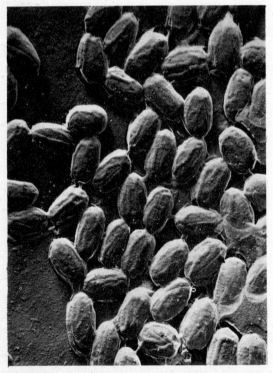

PLATE 2.8. A carbon replica of spores of *Bacillus licheniformis* showing characteristic grooves and ridges. × 5 250. (By courtesy of Dr D. E. Bradley and Editors of *Journal of General Microbiology*.)

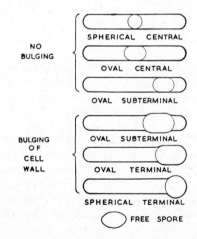

FIG. 2.7. The shape and situation of the spore in the bacterial cell.

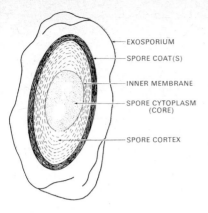

- EXOSPORIUM
- SPORE COAT(S)
- INNER MEMBRANE
- SPORE CYTOPLASM (CORE)
- SPORE CORTEX

FIG. 2.8. Cross-section of a bacterial spore. The core is surrounded by the inner spore membrane. The cortex, a laminated structure, invests the core and is protected by a more resistant layer or multiple layers forming the spore coat. In some cases, a loose outer covering (exosporium) can be defined and may give the spore a characteristically ridged appearance (see Plate 2.8).

of the vegetative form. The marked resistance of spores has been attributed to several factors in which they differ from vegetative cells: the impermeability of their cortex and outer coat, their high content of calcium and dipicolinic acid, their low content of water (maybe 5–20 per cent) and their very low metabolic and enzymic activity.

Germination of the spore occurs when the external conditions become favourable to growth by access to moisture and nutrients, in particular to trigger nutrients such as L-alanine, inosine or glucose in certain *Bacillus* species. It is irreversible and involves rapid degradative changes. The spore successively loses its heat resistance and its dipicolinic acid; it loses calcium, it becomes permeable to dyes and its refractility changes. Spores that have survived exposure to severe adverse influences such as heat are found to be much more exacting than normal spores in their requirements for germination. For this reason, specially enriched culture media are used when testing the sterility of materials, such as surgical catgut, that have been exposed to disinfecting procedures. In the process of germination, the spore swells, its cortex disintegrates, its coat is broken open and a single vegetative cell emerges.

Activation. The mature spore is characteristically inert towards a variety of exogenous substrates until germination is triggered. The initiation of germination is incompletely understood. It is clear that the degree of dormancy of spores may be altered by various treatments, including transient exposure to heat at 80°C for example, so that germination can then proceed more rapidly in the individual cells or more completely in a spore population. This alteration of the degree of dormancy is distinct from germination and is reversible if germination does not proceed. It is called *activation*.

Outgrowth. This term is used to denote the stage from germination up to the formation of the first vegetative cell and prior to the first cell division. The conditions required for successful outgrowth may differ markedly from those that allow germination.

Demonstration. In unstained preparations the spore is recognized within the parent cell by its greater refractility. It is larger than lipid inclusion granules and is often ovoid, in contrast to the spherical shape of the lipid granules. Mature ungerminated spores are 'phase-bright' in the phase-contrast microscope; immature or germinated spores are 'phase-dark'. When mature, the spore resists colouration by simple stains and Gram's stain, appearing as a clear space within the stained cell protoplasm. Spores are slightly acid-fast and may be stained differentially by a modification of the Ziehl-Neelsen method. The shape of the spore (spherical or ovoid), its size, judged by whether or not it 'bulges' the bacillus containing it, and its position in the bacillus (central, subterminal or terminal) are features that may be characteristic and important in the identification of a bacterial species. The simple observation that a bacterium is a *spore-former* limits its possible identity to species belonging to a very few genera.

Conidia (Exospores)

Some of the mycelial bacteria (*Actinomycetales*) form *conidia*, resting spores of a kind different from endospores. The conidia are borne *externally* (extracellularly) by abstriction from the ends of the parent cells (conidiophores) and are disseminated by the air or other means to fresh habitats. They are not specially resistant to heat and disinfectants.

Pleomorphism and Involution

In the course of growth, bacteria of a single strain may show considerable variation in size and shape, forming a proportion of cells that differ grossly from the normal, e.g. swollen, spherical and pear-shaped forms, elongated filaments and filaments with localized swellings. This pleomorphism occurs most readily in certain species (e.g. *Streptobacillus moniliformis*, *Yersinia pestis*) in ageing cultures on artificial medium and especially in the presence of antagonistic substances such as penicillin, glycine, lithium chloride, sodium chloride in high concentrations, and organic acids at low pH. The abnormal cells are generally regarded as degenerate or *involution* forms; some are non-viable, whilst others may grow and revert to the normal form when transferred to a suitable environment. In many cases the abnormal shape seems to be the result of defective cell-wall synthesis; the growing protoplasm expands the weakened wall to produce a grotesquely swollen cell comparable to a spheroplast (see below) that later usually bursts and lyses.

Spheroplasts and Free Protoplasts

If bacteria have their cell walls removed or weakened while they are held in a sufficiently concentrated solution such as 0·2–1·0 M sucrose with 0·01 M Mg^{2+} to prevent them imbibing water by osmosis, they may escape being lysed and, instead, may become converted into viable spherical bodies. If all the cell-wall material has been removed from them, the spheres are *free protoplasts*. If they remain enclosed by an intact, but weakened residual cell wall, they are called *spheroplasts*. Protoplasts, for example, are readily liberated from the Gram-positive bacillus, *Bacillus megaterium*, by dissolution of the cell walls with egg-white lysozyme. Spheroplasts are readily produced from Gram-negative bacilli such as *Escherichia coli* by growing the organism in the presence of a substance such as penicillin, bacitracin, oxymycin (cycloserine) or glycine, that specifically inhibits synthesis of the mucopeptide component of the cell wall. A similar result may be obtained by culturing certain bacteria on medium lacking a nutrient, e.g. diaminopimelic acid, lysine or a hexosamine

derivative, that they require specifically for cell-wall synthesis.

Protoplasts and spheroplasts are osmotically sensitive; they vary in size with the osmotic pressure of the suspending medium and if the medium is much diluted, they swell up, burst and perish by lysis. If maintained in an osmotically protective nutrient medium, they remain viable and continue to metabolize, synthesize and grow. Protoplasts enlarge but do not multiply. Spheroplasts, when kept on an osmotically protective agar medium containing a cell-wall inhibitor such as penicillin, may multiply by fission or budding and reproduce through many serial subcultures. The spheroplasts of Gram-negative bacilli, because they retain a residual wall structure, are not as osmotically sensitive as free protoplasts and are often capable of growing on an ordinary agar culture medium. Protoplasts have not been found capable of re-forming their cell walls and reverting to normal bacterial morphology, but spheroplasts commonly revert *en masse* when transferred to culture medium lacking the cell-wall inhibitor. Spheroplast cultures have sometimes been called 'unstable L-forms' on account of their resemblance in colonial and cellular morphology to the stable L-forms of bacteria (see below).

L-forms of Bacteria (or L-phase Organisms)

These are abnormal growth forms derived by variation, usually in the laboratory, from bacteria of normal morphology, e.g. cocci, bacilli or vibrios, and may be stable in the sense that special conditions of culture, such as the presence of penicillin, are not required to prevent their reversion to the parental bacterial forms. They differ from the parent bacteria in lacking a rigid cell wall and, in consequence, regular size and shape, but they are nevertheless viable and capable of growing and multiplying through an indefinite series of cultures on a suitable artificial nutrient medium. They are soft protoplasmic bodies, generally spherical or disk-like, but sometimes extremely variable in shape, and they range in size from minute bodies about 0·1 μm in diameter to large ones of 10–20 μm. The smallest *viable* forms are about 0·3 μm in diameter and can occasionally pass through bacteria-stopping filters. Some L-forms may be entirely devoid of a cell wall, and others, like spheroplasts, possess an intact cell wall that is weakened by absence of a strengthening component (mucopeptide).

Colonies of L-phase organisms on agar media are small and have a characteristic 'fried egg' appearance; they have a dark, thick centre, where many of the organisms embed themselves and grow within the agar, and a lighter peripheral zone with a lace-like texture consisting of organisms lying on the surface of the agar together with oily excretory droplets (probably containing cholesterol). In liquid media, growth is usually in the form of clumps. Because of their fragility, microscopical examination of L-forms is best done while they are *in situ* on the agar medium, a coverslip being applied to a block of agar bearing the growth. If desired, the organisms can be stained after fixation by a fixative that is allowed to diffuse through the agar.

Origin. Some bacteria, e.g. *Streptobacillus moniliformis* and *Bacteroides* spp., give rise spontaneously to L-forms even when grown in an optimal culture medium. In many other species, L-form growth may be induced by culture in the presence of an inhibitor of cell-wall synthesis, such as penicillin, or by deprivation of a nutrient essential for cell-wall synthesis, e.g. diaminopimelic acid, or by destruction of the cell wall with antibody and complement.

Maintenance. Though L-forms of some species may be grown on ordinary culture media and even in liquid medium, a special medium is generally essential, e.g. a soft agar medium containing meat infusion and 20 per cent horse serum. Agar apparently gives mechanical support to L-bodies embedding themselves and multiplying by budding within it. Some L-forms require a medium with a large content of sucrose or sodium chloride for osmotic protection, as described for the maintenance of spheroplasts.

Reversion to the bacterial form. True or stable L-forms, even if their origin was induced by exposure to penicillin or other cell-wall inhibitor, continue to reproduce as L-forms through repeated subcultures in the absence of cell-wall inhibitor, and do not give rise to revertants of normal bacterial morphology. Unstable L-forms, e.g. growths of penicillin-induced spheroplasts, generally revert *en masse* to the normal bacterial form within a few hours of culture in the absence of the inducing agent. Transitional L-forms give rise occasionally to small numbers of bacterial revertants.

Role. Although they have many resemblances to mycoplasma organisms, L-forms should probably be regarded as laboratory artefacts, degenerate growths that do not occur or survive to any important extent in natural habitats. This concept is still debated and it is possible that L-forms could account for bacterial persistence during therapy with certain antibiotics. L-forms are non-pathogenic to laboratory animals.

MORPHOLOGICAL STUDY OF BACTERIA

Microscopical examination is usually the first step taken in the identification of an unknown bacterium. The bacterium may be allocated to one or other of the major groups when its *morphology* and *staining reactions* have been observed. The morphological features of importance are the size, shape and grouping of the cells, and their possession of any distinctive structures such as endospores, flagella (sometimes inferred from the simple observation of motility), capsules and intracellular granules. Staining reactions are observed after treatment by special procedures such as the Gram and Ziehl-Neelsen stains, the different kinds of bacteria being shown in separate colours due to their different permeability to certain decolourizing agents. A preparation stained by one of these methods usually suffices for observation of the general morphology of the bacterium, but some morphological features can be demonstrated only by the application of further special stains.

The optical, or light microscope (employing visible light) is generally sufficient for making the observations of shape, staining reaction and special morphology that are required for the identification of a bacterium. The electron microscope, which has contributed much new information about the fine structure of the bacterial cell, is rarely required for bacteriological diagnostic work. It may be valuable, however, in enabling demonstration of certain structures of taxonomic importance, e.g. fimbriae, that cannot be demonstrated with the light microscope.

Unstained Preparations of Living Organisms

The morphology of bacteria can be studied in the first place by examining them microscopically in the unstained condition, suspended in a thin film of fluid between a glass slide and coverslip (i.e. in an 'unstained wet film'). In this way their general shape can be seen and their motility determined. Certain very slender bacteria, however, such as the spirochaetes, are so feebly refractile that they cannot be seen by the ordinary microscopic methods, and *dark-ground illumination* or *phase-contrast microscopy* is necessary for their demonstration. Phase-contrast microscopy may also be used to demonstrate motility, spores and intracellular granules (Chap. 1, Vol. II).

For the study of the development of individual organisms and the growth of bacteria in colonies, the 'agar-block' method of Ørskov, and the microscope-incubator may be used (Chap. 1, Vol. II). These methods enable living bacteria to be observed at intervals during their actual growth on a suitable substrate, and present a more natural picture than other procedures involving manipulations that may sometimes create artificial appearances. The application of time-lapse cine-photomicrography to such studies is a further refinement.

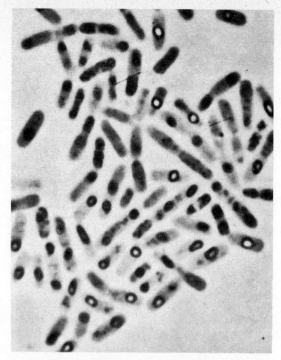

PLATE 2.9. *Bacillus cereus*. Bacilli from stationary-phase culture show spores (large refractile bodies with appearance of white centres) and lipid granules (dark bodies of variable size). Unstained wet film by phase-contrast microscopy. × 3 000.

Stained Preparations

The microscopical examination of fixed and stained preparations is usually an essential routine procedure. The bacteria are more readily discovered and studied when immobilized by fixation and darkly stained in contrast with the bright background. Methods for simple staining impart the same colour to all bacteria and other biological material, whereas methods for differential staining impart a distinctive colour only to certain types of bacteria (Lamanna and Mallette, 1965).

Simple staining is effected by the application of a watery solution of a single basic dye, e.g. methylene blue, methyl violet or basic fuchsin, or sometimes along with a mordant to allow better penetration. The coloured, positively charged cation of the basic dye combines firmly with negatively charged groups in the bacterial protoplasm, especially with the phosphate groups in the abundant nucleic acids. The stain is retained through a subsequent washing with water for the removal of excess dye from the slide. Acidic dyes, having coloured anions, do not stain bacteria strongly except at very acid pH values, and thus can be used for 'negative staining' (see below). Cells or structures that stain with basic dyes at normal pH values are described as *basophilic* and those that stain with acidic dyes as *acidophilic*.

Prior to staining, the film or smear of bacteria must be fixed on the slide. *Fixation* is usually effected by heat; the slide is first thoroughly dried in air and then heated gently in a flame. Vegetative bacteria are thereby killed, rendered permeable to the stain, stuck to the surface of the slide and preserved from undergoing autolytic changes. Chemical fixatives are used for sections of infected tissue and films of infected blood, since they cause less damage to the tissue cells; fixatives include formalin, mercuric chloride, methyl alcohol and osmic acid.

It should be noted that the bacterial cell wall is not stained by ordinary methods and the coloured body seen corresponds to the cell protoplasm only. This is usually much shrunken as a result of drying. Chains of stained bacteria thus show the coloured bodies separated by gaps that are the sites of unstained, connecting cell walls.

Beaded and bipolar staining. Certain bacteria do not colour evenly with simple stains. Thus, the diphtheria bacillus shows a 'beaded' appearance, with alternating dark and light bars. The plague bacillus shows 'bipolar staining', the ends being more deeply coloured than the centre. The uneven staining may be due to the manner in which the protoplasm shrinks when the cell is dried and fixed.

'Negative' or background staining is of value as a rapid method for the simple morphological study of bacteria. The bacteria are mixed with a substance such as India ink, or nigrosin, which, after spreading as a film, yields a dark background in which the bacteria stand out as bright, unstained objects.

Silver impregnation methods are utilized for the staining of spirochaetes, especially for demonstrating these organisms in tissues. The slender cells are thickened by a dark deposit of silver on their surface.

Differential staining reactions of bacteria are of the greatest importance in their recognition and identification. *Gram's staining reaction* has the widest application, distinguishing all bacteria as 'Gram-positive' or 'Gram-negative', according to whether or not they resist decolourization with acetone, alcohol or aniline oil after staining with a para-rosaniline (triphenyl-methane) dye, e.g. methyl violet, and subsequent treatment with iodine. The Gram-positive bacteria resist decolourization and remain stained a dark purple colour. The Gram-negative bacteria are decolourized, and are then counterstained light pink by the subsequent application of basic fuchsin, safranine, neutral red or dilute carbol fuchsin. In routine diagnostic work a Gram-stained smear is often the only preparation examined microscopically, since it shows clearly the general morphology of the bacteria as well as revealing their Gram-reaction. It should be noted that characteristically Gram-positive species may sometimes appear Gram-negative

under certain conditions of growth; thus, some show an increasing proportion of partly or wholly Gram-negative cells in ageing cultures on nutrient agar. On the other hand, characteristically Gram-negative species do not produce cells that stain Gram-positively in correctly treated smears. Gram-reactivity appears to reflect a fundamental aspect of cell structure and is correlated with many other biological properties. Thus, the different species of a single genus generally show the same reaction. Gram-positive bacteria are more susceptible than Gram-negative bacteria to the antibacterial actions of penicillin, acids, iodine, basic dyes, detergents and lysozyme, and less susceptible to alkalies, azide, tellurite, proteolytic enzymes, lysis by antibody and complement, and plasmolysis in solutes of high osmotic pressure. The walls of the Gram-positive bacteria contain more mucopeptide and are thicker and stronger than those of Gram-negative bacteria, a difference associated with the occurrence of a higher internal osmotic pressure in Gram-positive cells.

The mechanism of the Gram stain is not fully understood. Gram-positive organisms are able to retain basic dyes at a higher hydrogen-ion concentration than the Gram-negative species, showing an isoelectric point of pH 2–3 as compared with pH 4–5. The more acidic character of their protoplasm, which is enhanced by treatment with iodine, may partly explain their stronger retention of basic dye. Probably, however, the more important difference is in the permeability of the cell wall during the staining process. After staining with methyl violet and treatment with iodine, a dye-iodine complex or 'lake' is formed within the cell; this is insoluble in water but moderately soluble and dissociable in the acetone or alcohol used as the decolourizer. Under the action of the decolourizer, the dye and iodine diffuse freely out of the Gram-negative cell, but not from the Gram-positive cell, presumably because the latter's cell wall is less permeable (Salton, 1963). Gram-positive bacteria become Gram-negative when their cell wall is ruptured or removed.

The *acid-fast staining reaction*, as revealed by the Ziehl-Neelsen method is of value in distinguishing a few bacterial species, e.g. the tubercle bacillus, from all others. These 'acid-fast' bacteria are relatively impermeable and resistant to simple stains, but when stained with a strong reagent (hot basic fuchsin in aqueous 5 per cent phenol), subsequently resist de-colourization by strong acids, e.g. 20 per cent sulphuric acid. Any decolourized non-acid-fast organisms are counterstained in a contrasting colour with methylene blue or malachite green.

The acid-fast bacteria have an exceptionally rich and varied content of lipids, fatty acids and higher alcohols, and their acid-fastness has been attributed to this. When the lipids, including those firmly bound in the protoplasm, are re-moved by treatment with suitable solvents, the cells are no longer acid-fast. One of the lipids peculiar to acid-fast bacteria exhibits the pro-perty of acid-fastness in the free state; this is *mycolic acid*, a high molecular weight hydroxy acid wax containing carboxyl groups. The mere presence of such a substance in the cell is not by itself sufficient to explain acid-fastness, since the character is lost when the cell is ruptured by mechanical means or autolysis. Acid-fastness therefore depends on the structural integrity of the cell, its content of lipids and, possibly, a special anatomical disposition of the lipids.

REFERENCES AND FURTHER READING

DUGUID, J. P. (1951) The demonstration of bacterial cap-sules and slime. *Journal of Pathology and Bacteriology*, **63**, 673.

DUGUID, J. P. (1968) The functions of bacterial fimbriae. *Archivum Immunologiae et Therapie experimentalis*, **16**, 173.

DUGUID, J. P., SMITH, ISABEL W., DEMPSTER, G., & EDMUNDS, P. N. (1955) Non-flagellar filamentous appendages ('fimbriae') and haemagglutinating activity in *Bacterium coli. Journal of Pathology and Bacteriology*, **70**, 335.

DUGUID, J. P. & WILKINSON, J. F. (1961) Environmentally induced changes in bacterial morphology. *Symposia of the Society for General Microbiology*, **11**, 69.

GOULD, G. W. & HURST, A. (1969) *The Bacterial Spore*. London & New York: Academic Press.

GUNSALUS, I. C. & STANIER, R. Y. (1960) *The Bacteria*, Vol. I (Structure). New York: Academic Press.

HAROLD, F. M. (1966) Inorganic polyphosphates in biology: structure, metabolism, and function. *Bacteriological Reviews*, **30**, 772.

LAMANNA, C. & MALLETTE, M. F. (1965) *Basic Bacteriology*, 3rd edn, p. 125, Baltimore: Williams & Wilkins.

ROGERS, H. J. & PERKINS, H. R. (1968) *Cell Walls and Membranes*. London: E. F. & N. Spon Ltd.

SALTON, M. R. J. (1964) *The Bacterial Cell Wall*. Amsterdam, London, New York: Elsevier Publishing Co.

SALTON, M. R. J. (1963) The relationship between the nature of the cell wall and the Gram stain. *Journal of General Microbiology*, **30**, 223.

SHARON, N. (1969) The bacterial cell wall. *Scientific American*, **220**, 92.

STANIER, R. Y. & VAN NIEL, C. B. (1962) The concept of a bacterium. *Archiv für Mikrobiologie*, **42**, 17.

Symposium on the fine structure and replication of bacteria and their parts. (1965) *Bacteriological Reviews*, **29**, 277, 293, 299, 326, 345.

WILKINSON, J. F. (1958) The extracellular polysaccharides of bacteria. *Bacteriological Reviews*, **22**, 46.

3. Growth and Nutrition of Bacteria

When an inoculum of cells from a pure culture of bacteria is introduced into a suitable nutrient medium and incubated under appropriate conditions, almost all of the cells have the potential to grow at a very rapid rate. This growth, by which is meant an orderly increase in all the components of an organism, is normally associated with multiplication. The method of division of most bacteria is by binary fission—a new cell grows until it doubles its size when it divides into two halves. Very large populations of cells are normally involved and the individual cells do not all divide simultaneously. Equal proportions of the total population divide successively in unit periods of time so that growth and multiplication can be considered as synonymous in relation to time. This is not so for each single bacterium in which cell growth and cell division are clearly separately controlled variables. It is possible to produce a synchronously dividing population by artificial means such as a 'cold shock' so that the general relationship does not hold. However, such situations are not normally encountered and it is possible to use methods that measure increase in numbers (e.g. cell counts) or in mass (e.g. dry weight) as similar indices of mass gain, or 'growth'. It is important to realize the rapidity of growth under favourable circumstances when a cell may double every 20 min. If this rate were maintained for 24 h, the progeny of a single cell would be about 1×10^{21} cells and would have a mass of approximately four thousand tons. The conditions used for culture never permit such a rate of multiplication for more than a short time, generally because of an insufficiency of nutrients or of special growth factors.

When a comparatively small number of organisms are taken from a culture and inoculated into a fresh growth medium, the number of cells inoculated may multiply a million-fold or more during growth. If the number of cells present at different times after inoculation is measured, and the number is plotted in relation to the time (i.e. period of growth), the resultant plot is referred to as a batch growth curve. Two types of growth curve can be drawn according to the measurement of cell numbers that is used. (1) A *total count* is based on the number of cells present irrespective of whether they are living or not. In microbiology the definition of life can be only a practical one and an organism is considered living or viable if it is capable of continued multiplication; if it is not so capable it is called dead or non-viable. (2) On the other hand, a *viable count* measures only those cells capable of growing and hence of producing a colony on a suitable growth medium.

A typical growth curve is shown in Fig. 3.1. Four main phases of growth are generally recognized:

1. **Lag phase.** In this period there is no appreciable multiplication of cells although they may increase considerably in size and show marked metabolic activity. The duration of this phase varies according to the condition and number of cells in the inoculum and it can be looked upon as representing the time taken for the organism to adapt itself to growth in the fresh medium. The cells in an inoculum may be so depleted of enzymes, metabolic intermediates, and other factors, that some time is required for these materials to build up to their optimal

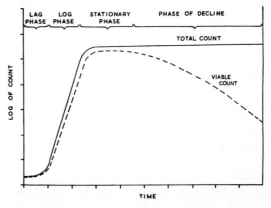

FIG. 3.1. Continuous line—total number of bacteria alive and dead. Interrupted line—total number of living bacteria.

levels. Alternatively, if the composition of the new medium differs significantly in composition from that in which the inoculum was growing previously, entirely new enzymes may require to be synthesized by the process of induction or by the selection of mutants.

2. **Logarithmic (log) or exponential phase.** In this period, the cells divide at a constant rate and, as a result of growth by binary fission, there is a linear relationship between time and the logarithm of the number of cells. It is important to realize the potential of this explosive growth. If the number of bacterial cells in a culture increases ten-fold in a given period of time, they will increase 100-fold in twice that time, 1 000-fold in three times the given period and so on, although the rate of division is much slower *in vivo*. Once an infection overwhelms the body defences and gets out of control, it becomes increasingly difficult to eradicate it as time goes on. In order to maintain such high rates of growth, bacteria must have a correspondingly high rate of metabolism. The actual rate of growth is directly related to the generation time (the time between divisions) of the bacterium under the particular environmental conditions that prevail. Some of the environmental factors that affect the rate of growth are considered later in this chapter.

3. **Stationary phase.** In due course, exponential growth is no longer possible and the rate of multiplication decreases until it ceases altogether and the cells pass into the stationary phase. It is theoretically possible to reach a stable number of cells by the establishment of an equilibrium between the rates of growth and death but the common situation is one in which neither growth nor death occurs but the cells remain in a state of suspended animation. Although the normal metabolism associated with biosynthesis and growth no longer occurs, there is usually some metabolic activity going on; this is known as endogenous metabolism and it probably acts to provide the cell with energy and intermediates required to maintain life. The cessation of growth in the stationary phase is most commonly caused by the exhaustion of an essential nutrient in the medium. Another factor may be the accumulation of toxic waste products; for example, organic acids are common end-products of fermentation and their accumulation can lead to a lowering of pH to a value inimical to growth.

Since a variety of factors can bring about the onset of the stationary phase, cells in this phase can exhibit a corresponding variation in morphology and physiology, both between themselves and in comparison with exponential-phase cells. Thus stationary-phase cells may have a high level of intracellular storage polymers such as polysaccharide (usually glycogen in bacteria) and lipid (usually poly-β-hydroxybutyrate in bacteria); these substances are often virtually absent in exponential-phase cells. Similarly a Gram-positive organism may become Gram-negative in the stationary phase. In routine studies of morphological characteristics it is usually important to observe young cells that are in a growing phase.

At the onset of the stationary phase, many species of bacteria produce *secondary metabolites*, i.e. natural products formed mainly or only by cells that have stopped dividing. These secondary metabolites are diverse in nature and each kind has a restricted taxonomic distribution. They include many antibiotics and exotoxins. In spore-forming species the initiation of sporulation typically occurs at the end of the exponential phase or early in the stationary phase, and since many antibiotic-producing and exotoxin-producing bacteria are sporing organisms there may be a relation between sporulation and the production of these secondary metabolites.

4. **Death or decline phase.** After a variable period of time in the stationary phase, the cells in a culture begin to die—they become incapable of growth when transferred to a fresh medium. This is reflected in Fig. 3.1 as an increasing divergence between the total count (living and dead cells) and the viable count (living cells only). The causes of this death or loss of viability are various, the main determinant being the nature of the factor that caused the cessation of growth at the onset of the stationary phase. If it is due to the accumulation of toxic products, there may be a very brief stationary phase followed by a rapid death rate. In some cases, there may be a rapid fall in the total count as well as the viable count because microorganisms are very prone to digest themselves so that they eventually lyse and liberate their cytoplasmic

contents into the environment; this process is known as *autolysis*. Associated with this tendency to autolysis is the common occurrence of bizarre cell shapes quite different from the normal range seen in exponential growth. Not all bacteria are subject to such rapid degeneration and death; some organisms under appropriate environmental conditions may stay in the stationary phase for days. Clearly the rapidity of the onset of the death phase is an important factor that may influence the spread of infection.

Growth of the type discussed above, in which an inoculum is placed in a culture vessel, is known as *batch culture* and is the usual method of growing bacteria in the laboratory. However, it is possible to use an 'open' system in which there is a continuous supply of fresh nutrients into the culture vessel and a continuous removal of grown bacteria by means of a constant level device. This method of culture—called *continuous culture*— is being used for both research and industrial purposes and it may correspond more truly with the situation occurring in some diseases of man and animals. The basis for most continuous culture systems in the laboratory is the *chemostat* which is represented in Fig. 3.2. In this system, the rate of growth is controlled by the rate of addition of fresh nutrient that is pumped from the medium vessel. This, in turn, controls the rate of removal of cells via the overflow device into the collector vessel. When equilibrium is reached, the rate of production of new cells by multiplication is equal to the rate of removal of grown cells into the collector vessel. This state can be continued indefinitely so as to provide a source of reproducible cells from an environment which can itself be varied by altering the nature or rate of addition of fresh medium. Another type of continuous-culture system is the *turbidistat* in which the addition of a measured volume of fresh medium is triggered when the turbidity in the growth vessel reaches a predetermined value that is monitored by a photoelectric cell. As a result of the addition, the cells are diluted and continue to grow until they again reach the critical turbidity and the process is repeated.

In order to identify and study a bacterial species, it is necessary to grow the organism under laboratory conditions and it is therefore essential to know its growth requirements. Two

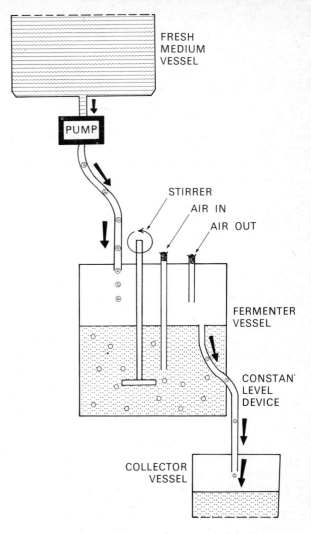

FIG. 3.2. Chemostat: an apparatus for the continuous culture of bacteria.

conditions must be fulfilled: (1) suitable nutrients must be supplied; and (2) the physical conditions must be as near optimum as possible for the organism under consideration.

Microorganisms differ widely in the nutritional factors and the physical conditions needed for their growth; these differences reflect the physiological characteristics of the organisms concerned. It is important, therefore, to understand some of the principles underlying microbial physiology.

PHYSIOLOGY OF MICROORGANISMS

The basic chemical composition of all microorganisms is essentially similar. Water is the major component making up about 80 per cent of the cell's weight. Typical figures for the other components are given in Table 3.1 for both a prokaryotic and a eukaryotic microorganism.

It must be emphasized that these figures are average and typical ones, the actual value varying with both the microorganism and the cultural conditions employed. For example, the mycobacteria are characterized by a high lipid content irrespective of the growth conditions, whereas most microorganisms grown in the presence of an excess of a carbon and energy source will have a high polysaccharide content due to the accumulation of storage polymers.

It is evident that polymers of high molecular weight make up a large proportion of the dry weight of microorganisms, as indeed they do with all living organisms. This fact is even more striking in prokaryotes where an appreciable part of lipid may be in the form of poly-β-hydroxybutyrate. Apart from normal lipid, the other low molecular weight components are co-enzymes, prosthetic groups, intermediary metabolites and inorganic salts.

The study of comparative biochemistry has shown that living organisms are similar in their component chemical units as well as in the mechanisms by which these components are formed—the process of metabolism. This concept is generally referred to as 'The Unity of Biochemistry'. Thus the nucleotide and amino acid components of nucleic acids and proteins are the same in bacteria as in mammals or higher plants. The types of enzymic reaction carried out and the coenzymes involved in them are virtually identical and in all organisms the adenosine diphosphate $\leftrightharpoons$ adenosine triphosphate (ADP $\leftrightharpoons$ ATP) system is used for energy conversions. The study of molecular biology has shown an even more striking picture of unity in the synthesis of protein and nucleic acid where the methods of transcription, translation and coding are almost identical. It is true that there are exceptions to this basic unity, a fortunate fact for the development of chemotherapy. As can be seen in Table 3.1, the mucopeptide is

unique to the prokaryotic cell wall as are its characteristic monomer components—N-acetyl muramic acid, diaminopimelic acid and some D-amino acids. Certain monosaccharides may also be specific and microorganisms are characterized by the wide variety of these that can occur in cell wall or capsular polysaccharides. The variety and the different methods of linkage involved partly explains why such a wide range of different antigenic types of organism can be seen in nature. There are also substances unique to eukaryotic cells such as sterols that are almost always absent from prokaryotes and are never synthesized by them.

Table 3.1. The composition of a typical prokaryotic and eukaryotic microorganism given as percentages of the dry weight.

		Prokaryote	Eukaryote
Polymers of	Nucleic acid	10	5
high	Protein	40	45
molecular	Polysaccharide	15	15
weight	Mucopeptide	10	0
	Lipid	15	20
Compounds of low molecular weight		10	15

Granted that all microorganisms have a remarkable resemblance in basic chemical composition, how far do they show a similar metabolism? A cell's metabolism can be conveniently divided into the following sections.

1. The conversion of the carbon of nutrients into basic 'building blocks' to be used in biosynthesis; and

2. The conversion of ADP to ATP by the energy-yielding metabolism.

These two processes can be considered together as comprising catabolism. Some non-parasitic microorganisms are able, like plants, to utilize carbon dioxide as the main source of carbon and are called autotrophs (or lithotrophs). Energy is obtained in these organisms by the oxidation of inorganic compounds (chemosynthetic autotrophs or chemolithotrophs) or from sunlight (photosynthetic autotrophs or photolithotrophs). However, the majority of microorganisms, including all those that are directly important in medicine, obtain their energy by the breakdown of suitable organic nutrients; they are called heterotrophs or chemoorganotrophs. In them, stages 1 and 2 are combined, the carbon and energy source being partly used to produce ATP and partly used to provide building blocks.

3. The building blocks are converted to monomers, eventually in an activated form.

4. These activated monomers are polymerized.

These two biosynthetic processes comprising anabolism require energy in the form of ATP.

5. The polymers are transported to the appropriate area of the cell for their proper functioning. For example, some proteins must be incorporated into the cytoplasmic membrane, others into the nucleus, others into ribosomes and so on. We know very little of this process, but there is no reason to believe that the basic mechanism in microorganisms differs from that in higher organisms.

Catabolism

Microorganisms differ widely in the range of organic compounds that can be used as a source of carbon and energy. Some bacteria are remarkably versatile, such as species of the genus *Pseudomonas*, and can utilize any one of over a hundred organic compounds (sugars, acids, alcohols, etc.) as the sole source of carbon and energy, whereas many bacteria are much more specific in their requirement. In general, all microorganisms seem to have certain fundamental metabolic pathways concerned in the interconversions necessary for the production of the basic 'building blocks' mentioned previously. Examples are the enzymes concerned in the glycolytic pathway, the pentose phosphate cycle and the tricarboxylic acid cycle; such enzymes are synthesized irrespective of the environmental conditions and form a group of the so-called *constitutive enzymes*. On the other hand, leading into these general metabolic sequences there are specific pathways concerned in the breakdown of a particular substrate. The enzymes concerned in these pathways are usually *inducible*, that is they are produced only in the presence of an inducer and this is generally the substrate itself. The obvious advantage of such a system to an organism like the pseudomonad

is one of economy; as there are hundreds of such specific enzymes that may be required it would be very wasteful to produce them all irrespective of what chemical compounds are present in the environment. A less well explained regulatory process is that of 'catabolite repression' in which a common carbon and energy source such as glucose actually represses the synthesis of a wide variety of enzymes that are not concerned with glucose breakdown.

Microorganisms differ considerably in the way in which the carbon and energy source is broken down to provide energy. This difference mainly concerns the involvement of oxygen as a terminal electron acceptor in the system. The majority of bacteria are described as *facultative anaerobes* because they are able to grow either aerobically, i.e. in the presence of air and free oxygen, or anaerobically, in its absence. Certain other species grow only in the presence of air or free oxygen, and are described as *strict* or *obligate aerobes*, whereas others that grow only in the absence of free oxygen and are usually killed in its presence are known as *strict anaerobes*. For the anaerobes the ultimate determining factor for growth is the state of oxidation of the environment, this being best described in terms of the oxidation-reduction, or 'redox' potential. It has been suggested that in the presence of oxygen a strict anaerobe is liable to produce toxic peroxides that it cannot destroy; many strict anaerobes lack catalase, an enzyme present in most aerobes and facultative anaerobes, and it has been tempting to link the 'toxic peroxides theory' with the lack of catalase as a unitarian explanation of anaerobiosis. However, the evidence for such a theory is lacking. Finally, there is a group of organisms that grow best in the presence of a trace only of free oxygen and often prefer an increased concentration of carbon dioxide; these are called *microaerophilic*.

The aerobic or anaerobic growth properties of a microorganism are related to the aerobic or anaerobic nature of their metabolism. Thus aerobes obtain most of their energy by a series of coupled oxido-reductions in which the ultimate electron-acceptor is atmospheric oxygen; in this *aerobic respiration*, the carbon and energy source may be completely oxidized to carbon dioxide and water. Energy is obtained by the production of energy-rich phosphate bonds and their transfer to adenosine diphosphate (ADP) to form adenosine triphosphate (ATP) during the passage of electrons through the electron-transport system. This process is known as oxidative phosphorylation. The electron-transport systems of microorganisms are often very similar to those occurring in higher organisms and involve pyridine nucleotide coenzymes, flavoproteins, cytochromes and cytochrome oxidases.

Anaerobes, on the other hand, oxidize compounds at the expense of some electron acceptor other than oxygen. In some instances, an inorganic compound capable of reduction such as nitrate or sulphate acts as the electron acceptor; this process is known as *anaerobic respiration* and energy is again produced mainly during the passage of electrons from the substrate to the inorganic electron acceptor. However, anaerobic growth probably occurs more commonly by a process in which the carbon and energy source acts both as the electron donor and the electron acceptor in a series of oxido-reductions. This process is known as *fermentation* and it leads to the formation of a variety of waste products such as ethanol in cultures of yeasts, and organic acids and alcohols in cultures of bacteria, e.g. lactic acid production by lactobacilli and streptococci, and formation of a mixture of lactic, acetic, formic and succinic acids by the enterobacteria. Carbon dioxide and, in some cases hydrogen, is commonly produced and therefore fermentation is usually accompanied by the production of both acid and gas. The nature of the fermentation product is also of significance in the classification of bacteria. During the process of fermentation, energy-rich phosphate bonds are produced by the introduction of inorganic phosphate into intermediates on the fermentation pathway, a process known as substrate-level phosphorylation. The energy-rich phosphate groups so produced are transferred on to ADP to form ATP under the influence of the appropriate phosphorylation enzyme. Facultative anaerobes may obtain their energy exclusively by fermentation (e.g. streptococci) or may be able to obtain it either by fermentation or respiration (e.g. enterobacteria). It should be noted that the amount of energy produced from a given amount of a carbon and energy source under anaerobic conditions is considerably less than that produced under aerobic conditions and therefore growth of a facultative anaerobe is usually much more abundant under aerobic conditions.

Anabolism

We have seen that the end-products of biosynthesis are very similar for all microorganisms. However, there are wide differences in the ability of cells to carry out the individual biosyntheses of essential monomers and coenzymes. Some are capable of synthesizing all their amino acids, nucleotides, monosaccharides, coenzymes, and so on from the building blocks produced by catabolism. Others almost completely lack such biosynthetic powers and, as is discussed later, depend entirely on their nutrient environment for the provision of such substances in ready-made form. Within these two extremes there is a wide spectrum of different biosynthetic abilities. With respect to the actual enzymes involved in particular pathways, there is very little difference in the intermediates and reactions involved in the whole range of living organisms. Just as the enzymes concerned in the specific utilization of carbon sources are subject to control by induction, enzymes catalyzing biosynthesis are subject to feedback inhibition and to repression. In feedback inhibition, the end-product inhibits the action of the *first enzyme* of the *specific* pathway and thus exerts a fine control over the action of enzymes already present. In repression the end-product inhibits the production of *all* the enzymes concerned in its specific biosynthesis. These two control processes between them prevent the synthesis of the enzymes and their products when the end-product is already present as a nutrient in the environment and they therefore contribute significantly to the economy of the cell.

Although microorganisms vary widely in their possession of enzymes that catalyse the biosynthesis of essential low molecular-weight compounds, all cellular forms of life must have a certain range of enzymes to catalyse the required polymerizations because it is not possible to incorporate an extracellularly provided polymer directly into the cell structure. In general, substances of high molecular weight cannot penetrate the cytoplasmic membrane. An exception to this rule is the acquisition of substantial lengths of DNA during genetic transfer (Chap. 7). Viruses are non-cellular, and have a completely different mode of reproduction from cellular forms of life; they are dealt with in separate chapters.

NUTRITION OF MICROORGANISMS

The growth of microorganisms is dependent on an adequate supply of suitable nutrients and the specific requirements vary according to the natural environmental adaptations of different species. Some species are able to grow under a wide range of conditions, but others, especially the more strictly parasitic such as the gonococcus, are very exacting and restrictive in their requirements. Whilst it is hardly possible to reproduce exactly the natural environmental conditions of pathogenic bacteria, suitable artificial culture media have been devised for the majority.

In view of the similarity of the chemical components of all microorganisms, the different nutrient requirements that are recognized must reflect different biosynthetic abilities. It is possible to view these different nutrient requirements in terms of the provision of bulk elements or in terms of the requirements for specific organic compounds. What are these requirements? The main elements required for growth are carbon, hydrogen, oxygen and nitrogen, with sulphur and phosphorus required in somewhat smaller amounts, and other elements such as sodium, potassium, magnesium, iron and manganese in considerably smaller amounts. Since hydrogen and oxygen can be supplied in the water that is essential for any growth, it is evident that carbon and nitrogen are the main bulk elements required.

CARBON AND ENERGY SOURCE. As already noted, a heterotroph must be supplied with a suitable organic compound or compounds that can be broken down to provide suitable building blocks and to convert ADP to ATP. The organic compounds that can be used generally reflect the normal environment of an organism; parasitic microorganisms will normally utilize organic compounds such as glucose and amino acids present in the tissue fluids of their hosts.

NITROGEN SOURCE. The main inorganic form of nitrogen used in biosynthesis is ammonia, usually in the form of an ammonium salt. It can be provided directly in the environment or it can be produced indirectly by the deamination of organic nitrogenous nutrients such as amino acids or by the reduction of nitrates. A few bacteria can utilize nitrogen gas as a nitrogen source and reduce it to ammonia by the process of nitrogen fixation. These nitrogen-fixing microorganisms are of no direct importance in medicine but their occurrence is of critical importance to agriculture and the maintenance of soil fertility.

OTHER INORGANIC SALT REQUIREMENTS. Microorganisms require a supply of inorganic salt for growth, particularly the anions phosphate and sulphate, and the cations sodium, potassium, magnesium, iron, manganese and calcium. Some ions such as cobalt are needed in such trace amounts that it is difficult in practice to demonstrate a requirement.

REQUIREMENT FOR ORGANIC COMPOUNDS. As mentioned previously, certain organic compounds such as amino acids, nucleotides, monosaccharides, lipids and coenzymes must be either synthesized by the microorganism or must be provided as nutrients in the environment. Microorganisms vary widely in their biosynthetic capacity and this variation is reflected in their nutrient requirements. Consider the amino acids as an example. Twenty amino acids must be provided for protein synthesis as well as perhaps three more for mucopeptide synthesis in prokaryotes. Some microorganisms can synthesize all of their amino acids for themselves from the carbon and energy source together with ammonium and sulphate ions. Other microorganisms are unable to carry out the biosynthesis of any of their amino acids and these therefore become essential nutrients that must be supplied in the growth medium. A complete range of biosynthetic abilities and, therefore, of nutrient requirements is found between these two extremes. It is interesting to note that man comes about midway on such a scale, being able to synthesize about half the total number of amino acids. A similar range of biosynthetic ability and nutrient requirement in the bacteria can be found for nucleotides and their component purines and pyrimidines and for co-enzymes. If a coenzyme or an essential part of a coenzyme is required as a nutrient, it is usually required in small catalytic amounts and is some-times known as a growth factor or microbial vitamin. Many of these substances are, of course, identical with the vitamins required for mam-malian nutrition, e.g. thiamine, riboflavine, nicotinic acid, pyridoxine, p-aminobenzoic acid, folic acid, biotin, cobamide, etc. Monosaccha-rides and lipids, however, are usually synthesized from the bulk carbon and energy source.

Permeability of the Cell to Various Nutrients

If any compound is going to be used as a nutrient, whether it is organic or inorganic, and be it a bulk carbon and energy source or a growth factor required in catalytic quantities, it has to pass through the cytoplasmic membrane in order to reach the cytoplasm where most further metabolism occurs. Since the cytoplasmic mem-brane is a semipermeable layer, active transport of these nutrients is essential and this is carried out by specific carriers or permeases which catalyse their entry. A considerable concentra-tion of a substance can occur within the cyto-plasm as a result. It is clear that a microorganism must have a number of permeases corresponding to the complexity of its nutrient requirements.

Microbiological Assay

If a microorganism requires a certain substance for its growth, then, provided that all other nutrients are present in excess, the final amount of growth will be proportional to the amount of the 'limiting substance' added. If the results are

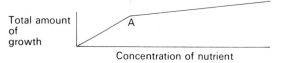

FIG. 3.3. The relationship between bacterial growth and the concentration of a limiting nutrient.

plotted, a graph similar to that shown in Fig. 3.3 should be obtained. Up to the point A on the graph, there is a linear relationship between growth and the concentration of the limiting nutrient and this fact is utilized in the method of microbiological assay. Amino acids or vitamins are commonly assayed in this way as in the determination of vitamin B12 with *Lactobacillus leichmannii*. The method has the advantage of specificity and high sensitivity that cannot be equalled by chemical assays. As little as 0·001 μg per ml of vitamins can be determined and some-times, as with biotin and vitamin B12, con-siderably less.

Nutritional Evolution

Bacteria differ widely in their requirements for amino acids, nucleotides and growth factors and therefore in their synthetic capacities. Some, especially among the non-parasitic species (e.g. *Klebsiella aerogenes*) have comprehensive syn-thetic abilities and are therefore *non-exacting* nutritionally; they are able to synthesize all their structural units from the carbon and energy source and inorganic salts. Other bacteria, in the course of evolution towards a strictly parasitic mode of life, have increasingly obtained their amino acids, nucleotides and growth factors from the tissues of their host, and have lost the power of synthesizing these compounds. Many species are thus nutritionally exacting (e.g. *Streptococcus pyogenes*) and can grow in a syn-thetic medium only if it contains a wide range of different amino acids, nucleotides and growth factors. Certain obligate intracellular parasites (rickettsia and chlamydia) have special cyto-plasmic membranes that allow the passage of nucleoside triphosphates from the host cell; these 'energy parasites' have come to depend on the uptake of preformed ATP. This process of nutritional evolution to increasing dependence upon nutrients in the environment can be paralleled in the laboratory by the selection of mutants. An enzyme catalysing a step in the synthesis of an amino acid, nucleotide or growth factor may be lost as a result of gene mutation and the variant strain thus becomes nutritionally exacting in respect of the substance which the parent strain can synthesize for itself.

MEDIA FOR THE GROWTH OF MICROORGANISMS

A variety of growth media have been devised for specific purposes in microbiology. Details of many of these are given in Volume II and here only the basic types of media will be considered.

1. **General laboratory media.** The purposes of a general laboratory medium are twofold. Firstly, it should support the growth of as wide a range of microorganisms as possible; in other words, it should contain a sufficiency of the generally required microbial nutrients. Secondly, it should be cheap and easy to produce. In practice, the most important substances required for microbial growth are amino acids, nucleotides, growth factors, a bulk source of carbon, energy and nitrogen and certain inorganic ions. In order to provide these components, most general laboratory media contain the following:

(a) A hydrolysate of a cheap protein, preferably prepared by the use of a proteolytic enzyme to prevent amino acid destruction. Such hydrolysates are called peptones and should contain all the essential amino acids.

(b) A source of growth factors and inorganic salts. This is usually provided by an extract of meat or of yeast. Sometimes a further enrichment is provided by the addition of special sources of growth factors such as blood, serum or egg.

(c) Usually sodium chloride is added for the growth of parasitic microorganisms to bring the osmotic pressure up to a figure comparable with that of host tissues.

It should be noted that such media have no single carbon and energy source, but instead a series of organic compounds such as amino acids are catabolized to produce building blocks (including ammonia) and energy; the remainder of these compounds may be incorporated directly into the cell.

2. **Synthetic media.** A synthetic medium is one in which all of the nutrients are specified and added separately to give a chemically defined product. Media of this type are used for various experimental purposes. A simple synthetic medium contains a suitable carbon and energy source (e.g. glucose or lactate), an inorganic nitrogen source (e.g. an ammonium salt) and various inorganic salts in a buffered aqueous solution. Such media provide the basic essentials for the growth of many non-parasitic heterotrophs but they will not support the growth of most parasitic microorganisms which require complex synthetic media incorporating the amino acids, purines, pyrimidines and growth factors. Synthetic media are designed to meet the particular requirements of the microorganism concerned; they are expensive and tedious to make and are therefore only used for special purposes such as in microbiological assay.

3. **Special media.** A variety of media have been developed for special purposes in microbiology. *Selective* media contain substances that inhibit or poison all but a few types of microorganism, thus facilitating the isolation of a particular species from a mixed inoculum. If a liquid medium favours the multiplication of a particular species, either by containing additional materials that selectively favour it or inhibiting substances that suppress competitors, derived from mixed inocula it is called an *enrichment* medium, and is commonly a first stage in the isolation of pure cultures by conventional plating-out methods. Clearly these cultures will not indicate the proportion of the species originally present in an inoculum. Certain media are referred to as *indicator* media; they contain some substance that is changed visibly as a result of the metabolic activity of particular organisms. Combinations of enriched media with selective agents and indicator systems are frequently used in the diagnostic laboratory.

PHYSICAL CONDITIONS REQUIRED FOR GROWTH

In order to double its size and divide within 30 minutes, a bacterial cell must be capable of synthesizing its own weight of cell material within that period. Accordingly, it must have a very rapid rate of metabolism together with a correspondingly rapid uptake of nutrients and disposal of waste products. It can do this only because of its small size, which gives it a very large surface for absorption and excretion in relation to its volume. But the very rapid growth that occurs in the log phase is possible only under certain restricted environmental conditions; it is most important to understand these thoroughly.

Influence of Oxygen

It is necessary to provide oxygen for a strict aerobe and to remove it completely from the environment of a strict anaerobe. A sufficiently low redox potential for the growth of strict anaerobes is usually provided by placing the culture in an atmosphere of hydrogen in the modern equivalent of a McIntosh and Fildes anaerobic jar.

The natural environment of a microorganism is determined accordingly. Thus a strict aerobe like the tubercle bacillus will grow best in a well aerated environment such as the animal lung, and a strict anaerobe like *Clostridium tetani* requires an anaerobic environment such as in dead tissue in a lacerated and infected wound.

Influence of Carbon Dioxide

It is now recognized that all bacteria require the presence of a small amount of carbon dioxide for growth, an amount normally provided by the atmosphere or by oxidation and fermentation reactions within the cell itself. Some bacteria (e.g. *Brucella abortus*, when first isolated from the body) require a much higher concentration of carbon dioxide (5 to 10 per cent), and this must be provided in the environment of the culture medium.

Influence of Temperature

1. *On growth.* For each species there is a definite temperature range within which growth takes place. The limits are the 'maximum' and 'minimum' temperatures, and an intermediate 'optimum' temperature can usually be recognized at which growth is most rapid. In the laboratory, bacteria are grown at this optimum temperature in a thermostatically controlled incubator. The optimum temperature of a bacterium is approximately that of its natural habitat, e.g. about 37°C in the case of organisms that are parasitic on man and warm-blooded animals. These, and many saprophytes of soil and water that grow best at between 25° and 40°C, are termed *mesophilic*. Some mesophiles have a wide growth temperature range (e.g. 5° to 43°C for *Pseudomonas pyocyanea* (*aeruginosa*), whereas others are more restricted (e.g. 30° to 39°C for *Neisseria gonorrhoeae*). None of them grows appreciably at temperatures below 5°C (as in a domestic refrigerator at 3° to 5°C), and few at temperatures above 45°C.

A group of soil and water bacteria, the *psychrophiles*, grow best at temperatures below 20°C, usually quite well at 0°C and in some cases, slowly, down to about −7°C on unfrozen media. Their importance lies in their ability to cause spoilage of refrigerated and frozen food, though none is pathogenic. Another group of non-parasitic bacteria, the *thermophiles*, grow best at high temperatures between 55° and 80°C, and have minimum growth temperatures ranging from 20° to 40°C (facultative thermophiles), or even above 40°C (strict thermophiles). These organisms are important as a cause of spoilage in under-processed canned foods, since many form spores of exceptionally high heat-resistance.

2. *On viability.* Heat is an important agent in the artificial destruction of microorganisms, the effect depending under moist conditions on the coagulation and denaturation of cell proteins, and under dry conditions, on oxidation and charring. Among the bacteria that are parasites of mammals, non-sporing forms in the presence of water generally cannot withstand temperatures above 45°C for any length of time. The time of exposure to heat that is necessary for killing is shorter the higher the temperature, and various other factors influence the exact amount of heating required. Thus, bacteria are more susceptible to 'moist heat', e.g. in hot water or saturated steam, than to 'dry heat', e.g. in a hot-air oven. They are rendered more susceptible to the lethal effect of heat by the presence of acid, alkali or any chemical disinfectant, and less susceptible by the presence of organic substances such as proteins, sugars and fats, and also by their own occurrence in large numbers. The *thermal death point* of a particular organism may be defined as the lowest temperature that kills it under standard conditions, and within a given time, e.g. 10 min. Under moist conditions, it lies between 50° and 65°C for most non-sporing mesophilic bacteria, and between 100° and 120°C for the spores of most sporing species (e.g. about 105°C for *Cl. tetani* and 115°C for *Cl. botulinum*).

The extreme limit of resistance to moist heat is shown by the spores of a non-pathogenic, strictly thermophilic bacillus, *B. stearothermophilus*, which is killed only after exposure to 121°C for 10 to 35 minutes. With dry heat, the 10-minute thermal death points of the different sporing bacteria are mostly between 140° and 180°C.

At low temperatures some species die rapidly, but the majority survive well. Cultures of the latter may be preserved for long periods at between 3° and 5°C in a domestic-type refrigerator, or in the frozen state at between −20° and −70°C in a 'deep freeze' cabinet. The process of freezing kills a proportion of the bacterial cells present, and this is least if freezing is effected rapidly, e.g. by use of solid carbon dioxide or if a stabilizer such as glycerol is added.

Influence of Moisture and of Desiccation

Four-fifths by weight of the bacterial cell consists of water and, as in the case of other organisms, moisture is absolutely necessary for growth. Drying in air is injurious to many microbes, and the different species vary widely in their ability to survive when dried under natural conditions, as in infected exudate smeared on clothing or furniture, and converted to dust. Thus, the gonococcus, *Treponema pallidum* and the common cold virus appear to die quickly, whereas the tubercle bacillus, *Staph. aureus* and the smallpox virus may survive for weeks or months. Bacterial endospores survive drying especially well; for instance the spores of *Bacillus anthracis*, when dried on threads, have survived for over sixty years.

Even delicate, non-sporing organisms may survive drying for a period of years if they are desiccated rapidly and completely, preferably while frozen, and thereafter maintained in a high vacuum (0·01 mmHg, or less) in a sealed glass ampoule stored at room temperature in the dark. This is the basis of the *lyophilization* or 'freeze-drying' process of preserving bacterial cultures in the laboratory (Chap. 6, Vol. II).

Influence of Hydrogen-ion Concentration

A suitable environmental pH is an essential factor in microbial metabolism and growth. The majority of commensal and pathogenic bacteria grow best at a neutral or very slightly alkaline reaction (pH 7·2 to 7·6). Some bacteria, however, flourish in the presence of a considerable degree of acidity and are termed *acidophilic*, e.g. *Lactobacillus*. Others are very sensitive to acid, but tolerant of alkali, e.g. *Vibrio cholerae*. Strong acid or alkali solutions, e.g. 5 per cent hydrochloric acid or sodium hydroxide respectively, are rapidly lethal to most bacteria, the mycobacteria (e.g. tubercle bacillus) being exceptional in resisting them.

Influence of Light and Other Radiations

Darkness provides a favourable condition for growth and viability. Ultraviolet rays are rapidly bactericidal, e.g. direct sunlight or radiation from a mercury vapour lamp. Even diffuse daylight, as it enters a room through window glass, significantly shortens the survival of microorganisms and may be of hygienic importance. Bacteria are also killed by ionizing radiations.

Influence of Osmotic Pressure

As a result of the presence of a semi-permeable cytoplasmic membrane, bacteria resemble other cells in being subject to osmotic phenomena. Relative to the cells of higher organisms, however, they are very tolerant of changes in the osmotic pressure of their environment and can grow in media with widely varying contents of salt, sugar and other such solutes. This is partly a reflection of the mechanical strength of their cell walls. For most species the maximum concentration of sodium chloride permitting growth lies between 5 and 12 per cent, though *halophilic* (or osmophilic) species occur that can grow at higher concentrations up to saturation. The latter are saprophytes whose importance lies in their ability to cause spoilage of food preserved with salt or sugar; they are not pathogenic. Sudden exposure of bacteria to solutions of high salt concentration (e.g. 2 to 25 per cent sodium chloride) may cause *plasmolysis*, i.e. temporary shrinkage of the protoplast and its retraction from the cell wall due to the osmotic withdrawal of water; this occurs much more readily in Gram-negative than in Gram-positive bacteria. Sudden transfer from a concentrated to a weak solution, or to distilled water, may cause *plasmoptysis*—i.e. swelling and bursting of the cell as a result of excessive osmotic imbibition of water.

Influence of Mechanical and Sonic Stresses

Although their cell walls have considerable strength and some elasticity, it is possible to rupture and kill bacteria by exposure to mechanical stresses. A bacterial suspension may be largely disintegrated by subjection to very vigorous shaking with fine glass beads, or to supersonic or ultrasonic vibration (9 000–200 000 and over 200 000 cycles per second, respectively). These measures are used in separating the large molecular components of the cell.

FURTHER READING

MANDELSTAM, J. & McQUILLEN, K. (1972) *Biochemistry of Bacterial Growth*. 2nd edn. Oxford: Blackwell.

4. Classification and Identification of Microorganisms with Special Reference to Bacteria

Microorganisms may be defined as living creatures that are microscopical in size and relatively simple, often unicellular in structure. The diameter of the smallest body that can be resolved and seen clearly with the naked eye is about 100 μm. All but a few of the microorganisms are smaller than this and a microscope is therefore necessary for their observation. The light microscope under optimal conditions can resolve bodies down to 0·2 μm in diameter; and this includes all microbes and largely excludes the viruses, most of which are smaller than 0·2 μm. Pox viruses, however, can be seen with the light microscope and influenza virus filaments by dark-ground illumination. The electron microscope has a limit of resolution smaller than 0·5 nm (0·0005 μm) and can resolve even the smallest viruses (0·01 μm diameter). When bacteria or fungi are allowed to grow undisturbed on a solid or semi-solid substrate, their numerous progeny accumulate locally to form masses, or colonies, that are readily visible to the naked eye.

The majority of microorganisms may be classified in the following large biological groups:

1. Algae.
2. Protozoa.
3. Slime moulds.
4. Fungi proper, or *Eumycetes,* including the moulds and the yeasts.
5. Bacteria, or *Schizomycetes* ('fission fungi').
6. *Rickettsiales.*
7. *Mycoplasmatales.*
8. Viruses, or *Virales.*

The algae (excluding the blue-green algae), the protozoa, slime moulds and fungi include the larger and more highly developed microorganisms; their cells have the same general type of structure and organization, described as eukaryotic, that is found in the cells of higher plants and animals. The bacteria and the closely related blue-green algae, the organisms of the mycoplasma and rickettsia and psittacosis-lymphogranuloma-trachoma (chlamydia) groups include the smaller microorganisms having a simpler form of cellular organization described as prokaryotic. The viruses are the smallest of the infective agents; the infectious virus particles, or virions, have a relatively simple structure that is not comparable with that of a cell, and their mode of reproduction is fundamentally different from that of cellular organisms. Accordingly, the view has been expressed that viruses are not microorganisms, but in terms of their infectivity and epidemiology, pathogenic viruses behave like other infective agents.

Since the algae and slime moulds contain no species of medical or veterinary importance, they will not be dealt with in this book. The main differential characters of the other groups are as follows:

Protozoa. These are non-photosynthetic unicellular organisms (a few are colonial) with protoplasm clearly differentiated into nucleus and cytoplasm (see Fig. 4.1). They are relatively large microorganisms, with transverse diameters mainly in the range of 2–100 μm. Their surface membranes vary in complexity and rigidity from a thin, flexible membrane in amoebae, that allows major changes in cell shape and the protrusion of pseudopodia in the movements of locomotion and ingestion, to a relatively stiff pellicle in ciliate protozoa that preserves a characteristic cell shape. Most free-living, and some parasitic species have the mode of nutrition typical of animals, that is called holozoic; they capture, ingest and digest internally solid masses or particles of food material. Many protozoa, for instance, feed on bacteria. Protozoa, therefore, are generally regarded as the lowest forms of animal life, though certain flagellate protozoa are very closely related in their morphology and mode of development to photosynthetic flagellate algae in the plant kingdom. Some free-living protozoa are saprophytic, absorbing soluble nutrient substances derived from dead plant or animal material, or from the excretions of plants and animals. Many protozoa are parasitic and live in and derive their nourishment from the body of an animal host; some of these parasites ingest masses of solid material whilst others absorb soluble nutrients through their cell surface. Malaria parasites, for instance, both absorb soluble nutrients from the host and ingest masses of host-cell cytoplasm. Protozoa reproduce asexually by binary fission or multiple fission (schizogony), and some also by a sexual mechan-

ism. Some species exhibit a definite life cycle with both sexual and asexual phases, and some form round, thick-walled resting cells, or 'cysts', which are important for the persistence and spread of the organism through the environment, where conditions may be unfavourable to survival of the vegetative forms.

Fungi. These are non-photosynthetic microorganisms possessing relatively rigid cell walls. They may be saprophytic or parasitic, and take in soluble nutrient substances by diffusion through their cell surfaces. When solid food materials are utilized, these are first broken down to soluble products by enzymes secreted extracellularly by the fungus. Except for the flagellate spores and gametes of the primitive aquatic species, fungi are non-motile. Moulds grow as branching filaments (hyphae), usually between 2 and 10 µm in width, which interlace to form a meshwork (mycelium). The hyphae are coenocytic (i.e. have a continuous multinucleate protoplasm), being non-septate or else septate with a central pore in each cross-wall. Moulds reproduce by the formation of various kinds of sexual and asexual spores that develop from the vegetative (feeding) mycelium or from an aerial mycelium that effects their airborne dissemination. Yeasts are ovoid or spherical cells that reproduce asexually by budding (see Fig. 4.1) and also, in many cases, sexually with the formation of sexual spores. They do not form a mycelium, although the intermediate yeast-like fungi form a pseudomycelium consisting of chains of elongated cells. The higher fungi of the class *Basidiomycetes* (mushrooms), which produce large fruiting structures for aerial dissemination of spores, play no part in infection of man or animals, although some species, e.g. *Amanita phalloides,* are poisonous when eaten.

Rickettsiales are simple unicellular organisms that are rod-shaped, spherical or pleomorphic. They are generally similar to, though smaller than bacteria, but they are still resolvable by the light microscope (i.e. over 0·2 µm in diameter). The majority are strict parasites that can grow only in the living tissues of a suitable animal host, usually intracellularly. A few exceptional species can grow in cell-free nutrient media containing body fluids. The organisms of psittacosis and trachoma, previously classed as viruses, are now included in the genus *Chlamydia.*

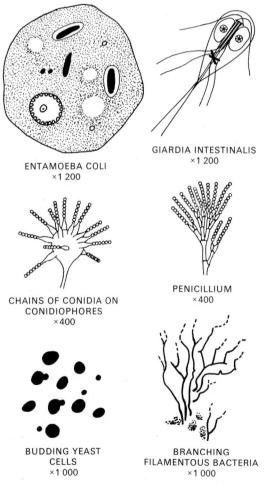

ENTAMOEBA COLI
×1 200

GIARDIA INTESTINALIS
×1 200

CHAINS OF CONIDIA ON CONIDIOPHORES
×400

PENICILLIUM
×400

BUDDING YEAST CELLS
×1 000

BRANCHING FILAMENTOUS BACTERIA
×1 000

FIG. 4.1. Examples of protozoa, fungi and filamentous bacteria.

Mycoplasmatales (pleuropneumonia-like organisms, or PPLO) are prokaryotic cellular organisms that differ from bacteria in their smaller size, their lack of a rigid cell wall, and their consequent extreme pleomorphism and great sensitivity to the osmotic tension of the environment. Cell size is variable and the viable elements range from 0·15 to over 1 μm in diameter, the smallest being capable of passing through bacteria-stopping filters. Mycoplasmas can be cultivated on artificial cell-free nutrient media enriched with serum and they are the smallest and simplest organisms capable of autonomous growth. Most are parasites of man or animals, but one known species is a saprophyte present in soil and sewage.

Viruses are the smallest and simplest of all the microorganisms and different species range in size from 0·01 to 0·3 μm in diameter. Most are 'ultramicroscopic' (i.e. are smaller than can be resolved by the light microscope, being less than 0·2 μm in diameter) and can pass through bacteria-stopping filters. All species are strictly parasitic and are capable of growing only within the living cells of an appropriate animal, plant or bacterial host; none can grow on an inanimate nutrient medium. A few bacteria and the rickettsiae resemble viruses in their inability to grow elsewhere than in living cells, but the viruses are distinguished from these organisms by having an entirely different method of growth and reproduction. The viruses that infect and parasitise bacteria are named *bacteriophages* or *phages*.

The bacteria and viruses predominate in the causation of human infective disease. Protozoal infections are more prevalent in tropical and subtropical countries, whilst the common fungal infections are mainly superficial (e.g. skin infections) and often of minor severity.

The remainder of this chapter and Chapter 3 will be devoted to the general biology of the bacteria.

MORPHOLOGICAL CLASSIFICATION OF BACTERIA

The main groups of bacteria are distinguished by microscopical observation of their morphology and staining reactions. Unstained bacterial cells are so feebly refractile that they are poorly visible with the light microscope unless special techniques such as phase-contrast microscopy are employed. It is therefore customary to stain smears of bacteria with simple stains or by more complex staining sequences. The *Gram staining* procedure, a complex sequence introduced by C. Gram in 1884, separates the bacteria into two great divisions: (1) *Gram-positive bacteria;* these appear purple because they retain the initially applied methyl violet stain which is complexed with iodine and potassium iodide during the staining procedure and then resists the decolourizing action of acetone or alcohol; (2) *Gram-negative bacteria* do not retain the Gram complex and are decolourized so that they then take up the pink colour of the fuchsin counterstain that is finally applied. The division afforded by the Gram reaction seems to be of wide biological significance (see p. 29). For example, Gram-positive bacteria share some general patterns of sensitivity to various classes of chemicals and antibiotics and these patterns are different from those of bacteria of the Gram-negative group.

Details of structure provide a basis for a separate division into the true bacteria and the filamentous bacteria that have some features in common with fungi; some produce a network, or *mycelium,* of branching forms and some have external sheath structures. Few of the filamentous bacteria are of medical interest as disease-producers (pathogens) in man, but some produce antibiotics. The medical bacteriologist is more directly concerned with the non-filamentous bacteria of which some are regularly associated with disease in man. The following simple classification is of practical use:

FILAMENTOUS BACTERIA
(Actinomycetes)

Sometimes referred to as 'the higher bacteria', these mycelial organisms include three main genera:

1. *Actinomyces.* Gram-positive, non-acid-fast, tending to fragment into short coccal and bacillary forms, and not forming conidia; anaerobic (e.g. *Actinomyces israelii*).

2. *Nocardia.* Similar to *Actinomyces,* but aerobic and mostly acid-fast (e.g. *Noc. farcinica*).

3. *Streptomyces.* Vegetative mycelium not fragmenting into short forms; conidia formed in chains from aerial hyphae (e.g. *Streptomyces griseus*).

TRUE BACTERIA

These simple, generally unicellular structures never occur in the form of a mycelium or sheathed filaments. They are classified on the basis of their shape:

1. Cocci—spherical or nearly spherical cells.
2. Bacilli—relatively straight rod-shaped (cylindrical) cells.
3. Vibrios—curved rod-shaped cells (comma-shaped).
4. Spirilla—spirally twisted, non-flexuous rods.

Cocci

The main groups of cocci are distinguished according to their predominant mode of cell grouping and their reaction to the Gram stain. The following groups correspond with biological genera:

1. *Streptococcus.* Cells mainly adherent in chains, due to successive cell divisions occurring in the same axis; Gram-positive (e.g. *Strept. pyogenes*).
2. *Staphylococcus amd Micrococcus.* Cells mainly adherent in irregular clusters, due to successive divisions occurring irregularly in different planes; Gram-positive (e.g. *Staph. aureus*).
3. *Sarcina.* Cells mainly adherent in cubical packets of eight, or multiples thereof, due to division occurring successively in three planes at right angles; Gram-positive (e.g. *Sarc. lutea*).
4. *Neisseria.* Cells mainly adherent in pairs and slightly elongated at right angles to axis of pair; Gram-negative (e.g. *N. meningitidis*).
5. *Veillonella.* Generally very small cocci arranged mainly in clusters and pairs; Gram-negative (e.g. *Veill. parvula*).

The different cocci are relatively uniform in size, about 1 μm being the average diameter. Some species are capsulate and a very few are motile. It should be noted that a pure growth will usually show, in addition to the predominant cell grouping (e.g. clusters or long chains), a number of single cocci, pairs and very short chains.

Bacilli

The primary subdivision of the rod-shaped bacteria is made according to their staining reactions by the Gram and Ziehl-Neelsen methods, and whether or not endospores are formed. Some of the groups thus distinguished include several biological genera, and these can be recognized only by study of their physiological characters in artificial cultures.

1. *Acid-fast bacilli.* In giving an acid-fast staining reaction by the Ziehl-Neelsen method, members of the genus *Mycobacterium,* including the tubercle bacillus, are distinguished from all other bacilli.
2. *Gram-positive spore-forming bacilli.* Apart from some rare saprophytic varieties, the only bacteria to form endospores are those of the genera *Bacillus* (aerobic) and *Clostridium* (anaerobic). They are primarily Gram-positive, but very liable to become Gram-negative in ageing cultures. The size, shape and position of the spore may assist recognition of the species; e.g. the tetanus bacillus is characterized by its bulging, spherical, terminal spore ('drum-stick' form).
3. *Gram-positive non-sporing bacilli.* These include several genera. *Corynebacterium* is distinguished by a tendency to slight curving and club-shaped or ovoid swelling of the bacilli, and their arrangement in parallel and angular clusters due to the snapping mode of cell division. *Erysipelothrix* and *Lactobacillus* are distinguished by a tendency to grow in chains and filaments, and *Listeria* by the occurrence of motility and flagellum formation.
4. *Gram-negative bacilli.* These include numerous genera belonging to the families *Pseudomonadaceae, Achromobacteraceae, Enterobacteriaceae, Brucellaceae* and *Bacteroidaceae. Pseudomonas* is distinguished by its polar flagellation, whereas motile members of the other families are peritrichously flagellate.

Vibrios and Spirilla

Vibrios are recognized as short, non-flexuous curved rods (e.g. *V. cholerae*) and spirilla as non-flexuous spiral filaments (e.g. *Sp. minus*). They are Gram-negative and mostly motile, having polar flagella and showing very active, 'darting' motility.

Spirochaetes

These organisms differ from true bacteria in being slender, flexuous spiral filaments. Their staining reaction, when demonstrable, is Gram-negative. They are distinguished from the spirilla in being capable of active flexion of the cell body and in being motile without possession of flagella. The different varieties are recognized by their size, shape, wave form and refractility, observed in the natural state in unstained wet films by dark-ground microscopy (see Fig. 4.2). The pathogenic species are classified in three genera:

1. *Borrelia*. Larger and more refractile than the other pathogenic spirochaetes, and more readily stained by ordinary methods; coils large and open, with a wavelength of 2–3 µm; by electron microscopy a leash of 8–12 fibrils, each about 0·02 µm thick, is seen twisted round the whole length of the protoplast (e.g. *Borr. recurrentis*).

2. *Treponema*. Thinner filaments in coils of shorter wavelength (e.g. 1·0–1·5 µm), typically presenting a regular 'corkscrew' form; feebly refractile and difficult to stain except by silver impregnation methods; by electron microscopy, a leash of 4 fibrils is seen wound round the protoplast within the cell wall (e.g. *Tr. pallidum*).

3. *Leptospira*. The coils are so fine and close (wavelength about 0·5 µm) that they are barely discernible by dark-ground microscopy, though clearly seen winding round two axial filaments by electron microscopy. One or both extremities of the spirochaete are 'hooked' or recurved, so that it may take the shape of a walking-stick, an S or a C (e.g. *L. interrogans*).

Biological Classification

Whilst observations of morphology and staining reactions are sufficient to distinguish the main groups, or *taxons* of bacteria, the biological classification of bacteria is based on a consideration of all kinds of demonstrable characters, including physiological, serological and ecological ones. Such a classification is not entirely compatible with a simple morphological classification, though morphological characters are mainly used to differentiate the major groups and other characters to differentiate the subgroups. At present no standard classification is universally accepted and applied. The older systems based solely on morphological characters are inadequate for detailed classification. For example, the term *Bacillus* was used in the past as a generic name for all rod-shaped bacteria, e.g. *Bacillus anthracis, B. tuberculosis* and *B. coli,* but in view of their heterogeneity the bacillary organisms clearly require subdivision into many separate genera. Thus the generic term *Bacillus* now applies only to those rod-shaped bacteria that are spore-forming and aerobic. It is, nevertheless, quite correct to use the term 'bacillus' as the common or vernacular name for any rod-shaped bacterium, and the common names such as 'anthrax bacillus', 'tubercle bacillus' and 'colon bacillus' in place of the international scientific names *Bacillus anthracis, Mycobacterium tuberculosis* and *Escherichia coli.*

STRAINS, ISOLATES AND CLONES. Since most of the tests used for identifying bacteria are inapplicable to single cells and require to be done on the large population of a culture, the ultimate unit to be identified is the *pure culture.* Pure cultures, e.g. young colonies, that are considered to consist exclusively of the progeny of a single cell and not to include any demonstrable mutant cells are described as *clones.* A 'line', or population of bacteria presumed to descend from a single ancestral bacterium, as found in a natural habitat and in primary cultures from that habitat and subcultures from the primary cultures, is called a *strain.* Thus, the cultures of typhoid bacilli isolated from 100 unrelated

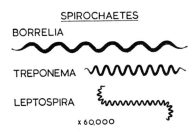

FIG. 4. 2. Spirochaetes.

patients with typhoid fever are said to include 100 different strains of the bacillus. Each primary culture isolated from a natural source is called an *isolate*. Thus, the cultures of a typhoid bacillus isolated from the same patient on ten successive days, or the cultures isolated at one time from ten patients known to have been infected with the same strain from a common source, are described as ten different isolates.

SPECIES. In the higher plants and animals the basic grouping of individuals, the *species,* is defined as a group of individuals that are generally similar in character (though commonly differing in minor characters, e.g. colouring), are adapted to a particular ecological niche and way of life, and are capable of continued fertile interbreeding. Species are designated by Latin binomials, the first term of which is the name of the *genus,* i.e. the next larger grouping, to which the species belongs.

Because bacteria do not reproduce by a sexual mechanism and only irregularly exchange genes, interfertility cannot be used for the definition of a species. The decision as to which of a series of generally similar strains with minor character differences should be included in the same species and which in different species is largely arbitrary. Ecological similarity is a criterion of some but limited value. Originally the medically important bacteria were grouped in species according to the diseases they caused. Thus all strains of bacilli causing diphtheria, even though they showed minor character differences such as in colony form, were allocated to the species *Bacillus diphtheriae,* all strains causing tuberculosis were allocated to the species *B. tuberculosis,* all causing plague to *B. pestis,* and so on. The power to cause such highly specific diseases is evidence of adaptation to a peculiar ecological niche and is a useful criterion for the definition of the species. Exception, however, must be made for the inclusion of non-pathogenic mutant strains along with the wild-type pathogenic strains in the same species. Some diseases, e.g. pneumonia, may be caused by any one of several widely different species of bacteria which may have different habitats. In these cases the value of the ecological criterion for the definition of species is minimal.

INTERNATIONAL CLASSIFICATION. The classification that has come to be generally accepted is one originally elaborated by American systematists and now given in Bergey's *Manual of Determinative Bacteriology,* 7th Edition. It conforms with accepted patterns of biological classification and is outlined in Table 4.1. The true bacteria are within the class *Schizomycetes* in the company of filamentous bacteria, spirochaetes and mycoplasmas. Moreover, it will be seen that the mycobacteria are here dealt with as filamentous bacteria, and the *Pseudomonas* genus is quite separate from other bacillary forms. Inevitably, microbiologists disagree among themselves regarding the pros and cons of any classification system and various amendments evolve.

In this book, for example, the above classification of the Enterobacteriaceae has been modified so that the genera conform more closely with the groups proposed by the Enterobacteriaceae Subcommittee of the International Committee on Bacterial Nomenclature and Taxonomy. The genera *Aerobacter* and *Paracolobactrum* are omitted and the following genera included:

Citrobacter, e.g. *Cit. freundii.*
Cloaca, e.g. *Cloaca cloacae.*
Hafnia, e.g. *Hafnia alvei.*

Thus, *Aerobacter aerogenes* is included in the genus *Klebsiella* as *Kl. aerogenes* and *Aerobacter cloacae* in the genus *Cloaca.* The *Paracolobactrum* organisms are regarded as lactose non-fermenting variants in the genera *Escherichia, Citrobacter, Klebsiella, Cloaca* and *Hafnia.*

Set apart from the class *Schizomycetes* on the ground of their smaller size and obligate parasitism, are the organisms in the class *Microtatobiotes* as follows:

CLASS MICROTATOBIOTES

This class contains the smallest of cellular organisms, all obligate parasites and capable of growth only in the living tissues of an appropriate host, usually intracellularly.

Rickettsiales

Individual organisms are over $0.2\ \mu m$ in diameter, resolvable by the light microscope and not filterable through bacteria-stopping filters,

Table 4.1. Class Schizomycetes

Order	Family	Genus	Species (one example given)
PSEUDO-MONADALES	Pseudomonadaceae. Cells are straight rods, occasionally coccoid. May form a water-soluble pigment (e.g. green or brown) or a water-insoluble pigment (e.g. yellow or red)	*Pseudomonas*	*Ps. aeruginosa* (*Ps. pyocyanea*)
	Spirillaceae. Cells are rigid, curved or spiral rods.	*Vibrio* *Spirillum*	*V. cholerae* *Sp. minus*
	Further families in this order include most of the photosynthetic and autotrophic species of bacteria		
	Achromobacteraceae. Cells rod-shaped and Gram-negative. Non-pigmented or forming yellow, orange or brown pigments. Grow well on ordinary peptone media. Few species can ferment sugars to give acid; glucose is usually attacked oxidatively if at all	*Alcaligenes*	*Alc. faecalis*
	Enterobacteriaceae. Cells rod-shaped and Gram-negative. Grow well on ordinary peptone media. Actively ferment glucose, and in many cases lactose and other sugars, producing acid, or acid and visible gas (CO_2 and H_2)	*Escherichia* *Aerobacter* *Klebsiella* *Paracolobactrum* *Serratia* *Proteus* *Salmonella* *Shigella*	*Esch. coli* *Aero. aerogenes* *Kl. pneumoniae* *Par. coliforme* *Serr. marcescens* *Pr. vulgaris* *S. typhi* *Sh. dysenteriae*
	Brucellaceae. Cells small, coccoid to rod-shaped, and Gram-negative. Obligate animal parasites. Many fail to grow on ordinary peptone media, requiring addition of body fluids. Many lack power to ferment sugars	*Pasteurella* *Bordetella* *Brucella* *Haemophilus* *Actinobacillus* *Moraxella*	*P. pestis** *Bord. pertussis* *Br. melitensis* *H. influenzae* *Actinobacillus lignieresi* *Morax. lacunata*
	Bacteroidaceae. Cells rod-shaped or filamentous and Gram-negative. Most are strict anaerobes and many require enriched culture media for growth. Parasites of mammals, especially of the alimentary canal	*Bacteroides* *Fusobacterium* *Sphaerophorus* *Streptobacillus*	*Bacteroides fragilis* *F. fusiforme* *Sph. necrophorus* *Streptobacillus moniliformis*
EUBACTERIALES	Micrococcaceae. Cells spherical and Gram-positive; occur singly and in pairs, tetrads, cubical packets and irregular clusters. Many form a non-water-soluble yellow, orange or red pigment. Mostly non-motile	*Micrococcus* *Staphylococcus* *Gaffkya*	*Micro. ureae* *Staph. aureus* *Gaff. tetragena*
	Neisseriaceae. Cells spherical to elliptical, and Gram-negative; occur mainly in pairs, with long axes parallel, or in clusters. Non-motile. Parasites of mammals.	*Neisseria* *Veillonella*	*N. meningitidis* *Veill. parvula*
	Lactobacillaceae. Cells are cocci or rods occurring singly, in pairs and in chains. Gram-positive. Mostly non-motile. Facultatively or strictly anaerobic. Actively ferment sugars with lactic acid as main product	*Diplococcus* *Streptococcus* *Peptostreptococcus* *Lactobacillus*	*D. pneumoniae* *Strept. pyogenes* *Peptostrept. putridus* *Lacto. acidophilus*
	Corynebacteriaceae. Cells rod-shaped or club-shaped; Gram-positive. Mostly non-motile	*Corynebacterium* *Listeria* *Erysipelothrix*	*C. diphtheriae* *List. monocytogenes* *Ery. insidiosa*

Table 4.1 (continued)

Order	Family	Genus	Species (one example given)
	Bacillaceae. Cells rod-shaped and usually Gram-positive. Form endospores. Many are motile	*Bacillus* *Clostridium*	*B. anthracis* *Cl. tetani*
	Mycobacteriaceae. Cells rod-shaped, but rarely filamentous or branching. Do not form conidia or other kinds of spores	*Mycobacterium*	*Myco. tuberculosis*
ACTINO-MYCETALES	Actinomycetaceae. Cells filamentous and branching. Grow as a mycelium which may fragment into short rod or coccoid forms, and reproduce by budding or by spores formed through fragmentation of the mycelium and in some cases from aerial hyphae	*Actinomyces* *Nocardia*	*Actinomyces israelii* *Noc. madurae*
	Streptomycetaceae. Cells filamentous and branching. Grow as a mycelium which does not fragment. Conidia are borne on sporophores, in many cases aerial	*Streptomyces*	*Streptomyces griseus*
SPIRO-CHAETALES	Treponemataceae. Cells slender flexuous spiral filaments (The small spirochaetes)	*Borrelia* *Treponema* *Leptospira*	*Borr. recurrentis* *Tr. pallidum* *L. interrogans*
MYCO-PLASMATALES		*Mycoplasma*	*M. mycoides*

* The genus *Pasteurella* is now divided into *Pasteurella*, *Yersinia* and *Francisella*. *P. pestis* is now re-classified as *Yersinia pestis*.

except for a few species with filterable phases. Gram-negative. Only a few species can grow on cell-free nutrient media.

Genera

Rickettsia, e.g. *R. prowazekii*
Coxiella, e.g. *Cox. burnetii*
Ehrlichia, e.g. *Ehrl. ovina*
Cowdria, e.g. *Cowdria ruminantium*
Chlamydia (Bedsonia), e.g. organisms of psittacosis, lymphogranuloma, trachoma and inclusion conjunctivitis
Bartonella, e.g. *Bart. bacilliformis*
Haemobartonella, e.g. *Haemobartonella muris*
Anaplasma, e.g. *An. marginale*.
The rickettsiae and related prokaryotic organisms have much in common with the bacteria in their cell wall and membrane components, their nucleic acid structure and their physiology, whereas the viruses are both structurally and functionally different and are now dealt with quite separately.
Medical microbiologists tend to avoid the conflicting arguments of the taxonomists; the simplified working system indicated in Table 4.2 involves many compromises but overcomes difficulties in a practical way.

Adansonian or Numerical Classification

In the international system of bacterial classification given above, the major groups, e.g. orders and families, are distinguished by characters, e.g. cell shape, Gram reaction, spore formation and flagellation, that are considered to be of major importance, and the minor groups, e.g. genera and species, by characters considered of less importance, e.g. fermentation reactions, nutritional requirements and pathogenicity. This system suffers from the weakness that decisions about the relative 'importance' of different characters, and thus about their priority in defining the major and minor groupings, must in many cases be purely arbitrary.

The uncertainties of the arbitrary choices made in drawing up the hierarchy of defining characters in the international system are avoided in the Adansonian system of taxonomy. This system determines the degrees of relationship between strains by a statistical coefficient that takes account of their similarities and differences in the widest possible range of characters, *all of which are weighted of equal importance*. It is clear, of course, that some characters, e.g. cell shape or the Gram reaction, represent a much wider and more permanent genetic commitment than other characters, e.g. lactose fermentation or the production of a particular exoenzyme which, being dependent on only one or a few genes, are relatively mutable. For this reason, the Adansonian method is most useful when used for classifying strains within a larger grouping that shares the major characters in common.

The different organisms are compared by scoring for a large number of phenotypic characters (score $+1$ if the character is present, -1 if it is absent). The classification thus depends upon total scores of as many similarities and differences as can be observed. It is possible to estimate a *similarity coefficient* when shared

Table 4.2. A simple classification of some microorganisms of medical importance

EUKARYOTIC ORGANISMS

PROTOZOA —Causative organisms of various diseases
FUNGI —Causative organisms of the deep mycoses
—Causative organisms of superficial infections:
—mould-like—*Epidermophyton, Trichophyton, Microsporum*
—yeast-like—*Candida* species

PROKARYOTIC ORGANISMS

FILAMENTOUS BACTERIA
(sometimes called 'higher bacteria') include *Streptomyces* and *Actinomyces*

TRUE BACTERIA
GRAM-POSITIVE BACILLI—{Aerobes —*Mycobacterium, Corynebacterium, Bacillus*
{Anaerobes —*Clostridium, Lactobacillus*

GRAM-POSITIVE COCCI —*Streptococcus*
Staphylococcus

GRAM-NEGATIVE COCCI —Aerobes —*Neisseria*
Anaerobes —*Veillonella*

GRAM-NEGATIVE BACILLI — { Aerobes— { ENTEROBACTERIA —*Escherichia, Klebsiella, Proteus, Salmonella, Shigella*

PSEUDOMONADS (polar flagella) —*Pseudomonas*

PARVOBACTERIA Small Gram-negative bacilli —*Haemophilus, Bordetella, Brucella, Pasteurella, Yersinia, Francisella*

Anaerobes —*Bacteroides-Fusiformis* group

GRAM-NEGATIVE VIBRIOS and SPIRILLA (related to Pseudomonads)—*Vibrio, Spirillum*

SPIROCHAETES *Borrelia, Treponema, Leptospira*

MYCOPLASMAS (formerly called pleuropneumonia-like organisms)

RICKETTSIA AND COXIELLA GROUP

CHLAMYDIA GROUP (formerly called *Bedsonia*)

VIRUSES

positive characters are considered, or a *matching coefficient* when both negative and positive shared characters (matches) are taken into account. Thus in a collection of strains in which the results of a large number of tests are compared between one strain and another, the degree of similarity of strain A to strain B is indicated by the *similarity index* (S):

$$S = \frac{Ns}{Ns + Nd} \times 100$$

where Ns is the number of shared (positive) characteristics and Nd is the number of differences detected. The observations can be analysed by computer to indicate degrees of similarity for a group of different organisms by the preparation of a *similarity matrix* in which the degree of similarity (similarity index) is indicated in decades (Figs. 4.3, 4.4, 4.5).

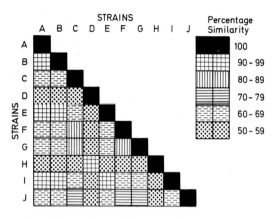

FIG. 4.3. A similarity matrix for ten strains A–J showing the degrees of similarity between them. By a process termed *cluster analysis*, the matrix is redrawn so that strains of equivalent similarity lie together.

All reproduced with slight modifications from P. H. A. Sneath (1962).

Biochemical Classification

The chemical constitution of the prokaryotic cell wall is different from that of eukaryotic cell walls. The framework structure of mucopeptide is composed of repeating units of *N*-acetyl glucosamine and *N*-acetyl muramic acid and these are cross-linked by peptide structures (see p. 16). The constituent amino acids vary, but include diaminopimelic acid and the 'unnatural' D-isomers of alanine and glutamic acid residues. *N*-acetyl muramic acid does not occur in eukaryotic cells and cell wall composition is an important differentiating feature of the prokaryotes. A further point is that the prokaryotic cell

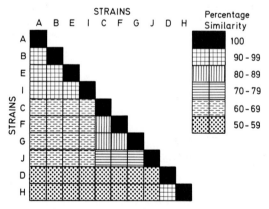

FIG. 4.4. The similarity matrix for strains A–J has been redrawn to show clusters of high similarity ('phenons') within the group. Thus, for the strains in Fig. 4.3, A, B, E, and I show high similarity and are linked into one group whilst strains D and H have high similarity and form a separate group. At the 80–89 per cent level, strains C, F and G are linked, and strain J is grouped with these at the 70–79 per cent level, and so on.

All reproduced with slight modifications from P. H. A. Sneath (1962).

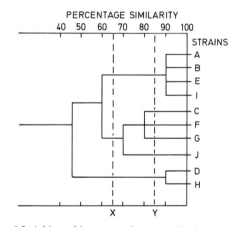

FIG. 4.5. A hierarchic taxonomic tree or 'dendrogram' prepared from the similarity matrix data for strains A–J. The broken lines X and Y indicate levels of similarity at which separation into genera and species might be possible.

Reproduced with slight modification from P. H. A. Sneath (1962).

membrane lacks sterols which typically occur in the membranes of eukaryotic cells, but mycoplasmas are an exception to this general rule.

Much is now known about the specific chemistry of the cell walls of various bacteria. Although the mucopeptide framework is common to all, there are differences in structure between the cell walls of Gram-positive and Gram-negative bacteria (Chap. 2). Moreover, there are individual differences in chemical constituents that are of taxonomic value. Gram-positive bacteria contain glycerol teichoic acid and ribitol teichoic acid in considerable amount and, in addition, a wide variety of monosaccharides including some that are relatively specific for the bacterial group, e.g. rhamnose for the *Streptococcus*, *Lactobacillus* and *Clostridium* genera, and arabinose for the *Corynebacterium*, *Mycobacterium* and *Nocardia* genera.

In the case of Gram-negative bacteria, the specificity of the outer lipopolysaccharide layer of the cell wall is a function of its polysaccharide moiety which carries a common (group specific) core of glucose, galactose, N-acetyl glucosamine, 2-keto-3-deoxyoctonate and a heptose, together with a highly specific side chain bearing a type-specific arrangement of sugars.

Chemical analyses employing chromatographic methods are now able to distinguish genera and species and sometimes multiple chemotypes and this knowledge supplements and extends serological classifications.

DNA Composition as a Basis for Classification

The hydrogen bonding between guanine and cytosine (G—C) base pairs in DNA is stronger than that between adenine and thymine (A—T) pairs. Thus the melting or denaturation temperature of DNA (at which the two strands separate) is primarily determined by the $G+C$ content. At the melting temperature, the separation of the strands brings about a marked change in the light absorption characteristics at 260 nm and this is readily detected by spectrophotometry. By measuring the $G+C$ content of a bacterial preparation in this way it can be shown that there is a very wide range of the $G+C$ component of the DNA in bacteria, varying from about 25 to 80 moles per cent in different genera. However, for any one species, the $G+C$ content

is relatively fixed or falls within a very narrow range and this provides a basis for classification (Table 4.3). Species grouped in this way are often adjacent to traditionally recognized close relatives, but some species within a single genus are widely separated—see members of *Clostridium*, *Bacillus*, *Proteus* and *Lactobacillus* for examples.

A geneticist's approach to classification (see Marmur, Falkow and Mandel, 1963) is to arrange individual organisms into groups on the basis of the *homology* of their DNA base sequences. Tests of DNA homology exploit the fact that double strands re-form from separated strands during controlled cooling of a heated preparation of DNA. This 'annealing' process can be readily demonstrated with suitably heated homologous DNA extracted from a single species, but it can also occur when a mixture of DNA from two related species is used; in the latter case, hybrid pairs of DNA strands are produced. These hybrid pairings occur with high frequency between complementary regions of two bits of DNA and the degree of hybridization can be assessed if labelled DNA preparations are used. m-RNA binding studies can also give information to complement these observations that provide genetic evidence of relatedness among bacteria.

Organisms with different $G + C$ ratios are very unlikely to show DNA homology. However, organisms with the same, or close, $G + C$ ratios do not necessarily show homology.

SYSTEM OF IDENTIFICATION OF BACTERIA

1. Morphology and staining reactions of individual organisms generally serve as a preliminary criterion, particularly for placing an unknown species in its appropriate biological group. A Gram-stained smear suffices to show the Gram reaction, size, shape and grouping of the bacteria, whether they possess endospores, and the shape, size and intracellular position of such spores. An unstained wet film may be examined with the dark-ground microscope for observation of the exact morphology of delicate spirochaetes, and an unstained wet film, or 'hanging drop' preparation is examined with the ordinary

Table 4.3.   DNA base compositions of bacteria

Moles per cent. Guanine plus Cytosine	Organism
30–32	*Clostridium welchii, Cl. tetani*
32–34	*Staphylococcus aureus*
34–36	*Bacillus anthracis,* *Staph. (epidermidis) albus,* *Streptococcus faecalis*
38–40	*Diplococcus pneumoniae, Strept. pyogenes,* *Haemophilus influenzae, Proteus vulgaris, Lactobacillus acidophilus*
40–42	*Neisseria catarrhalis*
42–44	*Bacillus subtilis, Coxiella burnetii*
46–48	*Vibrio cholerae*
48–50	*Neisseria gonorrhoeae*
50–52	*N. meningitidis, Salmonella typhimurium,* *Shigella sonnei, Proteus morganii*
52–54	*Corynebacterium diphtheriae*
54–56	*Klebsiella pneumoniae, Brucella abortus*
56–58	*Lactobacillus bifidus*
66–68	*Pseudomonas aeruginosa, Mycobacterium tuberculosis*
70–80	*Streptomyces spp.*

After Marmur J., Falkow, S. & Mandel, M. (1963).

microscope for observation of motility. When it is possible that the organism is a mycobacterium or a nocardia, a preparation is stained by the Ziehl-Neelsen method to demonstrate the acid-fast staining reaction.

In medical bacteriology the microscopic characters of certain organisms in pathological specimens may be sufficient for presumptive diagnostic identification, e.g. tubercle bacilli in sputum, or *Treponema pallidum* in exudate from a chancre. However, many different bacteria share similar morphological features, e.g. the meningococcus, gonococcus and *Neisseria catarrhalis,* and further tests must be applied, as below, to differentiate them.

2. Cultural characters, including the growth requirements and the appearance of cultures to the naked eye, are further criteria assisting identification.

The appearances of growths in liquid culture media such as nutrient broth are generally not distinctive. Much more value attaches to observations of the appearance of the discrete masses of growth, or colonies, that can be grown from isolated bacteria on the surface of solid culture medium such as nutrient agar. Attention is paid to the size of the colonies (diameter in mm), their outline (whether circular and entire, or indented, or wavy, or rhizoid, see Fig. 4.6), their elevation (low convex, high convex, flat, plateau-like, umbonate, or nodular, see Fig. 4.7), their translucency (clear and transparent, or translucent, or opaque), whether they are colourless, white or otherwise pigmented, and whether they produce any change in the medium (e.g. haemolysis in a blood-containing agar medium). However, simple observation of colonial morphology may be insufficient for the differentiation of a species. For example, different species of *Salmonella* produce colonies that are similar and are not even distinguishable on ordinary media from those of other enterobacteria. Attempts are then made to culture the bacterium on media of different compositions and incubated under a variety of conditions. The range of the conditions that support growth is characteristic of particular organisms.

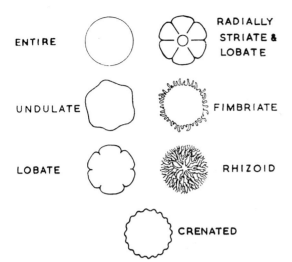

FIG. 4.6. Edges of bacterial colonies.

The ability or inability of the organism to grow on medium containing a selective inhibitory factor (e.g. bile salt, optochin, bacitracin, low pH, high pH, tellurite) may also be of diagnostic significance.

3. Biochemical reactions. Species that cannot be distinguished by morphology and cultural characters may exhibit distinct differences in their biochemical reactions. The most commonly used biochemical tests involve the observation of whether or not a growth of the bacterium in liquid nutrient medium will ferment particular 'sugars' (e.g. glucose, lactose, mannitol). There may then be production of acid, detected by

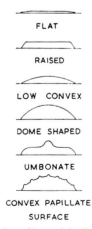

FIG. 4.7. The elevation of bacterial colonies.

change of colour of an indicator dye present in the medium, or of acid plus gas; gas production is detected by the collection of a bubble in a small inverted tube (Durham tube) immersed in the medium. Other tests determine whether the bacterium produces particular end-products, e.g. indole, H_2S, and nitrite, when grown in suitable culture media, and whether it possesses certain enzymic activities, such as oxidase, catalase, urease, gelatinase, collagenase, lecithinase, or lipase. Sometimes, more elaborate procedures for the analysis of end-products may utilize special techniques such as thin-layer chromatography and gas–liquid chromatography.

4. Antigenic characters. In bacteriology, species and types can often be identified by specific 'antibody reactions' observed in serological tests. These reactions depend on the fact that the serum of an animal immunized against a microorganism contains highly specific antibodies (for the homologous species or type) that react in a characteristic manner with the particular microorganism. Such antisera, for example, may agglutinate or clump the homologous organism in laboratory studies, and this effect can be observed with the naked eye. An unknown bacterium may thus be identified by demonstrating its reaction with one out of a number of standard known antisera.

5. Fluorescence microscopy and fluorescent-antibody (immunofluorescence) procedures. When certain dyes are exposed to ultraviolet light, they absorb energy and emit visible light. A dye rendered luminous in this way is a fluorochrome and is said to fluoresce. When tissue cells or organisms are stained with such a dye and examined with UV light in an adapted microscope, they are seen as fluorescent objects. The fluorescent dyes have partly selective staining affinities; for example, auramine can be used in this way as a useful stain for the detection of *Mycobacterium tuberculosis.*

Antibody molecules can be labelled by conjugation with a fluorochrome dye such as fluorescein isothiocyanate, which fluoresces green, or rhodamine which gives an orange-red colour. When fluorescent antibody is then allowed to react with homologous antigen exposed at a cell surface, this *direct immunofluorescence* procedure affords a highly sensitive method for the identification of the particular antigen. For the direct procedure it is necessary to have a specific antibody-conjugate preparation for each antigen. However, if the antigen is first exposed to specific antibody (immunoglobulin) prepared in a rabbit and then treated with a fluorescent antibody conjugate specific for rabbit globulin, this double-layer method allows unconjugated sera to be used in the first step. The diagnostic applications of immunofluorescence are numerous and they are referred to in detail in Volume II, Chapter 11.

6. Typing of bacteria. A single bacterial species with a particular set of pathogenic activities may nevertheless include strains of different types that are distinguishable in minor characters. Recognition of the type of a strain isolated from a patient may be of epidemiological value in tracing sources or modes of spread of infection in a community. The strain isolated may, for instance, be shown to be of a different type from that recovered from a suspected source of the patient's infection and the possible role of that source may then be discounted.

The 'typing' of strains may depend upon special biochemical or serological tests to distinguish respectively different *biotypes* and *serotypes* within the species. Identification of serotypes in certain genera, e.g. *Salmonella,* is now highly developed and can provide virtually absolute proof of identity of a species or of a serotype within a species.

Another important method of typing is by testing the susceptibility of the culture to lysis by each of a set of type-specific lytic bacteriophages, the *phage-type* of the culture being identified according to its pattern of susceptibility to the different phages. Methods of epidemiological tracing that exploit phage-typing have now replaced some serological procedures, e.g. in staphylococcal studies, or they may allow subdivision of a serological entity as in the case of serotype *S. typhi* which is divisible into 80 different phage-types.

In some other genera, however, serological and phage-typing methods have encountered problems and it has been necessary to develop different typing procedures.

The determination of *bacteriocine types* according to the ability of strains of bacteria to produce one or other of a series of bacteriocines is of considerable practical value, particularly for subdividing the serologically homogeneous *Shigella sonnei* subgroup and for typing *Pseudomonas pyocyanea* (aeruginosa) isolates. Bacteriocines are naturally occurring antibacterial substances elaborated by many members of the family Enterobacteriaceae and some other bacteria; they are active mainly against strains of the same genus as that of the producing strain. For example, indicator strains for the pyocine typing of strains of *Pseudomonas pyocyanea* are also members of the genus *Pseudomonas*.

Bacteriocines vary in their morphology and the large pyocines resemble phage-tail components but they do not possess a head and, like other bacteriocines, are not self-replicating. Other bacteriocines are much smaller and vary in size from particulate filamentous forms to smaller non-particulate or soluble forms.

7. Animal pathogenicity and toxigenicity. In the case of pathogenic organisms, such as the tubercle bacillus, that produce characteristic lesions in laboratory animals, the inoculation test provides a reliable method of identification.

In many cases, especially when a specific toxin is involved in the mechanism of pathogenesis, animal pathogenicity tests are controlled by the use of specific neutralizing antisera and the pathogenic organisms are thereby identified with a high degree of specificity. Thus, the final identification of a diphtheria bacillus may be made by injecting culture material intradermally into two guinea-pigs, one of which has been protected by prior injection of diphtheria antitoxin and the other is given partial protection with a small dose of antitoxin at the time of the test. The development of an inflammatory and necrotic skin reaction in the partially protected, but not in the protected animal identifies the culture as an organism producing diphtheria toxin. The tetanus bacillus is identified similarly by a test in mice that proves its production of the specific tetanus toxin. Strains of *Clostridium welchii* may be 'typed' by demonstration of the set of specific toxins they produce; in this case the culture fluid is mixed with specific antiserum before injection.

8. Antibiotic sensitivity. The organism is tested for its ability to grow on artificial nutrient media containing different antibiotic and chemotherapeutic agents in different concentrations. In the *disk diffusion test*, the culture to be examined is seeded confluently over the surface of an agar plate and 6 to 10 paper disks or tablets containing different antibiotics are placed on different areas of the plate. Antibiotic diffuses outwards from each disk into the surrounding agar and produces a diminishing gradient of concentration. On incubation the bacteria grow on areas of the plate except those around the drugs to which they are sensitive, and the width of each growth-free 'zone of inhibition' is a measure of their degree of sensitivity to the drug.

In a few cases, reactions are sufficiently uniform among the strains of a species, and distinctive from those of related species, to be valuable in the identification of the species (e.g. bacitracin sensitivity in *Streptococcus pyogenes*, and optochin sensitivity in the pneumococcus). Commonly, however, there are marked differences in antibiotic sensitivity between different strains of a species. Information about the sensitivity patterns of strains ('antibiograms') isolated from patients is required as a guide to the choice of drug for therapy and may also be used as an epidemiological marker in tracing hospital cross-infections.

Identification in Material containing a Mixture of Bacteria

Most of the identifying tests in the categories described above are valid only if made with a pure preparation or pure culture of a single kind of bacterium (i.e. a population of cells consisting exclusively of the progeny of a single ancestral cell). Certain kinds of materials collected for diagnostic purposes from the bodies of patients, e.g. specimens of faeces, sputum and throat secretion contain a wide variety of resident commensal bacteria besides any pathogens that may be present. Specimens of other materials, e.g. blood, pus, cerebrospinal fluid and urine, are free from a resident commensal flora and are likely to be infected with only a single pathogenic species, but these specimens are liable sometimes to contain other bacteria as a result of secondary infection from the body surfaces or contamination in the course of collection.

Useful information may be obtained from certain examinations made on mixed infective material. Thus, microscopical examination of direct smears reveals the morphology and staining reactions of the different organisms and also allows an assessment to be made of the relative numbers of each kind present; such an assessment is more reliable than one made from examination of a culture of the material because the conditions of culture may selectively favour the growth of some species and inhibit that of others.

When material containing a mixture of bacteria is cultured by 'plating', i.e. by inoculating it very thinly on the surface of a plate (Petri dish) of solid culture medium such as nutrient agar, the different bacteria are seen to grow as separate *colonies*, each of which is usually a *pure* culture descended from a single inoculated cell. Useful information relating to the identity of the different bacteria and their relative numbers in the specimen may be obtained by noting the appearances of the colonies. The occurrence and character of growth on a highly selective medium may suggest the identity of the bacteria, but it must be remembered that other kinds of bacteria incapable of growth on this medium may also be present in the specimen. Anaerobic bacteria will not grow or be recognized in cultures incubated aerobically.

Most other identifying tests can be performed only after the unknown bacterium has been isolated in pure culture. Isolation is generally done by careful subculture from a plate culture bearing well separated colonies (see Chapter 48). A single colony, suspected from its appearance of being that of a significant or pathogenic organism, is 'picked' with an inoculating wireloop and subcultured by itself in a tube or plate of fresh, sterile culture medium. If there is any doubt about the purity of a supposedly pure culture, it should be plated out again on fresh medium, the colonies in the subculture should be examined to confirm their uniform appearance and one of these colonies should be picked and subcultured to give, through a second purification, a final 'pure culture'.

The morphological and cultural characters of the organism should, where necessary, be confirmed in examinations of the pure culture which should then be used in definitive tests.

In some types of investigative work it is desirable to store pure cultures of strains for later reference. This is best done by the freeze-drying procedure. The organisms are held dried and *in vacuo* in a sealed ampoule and they remain alive, though not metabolizing or growing, for very long periods. Otherwise the organism should be subcultured on a suitable *maintenance medium* and stored under conditions, e.g. in the dark at room temperature or in a refrigerator at 4°C, conducive to their survival.

In addition to preliminary microscopical and cultural examinations, there are some special identifying tests that may be made directly on pathological specimens containing mixtures of bacteria. Use of the fluorescent antibody staining method makes it possible on microscopical examination to recognize and identify individual bacteria and viruses according to their antigenic character with a high specificity comparable to that of conventional serological tests. Material containing commensal bacteria as well as suspected pathogens, may be injected into a labora-tory animal where only the pathogen may be capable of producing a fatal infection. Anti-biotic sensitivity tests by the disk diffusion method are sometimes usefully performed on the primary diagnostic culture plate that grows the whole mixture of organisms present in the specimen; if this *primary sensitivity test* is made, results are more quickly available for reporting to clinicians.

REFERENCES

BREED, R. S., MURRAY, E. G. D. & SMITH, N. R. (1957) *Bergey's Manual of Determinative Bacteriology,* 7th edn. Baltimore: Williams and Wilkins.

MARMUR, J. FALKOW, S. & MANDEL, M. (1963) New approaches to bacterial taxonomy. *Annual Review of Microbiology,* **17,** 329.

SNEATH, P. H. A. (1962) The construction of taxonomic groups. In *Microbial Classification: 12th Symposium of the Society for General Microbiology,* edited by G. C. Ainsworth and P. H. A. Sneath, p. 289. Cambridge: Cambridge University Press.

5. Sterilization and Disinfection

Procedures that kill microorganisms have important applications in practical microbiology and in the practice of medicine and surgery. Thus, microbiological work with pure cultures requires the use of culture media and containers that have been freed from all live, contaminating microorganisms, whilst the need to avoid infecting patients requires the use of instruments, dressings, nursing equipment and parenteral drugs that have been freed from all live microorganisms or, at least, from all pathogenic ones.

Two terms, sterilization and disinfection, are used to describe the killing or removal of microorganisms and it is important to recognize the distinction between their meanings. The former is an absolute term, indicating the complete killing or removal of microorganisms of all kinds, whereas the latter is a relative term, applying to differing, helpful degrees of removal of pathogenic microorganisms.

applicable is by heating under carefully controlled conditions at temperatures sufficiently higher than $100^{\circ}C$ to ensure killing of even the most resistant microorganisms and spores. (2) *Filtration.* Bacteria-stopping filters are used to remove bacteria and all larger microorganisms from liquids that are liable to be spoiled by heating, e.g. blood serum and antibiotic solutions, and in which residual contamination with filter-passing viruses is improbable or unimportant. (3) *Irradiation* with ultra-violet or ionizing (e.g. gamma) radiation has special applications including the sterilization of disposable plastic equipment. (4) *Chemical disinfection.* This method is generally unreliable and unsuccessful in effecting sterilization. Only a few of the more toxic and irritant disinfectants, e.g. formaldehyde, glutaraldehyde and ethylene oxide, are capable of killing bacterial endospores, and they are effective only when used in an adequate concentration applied under carefully controlled conditions of temperature, moisture, etc.

STERILIZATION

Definition. Sterilization means the freeing of an article from all living organisms, including viruses, bacteria and their spores, and fungi and their spores, both pathogenic and non-pathogenic. Sterility is an absolute state. An article should never be described as being 'relatively sterile'; it is either sterile or unsterile.

Uses. Sterilization is required for culture media, suspending fluids, reagents, containers and equipment used in microbiology. It is also required for medical and surgical instruments and materials used in procedures that involve penetration into the blood, tissues and other normally sterile parts of the body, e.g. in surgical operations, intravenous infusions, hypodermic injections and diagnostic aspirations.

Methods. Four main methods are used for sterilization. (1) *Heat.* The only method of sterilization that is both reliable and widely

DISINFECTION

Definition. Disinfection means the freeing of an article from some or all of its burden of live pathogenic microorganisms which might cause infection during its use. The term is a relative one and disinfection may be described as being partially or highly effective according to the proportion of the pathogenic organisms killed or removed.

Uses. Disinfection, rather than sterilization, is attempted in circumstances in which sterility is unnecessary or sterilizing procedures are impracticable, yet there is still some value in obtaining a partial or complete removal of non-sporing pathogens. It is impracticable, for instance, to apply sterilizing procedures to bedpans, baths, wash-basins, furniture, eating utensils, bed-clothes and other fomites that might spread infection in hospitals, but because the pathogens that might be present on these articles and be capable of causing infection include none that forms spores, it is useful to disinfect the articles by procedures lethal only to vegetative organisms. It is similarly impracticable to apply sterilizing procedures to the skin, but because the bacteria most commonly infecting surgical wounds are non-spore-forming, it is a valuable pre-operative precaution to treat the skin around the operative site with a disinfectant that will kill many of the vegetative bacteria on it and so reduce the chances of some of them being carried into the wound.

Methods. Useful, though only partial disinfection is most readily obtained by the simple procedures of washing, cleansing and ventilation, which, if thoroughly done, may remove the majority of the harmful microorganisms from an article or room. More effective disinfection is obtained by the application, though to a less rigorous degree, of the same kinds of procedures as are used for sterilization. *Heat* may be used to disinfect eating utensils and clothing; thus, washing or rinsing such articles in water at 70 to 80°C for several minutes will kill the majority of the non-sporing pathogens present on them. Similarly, in the absence of means of sterilization, a glass hypodermic syringe or surgical instrument is best disinfected by boiling it in water at 100°C for at least 5 minutes. *Chemical disinfectants* provide for many purposes an even more convenient means of disinfection. Thus, a strong phenolic disinfectant may be added to faeces in a bed-pan or hypochlorite solutions may be used to rinse baths and wash-hand basins and to wipe contaminated floors and furniture. Chemical disinfectants, however, suffer from the drawback that they are very liable to be rendered inactive either by undue dilution or by contact with organic materials such as dirt, faeces, pus and blood.

STERILIZATION BY HEAT

Moist heat is much more effective than dry heat, sterilizing at lower temperatures in a given time or in shorter times at a given temperature. Moist heat kills microorganisms probably by coagulating and denaturing their enzymes and structural proteins, a process in which water participates. *Sterilization, i.e. killing of the most resistant spores, requires exposure to moist heat at 121°C for 10 to 30 minutes.* Dry heat is believed to kill microorganisms by causing a destructive oxidation of essential cell constituents. *Killing of the most resistant spores by dry heat requires a temperature of about 160°C for 60 minutes.* This high temperature causes slight charring of paper, cotton and other organic materials.

Factors Influencing Sterilization by Heat

The factors to be considered are the temperature and time of exposure, the number of vegetative microorganisms and spores present, the species, strain and spore-forming ability of the microorganisms, and the nature of the material containing the microorganisms.

1. THE TEMPERATURE AND TIME required for killing are inversely related, shorter times sufficing at higher temperatures. Thus, to sterilize, the heating must be 'hot enough for long enough'. Published findings on resistant spores show many discrepancies, but in practice the following may be taken as minimal sterilizing exposures (Table 5.1):

Table 5.1.   Minimal sterilizing exposures

Moist heat		Dry heat	
Temperature (Celsius)	Sterilizing time	Temperature (Celsius)	Sterilizing time
100°	20 hours	120°	8 hours
110°	2½ hours	140°	2½ hours
115°	50 minutes	160°	1 hour
121°	15 minutes	170°	40 minutes
125°	6½ minutes	180°	20 minutes
130°	2½ minutes		

For surgical and bacteriological sterilization, most authorities consider that a 10 to 12 minutes exposure of the organisms to moist heat at 121°C is sufficient. This ensures killing of all pathogenic sporing organisms and all saprophytes except for some strict thermophiles that cannot grow at less than 40°C.

The recommended minimal sterilizing times are the times for which the microbes themselves should be held at the given temperature, *and do not include heating-up time.* The total duration of the exposure should include time for the article to become heated up to the sterilizing temperature in addition to the recommended minimal sterilizing time at that temperature. The amount of time to be allowed for heating up (*heat-penetration time*) will be discussed later for the individual methods.

2. THE NUMBER OF MICROORGANISMS AND SPORES affects the rapidity of sterilization. The susceptibility and duration of survival on exposure to heat varies considerably among the individual cells, even in a pure culture. The number of survivors diminishes exponentially with the duration of heating, and the time for complete sterilization increases in relation to the number initially present. In practice it is usual to minimize the number of contaminating bacteria by cleansing procedures before applying heat for the purpose of sterilization.

3. THE SPECIES, STRAIN AND SPORE-FORMING ABILITY of the microbe greatly affect its susceptibility to heat. The amount of heat required to kill a given variety may be stated in terms of the temperature and time of exposure, either as the *thermal death point,* i.e. the lowest temperature to give complete killing in aqueous suspension within 10 min, or as the *thermal death time,* i.e. the shortest time for complete killing at a stated temperature. The tests are made under strictly standardized conditions, e.g. with sealed 9 mm diameter hard glass tubes containing 1 to 2 ml of a suspension of 5×10^7 organisms per ml in a defined phosphate buffer solution at pH 7·0. Because, however, thermal death point and time measurements depend on the killing of the variable tail of more resistant cells, a more reliable measurement is the *decimal reduction time,* or *D value,* which is the time (in minutes) required to achieve a tenfold reduction in viability of a bacterial population at a given temperature under standard conditions.

Susceptibility to Moist Heat

The vegetative forms of most bacteria, yeasts and fungi, and most animal viruses, are killed in 10 minutes by a temperature between 50°C (e.g. *Neisseria gonorrhoeae*) and 65°C (e.g. *Staphylococcus aureus*). Extreme susceptibility is shown by *Treponema pallidum* which is killed in 10 minutes at about 43°C; *Coxiella burnetii* is a markedly resistant vegetative organism, and extreme resistance is shown by thermophilic saprophytic bacilli, e.g. *Bacillus stearothermophilus*, whose vegetative forms can grow at temperatures approaching 80°C. A few animal viruses are more resistant than the majority; for example, that of poliomyelitis may require heating at 60°C for 30 minutes and that of serum hepatitis, when in serum, at 60°C for 10 hours. Many bacteriophages are more resistant than their host bacterium, and it is often possible to kill the latter by heating at 60°C for 15 to 30 minutes without affecting the phage; these phages are killed by temperatures in the range 65 to 80°C.

The spore forms of actinomycetes, yeasts and fungi are more resistant than the parental vegetative forms, though not as highly resistant as bacterial spores. The more susceptible kinds are killed at 70°C in 5 minutes and the more resistant at 80° to 90°C in 30 minutes.

The resistance of bacterial spores varies considerably between different strains of the same species. Thus, spores of most strains of *Cl. tetani* are killed by boiling at 100°C for 10 minutes, but exceptional strains resist boiling for 1 to 3 hours and these are the most resistant pathogens capable of infecting wounds; their degree of resistance thus determines the minimum standards for surgical sterilization: i.e. 121°C for 10 minutes or 115°C for 30 minutes, exclusive of heating-up time. The spores of some strains of *Cl. botulinum* resist boiling at 100°C at pH 7·0 for up to 8 hours and resist autoclaving at 115°C for 10 to 40 minutes; these limits determine the standards of heat processing employed in the preservation of non-acid canned foods (Vol. II, Chap. 12).

Susceptibility to dry heat. Dry heat at 100°C for

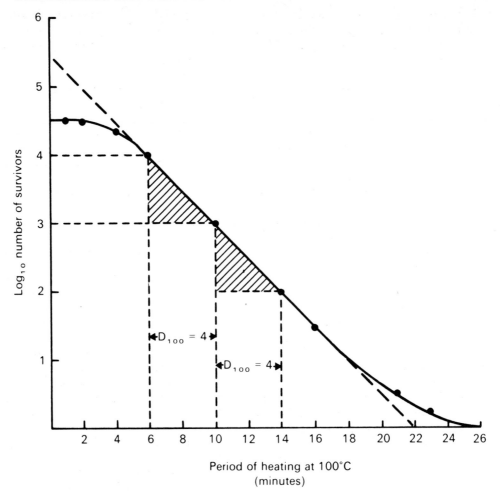

FIG. 5.1. The rate of inactivation of an inoculum of bacterial spores: a plot of results that might be obtained in a study of the decimal reduction time (D value) of heat-resistant spores at 100°C, showing the non-linear 'shoulder and tail' effects.

60 minutes is required to kill vegetative bacteria that would succumb to moist heat at 60°C in 30 minutes. Fungal spores are killed in hot air at 115°C within 60 minutes, and bacterial spores at temperatures in the range 120° to 160°C within 60 minutes.

4. THE NATURE OF THE MATERIAL in which the organisms are heated may affect the rate of killing. A high content of organic substances generally tends to protect spores and vegetative organisms against the lethal action of heat. Proteins, gelatin, sugars, starch, nucleic acids, fats and oils all act in this way. The effect of fats and oils is greatest with moist heat since

they prevent access of moisture to the microbes. The presence of an organic or inorganic disinfectant has the opposite effect and promotes killing by heat. The pH is important; the heat resistance of spores is greatest in neutral media (pH 7·0) and is diminished with increasing acidity or alkalinity. The effect of alkali has been used in the disinfection of metal instruments by boiling them at 100°C in water containing 2 per cent sodium carbonate; but this method is not as reliable as autoclaving.

The conditions under which sporulating bacteria are grown may influence the heat-resistance of the spores. Thus, the spores formed by soil bacteria and intestinal bacteria in artificial cultures are sometimes less resistant than those formed in the organism's natural habitat.

STERILIZATION BY DRY HEAT

1. RED HEAT. Inoculating wires, points of forceps and searing spatulas are sterilized by holding them in the flame of a Bunsen burner until they are seen to be red hot.

2. FLAMING. Direct exposure for a few seconds in a gas or spirit flame may be used for sterilizing scalpels and needles but it is destructive and uncertain. Needles, scalpels and basins are sometimes treated by immersing them in methylated spirit and burning off the spirit, but this method does not produce a sufficiently high temperature for sterilization.

3. HOT-AIR OVEN. This is the main means of sterilization by dry heat. The oven is usually heated with electricity and has a thermostat that maintains the chamber air constantly at the chosen temperature and a fan to assist circulation of air. Commonly, a temperature of 160°C is maintained for 1 hour.

The hot-air oven is used for sterilizing dry glassware, forceps, scalpels, scissors, throat swabs and syringes. It is also used for sterilizing dry materials in sealed containers, and powders, fats, oils and greases which are impermeable to moisture.

The sterilizing oven must not be overloaded and spaces must be left for circulation of air through the load. It may be cold or warm when loaded, and is then heated up to the sterilizing temperature in the course of 1 to 2 hours. The *holding period* of 1 hour at 160°C is timed as beginning when the thermometer first shows that the air in the oven has reached 160°C.

4. INFRA-RED RADIATION. Another method of sterilization by dry heat employs infra-red radiation. The infra-red rays are directed from an electrically heated element on to the objects to be sterilized, e.g. all-glass syringes, and temperatures of 180°C can be attained. Heating at or above 200°C by infra-red *in vacuo* has been employed as a means of sterilizing surgical instruments. Cooling is hastened and oxidation prevented during the cooling period by admitting filtered nitrogen to the chamber.

STERILIZATION BY MOIST HEAT

Killing by moist heat requires the microorganisms to be in contact with hot water or steam. If they are protected from wetting, as by grease or in a sealed impervious container, they will be subject only to the weaker effect of dry heat at the same temperature.

Moist heat may be employed: (1) at temperatures below 100°C; (2) at a temperature of 100°C; i.e. in boiling water or free steam; or (3) at temperatures above 100°C, i.e. in saturated steam under increased pressure in an autoclave. The first two procedures may be used for disinfection but only the third ensures sterilization and killing of highly resistant spores.

1. MOIST HEAT AT TEMPERATURES BELOW 100°C. In the pasteurization of milk, the temperature employed is either 63° to 66°C (145° to 150°F) for 30 minutes (the 'holder' method) or 72°C (162°F) for 20 seconds (the 'flash' method) and these processes usually destroy all the non-spore-forming pathogens such as *Mycobacterium tuberculosis*, *Myco. bovis*, *Brucella abortus* and various salmonellae that may be present in milk. *Coxiella burnetii*, the causative organism of Q fever, is heat-resistant and may survive pasteurization by the holder method. Unless large numbers of the organisms are present, the treatment usually reduces them to less than an infective dose.

Vaccines prepared from pure cultures of non-sporing bacteria may be inactivated in a special waterbath ('vaccine bath') at a comparatively low temperature; 1 hour at 60°C is *usually* sufficient. Higher temperatures may diminish the immunizing power of the vaccine.

Eating utensils, clothing, bed-clothes and some items of nursing equipment may be disinfected by washing in water for several minutes at 70° to 80°C.

2. MOIST HEAT AT A TEMPERATURE OF 100°C. *Boiling at 100°C*. Boiling at 100°C for 5 to 10 minutes is sufficient to kill all non-sporing and many, though not all, sporing organisms. The method does not ensure sterility, but has been found satisfactory for certain purposes in bacteriology and medicine where sterility is not essential or better methods are unavailable. When an instrument is removed from the boiling water, it should be allowed to dry before being

handled to prevent its working end, e.g. scalpel blade or syringe needle, from becoming contaminated with skin bacteria carried from the fingers in the film of water on its surface.

Steaming at 100°C. Pure steam in equilibrium with water boiling at normal atmospheric pressure (760 mm Hg) has a temperature of 100°C; at the lower pressures found at high altitudes the temperature is slightly less (95°C at 5000 ft). Sterilization of bacteriological culture media may often be effected by steaming in either of two ways:

(a) *By a single exposure at* 100°C *for* 90 *minutes.* The spores of some thermophilic and rare mesophilic bacteria can survive this treatment, but in practice it seldom fails to sterilize. The steaming period of 90 minutes includes the time required for the item to be heated up from room temperature to 100°C.

(b) *By intermittent exposure at* 100°C, e.g. *for* 20 *to* 45 *minutes on each of three successive days.* The method is used for culture media containing sugars that are decomposed at higher temperatures, and for gelatin media which after prolonged heating fail to solidify on cooling. The principle of this intermittent method of sterilization, or 'Tyndallization', is that the first exposure to heat suffices to kill the vegetative organisms; between the heatings the spores, being in a favourable nutrient medium, become vegetative forms which are killed during the subsequent heating. The duration of each steaming should be sufficient to heat up the medium to 100°C, i.e. 20 minutes for lots up to 100 ml and longer for larger volumes (see (a) above). Thermophilic, anaerobic and other bacteria whose spores will not germinate in the particular medium or under the conditions of storage between the heatings may escape being killed.

3. MOIST HEAT AT TEMPERATURES ABOVE 100°C. Saturated steam is a more efficient sterilizing agent than hot air, partly because it provides the greater lethal action of moist heat and partly because it is quicker in heating up the exposed articles and in penetrating porous materials such as cotton-wool stoppers, paper and cloth wrappers, bundles of surgical linen, and hollow apparatus. When the steam meets the cooler surface of the article, it condenses into a small volume of water and liberates its considerable latent heat to that surface; e.g. 1600 ml steam at 100°C and at atmospheric pressure condenses into 1 ml water at 100°C, liberating 518 calories of heat. The large contraction in volume brings more steam to the same site and the process continues rapidly until the article's temperature is raised to that of the steam. The condensation water ensures moist conditions for killing of the exposed microbes. Pure steam must be used and the presence of air avoided, since air hinders penetration by the steam.

When saturated steam is under pressures higher than atmospheric, temperatures higher than 100°C can be obtained and this additional advantage of steam as a sterilizing agent is exploited in the process known as *autoclaving.*

STERILIZATION IN THE AUTOCLAVE

Water boils when its vapour pressure equals the pressure of the surrounding atmosphere. This occurs at 100°C at normal atmospheric pressure (i.e. 760 mm Hg, 14·7 lb. per square inch absolute pressure or 0 lb/in² 'gauge pressure'). Thus, when water is boiled within a closed vessel at increased pressures, the temperature at which it boils, and that of the steam it forms, will rise above 100°C.

This is the principle employed in the pressure cooker and the autoclave, which subject articles to *moist* heat at temperatures *higher than* 100°C. Autoclaving is the method most widely used for sterilization of surgical supplies and bacteriological culture media.

In the autoclave, all parts of the load to be sterilized must be permeated by steam. The steam should be not only *saturated,* i.e. at the point of condensing to liquid water, but also *dry,* i.e. free from particles of liquid water. Once the whole of the load has been heated up to the temperature of the steam there is a minimum holding time at that temperature necessary for sterilization. The minimum holding times are 2 minutes at not less than 132°C (27 lb/in² gauge pressure); 12 minutes at not less than 121°C (15 lb/in² gauge pressure) and 30 minutes at not less than 115°C (10 lb/in² gauge pressure).

A 50 per cent safety period is usually added to these minimum holding times and they become 3, 18 and 45 minutes respectively.

IMPORTANCE OF AIR DISCHARGE. All the air must be removed from the autoclave chamber and the articles in the load, so that the latter are exposed to pure steam during the period of sterilization. There are three reasons for this: (1) the admixture of air with steam results in a lower temperature being achieved at the chosen pressure; (2) the air hinders penetration of the steam into the interstices of porous materials, surgical dressings especially, and the narrow openings of containers, syringes, etc.; and (3) the air, being denser than the steam, tends to form a separate and cooler layer in the lower part of the autoclave, and so prevents adequate heating of the articles there. For example, in an autoclave with no air discharge, a temperature of only 70°C was recorded at the bottom when that at the top was 115°C.

There is one exception to the necessity for complete air discharge from the load. Hermetically sealed bottles and ampoules containing *aqueous* solutions and culture media are satisfactorily sterilized in spite of the presence of some air in them. The contained water provides the conditions for moist-heat sterilization, making unnecessary the entry of steam for this purpose, and the contents are heated to the same temperature as the chamber steam, though to a higher pressure, by the conduction of heat through the container walls.

SIMPLE NON-JACKETED LABORATORY AUTOCLAVE. The simplest form of laboratory autoclave, the so-called 'pressure-cooker type' (Fig. 5.2), consists of a vertical or horizontal cylinder of gun-metal or stainless steel in a supporting frame or case. The size may be up to about 18 in (45 cm) in diameter and 30 in (75 cm) in length. The cylinder contains water up to a certain level (e.g. 3½ in for a vertical autoclave of 18 in internal height) and this is heated by a gas burner or electric heater below the cylinder. The bottles, tubes, etc., to be sterilized are placed on a perforated tray above the water level. The lid (or door) is fastened by screw clamps, being rendered air-tight by an asbestos gasket. At the top of the autoclave there is a discharge tap, a pressure gauge and a safety valve. The discharge tap is kept open for a few minutes after the water begins to boil to allow all the air in the chamber to be discharged in the stream of steam. The tap is then closed and when the pressure in the chamber rises to that chosen for autoclaving, e.g. 15 lb/in^2, the sterilizing period is timed as having begun. The safety valve is set to release steam at the chosen pressure, which is thereby automatically maintained throughout the period of heating. After the pressure has been held for the appropriate period, the source of heat is removed and as soon as the pressure is seen to have fallen to atmospheric the autoclave is cautiously opened. *If an autoclave is opened while still under positive pressure a serious explosion and scalding may be caused. If it is*

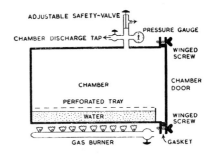

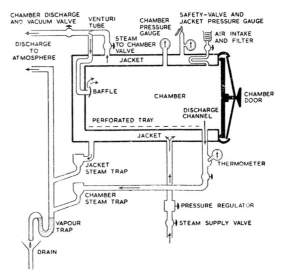

FIG. 5.2. Autoclaves. Above: Simple non-jacketed autoclave. Below: Steam-jacketed autoclave with automatic gravity discharge of air condensate and system for drying by vacuum and intake of filtered air.

left sealed after the pressure falls below atmospheric, there is excessive boiling and evaporation of aqueous media.

DEFICIENCIES OF THE SIMPLE AUTOCLAVE. The simple form of laboratory autoclave is effective when carefully operated, but has several disadvantages. The method of discharging air is inefficient, especially for a large and heavily loaded chamber, and it is difficult to decide when the discharge is complete. If, as a result, the discharge tap is closed and the holding period begun while there is still some air present in the chamber and load, the temperature produced at 15 lb pressure will not be as high as 121°C.

The simple autoclave also lacks means for drying the load after sterilization. Drying is desirable for apparatus wrapped in paper or cloth, and is essential for surgical linen and dressings. Although dry when put into the autoclave, these articles are moistened by the condensation of the steam. When damp, paper and cloth wrappings, even in several layers, are unable to prevent the entry of contaminating bacteria. *It is therefore important to avoid placing the sterilized articles in contact with unsterile objects until their wrappings are dry.*

A wide variety of autoclaves are manufactured that incorporate various devices to overcome these and other difficulties, some being specialized for particular purposes. Some autoclaves at present in hospitals and laboratories have been badly designed or wrongly installed, and cannot ensure sterilization. An increased interest in these problems was prompted particularly by the work of Bowie (1955) and Howie and Timbury (1956), and the Medical Research Council Reports of 1959 and 1960 are very comprehensive. The following description is given of an autoclave suitable for either laboratory or surgical purposes.

STEAM-JACKETED AUTOCLAVE WITH AUTOMATIC AIR AND CONDENSATE DISCHARGE. These may be horizontal metal cylinders but rectangular chambers are more conveniently loaded. A swing door is fastened by a capstan head that operates radial bolts and automatically remains locked while the chamber pressure is raised. A pressure-locked safety door is a valuable guard against the hazards of premature opening by the operator.

The autoclave (Fig. 5.2) also possesses: (1) a supply of steam from an external source; (2) a steam jacket that heats the side walls independently of the presence of steam in the chamber and so facilitates drying of the load; (3) a channel for discharging air and condensate by gravity from the bottom of the chamber, with a 'no-return' valve and a thermostatic valve ('steam trap') to control this discharge automatically; (4) a thermometer indicating the temperature in the discharge channel above the steam trap, i.e. approximately that of the lowest and coolest part of the chamber; (5) a vacuum system that may be used to assist drying of the load; and (6) an air-intake with a self-sterilizing filter for introducing warm sterile air into the chamber. It appears that glass fibre woven into sheet form provides the most reliable filter and that the working life of such a filter is at least one year (MRC Report, 1960).

Steam supply. The steam supplied to the autoclave should be *dry,* i.e. free from excess water in the form of suspended droplets, and *saturated,* i.e. not superheated above the phase boundary of equilibrium with water boiling at the same temperature and pressure.

Loading of chamber. When the jacket is heated, the load is packed into the chamber. Articles requiring different treatment should not be included in the same load, e.g. aqueous media in unsealed containers should be autoclaved on a separate occasion from wrapped goods requiring drying. The articles should be arranged loosely to allow free circulation of steam and displacement of air.

Heating-up and air-displacement period. The door is closed and steam allowed to enter the chamber through a baffle high up at the back. The steam tends to float as a layer above the cooler and denser air, and as more is introduced it displaces the air downwards through the articles of the load and out through the discharge channel at the bottom of the chamber. The condensation water formed on the cool load and cool chamber door also drains through this channel. The channel's thermostatic steam trap remains open while steam mixed with air and condensate passes through it but as soon as all air has been eliminated and the arrival of pure steam raises the temperature of the discharge to 121°C, the trap automatically closes and prevents further escape. About 5 or 10 minutes may be taken for this displacement of air by steam.

Holding period of sterilization. The holding period at 121°C is timed as starting when the thermometer in the discharge channel first shows that this temperature is reached. The exact duration of the holding period is decided according to the nature of the load. During the early part of the holding period some residual air may gradually be displaced from the interior of a porous load; this air together with excess condensate collects in the discharge channel above the steam trap, cools to 120°C or less, and so causes the trap to open momentarily and allow its escape.

A 'near-to-steam' trap is essential, i.e. one that opens when the temperature falls by only 1°C below that of pure steam. Control of the holding period by the temperature of the thermometer in the discharge channel ensures that autoclaving is carried out at the correct temperature, and is much preferable to control by pressure readings.

Cooling and drying period. At the end of the holding period the supply of steam to the chamber is stopped. The management of this stage depends on whether drying of the load is required, as for wrapped apparatus or surgical dressings, or whether it must be avoided, as for aqueous media in loosely stoppered containers.

HIGH PRE-VACUUM STERILIZERS. The most advanced surgical sterilizers are equipped with electrically driven pumps capable of exhausting the chamber to an almost perfect vacuum, e.g. to an absolute pressure of 20 mm Hg or less, by removing more than 98 per cent of the air. A 'high-vacuum' is drawn before admission of steam to the chamber and this enables the steam to penetrate to and heat up all parts of the interior of the load very rapidly. *Even a tightly packed load is heated rapidly and uniformly to the sterilizing temperature.* The rapidity of heating up makes it feasible to employ a higher sterilizing temperature for a shorter time, namely 135°C for 3 minutes (i.e. jacket and chamber steam at 30 lb/in^2 gauge pressure). The total operation time is greatly shortened and damage to heat-sensitive materials by exposure to air-steam mixtures or prolonged heating in the outer parts of the load is avoided. The load is finally dried within a few minutes by exhaustion of the chamber and the vacuum is then broken by admission of air through a filter.

Autoclave Control and Sterilization Indicators

Automatic process control. Modern autoclaves may be furnished with an automatic control system that carries through the whole sterilization cycle, including the heating-up, holding, cooling and drying stages, according to a preselected set of conditions. After the chamber has been loaded and the process started, no further attention is required until the load is ready for removal. Apart from saving the time of a skilled operator, automatic control is a valuable safeguard against error due to negligence or distraction. A monitoring system ensures that if the temperature at any time falls below that selected, the operation will be repeated.

In the absence of automatic control, a *recording thermometer* producing a graphic timed record of the temperature changes in the chamber discharge channel helps the operator to avoid errors in timing the holding period. A daily inspection of such a temperature record by a responsible person is of more value than more elaborate tests carried out at infrequent intervals.

Thermocouple measurement of load temperature. This is the method of discovering the heating-up time required for a given kind of load. A thermocouple is inserted deeply inside a test article in the autoclave chamber, e.g. a bottle of liquid or a pack of dressings, and its wire leads are carried out to a potentiometer which indicates the temperature inside the test article during the course of autoclaving.

These instrumental means of controlling the sterilizing cycle in the autoclave are of the greatest value, but there are some occasions when a test of overall efficiency is desirable. Two methods are available, one using chemical indicators, the other spore indicators.

Chemical indicators. These show a change of colour or shape after exposure to a sterilizing temperature. They may be placed inside the load. Browne's sterilizer control tubes contain a red solution that turns green when heated at 115°C for 25 minutes (type 1) or 15 minutes (type 2), or at 160°C for 60 minutes (type 3). They must be stored at less than 20°C to avoid deterioration and premature colour change. Bowie-Dick tape, which is applied to packs and articles in the load, develops diagonal lines when exposed for the correct time to the sterilizing temperature.

Spore indicators. A preparation of dried bacterial spores is placed within the load in the autoclave and after autoclaving is tested for viability on transfer to a culture medium. *Bacillus stearothermophilus,* a thermophile that requires to be cultivated at 55° to 60°C is a suitable test organism; its spores are killed at 121°C in about 12 minutes.

Successful chemical or spore tests give no assurance that the sterilizer and technique are reliable, since heating might be inadequate in other parts of the load or under different conditions of loading. The essential safeguard of sterilization is that the autoclave is correctly designed, installed and maintained, that its operation is carried out with careful attention to the correct procedure and that control is by an accurate thermometer in the discharge line and not by pressure readings.

STERILIZATION BY RADIATION

ULTRA-VIOLET RADIATION. The ability of sunlight to kill bacteria is mainly due to the ultra-violet rays that it contains. Visible light at the violet end of the spectrum at a wavelength of 400 nm and ultra-violet radiation are not markedly bactericidal until 330 nm is reached. Thereafter the effectiveness of ultra-violet light as a sterilizing agent increases with decrease in wavelength. These radiations induce thymine dimers in DNA and this interferes with replication. Other lethal effects are produced. On exposure to visible light, some of the thymine dimers produced in the irradiated bacteria or viruses dissociate spontaneously so that some of the apparently killed organisms may be *photoreactivated.* The shortest ultra-violet rays in sunlight that reach the earth's surface in quantity have a wavelength of some 290 nm, but even more effective radiations of 240 to 280 nm are produced by mercury vapour lamps.

Ultra-violet rays from suitably shielded lamps have been used to reduce the number of bacteria

in the atmosphere but for safety their intensity has to be restricted.

Ionizing Radiation. Ionizing radiations include high-speed electrons, X-rays and gamma-rays (short X-rays). In a sufficient dose these radiations are lethal to all cells, bacteria included, because they induce damage in DNA by various mechanisms including the production of free radicals. Bacterial species vary in their sensitivity to ionizing radiations and the degree of resistance varies during the growth cycle. Spores are generally more resistant than vegetative cells, but *Micrococcus radiodurans* is the most resistant bacterium known and it is not a spore-former. This paradox is attributed to the very efficient DNA repair mechanism that has evolved in this species. Sterilization by radiation is achieved in practice by the use of high-speed electrons from a machine such as a linear accelerator or by use of rays from an isotope source such as cobalt 60; a dose of 2·5 Mrad is generally adequate. The necessary apparatus is much too expensive for installation in a hospital. It is employed commercially for the sterilization of large amounts of pre-packed disposable items such as plastic syringes and catheters that are unable to withstand heat.

STERILIZATION BY FILTRATION

It is possible to render fluids, including bacterial cultures, free from bacteria by passing them through special filters with a pore size of less than 0·75 μm. The method is especially useful in making preparations of the soluble products of bacterial growth, such as toxins, and in sterilizing liquids that would be damaged by heat, such as serum and antibiotic solutions. Some types of filter with a smaller pore diameter can be produced and they are able to retain smaller microorganisms including many viruses. In general, however, even filters labelled 'sterilizing' must be regarded as rendering a liquid bacteria-free but *not* mycoplasma-free or virus-free. For many laboratory purposes this is perfectly satisfactory but such fluids, e.g. serum treated by Seitz filtration, must *not* be regarded as safe for clinical use and should not be referred to as sterile.

The various types of filter used in bacteriological work include: (1) earthenware candles

(Berkefeld, Chamberland), (2) asbestos and as-bestos-paper disks (Seitz), (3) sintered glass filters, and (4) cellulose membrane filters. Cellulose membrane filters have several advantages over the widely used Seitz asbestos filters. In particular, they are much less adsorptive and their rate of filtration is much greater. They have been used to separate viruses of different sizes by gradation of their pore size.

CHEMICAL DISINFECTANTS

Chemical antimicrobial agents for use in the environment or on the skin are often wrongly called sterilizing agents. They should be called *disinfectants* or *antiseptics*. These terms indicate the role of the agents in killing or inhibiting many pathogenic microorganisms without implying that they can be relied on to kill all micro-organisms and spores. The distinction between disinfectants and antiseptics is not clear-cut; it refers to the potency of the agent and some agents may be used as disinfectants in high concentration and as antiseptics in low ones.

Strong disinfectants are potent microbicidal but relatively toxic substances. They rapidly kill the vegetative forms of pathogenic organisms, though they are often ineffective against spores. They are suitable for application to inanimate objects but are generally too poisonous and irritant to be applied to the tissues or, other than momentarily, to the skin.

Mild disinfectants ('antiseptics') on the other hand, are substances sufficiently bland and non-toxic for superficial application to living tissues, e.g. to intact mucous membrane, broken skin or the interior of a wound. They may kill micro-organisms (microbicidal effect) or merely prevent their growth (microbistatic effect). Although they are sufficiently bland to be tolerated when applied to tissues, they may nevertheless damage tissues cells and kill phagocytes, so that in certain circumstances their beneficial action against infecting bacteria may be outweighed by their deleterious effect on the defences of the tissues (Fleming, 1945).

Mode and Conditions of Action of Disinfectants

Remarkably little is known about the mechanisms of action of many accepted antimicrobial chemicals. The protein-denaturing effects of acids and phenols, the oxidizing action of the halogens, the lipid-solvent properties of some organic solvents, and the detergent action of surface-active agents may account for some relatively non-specific antibacterial effects at the cytoplasmic membrane. Probably most disinfectants and antiseptics act by denaturing or altering proteins or lipids in the cytoplasmic membrane. Some antiseptics interfere with energy-yielding systems within the cell and some directly inhibit specific steps in biosynthetic pathways. It is known that mercuric salts combine with sulphydryl groups and that the antibacterial dyes combine with nucleic acids. This effect may be of practical use in the treatment of herpesvirus infections. Heterotricyclic dyes such as neutral red, proflavine and toluidine bind to the guanine bases of nucleic acids. Thereafter, on exposure to fluorescent light, the dye absorbs energy and this may cause single-strand breaks by excision of guanine. The effect is referred to as 'photodynamic action'.

In general, the rate of inactivation of a susceptible bacterial population in the presence of an antimicrobial chemical is dependent on the relative concentrations of the two reactants, the bacteria and the chemical, but there are other variables that must be controlled if disinfection is to be ensured. The principal factors determining effective disinfection are the *concentration* of the disinfectant in use and the *time* during which it is effectively applied. Thus it is essential that the application be 'strong enough for long enough'. The range of dilution over which a disinfectant is effective varies markedly with different chemicals and some disinfectants become quite inactive when diluted only several times beyond the correct dilution for use. Unless great care is taken in the preparation and replacement of 'in-use' dilutions, accidental over-dilution and thus failure of disinfection may occur.

The velocity of the reaction also depends upon the number of organisms present, the species involved and whether the organism is spore-forming or not. In general, chemicals have an uncertain action on bacterial endospores. The microbicidal action of disinfectants is usually increased by heat within the limits of the thermo-stability of the substance and it is preferable to use disinfectants under warm rather than under cold conditions.

Some antimicrobial effects are very dependent on the *correct pH* for their operation. Thus, the *reaction* of the suspending agent in any test of a disinfectant is very important. The 'hardness' of water may markedly interfere with the antimicrobial effect of surface-active agents with which it may be used. The presence of *organic matter* greatly influences the efficacy of many disinfectants and the neutralizing effect of proteins, e.g. in dirt, pus and blood, is well known. Water is pre-treated by filtration or precipitation to remove gross organic matter such as algal debris before chlorine is introduced to kill the potentially pathogenic microbes. Similarly, whenever possible, surfaces should be cleaned before disinfecting procedures are applied. In some cases this is not possible and the disinfectant chosen should then be of a kind that is relatively insusceptible to inactivation.

SELECTION OF A DISINFECTANT. Successful disinfection depends on (1) the selection of a disinfectant capable of performing the required task and (2) its careful use under appropriate conditions of concentration, duration of exposure, temperature, pH and absence of neutralizing substances. Unfortunately, disinfectants are frequently chosen which are unsuited to their task or are used under conditions in which they have no chance of being effective.

There are three main purposes for which disinfectants are correctly used:

1. *Decontamination of objects before disposal or re-use.* Faeces, urine, pus, sputum and other potentially infective discharges, whether in a container, e.g. bed-pan, or on dressings or clothing, may require to be disinfected before the container or soiled article is washed for reuse. Clinical instruments such as thermometers and specula for body orifices may require to be disinfected between use on different patients, although it is impracticable to sterilize them. The storage of cleaning mops, nail brushes and transfer forceps in disinfectant to prevent bacterial multiplication on them between different occasions of use is a similar application. In medical laboratories, contaminated slides, pipettes and other instruments are generally discarded into a jar of disinfectant; after several hours or days they are safely removed and

washed. The best disinfectants for these purposes, especially when there is heavy soiling with organic matter, are the phenolic disinfectants of the black fluid, white fluid and lysol types (but not the chlorinated phenols). Because they are cheap, have a wide spectrum of activity and are not very liable to become inactive in the presence of organic matter, these phenolic derivatives are the most commonly used general disinfectants. In the absence of heavy soiling with organic matter, hypochlorite solution, which is much less toxic and more easily washed away after disinfection, is recommended, but, since hypochlorite is readily inactivated by organic matter, care must be taken to ensure that only fresh, active solutions are used.

2. *Reduction of microbial contamination of the inanimate environment.* In hospitals, pathogenic staphylococci, streptococci, enterobacteria and pseudomonads may be present on the floors, walls and furniture of wards, surgical theatres and kitchens, and on baths, wash-hand basins and water-closets in the bathrooms used by patients. The risk of cross-infection of patients is probably lessened if the amount of this environmental contamination is reduced and disinfectants have a useful though limited role in doing this. In general, it is sufficient to clean floors, walls and furniture with warm water and detergent. A disinfectant is unnecessary except for areas known to have been soiled with an infected body discharge; these areas should be wiped with a cheap phenolic disinfectant. Rooms vacated by patients with smallpox or tuberculosis may be wholly disinfected by filling with formaldehyde vapour for 24 hours, but such terminal disinfection is rarely undertaken for other kinds of infection. Baths and wash-hand basins may be a source of cross-infection and should be regularly cleaned with a cleaning powder containing hypochlorite or with a mixture of hypochlorite and detergent. The seats, flushes and door handles in water-closets and working surfaces in kitchens should be wiped regularly with hypochlorite solution. If cheap, toxic phenolic disinfectants were applied to these surfaces they would have to be removed before use by careful cleansing. Hypochlorite is preferred as a *surface disinfectant* for relatively clean objects because it leaves no objectionable

residues. For small, relatively clean areas 70 per cent industrial methylated spirit or 70 per cent isopropyl alcohol is a pleasant and moderately effective, residue-free disinfectant.

3. *Disinfection of the skin of hands and operation sites.* Transient organisms that have been picked up by contact with outside sources and are lying on the surface of the skin are relatively easily removed by washing with soap and rinsing with a disinfectant. On the other hand, organisms such as *Staph. aureus* that are resident or growing in the depths of the skin are difficult or impossible to eliminate completely. Hands may be washed with liquid soap or detergent containing hexachlorophane (3 per cent) or rinsed with aqueous chlorhexidine (0·5 per cent). The skin of operation sites may be washed repeatedly with hexachlorophane soap and painted preoperatively with iodine (1 per cent) or chlorhexidine (0·5 per cent) or laurolinium (5 per cent) in 70 per cent ethyl alcohol (70 per cent industrial methylated spirit) or 70 per cent isopropyl alcohol.

PROPERTIES AND USES OF PARTICULAR DISINFECTANTS

The following disinfectants merit discussion in this chapter. A comprehensive account of the clinical aspects is given by Williams *et al.* (1966). ANTISEPTICS OF THE PHENOL GROUP. Phenol (carbolic acid) is powerfully microbicidal and the cheaper phenolic disinfectants derived from coal tar are widely used for decontamination of infective discharges, bathrooms, bed-pans and hospital floors. They are, however, too toxic and irritant to be applied to and left on objects that will come in contact with the skin. The preparations include Lysol (liquor cresolis saponatus) and other cresol fluids ('black fluid' and 'white fluid'). As they are active against a wide range of organisms and are not readily inactivated by the presence of organic matter, they are good general disinfectants.

Phenol itself is bactericidal at a concentration of 1 per cent, but its activity is drastically reduced by dilution, and it is virtually inactive at 0·1 per cent. It is used at a concentration of 0·5 per cent for preserving sera and vaccines. It is expensive and for general disinfection is replaced by cheaper preparations. Phenol and the coal tar derivatives are markedly toxic to man. Sudol is a less toxic substitute for Lysol; it contains xylenols and phenols, but must still be used with caution as a coarse disinfectant. Jeyes Fluid is a well-known proprietary preparation. This group of compounds can be used to treat faeces or sputum to render them safe before disposal.

The related chlorophenols and chloroxylenols marketed as Hycolin and Dettol are less toxic and irritant but also are less active and are more readily inactivated by organic matter. Hycolin is a green fluid containing a combination of synthetic phenols including 3 : 5-dimethyl 4-chlorphenol; 2-benzyl 4-chlorphenol; 2-hydroxy diphenyl sodium; 3-methyl 4-chlorphenol; and sodium pentachlorphenate. It can be incorporated in a liquid soap, a hand-cream or an antiseptic 1 per cent aqueous solution. Dettol contains 4·8 per cent chloroxylenol and is very widely used as a fluid and a cream. These compounds are relatively inactive against *Pseudomonas* species; indeed Dettol can be incorporated in a selective medium for the isolation of pseudomonads.

Hexachlorophane is an even blander agent and is incorporated in various antiseptic preparations for use on the skin. It is effective against Gram-positive organisms but much less so against Gram-negative organisms and it is ineffective against *Pseudomonas* species. Combined as a 3 per cent solution with a liquid detergent, it is marketed as Phisohex; it is also incorporated in a soap as Gamophen, but is less active in this form. In powder form it is available as Ster-Zac. These preparations have important applications in the control of pyogenic cocci in surgical and neonatal units in hospital. Their action is slow; and repeated use is necessary before they exert a significant effect on the skin flora. Frequent whole-body application of a detergent emulsion containing hexachlorophane 3 per cent to neonates or denuded surfaces, e.g. burns, may result in absorption of significant amounts into the blood. As hexachlorophane is potentially toxic, it should be used with care and whole body application should be followed by rinsing, but its efficacy in the prophylaxis of staphylococcal infection in paediatric, maternity and surgical units is so generally accepted that its *controlled use* and its good reputation are likely to survive recent public anxiety.

Chlorhexidine (Hibitane) is recommended as a relatively non-toxic skin antiseptic for general use. It is most active against Gram-positive organisms and fairly effective against Gram-negative bacteria. It is inactivated by soap and organic matter. A 0·5 to 1·0 per cent solution in 70 per cent isopropyl alcohol may be used for skin disinfection; aqueous solutions are used for the treatment of wounds.

THE HALOGENS. Chlorine and iodine are bactericidal and sporicidal. *Chlorine* has a special place in the treatment of water supplies, and combinations of hypochlorite and detergents are useful for cleansing and disinfection in the food and dairy industries. Various hypochlorite preparations have a usefully wide spectrum of activity against viruses. Chloros, Eusol and Milton are aqueous solutions of hypochlorite and other salts; their antibacterial and antiviral efficacy is limited because chlorine-releasing preparations are markedly inactivated by contact with organic matter. Chloros is a solution of hypochlorite yielding 100 000 parts per million of available chlorine. It is commonly used at a 1 in 100 dilution (yielding 1 000 parts/ 10^6 chlorine) for general disinfection and disposal of contaminated glassware such as microscope slides and pipettes, and at a 1 in 10 dilution (yielding 10 000 parts/10^6 chlorine) for disinfection of equipment visibly contaminated with blood. The working dilution must be made up freshly each day in a carefully cleansed container (Kelsey and Maurer, 1971) and may be tested at intervals with a starch-iodine paper to confirm by the demonstration of a dark-blue reaction that it is still active. Milton is used for the cleansing and disinfection of babies' milk-feed bottles. Hypochlorite should not be applied to metal, which it corrodes, or to cloth, which it may damage.

Iodine, like chlorine, is also inactivated by organic matter. Tincture of iodine (Weak Solution of Iodine BP: 2·5 per cent iodine and 2·5 per cent potassium iodide in 90 per cent ethanol) and iodine 2 per cent in 70 per cent isopropyl alcohol are powerful, rapid skin disinfectants and are valuable for preparation of the skin for surgery. A few individuals, however, are hypersensitive to iodine. Alcoholic solutions of iodine are too irritant for use on broken skin, and aqueous preparations are not as rapidly effective. The iodophors, containing iodine complexed with an anionic detergent, are less irritant; an example is Betadine, a water soluble complex of iodine and polyvinyl pyrrolidone (povidone). Betadine solution contains 1 per cent available iodine and can be used as a bactericidal antiseptic for intact skin and for disinfection of superficial wounds. It is only slowly sporicidal but it is rapidly effective against vegetative organisms including fungi and *Trichomonas*. A compress of povidone-iodine applied to abraded skin for 15 to 30 minutes markedly reduces the spore population; repeated applications of this type may, if need be, be used when operations are delayed for 2 or 3 days. Lilly and Lowbury (1971) found that disinfection of intact skin at an operation site for 2 minutes with povidone-iodine containing 1 per cent available iodine in 70 per cent ethyl alcohol reduced the resident flora to a similar degree as that achieved with alcoholic chlorhexidine (see above).

METALLIC SALTS AND METALLIC ORGANIC COMPOUNDS. Mercuric chloride (perchloride of mercury) is sometimes used as a disinfectant in a 1 in 1000 solution: mercuric salts are strongly bacteriostatic, but they are not effectively bactericidal. The use of these preparations as pre-operative skin disinfectants is no longer justified. 'Merthiolate', a proprietary name for sodium ethylmercurithiosalicylate, is used in a dilution of 1 in 10 000 for the preservation of antitoxic and other sera and for inactivation of some vaccines.

Silver nitrate enjoyed a vogue as an antibacterial agent. A drop of a 1 per cent solution placed in the eye in newborn babies was widely and successfully used in the prophylaxis of gonococcal ophthalmia. It has been largely replaced by more modern antiseptics such as chlorhexidine, but it may still retain a place in the treatment of extensive burns.

FORMALDEHYDE AND GLUTARALDEHYDE. Formaldehyde is highly lethal to all kinds of microbes and spores, killing bacterial spores almost as readily as the vegetative forms. It is applied as an aqueous solution or in gaseous form (Ministry of Health, 1958). It is cheap, and non-injurious to cloth, fabrics, wood, leather, rubber, paints and metals. In the gaseous form, it is used to disinfect rooms, furniture and a wide variety of articles liable to damage by heat, e.g. woollen blankets and clothing, shoes, respirators, hairbrushes, and gum-elastic catheters.

Commercial 'formalin' is a 40 per cent (w/v) solution of formaldehyde in water containing 10 per cent methanol to inhibit polymerization. A dilution containing 5 per cent formaldehyde in water is a powerful and rapid disinfectant when applied directly to a contaminated surface. *Glutaraldehyde* in 2 per cent aqueous solution is even more effective and somewhat less irritant. It is stable in acid solution but much more active in alkaline solution. Accordingly the commercially available preparation (Cidex) is supplied together with a separate alkaline buffer containing a rust inhibitor which is added before use. Cidex is bacteriocidal and sporicidal and effective against viruses. It is particularly useful for the sterilization of items of equipment that cannot be subjected to sterilizing temperatures, such as cystoscopes, anaesthetic equipment, plastic materials and thermometers.

Formaldehyde and glutaraldehyde are two of the few disinfectants that are sporicidal.

VOLATILE SOLVENTS. *Isopropyl alcohol* is not subject to Excise duty and is cheaper than *ethyl alcohol*. Both these alcohols are optimally bactericidal in aqueous solution at concentrations of 70 to 75 per cent, and have very little bactericidal effect outside this range, e.g. when 'absolute', i.e. undiluted with water, or when diluted too much. They are often used in skin disinfection before hypodermic injection, venepuncture, etc.; the skin should be dry before they are applied. Chlorhexidine (0·5 per cent) or iodine (1 to 2 per cent) or laurolinium acetate (5 per cent) in 70 per cent alcohol are used for the same purpose and such mixtures are superior to the alcohol alone.

Acetone and *ether* are only weakly antibacterial and are not effective alternatives to alcohol as skin disinfectants; they should not be used.

Chloroform has a limited use as a bactericidal agent in bacteriology. It is rapidly bactericidal to vegetative bacteria and readily removes itself from a treated medium or culture by evaporation.

SOAPS AND DETERGENTS. Ordinary *soaps* are anionic detergents and have a degree of antibacterial activity; they contribute greatly to hygiene by aiding the mechanical removal of organisms during washing. There is evidence that soaps of saturated fatty acids are mildly effective against some pathogenic intestinal bacteria and that soaps of long-chain unsaturated fatty acids are active against some of the respiratory pathogens.

Surface-active agents in general possess wetting and cleansing properties as well as some disinfectant activity. The synthetic *anionic detergents* such as the sodium alkyl sulphates inhibit Gram-positive bacteria to some extent, but they are much less effective against Gram-negative bacteria.

Among *cationic detergents* the quaternary ammonium compounds are most useful. They combine antibacterial properties with detergent activity and being relatively non-toxic and bland, they are popular cleansing agents in the treatment of accidental wounds. They are essentially bacteriostatic and are more active against Gram-positive than Gram-negative bacteria. They are inactivated by organic matter and soaps. *Pseudomonas pyocyanea* is notoriously resistant to them and this organism has been cultured from the corks of bottles of their solutions.

It is difficult to give a true assessment of the efficacy of the quaternary compounds. Commercially available preparations include Cetavlon (cetrimide), Roccal and Zephiran (benzalkonium chloride) and Laurodin (laurolinium acetate); there is interest in Laurodin as an effective skin antiseptic. Picloxydine is a biguanide with marked antibacterial activity. A 1 per cent solution in combination with octylphenoxypolyethoxy ethanol (11 per cent) and benzalkonium chloride (12 per cent) is marketed as Resiguard, which, at a dilution of 1 in 60, is active against both Gram-positive and Gram-negative organisms; it is relatively non-toxic and does not irritate the eyes or lungs. It may be used with a fogging or spraying machine for the disinfection of walls and other surfaces.

Tego compounds are bacteriostatic ampholytic surface-active derivatives of dodecyldi(aminoethyl)glycine. At a concentration of 1 per cent in water, they are said to be effective against a wide range of Gram-positive and Gram-negative organisms and some viruses, but the anti-microbial effect of Tego compounds is markedly reduced by a wide variety of substances including organic matter and even hard water. They cannot be recommended for general use. They have been recommended in the past for use in animal houses, partly on the basis of their good detergent properties and their relative non-toxicity, but there are many detergents on the market that are less expensive.

MISCELLANEOUS DISINFECTANTS. The aniline and acridine dyes are active against Gram-positive organisms but less active against Gram-negative organisms. The staining caused by *gentian violet* made it an unpopular remedy. Proflavine and acriflavine in aqueous solution are slowly bactericidal and effective in the presence of organic matter. They have been largely replaced by other antiseptics such as chlorhexidine.

The oxidizing agents, *hydrogen peroxide* and *potassium permanganate,* have been used as antiseptics in the past. They are readily inactivated by organic matter and they have no place in modern antiseptic practice. Boric acid has an interesting antibacterial activity; however, it can produce toxic reactions and it is now replaced by more effective agents. It is used as a bacteriostat in preserving samples of urine prior to examination for viable counts in the laboratory. *Sodium azide* is sometimes used as a preservative in biological preparations including experimental antisera. It inhibits esterification of inorganic phosphate and it can be used at low concentrations (e.g. 0·08 per cent). It is very toxic to man and animals.

Gaseous Disinfectants

Disinfection by formaldehyde gas. The gas is liberated by spraying or heating formalin, or by heating solid paraformaldehyde. The atmosphere must have a high relative humidity, over 60 per cent and preferably 80 to 90 per cent, and a temperature of at least 18°C. Moreover, the materials must be arranged to allow free access of the gas to all infected surfaces, since its penetration into porous fabrics is slow.

Small articles, such as instruments, shoes and hair-brushes, are disinfected by exposure for at least 3 hours to formaldehyde gas introduced into the air in a cabinet by boiling formalin in an electric boiler. Blankets and the surfaces of mattresses are disinfected similarly in a large cabinet, where they are hung unfolded. Folded blankets and clothing can be disinfected if they are packed in the chamber of a steam-jacketed autoclave and heated at 100°C for 3 hours in the presence of formalin vapour. The vapour may be used for the disinfection of premises; for example, after contamination by a patient with smallpox. Irritant residues of formaldehyde may be removed by exposure of the disinfected articles to ammonia vapour.

Ethylene oxide. This gaseous disinfectant is also highly lethal to all kinds of microbes and spores, but is capable of much more rapid diffusion into dry, porous materials. It is of particular value for sterilizing articles liable to damage by heat, e.g. plastic and rubber articles, blankets, pharmaceutical products and complex apparatus such as heart-lung machines (Kelsey, 1961). It must be used only in a special chamber or apparatus since it is toxic and forms an explosive mixture when more than 3 per cent is present in air. A non-explosive mixture of 10 per cent ethylene oxide in carbon dioxide or a halogenated hydrocarbon may be employed for sterilization. The sterilization time depends, among other factors, on the temperature of the reaction and the relative humidity, which should be between 20 and 40 per cent.

USE AND ABUSE OF DISINFECTANTS

Present hospital practice in Britain is far from satisfactory in the use of disinfectants. Ayliffe and his colleagues (Ayliffe *et al.*, 1969) visited 140 wards in 14 hospitals; the hospitals visited often had a different disinfectant policy, and the choice of disinfectants for similar purposes in the different hospitals varied considerably. A wide range of disinfectants was used and some were clearly unsuitable for the purpose for which they were employed. In dispensing the solutions of household disinfectants, members of staff apparently relied upon such measures as 'a tablespoonful to a bucket', 'until it looks enough' and 'depending on the smell'. The important principle of 'strong enough for long enough' was generally overlooked.

Floor cleaning mops were frequently found to be contaminated with potentially pathogenic Gram-negative bacteria. Cloths used for cleaning locker tops were commonly contaminated with a similar flora. Baths were usually contaminated with potential pathogens and so were bath mops and brushes. Wash-bowls contained Gram-negative bacteria. Holders for disposable bed-pans were occasionally found to be heavily contaminated with faecal organisms. Nail brushes regularly carried potential pathogens. Nineteen per cent of 213 thermometers were contaminated with Gram-negative bacilli. Antiseptic detergent creams and liquid soaps and hand creams provided sources of Gram-negative bacilli when communal jars were used. Toilet brushes and shaving brushes and equipment were usually contaminated.

These observations provide a timely reminder that antimicrobial chemicals must be properly applied if they are to be of service in medicine. Too often, their abuse provides a dangerously false sense of security. Each hospital should adopt a properly planned policy on the kind and concentrations of disinfectants to be used for particular purposes, a system of supervision to ensure that hospital staff are implementing this policy and a system of 'in-use' tests to be made by the bacteriologist on samples of the disinfectant dilutions actually being used in the different hospital areas to ensure that they are at the correct concentration and retain adequate activity. The problems of the use of disinfectants in hospitals are discussed by the Public Health Laboratory Committee (1965), and Kelsey (1970).

Comparative Tests of Disinfectants

The efficacy of a new disinfectant or antiseptic may be measured by comparison with that of phenol under given conditions. The 'phenol coefficient' is determined in parallel tests that compare killing times observed with suspensions of the typhoid bacillus exposed to known concentrations of the test substance and killing times observed with suspensions exposed to known concentrations of phenol (Rideal-Walker test). The phenol coefficient measured by the Rideal-Walker test does not, however, give any indication of how the test disinfectant will function under practical conditions, e.g. in the presence of much organic matter. Organic matter, in the form of dried yeast, is included in the test system in the Chick-Martin test, which therefore gives a more meaningful result.

'*In-use tests*'. The disinfectant or antiseptic should be tested in a model that bears some resemblance to the circumstances in which it is designed to operate and practical 'in-use tests' have been developed to meet this requirement. Thus, the liquid phase of disinfectant solutions in actual use in hospital practice, e.g. the dregs of solutions in containers, may be examined quantitatively for viable organisms and a use-dilution is then determined which only very rarely yields a positive culture (Kelsey and Maurer, 1966). The efficiency of a new surface disinfectant is judged in terms of its ability to inactivate a known number of a standard strain of a pathogenic staphylococcus on a given surface within a certain time. It is clear that the test conditions must be carefully defined and it is still difficult to make absolutely valid comparisons, but the results of such tests are generally more useful than those of the phenol coefficient test and its modifications.

One of the great problems of tests involving assessments of microbial inactivation is that, after exposure of a test population of organisms to an antimicrobial agent *in vitro,* a subsequent viability check must avoid carry-over of microbistatic traces of the agent. In some cases, the diluting effect of subculture is sufficient to reduce the concentration of the transferred disinfectant to an ineffective level. In other cases, a neutralizer must be incorporated in the test mixture or subculture medium so that residual effects are prevented. For example, a thiosulphate removes traces of chlorine. Alternatively, if a volatile agent is under test it may simply be driven off by heat. If a carry-over effect is not checked, the results greatly overestimate the efficacy of the antimicrobial substance.

REFERENCES

AYLIFFE, G. A. J., BRIGHTWELL, K. M., COLLINS, B. J. & LOWBURY, E. J. L. (1969) Varieties of aseptic practice in hospital wards. *Lancet*, **ii,** 1117.

BOWIE, J. H. (1955) Modern apparatus for sterilization. *Pharmaceutical Journal*, **174**, 473.

FLEMING, A. (1945) Antiseptics: The Lister Memorial Lecture. *Chemistry and Industry*, **3**, 18.

HOWIE, J. W. & TIMBURY, MORAG C. (1956) Laboratory tests of operating-theatre sterilizers. *Lancet*, **ii**, 669.

KELSEY, J. C. (1969) Sterilization by ethylene oxide. *Journal of Clinical Pathology*, **14**, 59.

KELSEY, J. C. (1970) Disinfectants for hospital use—an interim statement. *British Hospital and Social Service Journal*, **80**, 521.

KELSEY, J. C. & MAURER, I. M. (1966) An in-use test for hospital disinfectants. *Monthly Bulletin of the Ministry of Health and Public Health Laboratory Service*, **25**, 180.

KELSEY, J. C. & MAURER, I. M. (1971). *Health Trends*. Aug., pp. 147–149.

LILLY, H. A. & LOWBURY, E. J. L. (1971) Disinfection of the skin; an assessment of some new preparations. *British Medical Journal*, **iii**, 674.

MINISTRY OF HEALTH (1958) The practical aspects of formaldehyde fumigation. *Monthly Bulletin of the Ministry of Health and Public Health Laboratory Service*, **17**, 270.

PUBLIC HEALTH LABORATORY COMMITTEE ON THE TESTING AND EVALUATION OF DISINFECTANTS (1965) Use of disinfectants in hospitals. *British Medical Journal*, **1**, 408.

RUBBO, S. D. & GARDNER, J. F. (1965) *A Review of Sterilization and Disinfection (as Applied to Medical, Industrial and Laboratory Practice)*. London: Lloyd-Luke Ltd.

SYKES, G. (1965) *Disinfection and Sterilisation*. 2nd Edn. London: E. & F. Spon

WILLIAMS, R. E. O., BLOWERS, R., GARROD, L. P. & SHOOTER, R. A. (1966) Sterilisation or disinfection by chemicals. In *Hospital Infection*, 2nd edn, p. 311. London: Lloyd-Luke Ltd.

6. Antimicrobial Agents: Mode of Action Against Bacteria

Any chemical substance inhibiting the growth or causing the death of a microorganism is known as an antimicrobial agent. Although a wide range of chemicals have these properties if a sufficiently high concentration is used, the term is usually restricted to those substances that are effective at concentrations suitable for practical application. It is possible to subdivide antimicrobial agents into various groups according to the action and purposes for which they are employed. Unfortunately, there is not always general agreement on the strict definition of the terms used, but the following descriptions represent a consensus of opinions.

1. If the substance merely causes a cessation of growth of the microorganism which is reversed when the chemical is removed, it is called a *static* agent. If the substance kills the microorganism, it is called a *cidal* agent. This distinction is often a rather arbitrary one and in some instances depends on the concentration of the drug; a static agent may become cidal if the concentration is increased. In general, however, disinfectants have a cidal action whilst chemotherapeutic agents are often static at the concentrations used.

2. A further subdivision can be based upon the group of microorganisms affected. Thus agents acting on bacteria are called *bacteriostatic* or *bactericidal*, those acting on fungi are called *fungistatic* or *fungicidal,* and so on.

3. In practice it is useful to distinguish between antimicrobial agents acting at various levels in the relationship between potentially pathogenic microorganisms and their animal hosts.

(a) **Disinfectants.** This is a term applied to chemicals used to kill potentially infectious organisms. They are normally used in the treatment of inanimate objects, surfaces, waters, etc., and are not meant to come into direct contact with man. Because their potential toxicity to man may not be important, the main criteria used in the choice of a chemical as a disinfectant are its cheapness and its ability rapidly to kill a wide range of microorganisms (see Chap. 5).

(b) **Antiseptics (mild disinfectants).** This term refers to relatively non-toxic and non-irritant antimicrobial agents that may be applied topically to the body surface either to kill or to inhibit the growth of pathogenic microorganisms (see Chap. 5).

(c) **Chemotherapeutic agents.** This term describes the chemicals that are used to kill or inhibit the growth of microorganisms already established in the tissues of the body. In theory the name may be applied to any substance used for therapeutic purposes although in practice, it has tended to be restricted to chemicals used in the treatment of microbial infections. Another useful term that possibly expresses more clearly the function of this group of agents is *antimicrobial drugs.*

Chemotherapeutic agents need to act at a concentration that can be tolerated by the tissues of the host and therefore they must have a selective toxicity for the microorganism compared with the host. This selective toxicity is expressed in terms of the *chemotherapeutic index* which compares the maximum dose that can be tolerated by the host without causing death (the maximum tolerated dose) with the minimum dose that cures the particular infection (minimum curative dose).

i.e. Chemotherapeutic index
$$= \frac{\text{maximum tolerated dose}}{\text{minimum curative dose}}$$

The chemotherapeutic index provides a rough guide to the degree of selective toxicity and thus to the possible therapeutic value of a chemical; clearly as high a figure as possible is desirable, so that effective therapy may be given without danger of toxicity to the patient.

The most widely used chemotherapeutic agents are the *antibiotics,* which are defined as naturally occurring antimicrobial agents produced by microorganisms. The ability to produce antibiotics is particularly common among soil microorganisms and is presumed to give the producing organisms an advantage in the struggle for existence. The most common groups of antibiotic producers are the actinomycetes amongst prokaryotes and the fungi among eukaryotes. The antibiotics themselves represent a wide variety of chemical structures and the distinction between them and the synthetic chemotherapeutic agents is not a fundamental one since some antibiotics such as chloramphenicol (Chloromycetin) are now manufactured more cheaply by chemical synthesis than by cultivation of the antibiotic-producing microorganisms. Further, the mode of action of antibiotics is essentially similar to that of other chemotherapeutic agents.

Development of Chemotherapy

Many substances are antimicrobial, but very few of them are potential chemotherapeutic agents for the simple reason that mammalian cells and the intact animal are in general much more sensitive to chemical inhibition than are microbial cells. Microorganisms have a much simpler organization than animal cells, which renders them less susceptible to inhibition. Thus the substances commonly used as disinfectants are generally more toxic to the animal host than to microbes. In other words, the selective toxicity of most toxic chemical substances is likely to be in the wrong direction. How, then, can substances be found with the desired properties for chemotherapy? Initially, discovery depended upon a patient search through known chemical compounds and the synthesis and testing of new compounds. When a compound was found that showed some signs of having a positive chemotherapeutic index, then a whole series of new and related compounds with a

similar structure was synthesized in the hope that one of them would be more active against the microorganisms and less toxic to the human body. This type of search was initiated by Paul Ehrlich, in the early years of this century, but although he did discover drugs that could be used against trypanosome infections and organic compounds containing arsenic, such as arsphenamine (salvarsan), that were valuable in the treatment of syphilis, the majority of pathogenic bacteria evaded his search for the 'magic bullet'. Indeed, there was little progress in this 'hit and miss' process until the discovery of the sulphonamides by Domagk in 1935.

Sulphonamides. The discovery of the sulphonamides began with the finding that the red dye Prontosil was capable of curing infections with *Streptococcus pyogenes.* Surprisingly, Prontosil itself had no effect on the streptococci *in vitro*; the dye had to be broken down in the animal to form the effective compound, sulphanilamide. Sulphanilamide itself was effective in non-toxic doses and it was discovered that a series of even more effective drugs could be obtained by substitution of different organic groups (represented by the R group in the formula below. For example, the addition of a pyridine group gave sulphapyridine, a thiazole gave sulphathiazole and so on. In this way, thousands of derivatives called sulphonamides were produced and many of them were found to be effective antimicrobial agents. However, they all have the characteristic of only affecting a relatively restricted range of microorganisms. Consequently, relatively few of them have found a practical therapeutic use, particularly since the development of antibiotics. Indeed, in some respects their importance to chemotherapy lies in the indication they gave towards the design of antimicrobial agents by the discovery of their mode of action.

How do the sulphonamides act? The first clue came in the observation that many materials, including yeast and meat extracts, had the property of overcoming the inhibitory effect of sulphonamides on bacteria *in vitro*. The sulphonamide 'antagonist' in the extracts was isolated and shown to be para (*p*)-amino-benzoic acid (PABA), a compound not known to occur in living organisms at that time. However, it was soon shown that *p*-amino-benzoic acid was an essential metabolite in many organisms and was converted by them to dihydrofolic acid and then to tetrahydrofolic acid, which acted as an essential co-factor in reactions leading to the synthesis of nucleic acids. It was found that sulphonamides inhibit the first stage of the biosynthesis of dihydrofolic acid from p-amino-benzoic acid. The drug, trimethoprim, which was discovered and introduced to medicine at a much later date, inhibits the conversion of dihydrofolic acid into tetrahydrofolic acid.

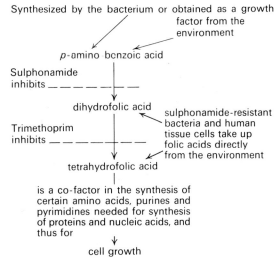

Prontosil SO$_2$NH$_2$

Sulphanilamide SO$_2$NH$_2$

Other sulphonamides SO$_2$NHR

p-amino-benzoic acid

The reason for the inhibition was not far to seek. Because of their similar structures, there was competition between the sulphonamide and the p-amino-benzoic acid for the active site on the surface of the enzyme initiating the conversion of p-amino-benzoic acid to dihydrofolic acid. For this *competitive inhibition* to be effective, a large number of sulphonamide molecules, of the order of a thousand, is required to inhibit the conversion of one molecule of p-amino-benzoic acid to folic acid. The need for comparatively large amounts of inhibitor is general in competitive inhibition and clearly represents problems for chemotherapy. Human tissues, cells and sulphonamide-resistant bacteria also require folic acid for the synthesis of nucleic acids, but are able to take up pre-formed folic acids from the environment and their growth is thus independent of the conversion of p-amino-benzoic acid into folic acid. This difference is the basis for the toxicity of sulphonamides towards the sulphonamide-sensitive bacteria as compared with human tissues.

These findings may be summarized as follows:

Synthesized by the bacterium or obtained as a growth factor from the environment

p-amino-benzoic acid

Sulphonamide inhibits ———

dihydrofolic acid

sulphonamide-resistant bacteria and human tissue cells take up folic acids directly from the environment

Trimethoprim inhibits ———

tetrahydrofolic acid

is a co-factor in the synthesis of certain amino acids, purines and pyrimidines needed for synthesis of proteins and nucleic acids, and thus for

cell growth

Antimetabolite programme. The discovery that sulphonamides acted by competitive antagonism with an essential microbial metabolite preventing its further utilization led to the hope that chemotherapeutic agents could be produced by a logical programme of antimetabolite synthesis. Many compounds were known to be microbial metabolites or essential nutrients and it was thought possible to produce the corresponding antimetabolites by the synthesis of chemical analogues. In this way a whole range of new drugs might be produced and, indeed, in the last thirty years or so many tens of thousands of analogues of such microbial nutrients as vitamins, purines, pyrimidines, amino acids and other metabolites have been synthesized and tested. Many of them are effective antimicrobial agents. Unfortunately, the hopes that some of them would also be good chemotherapeutic agents has been largely frustrated because most of them are too toxic to man and do not have the desired selective toxicity for microorganisms. The major reason for this lack of selective action is the principle stated in Chapter 3 that the metabolites and biochemical pathways of all living organisms, including man and microbe, are very similar. This similarity is particularly true of the low molecular weight monomers (amino acids, nucleotides) making up the protein, enzymes, co-enzymes and nucleic acids of living organisms. Most antimetabolites thus have an inhibitory effect on human cells as well as on microorganisms. Although there may be more specificity in the structure of proteins than in that of their constituent monomers, it is not practicable to synthesize protein antimetabolites. A further problem has been the presence of relatively large amounts of the metabolites in the circulating fluids of the body, which makes it impracticable to achieve the high level of antimetabolite required to exert a competitive inhibition. Ideally an antimetabolite is required that acts against a metabolite essential only to microorganisms and there are very few of these metabolites. Such microbe-specific metabolites as do occur are found mainly in the prokaryotic cell wall and many antibiotics act by inhibiting the biosynthesis of the bacterial cell-wall muco-peptide.

It has been assumed so far that the antimetabolite acts by inhibiting the enzyme reacting with the corresponding metabolite. This is often the case, but analogues may act in other ways. For example, there may be inhibition of a permease by competition at the active site on the specific protein. Such inhibition will affect the growth only of those microorganisms requiring the metabolite for growth. A more sophisticated example is the ability of some antimetabolites to inhibit the biosynthesis of the metabolite by affecting the control processes involved. This can occur by a pseudo-feedback inhibition of the first stage in the biosynthesis by an allosteric effect of the antimetabolite on the appropriate enzyme. Alternatively, there may be a pseudo-repression of all the specific biosynthetic enzymes by a combination of the antimetabolite with the repressor produced by the regulator gene (see Chap. 7). In either case, the antimetabolite interferes with the *formation* rather than the utilization of the metabolite.

Lethal synthesis following the biosynthetic incorporation of antimetabolites. Some antimetabolites are so similar to the natural substrate that they not only combine with the active site of the enzyme, but are further metabolized as though they were the substrate. For example, fluoracetate ($CH_2F.COOH$) is converted to fluoro-

citrate by the enzymes of the tricarboxylic acid cycle. However, fluorocitrate cannot be further metabolized and accumulates causing an antimicrobial effect. This process is often known as lethal synthesis and the most important and interesting examples are certain analogues of purine and pyrimidines. For example, 5-bromouracil acts as an analogue of thymine and is metabolized as though it were thymine into the corresponding nucleoside triphosphate which is finally incorporated in DNA in place of thymine. This leads to misreading of the code during transcription into DNA and lethal mutations result. In this instance the bromine atom is analogous to the methyl group of thymine. On 5-fluorouracil, the smaller fluorine atom is nearer in size to the hydrogen atom of uracil and the antimetabolite is metabolized as though it were uracil through the corresponding nucleoside triphosphate to RNA. Again this leads to misreading of the code, in this case in translation from m-RNA to protein.

Thymine

5-bromouracil

Uracil

5-fluorouracil

Lethal synthesis has not so far proved to be of great value in the chemotherapy of bacterial infections, but there has been some success in fungal infections and in the inhibition of virus and cancer growth where the high rate of nucleic acid synthesis compared with that in normal host cells allows for the exertion of some selective toxicity.

ANTIBIOTICS

The programme outlined above for the logical production of chemotherapeutic agents has so far been disappointing due to a lack of an understanding of the functioning of a cell at molecular level. However, in the 1940's attention became diverted by the discovery of the therapeutic value of penicillin which was much superior to that of any synthetic chemotherapeutic agents produced previously. Soon many other new antibiotics were found which allowed the successful treatment of the majority of microbial infections. These antibiotics exert their selective inhibitory or lethal effect on bacteria by affecting the synthesis of cell-wall substance, protein or nucleic acid.

Antibiotics inhibiting cell-wall synthesis. Mucopeptide is the component of the cell walls of bacteria responsible for their mechanical strength (Chap. 2). If synthesis of the mucopeptide is inhibited whilst synthesis of other cell components continues then the cell can be expected to lyse rapidly in normal osmotic environments. The prokaryotic mucopeptide contains monomeric components, namely, N-acetylmuramic acid, diaminopimelic acid and D-amino acids, not present in human and other eukaryotic cells. Further, the final polymer is produced by a unique type of cross-linking between amino sugars and amino acids. There is therefore the possibility of obtaining a chemotherapeutic agent that will act on the synthesis of this unique type of structure with consequently a selective toxicity to prokaryotic cells as compared with eukaryotic cells. Many antibiotics are now known to have this particular inhibitory property and the most important of them is penicillin.

It is often difficult to determine the reaction primarily inhibited by an antibiotic and it took about twenty years of intensive research in a large number of institutions to identify the exact reaction affected by penicillin. Early experiments had indicated an effect on cell-wall synthesis but this was not properly substantiated until it was shown that penicillin-sensitive bacteria could actually grow in the presence of 'lethal' concentrations of penicillin provided an osmotic stabilizer was added to the surrounding medium; under these circumstances the cells were converted into spherical protoplasts or spheroplasts as a result of the inhibition of the biosynthesis of the cell-wall mucopeptide responsible for cell shape and the support of the

soft cytoplasmic membrane against the high osmotic pressure of the cytoplasm (5 to 20 atmospheres). These osmotically fragile forms can survive only in an isotonic environment.

A further clue to the mode of action of penicillin was provided by the accumulation in the culture of sensitive cells, to which penicillin had been added, of a complex nucleotide—uridine diphosphate-N-acetyl muramic acid pentapeptide. This nucleotide contained similar components to the final mucopeptide and was shown to be an intermediate in the biosynthesis of the mucopeptide. Since it accumulated in the presence of penicillin only, it was suggested that the antibiotic inhibited some stage in its further metabolism.

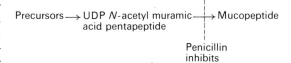

If the components of the nucleotide are compared with those of the mucopeptide, two differences in the content of amino sugars and amino acids are evident:

1. *The nucleotide contains no N-acetyl glucosamine.* It was found that the next stage in the metabolism of the nucleotide consisted of the transfer of the N-acetyl muramic acid pentapeptide from the nucleotide linkage to a lipid component of the cytoplasmic membrane. This was followed by the addition of an N-acetyl glucosamine unit on the transference of the whole unit into the growing cell wall, a process involving translocation from the inner to the outer surface of the membrane.

2. *The nucleotide contains two molecules of D-alanine per peptide chain whilst the mucopeptide contains only one.* If the effect of penicillin on mucopeptide biosynthesis is studied carefully, it is found that some mucopeptide can be produced in presence of penicillin, but it contains double the amount of D-alanine compared with the original mucopeptide. It also has little mechanical strength. The problem was clarified when it was shown that the final cross-linking stage in mucopeptide synthesis involves a transpeptidation reaction between adjacent peptide chains with the elimination of a molecule

of D-alanine per linkage. The cross-linking results in the product of a vast sponge-like macromolecule of considerable strength, but penicillin inhibits this final stage.

These stages in the biosynthesis of mucopeptide from the nucleotide are represented in Fig. 6.1 where the action of some other antibiotics is also given. However, the exact mechanism of the inhibition of a particular enzyme is usually not known although it is assumed to be due to the antibiotic being a competitive analogue. In one instance, the action is clear. D-cycloserine (oxamycin) is a structural analogue of D-alanine and inhibits the synthesis of the dipeptide D-alanyl–D-alanine which is a reaction in the final stage of the synthesis of the pentapeptide intermediate.

$$H_2C\!-\!\!-\!CH_2$$

D-cycloserine

D-alanine

D-alanine + D-alanine $\longrightarrow$ D-alanyl-D-alanine

D-cycloserine inhibits

UPD-*N*-acetyl muramic acid tripeptide +
D-alanyl-D-alamine → UDP-*N*-acetyl muramic
acid pentapeptide

It is interesting to note that penicillin is also thought to be a structural analogue, namely of D-alanyl-D-alanine; this would explain its effect on the final transpeptidation reaction involving the two terminal D-alanines on the pentapeptide.

Antibiotics affecting the synthesis of the prokaryotic mucopeptide would have no effect on the growth of bacterial L-forms, because these forms lack cell walls and are adapted to grow in certain protective environments without their support.

Antibiotics can also be obtained which inhibit the biosynthesis of certain eukaryotic cell walls. For example, griseofulvin, one of the few antimicrobial agents with a selective toxicity towards fungi, inhibits the production of chitin, a polymer responsible for the rigidity of the cell walls of many fungi.

Antibiotics affecting protein synthesis. A number of antibiotics are known to inhibit protein synthesis specifically; they include chloramphenicol, streptomycin, neomycin, kanamycin, tetracyclines, erythromycin and puromycin. Streptomycin was the first antibiotic to be introduced clinically after penicillin. Like penicillin, streptomycin shows a confusing variety of effects on growing bacteria, but there seems little doubt that the primary effect is on protein synthesis which is followed by an inhibition of respiration and nucleic acid biosynthesis and disruption of the cytoplasmic membrane. An important step in the further elucidation of the mechanism of its action was the discovery that not only could streptomycin-resistant mutants of a sensitive strain be found, but also that mutation could occur leading to a dependence on streptomycin for growth. Genetic analysis showed that sensitivity, resistance and dependence were due to allelic forms of the same gene. Comparison of the wild type with these two mutant forms provided an ideal system for the analysis of the mechanism of action of streptomycin because there seemed little doubt that the gene involved was concerned in some way with this action. For example, protein synthesis was inhibited by streptomycin in sensitive cells, was unaffected in resistant cells, whilst in dependent cells streptomycin was required for growth. A similar relationship could be shown in ribosomes separated from cell-free extracts where about one molecule of streptomycin per ribosome was found to be sufficient to inhibit protein synthesis. Streptomycin combined with the 30S component of the ribosome and this combination led to a malfunctioning ribosome in sensitive strains whilst it was required by dependent strains. In resistant strains, as in the ribosomes of eukaryotic cells,

FIG. 6.1. The action of some antibiotics on mucopeptide synthesis.

UDP	= Uridine diphosphate
UMP	= Uridine monophosphate
NAcM	= N acetyl muramic acid
NAcG	= N acetyl glucosamine
A1, A2, A3	= Amino acids 1 to 3
A4	= D alanine
Lipid ⓟ	= Membrane phospholipid
ⓟ	= Inorganic orthophosphate
→	= Inhibition

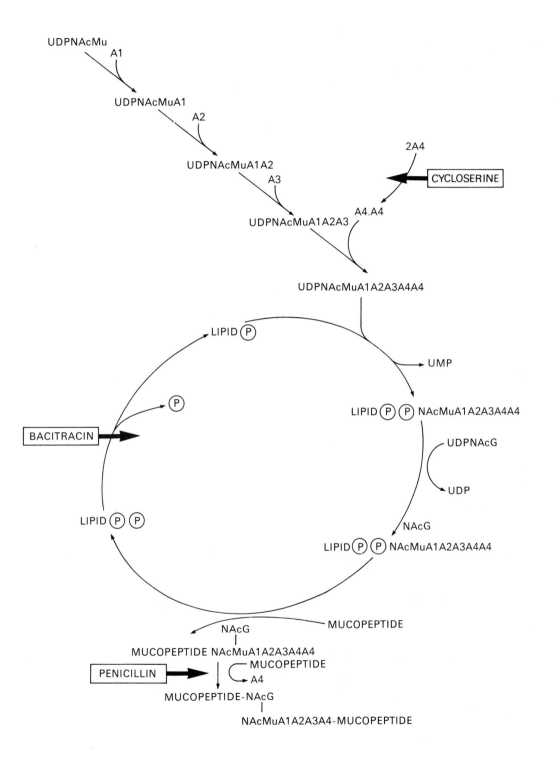

there was no combination. The effect of strepto-mycin on the ribosomes of sensitive cells is a misreading of the code so that the wrong amino acids are inserted into the growing polypeptide chain, non-functional proteins are synthesized and the cell eventually dies. Neomycin and kanamycin exert a similar effect on the 30S com-ponent of the ribosome whilst chloramphenicol and erythromycin seem to affect the 50S com-ponent of the ribosome.

Other stages of protein synthesis may also be affected. For example, tetracyclines interfere with the binding of *t*RNA to the ribosomes. In most cases, selective toxicity is due to inability to bind with the larger 80S ribosomes of eukary-otic cells although some drugs, such as chlor-amphenicol, may bind to the 70S mitochondrial ribosomes and by interfering with mitochondrial protein synthesis cause some toxicity to mam-mals. By contrast, the antibiotic cycloheximide inhibits the functioning of the 80S ribosome and therefore is of no value therapeutically. Puro-mycin is an analogue of *t*RNA, a component common in structure to both prokaryotic and eukaryotic cells; again, this antibiotic exerts no selective toxicity.

Antibiotics inhibiting nucleic acid synthesis. A few antibiotics combine with and alter the function-ing of nucleic acid although in general they are too toxic for therapeutic use. Actinomycin complexes with double-stranded, but not with single-stranded DNA, thus preventing RNA synthesis and, at higher concentrations, DNA synthesis. On the other hand, mitomycin links complementary strands of DNA, usually by guanine residues, which results in a blockage in DNA synthesis.

Antibiotics acting on the cytoplasmic membrane. A group of polypeptide antibiotics act on the cytoplasmic membrane, the best example being polymyxin, which acts essentially as a cationic detergent binding specifically to the membrane; as a result the semipermeable properties are lost and essential low-molecular weight intermedi-ates and coenzymes pass into the environment causing cell death. Because polymyxin will also combine with the membranes of eukaryotic cells, its selective toxicity is not great and it has to be used with caution.

Future development of chemotherapy. There is at present a range of antibiotics available for the treatment of bacterial infections. However, there are still two basic challenges to be faced in microbial chemotherapy.

1. Viruses remain essentially resistant to control by chemotherapy. The reason for this is only partly due to intracellular parasitism because some bacteria are also intracellular parasites and can be affected, albeit less satis-factorily than extracellular parasites, by anti-biotics. The great problem is that viruses rely almost entirely for their metabolic machinery on the host cell and any attempt to interfere with them usually results in inhibition and death of host cells as well. This problem is discussed in Chapter 13.

2. The development of resistance to chemo-therapeutic agents is becoming an increasingly pressing problem. Unfortunately, the possible occurrence of resistant variants is a consequence of the specific nature of the attack by chemo-therapeutic agents and thus of their selective toxicity; a simple mutation may suffice to confer resistance if there is only a single point of attack by an antimicrobial substance on the metabolism of the microbe. The position is made worse by the possibility of transferring plasmids that confer multiple resistance to a variety of antibiotics (see Chap. 7). How can the range of chemotherapeutic agents be increased over the present one? Unfortunately, it is unlikely that many new antibiotics remain to be discovered. There has already been an exhaustive survey of a vast number of microbial species from a wide variety of habitats for the ability to produce antibiotics and there can be little hope of many new substances being found which are wide-spectrum antibiotics. Another approach is to modify the structures of known antibiotics to produce substances with different properties. The synthesis of a range of new penicillins is an example of this approach. In many respects peni-cillin is an ideal chemotherapeutic agent, but it suffers from the fact that resistance to it is commonly conferred by the action of the enzyme penicillinase. However, the structure of peni-cillin can be so altered, e.g. to the forms of methicillin and cloxacillin, so that it becomes resistant to hydrolysis by penicillinase, but still exerts its antimicrobial effect. Further alterations can result in penicillins which are acid-resistant, e.g. phenoxymethyl penicillin, or have a wider

spectrum against the range of prokaryotic microorganisms, e.g. ampicillin. A further approach that may become more important is a return to the design of antimetabolites as previously outlined, but on the basis of a more sophisticated understanding of microbial biochemistry and molecular biology.

FURTHER READING

CROFTON, J. W. (1969) Some principles in the chemotherapy of bacterial infections. *British Medical Journal*, **ii**, 137 and 209.

GARROD, L. P., LAMBERT, H. P. & O'GRADY, F. (1973) *Antibiotic and Chemotherapy*, 3rd edn. Edinburgh: Churchill Livingstone.

7. Bacterial Genetics

The character of a cell is basically determined by the specific polypeptides that make up its enzymes and other proteins. The genetic information in bacteria, as in all cells, is contained in the specific sequence of nucleotides in the cell's deoxyribonucleic acid (DNA). The DNA acts as template for the replication of the DNA so that two copies are available at cell division and it also acts as template for the transcription of ribonucleic acid (RNA) for protein production within the cell. The sequence of nucleotides in the DNA determines the corresponding sequence of nucleotides in the RNA, and this is translated into the appropriate sequence of amino acids by ribosomes. The sequence of amino acids in the resultant polypeptide chain in turn determines the specific configuration into which this chain folds itself in forming the completed molecule of protein, and thus the specific enzymic or structural properties of the protein. Figure 7.1 illustrates this 'central dogma' of molecular biology; the model is generally true for prokaryotic cells, though there are some important variations, e.g. with certain viruses in eukaryotic cells.

A segment of DNA that specifies the production of a particular polypeptide chain is called a *gene* and the total complement of genes in a cell is known as the cell's *genome*.

Most bacteria contain enough DNA to code for the production of 1000 to 3000 different types of polypeptide chains—i.e. 1000 to 3000 genes. In the bacteria that have been most intensively studied, notably *Escherichia coli,* it has been found that the DNA is present as a single circular double-stranded molecule about 1000 to 1300 μm long. The DNA is not associated with protein or histones as in eukaryotic cell chromosomes. Since the DNA is about 1000 times longer than the cell, it is obvious that it is not arranged as a simple circle; electron microscopy of thin sections of bacteria shows the nuclear body as an irregular coiled bundle of DNA lying loose in the cytoplasm, like a skein of thread. The terms *nucleus* and *chromosome*

were originally restricted to the structures that could be seen in eukaryotic cells. There are many differences in detail between the organization and control of the DNA in prokaryotic and in eukaryotic cells, but it is accepted that the basic functions are the same, that the nuclear body is the functional equivalent of a nucleus and that its single circular molecule of naked DNA is the functional equivalent of a chromosome.

The prokaryotic cell has a single chromosome and, after replication, only a single molecule of DNA has to be directed into each daughter cell. The mechanism of this partition is not clearly understood but it may involve attachment of the DNA to a site on the cytoplasmic membrane or on the mesosome. Eukaryotic cells have multiple chromosomes held together in a nuclear membrane and they have a complex mitotic apparatus for separating the two sets of chromosomes after replication. The advantage of the eukaryotic type of organization is that it can handle much more genetic information; this has allowed the evolution of complex multicellular organisms with diploid chromosomes (i.e. two sets of chromosomes) and sexual methods of reproduction. Prokaryotic cells, which are normally haploid (i.e. with one set of chromosomes), have the advantages of simplicity, small size and rapid replication.

Genetic and Non-genetic Variation

As bacteria reproduce by asexual binary fission, the genome is normally identical in all the progeny. The DNA is a double helix with complementary nucleotide sequences in the two strands. At replication the strands separate and new complementary strands are formed on each of the originals so that two identical double helices are produced, each with the same nucleotide sequence and hence the same genetic information as the original. This process is very accurate, but occasional inaccuracies produce a

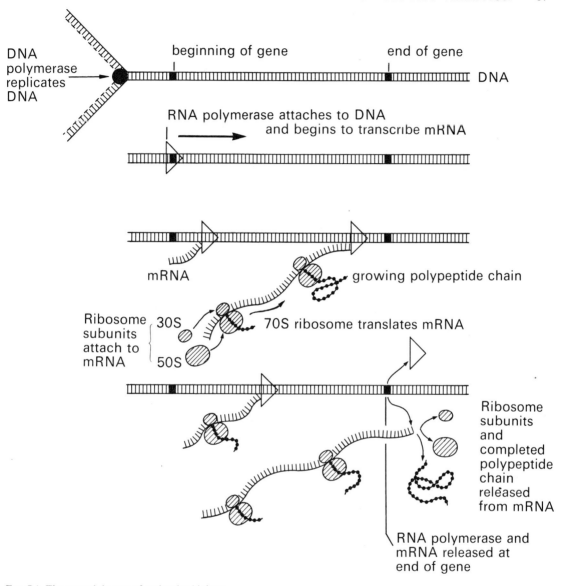

FIG. 7.1. The central dogma of molecular biology.

slightly altered nucleotide sequence in one of the daughter cells (a mutation, p. 88). One of the fundamental requirements for evolution is that although gene replication must normally be completely accurate to ensure stability there must also be occasional variation to produce new or altered characters that could prove to be of selective value to the organism. The mechanism of DNA replication has evolved not only to ensure accuracy of replication, but also to provide occasional 'mistakes'. Mutation is the commonest source of genetic variation in bacteria, but in addition the genome may occasionally be changed by acquisition of DNA from outside the cell; the various ways in which this can happen are detailed later in this chapter.

The characters that a bacterium shows at a

particular time (its *phenotype*) are determined not only by its genetic constitution (its *genotype*) but also by its environment. Because of the great rate at which bacteria multiply, laboratory cultures often show variation and it is important, though often difficult, to distinguish between genotypic and phenotypic variation. In the latter case the cell's genes are unaltered, but the *expression* of the genes is changed in response to alterations in the environment, e.g. the induction or repression of synthesis of certain enzymes. The main significance of the distinction between genotypic and phenotypic variation is that the former is heritable and maintained through changes in environmental conditions whereas the latter is dependent on the inducing environmental conditions, ceasing when these change.

MUTATION

Biochemically, a *mutation* is an alteration in the nucleotide sequence at some point in the organism's DNA. This may lead to the production of a protein that has an altered amino acid sequence. Such an alteration usually does not produce a readily observable change in the function of the protein. A small proportion of mutations lead to the production of a protein that is altered in a minor way so that its function is only slightly changed, e.g. an enzyme with altered specificity for substrates, inhibitors or regulatory substances. This is the kind of mutation that is most likely to be of evolutionary value to an organism; many examples of drug resistance acquired in the laboratory have been shown to be of this type. Occasional mutations alter a gene so that a non-functional protein is formed; if this protein is essential, the mutation is lethal.

Since mutation may occur in any of the cell's several thousand genes and different mutations in the same gene may produce different effects in the cell, the number of possible mutations is very large. Bacteria are normally haploid and therefore the effect of a mutated gene can be expressed immediately and is not masked by the presence of another copy of the gene as often happens in higher diploid organisms.

Particular mutations occur spontaneously at fairly constant rates, usually in the range of once per 10^4 to once per 10^{10} cell divisions. A large bacterial colony contains about 10^9 cells all derived from a single organism by repeated cell division. For many purposes it is valuable to consider such a colony as a clone of genetically identical cells, but it should be realized that after 10^9 cell divisions, many thousands of different mutations will have occurred, affecting very many of the genes in the cell. Thus any bacterial colony contains a small proportion of a variety of mutants, some of which are viable and might be selected by particular environmental conditions during subculture. For the same reason, in every infected patient, a variety of mutants arise spontaneously in the population of, say, 10^8 to 10^{14} progeny that soon grow from the single or few bacteria originally entering the body.

Selection of Mutants

Whether in culture or in a patient's body, a mutant will become sufficiently numerous to be observable and to produce significant effects only if its new character makes it better fitted to grow under the prevailing conditions in the culture medium or host's tissues than the parental bacteria and so enable it to outgrow and outnumber the latter. Thus mutation is significant only when conditions are selectively favourable to the mutant and bring about its natural or artificial *selection*. An antibiotic-resistant mutant, for example, will outgrow the sensitive parental bacteria in a culture medium containing antibiotic or in the body of a patient receiving antibiotic therapy. A mutant with enhanced ability to grow in the body of a particular host species, and thus with greater virulence for it, will be selectively increased in the course of a natural or experimental infection. A mutant with altered surface antigens will escape the restraining effect of immunity previously developed in an individual or a community against the parental form and so be able to cause a recurrence of the infection or a further outbreak.

Mechanisms of Mutation

The rate of mutation can be greatly increased artificially by exposing bacteria to irradiation by

X-rays or ultra-violet light or by growing bacteria in the presence of certain mutagenic chemicals that interfere with DNA replication, e.g. nitrogen mustard, acriflavin, mitomycin C, 5-bromouracil (a thymine analogue) and 2-aminopurine (an adenine analogue). Some chemical mutagens, such as nitrous acid and hydroxylamine, alter DNA bases *in situ* and this leads to mis-pairing during DNA replication. Mutations are normally permanent and stably inherited by the progeny, but further mutations may occur and these may occasionally restore the original nucleotide sequence. The rate at which such *back-mutation* can occur depends on the extent of the original mutation. The chance of a single nucleotide substitution being reversed is much higher than the chance of replacing a deleted sequence of a few amino acids, whereas mutations caused by deletion of a substantial portion of a gene are effectively irreversible by further mutation. Some organisms have particularly effective mechanisms for the repair of damaged portions of DNA.

The mutations first studied by bacteriologists were those producing effects that were detectable by the experimental methods then in use, e.g. mutations producing alteration in colonial morphology or pigmentation; variation in cell surface antigens or in sensitivity to bacteriophages or bacteriocines; loss of the ability to produce capsules, spores or flagella, or to utilize specific carbohydrates; or changes in virulence towards particular hosts. It was not originally possible to characterize these mutations in molecular terms. In some cases the mechanism is now understood; for example, in pneumococci a mutation leads to failure to produce a capsule. Loss of the capsule in this organism is directly related to failure to synthesize the type-specific (capsular) antigen, alteration of the normal smooth colony to a rough form (S–R variation) and loss of resistance to phagocytosis with consequent loss of virulence when the organisms are injected into mice. Thus a single mutation produces a variety of biological phenomena. The mechanism of biosynthesis of pneumococcal capsular polysaccharide is now known in some detail and it is possible to ascribe this mutation to the loss of a specific enzyme involved in polysaccharide synthesis (Fig. 7.2).

Many mutations, however, still cannot be characterized biochemically. The structure of normal bacterial cell walls is seldom well enough understood to permit a molecular description of altered somatic antigens or bacteriophage receptors. Some organisms have been subcultured in the laboratory for many generations until they have lost their virulence for man, e.g. in the production of live attenuated vaccines. Such strains have lost, by a series of mutations,

Type 3 pneumococcus capsule polysaccharide

| GLUCURONIC ACID | GLUCOSE | GLUCURONIC ACID | GLUCOSE | GLUCURONIC ACID | GLUCOSE |

The glucose and glucuronic acid subunits are derived from uridine diphosphate glucose (UDPG) and uridine diphosphate glucuronic acid (UDPGA) which are synthesized in the following steps:

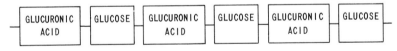

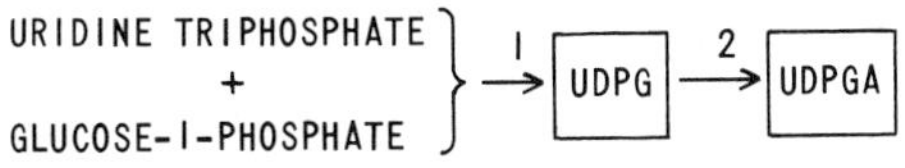

A mutation that prevents the formation of the dehydrogenase involved in step 2 blocks production of UDPGA and hence the synthesis of type 3 capsule polysaccharide

FIG. 7.2. A mutation preventing the synthesis of type 3 pneumococcus capsule.

characters that confer a selective advantage on the organism *in vivo*, but are of no advantage *in vitro*, e.g. aggressins, toxins or capsules that enable virulent strains of certain species to resist the actions of the body's phagocytes or other defence mechanisms. Mutants that no longer produce such factors can multiply a little faster *in vitro* since they do not waste nutrients and metabolites on the production of these unnecessary substances, and they may gradually outgrow the wild-type cells during repeated subculture. However, since the normal mechanisms of pathogenicity can seldom be described in molecular terms, it is usually impossible to identify the biochemical changes underlying the alterations in biological behaviour of the attenuated strains.

Great advances in bacterial genetics followed the realization during the 1940's that genes and mutations could be studied in precise biochemical terms (the 'one gene : one enzyme hypothesis' of Beadle and Tatum). Mutations may occur in any gene but, since many genes code for production of substances essential for cell survival and multiplication, many individual mutations are lethal. Other mutations affect gene products that are essential only under particular cultural conditions. Mutant cells have to be grown in the laboratory before they can be detected and considerable ingenuity may be required to devise conditions that promote growth of mutants defective in a particular function and that allow selection of small numbers of these mutants from the large numbers of unmutated cells in the culture.

Mutations that Affect Biochemical Pathways

Amongst the mutations that have been most studied are those in which the organism loses the ability to synthesize an essential metabolite (or regains it by back-mutation). Many organisms, e.g. *Esch. coli,* can grow in simple defined culture media because they have genes for the production of all the enzymes they require for the synthesis from simple nutrients of all the large variety of organic compounds essential for the construction and functioning of their cells. These are called *prototrophic* cells. Mutants that can no longer synthesize a particular essential metabolite, such as an amino acid, and are

unable to grow in a medium that does not contain the essential amino acid are called *auxotrophic* mutants. Studies of mutants blocked at different stages in a synthetic pathway (i.e. with mutations affecting different enzymes in the pathway) are very valuable in the elucidation of biosynthetic pathways.

.It is easier to select mutants that gain the ability to produce an enzyme than those that lose the ability to produce one. Auxotrophic cells that revert to the prototrophic state by back-mutation can be selected from the rest of the auxotrophic cells by culture in the simple defined medium; prototrophic revertants are the only cells able to grow in a medium that does not contain the essential metabolite. However, to select auxotrophic mutants from a prototrophic population, cells from a large number of colonies grown on a complex medium must be compared for the ability to grow on media with and without each of the specific metabolites of interest. This can conveniently be done by making replica plates with a velvet pad to sample the colonies and transfer a series of replicate inocula from a master plate to each test plate (Fig. 7.3). Colonies on the master plate that fail to be replicated on the plate that lacks a particular essential metabolite consist of auxotrophic mutants defective in the synthesis of that substance.

Mutations also occur that affect enzymes involved in the fermentation of sugars and the breakdown of a variety of other substances in the environment of the bacteria. Mutations in some of these genes can be detected by growing the cells on special media on which a distinctive colour is produced in or around colonies producing the enzyme. For example, the production of β-galactosidase can be demonstrated on media containing lactose as the only sugar and an indicator such as neutral red. Colonies producing β-galactosidase turn red as a result of the production of acid whereas colonies of mutants unable to ferment lactose because of a failure to produce normal β-galactosidase remain colourless.

Drug-resistance Mutations

Organisms with mutations that produce increased resistance to an antimicrobial drug can readily be isolated in the laboratory since resistant mutants grow in the presence of concentrations of the drug that inhibit the growth of normal drug-sensitive cells. Mutations can be found that produce increased resistance to almost any antimicrobial agent. The actual mechanism of resistance is related to the mechanism of action of the particular drug.

Sulphonamides are structural analogues of para-aminobenzoic acid (PABA) and inhibit the growth of sensitive bacteria by competing with PABA for the enzyme folate synthetase

(p. 78). Mutants that have acquired resistance to sulphonamides are readily detected in the laboratory, and it can be shown that several different mechanisms of resistance may be involved. Some owe their resistance to a decreased permeability for sulphonamide, presumably due to an alteration in specificity of, or a failure to produce, the permease that is necessary for the transport of sulphonamides through the cytoplasmic membrane. Others produce a folate synthetase whose substrate specificity is reversed so that it no longer accepts

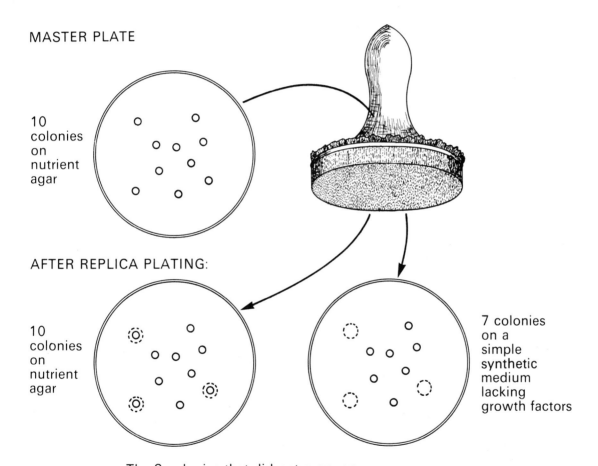

MASTER PLATE

10 colonies on nutrient agar

AFTER REPLICA PLATING:

10 colonies on nutrient agar

7 colonies on a simple synthetic medium lacking growth factors

The 3 colonies that did not grow on the simple synthetic medium are indicated here on the nutrient agar plate. These cells are auxotrophic mutants.

FIG. 7.3. The detection of auxotrophic mutants by replica plating. When 10 colonies were replica-plated from nutrient agar on to simple synthetic medium, the 3 colonies that failed to grow were auxotrophic mutants.

sulphonamide in preference to PABA. Other sulphonamide-resistant mutants have alterations in the regulatory mechanisms of the cell so that the level of PABA in the cell increases until the competitive inhibition by sulphonamide is overcome. Thus a variety of mutations that affect any of several genes may be responsible for increased resistance to a sulphonamide.

Streptomycin inhibits bacterial protein synthesis by binding to a single specific protein in the 30S sub-unit of 70S bacterial ribosomes (p. 82). In in-vitro protein-synthesizing systems the binding of streptomycin appears to cause misreading of the mRNA so that wrong amino acids may be incorporated into the polypeptide chain that is produced. *In vivo* a more important effect appears to be interference with the initiation steps of protein synthesis so that the 30S and 50S ribosome sub-units attach to the mRNA but cannot move along it. It seems that when streptomycin binds to a normal ribosome, the ribosomal protein is distorted so that it no longer functions properly in initiation or in accurate selection of the appropriate amino acyl-tRNA molecules for peptide chain elongation. Mutant cells that are resistant to streptomycin have ribosomes that function normally because they contain a ribosomal protein that can no longer be distorted by streptomycin. Other mutants can be found that have become not only resistant to streptomycin but also dependent on it for growth. In this case the mutant ribosome protein can function only when it is distorted back into the normal shape by the binding of streptomycin. Streptomycin does not affect the 80S ribosomes of eukaryotic cells and this is the basis of its selective toxicity for bacteria.

For many antibiotics, a particular mutation produces only a slight increase in resistance but a series of consecutive mutations can produce a stepwise increase in resistance. For some drugs, e.g. penicillin, such stepwise mutations are easily selected in the laboratory but the final level of resistance is still below the levels of antibiotic that are attainable in the tissues or body fluids during treatment of a patient. Many drug-resistant mutants produced in the laboratory grow less efficiently than the original drug-sensitive cells and may be less virulent. However, clinically important drug resistance in staphylococci has arisen largely by the selection

of spontaneous mutants with increased drug resistance. Resistance to many antibiotics can be produced only by the sequential selection of multiple 'small-step' mutations but resistance to streptomycin arises quite readily by a single 'large-step' mutation in a variety of species and it is probably because of this that acquisition of resistance to streptomycin by mutation is a serious clinical problem, e.g. in the treatment of tuberculosis.

Drug resistance of clinical significance is often found to be due not to mutation but to the production of inactivating enzymes. Penicillin resistance in staphylococci is due to the production of penicillinase (β-lactamase) and resistance to ampicillin, chloramphenicol, streptomycin and other aminoglycoside antibiotics in Gram-negative bacilli is often due to the production of enzymes that break down or modify the antibiotic. The origin of such resistance genes is unclear but they cannot be produced by simple mutation in a drug-sensitive cell.

Enzyme Regulation

The detailed function and regulation of many processes in the bacterial cell can be analysed by searching systematically for mutations that affect each separate step in a process. The evidence for the mechanism proposed by Jacob and Monod for the control of the inducible enzyme β-galactosidase in *Esch. coli* depends on the isolation and analysis of separate classes of mutant with defects in each part of the regulatory system. Many different types of regulation occur in the coordination of all the biochemical reactions that proceed inside a cell. The control of β-galactosidase production is described here to illustrate the sort of molecular mechanism involved in regulation and to show how it can be analysed genetically.

When *Esch. coli* is grown in the presence of lactose it can utilize the sugar as a source of carbon and energy for bacterial growth by producing β-galactosidase. The enzyme is formed only in the presence of lactose; its production is switched off when it is not required. β-galactosidase is said to be an *inducible* enzyme and lactose is described as the *inducer*. The production of two other enzymes involved in lactose metabolism, galactoside permease and transacetylase, is switched on and off in step with the production of β-galactosidase (coordinate induction and repression respectively). The genes for these three enzymes lie together in the chromosome and this functional unit is known as the lactose *operon* (*lac* operon). It is not uncommon to find that groups of related genes are clustered on the chromosome and coordinated by a common mechanism.

Regulation of enzyme levels in bacteria is produced by regulation of transcription of mRNA from DNA. Bacterial mRNA is short-lived and enzyme production ceases rapidly when transcription is stopped. The enzyme molecules themselves are relatively long-lived but, since they are progressively diluted in the cytoplasm as the cells continue to grow and divide, regulation of transcription is an efficient mechanism for controlling enzyme levels in bacteria. RNA polymerase has to attach to the DNA at a specific point and transcribes by moving along the DNA in a fixed direction. For transcription of the *lac* operon, the polymerase molecule has to attach to the *promotor* region and travel along the DNA to transcribe the structural genes in the order: β-galactosidase, permease, acetylase. The *lac* operon can be switched off by the attachment of a *repressor* molecule to a specific region of the DNA known as the *operator* which lies between the promotor and the first gene of the operon; the repressor blocks the movement of the RNA polymerase so that the structural genes are not transcribed. Production of the three enzymes can thus be switched off or on synchronously by attachment or removal of the repressor (Fig. 7.4).

The repressor molecule is a protein produced in the normal way by transcription and translation from a neighbouring gene (the '*i*' gene) and released into the cytoplasm of the cell. The repressor is an allosteric molecule with two active sites. One recognizes the operator region of the *lac* operon so that the repressor can bind to it to prevent transcription. The other recognizes the inducer—a molecule of lactose. When the inducer is present in the cell it combines with this site on the repressor. This produces an alteration in specificity at the other site; the repressor no longer binds to the operator and transcription is resumed. When the inducer has been metabolized by the resulting enzymes, the repressor is free again to attach to the operator and production of β-galactosidase is once more repressed. All these points can be demonstrated by isolating cells containing mutations that affect the various steps. The analysis and identification of each mutant requires considerable ingenuity and usually involves studying the interactions of two *lac* operons present in a partially diploid cell. This technical trick can be achieved by the use of an F-*lac* plasmid (p. 103). It can be shown that there are two classes of mutation that result in the loss of regulation— i.e. the continuing or *constitutive* production of β-galactosidase in the absence of lactose. Those with a defective operator site cannot be repressed by the absence of lactose even in the presence of a normal repressor produced from a second *lac* operon in the same cell. By contrast, those with a mutation that leads to the production of a defective repressor molecule still have a normal operator site that can be repressed normally in the presence of a second, normal, repressor gene. The mechanism of control of β-galactosidase production is very similar to that involved in the maintenance of lysogeny by temperate phage (p. 98).

It has been shown that the same basic regulatory system can be used not only for the induction of enzyme synthesis by exogenous substrates, but also for the repression of synthesis of the enzymes of a pathway when sufficient of the end-product of the pathway (e.g. an amino acid) has been produced. In this case the 'repressor' is normally inactive but is activated by the end-product; thus, only when the end-product is present in adequate concentration can the repressor combine with the operator and switch off transcription of the operon.

Phase Variation

A few examples of bacterial variation are readily reversible and occur with relatively high frequency in either direction, e.g. once per 10^3 cell divisions. The variation of certain Gram-negative bacilli between a fimbriate and a non-fimbriate phase, and the phase variation of flagellar antigens in *Salmonella* are of this kind. It has been suggested that the mechanism of phase variation differs from that of true gene mutation and represents a spontaneous repression or derepression of a gene, not dependent on environmental control.

GENE TRANSFER

A change in the genome of a bacterium may be due either to mutation in the organism's own DNA or to acquisition of DNA from an external source. Bacterial DNA may be transferred between bacteria by three mechanisms.

1. In some species free DNA, either extracted artificially or released by lysis from the cells of one strain, may be taken up directly by the cells of another strain. Alteration of a cell's

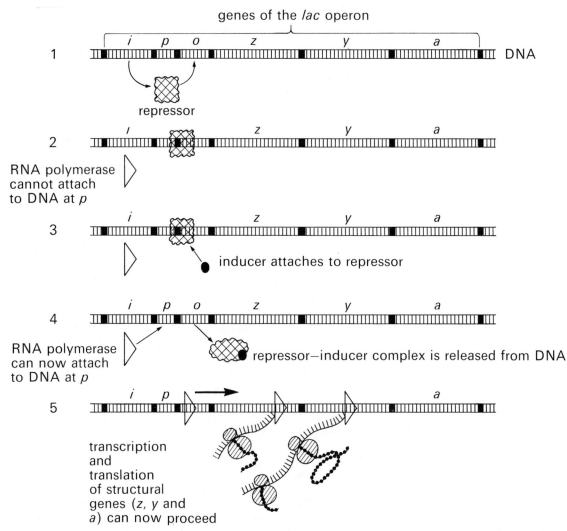

FIG. 7.4. The *lac* operon of *Escherichia coli*.
1. The *lac* repressor is produced from the *i* gene.
2. Binding of the repressor to the operator site (*o*) prevents transcription of the genes *z* (β-galactosidase), *y* (galactoside permease) and *a* (transacetylase).
3. The inducer (lactose) can bind specifically to the repressor.
4. The repressor molecule is thereby altered at its operator-binding site and the repressor-inducer complex is released from the DNA.
5. RNA polymerase can now attach to the promoter site (*p*) and transcribe the structural genes of the *lac* operon.

genome by DNA acquired in this manner is called *transformation*.

2. Bacterial genes may occasionally be transferred between bacteria by means of bacteriophage; this process is known as *transduction*.

3. DNA may pass between cells during *conjugation*, when there is direct contact with formation of a bridge between the cells.

All three mechanisms may occur in nature although normally at low frequency. This occasional transfer of genetic information between cells has probably been of some value in bacterial evolution, and there is no doubt that gene transfer has played an important part in the production of drug-resistant strains since the introduction of antibiotics some thirty years ago. It should be noted that the acquisition by bacteria of new properties by the mechanism of gene transfer, just as that by mutation, is observable and significant only if the new genetic forms are subject to favourable selection by the conditions under which the bacteria are growing.

In some cases an added piece of DNA is able to maintain itself in the cytoplasm as an independent extrachromosomal unit replicating synchronously with the chromosome (plasmids, p. 99). Normally, however, when a piece of DNA is introduced into a cell it has to become incorporated into the chromosome of the cell by a process of *recombination* in order to maintain itself in the cell and to be replicated successively in the progeny. When an added piece of DNA has sequences of nucleotides that are similar to those of the cell's DNA, the two pieces of DNA are said to have regions of *homology*. When two homologous pieces of DNA are present in the same cell they tend to come to lie together and recombination can occur between them; the two pieces break at matching sites and the ends rejoin to the opposite pieces (crossing over).

In eukaryotic cells, a single cross-over between two homologous chromosomes during meiosis

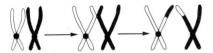

FIG. 7.5. Cross-over of chromosomes during meiosis in eukaryotic cells.

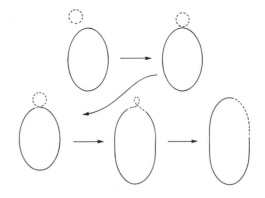

——— bacterial chromosome;
- - - - - added circular piece of DNA, e.g. phage or plasmid DNA.

FIG. 7.6. Insertion of a circular piece of DNA by a single cross-over.

leaves two complete chromosomes that have exchanged a portion of chromosome containing a number of genes (Fig. 7.5). Genetic transfer in prokaryotic cells usually involves the addition of a small extra piece of DNA to a cell containing a large circular DNA chromosome. If the extra piece of DNA is also circular (e.g. temperate phage and plasmids, see below) a single cross-over between the two pieces results in insertion of the added piece of DNA into the chromosome as a short linear segment (Fig. 7.6).

If the added piece of DNA is linear a single cross-over event between the two pieces would break the circle of the chromosome and the cell would not be viable. However, when two cross-overs occur, a linear piece of the added DNA is inserted into the circular chromosome and the net effect is that part of the added piece is substituted for the equivalent length of the original chromosome (Fig. 7.7). The distance between the two cross-overs may vary and when a long piece of DNA is added there may be multiple cross-overs resulting in the insertion of two or more portions of the added DNA. The pieces of DNA that are left unattached to the chromosome cannot be replicated with the chromosome and are lost during subsequent cell division.

Since the piece of DNA introduced into a cell by transformation or transduction may be long enough to contain between 10 and 100 genes there is a chance that several genes will be inserted together into the chromosome. The frequency at which any two introduced genes

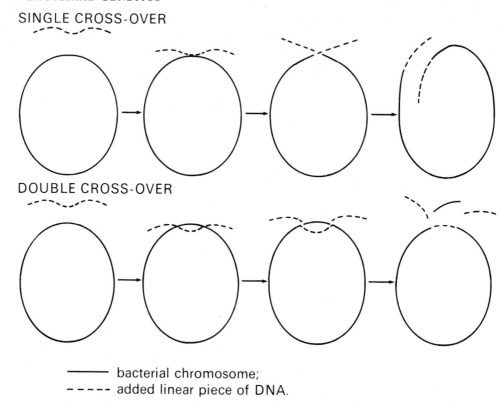

SINGLE CROSS-OVER

DOUBLE CROSS-OVER

———— bacterial chromosome;
- - - - - added linear piece of DNA.

FIG. 7.7. Insertion of a linear piece of DNA. A double cross-over is required to preserve the continuity of the chromosome.

can be found together in the progeny reflects the distance between the genes on the DNA—the closer together the genes the greater the chance that both will be incorporated in the chromosome. This is the basis of much *genetic mapping*. By determining the relative frequencies at which pairs of genes are acquired together, a map can be constructed showing the relative distances between the genes and their order along the chromosome.

Transformation

Most species of bacteria are unable to take up exogenous DNA and integrate it into the chromosome; indeed some bacteria produce nucleases that recognize and break down foreign DNA. The existence of such barriers to DNA transfer must be important in maintaining differences between evolving species. However, bacteria in a number of genera, e.g. pneumo-

cocci, *Haemophilus influenzae* and certain *Bacillus* species, have been found to be able to acquire new genetic characters by taking up free DNA directly from their surroundings. For transformation to occur, the DNA must have been derived from a closely related strain since pieces of DNA can undergo recombination with the chromosome only when there is adequate nucleic acid homology (p. 95).

DNA may be extracted from cells and purified chemically; the pieces of DNA involved in transformation are found to be large enough to contain about 10 to 50 genes. Cells are 'competent' for transformation only under certain conditions of growth, usually in late log phase or, in *Bacillus* species, during sporulation. The mechanism of DNA uptake is unclear, but it seems that competent cells must have specific receptors for DNA fragments on their surface and the physical state of the cell wall must be such that there are large enough pores for the

DNA to pass through. It is not known how these long molecules of DNA are transported through the cytoplasmic membrane.

Any gene may be transferred by transformation as any portion of the chromosome DNA may be taken up by the recipient cells. In *Bacillus* species a large number of auxotrophic mutations (p. 90) are available as genetic markers, but in *Haemophilus* and pneumococci far fewer genes have been identified. The classical experiments on transformation studied the genes controlling the production of specific capsular polysaccharides by pneumococci; these could be studied by immunological methods. In the original demonstration of pneumococcal transformation by Griffith in 1928, live rough cells derived from one capsular type (type 2) were transformed by mixing with killed smooth cells of a second type (type 1) in the peritoneal cavity of the mouse. The animals died of pneumococcal infection and the organisms recovered were smooth cells with type-1 capsules. It took nearly 20 years of work before Avery and his colleagues were able to report that the genetic information for type-1 capsule production had been transferred into the type-2 cells by a transforming material which was pure DNA. This was the first demonstration that genetic information was contained in DNA and it was the start of a major revolution in genetics and biology.

Generalized Transduction

Bacteriophages (phages) are viruses that multiply in bacteria. Most phages carry their genetic information (the phage genome) as a length of double-stranded DNA coiled up inside a protein coat. Other phages are known in which the phage genome consists of single-stranded DNA or double-stranded RNA, but the present discussion is limited to a consideration of transducing phages which all contain double-stranded DNA. During phage assembly, (Chap. 13), each phage head is normally filled with a phage genome, but with certain types of phage an occasional particle is formed (at a frequency of about 1 in 10^6) whose head has been accidentally filled with a similar length of host-cell DNA. When such a particle attaches to a second cell the DNA that enters the cell is not phage DNA capable of replicating and lysing the cell, but a short segment of chromosome from the first host; bacterial genes have been *transduced* by the phage into the second cell. Since these phages pick up any portion of the host chromosome at random they can transduce any gene at approximately the same frequency and this is described as *generalized transduction* (cf. restricted transduction).

Each transducing phage can pick up a piece of bacterial DNA of about the same size as its normal phage genome. Different types of phage may thus transduce pieces of bacterial chromosome long enough to contain anything from 30 to 150 genes. A number of these genes may then be incorporated into the host cell chromosome by recombination as discussed above (p. 95) and these transductants can be identified in the progeny by using appropriate selective conditions for the genetic markers under study. Comparison of the rates at which neighbouring genes are co-transduced into the same recipient is one of the basic tools of genetic mapping. It is the most widely applicable method of gene transfer as bacteriophages can be found that attack all species of bacteria. Not all bacteriophages are transducing phages, but as suitable genetic markers become available for new species, transducing phages can often be identified. For example, suitable phages have been isolated for transduction studies in *Escherichia, Shigella, Salmonella, Proteus, Pseudomonas, Bacillus* and *Staphylococcus* species. Genes can be transduced only between fairly closely related strains as each bacteriophage attacks a limited range of organisms with the same surface receptors. Transducing phages normally transfer chromosomal genes into the recipient cell but they may also pick up and transfer extrachromosomal DNA (plasmids, p. 99). The penicillinase gene in staphylococci is usually extrachromosomal and it may be transferred into other staphylococcal strains by transduction.

Restricted Transduction

Bacteriophages that lyse the host cell are known as *virulent* phages and are said to produce a lytic cycle of infection. However, *temperate* phages (Chap. 13) may become latent in the cell, which can still grow and divide normally. The progeny bacteria inherit the latent phage, which may later revert to the lytic cycle and kill the cell. Meanwhile, the cells are said to be *lysogenic* and the latent phage is called a *prophage*.

The molecular mechanism of lysogeny has been intensively studied in phage λ (lambda) of *Esch. coli*. When cells are infected by a temperate phage the majority are killed as the virus goes into the lytic cycle and multiplies in the normal way. However, in a small proportion of infected cells, the multiplication of the phage DNA is repressed. It can then be inserted into the host cell DNA so that it behaves like a small inactive portion of the bacterial chromosome. As long as it remains repressed it produces no phage components and is replicated only as part of the bacterial chromosome at cell division.

The mechanism of repression of λ phage is similar to that involved in the regulation of the *lac* operon in *Esch. coli* (p. 92). The phage DNA codes for the production of a specific repressor molecule that can attach to the phage DNA and prevent transcription of other phage genes that are essential for normal phage multiplication. Production of new phage is effectively switched off. The mechanism of the insertion of the phage into the bacterial chromosome is also understood in some detail. The λ phage DNA is linear inside the phage head but after it enters the bacterial cell the two ends are joined to form a circle. The phage genome can now be inserted into the chromosome by a single recombination event as previously described (p. 95).

In a small proportion of lysogenic cells, the repression is lifted spontaneously and the lytic cycle is resumed. The prophage is excised by a process that is the reverse of integration, phage proteins are produced again, the DNA is replicated and the cell is lysed in the normal way.

In a small proportion of cells, when the prophage is induced it is excised from the chromosome inaccurately so that a neighbouring portion of bacterial DNA is also removed (Fig. 7.8). Since the phage head can contain only a standard amount of DNA, a transducing phage that contains a few bacterial genes at one end of its DNA lacks a few phage genes at the other end, i.e. the phage genome is defective. When such a piece of DNA is transduced into a second cell, the defective phage can still integrate into its normal site on the chromosome, but it is unable to replicate normally to form more phage and lyse the cell. The result is that the added piece of bacterial DNA is carried into the chromosome by the defective phage DNA. The added bacterial genes are reproduced in the progeny of the recipient bacterium so that the new characters determined by these genes are expressed in all of the progeny. Since a temperate phage has a specific insertion site it can pick up and transduce only a short length of DNA containing a few genes on either side of this site; the variation is thus referred to as *restricted transduction*. Lambda phage is always inserted between the genes for galactose utilization (*gal*) and biotin synthesis (*bio*), and thus can transduce either the *gal* or the *bio* gene.

Lysogenic Conversion

The presence of prophage DNA in a cell constitutes a genetic alteration to the cell. Usually the only phage gene that is expressed is that which codes for production of the repressor, which switches off all the others. This in itself confers two new properties on the cell, superinfection immunity (Chap. 13) and the liability to revert to the lytic cycle with the production of new phage. It is worth noting that bacteriophages are not necessarily harmful to bacteria; temperate phages at least confer immunity to lysis by other phages of the same type. In practice, it is not easy to be certain whether any particular bacterial strain is lysogenic or not without fairly intensive investigation, but it is probable that lysogeny is quite widespread in nature.

In certain cases it can be shown that other prophage genes are also expressed so that the lysogenized cell has acquired other properties as well (*lysogenic conversion*). Non-lysogenized *Salmonella anatum* forms receptors that can adsorb phage ε^{15} but not phage ε^{34}. However, *S. anatum* lysogenized by ε^{15} forms different receptors that can adsorb phage ε^{34} but not ε^{15}. If the cells are now doubly lysogenized by the addition of phage ε^{34} to cells that are already lysogenic for ε^{15}, the receptors are changed again so that neither phage can be adsorbed. In this particular case the presence of a prophage directs the cell to alter its surface receptors so that the cell becomes resistant to that phage

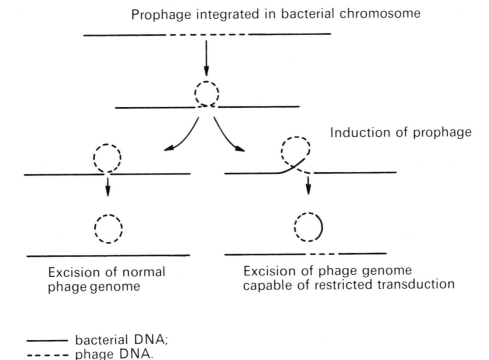

Prophage integrated in bacterial chromosome

Induction of prophage

Excision of normal
phage genome

Excision of phage genome
capable of restricted transduction

———— bacterial DNA;
- - - - - phage DNA.

FIG. 7.8. Restricted transduction.

(cf. the more normal superinfection immunity). This is a particularly interesting model as the effects of the prophages can be analysed in terms of the production of new phage-coded enzymes and the shut-off of host-coded enzymes involved in the synthesis of polysaccharide side chains on the bacterial surface. This allows a detailed analysis of the chemical structure of the cell surface components that make up the O-antigens and bacteriophage receptors of the cell. The system is also interesting in that such phage-coded alterations in the bacterial surface appear to be similar to the alterations in eukaryotic cell surface properties that occur after infection with integrated tumour viruses (Chap. 13). (ε = epsilon.)

Another example of lysogenic conversion has been found with *Corynebacterium diphtheriae*, which produces diphtheria toxin only when it is lysogenized by a specific phage (β phage). The activity of a prophage gene is required for the cell to produce toxin. It is probable that the production of certain toxins by staphylococci and streptococci is similarly dependent on the presence of a specific temperate prophage. In these cases, lysogeny not only gives the cell superinfection immunity, it also actively influences the virulence of the bacterium for man. One may speculate, with Hayes, to what extent we unjustly incriminate bacteria in general for the sins of their viruses!

Bacterial Plasmids

A *plasmid* is a small extrachromosomal piece of genetic material that can replicate autonomously and maintain itself in the cytoplasm of a bacterium for many generations; it is usually a circular piece of double-stranded DNA. It has many of the properties of a small chromosome and contains similar genetic information for controlling its replication and ensuring segregation of one copy into each daughter cell at cell division, but it differs in that it is much smaller than the chromosome (e.g. 50 to 100 genes) and the genes that it contains are not normally essential to the cell.

Plasmids have been found to be common in a number of species of Gram-negative bacilli, including *Escherichia, Shigella, Salmonella, Klebsiella* and *Proteus;* these plasmids are often loosely referred to as 'coliform' plasmids. Certain coliform plasmids can cause their host cell to conjugate with another cell and to transfer a copy of the plasmid into the second cell. Plasmids that contain the information for self-transfer to another cell by conjugation are described as *transmissible plasmids*. These transmissible coliform plasmids may be transferred between cells of different strains of the same species and also into cells of other species in this group of enterobacteria.

The plasmids of the coliform group of organisms have been intensively studied in recent years and have become of particular clinical importance since the discovery of transferable (plasmid-borne) drug resistance (p. 104). Many coliform plasmids have been found to contain genes that may be of value to the cell under particular circumstances—e.g. genes for bacteriocine production or antibiotic resistance. Genes that control several factors produced by certain enteropathogenic strains of *Esch. coli* (haemolysin, enterotoxin, surface antigen K88) may be present on transmissible plasmids. No doubt other types of gene will also be found to be extrachromosomal. Even the most intensively studied plasmids contain more DNA than is needed for the functions that are known at present.

A variety of plasmids have been detected in staphylococci, but as conjugation does not occur in staphylococci, all staphylococcal plasmids are defined as non-transmissible. This does not mean that they cannot be transferred by a mechanism other than conjugation—and they can indeed be exchanged between staphylococci by a transducing phage. The gene for penicillinase (β-lactamase) production is usually plasmid-borne in staphylococci, and those for erythromycin and tetracycline resistance are often so, although resistance to other antimicrobial drugs is usually chromosomal. Other plasmid-borne genes in staphylococci include determinants that confer increased resistance to certain heavy metal ions, e.g. mercury. Plasmids may

well be present in other genera of bacteria, but it is difficult to demonstrate the absence or presence of extrachromosomal genes when little is known about the genetic organization of the species.

Conjugation

During conjugation one cell, the *donor* or male cell, makes contact with another, the *recipient* or female, and DNA is transferred directly from the donor into the recipient. The ability to act as a donor in conjugation is determined by the presence of a transmissible plasmid in the cell; the transmissible plasmid contains the genetic information for conjugation of the host cell with a suitable recipient and for transfer of the plasmid DNA into it. Such a transmissible plasmid is known as a *transfer factor* or *sex factor*. Only cells that contain a sex factor are male and can act as donors; those lacking a sex factor are female and act as recipients.

Transfer of DNA between cells by conjugation requires direct contact between the donor and the recipient cell. Transfer factors contain genes that code for the production of a protein appendage on the surface of the donor cell—a specialized fimbria 1 to 2 μm long known as a *sex fimbria* or *pilus*. The tip of the pilus attaches to the surface of a recipient cell and holds the two cells together. The DNA of the transfer factor then passes into the recipient cell. The presence of a pilus is essential for the transfer of DNA, but it is unclear whether the DNA passes along it or is transferred across some other connecting bridge.

Many transmissible plasmids contain genetic markers such as genes for antibiotic resistance or colicine production and then the DNA transferred is not merely the basic transfer factor but also these associated genes. It is thought that one strand of the circular DNA of the transfer factor is nicked open at a specific point and the free end is passed through into the recipient cell. The DNA is replicated during transfer so that each cell receives a copy (Fig. 7.9). The analogy with sex is somewhat strained here as the recipient or female acquires a transfer factor and is converted into a male, able to conjugate with further females and convert them in turn! In this way a transfer factor may rapidly spread through a whole population of susceptible cells; this process is sometimes described as infectious spread of a plasmid, or 'infectious heredity'.

F FACTOR AND HFR DONOR STRAINS. The *F factor* (fertility factor) of *Esch. coli* was the first transfer factor to be discovered but in some ways it is not typical. It is unusual in that it can be inserted into the bacterial chromosome by a mechanism similar to that of the insertion of lambda (λ) phage into the chromosome (p. 98) and that it can then transfer chromosomal genes into recipient cells. This feature of its behaviour dominated discussion of the nature of transfer factors for many years. The more recent discovery of non-transmissible plasmids and of many transfer factors that carry genes for drug resistance but seldom, if ever, become associated with the chromosome, has led to a broader understanding of the general nature of plasmids. The classification and nomenclature of plasmids is discussed on p. 103.

The F factor is a transfer factor that contains the basic genetic information for extrachromosomal existence and for self-transfer, but does not normally contain other identifiable genetic markers such as drug-resistance genes. Cells that contain the F plasmid free in the cytoplasm (F^+ cells) have no unusual characters apart from the ability to produce pili and to transfer F to F^- cells by conjugation. In a very small proportion of F^+ cells F becomes inserted into the bacterial chromosome; such cells are able to transfer certain chromosomal genes into F^- cells with high frequency and cultures of these cells are known as *Hfr* strains. The F factor is a small circular piece of double-stranded DNA. When it becomes associated with the chromosome it may be inserted into it as a linear segment by a single recombination event. The F factor does not produce a specific integrase enzyme as does λ phage (Chap. 13); integration of F occurs simply by recombination between regions of genetic homology. Since there are several regions of homology between F and the chromosome of its normal host strain of *Esch. coli*, F may integrate at a number of different sites on the chromosome.

When F is integrated into the chromosome in the *Hfr* state, it is replicated as part of the chromosome and inherited by the progeny cells in the same way that λ prophage is inherited by lysogenized cells. The transfer functions of F are not repressed in the chromosome; it still directs the formation of pili on the cell surface so that *Hfr* cells can conjugate and transfer DNA. In this state they transfer not only the F factor DNA but also part of the chromosome to which it is attached. During conjugation one strand of the plasmid DNA is opened and a linear piece of DNA is transferred into the recipient cell. In

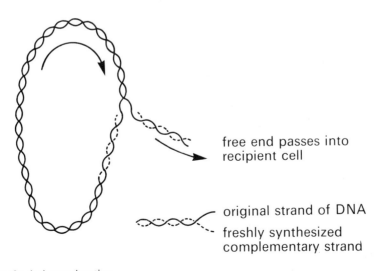

free end passes into recipient cell

— original strand of DNA
--- freshly synthesized complementary strand

FIG. 7.9. DNA transfer during conjugation.

this case F factor DNA is first transferred, followed by the part of the chromosome at one side of the site of insertion of F. As conjugation continues, more of the bacterial chromosome is pushed through into the recipient (Fig. 7.10). However, the chromosome tends to break randomly during transfer so that, on the average, only about 10 per cent is transferred, the whole chromosome entering the recipient only rarely.

All cells in a culture of a particular *Hfr* strain have F integrated at the same site in the chromosome. When *Hfr* cells conjugate with F^- cells, the recipients acquire the donor cell chromosomal genes in a specific order—the order in which they occur on the chromosome. Mating cells can be broken apart mechanically by vigorous shaking so that the piece of DNA that is being transferred is broken. If conjugation is interrupted at different times after the *Hfr* and F^- cells have been mixed, the order of the genes on the donor cell chromosome can be mapped by determining the time when each gene first becomes detectable in the recipient cells. It is found that 120 minutes is required for the whole chromosome to be transferred; thus the mating act in *Esch. coli* may last some three or four times the normal life-span! Since there is almost perfect homology between the recipient cell chromosome and the transferred portion of

chromosome, recombination occurs readily and there is quite a high probability that any introduced gene will be incorporated into the chromosome and inherited by the progeny. *Hfr* strains produce a high frequency of transfer of the early genes and thus a high frequency of recombination; hence the abbreviation *Hfr*.

Different *Hfr* strains have the F factor inserted at different sites. During conjugation, the genes are in the same order on the chromosome, but transfer starts at different points, and may proceed in either direction. Thus, as shown in the diagram (Fig. 7.11) one *Hfr* strain may transfer genes in the order ABCDE . . . while another transfers PQRST . . . and a third transfers JIHGF . . . Such experiments, using a number of *Hfr* strains, revealed that the genetic map of *Esch. coli* was circular before it was technically possible to demonstrate the circular nature of the chromosome DNA. The use of *Hfr* donors allows the study of much longer fragments of DNA than can be transferred between cells by transduction and it has made possible the construction of a circular map of the *Esch. coli* genome that locates the relative positions of some 300 genes. Transduction, by contrast, is particularly useful for analysing the detailed arrangement of genes that are closely clustered on the chromosome.

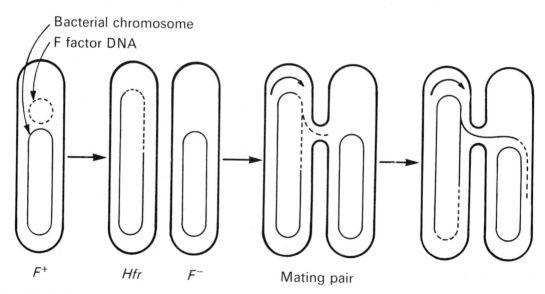

FIG. 7.10. Conjugation with *Hfr* donor.

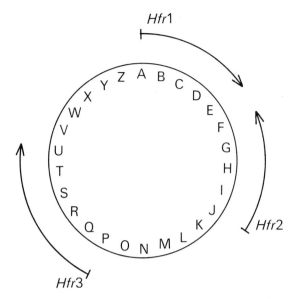

FIG. 7.11. Chromosome mapping by the use of *Hfr* strains. Circular chromosome of *Esch. coli* with hypothetical genes A–Z. Different *Hfr* strains (1, 2, 3, . . .) have the F factor integrated at different sites and transfer the chromosome into the recipient from different starting points. Different *Hfr* strains may transfer the genes in different directions.

F-PRIME FACTORS. In any culture of F^+ cells there is a small proportion of cells that have F integrated into the chromosome. Similarly, in any culture of *Hfr* cells there are a few in which F comes out of the chromosome again and reverts to the free state. This is similar to the situation with λ prophage where, in a small proportion of cells, the prophage is excised from the chromosome and phage replication is resumed (Chap. 13). As with λ phage, F is not always excised accurately and occasionally an F factor carries off some of the neighbouring genes when it leaves the chromosome. An F factor that has picked up a portion of the chromosome in this way is known as an *F-prime factor* (F^1). One well known example is the F-*lac* factor, which is an F^1 carrying the genes of the *Esch. coli lac* operon. When an F^1 factor transfers itself into another cell its associated genes function normally on the plasmid in the new host. Thus, non-lactose-fermenting organisms become lactose-fermenters when they receive F-*lac*. When F-*lac* is transferred into *Esch. coli,* the cells become diploid for the *lac* genes. The particular value of this sex factor is that it allows the study of interactions between different *lac* operon mutations within the same cell. This led to the discovery of the mechanism of control of inducible enzymes (p. 92).

Classification of Bacterial Plasmids

All bacterial plasmids contain the basic genetic information for extrachromosomal existence, i.e. for self-replication and segregation at cell division so that each daughter cell receives a copy of the plasmid along with its copy of the chromosome. In addition, plasmids may or may not contain a variety of other types of genetic information. Transmissible plasmids contain the information for production of a pilus and self-transfer to another cell by conjugation; they are known as *transfer factors* or *sex factors*. Many plasmids have been found that contain genes for resistance to antimicrobial drugs. These are known as *resistance factors* (R factors). R factors may be transmissible or non-transmissible; i.e. they may or may not also contain the genetic information for self transfer by conjugation. The term R factor is often used to refer only to transmissible R factors. The part of an R factor that codes for self transfer is a transfer factor, and is often known specifically as a resistance transfer factor (RTF). An RTF may exist either as part of an R factor or as a simple transfer factor, containing no resistance genes. Such a free transfer factor is able to recombine with a non-transmissible resistance plasmid to form a transmissible R factor. An R factor frequently contains several genes, each determining resistance to a different antibiotic.

The situation is similar with genes that determine the production of colicines. Many colicine genes are plasmid-borne. Some are found on transmissible plasmids and some are on non-transmissible plasmids but can be picked up by simple transfer factors. Particular transfer factors are often described as resistance transfer factors or colicine transfer factors according to the nature of the associated genes, but this is not an entirely satisfactory basis for classification as some transfer factors have no identifiable associated genes and others may carry both resistance and colicine genes.

The F factor (and a limited number of other plasmids) can be integrated into the host cell chromosome to produce *Hfr* strains. Such plasmids have been described as *episomes*. The term was introduced to emphasize the similarity between pieces of DNA such as the F factor and λ phage that show this reversible integration into the chromosome. However, it has limited usefulness in classification as it describes the behaviour of the phage or plasmid inside a particular host and this behaviour depends on the properties of the DNA of the host cell as well as of the plasmid or phage. When F is transmitted to cells of a species such as *Serratia* or *Proteus*, in which there are no regions of homology on the chromosome, F remains free in the cytoplasm. On the other hand, we cannot be certain that because a plasmid does not integrate into the chromosome of a number of species it could not integrate in any species. Similarly, λ phage is unable to lysogenize certain strains of bacteria in which it always behaves as a virulent phage. The terms episome and plasmid are often used as if they were freely interchangeable but it is better to use episome only when describing the reversible integration of a specific plasmid into the chromosome of a specific host.

TRANSFERABLE DRUG RESISTANCE

R factors were first demonstrated in Japan in 1959 when it was shown that resistance to several antibiotics could be transferred as a unit between strains of *Shigella* and *Esch. coli* by conjugation. Many surveys since then in all parts of the world have shown that R factors are now common and widespread. Resistance to sulphonamides, tetracycline, chloramphenicol, ampicillin, streptomycin, kanamycin, neomycin and furazolidone have all been found to be commonly extrachromosomal in enterobacteria and transferable to drug-sensitive organisms *in vitro* or *in vivo*. The actual incidence of drug resistance in particular species varies when different populations are studied, but is found to be increasing in most pathogenic species throughout the world; the incidence of strains with multiple resistance is similarly increasing.

It is not known how or where extrachromosomal (plasmid-borne) resistance genes originate, but whether they originate in chromosomal or in plasmid DNA, they are certainly liable to appear in R factors soon after a new antibiotic comes into general use. The exact way in which R factors are built up is the subject of some dispute, but it is clear that simple transfer factors that can pick up resistance genes are relatively common in enterobacteria and that such transfer factors can combine with non-transmissible resistance plasmids to produce transmissible R factors. R factors can recombine with non-transmissible resistance plasmids or with other R factors to produce complex R factors that contain genes for resistance to several antibiotics, so that under suitable conditions transferable multiple-resistance R factors can be built up. Resistance to as many as seven or eight different antimicrobial drugs has been found to be carried in a single R factor. This process need not occur in a single bacterial species. R factors and transfer factors can transfer themselves into a wide range of commensal and pathogenic bacteria *in vitro*, e.g. *Escherichia, Salmonella, Shigella, Klebsiella, Proteus, Serratia, Pasteurella, Vibrio* and *Pseudomonas*. Once drug resistance appears in any of these species it may be picked up and built into multiple-resistance R factors which may then be distributed to cells of other Gram-negative species.

It is relatively easy to study the build-up and spread of R factors *in vitro* under the selective pressure of antibiotics, but it is harder to analyse *in vivo*. Conditions in the normal gut are not very suitable for conjugation; alkaline pH, bile salts, fatty acids and anaerobic conditions may all inhibit conjugation; pili are better formed by actively growing cells than by stationary phase cells; and since the number of suitable recipient cells in the gut is considerably lower than that of other organisms such as *Bacteroides* and Gram-positive species, opportunities for a donor cell to come into contact with a suitable recipient are not frequent. It is often difficult to show spread of R factors to other bacterial species in the gut of a normal animal; the R factors are perpetuated mainly by linear transmission to the progeny at cell division. When an antibiotic is given, however, the numbers of drug-sensitive organisms are rapidly reduced, drug-resistant organisms are selected and multiply to take their place and opportunities for the transfer of R factors are improved. Any originally drug-sensitive organisms that receive R factors are also selected while those that do not are killed. It is much easier to show R factor spread *in vivo* when antibiotic selection is used; the result of giving an antibiotic may be a dramatic increase in the incidence of R factors in the gut flora. Although R factors may have been present originally in only a small proportion of the cells of a single species, antibiotic treatment may select for them so that they become present in a high proportion of cells in several species. Since R factors may contain multiple resistance genes the effect of giving a single antibiotic may be to ensure that the majority of the enterobacteria in the gut, commensal or pathogenic, come to contain an R factor that confers resistance, not just to the antibiotic given, but to several other drugs as well.

R factors were not demonstrated until 1959 in Japan, 1962 in Britain and 1966 in the United States, although many of the basic antibiotics had already been in use for many years before these dates. Whatever the reasons for this initial delay in appearance, R factors are now common in commensal and pathogenic drug-resistant enterobacteria from the gut, and from infections caused by organisms derived from the gut, e.g. urinary tract infection and Gram-negative septicaemia. R factors were almost unknown in 1960; now they are widespread. It seems that this is an inevitable consequence of the widespread use of antibiotics. The frequent exposure of a human or animal population to a variety of antibiotics leads to the appearance of extrachromosomal resistance genes in the gut enterobacteria. Transfer factors that can pick up these genes acquire a new survival value both to themselves and their host bacteria, and a continuing exposure to antibiotics leads to an increasing frequency of R factors in a variety of bacterial species. Infections caused by pathogens containing R factors may be very difficult to treat and as workers in human and animal medicine are faced with increasing drug resistance in pathogenic species, there is a tendency towards the administration of a greater range of drugs. In turn, this results in the build-up of more complex R factors that become more widely distributed to commensal and pathogenic organisms.

The potential dangers of transferable (infectious) drug resistance are obvious. If the incidence of multiple-resistance R factors continues to increase, infections by coliform organisms will become more difficult to treat. Many of these infections are usually mild and do not require antibiotic therapy, e.g. most cases of salmonella food poisoning and *Shigella sonnei* dysentery, but antibiotic therapy is of great importance in others. In typhoid fever, for example, treatment with chloramphenicol is often life-saving and if *Salmonella typhi* acquires chloramphenicol resistance, we have no effective substitute. Cholera and bacillary dysentery would become much harder to control if antimicrobial drugs were to lose their efficacy. The antibiotic treatment of *Esch. coli* enteritis in infants is becoming more difficult because of the increase in R factors in human enteropathogenic strains and drug resistance is a growing problem in the therapy of urinary tract infection. There is an increasing frequency of 'opportunist' infections caused by drug-resistant organisms that are normally of low virulence. These infections are liable to occur in patients who have a lowered resistance (e.g. because of uraemia, irradiation, immunosuppressive drugs, antitumour therapy) and who have already been treated with several antibiotics. Some opportunist pathogens belong to species that are naturally resistant to many antibiotics, e.g. *Pseudomonas* or *Candida,* but others are strains of Gram-negative species such as *Serratia* or *Klebsiella* that are normally drug-sensitive but have acquired R factors.

A further potential danger that has attracted a great deal of attention is the transfer to man of R factors evolved in farm animals. There is good evidence that R factors have spread to man from calves bred under intensive farming conditions. E. S. Anderson and others in the Enteric Reference Laboratory, London, studied strains of *Salm. typhimurium* isolated from calves during a succession of outbreaks of enteritis among calves in 1963–66. Infection spread rapidly because of overcrowding and poor hygiene as intensive rearing was introduced, and large amounts of antibiotics were used in unsuccessful attempts to control the outbreak. An increasing proportion of all salmonellae isolated from cattle were found to be *Salm. typhimurium* type 29 and these organisms acquired transferable resistance to increasing numbers of antibiotics as the outbreak progressed (Fig. 7.12). The multiple-resistance R factors became common not only in the infecting *Salm. typhimurium* type 29 but also in commensal *Esch. coli* from the same batches of calves. The outbreak was eventually brought under control only by alterations in the arrangements for breeding and transporting calves to reduce the amount of cross-infection between the animals.

Human infection with *Salm. typhimurium* is usually a result of food-poisoning; the main reservoir of infection is in farm animals and the disease is spread to man by contaminated meat or other food. The outbreak of infection in calves was paralleled by a rise in the incidence of human food-poisoning due to *Salm. typhimurium* type 29 containing the same R factors.

There is no doubt that these strains with multiple resistance were derived from the calves as many were resistant to furazolidone, a drug used only in veterinary practice, as well as to other agents used in both man and animals. There is a risk that such R factors, evolved in farm animals, will spread to human commensal *Esch. coli* and then be transferred to human pathogens that cause more serious infections than food-poisoning. The risk may be greater than at first appears as R factors may be transmitted to man by commensal bacteria from animals as well as by pathogens. The rate of transfer of food-poisoning salmonellae to man is considerable despite careful precautions in food preparation and handling; the rate of transfer of non-pathogenic organisms must be much greater.

R factors are common in *Esch. coli* and

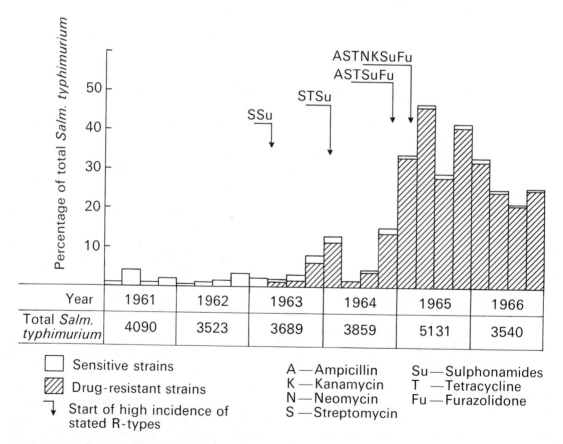

FIG. 7.12. Infections with type 29 *Salmonella typhimurium* as a percentage of total human and animal *S. typhimurium* infections, 1961 to 1966 [modified from Anderson, E. S. (1968) *Annual Review of Microbiology*, **22**, 163].

Salmonella strains isolated from pigs and chickens as well as from calves. Penicillin or tetracycline may be given to young animals as a feed supplement in order to produce a faster growth rate. The practice leads to the selection of R factors that contain genes for tetracycline resistance and for penicillinase production. Gram-negative bacilli are naturally resistant to penicillin but are susceptible to the semisynthetic penicillin derivative, ampicillin. Since ampicillin is also inactivated by penicillinase, the use of penicillin as a feed supplement leads to production of ampicillin resistance in the Gram-negative flora of the gut. The use of antibiotics as feed supplements is restricted by law in Britain to the administration of small amounts of penicillin and tetracyclines to pigs and chickens.

Antibiotics are also widely prescribed for the treatment of infections in farm animals and the drugs used in veterinary practice are largely the same as those used in man. In 1967 the total amount of antibiotic used in human medicine was estimated at 240 tons and the total amount in agriculture, both for therapy and feed supplements, was 170 tons. One of the main differences between veterinary and medical practice is a tendency for treatment of a whole animal population rather than an individual human patient. In certain cases the whole population is treated in the hope that the infected animals will be cured and infection will be prevented in the others. In other circumstances, farmers are accustomed to administer low doses of antibiotics to a whole population of animals that are judged to be under 'stress' and particularly liable to develop infection. When R factor resistance is present, the mass use of antibiotics fails to prevent the spread of infection or to cure infected animals and results in a very high incidence of the R factor in the gut flora of the whole batch of animals.

It is probable that sensible limitation of antibiotic usage in man and animals could prevent further increase in R factors and perhaps reduce their incidence. Many R factors are unstable and tend to lose resistance genes when the selective pressure is removed. R factors are lost spontaneously from a small proportion of cells in a culture since plasmid replication and segregation are not always precisely synchronous with chromosome replication and segregation. Cells that lose an R factor may have a slight metabolic advantage because they no longer have the burden of producing plasmid nucleic acids and proteins. In the absence of antibiotics, drug-resistant organisms have no selective advantage and may be slowly outgrown by drug-sensitive organisms. Moreover, R factors that evolve in one species may not thrive in another. An R factor that is well adjusted to existence in *Escherichia* may be unstable in *Proteus* strains and be lost at a high rate, or it may transfer itself to other organisms much less efficiently. Similarly, commensal or pathogenic organisms that are adapted to the gut of a calf, pig or chicken may not be established readily in man; they may be present only transiently and conjugate seldom with the human commensal flora. Such factors as these may be helping to contain the spread of R factors. The results of some experiments with populations of animals encourage the hope that R factors slowly disappear when no antibiotics are given.

Mechanisms of Increase in Drug Resistance

Discussion of the problem of drug resistance usually concentrates on the increasing drug resistance of species that were originally drug-sensitive, e.g. *Staph. aureus, Mycobacterium tuberculosis, Salmonella* and *Shigella*. This type of resistance is known as *acquired* resistance in contrast to the *natural* resistance of certain strains or species to particular antibiotics, e.g. that of *Pseudomonas* to most of the antibiotics that inhibit many other Gram-negative pathogens. The classic mechanism of acquired drug resistance is the selection by antibiotics of spontaneous mutants with increased resistance to the drugs (p. 88). This mechanism has been much studied in the laboratory. It is certainly of clinical importance in tuberculosis (Chap. 22) in which mutants resistant to any single drug, e.g. streptomycin or isoniazid, arise spontaneously and are likely to be present in the patient before the start of treatment. If only one drug is given to the patient, it kills many or all of the sensitive parental population of bacteria, but allows the few resistant mutant bacteria to multiply and eventually become so numerous as to cause a relapse of the disease. This occurrence is termed the 'fall and rise' phenomenon from the initial reduction and later increase in the number of viable bacteria demonstrable in the patient's body. It has been observed also in some cases of urinary-tract infections with Gram-negative bacilli under treatment with streptomycin. Combined therapy with at least two drugs to which the organism is sensitive is essential for the successful treatment of tuberculosis, so that each drug kills the few mutants that are resistant to the other drug. The frequency with which mutations to resistance to both drugs occur spontaneously in the same cell is so low as to be insignificant in clinical practice.

It is clear that in tuberculosis and some coliform infections the resistant mutants arise in the patient before the start of treatment and are selected and replace the sensitive parental forms during treatment, but it is more difficult to show that drug resistance may arise in this way in staphylococci. Strains of *Staph. aureus* occasionally develop high-level resistance to erythromycin or streptomycin by a single-step mutation and selection of the mutant may take place during a single course of antibiotic treatment, but for most antibiotics a more gradual multistep process occurs in a population of staphylococci that are being exchanged between a number of patients and carriers. In the majority of patients with resistant staphylococci the organisms have been acquired, already resistant, by cross-infection within the hospital. No doubt the resistance originally arises by mutation, but often the level of resistance to a particular drug has to be built up by sequential selection of multiple small-step mutations. This happens within a whole population of healthy carriers and infected patients who are receiving antibiotics for prophylaxis or therapy or are exposed to spilt antibiotic in the hospital environment. The resulting strain of *Staph. aureus* with multiple drug resistance is characteristic of the hospital, rather than of any particular patient. Such a strain is often known as a 'hospital staphylococcus' (Chap. 15). There is little argument for the use of combined drug therapy for the prevention of drug resistance in staphylococci. It is more important to minimize the use of antibiotics and to reduce the cross-infection that is the significant factor in the evolution of hospital strains.

Fortunately, not all bacterial species can become resistant to the antibiotics used against them. Mutation to penicillin resistance is rare; it has not occurred in *Strept. pyogenes* or pneumococci, although it is now beginning to present a clinical problem in gonococci. Acquired resistance to penicillin in staphylococci and to ampicillin in Gram-negative bacilli is not due to mutation but to the acquisition of a plasmid-borne penicillinase gene.

An increase in drug resistance in infections caused by a particular species is not always due to acquired resistance. There is evidence that the rise in incidence of sulphonamide-resistant meningococci is due to the selection of naturally resistant strains, rather than to the selection of resistant mutants. Similarly, the great, worldwide increase in the prevalence of penicillin resistance in staphylococci after the introduction of penicillin to general medical use reflected the selection of pre-existing penicillinase-producing strains (Chap. 15). The penicillinase gene is contained on a non-transmissible plasmid in staphylococci and it is probable that these plasmids were later transferred into new strains by transduction. Transduction of penicillinase plasmids can be shown to occur *in vivo* during experimental mixed staphylococcal infections in animals.

Plasmid-borne drug resistance also plays a very important part in the increasing acquired resistance of Gram-negative organisms; the actual and potential problems of transferable drug resistance are outlined earlier in this chapter. Genetic transfer allows an accelerated process of evolution as genes that evolve in different species under different pressures can be brought together in the same cell; they do not have to evolve sequentially in the same strain. The occasional occurrence of genetic transfer by transduction or conjugation gives bacteria some of the advantages that sexual reproduction confers on eukaryotic cells. Man's use of antibiotics has produced new selective pressures on bacteria and also new selective pressures on their plasmids. We do not know why resistance genes tend to occur on plasmids or what the role of transfer factors may have been before the antibiotic era, but our use of antibiotics in medicine and agriculture has suddenly conferred a new value on transfer factors that can pick up resistance genes. The ecology of bacteria and their plasmids has been dramatically altered so that certain types of R factor have become very much more widely distributed in Gram-negative bacteria than previously, and we do not know whether other genes may accumulate on plasmids. Some of the genes that have been identified on plasmids in coliform bacteria may be determinants of virulence, e.g. genes for production of enterotoxin and haemolysin by certain enteropathogenic strains of *Esch. coli*. If it were to be generally true that plasmids can accumulate genes that increase virulence, then the use of antibiotics could select for plasmids that confer not only multiple drug resistance but also increased pathogenicity.

REFERENCES

GARROD, L. P., LAMBERT, H. P. & O'GRADY, F. (1973) *Antibiotic and Chemotherapy*, 3rd edn. Edinburgh: Churchill Livingstone.

HAYES, W. (1968) *Genetics of Bacteria and their Viruses*, 2nd edn, Oxford and Edinburgh: Blackwell Scientific Publications.

WATSON, J. D. (1970) *Molecular Biology of the Gene*, 2nd edn, New York: W. A. Benjamin Inc.

8. Bacterial Pathogenicity: Sources and Spread of Infection in the Community

MICROBIAL PATHOGENICITY

Pathogenicity, or the capacity to initiate disease, is a relatively rare quality among microbes. It requires the attributes of *transmissibility* or communicability from one host or reservoir to a fresh host, *infectivity* or the ability to breach the new host's defences, and *virulence,* a variable factor that may enhance or reduce the capacity of the pathogen to cause overt disease. Virulence in the clinical sense is a manifestation of a complex parasite-host relationship in which an organism's capacity to harm the host is considered in relation to the host's resistance.

OPPORTUNISTIC PATHOGENS. Many commensal or non-pathogenic microbes are transmissible from person to person or are derived from the environment. They are present, often in large numbers, on the skin, in the upper respiratory tract, the intestines and the lower genito-urinary tract and as such they constitute the normal bacterial flora of the body and may play some part in the body's defences against invading pathogenic microbes. Their infectivity is low, since they are unable to overcome the defences of the healthy body and invade the tissues. However, this is a delicate balance. Some of the commensals are potential or opportunistic pathogens in the sense that they can initiate infection if they leave their natural habitat and gain access to other parts of the body, e.g. coliform bacilli are mostly harmless commensals in the gut but may cause infection in the urinary tract. Other commensals may produce disease in debilitated or damaged tissues where defence mechanisms have been rendered ineffective; for example, *Streptococcus viridans,* a common commensal in the mouth and oropharynx, may cause subacute bacterial endocarditis if it gets into the blood stream after a tooth extraction and settles on previously damaged or deformed heart valves. *Haemophilus influenzae* can maintain or aggravate a superimposed infection in a person with chronic bronchitis and *Clostridium welchii* can multiply and cause gas gangrene in locally damaged tissues.

TRUE PATHOGENS. Unlike the opportunistic pathogens, which can cause infection only when tissue resistance is lowered or the conditions are abnormal, the truly pathogenic species of microorganisms possess properties that enable them to overcome the body defences and infect the tissues of a normal healthy subject. Nonetheless, certain true pathogens are *more likely* to cause infection in the presence of predisposing conditions which depress the defence mechanisms. Several properties are essential for pathogenicity.

The transmissibility of a pathogen often involves an ability to grow profusely, or to be shed in large numbers, in body fluids or secretions capable of dissemination. The successful pathogen must also survive adverse environmental conditions, e.g. desiccation in dry dust, through which it may have to pass to reach a new host. Thus, factors of both quantity and quality may apply to the concept of transmissibility in which the viability of an effective number of organisms must be preserved en route to the new host, particularly if the route is indirect. Again, the outcome will depend on the mode and site of access to the new host, whether by direct contact, inhalation, ingestion or injection. The method of transfer may protect the pathogen as in the sexual transmission of venereal diseases or it may actually increase the dose as when viruses multiply in the insect vector; other pathogens such as the tetanus bacillus must depend on their own protective mechanism for survival between hosts.

Infectivity. Pathogenic microbes are able to initiate infection by penetrating the healthy body's first line of defences, that is, skin or mucous membranes to which they readily gain access. To do this they may have to run the gauntlet of protective barriers in the respiratory and alimentary tracts and no doubt only a few of the pathogens get through. The pathogen may initiate a localized lesion at the site of entry, e.g. a staphylococcal boil on the skin or a streptococcal pharyngitis in the throat. Frequently a restricted infection produces no obvious signs or symptoms of disease and this phenomenon is called a latent, symptomless or subclinical infection. Such a condition is often unnoticed and can be recognized only by laboratory tests demonstrating the presence of the pathogen or the development of specific antibodies to it; in some cases, a tissue hypersensitivity can be demonstrated by skin tests; for example, the tuberculin test has shown that a large proportion of the population may develop symptomless tuberculosis. The ratio of subclinical to clinical infection varies greatly in different diseases; in smallpox and measles, most of the susceptible population who contract the infection develop overt disease, whereas in poliomyelitis and meningococcal meningitis only a small proportion of the infected become clinically ill.

The capacity to initiate infection is often related to the dosage of the pathogen, its phase of growth and its endowment with 'virulence factors' (see below). Within the salmonella family, the infecting dose of *Salmonella typhi* may be very small whereas large numbers of the food-poisoning salmonellae must be ingested to produce acute vomiting and diarrhoea. Bacteria in the logarithmic phase of growth are more likely to overcome host resistance than those in the latent phase; for example, *Streptococcus pyogenes* is more infective when transferred directly from a person with sore throat than when it is inhaled after drying in dust particles. Because *Strept. pyogenes* is also well equipped with an antiphagocytic component, the capsular M protein, during the active phase of a sore throat infection, it is more infective in this form than in mutant forms containing less M protein which often replace the M-rich form in the throat during convalescence.

Virulence. Attempts to measure the virulence of a pathogen are often made by experiments with susceptible animals like the mouse and the guinea-pig which can be reasonably well standardized in terms of age, sex, weight, and some genetic factors; when death is the end-result, mortality rates are easily measured. The virulence of the pathogen under test is usually compared with that of a 'standard strain' (whose virulence has been repeatedly determined) and is expressed as the median lethal dose (LD50) or the numbers of the pathogen required to kill approximately half of the infected animals (see Vol. II, Chap. 14). Comparative tests of this kind have shown, *inter alia*, that strains of the tubercle bacillus isolated from Indian patients with tuberculosis are often less virulent for the guinea-pig than strains isolated in Britain; or that strains of specific pneumococcus types vary in their mouse virulence according to the amount of capsular substance they contain. However, assessments of virulence for animals are not necessarily applicable to virulence for man; indeed the fallacy of applying findings from mice to men was well demonstrated by *Salmonella typhi* which has a surface virulence (Vi) factor that largely determines its lethality for mice but which, when included in typhoid vaccines, has apparently little or no protective effect for man. Whether these findings indicate that the Vi factor is not involved in the organism's virulence for man, or whether it is merely poorly immunogenic in man, is not clear. It is even less possible to produce an experimental model that adequately reflects the many variables in human communities of age, sex, nutritional status and other factors that may affect natural or acquired resistance to infection. However, comparisons can be made from epidemiological data about the relative virulence of members of a particular microbial family; thus *Shigella dysenteriae*, group 1, and particularly the Shiga bacillus (type 1), causes much more serious infections than the group 4 (Sonne) members of the genus *Shigella*, whilst groups 2 and 3 are intermediate in virulence; the *gravis* strain of the diphtheria bacillus causes proportionately more deaths and serious complications than the *mitis* strain; type 1 poliovirus is much more likely to initiate epidemics of paralytic poliomyelitis than is type 2, and a type 3 pneumococcus pneumonia is ordinarily much more severe in the same age groups than a type 1 infection.

PATHOGENESIS

Toxigenicity

Pathogenic bacteria produce disease by virtue of one or other or both of two main attributes, toxigenicity and invasiveness.

Exotoxins. German and French workers were the first to prove that products of the diphtheria bacillus, diffused from a local infection or injected as bacteria-free filtrates of the cultured organism, could produce widespread systemic damage in guinea-pigs. Their findings explained why, in diphtheria, severe or fatal damage is done to heart muscle, nerves, adrenal glands and other organs despite the fact that the infecting bacilli remain localized in the throat; toxin produced in the throat is carried by the blood stream throughout the body (toxaemia). Later, it was shown that production of this toxin in broth culture proceeded *pari passu* with bacterial multiplication so that the poison was apparently secreted by actively growing bacteria and was therefore called an *exotoxin*. Other bacteria that actively secrete highly potent exotoxins are the clostridia of tetanus and botulism. The classical exotoxins have certain characteristic properties; they are thermolabile proteins of high molecular weight; purified preparations of tetanus and botulinal toxins are pharmacologically the most powerful poisons known to man. For example, 1·0 mg of tetanus or botulinal toxin is enough to kill more than one million guinea-pigs, and it is estimated that 3 kg of botulinal toxin could kill all the inhabitants of the world. However, the lethality of these exotoxins varies greatly for different animal species; diphtheria toxin is much more lethal for guinea-pigs, horses and man than for rats or mice; rabbits are 1000 times more susceptible to the Shiga bacillus 'neurotoxin' than are guinea-pigs.

The well documented exotoxins are produced mainly by Gram-positive bacteria (the Shiga bacillus neurotoxin and cholera enterotoxin are exceptions) and have affinities for specific tissues; for example, tetanus, botulinal and diphtheria toxins all affect different parts of the nervous system; tetanus toxin affects control mechanisms that govern the motor cells in the anterior columns of the spinal cord, botulinal toxin paralyses certain of the cranial motor nerves by blocking the transmission of effector messages from their endings, and diphtheria toxin has an affinity for peripheral nerve endings as well as for specialized tissues like heart muscle.

Exotoxins behave like enzymes and some have been identified as specific enzymes; for example, the α-toxin of *Clostridium welchii* is a phospholipase (lecithinase C) which acts on phospholipids in cell-membranes; diphtheria toxin inhibits cellular protein synthesis by interference with a transferase; and tetanus and botulinal toxins depress the formation and/or release of acetyl choline in different parts of the nervous system. Shiga neurotoxin, on the other hand, affects the CNS secondarily after a primary destructive action on the small blood vessels in the brain and spinal cord. The recently identified cholera enterotoxin induces excessive secretion of fluid into the small intestine without demonstrable damage to the intestinal mucosa. The exotoxin of the anthrax bacillus causes leakage of fluid through capillaries and shock.

Other important exotoxins react with phospholipids or other components of the surface membranes of cells and kill these cells either with or without lysis. The haemolytic, leucocidal and cytolytic toxins of pathogenic staphylococci, streptococci and clostridia are examples. Lysis of tissue cells makes extra nutrients available to the bacteria and killing of phagocytes protects the bacteria from phagocytosis.

Exotoxins, being proteins, are affected or destroyed by high temperature (e.g. 70° to 100°C), acid reaction and proteolytic enzymes. They are also affected by a variety of chemical reagents, the most important being formaldehyde which under suitable conditions partially denatures the toxin and so destroys its toxicity without affecting its antigenicity. This induced change converts the toxin to *toxoid* (*anatoxin* of French workers) which can then safely be used to produce specific *antitoxin* for active or passive protection against the lethal toxin.

Endotoxins. Toxins of a very different kind are released only after natural autolysis or artificial disruption of bacterial cells and are therefore called *endotoxins*. Typical endotoxins are particularly associated with Gram-negative bacteria (salmonellae, shigellae, escherichiae, neisseriae) and are distinguishable from exotoxins by the following properties: (1) they are an integral part of the outer layer of the bacterial cell wall (i.e. covering the rigid mucopeptide layer) and are complex phospholipid-polysaccharide-protein macromolecules; (2) they are heat-stable: (3) they are toxic but much less potent and less specific in their cytotoxic effects than exotoxins: (4) they are not convertible to toxoids: and (5) they are not rendered non-toxic when combined with homologous antibody. The complex molecule can be broken down by phenol extraction which separates a lipopolysaccharide moiety from the protein and most of the phospholipid fraction: the lipopolysaccharide can then be split into the polysaccharide fraction, containing various different sugars including those that determine the antigenic specificity of the endotoxin, and lipid A which is mainly responsible for the toxicity.

The specific antigenic character of the somatic (O) antigen of *smooth* (S) strains of Gram-negative bacteria is determined by the pattern of hexoses that compose peripheral O-specific polysaccharide chains attached to the endotoxic lipopolysaccharide molecule. Rough (R) strains, which commonly arise in the laboratory by mutation from the natural S strains, contain a lipopolysaccharide that lacks the O-specific chains but which, because it contains lipid A, is still fully toxic. Both 'smooth' and 'rough' lipopolysaccharides have an affinity for and tend to become incorporated in the lipoprotein membrane of tissue cells, e.g. leucocytes, platelets, vascular endothelium and RE phagocytes. They may exert their toxic effect by disturbing the function of these membranes.

Fever, or *pyrogenic effect,* is the toxic effect produced by the smallest doses of endotoxin. As little as $0.002\ \mu g$ endotoxin per kg body weight injected intravenously in a highly susceptible species such as rabbit or man, causes within 15 minutes an elevation of body temperature that lasts for several hours. The action of the endotoxin (an *exogenous pyrogen*) is to cause polymorph leucocytes, macrophages and perhaps other tissue cells to release a small molecular protein (*endogenous pyrogen*) which passes via the blood to, and acts on, the thermo-regulatory centre in the hypothalamus of the brain. If small pyrogenic doses of endotoxin are injected on several successive days, a state of *tolerance* to their effects is produced. Tolerance lasts for several days after the last injection and appears to be due to an induced enhancement of the power of the reticulo-endothelial (RE) system of phagocytes to remove endotoxin and other particulate matter from the blood. Single, larger doses of endotoxin have been shown to depress RE activity for the first few hours, apparently by damaging the phagocytes, but later, by 18 to 24 hours, to cause an enhancement of RE activity due to the multiplication of surviving phagocytes. This enhancement of RE activity is associated with a measure of increased non-specific resistance to a variety of bacterial infections.

The fever-inducing pyrogen sometimes found in fluid preparations used for therapeutic injections or intravenous therapy consists of endotoxin derived from saprophytic Gram-negative bacilli that have grown in small or large numbers in the water or other components of the preparation. Since this endotoxin is not inactivated by the autoclaving process used to sterilize infusion fluids, care must be taken to ensure the absence of bacterial contamination in their preparation, e.g. by the use of freshly distilled water and pure chemical ingredients and by thorough cleansing of glassware, etc. Care must also be taken to sterilize the fluid and protect it from subsequent contamination, as Gram-negative contaminants might readily multiply in the fluid during storage.

Endotoxic shock is caused by the intravenous injection of a large dose of endotoxin in experimental animals. It also occurs as a fatal, terminal condition in Gram-negative bacteriaemic infections in man. The LD50 of endotoxin for rabbits is in the range 1 to $100\ \mu g/kg$. The injected endotoxin causes vasomotor disturbances that within 4 to 18 hours bring about a drastic fall of blood pressure, collapse of the circulation and death. In the first few hours after the injection the animal shows fever, leucopenia and thrombocytopenia, and a marked intravascular deposition of fibrin, which is partly removed from the blood stream by the RE phagocytes. Later there is a leucocytosis and often there may be diarrhoea with blood-staining of the faeces. After death, there is often evidence of intravascular thrombosis and haemorrhagic necrosis, particularly in the intestinal mucosa.

Protein endotoxins. Whilst most endotoxins are lipopolysaccharides and share the toxic properties just described, a few Gram-negative pathogenic bacteria, e.g. *Pasteurella pestis* and *Bordetella pertussis* have been shown to produce an additional endotoxin that consists of protein, is present in the bacterial cytoplasm and has specific activities of a different kind from those of lipopolysaccharide.

Invasiveness

The other main attribute of pathogenic bacteria is invasiveness, that is, the capacity to invade and multiply in healthy tissues. The capacity of certain pathogens, such as the pneumococcus, to produce disease seems to depend almost entirely on this quality of invasiveness, just as that of the botulinus bacillus depends entirely on its toxigenicity, but most pathogenic bacteria usually possess in varying proportions both invasiveness and toxigenicity. Thus, the diphtheria bacillus must be initially invasive in order to establish itself in the tissues of the oropharynx where it manufactures its toxin; indeed, the greater virulence of *gravis* over *mitis* strains is probably related to the greater capacity of the former to invade and multiply in the tissues with a consequent greater production of toxin (see Chap. 21). *Strept. pyogenes* which is characteristically an invasive pathogen also produces an erythrogenic toxin which is responsible for the rash of scarlet fever. The production, moreover, of cytolytic and leucocidal toxins by organisms such as *Staph. aureus*, *Strept. pyogenes* and *Cl. welchii* contribute to their invasiveness by enabling them to breach tissue barriers and by protecting them against phagocytosis.

There are two categories of pathogenic bacteria that are predominantly invasive; (1) the pyogenic Gram-positive cocci initially attract phagocytes by chemotactic mechanisms but resist phagocytosis and are usually destroyed when they are ultimately engulfed by the phagocytes; (2) on the other hand, the tubercle, typhoid and brucella bacilli seem to be readily phagocytosed but are much more resistant to destruction when within the phagocyte; the latter become intracellular parasites and may depend to some extent on phagocytic mobility for their dissemination through the body. In infections with antiphagocytic bacteria, the fight between the parasite and the host is usually a short sharp affair, e.g. an attack of pneumococcal pneumonia, which when the outcome is favourable ends with a dramatic fall in temperature—the crisis—as specific antibodies acting as opsonins come to the aid of the phagocytes in destroying the invader. On the other hand, infection by intracellular parasites is often associated with a clinical illness that persists for some weeks with low fever before the patient recovers by a slow defervescence with a tendency to clinical relapses. The factors that determine whether the parasite or the host gains the upper hand in this kind of infection are not certainly known, but presumably the development of specific antibodies that facilitate intracellular destruction together with the appearance of phagocytes endowed with more actively bactericidal enzymes both play their part in the host's recovery. This is the field in which cell-mediated immunity is thought to be complementary to humoral defence mechanisms.

Capsules and pathogenicity. The role of capsules in conferring virulence on bacteria by enabling them to resist phagocytosis and bactericidal substances in body fluids is demonstrated by making comparative observations on capsulate and non-capsulate bacteria derived from the same strain. In this way, evidence has been obtained that capsulation is important for virulence in the pneumococcus, streptococci of groups A and C, the anthrax bacillus, the plague bacillus, *Klebsiella pneumoniae* and *Haemophilus influenzae*.

When a non-capsulate mutant or a decapsulated bacterium is injected into a laboratory animal that is highly susceptible to infection with the capsulate form, the non-capsulate strain is found to be non-virulent or, at least, much reduced in degree of virulence. For instance, in experiments in which group-C streptococci were injected intraperitoneally in mice, decapsulation of the cocci by the simultaneous injection of hyaluronidase decreased their virulence to the extent that their minimum lethal dose (MLD), i.e. the number of cocci that had to be injected to cause fatal infection, was *c.* 10 000 fold greater than that of the capsulate organisms. Similar results have been obtained in experiments with the type 3 pneumococcus decapsulated with an enzyme derived from a saprophytic bacillus.

Differences in virulence between the capsulate and non-capsulate forms of bacteria appear to be due mainly to differences in ability to resist capture and ingestion by phagocytes. Microscopical examination of smears of peritoneal exudate from infected animals shows that the non-capsulate bacteria are rapidly phagocytosed and, within a few hours, are mostly destroyed, whereas the capsulate bacteria remain free and soon multiply to large numbers. Similar differences in susceptibility to phagocytosis can be observed *in vitro* when capsulate and non-capsulate bacteria are added to normal blood, and smears show only phagocytosis when examined after the mixture has been incubated for $\frac{1}{2}$ to 1 hour. The mechanism of the anti-phagocytic property of capsulate bacteria is not known but it may be that the lipid-containing cell-membrane of the phagocyte's pseudopodia is inhibited from making contact with the hydrated capsule gel because of the surface charge. The shed excess capsular substance (specific soluble substance, or SSS) seems also to have a neutralizing effect on opsonin.

If the phagocytes and bacteria, instead of being suspended freely in fluid, are present on certain kinds of solid surfaces, e.g. on the wall of a lung alveolus or lymphatic vessel, or on a mass of fibrin, phagocytosis of capsulate organisms such as pneumococci may take place fairly readily. This *surface phagocytosis* occurs independently of the presence of specific opsonic antibodies and normal serum opsonins. When capsulate bacteria are exposed to specific antibodies and these combine with and coat the surface of the capsule, phagocytes can then capture, ingest and destroy the bacteria even when they are suspended freely in fluid and out of contact with a solid surface.

It must be emphasized that capsulation by itself does not necessarily confer resistance to phagocytosis and the property of virulence. Many harmless saprophytic bacteria are heavily capsulate, and certain non-virulent strains of the plague and anthrax bacilli are fairly sus-

ceptible to phagocytosis although they are capsulate.

Some pathogenic Gram-negative bacteria form outside their cell walls, a covering layer of acidic polysaccharide that is either not wide enough or not dense enough to be seen as a capsule. The Vi antigen of *Salmonella typhi* and the K antigens of many strains of *Escherichia coli* are of this type. There is evidence that the Vi and K antigens not only inhibit phagocytosis, but are also protective against the lytic attack of antibody and complement.

Other aggressins. Other protective or aggressive factors that are not toxins but may contribute to the ability of capsulate and non-capsulate pathogens to invade and multiply in the host's tissues include the following. (1) *Hyaluronidase,* or spreading factor, is an enzyme that dissolves the hyaluronic acid or cement-like substance that binds cells together and so allows pathogens like *Strept. pyogenes* to permeate through the tissues. But non-pathogenic bacteria and *Staph. aureus,* which characteristically causes localized lesions, also secrete hyaluronidase, and the pathogenicity of *Cl. welchii,* which produces hyaluronidase, is not affected by an anti-hyaluronidase serum. (2) *Coagulase,* a thrombin-like enzyme produced by all pathogenic staphylococci, may help to protect the pathogen in two ways: (a) by forming fibrin barriers around the staphylococci and the staphylococcal lesion and thus preventing phagocytosis, and (b) by inactivating a bactericidal substance present in normal blood serum. There is, however, some doubt about the validity of these claims. (3) *Fibrinolysin* or *kinase,* secreted by *Strept. pyogenes* (streptokinase) is invoked as a factor that may promote the spreading streptococcal lesion by breaking down barriers of fibrin deposited around areas of infected tissue; but again, the pathogenic staphylococci, although not associated with spreading lesions, also produce a fibrinolysin. (4) *Depolymerizing enzymes* such as mucinases, lipases, proteases, nucleases, are present in many pathogenic and non-pathogenic bacteria and may or may not contribute to virulence—some nucleases are very potent: *collagenase,* produced by *Cl. welchii,* may play some part in the pathogenesis of gas-gangrene; *neuraminidase,* a mucinase produced by many bacteria and viruses, catalyses the hydrolysis of mucoproteins at the cell surface and may facilitate attack on the cell.

Organotropism. An interesting but unexplained phenomenon associated with many pathogenic microbes is their affinity for specific tissues or organs (organotropism). Pneumococci and meningococci both have their natural habitat in the nasopharynx but the virulent pneumococcus has a predilection for lung tissue and the meningococcus for the serous membranes of the brain, whilst its cousin, the gonococcus, primarily affects genito-urinary mucous membranes. Experimental confirmation of this specific tissue affinity was demonstrated by Goodpasture and his colleagues (Goodpasture, 1938) in infected chick embryos; e.g. *Bordetella pertussis* attacked the bronchial mucosa only after ciliated epithelium developed on the 15th day of embryonic life; meningococci localized in the meninges; and *Streptobacillus moniliformis* (a causative organism in rat-bite fever in which arthritis is a feature) specifically attacked joint cavities. More knowledge of the nutritional requirements and of chemical substrates that specifically encourage the growth of pathogens will doubtless help to elucidate these tissue affinities. One such example is already known; the presence in the bovine placenta of erythritol, a growth factor for *Brucella abortus*, explains the localization of infection in this tissue in cows and the consequent occurrence of abortion. However *Cox. burnetii* and chlamydiae localize in the placenta but do not use erythritol. Both multiply in tissue that is essentially senile. An example of selective attack on the organs of one animal species and not on those of another is the development of multiple tubercles in the kidneys in rabbits but not in guinea-pigs after infection with the bovine tubercle bacillus, related presumably to the presence of the tuberculocidal polyamine, spermidine, in the guinea-pig kidney. Reference has already been made (Chapter 1) to another feature of many pathogens, viz. the characteristic pathological lesions they produce, related, in some part, to their tissue affinities; for example, the localization of the typhoid and tubercle bacilli in lymph-nodes with the production of a typically diagnostic pathology. The route of access of the pathogen to the host's tissues may determine the outcome; e.g. haemolytic streptococci or tetanus spores may produce dangerous infection if they are introduced through a skin wound but are likely to be harmless if swallowed.

VARIATION AND VIRULENCE

For many pathogenic bacteria, the maintenance of virulence requires frequent transfer of the pathogen from host to host. Virulence may often be enhanced by such frequent passage either naturally or artificially. Thus, it seems possible that scarlet fever became a dreaded infection with a high case fatality during the industrial revolution of the 18th and 19th centuries because of the population explosion resulting in overcrowding and poverty, and facilitating the rapid transfer of the haemolytic streptococcus; rheumatic fever as a sequel of streptococcal sore throat has a higher incidence (3 per cent) following cases of throat infection in crowded semi-closed communities such as army training camps where general outbreaks occur than in more dispersed populations where streptococcal infections occur more sporadically (0·1 to 0·3 per cent). Conditions that foster rapid transfer of infection presumably help to enhance the virulence or invasiveness of the streptococcus because, as long as there is an abundance of susceptible potential hosts, mutant forms of the bacterium will be selected that invade and multiply in the host more rapidly than the parental bacteria, and thus cause serious disease and the opportunity for rapid dissemination to further hosts. This phenomenon is illustrated experimentally when frequent mouse passage of a relatively avirulent, poorly capsulate pneumococcus sequentially exalts its virulence and quickly reduces the infecting dose from several hundreds to one or two capsulate cocci. Conversely, loss of virulence (attenuation) often occurs during the decline of an epidemic and during convalescence of a patient. The circumstances of the ending of an epidemic, when there is a scarcity of fresh susceptible hosts, are selective for mutant forms of the pathogen that are best suited to prolonged localized colonization of convalescent patients (carriers) and capable of avoiding elimination by the immune response. These mutant forms may be less virulent and invasive than the epidemic forms from which they were derived.

Virulence may be lost quickly during repeated culture of the pathogen on artificial culture medium. These conditions favour the selection of mutant forms of the organism capable of faster growth on the artificial medium than the parent form and these mutants may lack virulence factors that have no use except in the conditions of growth in the body. This loss of virulence is sometimes associated with changes in the colony appearance of the organism as in the classic examples of the *smooth→rough* (S→R) colonial variation in the salmonellae along with other changes such as to auto-agglutinability in saline, a form of S → R mutation may be demonstrated in the pneumococcus as a one-step mutation from the virulent capsulate to a non-capsulate variant so that after repeated subculture the rough variant, which grows more abundantly on the culture medium, becomes predominant. Similar genotypic S → R variation occurs with other capsulate bacteria. Another genotypic mutation concerns the toxigenicity of certain bacterial species, e.g. *Corynebacterium diphtheriae* and *Strept. pyogenes* which produce certain toxins only after being infected and rendered lysogenic with a temperate phage (see Chap. 7).

HOST FACTORS THAT CONTRIBUTE TO INFECTION

Various host factors affecting an individual or a community contribute to the occurrence of infection. Susceptibility is greatest in the very young and the very old, and this is related to inadequate cellular defences at the extremes of life (see Chap. 10). Malnutrition favours both a higher incidence and a greater severity of many infections, presumably for similar reasons, and is probably the major factor determining the high mortality from infections in poor communities (Scrimshaw *et al.*, 1959, 1968). Metabolic diseases like diabetes and hormonal upsets including those that accompany corticosteroid therapy predispose to infection. Haematological disorders such as leukaemia and drug-induced granulocytopenia, immunological deficiencies,

neoplasia and renal disease may all reduce host resistance to infection. In infections with some well-capsulated bacteria, e.g. pneumococci and klebsiellae, and in candida infections, there may be little or no mobilization of the host defences — a kind of silent invasion due, in part at least, to poor host resistance to pathogens that ordinarily are not highly invasive against healthy tissues.

Many nosocomial (hospital-acquired) infections are caused by opportunist organisms like staphylococci and Gram-negative bacilli attacking localized sites of lowered resistance; for example, the incidence of post-operative sepsis which is highest after gall-bladder, breast and upper abdominal operations and lowest after orthopaedic surgery, is affected by such host factors as age, obesity, size of wound and wound drainage, duration of operation and length of stay before and after operation. Tissue trauma and anaesthesia associated with surgery also upset host physiology. Foreign bodies like sutures, indwelling bladder catheters, tracheostomy tubes and cardiovascular prostheses considerably increase the risk of infection.

Antecedent diseases of particular tissues and systems lower resistance to infection, e.g. chronic skin diseases like eczema with superinfection by such viruses as the vaccinia and herpes viruses and psoriasis, chronic bronchitis and bronchiectasis, rheumatic heart disease, arteriosclerosis and paralytic diseases. Among the so-called iatrogenic diseases, the use of antimicrobial drugs, particularly the broad-spectrum antibiotics, upsets the normal bacterial flora and allows opportunistic organisms like candida and staphylococcus to invade and infect areas like the mouth and intestine which are deprived of their protective indigenous bacteria. Again, as a sequel to infection, toxic endogenous substances released from necrotic tissues, perhaps related to intravascular thrombosis, may contribute to the illness of the host.

Among community factors that may affect host resistance are the complex components of poverty (overcrowding, inadequate food, clothing and housing, hypothermia and poor personal hygiene); immigration and population movements including those in tourist camps; drug addiction and alcoholism; and large scale disasters (earthquakes, hurricanes, floods, etc.).

SOURCES OF INFECTION FOR MAN

The epidemiology of an infective disease depends to an important extent on the nature and distribution of the sources of infection. The term *source* of infection applies to the normal growth habitat of the microbe, e.g. a site in the body of the human or animal host. Objects contaminated with live but temporarily inactive microbes may act as, and should be called *vehicles* or *reservoirs* of infection, not sources of infection. Human disease may be acquired by mechanisms of *exogenous infection* from outside sources, e.g. from human patients with clinical infections, healthy human carriers of the pathogenic microorganism, animals with apparent or inapparent infection, or the soil. When the source of a clinical infection is within the patient's own body, the infection is said to be *endogenous*.

Exogenous Infection

1. *Patients.* Infections due to some microbial species are acquired mainly or exclusively from ill persons with active or manifest infection, e.g. pulmonary tuberculosis (human-type bacilli), leprosy, whooping-cough, syphilis, gonorrhoea, measles, smallpox, mumps and influenza. Some cases of the infection may be mild or atypical, and escape recognition as a source of danger, but healthy carriers of the diseases specified above are non-existent or so rare as to be unimportant. The life history and pattern of spread of the pathogen may be represented as being through a series of clinically diseased human patients (P) thus:

$$P \to P \to P \to P \to P \to P \to P \to$$

If the pathogen can be quickly eliminated by antimicrobial drugs, infections of this kind should be amenable to control, or even eradication, by the systematic practice of early diagnosis followed by isolation and/or antimicrobial therapy. This is currently the aim of the campaigns to control tuberculosis, syphilis, yaws and gonorrhoea by chemotherapy.

2. *Healthy carriers.* Many pathogenic species that typically cause overt disease are able to produce in certain individuals a limited or subclinical infection that is insufficient to give rise to the signs and symptoms of illness. Persons having such an inapparent infection are commonly capable of disseminating the causative microbes to other persons; they are then termed 'carriers' and constitute an unsuspected and thus especially dangerous source of infection. Some infectious diseases are contracted from carriers as frequently as, or even much more frequently than from patients, e.g. streptococcal, staphylococcal, pneumococcal and meningococcal infections, diphtheria, typhoid fever, bacillary dysentery and poliomyelitis. *Convalescent carriers* are persons in whom a limited, localized infection continues for a period of weeks or months after clinical recovery from a manifest infection. Other carriers suffer no more than subclinical infection from the time of first acquiring the pathogen; those of them who acquire the pathogen from a patient are termed *contact carriers* and those who acquire it asymptomatically from another carrier are termed *paradoxical carriers*. If carriage persists for more than an arbitrary period of time, e.g. one year in the case of typhoid infection, the person is called a *chronic carrier*.

In some carrier-borne infections, e.g. typhoid fever and bacillary dysentery, the number of carriers in a community in which the infection is epidemic may be either smaller than, or not much greater than the number of clinically ill patients, and the pathogen may be envisaged as spreading through a series of patients (P), convalescent carriers (PC) and contact or paradoxical carriers (C) thus:

$$C \to P \to PC \to P \to C \to PC \to P \to P \to C \to$$

In other carrier-borne infections, such as those due to the pyogenic cocci and the diphtheria bacillus, it is likely that the carriers in a community with endemic infection will greatly outnumber the clinically ill patients. A carrier: case ratio of about 50:1 has been estimated for *Strept. pyogenes* and the diphtheria bacillus in certain studies, and the carrier:case ratio for meningococcal infections may be much higher. Under these circumstances it is to be expected that many more infections will be acquired from carriers than from patients, and the spread of such pathogens may be shown thus:

$$C \to C \to C \to C \to P \to C \to C \to PC \to C \to$$

Infections of the kind that are mainly contracted from unrecognized healthy carriers are relatively insusceptible to control by isolation or treatment of the clinically ill persons, because these patients are only a minority of the potential sources of infection. Detection of carriers by microbiological tests and their isolation or treatment is not practicable if they are very numerous, as for instance the carriers of *Staph. aureus* who make up 30 to 40 per cent of an institutional community such as the medical and nursing staff in a hospital.

3. *Infected animals.* Some pathogens that are primarily parasites of a different animal species may in appropriate circumstances spread from the infected animal to man and so cause human disease. Such infections are called *zoonoses*. The pattern of spread of the pathogen through infected animals (A) and occasionally to man (P) as an 'end-host' in a zoonosis may be shown thus:

$$A \to A \to A \to A \to A \to A \to A \to A \to A \to A \to$$
$$\searrow P \qquad\qquad \searrow P$$

The control of these infections depends either on eradication of infection in the animals or on interruption of the means of communication of the pathogen from animals to man. Infections normally acquired from animals include bovine-type tuberculosis, salmonella food-poisoning, bubonic plague, anthrax, brucellosis, leptospiral jaundice, rabies and psittacosis. In these infections man is generally an end-host and there is rarely any secondary spread from the patient to other persons or back to animals. Exceptions are the man-to-man spread of pneumonic plague which may supervene on bubonic plague contracted by men from rodents, and arbovirus infections such as yellow fever in which man-to-man spread (urban yellow fever) may supervene on infection of man from an animal host (jungle yellow fever from monkeys).

4. *Soil.* A few infective diseases of man are caused by saprophytic microbes derived from the soil, vegetation and similar habitats, e.g. tetanus, gas-gangrene, maduromycosis and sporotrichosis. The main habitat of some of these opportunistic pathogens, e.g. *Cl. tetani* and *Cl. welchii* which are found as saprophytes in the soil, may be the intestines of animals from which they enter the soil in faecal droppings. The soil-derived infections are not infectious from one man to another.

Endogenous Infections

In the above examples, the infection is described as *exogenous*, i.e. from a source outside the body of the person becoming infected. In contrast, *endogenous* infection may occur in carriers of potentially pathogenic organisms when these previously harmless bacteria invade other surfaces or tissues in the carrier, e.g. *Escherichia coli* derived from the bowel, where it is harmless, may cause acute suppurative infection in the urinary tract; *Staph. aureus* from the nostrils may cause a boil in the skin or infection in a wound; and pneumococci from the naso-pharynx may cause bronchitis and broncho-pneumonia. The source of endogenous infection is thus the site in the patient's body (e.g. colon, skin or nasopharynx) where the organism grows harmlessly as a commensal. An infection that is commonly endogenous, as for instance staphylococcal sepsis of skin and wounds, may in certain circumstances become transmissible, as in hospital, where conditions may favour cross-infection between patients. Thus the cross-infected patients suffer exogenous infections. In general, however, patients with endogenous infections caused by organisms of low virulence are not likely to infect other persons, e.g. patients with bronchopneumonia due to pneumococci of the less virulent serotypes are not a danger to relatives, nurses or other patients, and there is no need to isolate them from other patients in hospital.

MODES OF SPREAD OF INFECTION

Some infections, e.g. respiratory and intestinal, can spread from host to host by a variety of mechanisms, whilst others, e.g. venereal and arthropod-borne blood infections, are normally transmitted by a single mechanism for which the parasite is specially adapted.

1. **Respiratory infections.** The causative microbes are mainly disseminated into the environment in masses of infected secretion, e.g. secretion transferred from the nose or

mouth on fingers, handkerchief, cups or spoons, or secretion expelled in spitting or blowing the nose; they are also discharged to a less extent in the droplet spray produced by sneezing, coughing and speaking, but hardly any are disseminated in normal breathing (Fig. 8.2).

Handkerchiefs, clothing, bedding, floors, furniture and household articles (fomites) become contaminated with the secretion and may act as vehicles or reservoirs of infection. The secretion dries and becomes pulverized into dust. When dried in dust, most kinds of respiratory microbes may remain alive for several days, and some even for several months if shielded from direct daylight, e.g. tubercle bacilli, diphtheria bacilli, streptococci, staphylococci and smallpox virus. Infection may therefore be passed to the recipient by contact, either (a) *direct contact,* i.e. touching of bodies as in handshaking, kissing and contact of clothing, or (b) *indirect contact,* involving an inanimate vehicle of infection, e.g. eating utensils, door handles, towels, and other fomites; the recipient may finally transfer the microbes with his fingers into his nose or mouth.

Infection may be *dust-borne* and take place by inhalation of air-borne infected dust particles. Very large numbers of such particles are liberated into the air from the skin and clothing during normal body movements, also from the dried parts of an infected handkerchief during its use, from bedclothes in bedmaking, from the floor when it is walked upon or swept, and from furniture during dusting. The larger infected particles settle within a few minutes on to the floor and other exposed surfaces, e.g. skin, clothing, wounds and surgical supplies. The smaller infected particles remain air-borne for up to 1 to 2 hours and may be inhaled into the recipient's nose, throat, bronchi or lung alveoli (Fig. 8.1). Air-borne infection is mainly a danger within the room of its origin; spread to other rooms in the same building is usually slight, though it may occur if the ventilating or convectional air currents move in the appropriate direction.

Droplet spray constitutes a third means of spread of respiratory infection. It is probably the least important means, except perhaps in the case of the pathogens that are rapidly killed by drying, e.g. meningococcus, whooping-cough bacillus and measles and common cold viruses.

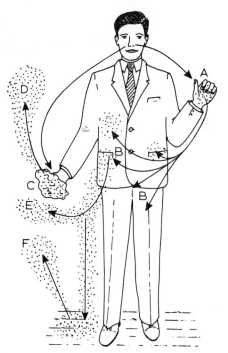

FIG. 8.1. Diagram showing infection of the air with dust particles derived from nasal and oral secretions contaminating hands, handkerchief, clothing and surrounding surfaces. A. Hand soiled with saliva and/or sputum from lips or nose-picking. B. Clothing contaminated by hand. C. Handkerchief soiled with dried nasal secretion, saliva or sputum. D. Infected dust from handkerchief. E. Infected dust from clothing (e.g. from near handkerchief pocket). F. Infected dust raised again into the air after settling on floor.

Sneezing, coughing, speaking and other forceful expiratory activities expel a spray of droplets derived almost exclusively from the saliva of the anterior mouth; this may be infected with small numbers of pathogenic microbes from the nose, throat or lungs. Very many droplets are expelled, but only a few are infected. The *large droplets,* those over 0·1 mm in diameter, fly forwards and downwards from the mouth to the distance of a few feet; they reach the floor within a few seconds, or bespatter the body surfaces, including the eyes, face, mouth and clothing, of persons standing immediately in front of the producer of the spray; but they probably cannot be inhaled. The *small droplets,* those under 0·1 mm in diameter, evaporate immediately to become minute solid residues, or 'droplet-nuclei' (mainly 1 to 10 μm in diameter), which remain air-borne in the manner of infected dust particles and may be inhaled into the nose, throat or lungs. It is thought that very few of the droplet-nuclei are likely to be infected with pathogenic microbes, but it is possible that certain virus infections are commonly spread by the larger droplet-nuclei, e.g. measles, chicken-pox and dog distemper (Fig. 8.2).

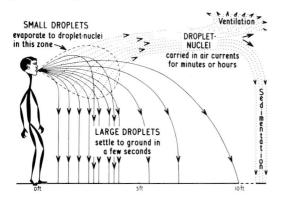

FIG. 8.2. Spread of respiratory infections by droplets and droplet-nuclei.

Because it is a spectacular mechanism which seems specially appropriate for the transmission of respiratory infections, there is a widespread tendency to overestimate the importance of droplet spray and, indeed, wrongly to regard it as *the* mode of spread of respiratory infections. Unfortunately, there is a general lack of evidence about the relative efficacy of contact, dust and droplets in spreading the different respiratory pathogens. The fullest observations have been made in the case of tuberculosis and for this infection the evidence strongly indicates that air-borne dried sputum particles are the main vehicle of infection. Chaussé, for instance, showed that many more infections were produced among guinea-pigs exposed to sputum-dust liberated into the air by shaking a patient's handkerchief than among guinea-pigs exposed to the spray of many coughs given by a highly infective patient. It is very convenient but very misleading to describe a respiratory infection as being 'spread by droplets'; it should be described as being 'spread by contact, secretion dust or secretion droplets'.

2. **Skin, wound and burn infections.** These superficial infections may be acquired by contact with infected hands, clothing or other articles, by exposure to sedimentation of infected air-borne dust or by contamination with droplet spray. Pathogenic streptococci and staphylococci derived from the respiratory tract are important causes of wound and burn infections.

3. **Venereal infections.** The venereal diseases are so-called because they are transmitted almost exclusively by sexual contact. An important reason for this limitation is that the causative organisms, e.g. *Trep. pallidum* and *N. gonorrhoeae*, are extremely susceptible to the lethal effects of drying and those of the other conditions encountered on potential vehicles whereby infection might be transmitted less directly than by intimate bodily contact. In urbanized and developed communities, therefore, the spirochaete of syphilis causes only the venereal form of syphilis. In less developed communities with low standards of hygiene, on the other hand, the spirochaete may be frequently spread by non-venereal means, e.g. by the use of common drinking vessels which carry the organism from the mouth of an individual with oral lesions to the mouths of others. This non-venereal, or *endemic*, syphilis commonly infects children, who thus become immune to reinfection before they reach the age of sexual activity. In a similar way, under unhygienic conditions of institutional living with communal use of towels and bathing facilities, the gonococcus has sometimes spread non-venereally in young girls and caused epidemics of vulvovaginitis.

4. **Alimentary tract infections.** Here, pathogenic microbes are discharged in the faeces of infected persons and are transmitted in various ways, the so-called *faecal-oral routes*, leading to their ingestion by the recipient. Most intestinal pathogens are poorly resistant to drying; they tend to die within a period of hours, though they may rarely survive on cloth or in dust for several days. They are more likely to be spread by moist vehicles such as water or food, in which they may survive for up to several weeks (e.g. typhoid and dysentery organisms). (a) *Water-borne infection* may occur when excreta contaminate a supply of water, e.g. a river or well, which is used, without purification, for drinking or culinary purposes. Water is a common vehicle of infection in those intestinal diseases, e.g. typhoid and cholera, for which the infecting dose may be small. Purification of

water rendering it non-infective is carried out on a large scale by storage, filtration and chlorination. Small amounts of water for drinking may be treated by boiling or by the addition of hypochlorite tablets. (b) *Hand infection*. A carrier tends to contaminate his hands with bacteria contained in traces of faeces that pass through moist or broken toilet paper; nurses may infect their hands in attending patients and in touching bed-pans. Such persons may handle and contaminate foodstuffs, eating utensils, wash-hand basins, baths, towels, door handles and other fomites. A recipient may eat or put into his mouth the contaminated foodstuffs or utensils, or he may pick up the microbes on his fingers and then transfer them into his mouth. (c) *Food-borne infection* may occur through a carrier handling the food, through preparation of the food in utensils infected by handling or washing in infected water, or through flies alighting on the food after feeding on exposed infected faeces. Conditions enabling growth of the bacteria and the production of enterotoxins in the contaminated food are prerequisites for 'bacterial food-poisoning', though not for 'food-borne infection', which may result from the ingestion of only a few pathogenic micro-organisms, e.g. in bacillary dysentery.

5. **Arthropod-borne blood infections.** In several systemic infections the causative microbes are abundantly present in the blood and are spread to other individuals by blood-sucking arthropods such as the mosquito (malaria, yellow fever), flea (plague), louse (epidemic typhus fever, European relapsing fever), tick (Rocky Mountain spotted fever, West African relapsing fever), mite (scrub typhus) and tsetse fly (trypanosomiasis). The parasite is adapted to multiply in, and be spread by, its particular arthropod vector and is rarely transmitted by any other means. Its adaptation to this method of spread includes its special ability to cause heavy, and often prolonged or relapsing infection of the blood of its human or animal host.

6. **Laboratory infections.** Laboratory workers occasionally become infected from artificial cultures or from infected diagnostic or necropsy materials collected from patients or experimental animals. Some organisms are especially liable to cause laboratory infections, e.g. the brucellae, rickettsiae and *Pasteurella tularensis*,

whilst others require to be handled with special care, e.g. tubercle bacillus, anthrax bacillus, freshly isolated typhoid and dysentery bacilli, pathogenic leptospires and borreliae, the psittacosis organism and the serum hepatitis virus. Especial danger attaches to the pipetting of infected liquids by mouth, leading to their accidental ingestion; an automatic pipette or a pipette fitted with a rubber teat or a mouth-piece containing two cotton-wool filters should be used for pipetting cultures and exudates. Accidental self-inoculation with a syringe may take place or the conjunctiva may be sprayed when the needle becomes loosened from a syringe during an injection. Many laboratory procedures atomize liquids and so may contaminate the air with infected droplet-nuclei, e.g. the expulsion of liquid from a pipette or syringe, the shaking of liquid in an open vessel, the use of mechanical blenders, the centrifugation of tubes bearing traces of liquid on their rim, and the breaking of liquid films as when a wetted stopper or a screw-cap is removed from a bottle or a drop is separated from an inoculating loop. When working with dangerous pathogens which are liable to cause airborne infection, such as the tubercle bacillus, it is recommended that all procedures be carried out within a specially ventilated 'protective cabinet' or 'ino-lation hood'.

For further discussion on the spread of infections in the community and within hospitals, see Vol. II, Chapter 16.

FURTHER READING

GOODPASTURE, E. W. (1938) Some uses of the chick embryo for the study of infection and immunity. *American Journal of Hygiene,* **28,** 111.

MUDD, S. (1970) *Infectious Agents and Host Reactions,* London: W. B. Saunders.

SCRIMSHAW, N. S., TAYLOR, C. E. & GORDON, J. E. (1959) Interactions of nutrition and infection. *American Journal of Medical Science,* 237, 367.

SCRIMSHAW, N. S., TAYLOR, C. E. & GORDON, J. E. (1968) *Interactions of Nutrition and Infection,* Geneva: W.H.O. Monograph Series No. 57.

SMITH, H. & PEARCE, J. H. (1972) *Microbial Pathogenicity in Man and Animals: Symposium 22 of Society of General Microbiology: London.* Cambridge University Press.

WEINBAUM, G., KADIS, S. & AJL, J. T. (1971) Microbial Toxins. In *Bacterial Endotoxins,* Vols 4 and 5, New York and London: Academic Press.

WILLIAMS, R. E. O., BLOWERS, R., GARROD, L. P. & SHOOTER, R. A. (1966) *Hospital Infection,* 2nd Edn. London: Lloyd-Luke.

9. Immunological Principles: Antigens, Antibodies and Antigen-antibody Reactions

An antigen is a substance capable of provoking the lymphoid tissues of an animal to respond by an immune reaction specifically directed at the inducing substance and not at other unrelated substances. The specificity of the response for chemical groupings—*antigenic determinants*—of the antigen molecule is an important characteristic. The reaction of an animal to contact with antigen—called the *acquired immune response* takes two forms (1) the *humoral or circulating antibody response* and (2) the *cell-mediated response,* and their characteristics are described in Chapter 10. Most of the information available on the specificity of the immune response comes from studies of the interaction of circulating antibody with antigen. An antibody directed against an *antigenic determinant* of a particular molecule will react only with this determinant or another very similar structure. Even minor chemical changes in the determinant with the resulting change in shape will markedly reduce the ability of antibody to the original structure to react with the altered material.

The term antigen, referring to substances capable of acting as stimulants of the immune response or reacting with antibody is used rather loosely by immunologists. Use is made of the functional classification of antigens into substances which are able (1) to stimulate *de novo* an immune response and are termed *immunogens* and (2) substances incapable of this but able to react with antibody formed to the substance attached to a carrier molecule which converts the material into an immunogen. Such substances are often low molecular weight chemicals or groupings and are termed *haptens.*

A common source of confusion with respect to the specificity of antibodies arises when an antibody to a particular antigen is found to be capable of combining with an apparently unrelated antigen. This raises the need to distinguish clearly between the structural specificity of an antigenic determinant and its distribution specificity. For example, the ubiquitous nature of the glucose molecule—present in many different types of macromolecule—must be distinguished from its specific chemical structure. An immune response against a glucose determinant in antigen A–G would be likely to react also with the glucose group in antigen B–G provided the two determinants were equally accessible. The antibody directed against the glucose determinant is not a non-specific type of antibody but is simply reacting with an identical chemical determinant in another antigen molecule.

A typical cross reaction is with pneumococcal polysaccharide type S8 which has a tetra-saccharide repeating unit containing cellobiuronic acid alternating with an isomer of lactose. Antisera to the polysaccharide cross reacts with oxidized cotton cellulose containing cellobiuronic residues. In laboratory practice cross reactions are a frequent source of difficulty and cross reactivity is often found between antisera to certain bacterial antigens and antigens present in cells such as erythrocytes. Antigens shared in this way are known as *heterophile antigens.* Antisera to such antigens will cross react with cell or fluids of different species of animal and with various microorganisms. The chemical determinants responsible for this cross reactivity are not known but are presumed to be similar or identical groupings possibly of muco-polysaccharide and lipid nature present in larger molecules which are part of the structure of the cells. The best known of the heterophile antigens is the Forssman antigen which is present in the red cells of many species as well as in bacteria such as pneumococci and salmonellae. Another heterophile antigen is found in *Escherichia coli* and human red cells of group B.

Chemical Nature of Antigens

Antigens are commonly classified as proteins, polysaccharides or lipids; this is however an oversimplified view since besides antigenic molecules of entirely protein, polysaccharide or lipid nature carbohydrate moieties frequently act as determinants of protein or lipid macromolecules or peptide units act as determinants on polysaccharide molecules.

The unravelling of the specific determinants of antigenicity of macromolecules has largely defied the efforts of immunochemists. So little information is available about the precise nature of the peptides acting as determinants in different protein molecules that immunologists still describe antigens in terms of the whole molecule, e.g. human serum albumin (HSA) rather than the individual determinants of specificity within the macromolecules.

ANTIGENIC DETERMINANTS

Degradation, Chemical Modification and Synthesis of Determinants

The number of determinants (sometimes referred to as its valency) in a molecule like bovine serum albumin (BSA) is probably in excess of 18 although only about six of these are exposed in the native intact molecule. The other (hidden) determinants can be identified only when the molecule is broken down by, for example, enzyme hydrolysis. Antibody produced in response to injection of the whole molecule is apparently able to react with the fragments produced by hydrolysis, which indicates that the molecule is broken down into similar fragments after injection, due possibly to the action of the digestive enzymes in phagocytic cells.

Attempts to identify the chemical nature of antigenic determinants have used this type of degradation procedure with some degree of success and some insight has been gained into the size and other features of the determinants. Two other approaches have also been used— chemical modification of known determinants and synthesis of polyaminoacid and polysaccharide antigens.

Degradation studies have been carried out on silk fibroin, a linear polypeptide chain of molecular weight between 50 000 and 60 000. The determinant site capable of reacting with antibody appears to consist of between eight and twelve amino acids (2·7 to 4·4 nm) with the C terminal tyrosine making a considerable contribution to the site. The important role of tyrosine is further supported by the finding that the poorly antigenic gelatin can be made antigenic by the addition of tyrosine in which the native molecule is very deficient, and which may confer rigidity on the gelatin molecule.

The protein coat of tobacco mosaic virus consists of identical subunits (approx. 2000) each with a molecular weight of about 16 500 consisting of 158 amino acids. The antigenic determinant site is present in the chain between position 108 and 112 and unlike fibroin contains no aromatic amino acids. The hydrophobic nature of leucine appears to be an important characteristic of their particular determinant site.

Some insight into the nature of the antigenic determinants of proteins has come from the studies of Sela in Israel. Synthetic polypeptide branched structures were built up with a non-antigenic backbone of polyalanine and polylysine to which were added amino acids such as tyrosine and glutamic acid (Fig. 9.1). Provided that these amino acids were attached at the outer ends of the branches they acted as antigenic determinants conferring antigenicity on the branched structure. If on the other hand the amino acids were attached at the inner ends of the branches as shown in the figure (Fig. 9.1) the complex remained non-antigenic.

A better understanding exists of the chemical nature of the antigenic determinants of blood group antigens. The blood group substances are mainly complex polysaccharides with polypeptides making up about 25 per cent of the molecule and these polysaccharides give their specificity to groups at the ends of the carbohydrate chains. Human blood group A substance for example owes its specificity to α-N-acetylgalactosaminoyl—(1–3)–galactose. The polysaccharide antigens of the coli-salmonella group present another situation in which the determinants of antigenic specificity have been defined. Specific sugars have been identified

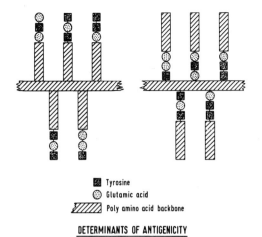

Tyrosine
Glutamic acid
Poly amino acid backbone

DETERMINANTS OF ANTIGENICITY

FIG. 9.1. The amino acids, tyrosine and glutamic acid can convert a non-antigenic polyamino acid branched structure (polyalanine and polylysine) into an antigen provided they are attached to the outer end of the branches (left); if attached at the inner end of the branches (right) the complex is not antigenic.

which play an important role in determining the specificity of the antigens and are important in determining the serological classification of the group in the Kauffmann-White scheme.

Transplantation or histocompatibility antigens present in the surface and internal membranous structures of tissue cells are likely to be similar to the blood group antigens and are probably glycoproteins associated with lipids. Although important in transplantation immunology their detailed chemical nature has yet to be unravelled. Antigens of the cell walls of bacteria such as streptococci, staphylococci, corynebacteria, etc. are rather less well-defined and appear to be complex mucopeptides sometimes associated with lipids. Capsulated microorganisms such as pneumococci have complex high molecular weight polysaccharides in their capsules; the chemical structure of these polysaccharides is not fully known, but similar structural units are present in blood group substances.

GENERAL PROPERTIES OF ANTIGENS

A substance that acts as an antigen in one species of animal may not do so in another because it is represented in the tissues or fluids of the second species. This underlines the requirement that an antigen must be a foreign substance to elicit an immune response; for example, egg albumin, whilst an excellent antigen in the rabbit, fails to induce an antibody response in the fowl. The more foreign a substance is to a particular species the more likely it is to be a powerful antigen. A good antigen need not contain different building blocks, e.g. amino acids of a protein, but their arrangement should be such that at least part of the surface of the molecule presents a configuration which is unfamiliar to the animal. Since macromolecules have a three dimensional structure, it is easy to visualize how they could become unfolded by denaturation so as to present new and unique surface arrangements. For example, RNAase molecules after oxidation become unfolded and the change in shape prevents the interaction of the molecule with antibody to native RNAase.

A widely recognized requirement for a substance to be antigenic in its own right without having to be attached to a carrier molecule is that it should have a molecular weight in excess of 5000. It is possible to induce an immune response to substances of lower molecular weight, for example glucagon of mol. wt. 3800, but this can only be achieved if special measures are taken such as the use of an antigen adjuvant (Chapters 10 and 58) which gives an additional stimulus to the immune system. Very large proteins such as the crustacean respiratory pigment haemocyanin are very powerful antigens, and are widely used in experimental immunology. Polysaccharides vary in antigenicity, for example dextran of mol. wt. 600 000 is a good antigen, whereas a dextran of mol. wt. 100 000 is not. Yet the two materials are made up of identical building blocks and do not differ as far as the type of antigenic determinant is concerned.

Some low molecular weight chemical substances appear to contradict the need that an antigen be a large molecule. Among these are included picryl chloride, formaldehyde, drugs such as aspirin, penicillin and sulphonamides. These substances are highly antigenic particularly if applied to the skin. The reason for this appears to be that such materials form complexes by means of covalent bonds with tissue protein and the complex of these substances,

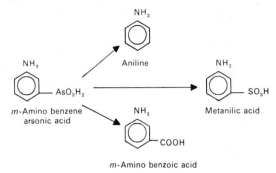

FIG. 9.2. Rabbit antisera to azoproteins containing any of the above acid radicals as antigenic determinants react only with the inducing azoprotein and not with any of the others. Even azoproteins obtained by changing the COOH of *m*-amino benzoic acid or the $-SO_3H$ of metanilic acid to the ortho or para positions do not react with antisera to the original determinant. Methyl and halogen radicals substituted in the benzene ring instead of the acid radicals shown in the figure are less effective as determinants of specificity and considerable cross reactions are found in precipitin tests.

acting as haptens, with a tissue protein carrier forms a complete antigen. This phenomenon has important implication in the development of certain types of hypersensitivity (Chap. 11).

Antigenic Specificity

Foreignness of a substance to an animal can depend on chemical groupings which are not normally present in the animal's environment. Arsenic acid, for example, can be introduced by diazotization into a protein molecule, and, as a hapten, acts as a determinant of antigenic specificity of the molecule. This type of chemically defined determinant enabled Karl Landsteiner early in this century to study antigenic specificity in fine detail. By slight chemical modifications of the antigenic determinant he was able to demonstrate how critical and precise was the fit between antibody and an antigenic determinant. Thus, changes as minor as the replacement in the benzene ring of the AsO_3H_2 group by a COOH or a SO_3H group were sufficient to affect substantially the ability of the determinant to react with antibody to the original hapten (Fig. 9.2).

Further evidence for the high degree of specificity comes from Landsteiner's studies on the ability of antibody against the various isomers of tartaric acid (linked to a carrier protein) to react with the different isomeric forms of the antigen. Rabbit antibody against, for example, *laevo*-tartaric acid whilst giving a heavy precipitate with the inducing antigen would not precipitate *dextro*-tartaric acid antigen and would only form a slight precipitate with *meso*-tartaric acid.

There are many other examples which have validated Landsteiner's classical studies including experiments with simple sugars coupled to proteins. The antisera produced by immunizing animals were found to be able to distinguish between glucose and galactose differing only by the interchange of H and OH on one carbon atom.

The ability of antibody to form a strong bond with an antigen depends on intermolecular forces which act strongly only when the two molecules come together in a very precise manner. The better the fit the stronger the bond. An antibody molecule directed against a particularly shaped antigenic determinant might be able to react with another similar but not quite identical determinant as shown in Fig. 9.3. This type of cross reaction occurs but the strength of the bond between the two molecules will be diminished in the case of the non-identical determinant.

It was concluded from studies of this type (a) that acidic and basic groups are very important in regulating the specificity of an antigenic determinant; (b) that spatial configuration of haptens is important; (c) that terminal groups in

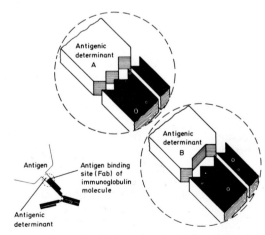

FIG. 9.3. Diagrammatic view of cross reaction with antigen B between antigen-binding site of antibody to antigen A.

an antigen are often important determinants of specificity, and (d) that interchange of non-ionic groups of similar size had little effect on specificity of a determinant.

THE IMMUNOGLOBULINS

The recognition towards the end of the 19th century by Von Behring and Kitasato in Berlin, that the blood-serum of an appropriately immunized animal contained specific neutralizing substances or antitoxins able to inactivate tetanus and diphtheria toxins, was the first demonstration of the activity of what is now known to be an antibody or immunoglobulin. This substance is induced as a consequence of the response of an animal's lymphoid tissues to the antigen and is specific for the inducing antigen. Thus diphtheria antitoxin has no effect on tetanus toxin and *vice versa*. Very shortly after the discovery of antitoxins, Pfeiffer using the cholera vibrio showed that the microorganisms themselves, not just their toxins, could be destroyed by serum from an immune animal. This observation was soon followed by the recognition of clumping or agglutination of microorganisms and of the precipitation of soluble antigens by the serum of immunized animals. The clinical application of the agglutination reaction in the diagnosis of enteric fever was made by Widal in 1896 utilizing the specificity of antibodies for their inducing antigen. The injection of antiserum for therapeutic purposes from an immune individual or immunized animal to a non-immune patient led to widespread use of serotherapy in bacterial infections but with the advent of antibiotics this form of treatment is largely restricted to the use of antitoxins.

Besides its important role in clinical medicine immunology bears directly on some very fundamental biological problems; for example, the nature of the mechanisms by which cells and molecules recognize one another, the way an animal maintains its cell population free from undesirable mutants; the manner in which genes are expressed in higher organisms, and the origin of diversity in the structure of protein molecules. An understanding of these problems requires knowledge of the structure of antibodies and the relationship of structure to function of the molecules.

Enormous advances have been made in the last decade in knowledge of the chemical structure of immunoglobulins and the relationships of the structure to the biological activities of the molecule. As a result immunologists have agreed internationally on a nomenclature that distinguishes a number of different classes of immunoglobulin based on structural rather than functional characteristics. It was the practice to refer to an antibody as an agglutinin, or as a neutralizing or a precipitating antibody without knowing that each of these activities could be exhibited by a chemically heterogeneous population of molecules and could be shared by the same molecule. Other classifications were dependent on the behaviour of the molecules in electrophoresis which did little more than split the population up into still heterogeneous proteins differing only in their overall charge and molecular size.

Methods have been developed for the fragmentation of the immunoglobulin molecule by chemical cleavage in Edelman's laboratory, and by pepsin digestion by Nisonoff in the United States. Porter in Britain, using pepsin digestion, was the first to achieve cleavage with retention of biological activity of the fragments. These studies gave impetus to the work that has enabled immunologists to distinguish five main classes of immunoglobulin each based on a similar polypeptide chain structure consisting of two pairs of 'heavy' and 'light' chains joined by disulphide bonds, sometimes occurring as multiples of this basic unit.

It is considered that the molecule is based on a 12-unit structure, each unit consisting of a polypeptide chain with 110 amino acids of mol. wt. 12 000. Most primitive vertebrates appear to have fully developed heavy and light chains. By partial gene duplication a gene capable of coding for a complete light chain evolved and similarly genes evolved for the K and L forms of light chain (see below). Presumably by gene duplication a gene was formed, capable of coding for a peptide chain twice the length of the light chain—the primitive heavy chains which seem to have appeared with the cyclostomes some 400 million years ago. The early form has since become considerably diversified represented by the variety of forms of the basic structure seen today. Each light chain of mol. wt. 25 000 consists of two of the basic units and each heavy chain four basic units. Heterogeneity of immunoglobulin struc-

ture occurs within this general framework with some of the basic units being affected more than others. A picture of the immunoglobulin molecule has been built up and is represented in Fig. 9.4. The general arrangement has been confirmed by electron microscopic examination of the molecule.

On the basis of marked antigenic differences in the heavy chains it has been possible to define the existence of the five classes of human immunoglobulin, using the technique of immunoelectrophoresis. These are referred to as IgG, IgM, IgA, IgE and IgD (Table 9.1, Fig. 9.4).

Immunoglobulin G or IgG

This is the major immunoglobulin component of serum making up 75 per cent of the total and having a molecular weight of 150 000 in man. The molecule has two antibody combining sites as shown in Figure 9.4. on what are termed the Fab (antigen binding) portions of the molecule and involving part of both the heavy and light chains. The amino acid sequences have been worked out in whole or part for a small number of light and heavy chains in various species by the analysis of myeloma proteins. These abnormal proteins are present as a homogeneous population in the serum of individuals with plasma cell tumours in sufficient quantity to enable studies of this type to be made. The light chains consist of two parts joined together, one with a constant sequence of amino acids at the C terminal of the chain common to the light chains of the species under study, and the other at the N terminal in which variation occurs in the sequence of the 107 amino acids differing between one myeloma and another, being similar only within a particular myeloma. Up to 50 per cent of the positions in the N terminal portion have been found to be variable. This leads to an enormous number of different permutations of sequence and thus in antibody specificity. Similar variation has been found in rather more limited studies of the N terminal of the heavy chain. The variable portion of the light and heavy chains are contained in the Fab portion of the molecule and it is here that the antibody combining site is present. The light chains are of two distinct types known as K or L (κ or λ) chains.

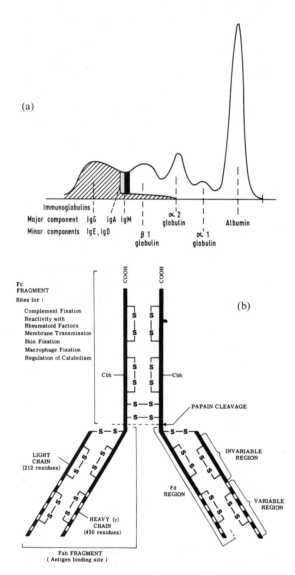

FIG. 9.4. (a) Electrophoretogram obtained by UV scanning of paper electrophoresis strip and showing diagrammatically the main components of human serum and the immunoglobulin classes.

(b) Structure of IgG molecule. (Reproduced with permission from Stanworth and Turner, *Handbook of Experimental Immunology*, Ch. 10. Edited by D. M. Weir, Blackwell.)

No species specific amino acid residues have so far been found in the variable portion and this suggests that during embryogenesis a single gene controls the development of the entire range of variability in the light chains. This gene probably arose early in evolution and the survival value associated with diversification of the antigen-binding site has ensured its maintenance since then.

In any one individual, both K and L chains are produced but they are not found together in the same immunoglobulin molecule. K and L chains are present in a ratio of about 2:1 in any one individual. Two intra-chain disulphide bonds (Fig. 9.4) occur in almost exactly the same position in both K and L chains and both chains have cysteine as the terminal amino acid at the carboxyl end. This serves for the attachment to the heavy chains. These facts suggest a common genetic origin of K and L chains which although they have diverged during evolution have retained many common structural characteristics. The heavy chains are however specific for each class; in the human IgG molecule the heavy chain or γ chain exists in four different forms, IgG1, IgG2, IgG3 and IgG4, which can be distinguished by specific antisera able to detect differences in the Fc fragment of the heavy chains. Sixty-five per cent of the IgG molecules in human serum are of the IgG1 sub-

group, 23 per cent of the IgG2 and 8 per cent and 4 per cent IgG3 and IgG4 respectively. Allotypes or Gm and Inv factors of immunoglobulin have been detected. The antigenic groupings determining the Gm group are present only in the γ chains of the IgG molecule whereas the Inv factors are present in the light chains of each of the major immunoglobulin classes. Twenty-six genetically determined allotypes have been described. These globulin differences between individuals can be compared to the blood groups but instead of involving antigenic differences in the red cell surface they depend on antigenic differences in the light and heavy chains of the immunoglobulin molecule.

IgM, IgA and IgD

Like IgG globulin each of these classes of immunoglobulin in man have been found to contain K and L light chains. The heavy chains on the other hand are unique for each of these types of immunoglobulin; IgM contains μ chains, IgA α chains and IgD δ chains and these differences enable them to be distinguished one from another. The Gm factors found in the Fc region of IgG have been found to be absent from a number of IgM and IgA globulins. IgM globulin with a molecular weight of about 900 000 can be split by reduction of disulphide

Table 9.1 Human immunoglobulins
(Levels vary widely, males tend to have slightly lower levels of IgG and IgM but higher IgA)

Immunoglobulin class	Serum concentration mg/100 ml	Molecular weight	Half life days	Light chains	Heavy chains	Characteristic properties
IgG	900–1800	160,000	18–23	K and L	γ	Precipitins Antitoxins Complement fixation Late antibody
IgA	156–294	170,000 and polymers	5–6·5	K and L	α	Surface protection
IgM	67–145	960,000	5	K and L	μ	Agglutinins Opsonins Lysins, complement fixation Early antibody
IgD	0·3–40	184,000	2·8	K and L	δ	Not known
IgE	10–130 (μg)	188,000	2–3	K and L	ε	Reaginic antibody

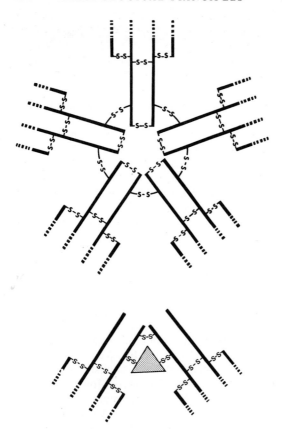

FIG. 9.5. Diagrammatic view of IgM (top) and IgA (bottom) molecules. The triangular structure joining the two IgA components together is known as the secretory piece. In the IgM molecule five similar subunits are joined by disulphide bonds to form the large IgM molecule with multiple binding sites. (Reproduced with permission from Stanworth and Turner, *Handbook of Experimental Immunology*, Ch. 10. Edited by D. M. Weir, Blackwells.)

bonds into five subunits. These subunits have a molecular weight of 180 000 daltons and are believed like IgG to have two heavy and two light chains.

Until recently most studies on the number of antigen-binding sites of IgM antibody showed that the molecule had only five binding sites despite the fact that theoretically ten were present. Both human and rabbit IgM however have now been shown to have the ten sites and it is believed that the two binding sites on each are unable to combine with antigen with similar efficiency thus making it difficult to demonstrate

all ten sites. The molecular structure of some of these immunoglobulins is shown in Fig. 9.5.

STRUCTURE AND FUNCTION OF IMMUNOGLOBULIN

Knowledge gained from the structural studies discussed above has gone some way towards an understanding of the biological activities of the immunoglobulin molecule and it is now possible to pinpoint areas of the molecule responsible for different activities. In the Fab portion, the heavy chain component (Fd portion) seems in some studies to contain as much as 85 per cent of the antigen-binding ability. The light chain component, although usually inactive alone, seems to act together with the heavy chain to form a stable antibody-combining site.

Complement Activation, Toxin Neutralization and Agglutination

The Fc portion of the molecule appears in IgG molecules to be the major component responsible for activating the complement system, although activation does not occur unless two or more molecules of IgG are brought into close apposition. It is not quite certain what changes in molecular configuration or other effects take place when the molecules come close together but isolated Fc fragments do not activate complement and will do so only if aggregated first. One suggestion is shown in Figure 9.6 in which IgG that has not combined with antigen is represented as folded so that the Fc portion is partly hidden. On combination with antigen the molecule springs open at the hinge region thus exposing the Fc portion which can then activate complement. It has been calculated that a single IgM molecule attached to a red cell by multiple combining sites can bring about lysis whereas 1000 IgG molecules are required for the same effect. It was therefore assumed that as two IgG molecules must come together for complement activation, a large number of IgG molecules would be required for this to occur as the antigenic determinants are spread

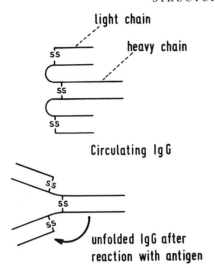

light chain

heavy chain

Circulating IgG

unfolded IgG after
reaction with antigen

Fig. 9.6. Possible molecular forms of IgG before and after combination with antigen (see text).

evenly over the surface of the red cell. Agglutination is brought about by the linking of particulate antigens such as red cells or bacteria by the two Fab fragments of the immunoglobulin molecule. As might be expected from knowledge of the structure of the IgM molecule its five to ten combining sites make it a very efficient agglutinating antibody molecule and rabbit IgM antibacterial antibody is known to be 22 times as active as IgG antibody (mol for mol) in bringing about bacterial agglutination. Because of its large molecular size IgM is largely confined to the bloodstream and probably plays an important role in protection against blood invasion by microorganisms. Septicaemia is often associated with deficiency of IgM. IgG antibodies on the other hand are more effective than IgM antibodies at neutralizing diphtheria toxin, lysozyme or viruses such as poliovirus. Whilst some of this activity was present in isolated Fab fragments the evidence with virus neutralization indicates that the Fc fragment may assist the Fab fragments in neutralization of virus infectivity. The molecular basis for such effects has yet to be elucidated.

Tissue Fixation and Opsonization

The ability of immunoglobulin to attach to tissue cells, which appears to be a well marked

feature of the IgE class of immunoglobulin responsible in humans for various forms of the hypersensitivity reaction may be dependent on the activity of the Fc portion of the molecule. This is suggested by studies on the ability of immunoglobulin fragments to adhere to guinea-pig skin and produce a particular form of hypersensitivity reaction known as passive cutaneous anaphylaxis (Chap. 11). Immunoglobulin antibody specific for particular antigens such as bacteria plays a valuable role by coating the surface and making the antigen more susceptible to phagocytosis. These are known as opsonizing antibodies and IgM antibodies perform this role particularly well. In the rabbit it has been shown that IgM salmonella antibodies are some 500 to 1000 times more effective than IgG antibodies as opsonizing agents. How opsonization is brought about is not clear; it is possible that alteration in the surface properties, such as the surface charge of a particulate antigen, might be effected by antibody and thus prevent possible electrostatic repulsion between the phagocyte and the antigen. It is also conceivable that the Fc fragments of the antibody might have an affinity for the surface of the macrophage and thus link the particulate antigen, attached by means of the antibody combining sites, to the macrophage via the Fc fragment. In support of this possibility, antibody with the ability to attach to macrophages by means of the Fc fragment has been described in the guinea-pig and is known as cytophilic antibody.

Selective Transport

In women, IgG globulins have the ability to pass through the placenta and reach the foetal circulation; this is not a simple filtration process but is due to selective transfer of the molecules brought about by a part of the Fc fragment of IgG heavy chains. This property is a feature only of the γ chain of IgG and has not been found in the μ and α chains of IgM and IgA. This mechanism seems to be limited to primates whereas in ruminants immunoglobulin from the colostrum is absorbed through the intestinal epithelium.

Another selective transport mechanism is found with IgA globulins which are selectively secreted into saliva and respiratory and intestinal mucous secretions as well as into the colostrum. The IgA found in these secretions is manufactured locally and has an attached secretory or transport piece not found in serum IgA. It seems likely that this piece is added to the molecule during its passage into the mucous secretions from the lamina propria, underlying the mucous membranes of the gut and respiratory tract. At the same time as the secretory piece is added the monomeric IgA molecule is turned into a dimer. Salivary and colostral IgA, probably because of the attached secretory piece, appears to be relatively resistant to digestion by proteolytic enzymes in contrast to other immunoglobulins; the secretory immunoglobulin would thus remain active and able to perform a protective role in the intestinal tract. The dimer form of IgA acquires the ability to fix complement and after attaching to Gram-negative organisms when the complement system is activated the IgA can be shown *in vitro* to allow the enzyme lysozyme to digest the mucopolysaccharides of the microorganism's cell wall. The monomeric form of IgA can also pass from the lamina propria to the bloodstream via the lymphatics so that gut infections can lead to increased serum IgA levels. Much effort is being expended in studying the role of IgA as a protective mechanism at the mucous surface and the possible future use of locally applied vaccines designed to stimulate this form of antibody response may be of considerable value, e.g. in respiratory and intestinal infections.

INTERACTION OF ANTIBODY WITH ANTIGEN

An antibody is an immunoglobulin molecule secreted into the tissue fluids from lymphoid cells that have been exposed to a foreign substance—an antigen. An antigen may be potentially harmful, such as a bacterium or virus, or it may be a harmless bland substance such as foreign serum protein. When molecules of antibody and antigen are brought together in solution, they interact with each other by the formation of a link between an *antigen binding* site on the immunoglobulin molecule—part of the Fab fragment—and the particular chemical groupings which make up the *antigenic determinant* of the antigen molecule. The molecules are held together by non-covalent intermolecular forces which are effective only when the antibody-combining site and the antigenic determinant group are able to make close contact. Antibodies vary in their combining quality and the overall tendency to combine with antigen is the average ability of the antibodies to combine with antigen or the average intrinsic association constant. This can be calculated experimentally by application of the concepts of chemical equilibria to antigen-antibody interactions. Studies of this type have shown that the affinity of antibodies increases as immunization proceeds and that the dose of antigen can influence the quality of antibody.

The methods used for the detection of antigen-antibody reactions in the laboratory fall into two functional groups: first, procedures designed to elucidate the cytodynamics of antibody formation which involve the study of the behaviour of single cells or small populations of cells; the second group, which is the subject of the present discussion, concerns the detection and quantitation of *secreted antibody* circulating in the blood or present in the tissue fluids.

The methods used here range in their application from highly specialized studies of the physico-chemical aspects of antigen-antibody interaction to widely used procedures designed to aid in the diagnosis of disease.

In practical terms, the union of antibody with antigen can be detected at different levels. The first level follows *primary union* of the two reactants and usually requires that one or other reactant is labelled with a suitable marker such as a fluorescent dye or a radioactive isotope. A simple example of this is the microscopic localization in a tissue of a particular microorganism by mixing it with an antiserum prepared against the microorganism and labelled with a dye that fluoresces under ultraviolet light.

The second level at which antigen-antibody combination can be detected depends on the development, after primary union, of certain changes in the physical state of the complex, resulting in precipitation or agglutination of the components or, alternatively, in the activation of non-antibody components such as serum complement or histamine from mast cells. Reactions of this type occurring subsequent to primary union are termed *secondary phenomena*. This text is concerned with the principles and practice of a few of these secondary phenomena which are in common use in medical microbiology.

These reactions will be considered individually in Volume II; however, it is important to be aware of the difficulties in interpreting results of such tests. The initiation and development of the secondary phenomena constitute a complicated series of events involving many variables such as the type of antibody taking part, the relative proportions of antibody and antigen, characteristics of the antigen molecule, presence of electrolytes, inhibitory substances and unstable components.

Despite these formidable difficulties, the widely used secondary phenomena such as precipitation, agglutination and complement fixation have an important role to play as aids in the diagnosis of disease and in the identification of microorganisms. They are used in tests to demonstrate the presence of antibody in the sera of patients suffering from infectious disease, or the production of an antibody response to cell antigens as might occur after prophylactic vaccination, incompatible blood transfusion, tissue grafting or in autoimmune states. Reactions of this type can also be used to identify antigens in the tissues or body fluids and are utilized for blood grouping, tissue typing or the identification of microorganisms.

Among the most important of these reactions are *precipitation,* which occurs between antibody and antigen molecules in soluble form; *agglutination,* in which the antibodies directed against surface antigens of particulate materials such as microorganisms or erythrocytes link them together in large clumps or aggregates; *complement fixation* in which antibody molecules, after reaction with antigen, activate the complex blood components which make up serum complement, *neutralization* tests used in virus identification, *immobilization* tests with motile bacteria and protozoa and *intradermal* tests for the reaginic antibody characteristic of hypersensitivity states.

10. Natural and Acquired Immunity

INNATE IMMUNITY—NON-SPECIFIC DEFENCE MECHANISMS

The healthy individual is able to protect himself from potentially harmful microorganisms in the environment by a number of very effective mechanisms present from birth which do not depend upon his having previous experience of any particular microorganism. The innate resistance mechanisms are non-specific in the sense that they are effective against a wide range of potentially infective agents. The main determinants of innate immunity seem genetically controlled, varying widely with the species and strain of the host and to a less extent between individuals. Age, sex, nutritional factors and hormone balance also contribute. In comparison, acquired immune mechanisms depend upon the development of an immune response to individual microorganisms that is specific only for the inducing organism.

DETERMINANTS OF INNATE IMMUNITY

Species and Strain

Marked differences exist in the susceptibility of different species to infective agents. The rat is strikingly insusceptible to diphtheria whilst the guinea-pig and man are highly susceptible. The rabbit is specifically susceptible to myxomatosis and man to syphilis, leprosy and meningococcal meningitis. Susceptibility to an infection does not always imply a lack of resistance; for example, man is highly susceptible to the common cold but he overcomes the infection within a few days. In some diseases, it may be difficult to initiate infection but once established the disease can progress rapidly. For example, rabies occurs in both man and dog but is not readily established as the virus does not ordinarily penetrate healthy skin. Once infected, however, the host lacks the resistance mechanisms to overcome the disease. Marked varia-

tions in resistance to infection have been noted between different strains of mice and it is possible to breed by selection from the same parental stock distinct strains of rabbits of low, intermediate and high resistance to experimental tuberculosis.

In man, the habits and environment of a community may enhance the ability to resist particular infections due to the development of specific immunity early in life. This environmentally determined type of immunity is easily confused with the genetically controlled innate resistance and makes it difficult to establish differences in innate immunity in different communities. It is, however, fairly clear that the American Indian and the Negro are genetically more susceptible to tuberculosis than are Caucasians. It seems reasonable to assume that certain interspecies and interstrain differences have arisen by a process of natural selection and that communities that have been highly exposed to a specific infection through many generations have been subject to genetic selection for enhanced innate immunity.

Individual Differences and Influence of Age

The role of heredity in determining resistance to infection is well illustrated by studies on tuberculosis in twins. If one homozygous twin develops tuberculosis, the other twin has a three to one chance of developing the disease compared to a one in three chance if the twins are heterozygous. Sometimes genetically controlled abnormalities are an advantage to the individual in resisting infection as, for example, in a hereditary abnormality of the red blood cells (sickling) which cannot be parasitized by *Plasmodium falciparum* thus conferring a degree of resistance to malaria.

Infectious diseases are often more severe in early childhood and in the young animal; this high susceptibility of the young appears to be associated with immaturity of the immunological mechanisms affecting the ability of the lymphoid system to deal with and react to foreign antigens. In the elderly, besides a general diminution in resistance and a probable waning of the activity of the immune mechanisms, physical abnormalities (e.g. prostatic enlargement leading to stasis of urine) or bad habits (e.g. smoking) are common causes of increased susceptibility to infection.

Hormonal Influences: Sex

There is decreased resistance to infection in diseases such as diabetes mellitus, hypothyroidism and adrenal dysfunction. The reasons for this decrease have yet to be clarified but may be related to enzymic activities; thus it is known that the glucocorticoids are anti-inflammatory agents, decreasing the ability of phagocytes to digest ingested material (probably by stabilizing the lysozome membranes). They also have the beneficial effect of interfering in some way with the toxic effects of bacterial products such as bacterial endotoxin. Cortisone, given therapeutically, may reduce resistance to tuberculous infection.

There are not marked differences in susceptibility to infection between sexes. Although the overall incidence and death rate from infectious diseases is greater in the male than in the female, both infectious hepatitis and whooping cough have a higher morbidity and mortality in females.

Nutritional Factors

The adverse effect of poor nutrition on susceptibility to infectious agents is not now seriously questioned. Experimental evidence in animals has shown repeatedly that inadequate diet may be correlated with increased susceptibility to a variety of bacterial diseases, associated with decreased phagocytic activity and leucopenia. In the case of infective agents such as viruses which depend upon the normal metabolic function of the host cells, malnutrition, if it interfered with such activities, would be expected to hinder proliferation of the potentially infective agent. There is experimental evidence in support of this view in a number of animal species which when undernourished were less susceptible than normal animals to a variety of

viruses including vaccinia virus and certain neurotropic viruses, e.g. polioviruses. The same may be true of malaria infections in man. The parasite requires para-aminobenzoic acid for multiplication and this may be deficient when a low level of nutrition exists. The exact role of nutritional factors in resistance to infectious agents in man is difficult to determine by epidemiological data. Poor diet is often associated with poor environmental conditions and increased incidence of infection can correlate with poor sanitary conditions.

MECHANISMS OF INNATE IMMUNITY

Mechanical Barriers and Surface Secretions

The intact skin and mucous membranes of the body afford effective protection against nonpathogenic organisms and a high degree of protection against pathogens (Fig. 10.1). The skin is a more resistant barrier because of its outer horny layer consisting mainly of keratin, which is indigestible by most microorganisms; and thus shields the living cells of the epidermis from microorganisms and their toxins. The relatively dry conditions on the skin, and the high concentration of salt in drying sweat are inhibitory or lethal to many microorganisms. Furthermore, the sebaceous secretions and sweat of the skin contain bactericidal and fungicidal fatty acids and these constitute an effective protective mechanism against many potentially pathogenic microorganisms. The protective ability of these secretions varies at different stages of life and some fungal 'ringworm' infections of children disappear at puberty with the marked increase of sebaceous secretion.

The sticky, mucous secretion covering the mucous membranes of the respiratory tract acts as a trapping mechanism and the action of the hair-like processes or cilia sweeps the secretion containing the foreign particulate material towards the oropharynx so that it is swallowed; in the stomach the acid secretion destroys most of the microorganisms present. Nasal secretions and saliva contain mucopolysaccharides capable of inactivating some viruses and the tears and the mucous secretions of the respiratory, alimentary and genitourinary tracts

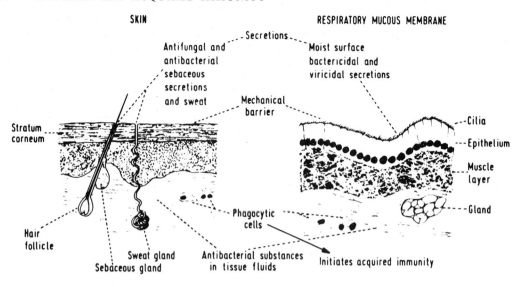

FIG. 10.1. Innate immune mechanisms.

contain lysozyme, particularly active against some Gram-positive bacteria.

Bactericidal Substances of the Tissues and Body Fluids

Lysozyme. This is a basic protein of low molecular weight found in relatively high concentration in polymorphonuclear leucocytes as well as in most tissue fluids except CSF, sweat and urine. It functions as a mucolytic enzyme, splitting sugars off the structural mucopeptide of the cell wall of many Gram-positive bacteria and resulting in their lysis. It seems likely that lysozyme may also play a role in the intracellular destruction of some Gram-negative bacteria. In many pathogenic bacteria the mucopeptide of the cell wall appears to be protected from the access of lysozyme by other wall components, e.g. lipopolysaccharides, and the action of other enzymes of phagocytes or that of complement may be needed to remove this protection and expose the mucopeptide to the action of the lysozyme. Lysozyme was described in 1922 by Fleming who was able to measure its effect on a particular Gram-positive organism *Micrococcus lysodeikticus.* Human tears contain a large

quantity of lysozyme and egg white is a rich commercial source.

Basic polypeptides. A variety of basic proteins, derived from the tissue and blood cells of animals damaged in the course of infection and inflammation, have some antibacterial properties. This group includes the basic proteins called spermine and spermidine which kill tubercle bacilli and some staphylococci, and the arginine and lysine-containing basic proteins protamine and histone. The bactericidal activity of basic polypeptides probably depends on their ability to react non-specifically with acidic polysaccharides at the bacterial cell surface.

Phagocytosis and the Inflammatory Response

Microorganisms or inert particles such as colloidal carbon entering the tissue fluids or blood stream are very rapidly engulfed by various circulating and tissue-fixed phagocytic cells. These cells are of two types, the polymorphonuclear leucocytes or microphages of the blood and the mononuclear phagocytic cells or macrophages distributed throughout the body, both circulating in the blood and fixed in the tissues—the latter include the cells of the reticulo-endothelial system or RES, present particularly in the liver sinuses (Küpffer cells), red bone marrow, spleen and lymph nodes. Macrophages in the blood are known as monocytes, those in the connective tissues as histiocytes, those in the spleen, lymph nodes and thymus as the sinus-lining macrophages (sometimes called littoral cells).

It is now established that the macrophages of connective tissues are derived from peripheral blood monocytes as are the Küpffer cells of the liver, the alveolar macrophages of the lungs and the macrophages of the spleen, lymph nodes and bone marrow. The term *mononuclear phagocyte system*, to describe actively phagocytic cells, is now gaining favour as a more satisfactory description of the function, origin and morphology of phagocytes than the older RES classification which included both actively and poorly phagocytic cells.

The three essential features of these cells are (1) that they are actively phagocytic; (2) that they contain digestive enzymes to degrade ingested material; and (3) that they are an important link between the innate and the acquired immune mechanisms. Their role in regard to acquired immunity is partly that they pass on antigens or their products to the lymphoid cells and partly that they retain a large proportion of the antigen to ensure that the lymphoid cells are not overwhelmed by excess antigen.

The process of phagocytosis is undoubtedly one of the earliest accomplishments of living cells. At the beginning of this century Metchnikoff first appreciated the continuity of this scavenging function through evolution and the important role of this activity in resistance to infectious agents. The role of the phagocyte in innate immunity is to engulf particulate (phagocytosis) or soluble material (pinocytosis), and either to digest it—and thus kill it if it is a living microorganism—or if indigestible to store it away so that it no longer serves as a local irritant, e.g. carbon particles from a polluted atmosphere.

The macrophages of the reticulo-endothelial system present in the walls of capillaries and vascular sinuses in spleen, liver, lungs and bone marrow serve a very important role in clearing the blood stream of foreign particulate material such as bacteria. The efficiency of this process can be dramatically illustrated by injecting colloidal carbon into the circulation of a mouse. Samples of blood taken at short intervals thereafter show that there is a very rapid removal of most of the particles within a few minutes after injection and the blood is cleared within 15 to 20 minutes. Dissection of the animal will show massive localization of the carbon particles, particularly in the liver (Küpffer cells), spleen (sinus-lining macrophages) and in the macrophages of the lungs. This system of phagocytic cells has an enormous capacity to take up material from the blood and the finding of free microorganisms in the blood stream usually indicates that there is a continuing release of organisms from an active focus such as an abscess or the valve vegetations found in bacterial endocarditis. The ability of animals to ingest and destroy different kinds of microorganisms can be impaired or enhanced by depression or stimulation of the phagocytic system. The destruction of phagocytic cells by chemical agents in the rabbit makes the animal temporarily susceptible to a normally non-virulent strain of pneumococcus. The enhanced ability of macrophages from animals infected with tubercle bacilli and listeria to resist these and other infective agents is discussed later. Some microorganisms such as tubercle bacilli and brucellae can resist intracellular digestion by normal macrophages, though they may be digested by 'activated' ones.

Phagocytosis may occur in the absence of serum antibodies, especially on surfaces such as those of the lung alveoli (surface phagocytosis). On the other hand, antibodies to the surface antigens of bacteria that are relatively resistant to phagocytosis can markedly enhance the activities of phagocytic cells on these bacteria and may even improve their intracellular digestion. Such antibodies are known as opsonins. Injury to tissue excites an inflammatory response consisting of dilatation of local capillaries, slowing of the blood flow and exudation of fluids (oedema); phagocytic cells initially stick to the capillary walls and then pass through them into the tissue spaces. Once outside the capillaries the phagocytic cells, which initially are mainly the polymorphonuclear leucocytes of the blood, migrate to the source of the irritation. This leucocyte attraction phenomenon is known as *chemotaxis* and can readily be induced by microorganisms entering the tissues, by the breakdown products of damaged tissue cells and by various irritant substances, possibly because they cause damage to cells. The precise mechanisms of chemotaxis are not understood but it is known that complexes of antigen and antibody generate the production of a diffusible factor which acts in this way; this phenomenon requires the participation of complement components.

After the initial polymorph infiltration in an inflammatory response, the mononuclear cells (blood macrophages) can be seen to enter the area but the nature of the mechanisms that lead to this macrophage aggregation is not understood; it seems to be quite distinct from that responsible for polymorph migration.

Once ingested, susceptible bacteria disintegrate within an hour or two, probably due to the secretion of acids and digestive enzymes secreted into the vacuole surrounding them. The cytoplasmic granules (lysosomes) of polymorphs contain many enzymes including acid and alkaline phosphatases, β-glucuronidase and ribonuclease. The antibacterial agents lysozyme and phagocytin are also present. These lytic effects occur after the fusion of the lysosomes with the vacuole containing the microorganism.
Phagocytin. Extracts of the cytoplasm of polymorphonuclear leucocytes from several species have been found to contain an acid-soluble protein (phagocytin) which is bactericidal mainly to Gram-negative bacteria and also to a few Gram-positive organisms. Phagocytin is present together with other antibacterial substances in the granules of polymorphs.

Temperature

The temperature dependence of many microorganisms is well known and tubercle bacilli, pathogenic for mammalian species, will not infect cold-blooded animals. Conversely, the mycobacteria parasitic on cold-blooded animals, e.g. *Myco. marinum,* cannot cause deep or systemic infections in man. Fowls which are naturally immune to anthrax can be infected if their temperature is lowered. Gonococci and treponemes are readily killed at temperatures over 40°C and fever therapy was used in chronic

gonococcal infection and cerebral syphilis before the introduction of antibiotics. The neisseriae and treponemes are also susceptible to temperatures around freezing point. The smallpox virus, which has a ceiling temperature of 38·5°C, grows mainly in the cooler skin, causing a rash, during the febrile phase of the infection, though it grows internally, probably in the respiratory tract during the afebrile incubation period.

It is therefore apparent that temperature is an important factor in determining the innate immunity of an animal to some infective agents and it seems likely that the pyrexia which follows so many different types of infection can function as a protective response against the infecting microorganisms.

THE COMPLEMENT SYSTEM

The existence of a heat-labile serum component with the ability to lyse red blood cells and destroy Gram-negative bacteria has been known for the last 50 years or so. The chemical complexity of the phenomenon was not appreciated by early workers who ascribed the activity to a single component, called complement. It is now known that complement is in fact an extremely complex group of serum proteins present in low concentration in normal serum. Collectively the complement system is the effector mechanism responsible for the biological activity of complement-fixing antibodies.

Complement components have the characteristics of interacting with certain antibody molecules once these have combined with antigen. These components are best known for their ability to combine with anti-erythrocyte antibody attached to the red cell membrane, the effect of complement being to bring about lysis of the red cell by what appears to be enzymic digestion of small areas of the cell membrane. Much of what is known today about the complement system comes from studies of immune haemolysis.

The erythrocyte—usually sheep red cells—(E) is coated with rabbit anti-sheep cell antibody (A). These 'sensitized' erythrocytes (EA) react with the first component of complement (C1). C1 is a complex globulin of high molecular weight existing in serum as an enzyme precursor.

The three components of the complex are held together by calcium ions and are known as C1q, C1r and C1s. They can be separated by chromatography and gel filtration methods. The C1q component combines with a receptor on the antibody molecule. The inability of some immunoglobulins (e.g. IgA) to activate complement is due to the absence of the appropriate receptor. This precursor is converted after interaction with EA into an active enzyme C1 esterase (or C1a) in the presence of calcium ions. The complex thus becomes EA C1a. The next component of complement to enter the reaction is known as C4 which is β-globulin. The complex then becomes EA C1a4. It seems that C4 reacts with a portion of the red cell membrane altered by the enzymic effect of C1a. The next step is the interaction of EA C1a4 with another β-globulin component C2, which is believed to attach to a receptor on C4 and is then acted upon by C1a to form a new enzyme C2a. Six additional complement components are necessary to bring about haemolysis of the complex and in human serum these are known as C3, C5, C6, C7, C8 and C9. Until a few years ago the individual components of this group of β-globulins had not been differentiated and the activity of the complex was referred to as C3 activity. The biochemical events associated with the interaction of these components with the EA C′1a4,2a complex are thought to be due to an effect on a phospholipid component of the cell membrane. The result is the production of nearly circular holes 8 to 10 nm in diameter in the red cell membrane with the resulting lysis of the cell. Recently, a new pathway, the alternate or bypass pathway for complement activation has been described. The C1, C4 and C2 components are not involved, activation starting at C3 and going on to the later components. The mechanism of activation does not depend upon the same part of the immunoglobulin molecule as the classical pathway and can be activated by aggregated immunoglobulins and various polysaccharides including bacterial endotoxin. This pathway is phylogenetically more ancient than the classical pathway as the late components of complement have been found in invertebrates. The classical pathway does not appear until the vertebrate period.

Red cell lysis, whilst the most intensively studied complement activity, is by no means the only role played by the complex. Complement action is of considerable importance because of its ability to 'neutralize' various types of cell such as Gram-negative bacteria or human cells after they have interacted with antibody. Complement appears to render the bacteria susceptible to lysozyme by digesting holes in the lipopolysaccharide which protects the inner lysozyme-sensitive layer of mucopeptide in the cell wall.

Again leukaemic tumour cells can survive indefinitely in the presence of antibody but on the addition of complement the cells develop blebs in the membrane, become fragile, lose many of their intracellular constituents and die. Complement also plays an important role in the attraction of polymorphonuclear phagocytes to sites of antigen–antibody interaction. This chemotaxis appears to depend on the components C5, 6 and 7 interacting with the C1a,4,2,3 complex. In hypersensitivity states complement activity results in the formation of a group of substances known as *anaphylotoxins* which appear after C3 and C5 activation and are responsible for bringing about the release of histamine leading to increased vascular permeability and smooth muscle contraction. The formation of the plasma kinins which are also active in hypersensitivity states, appears to depend upon complement activation. The C3a fragment bound to the surface of a cell, microorganism or antigen–antibody complex promotes phagocytosis and adherence to certain lymphocytes and may be of importance in the initiation of the immune response by localizing antigen in the lymphoid tissues. In laboratory practice complement fixation tests have wide and important applications (Vol. II).

ACQUIRED SPECIFIC IMMUNITY

Microorganisms that overcome or circumvent the innate nonspecific resistance mechanisms are faced, generally after an interval required for its activation, by the host's second line of defence. To give expression to this acquired form of immunity it is necessary that antigens of the invading microorganisms should come in contact with cells of the immune system (macrophages and lymphocytes) and so initiate a specific immune response. This response takes two forms which usually develop in parallel.

Humoral immunity depends on the appearance in the blood of globulins known as antibodies or immunoglobulins. These combine specifically with antigen of the kind that stimulated their production and this union can lead to some remarkable consequences. For example, the antigen molecules or particles of bacteria may be clumped, their toxins may be neutralized and their uptake by phagocytes and subsequent digestion facilitated whilst cellular antigens such as red blood cells or bacteria may be lysed as a result of the activation of complement.

Cell-mediated immunity depends on the development of lymphoid cells which are specifically sensitized to the inducing antigen and which react directly with the antigen to bring about cytotoxic effects as, for example, on cells containing viral antigens or on foreign cells from a graft. The precise manner in which the sensitized lymphoid cells perform this function is not understood. Development of 'activated' macrophages can also result from this process.

It is important to note that the antibody response is a physiological reaction to the introduction into the body of foreign material, irrespective of whether it is harmful or not. Further, antibodies may be formed against internal antigens that have been liberated from disintegrated microorganisms; in the intact microorganisms these antigens are inaccessible to the antibody which therefore cannot perform a protective role. In contrast to innate immune mechanisms which vary greatly between species, the acquired response is little different between species and the main detectable differences occur between individuals.

Specific immunity may be acquired in two main ways: (1) it may be induced by overt clinical infection, inapparent clinical infection or deliberate artificial immunization. This is *actively acquired immunity* and contrasts with (2) *passively acquired immunity* which is the transfer of pre-formed antibodies to a non-immune individual by means of blood, serum components or lymphoid cells.

Actively acquired immunity due to infectious agents falls into two general categories. Some infections, such as diphtheria, whooping cough, smallpox and mumps, usually induce a long-lasting immunity. Others such as the common cold, influenza and pneumococcal pneumonia confer immunity lasting only for a short time. Failure of the second group of infections to induce long-lasting immunity is due particularly to the fact that different serotypes of the same species of organism may be involved and the acquisition of immunity to one serotype may not prevent infection by another serotype of the same organism because of differences in their surface antigens, e.g. pneumococcus capsules.

Passively acquired immunity. Administration of immune serum usually from another species, e.g. the horse, is a therapeutic procedure in diphtheria and tetanus and was used in lobar pneumonia and gas gangrene until the advent of antibiotics. Tetanus antitoxin is used prophylactically in accidental wounds that may be contaminated with tetanus spores. Passive immunity due to maternal antibody may be transferred to the foetus by the passage of maternal antibody across the placenta in some species, such as man and rabbit, where a particular part of the immunoglobulin polypeptide chain has been found to be necessary for effecting the transfer. In other species such as the rat and dog antibodies are transmitted through the colostrum via the intestine as well as via the placenta. Other animals, notably the lamb and calf, receive this form of immunity only by means of the colostrum. Pooled human immunoglobulin is also used as a source of antibody in a number of infections including measles, smallpox and infectious hepatitis, when it is given during the incubation period to modify or prevent the attack. Human immunoglobulin is also

METHODS FOR DETECTING ANTIBODY FORMATION BY SINGLE CELLS

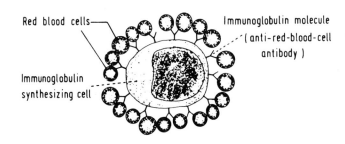

IMMUNO-CYTO-ADHERENCE — Rosette technique

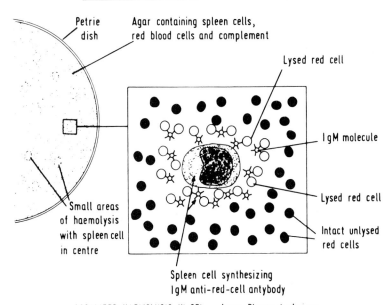

LOCALIZED HAEMOLYSIS IN GEL — Jerne Plaque technique

FIG. 10.2. Two methods for demonstrating antibody formation by single cells. In the immuno-cyto-adherence test spleen cells from an animal immunized with, for example, sheep red blood cells, are mixed with the red cell antigen and after a period of incubation 'rosettes' are formed as shown. The red cells often completely surround the antibody-producing spleen cell. In the Jerne plaque technique, the spleen cells from the sheep-cell immunized animal are mixed with the red cell antigen in soft agar and when complement (guinea-pig serum) is layered on the surface, lysis of the red cells occurs. This happens because the antibody produced by the spleen cell has diffused into the surrounding agar and coated the red cells. This enables the complement system to be activated with the resulting lysis of the red cell.

given to patients with a congenital inability to make antibody globulin.

THE IMMUNE RESPONSE

IMMUNOGLOBULIN PRODUCTION—THE HUMORAL ANTIBODY RESPONSE

The antibody response resulting from exposure to antigenic substances has certain well defined characters. After first contact of tissues with the antigen there is an interval of about two weeks before antibody can be found in the blood and during this initial period there is intense activity in the antibody-forming tissues. This can be shown by studies with isotope-labelled precursors of cell components, for example, studies with tritiated thymidine to show DNA synthesis and studies with carbon-14 labelled amino-acids to show protein synthesis. After antigenic stimulation there is a rapid increase in cell proliferation and in the synthesis of protein in the cells of the lymphoid organs. In a mouse, immunized for instance with sheep red blood cells, lymphocytes taken from the spleen or lymph nodes can be shown to have synthesized sheep-cell antibodies because sheep red cells, after being mixed with the cells of spleen or lymph node aggregate round individual lymphocytes giving a rosette appearance when examined microscopically (Fig. 10.2). The red cells become attached to the surface of lymphocytes by means of antibody located at the cell membrane, these bone-marrow derived cells are referred to as B lymphocytes. The antibody which eventually

can be detected in the blood—during the so-called 'primary immune response'—does not reach a high level and does not persist unless a second dose of antigen is given (Fig. 10.3). When this happens, any remaining antibody will be rapidly mopped up by combination with the antigen reflected by an initial fall in detectable antibody in the blood; then after only a day or two a remarkable rise in the level of antibody begins and within a few days reaches a peak which can be from 10 to 50 times higher than that of the primary response. This 'secondary response' is maintained at a high level falling slowly over a period of months. The response can be boosted to even higher levels by a further injection of antigen (booster or recall dose) until a stage is reached when no further increase occurs. Once an animal has responded to a *single* dose of a live attenuated (e.g. smallpox or polio vaccine) antigen, the animal retains a 'memory' of the antigen so that months or years later it responds with a rapid mobilization of antibody-forming cells. Vaccination with even a non-living agent such as tetanus or diphtheria toxoid, if given in two spaced doses provides several years of useful protection against infection even though soon after vaccination the level of antibodies falls to a low level, the memory is retained.

To obtain a maximum response, the interval between the primary and secondary injection should not be too short and an interval of less than ten days is likely to reduce the level of the secondary response; a spacing of at least 6 to 8 weeks is required for an optimal response. This allows time for a maximal increase in the numbers of antibody-forming cells which can be stimulated by subsequent injections. The nature of the antigen, the form in which it is presented, the route of injection and the dose all have marked effects on the antibody response.

DETERMINANTS OF ACQUIRED SPECIFIC IMMUNITY

Form, Dose and Route of Entry of Antigen

The natural ability of an antigen to induce an immune response may be enhanced by altering it or mixing it with another substance, called an

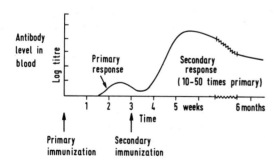

FIG. 10.3. The antibody response.

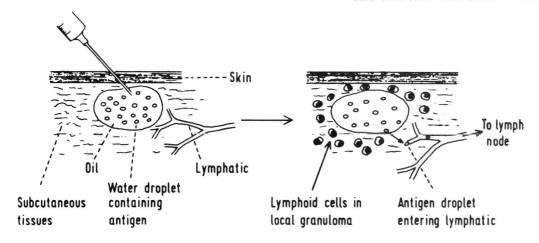

FIG. 10.4. Water in oil adjuvant (depot forming adjuvant).

adjuvant. A procedure of much practical value is to alter the physical state of the antigen by absorbing it on to a mineral gel such as aluminium hydroxide or aluminium phosphate. These alum-precipitated antigens are widely used as immunizing agents for man. Such particulate forms of antigens seem to be able to initiate antibody production much more effectively than the same antigens in non-particulate form. The effect is not fully understood but may be due to a direct effect of the particulate material on the lymphocyte cell membrane leading to more effective transformation of the cell for antibody formation than can be brought about by antigen in solution. An additional factor which may be important for some types of antigen is that particulate material is more readily phagocytosed by macrophages. These cells have been shown in certain situations to make a contribution by serving as a store of antigen for later release and stimulation of lymphocytes. It has also been suggested that macrophages may improve the antigenicity of weak antigens by altering them in some way before passing them on to lymphocytes. It is conceivable also that the phagocytes by removing antigen from the circulation protect the lymphocytes from the effects of excess antigen which would be likely to paralyse the lymphocytes rather than initiate the production of antibody.

For a protein antigen a dose of a few hundred micrograms is required to stimulate the production of detectable circulating antibody. The increase in antibody response is small in proportion to the increase in dose of antigen given and is proportional approximately to the square root of the increase in antigen administered until an upper limit is reached when no further increase can be induced. An increase above this level can result in specific paralysis of the antibody-forming tissues; or 'immunological tolerance'. This form of inhibition is specific for the antigen which caused it; the lymphoid tissues remain normally responsive to other antigens.

Other methods have been developed to enhance the antibody response, of which the most important consists of the preparation of a water-in-oil emulsion (Fig. 10.4); an aqueous solution of antigen is emulsified in a light mineral oil so that tiny drops of antigen solution are dispersed throughout the oil. The emulsion forms a depot of antigen in the tissues, from which small quantities of antigen are continually released, sometimes for a year or more. An influenza vaccine in this form has been used successfully in man. New possibilities have been opened up by the development in Edinburgh of a multiple form of emulsion, in which the aqueous solution is first dispersed in oil and the oil is finally dispersed in a water phase (Herbert, 1973). These emulsions are stable and being much less viscous are less difficult to inject than the water-in-oil type.

Excellent responses have been achieved in experimental animals when killed tubercle bacilli are included in the oil emulsion; a wax constituent of the bacterial wall is responsible for this effect, and the mixture is called Freund's adjuvant after the originator.

The advantage of these 'adjuvant' methods of immunization is that a kind of combined primary and secondary immune response is achieved by the first injection of antigen and that after a second dose of plain or adjuvant vaccine the peak level of antibody is maintained over a long period, presumably by the small quantities of antigen released from the depot.

If an antigen is given intravenously most of the antibody is produced by the spleen, and some in the lung and bone marrow; on the other hand, if given subcutaneously or intradermally, the antigen travels via lymphatics to the local lymph nodes where antibody production is initiated. When antigen is given with adjuvants, there is a local accumulation of inflammatory cells, and antibody production occurs in the resulting granulomatous tissue as well as in the draining lymph nodes.

CELL-MEDIATED ACQUIRED IMMUNE RESPONSE

In the immunologically mature individual, contact with an antigen leads not only to the production of circulating antibody, but also to the development of a separate cell-mediated form of response. In both types initial contact with the antigen is necessary and the response is specific for the antigen. Cell-mediated immunity occurs particularly in infections by microorganisms that enter and grow within tissue cells, such as viruses, tubercle bacilli, brucellae and some salmonellae. The sequence of steps leading to this form of immunity manifested often as delayed hypersensitivity is essentially no different from that leading to the antibody response. Although the response is initiated in different areas of the spleen and lymph nodes (white pulp around the central arterioles of the spleen and the paracortical areas of the lymph nodes), these areas are under the control of the

thymus and the lymphocytes are referred to as T cells.

A characteristic of these thymus-dependent lymphocytes is that they can be stimulated to differentiate and divide by plant extracts known as phytohaemagglutinins (PHA) and by certain extracts of microorganisms such as streptolysin S from streptococci. These substances, sometimes referred to as *mitogens*, appear to act on the small lymphocytes of all vertebrates so far examined and induce enlargement of the cells, increased synthesis of RNA followed later by DNA synthesis. This process is known as *lymphocyte transformation* and can be induced in sensitized lymphocytes on subsequent exposure to the sensitizing antigen. Transformation is readily measured *in vitro* by culturing the cells in the presence of labelled precursors of nucleic acids, e.g. ^{14}C thymidine for DNA synthesis or ^{14}C uridine for RNA synthesis. The test can be used to detect sensitization to an antigen and the non-specific plant mitogens are used as a test of the competence of the cell-mediated immune system. Lymphocytes from an individual with, for example, an immune deficiency state with thymic aplasia and consequent defective cell-mediated immunity would be unable to transform in the presence of PHA. Transformation of lymphocytes by PHA is reduced in certain virus infections.

This lymphocytic response is usually recognized by means of a skin test with the antigen which in an individual who has developed a cell-mediated immune response results in a delayed-type inflammatory reaction at the injection site. When examined histologically the tissues at the injection site are seen to have been infiltrated by mononuclear cells, mainly lymphocytes and a few macrophages.

A number of as yet uncharacterized non-antibody lymphocytic factors referred to as 'lymphokines' have recently been described. The best known of these is released from sensitized lymphocytes in contact with antigen and has the property of preventing the *in-vitro* migration of macrophages on a glass surface. Macrophages can be set up in culture in small capillary tubes and will normally migrate out of the open end of the tube into the culture fluid (Fig. 10.5). A factor released from lymphocytes exposed to antigen will prevent this migration

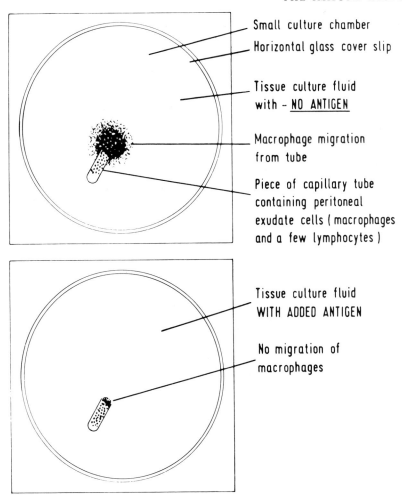

Small culture chamber

Horizontal glass cover slip

Tissue culture fluid
with - NO ANTIGEN

Macrophage migration
from tube

Piece of capillary tube
containing peritoneal
exudate cells (macrophages
and a few lymphocytes)

Tissue culture fluid
WITH ADDED ANTIGEN

No migration of
macrophages

FIG. 10.5. Macrophage migration inhibition test.

by causing the macrophages to stick together. This factor is likely to be released also *in vivo* and may be responsible for the accumulation of macrophages in cell-mediated immune reactions. Another factor released from sensitized lymphocytes after exposure to antigen causes stimulation and proliferation of normal unsensitized lymphocytes; this is known as mitogenic factor. Yet another lymphokine has a chemotactic effect on macrophages attracting them to the site of the inflammatory response. A cytotoxic effect, apparently due to a lympho-

kine (lymphotoxin), has also been demonstrated with a damaging effect on different types of cell. A factor which increases capillary permeability (skin reactive factor) can also be shown to be released by sensitized lymphocytes. The overall contribution of these factors in the cell-mediated immune response is still not clear nor has their chemical identity or mode of action been established. However, it is widely believed that the lymphokines are the main effector mechanism in the cell-mediated responses.

It seems likely that the cell-mediated immune

response is involved in protection against various infective agents, particularly those causing intracellular infections. It may also serve an important physiological role in the normal individual by the elimination of spontaneously arising neoplastic cells which might represent a potential threat. In support of the existence of such an *immunological surveillance* mechanism it has been found that the incidence of tumours is highest at the two extremes of life when the immunological mechanisms are least efficient. The cell-mediated immune system is under the influence of the thymus and after thymectomy in mice the incidence of tumours induced by chemical carcinogens and viruses is significantly higher than in sham-thymectomized control animals. In certain rare immune deficiency states of children when the thymus is absent there is a deficiency of lymphocytes from the areas of spleen and lymph nodes under thymic control and cell-mediated immune reactions are absent with a resultant inability to cope with virus infections.

The cell-mediated immune mechanism is likely to have arisen early in evolution with the development of multicellular organisms and would have additional survival value in that it would also be effective against exogenous parasites.

TISSUES INVOLVED IN IMMUNE REACTIONS

The lymphoid tissues that are predominantly engaged in the immune response are the lymph nodes, spleen and bone marrow. Whilst the lung and to a smaller extent the liver can both take part in the immune response, their contribution is much less than that of the other tissues. The large overall contribution of the bone marrow is a reflection of the mass of this tissue throughout the skeleton. However, weight for weight

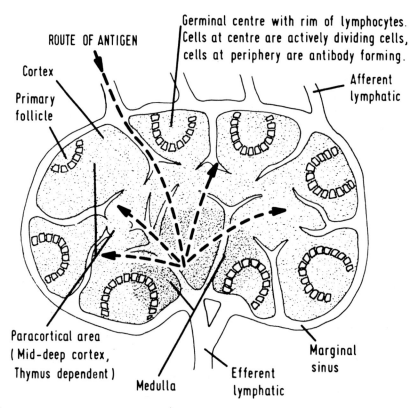

FIG. 10.6. Diagrammatic view of lymph node structure.

the spleen and lymph nodes by far exceed the capacity of the bone marrow. For this reason much effort has been expended in attempting to unravel the way in which the specialized lymphoid organs, the spleen and lymph nodes take up foreign antigens and initiate the immune process.

Gross Structure

The lymph nodes of man are structures of the shape and approximate size of a bean. In a small animal such as a mouse, the lymph nodes, whilst of the same general structure, are correspondingly smaller. The lymph flows from the limbs and organs through the lymph nodes on its way to the main lymphatic vessels of the neck and their union with the veins. The afferent lymphatics enter the capsule of the node (Fig. 10.6) and the lymph leaves via the efferent lymphatics of the hilum. Trabeculae extend radially into the node from the capsule passing

from the marginal sinus through the cortex to the medulla. The tissue of the gland consists of a meshwork of reticular cells in which large numbers of lymphocytes are embedded. These cells are grouped in nodules or follicles in the cortex and form interconnected cords in the medullary area sometimes called medullary cords. Around each nodule in the cortex is a condensation of reticular cells and macrophages with cytoplasmic extension or dendritic processes. Macrophages are present throughout the gland, many being found in the medullary area. Plasma cells and their precursors are also found particularly at the cortico-medullary junction.

The spleen (Fig. 10.7) like the lymph nodes is enclosed by a capsule and divided by trabeculae into communicating compartments. The tissue consists of (a) the white pulp—around the branches of the splenic artery which are surrounded by peri-arterial lymphatic sheaths and lymphatic nodules or Malpighian bodies, and (b) the red pulp—splenic sinuses filled with

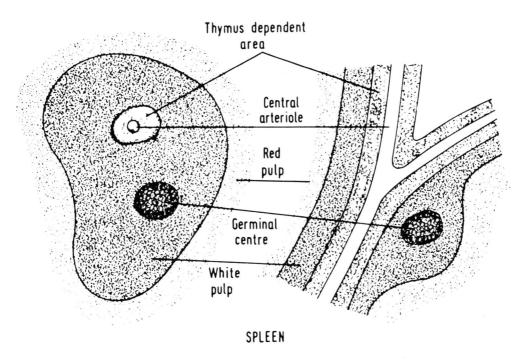

SPLEEN

FIG. 10.7. Structure of Malpighian corpuscle. Transverse section of part of spleen showing area of white pulp related to central arteriole and considered to be thymus-dependent.

blood and splenic cords. The cords make up bands of tissue—reticulum cells, erythrocytes, lymphocytes and granulocytes—lying between the sinuses which are themselves lined by 'sinus-lining cells' held together by a network of reticular fibres. The blood leaves the white pulp via capillaries and enters the red pulp passing into the sinuses and is collected up into venules and veins leaving by the splenic vein. The precise details of the blood circulation in the spleen are not yet fully elucidated, but particulate material and cells undoubtedly can pass through the walls of splenic vessels or be discharged directly into the splenic tissue. The lymph nodes and spleen can be regarded as a complex organization of three types of cell involved in the initiation of the immune reaction —lymphocytes, plasma cells and phagocytic cells of the reticulo-endothelial system.

The structure and histological detail of the spleen and lymph nodes whilst important must not obscure the fact that many of the cells in these organs are part of a mobile population circulating between the blood and lymphoid tissues.

Development

The lymphoid tissues responsible for humoral antibody production are associated developmentally with the gut and consist of lymphocytes and plasma cells of the lymph nodes and spleen. In both the spleen and lymph nodes there are areas of lymphoid tissues under the influence of the thymus, the so-called thymus-dependent areas (Fig. 10.7), lying adjacent to the central arterioles in the spleen and the post-capillary venules in the medulla of the lymph node. After experimental neonatal thymectomy these areas do not develop properly and cell-mediated immune reactions are absent. There is a rare human condition (Di George's syndrome) where this occurs in the absence of thymus function. Histological examination of the spleen and lymph nodes shows that the areas described are deficient in cells.

In the humoral immune response, immuno-globulins are secreted into the blood by lymphoid cells, predominantly plasma cells situated in the spleen and lymph nodes. In contrast the cell-mediated response when it occurs peripherally (e.g. in the skin) is effected by migration of the stimulated cells themselves from the lymphoid tissue via the efferent lymphatics to the blood stream. Some of the cells leave through the capillary endothelium, and pass into the tissue fluids ready to interact with foreign antigenic material. These cells are then collected by the afferent lymphatics and recirculate. Organized lymphoid tissues are absent in invertebrates and the most primitive of the vertebrates, the hag fish. This system develops late in phylogeny and the first vestiges appear in the lamprey. Both the hag fish and the lamprey are able to give a restricted immune reaction to some antigens. The classified complement system, which appeared some time later in evolution, is developed in the jawed vertebrate, the paddle fish. With increasing structural complexity of animal species the immune reaction has become more diversified and effective. However, once components of the immune system appear in evolution they are maintained with a remarkable constancy both at the molecular and functional level.

In man, lymphoid tissue appears first in the thymus at about eight weeks' gestation. Peyer's patches are distinguishable by the fifth month and immunoglobulin secreting cells appear in the spleen and lymph nodes at about 20 weeks. From this period onwards both IgM and IgG globulins are synthesized by the foetus with IgM predominating. At birth the infant has a blood concentration of IgG comparable to, or sometimes higher than, that of maternal serum having received IgG but not IgM via the placenta from the mother. The rate of synthesis of IgM in the infant increases rapidly within the first few days of life but does not reach adult levels until about a year. This compares with the much slower rise in IgG and IgA globulins which do not reach adult levels until between the sixth and seventh years of life. Cell-mediated immune reactions can be stimulated at birth but these reactions (e.g. homograft rejection) may not be as powerful as in the adult.

Cells Concerned in Antibody Production

A simplified picture of the cellular mechanisms leading to antibody formation takes the view that antibodies of different specificities are made by different families or clones of cells, each family being genetically programmed to make only one particular specificity of antibody. There is evidence to show that the cells carry at least part of the molecule of their particular antibody exposed on the cell membrane as a receptor for antigen. Then when an antigen is injected into the body and comes in contact with lymphoid cells it combines with those exposed antibody receptors which are best able to fit the determinant groups of the antigen molecule.

If isotope-labelled antigen is injected into an animal it is rapidly localized in the sinus-lining macrophages in the marginal zone around the Malpighian bodies in the spleen or the medullary macrophages of the lymph nodes (Fig. 10.6), depending on the route of injection. After this localization, plasma cell precursors (probably small lymphocytes) at the cortico-medullary junction are triggered to proliferate into antibody-producing cells. This triggering mechanism may be initiated by antigenic fragments passed on to the lymphocytes after partial degradation in the macrophage. It is also possible that some antigens can react directly with the lymphocytes themselves. This stimulation and proliferation leads to the development of localized collections of active lymphoid cells called lymphoid follicles taking part in the primary immune response. Subsequent contact with antigen now results in a rather different pattern of localization influenced by the presence of secreted antibody; antigen although still taken up by medullary macrophages is also localized on the surface of dendritic macrophages (macrophages with cytoplasmic extensions) which interdigitate with each other and with the lymphoid cells of the lymphoid follicles or Malpighian bodies. The localization seems to depend on antibody at the surface of the macrophage. Lymphocytes themselves may also come directly in contact with antigen as they can be shown to have at least portions of the immunoglobulin molecule on their surface because they can readily be stimulated to respond to contact with antibodies directed at various parts of the immunoglobulin molecule. The function of the antigen at the surface of the lymphocyte is to induce it to transform and proliferate into active antibody-producing cells. The mechanism whereby this change is brought about is not clear but certain

antigens, e.g. bacterial flagella and keyhole limpet haemocyanin, are apparently able to induce lymphocyte transformation leading to antibody production. Other antigens are less active and must be taken into macrophages and processed in such a way that they can then influence lymphocytes. Some antigen may be retained at the surface of macrophages where it serves as a depot of antigen for the maintenance of the immune response. It is also possible that some antigen retained within the macrophage will function in this way although antigen can also be catabolized within the macrophage and later eliminated from the body as breakdown products. Another possible result of the interaction of certain types of antigen, e.g. soluble protein antigens, with the surface of lymphocytes is that the cell is prevented in some way from transforming for antibody production and is thus functionally eliminated from further participation in the immune response. This phenomenon is known as *immune tolerance* and is specific for the inducing antigen. The phenomenon was first described, by Medawar and his colleagues, in mice injected neonatally with cells from another strain of mice and thus containing transplantation antigens. The injected mice were then found to be able to accept grafts from the strain of mice that had donated the original injected cells. Tolerance has since been found to be readily inducible to a large variety of antigens injected neonatally. It may also be induced in the adult provided more antigen is given to take into account the maturity of the lymphoid system, the larger size of the lymphoid organs and hence the more cells to paralyse. A notable advance was made in this field when Mitchison using serum protein antigens showed that there was another form of tolerance inducible by very small doses of antigen. This was termed *low zone tolerance* in contrast to the high zone tolerance previously described. Doses between these two levels were found to immunize. Other workers have confirmed these findings with different types of antigen. Immunologists do not as yet understand the mechanisms underlying tolerance induction but the phenomenon has important implications, particularly in its low zone form, for transplantation immunology.

Cell co-operation between thymus dependent

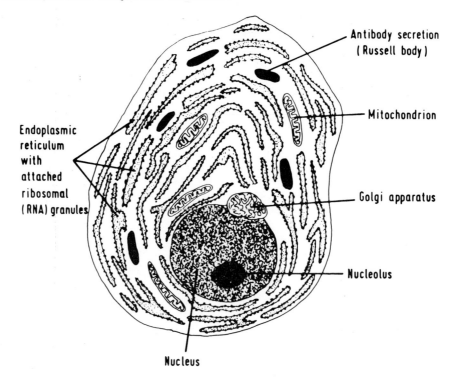

FIG. 10.8. Plasma cell.

(T) lymphocytes and bone marrow derived (B) lymphocytes has been shown to occur. The T lymphocytes assist the B lymphocyte in some as yet undefined way, possibly by concentrating antigen on their surface and presenting it to B cells or perhaps by releasing a lymphocyte activation product (lymphokine) to stimulate the B cell to respond to the antigen.

After the initial changes of transformation of lymphocytes have been set in motion, the actual synthesis of large amounts of immunoglobulin takes place. Two types of cell have been shown to be engaged in this process: (1) cells of the plasmocytic series and (2) cells of the lymphocytic series (small, medium and large lymphocytes). Of these two types the plasma cell line makes the larger contribution to immunoglobulin production and when single cells from immunized animals are examined in microdrops it can be shown that two-thirds of the antibody-producing cells are of this type (Fig. 10.8). An important characteristic of any cell making immunoglobulin is the presence of a rough endoplasmic reticulum; the lymphocytes contain less of this than do plasma cells. The immunoglobulin is localized in the spaces of the endoplasmic reticulum sometimes forming distinct aggregates termed Russell bodies.

In the spleen the cells engaged in antibody production tend to be found in the red pulp and in the lymph glands in germinal centres of the cortex.

Individual immunoglobulin-producing cells appear to be able to synthesize the whole molecule, both heavy and light polypeptide chains. Individual cells make only one class of immunoglobulin and the light chains are restricted to one of the two types (K and L). T and B lymphocytes are morphologically indistinguishable until they transform after antigenic stimulation. The cytoplasm of transformed B lymphocytes is packed with rough endoplasmic reticulum and later with intracytoplasmic vesicles of antibody whereas the T cells contain numerous polyribosomes only. Initially the B cells produce IgM antibody and then switch to IgG production, coincident with this change the surface receptors for antigen on B cells change from IgM to IgG type.

CELLULAR PROCESSES INVOLVED IN ANTIBODY FORMATION

The outstanding feature underlying these mechanisms is that the immune response is a *learning process* involving the cells of the lymphoid tissues.

After initial contact with an antigen the cells of the immune system retain a 'memory' which can be evoked on subsequent contact with the antigen, and furthermore, like other learning processes, the immune system becomes increasingly skilled with continued experience of a particular antigen. The antibody which is synthesized becomes more effective in binding with antigen, as those cells which are best able to produce a 'good fitting' (avid) antibody molecule are selected from the population of antibody-forming cells. At the same time increasing numbers of committed cells are added to the immune system on repeated contact with antigen, and the response is magnified. This increase in quantity and avidity of antibody can lead for example to increased efficiency in neutralizing an infective agent or its toxic products so that a well immunized animal would be able to withstand a dose of the agent that might be lethal to a poorly immunized animal.

Two main theories have been evolved to account for antibody synthesis and are referred to as *directive* and *selective* theories. The *directive* theory was formulated by Haurowitz, Mudd and Alexander in the early 1930's and later modified by Pauling. The antigen is visualized as a mould or template which can enter any immunoglobulin-producing cell and cause the pattern of amino acids laid down to be modified so that it will fit the template, resulting in the synthesis of a molecule with a spatial configuration complementary to that of the antigen molecule. To account for the continued production of antibody it is assumed that the antigen, or part of it, remains in the cell to direct future antibody production. Alternatively, it is proposed that the antigen modifies the genetic information in the DNA of the cell so that it and its daughter cells continue to produce the specific immunoglobulin.

In contrast, the *selective theories* propose that antigen selects, from the population of cells capable of making antibody, only those few cells that already have the inherent ability to make an immunoglobulin specific for the antigen. The antigen serves simply as a trigger on reacting with antibody receptor sites at the lymphocyte cell membrane. The *clonal selection theory* of Burnet is the best known of the selective theories and was formulated and modified over the years to take account of the hitherto unexplained phenomenon of recognition by the normal individual of tissue antigens as part of *self* and distinguishing these from foreign *non-self* antigens. Such an explanation became necessary with the description of human diseases where self recognition breaks down and self antigen is treated as if it were foreign antigen —resulting in so-called 'autoimmune disease' (Chap. 11). The theory proposes that the cells of the antibody-forming system have arisen by random mutation resulting in the emergence of small numbers of cells or clones of cells differentiated so as to be capable of producing one or a very small number of specific antibodies. Contact by such differentiated cells during foetal life before the cells have reached maturity, with self or foreign antigenic material, would lead to suppression rather than stimulation of antibody formation against the particular antigen concerned—immune tolerance.

The result of the early contact with self antigens results in the individual developing an immune system which is suppressed or is tolerant towards self antigens. The unblocking of a cell inherently capable of producing antibody against self antigen would explain autoantibody formation (Chap. 11). It is for this aspect of immunity in particular that the clonal selection theory provides a more plausible explanation than the directive theory which requires that all antibody-forming cells are blocked by every self antigen rather than only those cells destined to respond to the antigen concerned. The other main characteristics of antibody formation—the specificity of antibody for antigen and the differences between the primary and secondary responses—can be explained equally well by either theory; the clonal selection theory is however the more complete attempt so far to take into account all the known facts of antibody production. In view of the fact already discussed in chapter 9 that the specificity of the antibody molecule for antigen depends on the amino acid sequences in the variable portions of the polypeptide chains, it is unlikely that antigen could play any role in determining such sequences as envisaged in the template theory. The shape of the antigen binding site will depend not on the influence of antigen but upon the constituent amino acids and their order in that portion of the immunoglobulin molecule. This information will be encoded in the gene determining the variable portion.

A number of variations of Burnet's original selective hypothesis have been proposed in the last few years but all maintain the assumption that the cell is already programmed to produce the antibody induced by contact with antigen. It has been postulated, for example, that each potentially immunologically competent cell carries in its chromosomal DNA, genes for a large variety of different types of antibody and is thus capable of reactions to many antigens. An alternative proposal is that all antibody-producing cells may initially make identical immunoglobulins but during the lifetime of the individual variability of amino acid sequence appears due to crossing over of nucleotides during mitosis, such nucleotides being responsible for coding of the amino acid sequence of the Fab portion of the molecule. There is a clear survival value in such a variation-producing mechanism resulting in the production of immunoglobulins capable of reacting with environmental antigens. Similarly there is survival value in the maintenance of those parts of the gene carrying the nucleotide sequences for the constant parts of the immunoglobulin molecule which maintain its structural integrity.

ROLE OF THE THYMUS IN IMMUNE REACTIVITY

The thymus in mammals arises from the endoderm of the third and fourth branchial clefts and is the tissue in which lymphocytes can first be recognized. The thymus gland increases in size until puberty and then slowly atrophies although it is still readily recognizable in the adult. The cells of the thymus are of three main types, thymocytes morphologically similar to blood lymphocytes, phagocytic reticulum and reticular epithelial cells. The general organization is like that of other lymphoid organs; a central medulla contains a high proportion of reticular cells and a peripheral cortex contains the thymocytes with some surrounding reticular cells. Unlike the spleen and lymph nodes the thymus has no germinal centres and no plasma cells. Thus under normal physiological conditions the thymus cells do not make antibody. Plasma cells will appear only if antigen is injected directly into the organ. Hassall's corpuscles are a feature peculiar to the medulla of the thymus and consist of groups of reticular epithelial cells sometimes flattened and concentrically arranged around a central core of nuclear debris.

The thymus can be shown, by tritiated thymidine incorporation studies, to be actively engaged in lymphopoiesis, there being a higher proportion of primitive actively dividing lymphoid cells than in any other lymphoid tissue. Evidence suggests that the stimulus for thymocytes to divide arises in some way from the reticular epithelial cells. The primitive cells in the thymus are slowly replaced by cells derived from the bone marrow that migrate via the blood stream into the thymus. A small proportion of these cells leave the thymus and find their way to the peripheral lymphoid tissues.

If the thymus is removed during the neonatal period, it is possible to find lymphocyte-deficient areas in the white pulp of the spleen around the central arterioles and in the paracortical area of the lymph nodes. These areas have been termed 'thymus-dependent' areas of the lymphoid tissues. Associated with this localized lymphocyte deficiency, neonatally thymectomized animals also have a considerably impaired cell-mediated immune effector mechanism affecting graft rejection and other forms of cell-mediated immunity such as delayed hypersensitivity reactions; humoral immune activity is much less affected.

Studies in mice of cell turnover in the adult thymus show that the thymic population of lymphocytes is replaced every three or four days but that most cells never leave the organ and die there. The reasons for this intense lymphopoiesis is unknown. In the adult it seems that the thymus enables repopulation of lymphoid tissues depleted by X-irradiation or other methods. However, studies with chromosome markers have shown that the new cells are not derived directly from the thymus but are lymphoid cells from elsewhere in the body, probably from the bone marrow. The role of the thymus in this situation appears to be the production not of thymus-derived cells but of a humoral factor which restores immunological reactivity to remaining lymphoid cells. This was strongly suggested by experiments in which thymus implants were placed, in millipore diffusion chambers, in the peritoneal cavity of thymectomized mice. Immunological capacity was restored to the recipients, which recovered the ability to reject skin grafts although the chambers were impermeable to cells, and were on later recovery shown to contain only reticular epithelial and reticular cells and no lymphocytes.

The essential functions of the thymus can be summarized as (a) the differentiation and proliferation of primitive lymphoid cells derived from bone marrow and (b) the production of a humoral factor with the ability to induce immunological competence in lymphocytes. The exact mechanisms of interactions between the gland and the peripheral lymphoid tissues are still not understood.

The thymus appears to control the cells of the cell-mediated immune system (T cells) probably by providing facilities for the maturation of immature bone marrow cells. The cells of the immune system concerned with producing circulating antibodies (B cells) reside mainly in the cortico-medullary junction and medullary cords of lymph nodes and the red pulp of the spleen. These cells, in contrast to those responsible for cell-mediated immunity, appear to be influenced not by the thymus but by lymphoid tissues associated with the intestine—namely in Peyer's patches and the appendix.

The first evidence that this might be so came from phylogenetic studies in neonatal chickens which failed to develop normal immunological capacity after removal of the gut-associated organ known as the bursa of Fabricius. Thymec-

tomized chickens fail to develop cell-mediated immune processes but are capable of a humoral immune response. In striking contrast, bursectomized chickens fail to make immunoglobulins and have no plasma cells or germinal centres in the lymphoid organs. Their cell-mediated mechanisms are, on the other hand, intact. Evidence is now emerging which suggests that there is a traffic of bursal lymphocytes to germinal centres in the spleen and lymph nodes comparable to that described in the thymus. The evidence so far accumulated suggests that in mammals, lymphoid tissues of the appendix, Peyer's patches and perhaps the tonsils, may perform this function.

Knowledge of immune reactivity which is either thymus-dependent or bursa-dependent has led to the concept of separate *central* and *peripheral* lymphoid tissues. The central organs, the thymus and the bursa of Fabricius (or its equivalent gut-associated tissue in mammals), are responsible for development and control of the peripheral lymphoid tissues, the spleen and lymph nodes.

A tentative scheme showing the possible inter-relationships of central and peripheral lymphoid tissues is given in Fig. 10.9. Recent work, based on repopulation of irradiated animals by lymphoid cells from different origins, indicates that for the expression of at least some forms of immune response, there may be cooperation between cells in the peripheral lymphoid tissues derived directly from the bone marrow and lymphocytes derived from the thymus. The former cells are referred to as B cells and the latter T cells. The B cells are believed to be responsible for immunoglobulin synthesis and can either react to direct contact with antigen or co-operate with T cells which act as helper cells leading in some way to an immune response by the B cells.

CELLULAR TRAFFIC IN OTHER LYMPHOID TISSUES

Consideration has already been given to the traffic of lymphocytes from the bone marrow via the thymus to the lymph nodes. This journey, during which the cells are maturing and proliferating, probably goes on over a period of weeks. Another form of lymphocyte traffic also exists

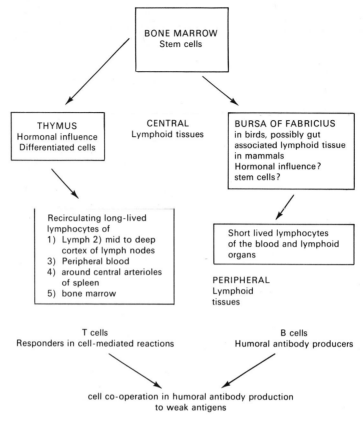

FIG. 10.9. Scheme illustrating possible relationship between central and peripheral lymphoid tissues.

involving a non-dividing population of small lymphocytes with a potential life span of many months and derived mainly from the thymus. This journey is measured in hours rather than days (Fig. 10.10) and this takes the form of a recirculation of small lymphocytes between the blood and lymphoid tissue, each small lymphocyte may be exchanged between these two compartments very many times during its lifetime. One of the main advantages to the individual of such a recirculation process is that during the course of a natural infection the continual traffic of lymphocytes would enable very many different lymphocytes to have access to the antigen as a result there would be a good chance that a lymphocyte carrying antibody receptor for the particular antigen would come across it and initiate an immune reaction. Another possible role of this recirculation

process is that it can be used to replenish the lymphoid tissue of, for example, the spleen which might have been depleted by infection, X-irradiation or trauma.

There is convincing evidence that lymphoid tissues can recruit lymphocytes from the recirculating pool. If a rat spleen is irradiated immediately after an intravenous injection of sheep red cells the antibody response is only slightly delayed. However, if whole body irradiation is given after the initial splenic irradiation there is complete suppression of the anti-sheep cell response. It thus seems likely that without whole body irradiation the irradiated spleen is able to recruit a fresh supply of lymphocytes from the circulating pool. Another situation in which recirculation of lymphocytes could be helpful in the induction of an immune response is where the local concentration of antigen

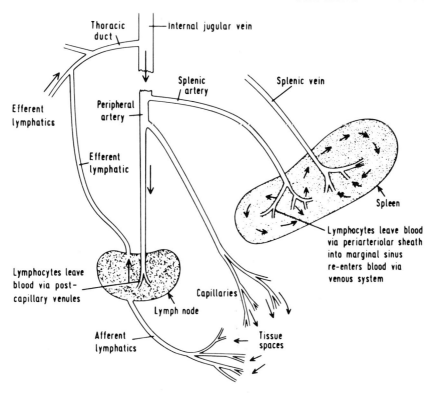

Fig. 10.10. Schematic view of main pathways of lymphocyte circulation.

might be sufficient to induce tolerance rather than immunity in a static cell population. The passage of lymphocytes through an area where antigen had been localized and concentrated on the dendritic processes of macrophages might facilitate the induction of immunity.

Routes of Lymphocyte Recirculation

There are three main areas where the migration or transfer of lymphocytes from the blood takes place; the lymph nodes and Peyer's patches, the spleen and the peripheral blood vessels. Most is known about the mechanism of transfer in the lymph nodes where studies with the electron microscope show that small lymphocytes actually penetrate and traverse the cytoplasm of the cuboidal endothelial cells of the post-capillary venules. These post-capillary venules are confined to the deep and mid-zones of the lymph node cortex and are unusual in that their endothelial cells are hypertrophied and cuboidal in appearance in comparison with the flattened

endothelium of normal post-capillary venules found elsewhere, From the lymph node cortex the lymphocytes pass through the node to the medullary sinuses and then to the efferent lymphatics.

The precise routes of lymphocyte migration in the peripheral blood circulation are not clear but the migration seems to be on a much smaller scale than in lymphoid tissues and almost certainly takes place across capillary walls. The flow can be increased if, for example, a local granuloma is formed in response to some foreign agent; then the migration from blood to lymph can be as great as in the lymph nodes themselves.

In the spleen, post-capillary venules have not been described and small lymphocytes seem to enter the periarteriolar sheath from the blood, passing between the cells rather than through them as in the post-capillary venules. The cells later re-enter the blood within the spleen rather than leave via the lymphatics.

PROTECTION AND IMMUNITY

The mechanisms and characteristics of acquired specific immunity, both cell-mediated and humoral, and the interactions between antibody and antigen have already been discussed. It must however be emphasized that neither the production of antibody to the antigens of an invading microorganism nor even the combination of the antibody with such antigen is in itself any guarantee that the infective agent will be inactivated or eliminated from the body. Microorganisms have numerous ways of protecting themselves from, and side-tracking, the immune reactions of the host. For example, the pneumococcus secretes large quantities of capsular polysaccharide which neutralizes natural opsonin and mops up acquired antibody as it is produced, thus allowing the pneumococcus to proliferate unhindered for some time. Trypanosomes appear to change their surface antigenic make-up from one generation to the next, so that the antibody made in response to the antigens of the original organism is inactive against the second generation of organisms. Many microorganisms, particularly tubercle bacilli, brucellae and viruses, disappear inside tissue cells before sufficient antibody is produced to act against them. Leprosy bacilli may have the ability to destroy the cells in the thymus-dependent areas of the lymphoid tissues, and thus prevent the mounting of a cell-mediated immune response against the invading organisms so that its proliferation is unhindered. The same appears to be true for cutaneous leishmaniasis where instances have been described of a loss of cell-mediated immunity. In short, a particular microorganism may be pathogenic because in some way it is able to circumvent, at least initially, the immune response of the host.

IMMUNITY IN BACTERIAL INFECTIONS

Antibody Mediated Immunity

Some microorganisms owe their pathogenic abilities to the production of exotoxins. Amongst diseases dependent on this type of mechanism are diphtheria, tetanus, gas gangrene and botulism. Antibodies either acquired by immunization or previous infection or given passively as antiserum are able to neutralize these bacterial toxins. To give protection, antibodies must either be present in sufficient quantity, as they would after administration of antiserum, or be produced faster than the toxin is produced by the microorganism. This active response is most likely to occur if the individual had previously been exposed to the organism or its products by natural infection or artificial immunization. The previously exposed individual has an 'immunological memory' of the toxin and has a population of cells ready to respond rapidly to the slightest stimulus from the exotoxin. The infected individual with no 'immunological memory' may have to be given antibody prophylactically in order to tide him over the first stages of infection.

Bacterial toxins have been largely identified as enzymatic in nature and the antibody in some way is able to interfere with the ability of the enzyme to interact with its substrate. The antibody probably does not interact with the active site of the enzyme but the nearer it reacts to this site the more effective is its neutralizing power likely to be. The most probable explanation of the inhibitory effect of antibody is that it produces what is called 'steric hindrance', which simply means that it gets in the way and physically prevents the enzyme from coming in close apposition to its substrate (Fig. 10.11). This idea is supported by the finding that antibody is much more effective against enzymes which have substrates of high molecular weight than it is against those with low molecular weight substrates. Figure 10.11 shows how a substance of low molecular weight can come in contact with the active site of the enzyme even in the presence of antibody.

Where a microorganism does not secrete exotoxins, the protection afforded by antibodies depends on the direct effect of antibodies attached to the surface of the microorganism. The most important effect of this attachment is to encourage phagocytosis by blood macrophages or polymorphs (opsonization). The antibody in some way, perhaps by altering the surface charge, changes the surface characteristics of the microorganism, so making it more susceptible to phagocytosis. The phagocytic

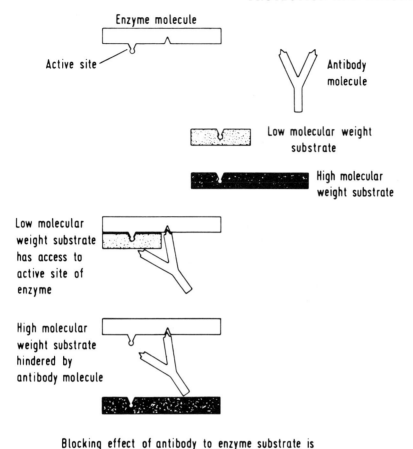

Enzyme molecule

Active site

Antibody molecule

Low molecular weight substrate

High molecular weight substrate

Low molecular weight substrate has access to active site of enzyme

High molecular weight substrate hindered by antibody molecule

Blocking effect of antibody to enzyme substrate is effective only if enzyme substrate is of high molecular weight.

FIG. 10.11. Diagrammatic view of the possible 'steric hindrance' effect of antibody against an enzyme toxin. A low molecular weight substrate avoids the blocking effect of the antibody molecule. The closer the antibody is attached to the active site of the enzyme the more effective will be its blocking action.

cell then in many instances can digest the microorganisms by a variety of digestive enzymes carried in the intracellular lysosomes. However, some microorganisms, such as *Strept. pyogenes,* the typhoid bacillus and *Mycobacterium tuberculosis,* are able to resist intracellular digestion. The streptococcus carries, as part of its cell wall, a substance known as M protein, which confers the ability to resist digestion by the enzymes. If immunity exists to the M protein, by previous exposure or artificial induction, the streptococcus is then susceptible to intracellular digestion. Rough (avirulent) strains of salmonellae are susceptible to intracellular digestion whilst the smooth (virulent) strains are able to resist digestion in some way. In the case of enteric infections such as those due to salmonellae, antibodies can be secreted into the intestinal lumen and attack the organism before it invades the intestinal mucosa. These antibodies secreted by an immune individual are known as copro-antibodies and may be predominantly IgA immunoglobulin which is selectively produced in intestinal and respiratory mucous membranes. Other effects of antibody attachment to the surface of the microorganisms include the lysis of Gram-negative bacteria brought about by the activation of the complement system. Its effect is to digest the cell-wall lipopolysaccharide so that the structural mucopeptide is exposed to attack by lysozyme. Attachment of bacteria to the host's red blood cells in the presence of antibody and complement is another way in which phagocytosis is encouraged. The rationale of this phenomenon, known as 'immune adherence', is not clear.

Apart from the clumping effect on the bacteria, agglutination seems to have little effect on the viability or respiratory activity of the organism although bacteria at the centre of a large mass of clumped organisms could have limited metabolic activity simply by a lack of sufficient nutrient material.

Precipitation of antibody on the surface of certain parasitic nematodes has been proposed as a mechanism whereby the excretory orifices of the worm are blocked, thus interfering with its metabolism.

Acquired Cellular Immunity

The interrelations of antibody-mediated immune mechanisms and acquired cellular immunity are not yet clearly defined. It is known, however, that macrophages from animals immune to tubercle bacilli are more actively phagocytic than those taken from a normal animal. Enhancement of cellular immunity has been reported with macrophages from brucella-infected animals; such cells restricted the intracellular growth of brucellae although the activation was dependent on the initial immunization with a living virulent strain of the organism. The same phenomenon has been found after *Listeria monocytogenes* infection in mice whose macrophages isolated from the peritoneal cavity acquire an increased intracellular activity not only to listeria but also to tubercle bacilli and brucellae: that is, the increased intracellular resistance is non-specific in being directed at species of intracellular parasites other than that responsible for the initial infection.

The non-specific enhancement of macrophage activity, including their ability to kill microorganisms and spread themselves throughout the peritoneal cavity to mop up an infectious agent, appears to depend partly upon the transfer of an as yet undefined stimulus from lymphoid cells which have reacted immunologically to the initial injection of microorganisms. Thus the first part of the response depends on a specific immune reaction on the part of lymphoid cells to an agent such as *L. monocytogenes*; these cells proliferate and in turn activate the macrophages which not only handle listeria more effectively but also other bacterial species. This phenomenon can be shown quite clearly by transferring stimulated mouse lymphoid cells to an unstimulated recipient whose macrophages then assume enhanced bactericidal properties.

IMMUNITY IN VIRUS INFECTION

Antibody-mediated Immunity

In virus infections the efficiency of antibody depends largely on whether the virus passes through the blood stream in order to reach its target organ. A well known example of a virus that follows such a route is the poliovirus; this crosses the intestinal wall, enters the blood stream and passes on rare occasions to the spinal cord and brain where it proliferates. Small amounts of antibody in the blood can neutralize the virus before it reaches its target cells in the nervous system. A number of other viruses behave in the same way and pass through the blood stream on their way to their target organ; examples are the viruses of measles, smallpox, mumps, rubella and chickenpox. Disease caused by these viruses is characterized by a prolonged incubation period. In comparison, in another group of virus diseases with a short incubation period such as influenza and the common cold the viruses do not pass through the blood stream, as their target organ is their site of entry to the body, namely the respiratory mucous membranes. In this type of infection a high blood level of antibody will be less effective against these viruses in comparison with its effect on the blood-borne viruses. For this antibody to act on such respiratory viruses it must pass through the mucous membranes into the respiratory secretion. Examination of the antibody content of mucous secretion has shown that in contrast to the blood there is very little IgG antibody and often no IgM; it thus appears that the mucous membranes are not very permeable to antibodies of these classes. The predominant immunoglobulin in these secretions is IgA manufactured by plasma cells in the lamina propria of the mucous membranes, and IgA derived from nasal secretions is responsible for most of its neutralizing activity against common cold viruses. It may be concluded from these data that conventional immunization methods for stimulating local blood levels of antibody are less likely to be effective against viruses that attack the mucous membranes, than methods for stimulating local IgA antibody production in the mucous membranes themselves. An example of this is the intranasal administration of a live attenuated influenza virus which has been used in the Soviet Union apparently with some success. Again the high degree of immunity provided by the oral polio vaccine may be due in part to locally produced antibody in the gut neutralizing the virus even before it reaches the blood stream. After oral vaccination IgA antibody against polio virus has been demonstrated in the faeces, in duodenal fluid and in saliva, whereas no such antibodies could be found after injection of inactivated virus vaccine. The nasopharyngeal antibodies persist for at least 300 days and afford long term protection. The levels of IgA anti-polio antibody were lower in tonsillectomized children.

Cell-mediated Immunity

The humoral immune response is probably the predominant form of immunity responsible for protection from reinfection by viruses. For this reason immunization procedures aim at producing circulating or mucous membrane antibody. In primary virus infections some form of cell-mediated immunity is probably involved. Thus, children with congenital hypogammaglobulinaemia can recover from virus infections without producing any demonstrable virus-neutralizing antibody. Although these children may be producing small amounts of neutralizing antibody, it is significant that the capacity to resist virus infection is associated with normal cell-mediated immune reactions. These subjects are able to develop normal delayed hyper-

sensitivity reactions to bacterial and viral antigens and contact sensitivity to simple chemicals. In patients with Swiss-type agammaglobulinaemia who have an additional cell-mediated immune deficiency, susceptibility to virus infection is very great and death often follows the development of severe generalized vaccinia after routine inoculation of live vaccine. Some viruses, e.g. measles virus, may interfere with the normal activity of lymphocytes as judged by the inability of such cells from infected individuals to respond to the plant mitogen PHA. The phenomenon can be reproduced in normal lymphocyte cultures infected *in vitro* with virus, and may be of some importance in the pathogenesis of certain virus diseases. Certain viruses are able to replicate in macrophages (e.g. arboviruses, murine hepatitis, lactic dehydrogenase virus and herpes simplex virus) and others do so in lymphocytes (e.g. lymphocytic choriomeningitis virus). The effects on the immune response have been studied mainly in mice which show selective depression of some aspect of the immune response (e.g. depression of IgG after Friend virus infection or an impaired ability to reject grafts in Gross leukaemia virus infections).

Further evidence that cell-mediated immune reactions are involved in resistance to viruses comes from the finding that cell-mediated reactions of the delayed hypersensitivity type (Chap. 11) can be demonstrated after many types of virus infection. Examples of this are the 'immune' or 'accelerated' reaction sometimes seen after revaccination with vaccinia virus and the Frei skin reaction in lymphogranuloma venereum (q.v.).

A quite distinct type of resistance mechanism in virus infection is the production of a substance by the infected host cells known as 'interferon' which interferes with the synthesis of new virus by tissue cells of the host (Chap. 13).

Immunity to Protozoa and Helminths

The life cycles of organisms in this category are complicated and the immune response to be effective has to interrupt the cycle at a stage when the parasite is accessible to the immune processes.

Malaria infections are initiated by sporozoites which transform into exoerythrocytic schizonts in the liver, and at this stage there is no recognizable immunity. The schizonts rupture and discharge their merozoites into the peripheral circulation where they invade erythrocytes. There appears at this stage to be an alteration in the permeability of the red cell membrane so that immunoglobulin molecules can enter and attack the parasite. Antibodies are readily detectable in the serum and increase until the crisis 7 to 10 days later and then slowly decline. Because these antibodies are able to get access to the parasite only during a relatively short period of its life cycle, immunity is incomplete and the host usually fails to eliminate the parasite completely. Plasmodia like trypanosomes are subject to antigenic variation and antigenically distinct forms may appear after each relapse, Immunity probably depends on a gradual build up of antibodies to a group antigen common to all variants. The state in which the organisms persist in small numbers in the tissues in the presence of an immune reaction is called 'premunition' by parasitologists.

The adaptive phenomenon of antigenic variation seen in trypanosomes means that the immune response has great difficulty in coping with these parasitic variations so that in African sleeping sickness the parasite does not induce an effective immunity and the infected subject develops a progressive infection with invasion of the central nervous system leading to death. Trypanosomiasis is associated with high levels of IgM immunoglobulins in both the blood and CSF. It is not certain if this is due to the repeated new antigenic stimuli resulting from changes in the organism or if the parasite in some way influences directly the cells of the immune system. Increased immunoglobulin production is a common finding in protozoal infections and often affects all classes of immunoglobulins. Because usually less than five per cent of the total immunoglobulin appears to react specifically with the inducing parasite it is probable that protozoa stimulate the lymphoid cells in a non-specific way to overproduce immunoglobulins (called *paraglobulins*).

Helminths like protozoa go through a complex life cycle and protective immune mechanisms probably act only at an early stage in the cycle. The main stimulus seems to be due to antigens derived from the adult worm and the immune mechanisms act on new parasites entering the body. A noteworthy feature of these infections is the appearance of IgE (reaginic) antibodies with pulmonary eosinophilia, and it seems likely that immediate hypersensitivity reaction of the anaphylactic type (type 1) is involved in the pathogenesis of helminth infection.

SAPROPHYTIC FUNGI AND RESPIRATORY DISEASE

Examples of pulmonary hypersensitivity to inhaled fungal antigens have been reported in recent years, and precipitating antibodies have been found in the patient's serum. The first of these disorders to be recognized was Farmer's Lung disease in which precipitating antibodies could be demonstrated against antigens derived from mouldy hay later identified as *Micropolyspora faenii*. Subsequently precipitins have been demonstrated against *Aspergillus clavatus* in malt-workers exposed to high concentration of *A. clavatus* spores from contaminated barley and to *Coniosporium corticale* in the serum of maple bark strippers. It is likely that after exposure to high concentrations of any of a variety of fungal spores individuals would produce precipitating antibodies and thus this form of pulmonary hypersensitivity may be more widespread than has so far been identified. The hypersensitivity reaction induced by the presence of precipitating antibodies would be of the toxic-complex (type 3) form inducing a diffuse pulmonary interstitial pneumonitis which has been termed allergic alveolitis. Some of the antigens responsible for this form of hypersensitivity can also provoke in susceptible individuals the anaphylactic (type 1) response exemplified by pulmonary asthma. There is no direct evidence that the antibodies hinder the spread of fungal infections once they are established. That such antibodies play a useful role is suggested by the fact that individuals with immune deficiency states are unduly prone to fungal infections.

Defects in Immunoglobulin Synthesis and Cell-mediated Immune Reactivity

The immunologically competent cells of the lymphoid tissues derived from, renewed and influenced by the activity of the thymus, bone marrow and probably gut-associated lymphoid tissues may be functionally deranged due either to defects in one of the components of the complex itself or secondarily to some other disease process affecting the normal functioning of some part of the lymphoid tissues. In 1953 Bruton first described hypogammaglobulinaemia in an 8-year-old boy who developed septic arthritis of the knee at 4 years of age followed by numerous attacks of otitis media, pneumococcal sepsis and pneumonia. Electrophoretic analysis of the serum proteins showed almost complete absence of the gamma-globulin fraction; e.g. the child was unable to give an immune response to typhoid and diphtheria immunization. It is now recognized that this form of deficiency is only one of a group of specific deficiencies affecting the lymphoid tissues of both sexes, and all ages, and be either genetically determined or arise secondarily to some other condition.

Primary Defects

In the first category are the congenital defects affecting immunoglobulin synthetic mechanisms, cell-mediated immune mechanisms or sometimes both. Deficiency of immunoglobulin synthesis is complete in Bruton type agammaglobulinaemia, an X-linked recessive character found in boys, in which the IgG level is reduced about tenfold and the IgA and IgM about a hundredfold of normal values. Cell-mediated immune mechanisms function normally in these patients who can reject grafts and develop delayed hypersensitivity reactions to tuberculosis. However, they do not give the normal circulating antibody response to bacterial vaccines and are thus very susceptible to pyogenic infections. The lymphoid tissue in the appendix and Peyer's patches is somewhat reduced, and patients do not develop plasma cells and germinal centres in lymph nodes.

Partial defects in immunoglobulin synthesis have been described affecting one or more of the main immunoglobulin classes. For example
(a) the IgG or IgA levels may be reduced and the IgM level raised;
(b) the IgA and IgM may be reduced and the IgG level be normal or
(c) the IgA level may be reduced and the others normal.

In (a), which is also inherited as an X-linked recessive character, the lymphoid tissues appear normal histologically although the plasma cells appear to be making predominantly IgM. Patients are susceptible to pyogenic infections and the condition is often associated with anaemia, thrombocytopenia and neutropenia. In (b) even the IgG which is produced in normal quantity is thought to be abnormal in some way and unable to combine with antigen. Defect (c) occurs in 80 per cent of patients with a condition known as hereditary ataxic telangiectasia; they have increased susceptibility to infections of the upper and lower respiratory tract and the disease is probably due to lack of protection at the level of the respiratory mucous membranes normally brought about by IgA secretion. There is also a deficiency in plasma cells in the mucous membranes of the intestinal tract, where IgA is known to be produced in normal individuals.

Both *cell-mediated* immune mechanisms and *immunoglobulin synthesis* are deficient in an X-linked disease of male children known as 'Swiss type agammaglobulinaemia'. There is almost complete absence of lymphoid tissue in the body, the thymus is very small and the lymphoid tissues of the appendix and Peyer's patches are absent. Children with this condition cannot make antibodies or develop cell-mediated immune reactions, and they suffer from progressive bacterial and/or viral infection and die within two years of birth.

In another type of deficiency state only the cell-mediated immune response to infective agents is affected; here, there is thymic dysplasia and deficiency of lymphoid cells from those areas of the spleen and lymph nodes which are under thymic control. Although children with this rare type of deficiency can produce circulating antibody their inability to develop cell-mediated immunity renders them highly susceptible to virus infection. One form of this condition associated with thymic dysplasia and absence of parathyroid glands is known as Di George's syndrome.

Secondary Defects

Acquired deficiencies of the immunological mechanisms can occur secondarily to a number of disease states affecting the lymphoid tissues such as Hodgkin's disease, multiple myeloma, leukaemia and lymphosarcoma. Deficiency of immunoglobulins can also be brought about by excessive loss of protein through diseased kidneys or via the intestines in protein-losing enteropathies. In contrast to these deficiencies, raised immunoglobulin levels are found in certain disorders of plasma cell function, which amount to malignant proliferation of a particular clone or family of plasma cells. In this condition known as multiple myeloma, a malignant clone is found to produce one particular class of immunoglobulin usually IgG or more rarely one of the other classes. There is usually a decreased synthesis of normal immunoglobulins associated with a deficient immune response to infective agents. On electrophoresis of serum a distinct band can be seen in the immunoglobulin area. This abnormal band is produced by the raised levels of the myeloma immunoglobulin which is termed an M-type protein. In about 20 to 30 per cent of patients with multiple myeloma immunoglobulin light chains are found in the urine. These occur as dimers and are known as Bence-Jones protein. The condition is also associated with excess numbers of plasma cells in the bone marrow and X-ray evidence of myeloma cell deposits in bone.

Clinical Aspects

Increased susceptibility to many types of infection is the outstanding feature of the immunological deficiency states. The age of onset of the congenital types is rarely earlier than 3 to 4 months of age due to the protective effects of maternal antibody. The most frequently affected site is the respiratory tract which is attacked by pyogenic bacteria or fungi. Lack of IgA antibody leads in particular to susceptibility of the respiratory tract to chronic infection.

When there is deficiency of the cell-mediated immune mechanisms resistance to virus infections is diminished, e.g. in the severe tissue necrosis after smallpox vaccination. Rarely BCG vaccination has been followed by generalized tuberculosis in such individuals.

Investigation of suspected immunological deficiency states should include family studies for any abnormalities of immune function, quantitative determination of immunoglobulin levels and estimation of the response to immunization with standard antigens. Peripheral blood counts and X-rays of the thymus region may also prove useful.

Treatment of deficiency states includes use of an appropriate antibiotic and regular administration of pooled human immunoglobulins. Closely matched sibling bone marrow has been used successfully in some cases and a graft of foetal thymus has been used in the case of thymic aplasia.

Defective Phagocytic Mechanisms

These defects take two forms: (1) Where there is a *quantitative* deficiency of blood leucocytes which may be *congenital* (e.g. infantile agranulocytosis) or *acquired* as a result of replacement of bone marrow by tumour tissue or the toxic effects of chemicals. (2) Where there is a *qualitative* deficiency in the functioning of neutrophil leucocytes which whilst ingesting bacteria normally fail to digest them because of an enzymic defect. The clinical form of this defect is known as chronic granulomatous disease and is a sex-linked recessive condition characterized by increased susceptibility in early life to infection by microorganisms of low virulence to the normal individual.

FURTHER READING

Bacteriological Reviews (1960) Symposium on mechanisms of non-specific resistance to infection, **24**, 1.

BARRETT, J. T. (1970) *Textbook of Immunology*. London: Kimpton.

BURNET, F. M. (1969) *Cellular Immunity*. Cambridge University Press.

COHEN, S., HUMPHREY, J. H. & COOMBS, R. R. A. (1967) Antibodies structure and biological function. *Proceedings of the Royal Society of Medicine*, **60**, 589.

COHEN, S. & MILSTEIN, C. (1967) Structure and biological properties of immunoglobulins. *Advances in Immunology*, **7**, 1.

DRESSER, D. W. & MITCHISON, N. A. (1968) The mechanism

of immunological paralysis. *Advances in Immunology*, **8**, 129.

EDELMAN, G. M. (1970) The structure and function of antibodies. *Scientific American*, **223**, 34.

FORD, W. L. & GOWANS, J. L. (1969) The traffic of lymphocytes. *Seminars in Haematology*, **6**, 67.

VAN FURTH, R. (1970) *Mononuclear Phagocytes*. Oxford & Edinburgh: Blackwell.

GOOD, R. A., FINSTAD, J., GEWURZ, H., COOPER, M. D. & POLLARA, B. (1967) The development of immunological capacity in the phylogenetic perspective. *American Journal of Diseases of Children*, **114**, 477.

HARKNESS, D. R. (1970) Structure and function of Immunoglobulins. *Postgraduate Medicine*, **48**, 64.

HERBERT, W. J. (1973) Methods for the preparation of water-in-oil and multiple emulsion for use as antigen adjuvants, and notes on their use in immunization procedures. In *Handbook of Experimental Immunology*, Vol. 3, 2nd Edn. Edited by D. M. Weir. Oxford: Blackwell.

HOBBS, J. R. (1970) Immune globulins in some diseases. *British Journal of Hospital Medicine*, **3**, 669.

HOLBOROW, E. J. (1968) *An ABC of Modern Immunology*. London: Lancet.

HOWARD, J. G. (1963) Natural immunity. In *Modern Trends in Immunology I*. Edited by R. Cruickshank. London: Butterworths.

HUMPHREY, J. H. (1969) The fate of antigen and its relationship to the immune response. In *The Immune Response and its Suppression*. Edited by E. Sorkin. Basel: Karger.

HUMPHREY, J. H. & WHITE, R. G. (1970) *Immunology for Students of Medicine*, 3rd Edn. Oxford: Blackwell.

KABAT, E. A. (1968) *Structural Concepts in Immunology and Immunochemistry*. New York: Holt, Rinehart & Winston.

MACKANESS, G. B. & BLANDEN, R. V. (1967) Cellular immunity. *Progress in Allergy*, **11**, 89.

MARTIN, N. H. (1970) The paraproteinaemias. *British Journal of Hospital Medicine*, **3**, 662.

MIESCHER, P. A. & GRABAR, P. (1968) Complement. In *Immuno-pathology*, Vol. 5. Basel: Schwabe.

MITCHISON, N. A. (1968) Immunological paralysis as a dosage phenomenon. In *Regulation of the Antibody Response*, p. 54. Edited by B. Cinader. Springfield, Illinois: Thomas.

MÜLLER-EBERHARD, H. J. (1968) Chemistry and reaction mechanisms of complement. *Advances in Immunology*, **8**, 2.

NELSON, D. S. (1968) *Macrophages and Immunity*. Amsterdam: North Holland.

NOSSAL, G. J. V. (1967) Mechanisms of antibody production. *Annual Review of Medicine*, **18**, 81.

OSABA, D. (1968) The regulatory role of the thymus in immunogenesis. In *Regulation of the Antibody Response*, p. 232. Edited by B. Cinader. Springfield, Illinois: Thomas.

PINCHUCK, P. & MAURER, P. H. (1967) Genetic control of the immune response. In *Regulation of the Antibody Response*, p. 97. Edited by B. Cinader. Springfield, Illinois: Thomas.

ROGERS BRAMBELL, F. W. (1970) *The Transmission of Passive Immunity from Mother to Young*. Amsterdam: North Holland.

SCHUR, P. H. & AUSTEN, K. F. (1968) Complement in human disease. *Annual Review of Medicine*, **19**, 1.

SMITH, R. T. & GOOD, R. A. (1969) *Cellular Recognition*. New York: Appleton, Century & Crofts.

SMITHIES, O. (1968) Perspectives: mutation and selection in the immune system. In *Regulation of the Antibody Response*, p. 151. Edited by B. Cinader. Springfield, Illinois: Thomas.

SOOTHILL, J. F. (1968) Immunity deficiency states. In *Clinical Aspects of Immunology*, 2nd Edn. Edited by P. G. H. Gell and R. R. A. Coombs. Oxford: Blackwell.

SORKIN, E. (1968) *The Immune Response and its Suppression*, Basel: Karger.

TURK, J. L. (1969) *Immunology in Clinical Medicine*. London: Heinemann.

WALDENSTROM, J. G. (1968) *Monoclonal and Polyclonal Hypergammaglobulinemia—Clinical and Biological Significance*. Cambridge University Press.

WEBB, T. & GOODMAN, H. C. (1967) The structure and function of immunoglobulins. In *Modern Trends in Immunology*, Vol. 2, p. 151. Edited by R. Cruickshank and D. M. Weir. London: Butterworth.

WEIR, D. M. (1973) *Immunology for Undergraduates*. 3rd Edn. Churchill-Livingstone.

WHITE, R. G. (1967) Antigen adjuvants. In *Modern Trends in Immunology*, Vol. 2, p. 28. Edited by R. Cruickshank and D. M. Weir. London: Butterworth.

WIGZELL, H. (1967) Studies in the regulation of antibody synthesis. *Cold Spring Harbour Symposia on Quantitative Biology*, **32**, 507.

WILSON, G. S. & MILES, A. A. (1964) *Topley and Wilson's Principles of Bacteriology and Immunity*, 5th Edn. London: Arnold.

WOLSTENHOLME, G. E. W. & KNIGHT, J. (1970) *Hormones and the Immune Response*. Ciba Foundation Study Group No. 36. London: Churchill.

11. Hypersensitivity and Autoimmunity

Because immunity was first recognized as a resistant state that followed infection, immunology developed primarily as an aspect of medical bacteriology with emphasis on acquired specific resistance to invasion by microorganisms as a means of protection against infection. The term immunity, meaning safe or exempt, has now been extended far beyond its early meaning and includes reactions to foreign material such as grafted tissues, blood products and various bland chemical substances none of which bears any relation to infectious agents. Some forms of immune reaction instead of providing exemption or safety to the affected individual can occasionally produce severe and occasionally fatal results. These are known as 'hypersensitivity reactions' and in the main are due to tissue damage caused by effects of pharmacologically active agents, such as histamine, that are formed under certain conditions of antigen–antibody combination.

The term *allergy* was originally coined by von Pirquet to describe the altered reactivity of an animal after exposure to a foreign antigen, and included both immunity and hypersensitivity. The term, however, has over the years become restricted to refer only to the hypersensitivity which may be associated with the development of the immune response to a foreign substance. *Autoallergic* or *autoimmune* reactions refer to the situation where the immune system fails to distinguish between foreign antigens and self antigens. This form of hypersensitivity can have serious consequences for the individual.

There are two main forms of hypersensitivity reaction: *immediate* and *delayed* (Fig. 11.1). The immediate form appears rapidly after exposure of the sensitized person to a further dose of antigen and usually depends on the liberation of pharmacologically active mediator substances by interaction of the antigen with humoral antibody. The delayed form appears more slowly (usually after 24 hours) and depends on immunologically activated lymphoid cells which on reaction with antigen appear to release substances with a variety of activities on other cells, including cytotoxicity and effects on vascular permeability.

Various classifications of hypersensitivity reactions have been proposed and probably the most widely accepted is that of Coombs and

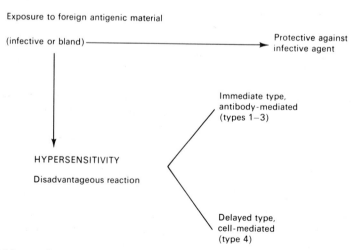

FIG. 11.1. Hypersensitivity reactions.

Gell. This recognizes four types or categories of hypersensitivity reactions, three of which come under the heading of immediate reactions: type 1, *anaphylactic* reactions; type 2, *cytolytic* or *cytotoxic* reactions; and type 3, *toxic-complex* syndrome. The fourth type is the *cell-mediated, delayed* hypersensitivity form of reaction.

Anaphylactic Reactions of Type 1

If a guinea-pig is injected with a small dose of an antigen such as egg albumin, no adverse effects are noted. If, however, a second injection of the egg albumin antigen is given intravenously after an interval of about 10 days a condition known as 'anaphylactic shock' is likely to develop. The animal becomes restless and starts to chew and rub its nose with its front paws; then with respiration becoming laboured, the animal becomes cyanosed and may develop convulsions and die. The initial injection of antigen is termed the 'sensitizing dose' and the second injection the 'shocking dose'. During the interval between the two injections the animal has formed antibody and anaphylaxis is the result of interaction of the shocking dose of antigen with the newly formed antibody on the surface of cells. This interaction triggers the release of pharmacologically active substances which increase capillary permeability and cause contraction of smooth muscle in many parts of the body. In the guinea-pig this reaction particularly affects the smooth muscles of the bronchioles causing bronchospasm and thus respiratory embarrassment of the type present in asthma in man; the asphyxiating effect of the bronchospasm is increased by peribronchial oedema caused by the increase in capillary permeability.

Four pharmacologically active substances have been implicated in anaphylactic reactions; predominant amongst these and responsible for many of the symptoms of anaphylactic shock is *histamine,* which can be shown to be liberated *in vitro* from antibody-sensitized pieces of tissues, including uterine muscle, lung and intestine, exposed to contact with antigen. Sensitization may be induced by prior injection of antigen into the animal supplying the tissue which makes antibody as described above, or the tissue may be sensitized passively by the addition of antibody produced in another animal. The typical contractions induced in this way in isolated strips of uterus and intestine are called Schultz-Dale reactions after the originators. The histamine is derived from the granules of mast (basophil) cells where it exists as its precursor histidine, in combination with heparin; these substances are released by the interaction of antigens with antibody via other pharmacologically active substances, anaphylatoxins, acting together with serum complement components.

The eosinophil is thought to play an important part in anaphylaxis, many of these marrow-derived cells being found in the blood and tissues during an anaphylactic reaction. Although their role is uncertain, these cells may be attracted by released histamine and take part in its detoxification.

The other pharmacological mediators of immediate hypersensitivity reactions are: 5-hydroxy-tryptamine, or serotonin, which causes contraction of plain muscle and increased capillary permeability; it has an uncertain role in anaphylaxis, although it may be involved in intestinal food allergies; slow-reacting substance (or SRS-A) which has a contracting effect on plain muscle and acts, unlike histamine, on the larger, rather than the smaller, blood vessels. SRS-A has a marked constricting effect on bronchial muscle in man and is probably the predominant pharmacological agent in human asthma. The remaining substances—the plasma kinins, the best known example of which is bradykinin—are simple peptides formed from plasma α-globulins (kininogens) by kinin-forming enzymes; they depend upon the activation of complement by antigen–antibody complexes. Bradykinin has histamine-like effects on smooth muscle and capillaries and is present in the bloodstream in many animal species in the early stages of an anaphylactic reaction although it has an uncertain role in human relations.

In man there are two types of anaphylactic reaction—*systemic* and *local*—which are related to the mode of entry to the body of the shocking dose of antigen. If the antigen is injected parenterally, as in the case of foreign serum (e.g., horse anti-tetanus serum), a drug such as penicillin, or perhaps by the bite of an insect, the systemic form of anaphylaxis is likely to develop.

ANAPHYLAXIS (Type 1)

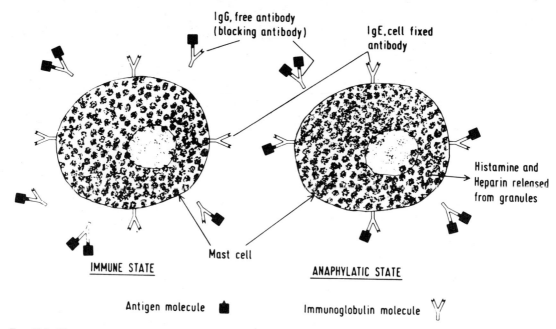

FIG. 11.2. Diagrammatic view of the possible difference between an 'immune state' (i.e. when immunized animal will not develop anaphylaxis on challenge with antigen) and an 'anaphylactic state'. Here there is insufficient antibody free in the tissue fluids to mop up the antigen thus allowing it to combine with reaginic antibody (IgE) attached to cell. The interaction triggers the release of histamine and heparin from mast cell granules.

The symptoms include dyspnoea with broncho-spasm and peribronchial and laryngeal oedema, sometimes skin rashes, a fall in blood pressure and occasionally death. If, on the other hand, the antigen comes primarily in contact with respiratory mucous membranes, then in a sensitized individual, the local form of anaphylaxis will develop, i.e. hay fever or asthma. If the appropriate antigen (e.g. nuts, fish or straw-berries), comes in contact with the intestinal mucous membrane of a susceptible individual, a mixed form of reaction may develop, with intestinal symptoms, skin rashes (urticaria) and sometimes the symptoms of asthma.

Antibodies involved in Anaphylactic Reactions

In man the antibodies that sensitize the tissues for anaphylactic reactions have been known for many years as *reaginic* antibodies. These anti-bodies have a strong affinity for tissues and can

readily be detected in the serum of a sensitized individual by injecting a small quantity of the serum into the skin of a normal recipient and, 24–28 hours later, introducing the appropriate antigen into the injection site. Within about 20 minutes a 'wheal-and-flare' erythematous reaction develops at the injection site, just like the response to an injection of histamine. This reaction is called the Prausnitz-Küstner (or PK) test after its originators.

The nature of reaginic antibody was not elucidated until 1967 when a hitherto un-described form of myeloma protein was dis-covered in Sweden. By use of an antiserum prepared in a sheep to the myeloma globulin a new class of immunoglobulin was shown to be present in normal serum. Its concentration was very low, 0·0001 to 0·0007 mg/100 ml of serum, compared with 800 to 1680 mg of IgG/100 ml serum. The skin-sensitizing activity of reaginic antibody could readily be neutralized by means of the antiserum to this new immunoglobulin which has been named IgE (see Chap. 9). The concentration of IgE in patients with allergic asthma has been found to be much higher than in normal individuals. The comparatively low levels of IgE found in serum presumably reflect the affinity of this immunoglobulin for tissues so that freshly made IgE is very soon removed from the blood when it comes in contact with the appropriate cell receptors on mast cells and possibly elsewhere.

Immunological Approaches to the Prevention of Anaphylaxis

Consideration of the mechanism of systemic anaphylaxis makes it seem likely that if the parenterally injected antigen could be prevented from reaching the tissue-fixed IgE then anaphyl-axis would not develop. This desirable state of affairs can be achieved by the simple expedient of injecting frequent small doses of the antigen to which the patient is sensitized; this induces the formation of increasing levels of IgG anti-body which, by circulating in the blood and tissue fluids, mops up the injected antigen so that it does not reach the tissue-fixed IgE (Fig. 11.2). This IgG antibody has been termed *blocking antibody* and its induction is the basis of desen-sitization treatment in allergic individuals. This procedure is naturally much more effective in preventing systemic anaphylactic reactions than local anaphylaxis, where the antigen does not enter the bloodstream. To prevent the latter form blocking antibody would need to be pre-sent in the mucous secretions and parenteral injection of antigen is not the best way to achieve this although desensitization to pollens which cause hay fever and asthma may be achieved by prophylactic courses of pollen antigen injec-tions.

For pollen or seasonal allergies desensitizing injections are given before the onset of the pollen season and clinical benefit is claimed in about 70 per cent of cases. Symptomatic treatment of allergies commonly involves the use of anti-histamines and more recently of disodium chromoglycate which is effective in blocking histamine release if the drug is present before challenge with antigen.

Cytolytic or Cytotoxic Type-2 Reactions

Reactions of this type are initiated by an anti-genic component that is either part of a tissue cell or closely associated with a cell (e.g. a drug attached to the cell wall) (Fig. 11.3). The antibodies directed against such a cell-associated antigen bring about a cytotoxic or cytolytic effect usually involving the participa-tion of complement. Reactions of this type include the cytolytic effect of antibodies on foreign red cells induced by incompatible blood transfusion. Haemolytic disease of the newborn has a similar mechanism as do certain forms of autoimmune haemolytic anaemia in which the patient forms antibodies against autologous red cells. There are many examples of these cyto-toxic or cytolytic reactions brought about by an immune reaction to a foreign substance which becomes attached to the cell membranes of erythrocytes, leucocytes or platelets. One of the best known is Sedormid purpura which is due to the union of the drug Sedormid with platelets; as a result an antibody response against the platelet-adsorbed drug brings about destruction of the platelets and thus causes purpura. Sedormid has therefore been withdrawn from use. This type of reaction may be more wide-spread than is generally suspected.

A variety of infectious diseases due to salmonella organisms and mycobacteria are associated with haemolytic anaemia and from studies in salmonella infections, the haemolysis is apparently due to an immune reaction against a lipopolysaccharide bacterial endotoxin which becomes coated on to the patient's erythrocytes. A detailed study of *Salm. gallinarum* infection in chickens has shown conclusively that the red cells are coated and have a shorter life in the circulation due to haemolysis and that the development of haemolysis directly parallels the level of the anti-lipopolysaccharide antibody.

Toxic-complex Syndrome Type-3 Reaction

These reactions are due to the combination of antigen with circulating antibody leading to formation of microprecipitates in and around small blood vessels with consequent inflamma-tion and sometimes mechanical blockage of the

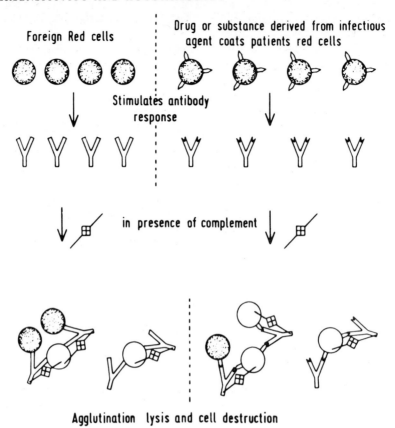

FIG. 11.3. Cytolytic and cytotoxic (type 2) reactions.

vessels, causing interference with the blood supply to surrounding tissues. There are two types of reaction that fall into this category; a systemic form or *serum sickness,* and a local form, the *Arthus reaction.* 'Serum sickness' develops in individuals given injections of foreign serum and was first described soon after the introduction of parenteral administration of horse diphtheria antitoxin for therapeutic purposes. Foreign serum protein is eliminated from the circulation over a period of a few weeks and after the injection of 10 to 20 ml a large amount will still be present when antibodies to the foreign protein develop. The consequent formation of antibody–antigen complexes may cause a wide variety of symptoms ranging from anaphylactic reactions such as asthma or laryngeal oedema, in which IgE antibody attached to mast cells is involved, to

symptoms dependent on the deposition of immune complexes (antigen + IgG antibody) in blood vessels which activate complement and cause inflammatory changes. The organs affected include the kidney in which glomerulonephritis may develop, the heart in which there may be myocarditis and valvulitis, and the joints which become swollen and painful. Urticaria frequently develops and the patient becomes pyrexial. The symptoms disappear whenever all the foreign serum protein is eliminated. Nowadays, the most likely causes of serum sickness are drugs such as penicillin which form drug-protein complexes in the host.

The Arthus reaction, like serum sickness, is brought about by the formation of antibody–antigen complexes but in this case the phenomenon is a local one at the site of injection of antigen. The Arthus reaction occurs in the walls of small blood vessels in the presence of large quantities of IgG antibody which forms microprecipitates with antigen. Vasculitis develops a few hours after injection of antigen and persists for 12 to 24 hours. With the fluorescent antibody technique, immune complexes can be seen in the vessel wall and there is a massive infiltration of granulocytes due to a chemotactic effect generated by the antigen–antibody complex. Liberation of the vasoactive amines such as histamine causes an increase in vascular permeability and consequent oedema. These reactions are of relatively minor clinical importance; they may occur in diabetics who have received many injections of insulin and have developed high levels of IgG antibody to antigenic constituents in the insulin preparation.

Delayed Hypersensitivity, Type-4 or Cell-Mediated Hypersensitivity

This form of hypersensitive reaction may be defined as a specifically provoked, slowly evolving (24 to 48 hours) mixed cellular reaction involving particularly lymphocytes and macrophages. The reaction is not induced by circulating antibody but by sensitized lymphoid cells and can be transferred in experimental animals by such cells, but not by serum. The classical example of this type of reaction is the tuberculin response which occurs when an individual previously or currently infected with tubercle bacilli is given an intradermal injection of 0·1 ml of a 1 in 1000 dilution of a protein extract of tubercle bacilli (purified protein derivative or PPD): 24 to 48 hours later an indurated inflammatory reaction of variable size can be seen in the skin. The injection site is infiltrated with large numbers of mononuclear cells, mainly lymphocytes, with about 10 to 20 per cent of macrophages. Most of these cells are in or around small blood vessels. Despite intensive investigation of the delayed hypersensitivity reaction, its underlying mechanisms are poorly understood. A possible explanation is that amongst the continuous traffic of lymphocytes passing through the tissues there are some sensitized cells with antibody-like receptors on their surface. These cells interact with the antigen they meet and, in some unknown way, influence other lymphocytes to migrate to the area. Macrophages in delayed hypersensitivity reaction sites may contribute lysosomal enzymes from their intracellular granules and thus cause further inflammatory changes. When they come into contact with antigen the sensitized lymphocytes release a number of non-antibody factors (termed lymphokines) which include a factor inhibiting macrophage migration, a chemotactic factor and a cytotoxic factor, but the role of these substances in delayed hypersensitivity is not yet clear (Chap. 10).

Delayed hypersensitivity reactions are characteristically induced by intracellular infectious agents including salmonellae, brucellae, mycobacteria, pathogenic fungi, and a wide range of viruses including those of measles, mumps, vaccinia and herpes simplex. A virus reaction with clinical relevance may occur in vaccinia, the so-called 'reaction of immunity' developing within 24 to 72 hours after vaccination (see Chap. 30). Delayed hypersensitivity reactions sometimes develop after sensitization to a variety of metals such as nickel and chromium, to simple chemical substances such as dye stuffs, potassium dichromate (affecting cement workers), primulin from primula plants, poison ivy and chemicals such as picryl chloride, dinitrochlorobenzene, and paraphenylene diamine (from hair dyes). Skin-sensitization to penicillin is not uncommon after the topical application of the antibiotic in ointments or creams. These substances are not themselves antigenic and only become so on combination by covalent bonds with proteins in the skin. The clinical signs induced in these 'contact hypersensitivity' reactions (contact dermatitis) include redness, swelling, vesicles, scaling and exudation of fluid.

AUTOIMMUNITY

A fundamental characteristic of an animal's immune system is that it does not under normal circumstances react against its own body constituents. There exists a mechanism that enables the cells of the immune system to recognize what is 'foreign' and what is 'self'. Attempts to explain the absence of reactions against self go back to the early days of immunology when Paul

Ehrlich enunciated his well known doctrine of 'horror autotoxicus'. Ehrlich and Morgenroth in 1900 after immunizing a goat with red blood cells of other goats found that although the animal readily made antibodies against the red cells of other goats these antibodies failed to react with the animal's own red cells. It was thus clear that in some way the immunological response to self antigens was prevented. Because of Ehrlich's high standing as an immunologist, it seemed inconceivable that the rule of 'horror autotoxicus' could be broken and this view persisted despite clinical evidence of the existense of diseases in which the patient was apparently destroying his own cells.

The main reason that observations of this type failed to achieve recognition was the absence of serological techniques capable of demonstrating convincingly the existence of antibodies able to react with the host's tissue eells or of the presence of such antibodies actually attached to cells. Then in 1946 Coombs, Mourant and Race described a technique which detected the presence of antibody globulin on red blood cells by the simple expedient of adding an antiglobulin serum which, after reacting with the globulin coating the cells, linked the cells together and agglutinated them. This method was particularly valuable for showing the presence on cells of antibody globulin that was in itself unable to agglutinate the cells. This technique is commonly known as the 'Coombs' or 'antiglobulin' test: many, sometimes rather complicated, variations of the antiglobulin technique were subsequently developed. Amongst the more important of these is the fluorescent antibody technique in which a commonly used procedure is to label an antiglobulin serum with a fluorescent marker (fluorescein isothiocyanate) so that the reaction of the labelled antiglobulin with, for example, globulin-coated cells can be visualized under UV light microscopy. Under these conditions the site of attachment of the fluorescein-labelled antiglobulin shows up as bright apple-green fluorescent areas.

These methods allowed a breakthrough in the recognition of a variety of human and animal diseases in which antibodies capable of reacting with a number of different antigens of the individual's own tissues could convincingly be demonstrated in his serum. The first of these discoveries was the demonstration that in some types of haemolytic anaemia in man the red blood cells were coated with antibody globulin. This was soon followed by the finding of an autoantibody serum factor in the blood of patients with a severe connective tissue disease called systemic lupus erythematosus (SLE), and because the factor was an antibody for the nuclei of tissue cells, it was called anti-nuclear factor (ANF). About the same time the presence of an antibody to thyroglobulin was demonstrated in patients with a particular form of interstitial thyroiditis known as Hashimoto's disease.

An early clinical description of acquired haemolytic anaemia was given in 1898 in France, and in 1908 haemolytic activity against red cells was found in the serum of patients in whom intense haemolysis was taking place *in vivo*. These early observations were neglected until 30 years later when Damashek and Schwartz again reported haemolysins in patients suffering from haemolytic anaemia. With the introduction of the Coombs test in 1946 the immunological basis of the disease was put on a firm foundation.

Associated with the accumulating evidence on the autoimmune nature of the haemolysins in acute haemolytic anaemia, there arose the need to consider the meaning of foreignness and self-recognition and the mechanisms underlying the ability of the body to differentiate between 'self' and 'non-self'. A solution to the problem this created in immunological theory was offered by Burnet and Fenner in 1949, who, whilst accepting the validity of the direct template theory (see Chap. 10), included the notion of 'self-markers' attached to body components by which antibody-forming cells were able to recognize them and render them immunologically inert. They also predicted that an equivalent tolerance to foreign antigens should be demonstrable if these antigens had been introduced at an appropriate stage in embryonic life while the animal's immune system was in the process of learning to recognize the 'self-markers' of its own tissues. This prediction was later confirmed experimentally by Medawar and his colleagues who showed that if neonatal mice were injected with transplantation antigen from another strain of mice, they would later be able to accept skin grafts that an animal not injected neonatally would rapidly reject. Burnet soon followed his 'self-marker' theory by the more generally acceptable 'clonal selection' theory, in which the capacity to produce a given antibody was regarded as a genetically determined quality of certain clones or families of mesenchymal cells; the function of the antigen was to stimulate cells of these clones to proliferation and antibody production. The theory postulated that in the early stages of embryonic development, mutation of cells led to a variety of random arrangements in the globulin molecules so that a very large number of clones was generated which could correspond to potential antigenic determinants. To explain the inability of the antibody-forming system to react with self, Burnet proposed that the immature cells were destroyed at this early stage if they met the antigens with which they could react. Tolerance would result from the elimination or inhibition of all cell clones which had the ability to react with antigenic determinants present in the body. After birth when foreign antigen entered the tissues, antibody to it would be produced by specific stimulation of those cells in clones pre-adapted to react with the corresponding antigenic determinants. On the basis of this theory Burnet accounted for the development of autoimmune disease as a failure of the maintenance of the 'non-self' reactive population of antibody-forming cells.

Possible Mechanism involved in the Development of Autoimmunity

The question now arises as to how the normal controlling mechanism fails with the resulting

---

Table 11.1. Mechanisms of antibody formation

---

1. EVASION of normal tolerance to 'self' antigens
   (a) Hidden antigens
   (b) Altered antigens—
       chemicals, drugs,
       infectious agents

2. BREAKDOWN of tolerance mechanism
   (a) Agents affecting antibody forming cells—
       chemicals, drugs,
       infectious agents
   (b) Genetically determined lack of efficiency
       of tolerance control mechanisms.

---

inability to maintain self-recognition manifested by immune reactions against self.

There are two main ways (Table 11.1) in which this mechanism for maintaining tolerance could conceivably be overcome. The first involves evasion or circumvention of a normal functioning mechanism and the second failure of the mechanism itself.

In the first category evasion may occur in two possible ways: (1) because a particular body antigen is not normally accessible to the cells of the immune system as the antigen is hidden within a cell or tissue; these antigens are known as *sequestered antigens*: (2) because a tissue antigen is altered in some way by a chemical agent, a drug or an infectious agent—*altered antigens*.

Hidden or sequestered antigens do seem to exist and the best examples of these are sperm antigens and lens antigen of the eye. Sperm can be shown to acquire an antigen during maturation which is absent from the immature germinal cells and antibodies can be induced in the guinea-pig by immunizing with autologous sperm, showing that the immune system fails to recognize the sperm as part of self. Orchitis can be induced by combining the sperm with an adjuvant which gives a boost to the immune response and at the same time allows the stimulated lymphoid cells and antibody to gain access to the sperm-forming tissues. Orchitis in man is a rare complication of mumps infection in which it is assumed that the virus damages the basement membrane barrier of the seminiferous tubules and the cells of the immune system are thus allowed entry to initiate an immune response.

As for the lens antigen, a rabbit which is given an injection of bovine lens material develops antibodies that react with its own lens *in vitro*. Occasionally the extraction of a lens for cataract is succeeded by inflammatory changes in retained lens substance sometimes affecting the other remaining lens; the same phenomenon can be induced experimentally in animals. However, such observations should be regarded at present as speculative evidence to support the concept of sequestered antigens as an initiating factor in autoimmune disease.

Evidence in support of the second proposed way in which normal tolerance mechanisms are circumvented is more concrete. Experimental studies of tolerance evasion by altered antigens have been carried out with purified proteins, conjugates of hapten and protein, and with cellular antigens. Some of the most definitive work was carried out in America by Weigle who showed that rabbits made tolerant of bovine serum albumin (BSA) and then immunized with the cross-reacting human serum albuin (HSA) eventually made antibodies that would react with BSA. The same result was obtained with chemically modified BSA. A closer approximation to autoimmune disease in man is provided by experiments with thyroglobulin in rabbits; not only are rabbit thyroglobulin antibodies induced by injection of altered thyroglobulin but inflammatory lesions are also produced in their thyroid glands as a result of the immunizing procedure.

There has developed considerable interest in the role of microorganisms as a source of cross-reacting antigens sharing antigenic determinants with tissue components. The ability of viruses to bring about alterations of cell membranes has been suggested by studies on the effect of herpes and rabies viruses on tissue culture cells. New cell surface antigens, which appear to act as transplantation antigens, have been found in mouse cells injected with herpes and polyoma viruses.

In the human colon an antigen exists, extractable from even sterile foetal colon, which is similar to a polysaccharide antigen present in *Escherichia coli* O14. It is conceivable that the inflammatory condition of the colon known as ulcerative colitis, in which anti-colon antibodies are found, is due to an immune reaction initiated by the cross-reacting bacterial antigen. Similarly group A streptococci, which are closely associated with rheumatic fever, have an antigen in common with a human heart antigen: anti-heart antibody is found in just over 50 per cent of patients with rheumatic heart lesions. Again, nephritogenic strains of type 12 group A streptococci carry surface antigens similar to those found in human glomeruli and infection by these organisms has been associated with the development of acute glomerulonephritis.

Drugs can act as haptens (Chap. 9) which bind to tissue proteins. The resulting complex may be antigenic and result in an immune reaction which damages cells coated with the drug. Examples of this are a metabolic breakdown product of the drug α-methyldopa, used in the treatment of hypertension and a breakdown product of penicillin, each of which can bind to the surface of red cells. The immune response generated by these drug-altered cells can then result in haemolysis of the affected cells.

The second main category of mechanisms by means of which autoimmune reactions may develop (Table 11.1) are those due to alteration in the cellular processes on which maintenance of normal tolerance depends. This could occur by the direct effect of a chemical, a drug or an infectious agent on the lymphoid tissues. Alternatively, the loss of normal tolerance control could be due to an inherited defect or lack of efficiency in the lymphoid cell population.

There is much speculation on the role of infectious agents acting *directly* on the lymphoid tissues as a cause of autoimmune disease. This stems from the experimental evidence on the induction of autoimmune disease by injection of tissue antigens combined with Freund's complete adjuvant. This water-in-oil emulsion owes its powerful stimulating effect on the lymphoid tissues to killed mycobacteria incorporated in the oil. Rabbits given injections of *Mycobacterium tuberculosis* alone have been shown to develop autoantibodies against a wide range of autologous tissues. The same phenomenon is found in a number of chronic infections in man such as syphilis, actinomycosis and chronic tuberculosis. Infection with *Mycoplasma pneumoniae* associated with a primary atypical pneumonia may cause the development of IgM agglutinins which in the cold will react with the patient's own red cells and may produce haemolytic anaemia.

A leukaemia virus has in the last few years been found in a strain of mice (New Zealand Black or NZB mice) that induces the early development of autoimmune disease including autoimmune haemolytic anaemia and immune complex nephritis. The virus has been found in many body tissues and in the blood and may be seen in lymphoid organs attached to the surface of lymphocytes. Similar virus particles have been found in embryos of the NZB strain suggesting that it is passed through the placenta or is associated with the germ cells. The association of the virus with lymphocyte membranes has led to the speculation that the presence of the virus might interfere with normal lymphocyte reactivity to antigens. It is known that antigens can react with the lymphocyte surface and that this is probably one stimulus to immune transformation of these cells. The virus could conceivably upset the mechanisms controlling lymphocyte reactivity so that they respond abnormally to antigens to which they should remain tolerant. This idea receives some support from experiments in which animals stimulated with certain microorganisms (e.g. tubercle bacilli or corynebacteria) or the products of organisms (e.g. bacterial endotoxin) do not develop the expected immunological tolerance to antigens administered in a way which would induce tolerance in normal animals. Recent evidence suggests that B lymphocytes lose tolerance more readily than T lymphocytes and that T cells tolerant to self may be bypassed by presenting autoantigens to B cells in a sufficiently immunogenic form, perhaps combined with adjuvants as discussed above.

PATHOGENESIS OF AUTOIMMUNE DISEASE

There is much uncertainty about the mechanism of pathogenesis in autoimmune disease. The immune reactions, as a form of hypersensitivity, may bring about severe and sometimes fatal reactions affecting the individual's own tissues and cells. Three of the four types of hypersensitivity reactions are involved in autoimmune reactions.

Cytolytic or Cytotoxic Type-2 Reactions

The foremost of the autoimmune conditions in this category is autoimmune haemolytic anaemia. Here the antibodies are of two main types; (1) antibodies of the IgM type which agglutinate the patient's own red cells in the cold; (2) antibodies of IgG type which do not usually bring about direct agglutination of the red cells but can be detected by the Coombs test with an antiglobulin serum.

The anaemia is caused largely by the removal of antibody-coated cells in the spleen or the liver. Only rarely does lysis or agglutination take place to any extent in the circulation and involve the uptake of serum complement. Whilst normal red cells survive with a half life in the circulation for just over three weeks, in this form of anaemia their half life rarely exceeds one week.

Other forms of haemolytic anaemia include drug-induced types and those involving infective agents such as mycoplasma. Drugs involved include penicillin, phenacetin, quinine and α-methyldopa. The anaemia is brought about by reaction of antibody with the drug linked as a hapten to the red cell surface resulting in haemolysis. The precise details of the haptenic groups responsible for antigenic stimulation and their linkage to the red cell surface are uncertain. In mycoplasma infections the IgM cold agglutinins react with a common red cell antigen known as the I antigen.

Drug-induced granulocytopenia and thrombocytopenia have also been described in which the cells are destroyed by antibody directed at a complex of the drug and cell surface structures. Sedormid purpura has already been mentioned.

Toxic-complex Type-3 Reactions

Complexes of antibody and tissue antigens, particularly nuclear antigens, are the cause of glomerulonephritis in a number of autoimmune states and notably in systemic lupus erythematosis where a wide range of anti-tissue antibodies is found, and in the similar type of disease of NZB mice. Complexes of antinuclear antibody and nuclear antigen together with complement can readily be demonstrated in the glomerular capillaries. The glomerular basement membranes become thickened and secondary changes develop in the renal tubules with progressive renal failure.

Cell-mediated Type-4 Reactions

There is no doubt that in both man and experimental animals the development of a number of autoimmune states is paralleled by the existence of cell-mediated reactions of the delayed hypersensitivity type as demonstrated by skin tests with tissue antigens. Whether the diseases are actually caused by immune reactions mediated by lymphoid cells is a matter of conjecture. Support for the role of cells in the disease process comes from studies in an experimental autoimmune disease known as autoimmune allergic encephalomyelitis. This disease follows immunization of animals with brain homogenate in Freund's complete adjuvant and is associated with demyelination of motor nerve fibres. The disease can be transferred to inbred strains of rats by the injection of lymphoid cells from affected animals to normal animals. The same type of transfer has been performed in autoimmune thyroiditis. In the latter condition it is suggested that the sensitized lymphocytes produce a surface injury to the cells of the thyroid acini and thus allow the cytotoxic antibody frequently present in the serum of affected subjects to enter the cell and react with intracellular antigens.

That there may be an association between the reactions of cell-mediated immunity and humoral antibody is emphasized by work on autoimmune orchitis in guinea-pigs. Animals given injections of a purified testis homogenate in Freund's complete adjuvant develop cell-mediated immunity, as shown by the development of delayed hypersensitivity on skin testing, but there is no circulating antibody or testicular lesion. When these animals are given injections of testis antibody from a guinea-pig injected with testis homogenate in incomplete Freund's adjuvant (i.e. without tubercle bacilli), orchitis develops. This association is supported by the finding that testis antibody enters the seminiferous tubules (as shown by indirect immuno-fluorescent) at the same time as cell-mediated immunity first appears.

OTHER DISEASES ASSOCIATED WITH AUTOIMMUNE STATES

There is a large reservoir of diseases in which some form of autoantibody has been found but where neither the stimulus for autoantibody formation nor the role, if any, of immune reactions has been elucidated.

Among these conditions is rheumatoid arthritis in which an IgM antibody called rheumatoid factor is present in the serum. This antibody is detected *in vitro* by its ability to agglutinate red cells or latex particles that have been coated with IgG globulin. The rheumatoid factor does not appear to be involved in the pathogenesis of the disease which is still unresolved. There is the possibility that infective agents such as myco-plasma or other microbial agents are involved and there are reports of the isolation of such agents from rheumatoid joints in arthritis in man and in a number of other species. Experimental arthritis can be induced in rats by the injection of Freund's complete adjuvant containing killed tubercle bacilli. This is a polyarthritis with mononuclear infiltration similar to the arthritis found in Reiter's syndrome, the main features of which are urethritis and arthritis and which may be related to mycoplasma infection.

ANTIBODIES AS A CONSEQUENCE OF TISSUE DAMAGE

In considering the role of autoantibodies as a possible cause of autoimmune disease it should be remembered that antibodies of IgM type directed at subcellular antigens can readily be induced by various forms of tissue damage. These arise secondarily to the damage and appear to have no role in perpetuating it. Antibodies of this type have been induced in rats by the injection of the hepatotoxic agent carbon tetrachloride; it was subsequently found that normal rats, mice and hamsters have some IgM anti-tissue antibody in their serum. A possible physiological role for these antibodies is suggested by the finding of a chemotactic effect *in vitro* on rat polymorphs of a mixture of the anti-tissue antibody and its antigen. Thus the antibody might be responsible for initiating a phagocytic cell clearing process to deal with the breakdown products of normal cell turnover. All autoantibodies are therefore not necessarily autoaggressive although the history of immunity and protection inculcates the idea of antibodies acting solely as aggressive agents.

FURTHER READING

ASHERSON, G. L. (1968) The role of micro-organisms in autoimmune responses. *Progress in Allergy*, **12**, 192.
ASHERSON, G. L. (1968) Autoantibody production as a

breakdown of immune tolerance. In *Regulation of the Antibody Response*, p. 68. Edited by B. Cinader. Springfield, Illinois: Thomas.

BROSTOFF, J. (1973) Atopic allergy. *British Journal of Hospital Medicine*, **9**, 29.

BUCHANAN, W. W. & IRVINE, W. J. (1967) Symposium on autoimmunity and genetics. *Clinical Experiments in Immunology*, **2**, Suppl.

BURNET, F. M. (1959) *The Clonal Selection Theory of Acquired Immunity*. Cambridge University Press.

CREAM, J. J. (1973) Immune complex diseases. *British Journal of Hospital Medicine*, **9**, 8.

EAST, June (1969) Viruses and autoimmunity. *Vox Sanguinis*. **16**, 318.

GLYNN, L. E. & HOLBOROW, E. J. (1964) *Autoimmunity*. Oxford: Blackwell.

HUMPHREY, J. H. & WHITE, R. G. (1969) *Immunology for Students of Medicine*, p. 600. Oxford: Blackwell.

IRVINE, W. J. (1967) Immunobiology of the thymus and its relation to autoimmune disease. In *Modern Trends of Immunology*, Vol. 2, p. 250. Edited by R. Cruickshank and D. M. Weir, London: Butterworth.

PERLMANN, P. (1969) Bacteria and autoimmunity. *Vox Sanguinis*, **16**, 314.

ROITT, I. M. (1969) Humoral immunity and autoimmune disease. *Vox Sanguinis*, **16**, 314.

SAMTER, M. (1971) *Immunologic Diseases*. 2nd Edn. Boston: Little Brown.

TRENTIN, J. J. (1967) *Cross-reacting Antigens and Neoantigens (with implications for Autoimmunity and Cancer Immunity)*. Baltimore: Williams and Wilkins.

TURK, J. L. (1969) *Immunology in Clinical Medicine*. London: Heinemann.

TURK, J. L. (1969) Cellular immunity and autoimmune diseases. *Vox Sanguinis*, **16**, 341.

WEIR, D. M. (1969) Altered antigen and autoimmunity. *Vox Sanguinis*, **16**, 304.

WHALEY, K. & DICK, W. C. (1969) Rheumatoid arthritis: aetiological and pathogenic considerations. *British Journal of Hospital Medicine*, **2**, 1916.

12. Viruses: Structure, Composition, Classification

Among the common contagious illnesses of man and animals there are many for which no bacterial cause has been found. These diseases have been known clinically throughout the centuries; smallpox has been recognized as a deadly infection since pre-Christian times and Hippocrates was perfectly familiar with the swollen neck in mumps. At the beginning of the present century it was realized that an agent present in the tissues or blood of such cases could transmit the infection in the absence of bacteria. Pasteur in 1884, when he failed to detect bacteria in infective material from rabid dogs, said that he was tempted to believe that the cause of the disease was 'a microorganism infinitesimally small'. In 1892 Pasteur's theory was confirmed, though in a different disease, by Iwanowsky, who showed that the mosaic disease of tobacco plants was caused by a minute agent which was so small that it was ultramicroscopic and would pass through the pores of a filter that would not permit the passage of any known bacterium. In 1898 the vesicle fluid from cases of foot and mouth disease in cattle was shown by Loeffler and Frosch to contain an infectious agent that was similarly filterable. In 1901 it was proved that yellow fever in man was caused by a filterable virus carried by mosquitoes. From these discoveries it soon became apparent that there were a number of viral agents which could pass through bacteria-stopping filters and still retain their powers to cause disease in animals and human volunteers. Viruses were therefore originally recognized as ultramicroscopic and filter-passing.

During the years that followed, many similar minute filter-passing organisms were found to be widely distributed throughout the animal and plant kingdoms, causing mild as well as severe diseases and often being carried latently in their hosts without giving rise to any obvious signs of harm. In man it was shown that viruses cause not only such serious illnesses as smallpox, poliomyelitis, encephalitis and infectious hepatitis but are also responsible for many familiar and less serious infections including the common cold, influenza, mumps, measles and chickenpox, and a whole host of other conditions. Amongst the many important virus diseases of animals are foot and mouth disease and rinderpest in cattle, distemper and rabies in dogs, and fowl pest in poultry.

Not only do viruses cause many infectious illnesses, but it has been gradually realized that they also play a part, perhaps with the aid of other factors, in the production of certain types of tumours. Rous in 1911 discovered that certain sarcomata in fowls could be transmitted with cell-free filtrates of the tumours and since that time an impressive list of animal tumours has been compiled in which viruses undoubtedly play a causative role. These *oncogenic viruses* include the agents that cause warts in man, fibromas, papillomas and related tumours in rabbits and other mammals, mammary carcinomata, leukaemias, and parotid tumours (polyoma virus) in mice, and leucosis in poultry.

Many insects suffer from virus diseases, e.g. epizootics of jaundice in silk worms and sac brood in bees have been the cause of much economic loss. Insects are, however, more notorious as the *vectors* of viruses that attack man, animals and plants. Some viruses can multiply within their bodies without harming them and often the virus is carried through the whole of the life cycle of the insect. Thus lice, ticks, flies and mosquitoes transmit viruses within human and animal communities and can carry infection from plant to plant. Again, nematode worms that are parasitic in pigs spread the swine influenza virus, and other nematodes that infest plants play an important part in the transmission of infection to vines and cereals.

When plants are affected by viruses, one of the characteristic effects is a mottling, or 'mosaic', of the leaves, which may be followed by withering and death of the plant. There are more than three hundred viruses recognized as pathogenic for plants and many, for example the tobacco mosaic virus, the tomato bushy stunt virus and the virus of 'X' disease of potatoes, are of great economic importance. One plant virus, the tulip mosaic virus, however, is virtually harmless and is responsible for the beautiful coloured mottlings and pencillings on the petals of tulip flowers.

That bacteria too are subject to infection by viruses was realized when Twort in 1915 and d'Herelle in 1917 independently observed the phenomenon of the transmissible lysis of bacteria. This was demonstrated by d'Herelle in the following way: a few drops of liquid faeces from a case of bacterial dysentery were added to a tube of broth which was incubated overnight; filtration of this culture through a porcelain candle yielded a bacteria-free filtrate which, when added in very small quantities to a young culture of *Shigella shigae*, produced clearing and lysis of the bacteria after incubation for several hours. D'Herelle was able to show that this lysed culture possessed a similar lytic property towards a fresh culture and he was able to carry the effect through more than fifty successive transfers; he thought the effect was caused by 'an invisible microbe that is antagonistic to the dysentery bacillus' and suggested that this was a minute parasite of bacteria propagating and multiplying at the expense of the bacterial cells. He called the microbe 'bacteriophage', a name now frequently abbreviated to *phage*, and his view that it was a virus has been fully confirmed. Bacteriophages are also recognized by their ability to produce a clearing of an area when 'spotted' on to a confluent growth of the host bacterium on an agar plate. The clear area is known as a *plaque*; it is often produced by a single phage particle and is therefore analogous to a bacterial colony. Bacteriophages have the great advantage that they can be easily propagated and counted, and moreover their hosts, the bacterial cells, lend themselves readily to study at biochemical and genetic levels. Because of this, knowledge of the mechanisms of phage infection and reproduction is far more advanced than knowledge of the corresponding mechanisms in animal viruses. There is therefore a tendency to regard phages as model viruses and to adapt the methods used successfully in their study to the more complex relationships between the animal virus and its host cell.

DEFINITION OF A VIRUS

From the many previous attempts that had been made to define viruses formally, Luria in 1967 produced a composite definition incorporating all the accepted essential features of viruses:

'Viruses are entities whose genome is in an element of nucleic acid, either DNA or RNA, which reproduces inside living cells and uses their synthetic machinery to direct the synthesis of specialized particles, the virions which contain the viral genome and transfer it to other cells'.

The two cardinal features of viruses expressed here are first that they possess genetic material which when it is within the host cell behaves as part of the cell, and second that they also exist in an extracellular form which is the product of the host cell under the genetic control of the virus itself. The extracellular form—*the virion*—serves as a vehicle to carry the viral genome to other cells.

Viruses can reproduce only when they are within their host cells and are of necessity intracellular parasites. They have no ribosomes and are devoid of enzymes to generate high energy bonds. They have no mitochondria or other organelles, and they lack a rigid cell wall. Thus there is no muramic acid in their outer coverings and they are unaffected by most of the antimicrobial drugs. Indeed, viruses have no real cell structure and it is difficult to regard them as microorganisms at all. True microorganisms multiply by binary fission and synthesize the macromolecules that they require, but viruses can do neither of these things (see Table 12.1).

A complete infective virus particle is called a *virion* and the genome is in a core and consists of *either* deoxyribonucleic acid (DNA) *or* of ribonucleic acid (RNA) *but not both*. The nucleic acid is enclosed within an outer shell of protein often known as a *capsid*. The protein and nucleic acid are closely integrated to form a *nucleocapsid* of strictly defined symmetry.

Some virions during the late phases of their maturation acquire an extra covering in the form of a lipoprotein *envelope* which is derived, for the most part, from the host cell membrane (Fig. 12.1).

When a virion enters its host cell its protein

Table 12.1.   Distinctive characters of viruses and other microorganisms

	Bacteria	Mycoplasmas	Rickettsiae	Chlamydiae	Viruses
Growth on inanimate culture media	+	+	−	−	−
Multiplication by binary fission	+	+	+	+	−
DNA or RNA	Both	Both	Both	Both	Either but not both
Presence of ribosomes	+	+	+	+	−
Energy-producing enzymes	+	+	+	+	−
Sensitivity to antibiotics	+	+	+	+	−
Sensitivity to interferon	−	−	−	+	+

capsid is stripped off and its nucleic acid is liberated within the host cell. At this stage it ceases to exist as a particle although its nucleic acid is still present and intact. Component parts are still detectable. This stage in viral multiplication is known as the *eclipse phase*. All true viruses have an eclipse phase in their reproductive cycles.

CLASSIFICATION OF ANIMAL VIRUSES

With the rapid progress of knowledge in all the sciences that bear on virology new information enforces the continual review and revision of virus nomenclature. Seven or eight different schemes of classification for viruses have been produced by different authors in an attempt to introduce a scientific and logical taxonomy. These are reviewed by Lwoff and Fournier (1971) and the present position has been set out by the International Committee on Nomenclature of Viruses (Wildy, 1971).

Animal viruses may be arranged into named groups, many of which have the taxonomic status of genera; the names of these groups end in the suffix *-virus*, e.g. adenovirus, herpesvirus and poxvirus. Members of these groups share similar features and can constitute families

ending with the suffix *-idae*, i.e. the family *Herpesviridiae* would have as its type genus *Herpesvirus* which is a group that contains the herpes simplex, varicella-zoster and cytomegaloviruses together with some others (see Table 12.2).

Of the many criteria that have been used in distinguishing the groups of animal viruses the following are some of the most important: (1) type of nucleic acid; (2) chemical composition;

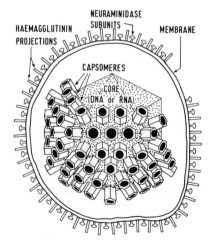

FIG. 12.1. A schematic representation of a hypothetical virion indicating the structures that it may possess.

(3) susceptibility to physical and chemical agents; (4) size measurement; (5) design and construction; (6) antigenic characters.

The properties of tissue and cell affinity, clinical and pathological effects and natural modes of transmission were much used in the early attempts at taxonomy. Currently, molecular biology, biochemistry and genetics are contributing valuable data that advance the evolution of viral nomenclature.

Deoxyriboviruses are at present placed in five groups (Table 12.2) and riboviruses in nine groups (Table 12.3).

There are many viruses that do not fit neatly

Table 12.2.   Basic features of Deoxyriboviruses

Group	Representative viruses	Important characters	Pathogenic qualities
Poxvirus	Variola, vaccinia, molluscum contagiosum. Various viruses of animal and avian pox diseases. Fibromatosis and myxomatosis of rabbits	Large brick-shaped particle 230 to 300 × 200 to 250 nm visible by the light microscope. Resists drying indefinitely. If dried, survives 10 min at 100 °C. Multiply in chick embryo Intracytoplasmic eosinophillic inclusions form. Produces a lipoprotein haemagglutinin which reacts with erythrocytes of some fowls and is smaller and separable from the virion itself	Smallpox, vaccinia, molluscum contagiosum, cowpox, milker's nodes. Localized skin lesions and generalized rashes. Animal and avian pox diseases some of which, e.g. cowpox, are transferable to man. Myxomatosis in rabbits
Herpesvirus	Herpes simplex virus, varicella-zoster virus, Epstein-Barr virus; Cytomegalovirus feline, canine, bovine, avian strains. Virus B	Enveloped icosahedral nucleocapsid—162 capsomeres. Multiplies within the nucleus. Covered by an ether-sensitive envelope. Intranuclear Cowdry type-A inclusions formed. Labile at room temperature. No haemagglutinin	Vesicular skin lesions. Prolonged latency and repeated recrudescences. Stomatitis. Encephalitis. Chickenpox and shingles. Glandular fever. Virus B causes stomatitis in monkeys and fatal encephalitis in man
Adenovirus	Many serotypes causing human infection, also numerous bovine, simian, porcine, avian, murine and canine strains	Naked icosahedron has 240 hexamers and twelve pentamers with fibres and knobs attached. Multiply in nucleus. Ether-resistant. Serotypes distinguished by neutralization. One CF group antigen common to all serotypes. Haemagglutination of rat, mouse, human O and rhesus erythrocytes by some types	Ubiquitous agents of latent infections of lymphoid tissue. Intussusception and bronchiectasis. Feverish pharyngitis and mild respiratory disease. Pneumonia, conjunctivitis and keratitis. Hepatitis in dogs. Some serotypes are oncogenic
Papovavirus	Shope papilloma virus of rabbits, human warts, bovine, canine and equine papilloma virus, vacuolating viruses of monkeys and rabbits	Icosahedral. Multiply in nucleus. Slow growth cycle. Ether-stable. Resist 56 to 65 °C. Many species of erythrocytes haemagglutinated	Human warts and papillomata (PA) of rabbits, dogs, bovines and other mammals. Polyoma (PO) (malignant parotid tumour of mice). Vacuolating agent (VA) SV40 of healthy monkeys. All are potentially oncogenic
Parvovirus	Minute virus of mice, Kilham rat virus (RVM), adeno satellite viruses	Very small. 18 to 22 nm in diameter Ether-resistant	Minute viruses of mice and rats. Natural history not yet known

Table 12.3.   Basic features of Riboviruses

Group	Representative viruses	Important characters	Pathogenic qualities
Orthomyxovirus	Influenza viruses A, B and C, swine influenza, fowl plague	Spherical or filamentous with a coiled tubular nucleo-capsid whose inner ribonucleoprotein helix is 8 nm in diameter. Enveloped with a lipoprotein membrane which is studded with haemagglutinin or neuraminidase subunits. Marked antigenic variation in some members. Matures at cell membrane. Ether-sensitive	Epidemic and endemic influenza, pneumonia, bronchitis, fowl plague, swine influenza
Paramyxovirus	Parainfluenza viruses 1 to 4. Measles, distemper, rinderpest, mumps, Newcastle, SV5	Similar to myxoviruses, but larger and more pleomorphic. RNA helix double the diameter, e.g. 18 nm	Acute respiratory infections, colds, croup, measles, mumps, fowl pest, SV5 of doubtful pathogenicity in the monkey
Rhabdovirus	Vesicular stomatitis, rabies, and some plant, insect and fish viruses	Large enveloped bullet-shaped virions with helical cores. Ether-sensitive. Mature at cytoplasmic membrane. Some members haemagglutinate	Rabies in mammals, vesicular stomatitis in cattle, diseases of trout, insects and plants
Togavirus	Yellow fever, sindbis and dengue viruses	Icosahedra enveloped by a lipid-containing envelope which contains a protein haemagglutinin. Arthropod vectors. Antigen-sharing in several groups	Meningo-encephalitis, lymphadenopathy, bleeding and purpuric rashes, yellow fever
Arenavirus	Lymphocytic choriomeningitis viruses and others	Enveloped and ether-sensitive. Grows in cytoplasm	Benign meningitis, encephalitis
Reovirus	Three mammalian and five avian serotypes	Naked icosahedra with cores of double-stranded RNA. Ether-resistant	Mild respiratory and enteric diseases
Picornavirus	Enterovirus groups: Contains 3 polio, more than 24 ECHO and some 30 Coxsackie viruses, rhinoviruses, foot-and-mouth disease viruses	Small naked icosahedra, cubical symmetry, ether- and acid-resistant, stabilized by MgCl to heat inactivation. Rhinoviruses are acid-labile at pH 5·3. Stable at atmospheric temperatures for several weeks	Neuronal damage and paralyses (mainly polio 1 and 3 viruses), aseptic meningitis, epidemic myalgia (Bornholm), herpangina, myocarditis and pericarditis, common colds, foot and mouth disease
Leukovirus	Avian leucosis group. Rous sarcoma, murine leukaemia group, murine mammary tumour virus (Bittner) agent, feline leukosis	Induce malignant transformation of cells with formation of new antigens and enzymes and loss of contact inhibition. Oncogenic. Not cytocidal	Leukaemia, myoblastosis and sarcomata in fowls; leukaemia, sarcomata and mammary carcinomata in mice
Coronavirus	Human, murine and avian viruses	Elliptical or spherical with club-shaped surface projections about 20 nm long. Ether-sensitive. Grown in cytoplasm of embryonic human epithelial cells	Colds and acute respiratory infections, avian bronchitis, mouse hepatitis and rat pneumonia

into these groups. This is particularly true of the 150 or more viruses at present placed in the group *Arbovirus* because they are thought to be transmitted by biting arthropods. Many members of this group have no other features in common and present opinion would subdivide them, e.g. into (a) togaviruses which would form a group including all those that had enveloped icosahedral capsids and shared antigens; (b) arenaviruses containing the Tacaribe, Junin, Machupo and several South American encephalitis viruses together with the lymphocytic choriomeningitis (LCM) virus; whether arthropods play a role in the transmission of these viruses is doubtful but all share a group specific antigen: (c) other members at present classified as arboviruses that would be more properly included in the reovirus or rhabdovirus groups.

Type of Nucleic Acid

The genome and the infectivity of viruses is carried in their nucleic acid, either DNA or RNA. The molecular weight and type of nucleic acid are characteristic for each group of viruses. Nucleic acids are very large polymers constructed from nucleotide units. Each nucleotide is formed from a molecule of pentose sugar joined to a molecule of phosphoric acid and to bases which can be adenine, guanine, cytosine and for DNA thymine, or for RNA uracil (Newton and Waterson, 1967). The combination of bases in different viral nucleic acids varies greatly from one major group to another and amongst the individual viruses within the groups. Each virus has its own characteristic ratio of these bases (see Table 12.4).

Most deoxyriboviruses have linear double-stranded DNA, although in the parvoviruses the molecule is single-stranded. The great majority of riboviruses contain one molecule of single-stranded RNA. Reoviruses, however, are an exception and contain double-stranded RNA. Also the RNA may be present not as a single molecule but in multiple pieces.

Although viral nucleic acids are very fragile when their protective capsids are removed,

Table 12.4.   Nucleic acids of major groups of animal viruses

Group	Type and molecular wt. of N.A. ×10⁶ daltons	Configuration of strands	Proportion (%) of bases in N.A.					Approx. no. of genes
			A	T	U	G	Cy	
Deoxyriboviruses								
	DNA							
Poxvirus[1]	160	DS	31·5	31·5		18	19	400
Herpesvirus[2]	99	DS	14	13		38	35	250
Adenovirus[3]	23	DS	22	21		28	29	60
Papovavirus[4]	3·5	DSC	26	26		24	24	7
Parvovirus	2	SS	25	35·5		18	21·5	10
Riboviruses								
	RNA							
Orthomyxovirus[5]	5	SS	22–25		30–33	18–20	24–25	15
Paramyxovirus[6]	7·5	SS	24		30	22	24	35
Rhabdovirus[7]	6	SS	27		31	20	22	25
Togavirus A and B[8]	2·3	SS	29·6		19·7	25·8	24·9	15
Reovirus	10	DS	28		28	22	22	35
Picornavirus[9]	3	SS	29		25	24	22	14
Leukovirus[10]	10	SS	22·1		22·4	28·3	24·2	50
Coronavirus	?	SS	?	?	?	?	?	?

N.A., nucleic acid; DS, double stranded; SS, single stranded; C, circular; A, adenine; T, thymine; U, uracil; G, guanidine; Cy, cytosine; 1, Vaccinia virus; 2, Herpes simplexvirus; 3, type 4 adenovirus; 4, polyoma virus; 5, influenza virus A; 6, type 1 para-influenza virus; 7, Vesicular stomatitis virus; 8, Sindbisvirus; 9, Polio virus (all 3 types); 10, Rous sarcoma virus.

some retain their infectivity for a time and it is possible to view them and measure them in the electron microscope without disrupting them. Most of them are linear, but some are circular as in papovaviruses whose DNA takes the form of a double-stranded circle. Quite often a circular nucleic acid may be twisted into a number of convolutions. Infectious nucleic acid can not be extracted from viruses that contain RNA transcriptase because this enzyme is destroyed by the processes of extraction.

Chemical Composition

Proteins are the main component of all viruses. Of their several functions the most important is to provide a protective shield for the underlying frail nucleic acid molecules (see Table 12.5). The surface proteins of the virion have special affinities for specific receptor sites on the host cell and provide a means of attachment of the particle to a position where it can enter the host cell and initiate the process of infection.

Proteins also contain the viral antigens that stimulate the host's immune responses during infection. They confer on a virus its distinctive serological characteristics from which is possible the recognition of each individual strain and its mutants.

The capsomeres of most pathogenic viruses contain several different polypeptides; simple viruses have only one or two in each capsomere but complex viruses may have as many as twenty. Polypeptides make up the surface configurations of newly matured virions. They constitute the haemagglutinin prickles of ortho and para-myxoviruses and the neuraminidase subunits that are situated in a strategic position to attach the virus to its host cell and to aid the transference of nucleic acid through the cell membrane. They also form a part of the mushroom-shaped projections of neuraminidase (Fig. 12.1).

VIRAL ENZYMES. There are many examples of enzymes being coded in the viral nucleic acid but in only a few instances are they actually carried within the virion as for example neuraminidase in myxoviruses, or the muraminidase of the T2 coliphage. Some viruses carry DNA- or RNA-dependent transcriptase polymerases

Table 12.5. Chemical composition of major groups of animal viruses

Group	Proteins		Nucleic acid	Carbohydrate	Lipid	Ether resistance (R) or sensitivity (S)
	*No. of polypeptides	per cent	per cent	per cent	per cent	
Deoxyriboviruses		DNA				
Poxvirus	About 20	89	5·6	?	5–7	~R
Herpesvirus	At least 27	70	6·5	1·6	22	S
Adenovirus	9–10	88	12	—	0	R
Papovavirus	2 or 3		7–10	—	0	R
Parvovirus	?	?	?	—	0	?
Riboviruses		RNA				
Orthomyxovirus	7	60–70	0·86	3·8	24–30	S
Paramyxovirus	6		10	—	+	S
Rhabdovirus	6	?	—	—	+ +	S
Togavirus. A and B	3	40	4·4	3–8	54	S
Reovirus	7	85	14·6	—	—	R
Picornavirus	4	70–80	20–30	—	—	R
Leukovirus	4		1.42	—	47	S
Coronavirus		UNDETERMINED				S

*Approximate number of different virus-coded polypeptides in virion.

which play an important role in the early phases of the establishment of viral replication within the host cell (see Chap. 13).

LIPIDS. When some mature viruses are liberated by a process of budding from nuclear and cytoplasmic membranes they acquire a surface layer of lipoprotein derived in part from the host cell. The lipids may serve to cement virus-coded proteins in viral envelopes. Such viruses are readily inactivated by lipid solvents such as ether, chloroform or bile salts.

CARBOHYDRATE. Some viruses contain minimal amounts of carbohydrate in addition to the sugar in the nucleic acid molecule. Ortho and paramyxoviruses and togaviruses, for example, have glycoproteins in the prickles that protrude from the viral envelopes.

Susceptibility to Physical and Chemical Agents

Outside the body, and at room temperature, many viruses are extremely labile and may survive for only a few hours. Such is the case with the viruses of influenza, mumps and measles, and in these diseases great care must be taken to ensure that the specimens under investigation are frozen with a minimum delay. Other viruses, such as those of smallpox and poliomyelitis, are much hardier and may survive under ordinary atmospheric conditions for many days, weeks or even months.

HEAT AND COLD. The viruses causing disease in man and animals are in general readily inactivated by moderate heat (56° to 60°C for 30 min) though there are some notable exceptions, e.g. serum hepatitis and poliomyelitis viruses. Like bacteria, viruses are resistant to extremes of cold; freezing at $-35°C$ or $-70°C$ is a satisfactory method for their preservation and is much used in the laboratory. The majority of viruses are also well preserved when dried from the frozen state by the method of freeze-drying. By this means, virus vaccines are preserved in an active form for long periods before use to immunize against such diseases as smallpox and yellow fever.

pH VARIATION. Viruses remain viable as a rule within the range of pH 5 to 9, but are destroyed by extreme acidity or alkalinity. Certain of their properties, however, like haemag-glutination (*vide infra*) may be profoundly disturbed by variations of a few tenths of a pH unit.

GLYCEROL. In a 50 per cent solution of glycerol, ordinary non-sporing bacteria are killed comparatively quickly, but many viruses remain alive in this fluid for several months or even years. The preservation of the vaccinia virus used prophylactically against smallpox is accomplished by means of glycerol. Other viruses that can be kept for long periods in glycerol at 4°C, or lower temperatures, are those of poliomyelitis, rabies and herpes simplex. On the other hand, some viruses, e.g. the rinderpest virus, do not tolerate glycerol as well as certain bacteria.

VIRUCIDAL AGENTS. The most efficient disinfectants for use against viruses are oxidizing agents such as hydrogen peroxide, potassium permanganate and hypochlorites, and organic iodine derivatives. Formaldehyde (a reducing agent) is slower in action but is valuable in defined concentrations in the preparation of inactivated poliomyelitis vaccines. Glutaraldehyde has an important role in the disinfection of apparatus used in renal dialysis units. This agent is also a particularly valuable fixative for tissues that are to be embedded and examined by electron microscopy. Phenol and certain cresol disinfectants such as lysol are active against only a few viruses and are not to be recommended for material contaminated with the poliomyelitis or smallpox viruses.

ETHER. The possession of a lipid-containing envelope renders a virus sensitive to ether (see Table 12.5). Thus the herpes, orthomyxo and paramyxo, rhabdo, corona and leuko viruses are all inactivated by ether whereas the naked polio, echo, coxsackie, adeno, papova and parvo viruses and some poxviruses are resistant.

BILE. Practically all enveloped viruses, except the vaccinia virus, are sensitive to bile, but naked viruses are resistant.

VITAL DYES. Acridine orange, neutral red and toluidine blue permeate the nucleic acid and render virions vulnerable to ultraviolet light. Viruses may vary in the degree to which they are affected; for example, herpes simplex and vaccinia viruses are more severely damaged than polioviruses. Double-stranded DNA viruses stained with acridine orange fluoresce with a yellow colour when viewed in the ultra-violet light microscope, whilst single-stranded DNA viruses fluoresce red. Single-stranded RNA viruses are also red, but double-stranded RNA viruses fluoresce yellow. When these reactions in infected cells are compared with enzyme-digested preparations and normal controls, it is then possible to determine the types of viral nucleic acids.

MAGNESIUM, ALUMINIUM AND SODIUM SALTS. Molar concentrations of these salts are used to stabilize suspensions of certain viruses and may enable virions to withstand heating for an hour at 50°C. In this way the potency of a preparation may be preserved for several weeks at atmospheric temperatures even in the tropics. Unwanted viral contaminants can be eliminated by heating a suspension in the presence of selected salts. For example, it is possible to rid poliovirus suspensions of such simian viruses as the SV40 and foamy agents by heating them in molar MgCl$_2$ at 50 to 55°C.

ANTIBIOTICS AND CHEMOTHERAPEUTIC SUBSTANCES such as sulphonamides, peni-cillin, streptomycin and the tetracyclines have no effect on true viruses. The fact that the agents of the psittacosis-lymphogranuloma group are susceptible to these drugs has been an important consideration in their being classified as rickett-siales instead of as viruses. Originally, viruses were 'purified', i.e. separated from bacteria in contaminated fluids such as sputum or faeces, by filtration through a bacteria-retaining filter, but it is easier to use antibiotics; these (e.g. penicillin and streptomycin) are added to the material to kill the bacteria and they leave the viruses unharmed.

Size and Measurement

The unit used for the measurement of viruses is the nanometre (nm); it is 10^{-9} metre, i.e. a one-thousandth part of a micrometre (μm) or a one-millionth part of a millimetre. For very small objects such as the component parts of viruses and macromolecules, the Ångström unit (Å), which is one-tenth of a nanometre may be used. The Ångström is the unit used in measuring the wave-length of light in microscopy.

Virions vary in diameter from 300 to 18 nm. The largest are nearly half the size of small bacteria and can just be seen with a good optical microscope (Fig. 12.2). Most viruses, however, can be seen only by electron microscopy which is also the most commonly used method for measuring the size of viruses. Viruses that are far beyond the limits of the resolution of the light microscope can be seen and photographed in the electron microscope which is capable of resolving objects as, small as 0·3 nm (3Å) in diameter (see Chap. 1, Vol. II). One method of making the measurements is to include in a suspension of purified virus some latex particles of known size (e.g. 88 nm); in electron micro-graphs the known and the unknown particles can be measured with accuracy and the size of the virus is determined with precision. One advantage of electron-microscopical examina-tion of viruses is that the shape as well as the size of the virions can be determined. In this way it was found that the vaccinia virus particles are brick-shaped, that influenza viruses have a filamentous as well as a spherical form, and that some bacteriophages have a sperm-like mor-phology, with a polyhedral head and a tail.

Originally viruses were measured by their capacity to pass through filters. Many types of filter have been used for this purpose, but the best are made from collodion (cellulose mem-brane filters). Filtration methods, however, have not a high degree of precision in virus measurement and have for the most part been replaced by newer techniques. Nevertheless, filtration does have a special use in measuring a very small virus when it is contained in a material contaminated with so much host cell protein that other methods cannot be used.

A third method of determining virus size is to estimate the rate at which the particles fall in a suspending fluid; large particles, being heavier, fall faster than small ones. This relationship between particle size and rate of sedimentation follows Stokes' law and holds good even when forces many times greater than that of gravity are applied to a virus preparation in a fast-moving centrifuge. From values for the density and viscosity of the medium, the distance from the axis of rotation and the speed in rev/min, the diameter of the virus particle can be calculated (Chap. 14, Vol. II).

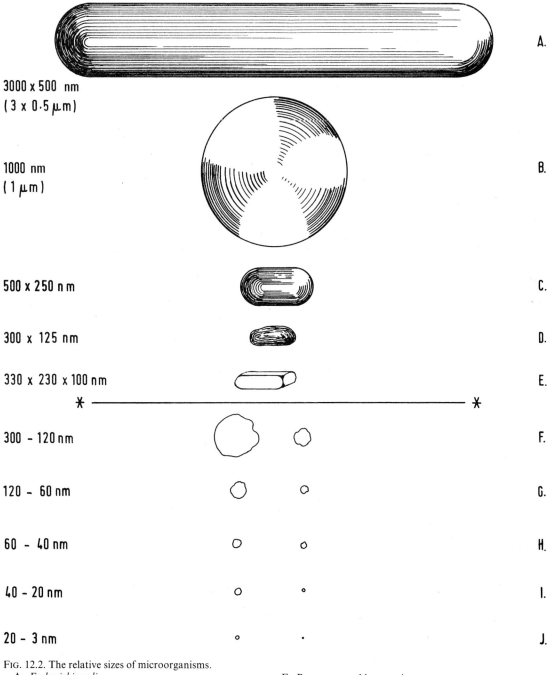

3000 x 500 nm
(3 x 0·5 μm)
     A.

1000 nm
(1 μm)
     B.

500 x 250 n m
     C.

300 x 125 nm
     D.

330 x 230 x 100 nm
     E.

＊————————————————————＊

300 – 120 nm
     F.

120 – 60 nm
     G.

60 – 40 nm
     H.

40 – 20 nm
     I.

20 – 3 nm
     J.

FIG. 12.2. The relative sizes of microorganisms.

A. *Escherichia coli.*
B. *Staphylococcus aureus.*
C. *Coxiella burnetii.*
D. *Mycoplasma.*
E. Vaccinia virus.

F. Paramyxo and herpes viruses.
G. Influenza and adeno viruses bacteriophages
H. Reo, toga and papova viruses.
I. Picorna and parvo viruses.
J. Haemoglobin and albumin molecules.

＊————————————————————＊

Microorganisms above this line are visible in the optical microscope.

Design and Construction of Viruses

A virion in its simplest form is a single molecule of nucleic acid enclosed within a protein capsid. The shape taken by the capsid is that of a rigid spherical cage or of a tube of varying flexibility and length and its main purpose is the protection of the fragile nucleic acid core. There is a specific relationship in the way the nucleic acids are linked to the polypeptides of the outer shell.

Viral capsids are built from large numbers of small 'morphological units' or *capsomeres* that are attached to each other by non-covalent bonds. Electron microscopy shows that the capsomeres are disposed in regular solid geometrical figures to form capsids of either cubical or helical symmetry.

At first sight the capsomeres often seem to be spherical but on close scrutiny at very high resolving powers they are frequently found to be hollow and pyramidal in shape, and to consist of aggregates of even smaller 'structural' (or 'chemical') units. These structural units consist of differing polypeptide chains and a capsomere may contain several of them or only one. For instance, the capsomeres of the tobacco mosaic virus are known as 'monomers' because they contain only one structural unit, a polypeptide chain of a molecular weight of 20 to 30 million *daltons*. Capsomeres of the poliovirus are oligomers and contain four different polypeptides.

The fitting of the capsomeres and their components together to construct the capsid is precisely accurate and symmetrical because an impenetrable shield has to be formed to protect the nucleic acid from damage by enzymic actions and destructive mechanisms of the host.

CUBICAL CAPSIDS. Viruses with cubical symmetry take the form of an icosahedron, one of the classical polyhedral bodies of solid geometry. An icosahedron has 20 facets, each an equilateral triangle, and 12 vertices or corners. An axis entering at one of these vertices and passing through the centre of the figure enables the icosahedron to be rotated through five new positions in each of which the same appearance is presented. If the axis enters through the centre of any one of the equilateral triangles only three identical positions can be obtained and if the point of entry is through the centre of any of

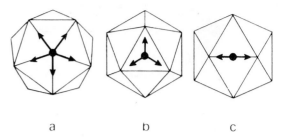

FIG. 12.3. An icosahedron viewed along its (a) fivefold, (b) threefold and (c) twofold axes of symmetry.

the edges of the triangular facets there can only be two such positions (see Fig. 12.3). Thus any icosahedron is said to have a 5.3.2 rotational symmetry.

The arrangement of capsomeres in the icosahedral capsids follows the rules of crystallography. The minimum number is 12, one capsomere being placed at each vertex. The next permissible numbers are 32, 42, 72, 92, 162, 252, and 812. Capsomeres have to conform to the symmetry of the icosahedron and those placed at the vertices touch only five neighbours and are

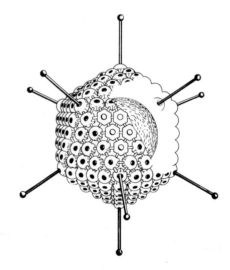

FIG. 12.4. A diagram of an icosahedron of an adenovirus. The core of DNA is represented by a circular mass. Some of the pentamers at the twelve vertices have been indicated with protruding fibres and terminal capsomeres. The remaining 240 hexamer capsids are, for the most part, shown as compressed into hollow spheres linked to each other by diavalent bonds. The hexagonal shape of a few of the capsomeres is seen in the centre of the diagram.

pentagonal. They are often referred to as *pentons*. All the other capsomeres touch six neighbours and are hexagonal. They are called *hexons* and acquire this shape in conforming to the 5.3.2 rotational symmetry of the capsid (see Fig. 12.4).

The twenty triangular facets of the icosahedron can be further subdivided into smaller triangles and the resulting solid is then an icosadeltahedron. In architecture it is well known that a dome or sphere derives much of its strength and stability from such a surface lattice.

The number of small equilateral triangles (T) that can be contained in the area defined by three adjacent axes of five-fold symmetry can be calculated by the formula $T = H^2 + HK + K^2$ where H and K are any pair of integers that share no common factor.

On any one of the very small triangles three asymmetrical chemical units can be accommodated, but they may cluster together with their neighbours in a number of different ways. Commonly the units aggregate to form hexamer or pentamer capsomeres. When this happens, the simple formula $10T + 2$ gives the total number of capsomeres in the capsid. T values (small triangle numbers) for the various major virus groups are given in Table 12.6, e.g. for the herpes simplex virus T = 16 so this virus has $10 \times 16 + 2 = 162$ capsomeres. Another method to calculate the total number of capsomeres is to use the formula $10(n-1)^2 + 2$ where n is the number of capsomeres seen by the electron microscope to be situated along the edge of one equilateral triangle, e.g. for the herpes simplex virus, $10(5-1)^2 + 2 = 162$. Values for T appear in Table 12.6. The total number of polypeptide molecules in any capsid is always 60T.

Some icosahedral virions have unusual features. For instance, members of the adenovirus group are naked icosahedra constructed from 240 hexons that are hollow polygonal structures and 12 pentons, from whose bases protrude fibres of variable length bearing knobs at their ends (Fig. 12.4). The fibres of the pentons have been purified and have been shown on immunological evidence to contain at least two distinct proteins.

Reoviruses differ from other icosahedral viruses in that their capsids are constructed of

Table 12.6.   The structure of the main groups of animal viruses

Group	*Virion diameter (nm)	Nucleo-capsid symmetry	Total number of capsomeres or length of helix (nm)			Nucleo-capsid diameter (nm)	Triangulation no. (T)	Virion enveloped or naked
			Penta-mers	Hexa-mers	Total			
Deoxyriboviruses								
Poxvirus	100 × 230 × 300	Complex						Complex coats
Herpesvirus	150–250	Icosahedral	12 +	150 =	162	100	16	Enveloped
Adenovirus	70–80	Icosahedral	12 +	240 =	252	70–80	25	Naked
Papovavirus	45–55	Icosahedral	12 +	60 =	72	45–55	7	Naked
Parvovirus	18–24	Icosahedral	12 +	20 =	32	18–24	3	Naked
Riboviruses								
Orthomyxovirus	80	Helical			600–1 000 nm	6–9	—	Enveloped
Paramyxovirus	120–200	Helical			1 000 nm	18	—	Enveloped
Rhabdovirus	175 × 68	Helical			3 500–4 000 nm	5	—	Enveloped
Togavirus. A and B	40–60	Icosahedral			?	35	—	Enveloped
Reovirus	54–75	Icosahedral			92 or 180	?	9	Naked
‡Picornavirus	22	Icosahedral			60	?	3	Naked
Leukovirus	100–120	Helical			?	?	—	Enveloped
Coronavirus	80–160	Unknown			?	?	—	Enveloped

*nm = Nanometres.
† n = Number of capsomeres on one side of each equilateral triangle.
‡   = in the form of a rhombic triacontahedron.

two layers of capsomeres; the inner layer conforms closely to the symmetry of the outer layer. The nucleic acid of reoviruses is double-stranded RNA.

HELICAL CAPSIDS. The symmetry of a helix is much simpler than that of an icosahedron because it has only the one rotational axis of symmetry which coincides with the axis of the cylindrical molecule of nucleic acid. The capsomeres are monomers that are wedge-shaped and bound together in the form of ribbons. Being thicker at one end than the other, the capsomeres make the ribbon twist into a spiral. The number of capsomeres is not always constant for each turn of the helix.

Stability is conferred by bonds between neighbouring capsomeres, both those placed side by side and also those above and below on each adjacent turn of the helix. In this way a hollow cylinder is formed which is usually flexible enough to be folded repeatedly on itself in the shape of an irregular rounded mass (see Fig. 12.5 and 12.6).

ENVELOPES. During the final phases of their reproductive cycle, nucleocapsids of some viruses acquire a covering of lipoprotein derived

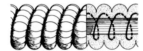

FIG. 12.5. Part of the nucleocapsid of a helical virus. It has been formed from capsomeres attached to the helical core of RNA which is represented by a coiled heavy dashed line. It is a hollow flexible filament in e.g. ortho and paramyxoviruses.

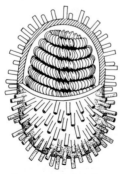

FIG. 12.6. An ortho or paramyxovirus with helical symmetry and a covering membrane and projecting haemagglutinins.

from the cytoplasmic membrane of the host cell. These viral envelopes are not simply unaltered host cell membrane for their protein content consists of virus-specified monomers that can be seen in electron-micrographs as projecting prickles. These morphological appearances are clearly seen in the influenza viruses where the coiled helix of the nucleocapsid is seen to be enclosed within a loosely fitting envelope from which numbers of two sorts of prickles protrude. Both kinds have hydrophobic tips that are embedded in the lipid of the viral envelope; their other ends are hydrophilic and project to the exterior (Fig. 12.1). One type of prickle—the haemagglutinin—is 10 nm long and is triangular in cross-section; it is a polymer of identical viral protein molecules linked to cellular carbohydrate. The other type is neuraminidase which is mushroom-shaped and composed of a viral protein quite distinct from enzymes found in some normal cells.

Cubical capsids of some viruses may also acquire envelopes. For example, the herpes simplex virus begins its reproductive cycle in the nucleus of its host cells and as it matures it acquires a covering layer from the altered nuclear membrane as it passes into the cytoplasm.

Some viruses, however, do not have any covering at all. The helical rod-shaped nucleocapsids of the tobacco mosaic virus are naked as also are the icosahedral virions of the adeno- and polio-viruses.

COMPLEX VIRUSES. There are a number of viruses whose structure is far more complex than any so far described. Their symmetry has not yet been determined, but they do possess internal components such as nucleoid bodies. The vaccinia virus, a poxvirus, is one of the best studied and the virion contains an oval central core which is indented by two spherical 'lateral' bodies so that it has the appearance of a dumb-bell. This core is composed of DNA, and is probably a single molecule 80 nm in length corresponding to a molecular weight of about 160 to 200 million daltons. On the surface are loops of hollow cylindrical threads of protein about 9 nm in diameter; they cover most of the virion conferring on it a rugged ridged appearance. The whole nucleocapsid is enveloped by two or more membranes (see Fig. 12.7A).

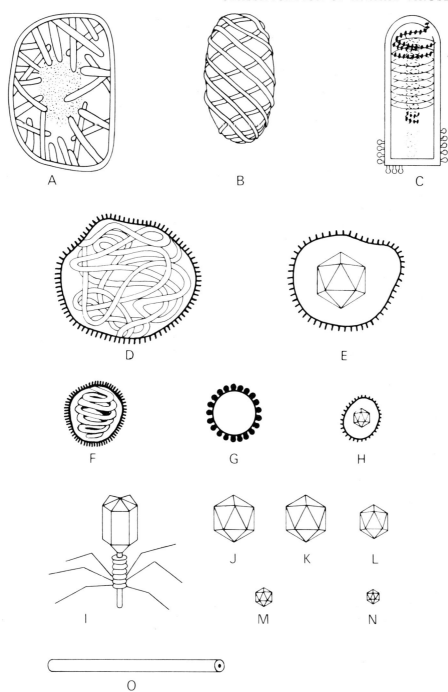

FIG. 12.7. Morphology of viruses.

A. Poxvirus.
B. Orf virus.
C. Rhabdovirus.
D. Paramyxovirus.

E. Herpesvirus.
F. Orthomyxovirus.
G. Coronavirus.
H. Togavirus.

I. T-even coliphage.
J. Adenovirus.
K. Reovirus.
L. Papovavirus.

M. Picornavirus.
N. Parvovirus.
O. Tobacco mosaic virus.

Bacteriophages exhibit a wide variation in structure ranging from the small icosahedral particles of the single-stranded RNA phage f2 or the single-stranded DNA phage $\phi \times 174$ to the complex structures of the double-stranded DNA coliphages of the T even (T2, T4, T6) series.

The smallest phages have polyhedral symmetry with a diameter of about 25 nm. Phages of this type may contain either single-stranded RNA (phage f2) or single-stranded DNA (phage $\phi \times 174$) as their nucleic acid. Filamentous phages, such as fd, have helical symmetry; the length of the virions is 800 to 850 nm, and the diameter is 6·5 nm. The nucleic acid of these phages is single-stranded DNA, which is believed to be in the form of a closed circle pulled out so that the strands are parallel and close together. This stretched loop of DNA is enclosed within the protein of the capsid to give the filamentous appearance.

More complex structure is seen in the double-stranded DNA phages with polyhedral heads. The outline of the head structure of this type of phage is illustrated in Fig. 13.3. The ends and the intermediate part of the head all appear to have triangular facets. In addition phages are known that possess varying lengths of tail attached to a head structure as described. The head of phage T4 has a diameter of 65 nm and is 100 nm long. The tail is 100 nm in length and 25 nm in diameter and consists of a central, hollow core or tube (7 nm thick) surrounded by a contractile sheath attached to a collar at the base of the head, and terminating in a hexagonal base plate. A short pin or spike is located at each corner of the base plate, along with a tail fibre 130 nm long. This is the most complex form of tail structure. Phage λ and the T-odd coliphages are also tailed phages of the same general construction, although their tails vary in length and are non-contractile.

Antigenic Classification

Antigenic characters usually reside in the surface structures of the virions. Some antigens are constant and stable and thus provide valuable criteria for taxonomy. For example, the adenoviruses all possess a common group antigen, and all the influenza A viruses share a common complement fixing antigen. But individual viruses often possess other special antigens of their own. Each virus strain possesses an individual pattern of antigens including those of the whole group together with others that confer type specificity.

Antigenic patterns provide bases for the classification of animal viruses into their major groups. Thus the adenoviruses which all possess the same group antigen are subdivided into 32 serotypes according to their other antigens, and the enteroviruses are arranged in groups such as polioviruses, echoviruses and coxsackie viruses, each of which contains its own number of serotypes.

Virus Haemagglutination

Many different viruses can agglutinate red blood cells. When virions and erythrocytes in a suspension collide they adhere to each other; the cells become speckled with attached virions and they are bound to each other by viral bridges. Considerable numbers of cells are clumped together to form sticky heavy agglutinated masses that sink through the suspending fluid to be deposited in an irregular ragged pattern. Although different viruses agglutinate the erythrocytes of a diversity of animal species and the physical conditions necessary for the reaction to take place may vary from one virus to another, it is true to say that in general haemagglutination is similar in all cases.

MYXOVIRUS HAEMAGGLUTINATION. A great deal of attention has been paid to the way influenza viruses combine with red blood cells because this mechanism may be analogous to that employed by the virus to attach itself to epithelial cells when it is inhaled and enters the human respiratory tract. The haemagglutinin is located in prickles that protrude from the surface of the virion and is composed of a glycoprotein that has a special affinity for another but different glycoprotein situated in 'receptor areas' located in the envelope of the cell. A virus will unite with erythrocytes of any species provided they carry the complementary receptor areas. The structure of the receptors is that of complementary conjugated proteins with prosthetic groups of oligosaccharides at whose ends are residues of neuraminic acid.

The complexity of the mechanics of influenza virus haemagglutination is increased by the virions possessing an enzyme, 'neuraminidase', close to or in between the haemagglutin in prickles. This enzyme reacts with N-acetyl-neuraminic acid which is a member of the group of sialic acids and a component of the receptor areas. It can therefore disrupt the neuraminic acid residues on the end of the prosthetic groups and liberate the virions from attachment to the cell. This process of 'elution' occurs only when physical conditions are right; the enzyme cannot act if the temperature is too low (4°C) or if the pH is too high or too low. After elution the receptors are irretrievably damaged and cells are no longer agglutinable by that particular virus. The free virions however, are, unharmed.

Neuraminidase (sialidase) plays no part in the attachment to or the entry of virions into cells. Viruses whose enzymic activity has been destroyed by heat can still attach to cells or if the cell receptor is destroyed by periodate treatment the virions can nevertheless attach to the cell. N-acetyl-neuraminic acid is also present in the mucopolysaccharides of a variety of tissues and secretions and these may compete with the erythrocyte receptors for the viral enzyme; it is found in serum, urine, saliva, sputum, egg-white, red cell stroma, ovarian cyst mucin, allantoic fluid and membrane, and is often referred to as the non-specific, or Francis inhibitor.

Cholera vibrios and *Clostridium welchii* also possess an enzyme which reacts with sialic acid derivatives; it is known as the receptor-destroying enzyme (RDE) and it can be obtained in a purified concentrated form. It provides a valuable means of removing the unwanted non-specific inhibitors found in serum or egg fluids.

The haemagglutination reaction is important in laboratory work because it provides a simple and rapid method for the detection of viruses in egg or tissue culture fluids. Haemagglutination is also the basis of a useful method for virus purification. Virions in crude cellular extracts or in culture fluids are absorbed on red cells which are then sedimented; after removal of the supernatant, the agglutinated cells are rinsed with ice-cold saline and then the virions are eluted at 37°C into a small volume of clean fluid. The red blood cells are now removed by slow centrifugation and usually about a four-fold concentration of the virus has been achieved.

POXVIRUS HAEMAGGLUTINATION. Extracts of cells infected with the vaccinia virus are able to agglutinate fowl red blood cells. Only about 50 per cent of fowls, however, have sensitive cells. The haemagglutinin is distinct from the virions from which it can be separated by slow speed centrifugation or by elution from a diethylamino-ethyl-cellulose column. It is 65 nm in diameter (the vaccinia virion measures $240 \times 200 \times 100$ nm) and is not infective. The haemagglutinin has two components—one heat labile and the other heat stable. The former is a lipoprotein and is sensitive to lecithinase. Once attached to the red cell surface it does not elute spontaneously. The vaccinia haemagglutinin attaches readily to the surfaces of red cells that have been treated with myxoviruses. This mechanism of haemagglutination is thus quite different from that of the myxoviruses.

During convalescence after vaccinia or smallpox infections, antibodies to the haemagglutinin appear in the patient's serum. They are distinct from the viral neutralizing and the complement-fixing antibodies, but nevertheless it is useful to demonstrate their presence because they appear very soon—five or six days—after the onset of infection. Antihaemagglutin antibody tests are more sensitive than tests for other antibodies to the poxviruses.

HAEMAGGLUTINATION BY OTHER VIRUSES. A third group of viruses, the togaviridiae which cause such infections as yellow fever, dengue and various types of encephalitis, also possess haemagglutinins. The reaction appears to be a reversible state of equilibrium between virions and erythrocytes and is inhibited by lipids and slight variations in pH. Togaviruses have no enzyme analogous to the neuraminidase of myxovirus and virions do not elute from the cell surfaces. Some of these viruses are able to lyse the erythrocytes of one-day-old chicks.

A fourth group of haemagglutinating viruses contains many members of the echo and coxsackie viruses. Here the infective and haemagglutination properties of the virions cannot be separated and little is known of the nature of the attachment of virus to the cell.

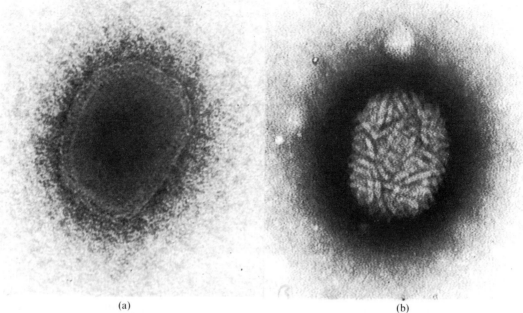

(a)   (b)

PLATES 12.1a and b. (a) Vaccinia virus particle. (b) Vaccinia virus showing internal structure. (Phospho-tungstic acid. × 150 000.)

CULTIVATION OF VIRUSES AND THEIR HOST CELLS

Viruses can reproduce only within living cells, where they gain access to the energy-producing systems and protein synthesizing machinery which they lack. Within the infected cell, nucleic acid is replicated and structural proteins for the virus are made. The relation between virus and host cell is very intimate and a variety of effects on the cell may result. One possible outcome is the complete destruction of the host cell but another possibility is that both cell and virus can survive and that the behaviour and properties of the host cell may be changed.

Before a study can be made of the interaction of virus and cell, we must be able to grow and maintain the appropriate cells in culture in the laboratory. Bacteria can be grown easily, and are less complex than eucaryotic cells; the result is that bacterial viruses have been studied in greater detail than viruses that grow in mammalian cells.

An increasing understanding of the processes of animal virus replication has depended on improvements in methods of culturing animal cells and developments in techniques of extraction, purification and concentration of animal viruses. The use of the electron microscope, in particular the examination of ultra-thin sections of infected cells, has yielded much information on the events occurring during virus growth. It is now apparent that animal and bacterial viruses may differ in some respects in their interactions with cells but they have many similarities. Indeed, the more detailed knowledge of bacterial viruses has repeatedly been used to suggest lines of investigation of the animal virus-cell interaction.

The study of the growth of viruses requires not only suitable cell cultures but also adequate systems for the growth, detection and assay of the viruses themselves.

GROWTH AND ASSAY OF BACTERIAL VIRUSES

Bacteriophages were first detected when cell lysis occurred in cultures of bacteria. Virus stocks can be obtained by inoculation of a virus seed into an exponentially growing suspension culture of bacteria and continuing incubation. After one or two hours, the bacterial culture may clear as the cells lyse, or may be lysed by a brief exposure to chloroform bringing about the release of the progeny virions. The number of infectious virus particles in a preparation can be determined by means of a *focal assay*—in which one infectious virus particle gives rise to one hole or plaque in a lawn of bacteria on a culture plate. To perform a phage titration, measured volumes of increasing dilutions of the virus suspension are added to fresh host bacteria in molten agar and poured on to the surface of the medium in an ordinary culture plate (see Fig. 13.14). Alternatively, standard drops of the virus suspensions are dropped on to the surface of a culture plate that has already been seeded with the host bacterium. When the inoculated plate is incubated, the host cells multiply to produce an even growth or lawn over the whole surface of the plate, except where a phage particle has infected a cell. At these sites, the virus grows within the infected cell and is released after lysis of the cell. The progeny virions can infect cells only in the immediate vicinity, and as a result an enlarging hole or plaque is produced in the bacterial lawn. The number of plaques produced by inoculation of a measured volume of a known dilution of the virus suspension can be counted and simple calculation gives the titre of the phage stock in plaque forming units per ml (p.f.u./ml.).

GROWTH AND DETECTION OF ANIMAL VIRUSES

Living cells can be provided for the growth of animal viruses in three main ways. Historically the first method available was the inoculation of *live animals* to produce disease or death. Apart from ethical considerations, use of animals in virology is restricted nowadays because animals are expensive to buy and maintain and may be difficult to handle; they vary in their response to the inoculation of virus and can respond to infection with their own defence mechanisms. In addition, the animals may be latently infected with their own viruses which may contaminate virus stocks derived from animal tissues. Obviously, the use of whole animals does not allow a study of the interaction of virus with defined cell types under controlled conditions.

A considerable advance in the ease of growing and detecting some types of viruses was possible when the methods of inoculation into the embryonated hen's egg were developed. Fertile eggs are much easier to handle than animals, are cheap and readily available, and suitable cells for virus growth are present in the embryo and its membranes. The chick embryo does not have well-developed defence mechanisms but may be contaminated with latent fowl viruses. Viruses may kill the chick embryo or they may produce evidence of specific viral activity such as visible lesions on the chorioallantoic membrane (CAM). The haemagglutinating activity in amniotic or allantoic fluid may reveal the presence of influenza or related viruses. Inoculation onto the CAM has been of value both in the isolation of viruses from the lesions of patients, e.g. smallpox and as a focal assay for infectious virus. One lesion (or pock) may arise from one infectious virus particle, hence poxviruses may be assayed by the pock forming units per ml of a virus suspension. Despite its many advantages, this method of cultivation does not permit a controlled study of virus-cell interaction and there are many viruses that fail to multiply on primary inoculation into eggs.

More precisely defined conditions became available with the development of methods for growing and maintaining animal cells in culture in the laboratory. The handling of cultured cells has been facilitated by a growing knowledge of their nutritional requirements and the incorporation of antibiotics in culture media to control bacterial contamination. Cell cultures can be initiated from many different cell types, and may be classified on the basis of their behaviour into primary or established cell lines.

Primary cell cultures may be prepared from tissues by disaggregation with a proteolytic enzyme such as trypsin. This treatment produces a suspension of detached cells which may be counted and sown in growth medium in a culture vessel where the cells settle and adhere to the glass. If the culture conditions are suitable, the cells begin to divide and spread over the surface of the glass, usually in regular orientation, e.g. fibroblasts in parallel array, until a single layer of cells or monolayer is produced. At this stage DNA synthesis declines and cell division ceases —the phenomenon of *contact inhibition*. If the cells are detached from the glass with trypsin or a chelating agent such as EDTA (ethylene-diamine-tetra-acetic acid) they can be resown in a fresh culture vessel and are designated a *secondary cell culture*. Such a culture retains many of the properties of the parent cells, continues to divide and may be subcultured repeatedly; but after a variable period of time, the rate of growth declines, and the cells eventually die. Occasionally, these cell cultures do not decline, but may alter in behaviour, either slowly or suddenly, and after perhaps 70 subcultures, may be called an *established cell line*. This process has been called *transformation* or cell alteration. The transformed cells grow more rapidly than the cell of origin, show less orientation and are not so subject to contact inhibition. Transformation may occur spontaneously or it may be induced by an oncogenic (tumour producing) virus or treatment of the cells with chemical carcinogens. If the primary cell culture is prepared from tumour tissue these cells may behave as transformed cells from the first.

Organ and tissue cultures are other methods of maintaining cells in the laboratory. Tissue cultures are made by placing small pieces of tissue in media and allowing cells to migrate out from the tissue fragments. Organ cultures have the virtue of preserving the organization of small pieces of organs in which the cells are situated, e.g. pieces of ferret trachea can be grown and maintained in Petri dishes, and the rhythmic movement of the cilia of the epithelial surface observed directly with the microscope.

Growth and Detection of Animal Viruses in Cell Cultures Grown in Test Tubes

After inoculation into monolayer cell cultures, a virus in some instances causes degeneration of the cell sheet. The progress of the infection can be followed by examination of the inoculated cultures with the low-power objective of a light microscope. By this means, the cell degeneration or cytopathic effect (CPE) may be studied. The appearance of the CPE varies with different viruses, e.g. cells may become rounded and shrivelled, or ballooned, or may be fused together to form multinucleate

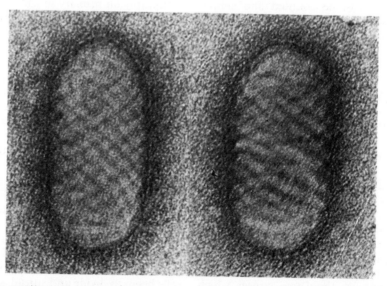

PLATE 12.2. An electromicrograph of two orf virus particles seen in swabs from the lesions from the mouth of a sheep. Notice the criss-crossing nucleoprotein strands and the double layered outer covering membrane. (Phosphotungstic acid. × 160 000.) (From Swain and Dodds, *Clinical Virology*, 1967.)

syncytial masses. Eventually all the cells of the culture are affected and detach from the glass. This process may take only a few hours or as long as several weeks, depending on the virus inoculum. Histological examination of stained infected cells may reveal in more detail the effects of viruses on cells. Frequently, the histological picture is characteristic of the virus present. Changes may include the appearance within the cells of *viral inclusion bodies*. These inclusions vary in size from 0·5 to 7 or more μm and may either be in the cytoplasm or the nucleus; they may be seen not only in cultured infected cells, but also in the organs or tissues of infected animals or man. The location and staining properties of the inclusion may be characteristic of one particular virus or virus group. In some instances, the inclusion body seems to be the site where new virions are synthesized within the cell.

Not all viruses produce a CPE, although they may be present and replicating in infected cells. The presence of virus in cells may be inferred in several ways. Some viruses can adhere to the surface of certain species of red blood cells and hence cause the red cells to clump or agglutinate. This is known as *haemagglutination*. It is possible to detect such viruses by testing the cell culture fluids for haemagglutinating ability. Also, many haemagglutinating viruses are assembled at the host cell cytoplasmic membrane, and this phenomenon may be detected by the addition of a suspension of the appropriate red blood cells to the infected cultures. After a short period of contact, microscopic examination reveals that red blood cells are adhering to the surface of some of the cells. This property of *haemadsorption* allows the detection of the virus. These methods are especially useful with members of the myxovirus, paramyxovirus and togavirus groups.

Another indirect method of detecting virus is by means of *viral interference* phenomenon test. This occurs when a cell infected with one virus is unable to support the growth of a second or challenge virus. In practice, after initial incubation of the inoculated culture to allow time for virus growth to occur, a challenge dose of virus, known to cause a CPE in a few days, is added. If the test cultures contain many surviving cells despite the inoculation of the challenge virus it may be assumed that an interfering virus is present. As will be discussed in the next chapter, viral interference may occur at the host cell membrane or, more usually, at an intracellular stage in the growth of a virus.

Immunological methods may be applied to the detection of virus particles or virus antigens within infected cells. Any immunological method relies on the availability of a specific, potent antiserum to the virus under study. Thus gel precipitation studies with infected cell extracts as antigen may reveal the presence of virus or viral products, and the technique of *immunofluorescence* (Chap. 1, Vol. II) has been of great value in the detection of virus antigens during the time sequence of events in the virus growth cycle.

AUTORADIOGRAPHIC TECHNIQUES can be used to locate sites of virus nucleic acid and protein synthesis within cells. To perform such a test, virus-infected cells are exposed for a short time to a radioactive labelled precursor, e.g. tritiated thymidine, to detect DNA synthesis. After washing, the cell preparation is fixed and a photographic emulsion placed in close contact. After a period of days, development of the emulsion shows dark silver grains located over those sites in the cell where synthesis of the component, e.g. DNA, was occurring during the period when the labelled precursor was present in the culture.

ELECTRON-MICROSCOPICAL examination of ultra-thin sections of infected cells can be applied to the detection of virus. But, in view of the relative sizes of virions and cells and the many structures within them, it may be very difficult to locate virions. However, in combination with growth studies, electron microscopy has been invaluable in studying the events of the virus growth cycle.

Infection of cells with some viruses, e.g. oncogenic or tumour viruses, is not always followed by a productive or cytolytic virus growth cycle. In some instances, *transformation* may occur in the behaviour of the cells in that they do not show contact inhibition and do not grow in an orderly fashion. The sites of infection, if transformation has occurred, may be detected in monolayer cultures as clumps or foci of cells heaped on top of each other.

Assay of Animal Viruses

The following methods of growth and detection may be used to estimate the numbers of infectious particles in a suspension. Monolayer cell cultures growing in Petri dishes may be inoculated to perform a *focal assay* of a virus suspension. The principle is identical to that described for the focal assay of bacteriophage. To perform a titration, small measured volumes of varying dilutions of the virus stock are inoculated on to drained monolayer cultures of sensitive cells in Petri dishes. After one to four hours' adsorption, excess virus is removed by washing and an overlay medium added. The overlay is necessary as the cells require medium for survival. Virus released from infected cells could diffuse readily through a fluid medium to produce a diffuse CPE. The virus can be confined and focal lesions produced if the overlay medium is solidified with agar. The cell culture can survive these conditions, and a focal assay of the virus obtained, as released virus can only reach immediately adjacent cells to produce expanding local lesions or plaques. A similar effect may be obtained for the larger viruses by rendering the overlay medium viscous by the addition of methyl cellulose (methocel). An alternative method is the incorporation of specific antiserum to the virus in the medium. This neutralizes free virus in the medium, but plaques can still develop if newly released virus immediately attaches to and enters neighbouring cells. Plaques may be visualized by draining the Petri dish and staining the cells with a dye such as methyl violet. As with bacteriophages, the titre of animal viruses is expressed in plaque forming units (p.f.u.) per ml based on the number of plaques produced from a measured volume of a known dilution of the virus suspension.

An alternative method is the *quantal assay*, which is not as accurate as the focal type. This method may be valuable if a virus cannot be made to produce plaques. In a quantal test, identical numbers of animals or cultures are inoculated with measured volumes of equally spaced virus dilutions. After a period of incubation the animals or cultures are examined for signs of disease or CPE. By a mathematical treatment, the LD50 or TCID50 of the original virus suspension is calculated (see Vol. II, Chap. 14). This represents the greatest dilution of the virus suspension that causes signs of infection in 50 per cent of the inoculated animals or cultures A quantal assay is far less reproducible than a focal assay, the important limitation is the susceptibility and the number of animals or cultures required.

The phenomenon of *metabolic inhibition* offers a special method of detecting the presence of virus in an inoculated culture. Some viruses, e.g. poliovirus, have a marked early inhibitory effect on infected cells. The result of infection is that the metabolism of the cells declines rapidly after infection, and no acid metabolites are produced. In a balanced medium containing an indicator, normally respiring cells produce an acid pH change. In a quantal titration of a virus suspension, inoculated cell cultures are scored as positive for virus if the cultures do not show an acid pH shift because their metabolism has been inhibited by the virus.

Focal and quantal assays of virus suspensions give an indication of the number of infective virus particles present. The resulting titres are usually much lower than the total number of virus particles present. An estimate of the total number of virus particles (viable and non-viable) present can be made with the electron microscope by counting the number of particles demonstrable in a negatively stained preparation. To do this, virus in suspension is mixed with latex or polystyrene particles of known concentration and dried on an electron-microscope grid with negative stain, usually phosphotungstic acid. On examination, the relative numbers of virus and latex particles in several fields are determined and the number of virus particles per unit volume calculated. The lowest total particle: infective virus ratios are obtained with some bacteriophage preparations when a ratio of $1:1$ may occur. When animal virus preparations are examined, the ratio is much higher and often several hundred particles are seen for every infectious unit detected. This preponderance of non-infectious particles may be important in growth and serological studies. Variation in the ratio may occur in different preparations of a virus, and may cause varying degrees of interference with virus growth, since non-infectious particles may still have effects on cells.

A rough estimate of the number of virus particles in a suspension may be derived from a haemagglutinin titration. This method applies only if the haemagglutinin is an integral part of the virion. The titration is performed by preparing serial dilutions of the virus suspension, adding the appropriate red blood cells and incubating until agglutination is complete. The end point of the titration is the highest dilution of the virus suspension that causes complete agglutination. This assay does not measure the infectivity of the virus, but may be a quick and convenient assay in some circumstances.

FURTHER READING

FENNER, F. (1968) *The Biology of Animal Viruses,* Vol. 1 and 2. London: Academic Press.

LURIA, S. E. & DARNELL, J. E. (1967) *General Virology.* 2nd Edn. New York: John Wiley & Sons Inc.

LWOFF, A. & FOURNIER, P. (1971) *Remarks on the Classification of Viruses in Comparative Virology.* Edited by K. Maramorosch and E. Kurstak. New York: Academic Press.

NEWTON, A. & WATERSON, A. P. (1967) Chapter 2. In *Viral and Rickettsial Infections of Animals.* Edited by A. O. Betts and C. J. York, Vol. 1. London: Academic Press.

RHODES, A. J. & VAN ROOYEN, C. E. (1968) *Textbook of Virology.* Baltimore: Williams and Wilkie.

WILDY, P. (1971) *Classification and Nomenclature of Viruses.* Basel: Karger.

13. Virus-cell Interactions: Virus Genetics: Antiviral Agents

Titration methods aided by electron microscope examination and many biochemical assay techniques, have led to the description of a range of virus-cell interactions of which there are three main categories—*lytic*, *steady state* and *integrated*. It is now known that viruses may infect and replicate within cells, and as a result cause the infected cells to lyse when the progeny virions are released. This lytic or cytocidal cycle results from infection with a virulent virus. In addition to cytocidal infective cycles, a steady-state, non-cytocidal interaction may occur. In this form, virus is produced over a period of time, and the infected cells survive. The third category of interaction is the nonproductive, latent or lysogenic state in which the viral genome remains within the host cell and replicates in association with the host cell chromosomes without the production of virions.

The Lytic or Cytocidal Growth Cycle

The quantitative aspects of the growth curve were first determined with bacterial viruses, but similar results may also be obtained with animal viruses. The one-step growth curve is the name given to the graph which is derived from the study of a single cycle of virus infection when the cells of a culture are infected synchronously and the culture is sampled at intervals to determine the content of infectious virus by titration. Two forms of growth curve can be described, depending on the treatment of the samples from the infected culture, that is, whether the cells are lysed or not. The duration of the growth cycle varies from about 30 minutes for a bacterial virus to 5 to 20 hours for an animal virus.

1. *Artificial lysis*. In this study, a culture of cells is inoculated with sufficient virus particles to infect most of the cells. Samples are removed at intervals thereafter, and are treated so that all the cells are lysed; the resulting suspensions are titrated for infectious particles. Under these

artificial conditions of lysis the type of growth curve obtained is illustrated in Fig. 13.1. This curve may be divided into three stages. During stage 1 decreasing amounts of virus are demonstrated in the lysed culture samples; later (2) no virus at all may be recovered; then (3) at longer intervals after infection increasing amounts of virus are detected.

The early part of the cycle (1) is the stage of adsorption and penetration. Virus comes into contact with cells by random collision and may then attach to or adsorb to them. With some viruses, adsorption has been shown to depend on the presence of specific receptor sites on the host cell membrane (see below). Once a virus has adsorbed to a cell either the viral nucleic acid alone may penetrate the host cell or the intact virion may be taken in. Bacterial viruses transfer their nucleic acid and some protein into cells, whereas the whole animal virus particle is usually taken into cells before the nucleic acid is released. When the viral nucleic acid is free within the cell, it is vulnerable to attack by nucleases liberated by lysosomes. Probably for this reason decreasing numbers of infective

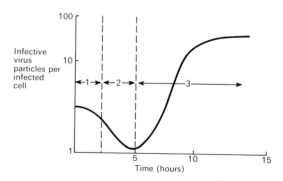

FIG. 13.1. Diagram of the multiplication curve of a virus. Samples are removed from an infected culture at intervals and assayed for the total content of virus. Stages: (1) adsorption and penetration; (2) eclipse; and (3) maturation and release.

virions are demonstrated as the next stage of the growth cycle commences.

Stage 2 when no virions can be detected within infected cells is known as the *eclipse phase* and is a distinctive character of the virus growth cycle. It can be shown only if the samples removed from the culture are treated to lyse the cells; then unprotected viral nucleic acid is degraded by nucleases and no infectious virus can be found. During the eclipse period, virus enzymes, nucleic acid and structural proteins are synthesized and these are then assembled into new virion progeny. At stage 3 the viral nucleic acid is once more protected from degradative enzymes, so that increasing amounts of virus can be detected within cells. The *assembly phase* is followed by the release of the virus particles by lysis of the cell. Due to the rapidity of phage infection, it may not be possible to define the early stages of adsorption and penetration, but the end of the eclipse phase and virus maturation can be demonstrated (Fig. 13.2B).

2. *Without artificial lysis.* When a comparable study is performed, but each sample is treated to avoid artificial lysis of the cells, a growth curve as illustrated in Fig. 13.2A results. Under these conditions, there is no clearly defined stage of adsorption and penetration or eclipse, related to the fact that the early samples contain only infected intact cells, each of which gives rise to a single plaque when the samples are diluted and titrated on fresh susceptible host cells. If each infected cell contains one or more virus particles, or viral genomes, only one plaque will result on titration, because despite replication within the infected cell, the progeny virions are all released at one site on the titration plate and they can infect fresh cells only at the point of release. Hence the apparently steady level of virus in the early part of the growth cycle is equivalent to the number of infected cells present in the culture. Later, a rapid increase in virus content occurs due to the natural lysis of the infected cells with release of the newly formed virions each of which can give rise to one plaque. The time interval between inoculation and this sudden increase in extracellular virus is called the *latent period*. The ratio of the final virus titre to the number of infected cells measures the average yield of infectious virus

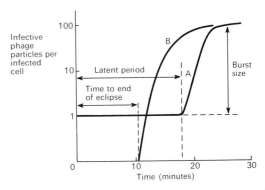

FIG. 13.2. Bacteriophage growth curves: without (A) and following (B) artificial lysis of the infected cells. The interval to the first appearance of virus within an infected cell measures the time to the end of the eclipse period. The latent period is the time to spontaneous release of virus. The ratio of the total yield of virus to the number of infected cells measures the average yield of virus from each infected cell (burst size).

particles from each infected cell—the *burst size* or yield for lytic viruses.

These growth studies were first performed with bacterial viruses but experiments confirm that similar events occur in the growth cycle of animal viruses. The duration of the latent period varies considerably. Bacterial viruses have short latent periods, under optimal conditions as short as 10 to 15 minutes. The replication of animal viruses is slower than that of bacteriophages and more variable in duration. Thus, with RNA animal viruses, latent periods range from 3 hours for some picornaviruses to 10 hours for the leukoviruses. Among the DNA animal viruses, periods range from 5 hours for some herpesviruses and poxviruses through 15 hours for adenoviruses up to 20 hours for papovaviruses.

Mechanisms of Adsorption and Penetration of Virus

The initial contact between virus and cell occurs by random collision, and therefore the rate of collision will depend on the relative concentrations of viruses and cells. Similarity of surface charge may tend to keep virus and cell apart; consequently the ionic composition of the suspending fluids, particularly the cation concentration, may affect virus adsorption.

Growth studies with bacterial viruses are usually performed with both virus and bacterium in suspension. With animal viruses, the cells are often infected as monolayer cultures; under these conditions collisions between virus and cell are less likely to occur than in suspension. The efficiency of adsorption of virus to cells in monolayers is increased if the virus is contained in as small a volume of fluid as will cover the cell sheet and kept in contact with the cells for a period of 1 to 4 hours. Conditions resembling the phage system can be obtained with some viruses and animal cells by shaking virus and cells together in suspension before plating on glass or plastic.

Attachment of the virus to the cell surface depends on the interaction of complementary steric groups on the surfaces of each. Thus not all collisions between virus and cell will be successful as the virus may not make contact with a specific receptor site. Some bacteriophages require the presence of cofactors before adsorption is accomplished. For example, T4 phage requires the presence of six molecules of tryptophan for each virion before the tail fibres unfold and attach to the host cell wall. Animal viruses do not possess comparable tails and probably attach by a specific part of the capsid, e.g., projecting fibres and knobs of the adenoviruses. Similarly, the projecting haemagglutinin spikes of myxoviruses attach to receptors containing neuraminic acid on the host cell membrane.

Adsorption of virus to susceptible cells may be prevented by specific antibody, thus neutralizing the virus or preventing the infection. Failure of adsorption under these conditions may be due to a structural distorting change in the virus capsid or simply to the masking of the viral attachment sites, e.g., antibody with specificity limited to the tail structure of T-even phages has this neutralizing effect.

Knowledge of the host cell receptor sites is limited. The specific receptor sites for T phages of *Escherichia coli* are located at different levels of the bacterial cell wall and small changes in its chemical composition can render a susceptible cell resistant. Such alterations may arise by mutation, or from previous infection of the cell with a virus which alters the receptors in the host cell wall (resistance to superinfection).

In some instances the receptor substances have been isolated and characterized; T5 coliphage adsorbs to a protein-lipopolysaccharide constituent of *Escherichia coli* cell walls. Other phages can adsorb only to special bacterial structures; the small icosahedral viruses MS2 and f2 attach to the sides of the F fimbriae (F pili) of male *Esch. coli* cells and filamentous phages such as F1 adsorb only to the tips of the fimbriae (Chap. 2).

The cellular receptors of animal viruses have been investigated in a few instances. The best studied are those of the orthomyxoviruses and paramyxovirus groups which require specific neuraminic acid-containing glycoproteins for attachment. Destruction of these sites by previous treatment of cells with the enzyme neuraminidase (sialidase) renders the cells insusceptible to infection. Paradoxically, these viruses also possess the neuraminidase as short projecting spikes on the lipoprotein envelope, and so can elute from their own receptor sites. The phenomenon is illustrated in the interaction of viruses with red blood cells in which haemagglutination first occurs by a mechanism probably similar to the attachment of the virus to a host cell followed by elution. In nature, the viral neuraminidase probably liberates virus from mucoproteins in mucus films or from the cell surface on maturation.

Poliovirus is known to attach to specific lipoprotein sites on the surface of susceptible cells. The species specificity of poliovirus, namely that it can infect many primate cells when established in culture, but not non-primate cells is believed to arise because cells of non-primate species do not possess these receptors.

The requirement for specific receptors on the cell membrane can be bypassed, experimentally at least, by infection with extracted viral nucleic acid. By this method, normally resistant cells may be infected as no specific adsorption of virus capsid to cell wall is involved. Thus, chick fibroblasts may be infected, for one cycle, by poliovirus ribonucleic acid; the virions produced are not infective for other chick fibroblasts as there are no receptors for the poliovirus capsid protein.

Penetration and uncoating. Once a virion has attached to a cell surface, the next stage is the entry of the viral nucleic acid into the cell.

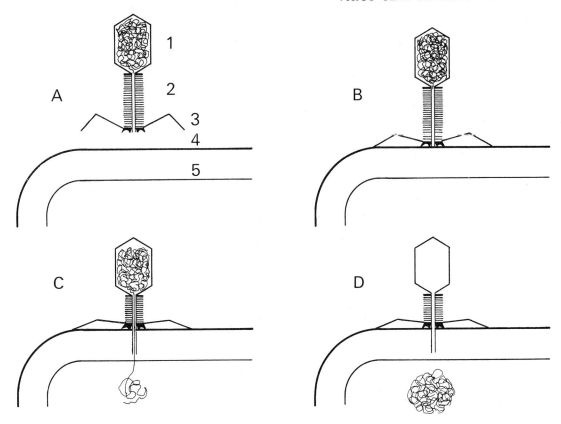

FIG. 13.3. Entry of T-even phage DNA into a host cell.
  A. Free phage with (1) head containing DNA, (2) sheath with central core, (3) base plate with short spikes and fibres, (4) bacterial cell wall, and (5) cytoplasmic membrane.
  B. Phage attaches to cell wall with fibres, base plate in close contact with outer layers of cell wall.
  C. Sheath contracts and central core is pushed through the cell wall and DNA transfer begins.
  D. Transfer of DNA completed. Phage head is now empty and early events of phage growth cycle can commence in the cell.

The process differs with bacterial and animal viruses as the bacterial cell wall is thicker and more complex than the animal cell membrane. Once again, the most detailed knowledge concerns the mechanism of penetration of the T-even series of coliphages (Fig. 13.3) which seem especially well adapted to penetrate the rigid bacterial cell wall. After the phage attaches to the cell wall by means of the tail fibres, the tail sheath contracts, pulling the collar and head of the phage closer to the base plate. As a result, the central hollow core or tube is pushed first through the base plate, and then through the cell wall, already weakened by the action of a phage muramidase present on the base plate. The tube does not penetrate the cell membrane of the bacterium, but the viral nucleic acid passes down the core tube and does so. Virtually all the phage capsid and other protein remains on the outside of the cell and only a small proportion enters the cell in association with the viral nucleic acid.

The injection process is typical of the T-even phages. T5 coliphage requires host cell protein synthesis before transfer of viral nucleic acid can occur. The filamentous phages attach to the tip of the F pili of male *Esch. coli* and may be sufficiently slender to penetrate down the central pore of the F pilus. How the protein and nucleic acid are separated is not known but there

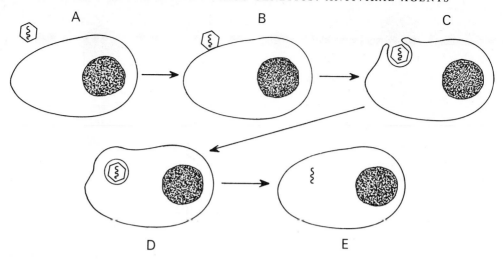

FIG. 13.4. Entry of an animal virus into a host cell.
  A.   Free virus containing nucleic acid collides with susceptible cell.
  B.   Virus adsorbs to cell surface.
  C.   Cell begins to engulf virion.
  D.   Virion within cell, still intact, contained within vesicle.
  E.   Vesicle breaks down and capsid disrupted, releasing viral nucleic acid.

is evidence that only the nucleic acid enters the cell.

The mechanism of penetration of cells by animal viruses is essentially that of phagocytosis. As a result, almost all the viral protein is taken into the cell along with the nucleic acid (Fig. 13.4). There is evidence that the lipoprotein outer covering of some enveloped viruses fuses with the host cell membrane, thus releasing the viral nucleoprotein directly into the cell cytoplasm. After engulfment, non-enveloped viruses are contained, apparently intact, within vesicles (phagosomes) in the cytoplasm. Little is known of the mechanism whereby the virus escapes from the vesicle and releases its nucleic acid. Enzymes secreted in the vesicle fluid when the lysosomes fuse with the phagocytic vesicle may be important in weakening the capsid so that the nucleic acid is liberated when the vesicle breaks down. Release of the adenovirus genome could occur through the gaps left in the capsid if some of the 12 penton units including the fibres are lost during adsorption and penetration.

The penetration and uncoating of vaccinia virus, a member of the poxvirus group is a complex process (Fig. 13.5). The early stages of adsorption and penetration of this virus seem to be similar to those of other animal viruses. However, after the first stage of the uncoating process, viral nucleic acid is not released and is still associated with the virion core. Before the release of the viral nucleic acid, or second stage uncoating, can occur there is a requirement for DNA transcription and protein synthesis; this is indicated by experimental inhibition of the process with actinomycin D or puromycin which block respectively viral transcription and translation (protein synthesis). The vaccinia virion is known to contain virus-coded DNA-dependent RNA polymerase that can transcribe messenger RNA (mRNA) from the viral DNA while the latter is still within the core structure. This viral mRNA is then translated on host cell ribosomes to produce the enzymes necessary to complete the uncoating process.

Events Following Release of Viral Nucleic Acid

When the viral nucleic acid is free within the cell, information is transcribed and diverts the host-cell's energy stores, precursor pool and protein synthesizing machinery to produce viral enzymes and regulator proteins, and subsequently

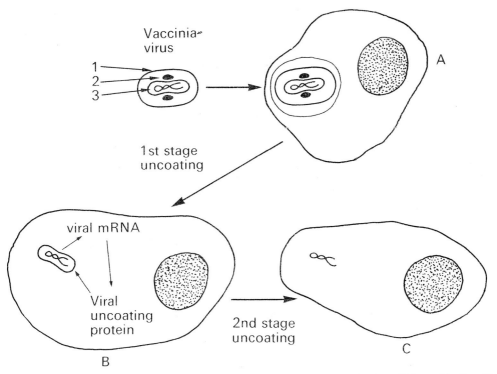

Fig. 13.5. Diagram of the entry and uncoating of vaccinia virus. (1) Outer layers of virion. (2) Lateral bodies. (3) Core containing viral DNA and RNA transcriptase.

At stage A, virus lies within a vesicle in cell cytoplasm.

At stage B, outer layers and lateral bodies have been removed, and the core lies in cytoplasm (1st stage). At this time, a virus-specified uncoating protein is synthesized, and the remaining virus protein is removed (2nd stage) leaving viral DNA free within cell.

viral nucleic acid and viral structural proteins. Unlike bacterial viruses, synthesis of nucleic acid and assembly of animal viruses can take place either within the cytoplasm or in the nucleus of the infected cell or different parts of the cell may be used for these activities at different stages of the cycle. Thus the entering viral nucleic acid may have to traverse a large and highly organized cell to reach its replication site. The retention of some protein in association with the animal virus genome may be important in protecting the nucleic acid until the replication site is reached. Adenovirus DNA, for example, has to reach the host cell nucleus, and the viral genome may be associated with protein until it reaches the safety of the nuclear membrane and nucleus. The DNA of herpesviruses and adenoviruses is replicated and enclosed within capsids only inside the nucleus. However,

not all DNA viruses replicate within the nucleus; members of the poxviruses, e.g. vaccinia virus, synthesize components and are assembled within the cytoplasm (in so called 'factories'). Similar discrete cytoplasmic sites are found with the RNA enteroviruses. Bacterial viruses may be synthesized and assembled throughout the simpler prokaryotic cell and at the end of the growth cycle the virions may represent almost the entire contents of an infected cell. By comparison, animal viruses occupy a much smaller proportion of the cell and may comprise only about 5 per cent of the cell constituents. As a result the synthesis and assembly of virions usually takes place within localized regions of the cell. However, during myxovirus replication the internal nucleoprotein is synthesized in the nucleus and various envelope proteins in the cytoplasm; these components are finally assembled into a virion which buds from the cytoplasmic membrane. As mentioned in Chapter 12 the amount of nucleic acid contained in virions varies considerably from about 2×10^6 daltons to 160×10^6 daltons. The coding capacity, therefore, is very different and the number of virus coded proteins varies from about 3 for the smallest to several hundred with the largest viruses. The extreme example is the small cubical RNA bacteriophage which can only code for three polypeptides. Two of these are incorporated into the capsid, one as the basic structural unit and the other as the attachment protein, whilst the third is the virus-specified RNA polymerase. The degree of dependence of the virus on the host cell for the synthesis of viral enzymes, regulator and structural proteins will therefore be very different for small and large viruses.

Viral macromolecular synthesis. The genes of DNA bacterial and animal viruses are transcribed and translated in a manner resembling that of the genetic material of other biological systems. The RNA viruses, particularly the leukoviruses, exhibit some unique properties (see below).

After virus infection, new types of nucleic acid and protein can be detected in the cell and identified as being of viral origin by sedimentation and hybridization studies and by their serological specificity as proteins or nucleoproteins. Chemical inhibitors have proved to be extremely useful in growth studies by interrupting various stages of the cycle. Chloramphenicol, an inhibitor of protein synthesis on bacterial ribosomes, can be used to study the stages at which protein synthesis is necessary for bacterial virus replication. Similarly, in mammalian cells, cycloheximide, parafluorophenylalanine and puromycin can be employed to interrupt normal protein synthesis. Actinomycin D prevents mRNA transcription from the DNA of the host cell or of a DNA virus; the addition of this compound at intervals after virus inoculation will indicate the requirement for viral mRNA synthesis, or in studies with RNA viruses, 'clear' the ribosomes of host mRNA. Mitomycin C which cross-links complementary strands of DNA can be used to prevent DNA replication. The halogenated deoxyuridines, especially the 5′-fluoro-2-deoxyuridine (FUdR)

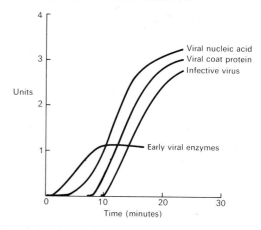

FIG. 13.6. Time sequence of synthetic events during a phage growth cycle. After the appearance of early virus enzymes, viral nucleic acid is replicated, synthesis of early enzymes is stopped, viral coat protein is made, and finally nucleic acid and protein are assembled into mature virions.

derivative also inhibit DNA synthesis by preventing the incorporation of thymidine into nucleic acid.

The synthesis of macromolecules in a virus infected cell can be summarized as in the diagram (Fig. 13.6). The time scale illustrated is for a bacterial virus but the same series of events, in the same order, occurs with all viruses. The earliest event depicted in the diagram is the synthesis of virus-coded 'early proteins'; this takes place from the incoming viral genome of a DNA virus which is transcribed, a viral mRNA is produced and translated on host ribosomes. These early proteins initiate and maintain viral nucleic acid synthesis; also in many instances, early proteins have an inhibiting effect ('switch off') on a variety of host cell functions. After early enzyme production, viral nucleic acid replication can commence. As a pool of new nucleic acid molecules builds up, these are transcribed in turn and 'late proteins' are synthesized. The late proteins have a function in regulating the production of early enzymes, although the mechanisms are not yet clear, and also include most of the structural proteins for the new virions. In addition, late proteins may be involved in the process of assembly and in the release of the new virions from the cell. The diagram (Fig. 13.7) summarizes the events of the virus growth cycle.

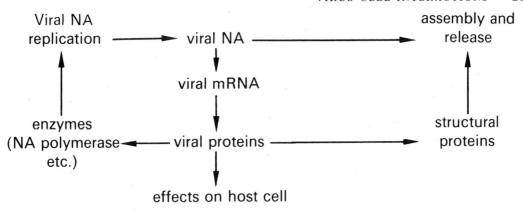

FIG. 13.7. Diagram of the events in the replication of a virus. NA = Nucleic acid.

Viral mRNA synthesis. The presence of viral mRNA was first demonstrated in a bacterial virus system, but similar products may be detected in cells infected with animal viruses. Their viral origin may be demonstrated by molecular hybridization experiments with DNA extracted from purified virions. Fig. 13.8 illustrates the results that are obtained with vaccinia virus when susceptible cells are synchronously infected at high multiplicity; two peaks of RNA synthesis (1 and 2) occur. If replication of the viral DNA is prevented by the addition of FUdR, only the first peak is found and represents the production of mRNA from the incoming or *parental* strands of DNA; whilst the second peak (2) represents mRNA transcribed from *progeny* DNA strands. The function of the DNA-dependent RNA polymerase in the core of vaccinia virions has been mentioned in the discussion of 'uncoating'. If complete uncoating of the DNA is prevented by an inhibitor of protein synthesis, early viral mRNA continues to be produced to a greater level than normal, but no later peak of viral mRNA is detected.

Only vaccinia has been shown to contain a DNA-dependent RNA polymerase within the virion. Other DNA viruses presumably rely on a host cell polymerase for the production of early mRNA before new virus enzymes can be made (Fig. 13.9).

The riboviruses are unique in that they rely on RNA both to contain their genetic information and to act as mRNA. The synthesis of viral protein occurs in the same way as for host cell protein; viral nucleic acid is transcribed by a polymerase or transcriptase enzyme and the mRNA is then translated on host cell ribosomes with the participation of transfer RNA (tRNA). A host enzyme cannot be used for RNA production as none is known which could make mRNA on an RNA template. This enzyme must therefore be virus-coded and either carried into the

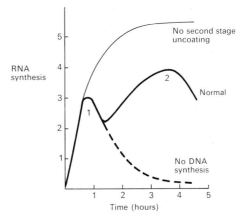

FIG. 13.8. RNA synthesis in cells infected with large numbers of vaccinia virus particles shows two peaks of activity. Transcription of the infecting parental DNA results in peak 1, while the progeny strands are responsible for peak 2. If uncoating is blocked, RNA continues to be synthesized on the viral DNA by means of the RNA polymerase present in the virion core. If viral DNA replication is prevented, RNA synthesis from the input strands declines, and no peak 2 is seen as no progeny DNA is produced.
(From Woodson, B. (1967) *Biochemical and Biophysical Research Communications,* **27,** 169.)

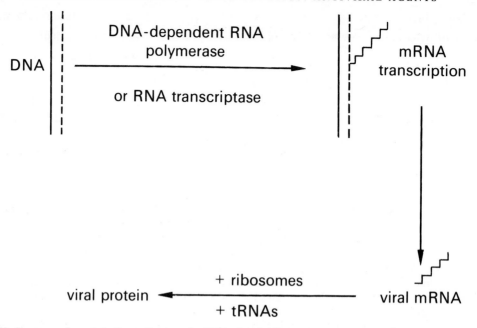

FIG. 13.9. Sequence of events in the replication of a DNA virus leading to the synthesis of viral proteins.

cell in the virion or synthesized early in the growth cycle by direct translation of the infecting RNA strands. Both mechanisms obtain. RNA polymerase activity has been detected in the virions of reoviruses, vesicular stomatitis virus (rhabdoviruses), influenza virus and paramyxo viruses and seems to have a transcriptase function (Fig. 13.10). On the other hand the poliovirus virion has not been shown to contain a polymerase enzyme but activity can be demonstrated in infected cells after translation

of the viral genome. As opposed to the larger viruses with well-defined early and late functions, the poliovirus genome acts as a polycistronic message (Fig. 13.11), and is translated to produce a single large polypeptide which has to be broken down to produce the required proteins.

Viral Nucleic Acid Replication

The replication of viral double-stranded DNA occurs in the same way as other DNA molecules.

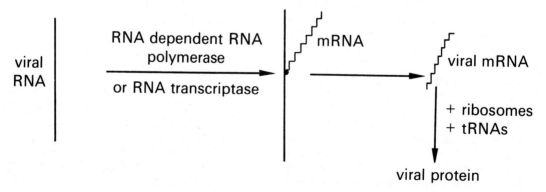

FIG. 13.10. Diagram of the events leading to viral protein synthesis with RNA viruses that contain RNA dependent RNA polymerase activity.

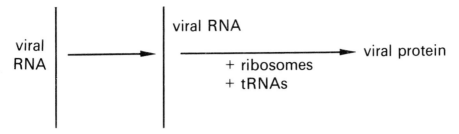

FIG. 13.11. Diagram of events leading to viral protein synthesis with an RNA virus with no virion RNA transcriptase activity.

This is by semiconservative replication in which each strand of DNA can serve as a template for a new strand and can combine with this new strand to form a double-stranded molecule. A new viral DNA polymerase is often produced to aid this process. The replication of the DNA of some bacterial viruses may be accompanied by considerable breakage and reunion of strands, a phenomenon which is probably related to a high rate of genetic recombination. Special mechanisms may be involved in the replication of nucleic acids unique to viruses, viz., single-stranded DNA and single- and double-stranded RNA. Double-stranded RNA molecules are probably replicated in an analogous manner to double-stranded DNA, with the help of the appropriate enzyme, i.e., RNA-dependent RNA polymerase (RNA synthetase). With single-stranded viruses many identical copies of the single strand have to be produced. By the usual base pairing method these progeny strands would have to be synthesized on a strand of nucleic acid complementary to the incoming viral genome. Thus, the first stage in viral replication would be the production of a double-stranded molecule by the synthesis of a complementary strand on the incoming strand. The name 'replicative form' or RF has been given to this double-stranded molecule. The next step is the production of many copies of the viral genome via the complementary strand in this RF. In poliovirus-infected cells, large RNA molecules can be detected, which have been called replicative intermediate complexes and are probably composed of the RF core and several attached pieces of single-stranded RNA in various stages of synthesis; their significance is still uncertain.

Another mechanism has been proposed for the replication of single-stranded DNA, and perhaps also for single-stranded RNA; the 'rolling circle' hypothesis. In this method the incoming strand is circularized, and a complementary circular strand made. A long chain consisting of many copies of the parental strand can be 'rolled off' this molecule. If this chain is then severed by specific enzyme action at appropriate points, then many copies of the viral genome are produced. Virus-coded enzymes (RNA polymerases) are involved in the stages of RNA replication, first in synthesizing the complementary strand and then, in producing the multiple copies of the viral genome. These two reactions could be catalysed by distinct enzymes, or by one enzyme with two separate functions.

Single-stranded DNA bacterial viruses apparently rely on a host cell enzyme for the synthesis of the complementary strand, but they produce their own DNA polymerase or synthetase for the second stage.

Viral Protein Synthesis

Virus-coded proteins are required as outlined, as polymerases, regulators of host or viral syntheses, as structural proteins or enzymes in virions, or to effect release from the cell. The functions of these proteins at different stages of the growth cycle have been discussed. Of particular interest is the special substrate specificity of the virus-coded polymerases and regulator proteins. The specificity of the enzyme might arise either by the complete synthesis of the enzyme protein from a viral mRNA, or by modification or incorporation of a small virus-coded polypeptide into a cellular enzyme with consequent alteration of its substrate specificity. An example of the latter method is the alteration of specificity of initiation and termination of transcription by the RNA polymerase of *Esch. coli* by the insertion of new sigma (σ) and rho (ρ) factors. In some instances an infecting virus may stimulate synthesis of host cell enzymes, thus producing increased activity. This effect has been noted with some of the small DNA tumour viruses (Papova viruses) which have limited genetic information and might therefore code for sigma and rho factors rather than complete enzymes. Within a few minutes after infection of a cell, new viral enzymes (early proteins) may be detected which are synthesized before viral nucleic acid or structural components. Some of these have been characterized. In the case of the T-even phages, in addition to a DNA polymerase, a series of enzymes are produced that are necessary for the synthesis of the unusual base hydroxymethylcytosine present in the phage DNA instead of cytosine. A DNA nuclease is also made and this is probably involved in the breakdown of host cell DNA demonstrable very soon after infection. No structural proteins of the capsid are detectable at this early stage, but an internal head protein can be found. Coat proteins are synthesized after viral DNA replication

has commenced and the different head, sheath and tail subunits accumulate before assembly takes place, perhaps with the aid of further non-structural proteins (Fig. 13.6).

As with bacteriophage, there is good evidence that animal viruses also regulate the time sequence of protein synthesis. In vaccinia and herpesvirus infected cells, new DNA polymerase, DNA nuclease, and thymidine kinase activities appear early in the cycle. Structural proteins are usually synthesized late in the cycle, although some poxvirus internal and surface proteins are detectable early in infection. In infection with vaccinia virus (Fig. 13.12), the level of thymidine kinase activity within cells reaches a plateau about 4 hours after infection. This plateau effect depends on the stability of both the enzyme and the mRNA coding for the enzyme. If the synthesis of viral mRNA is prevented, then no switch-off effect is seen and increased enzymic activity can be detected over a period of several hours.

Modification of host cell function. Viruses vary considerably in the degree to which they affect the host cell. In cytocidal infections, interruption of host cell functions can usually be demonstrated early in the growth cycle. T-even phages cause the breakdown of *Esch. coli* DNA within a short time. Poliovirus breaks up host cell polysomes, and the released ribosomes are then utilized for viral protein synthesis; it also interrupts the synthesis and release of host RNA. Other viruses may not have such an early direct effect on the host, although a gradual decline in synthetic activity can be demonstrated. In non-cytocidal infection, if the infecting virus can transform the cell, there may be increased cell DNA and enzyme synthesis, in keeping with the increased rate of growth seen in the transformed cell.

Site of protein synthesis. Despite the site of animal virus replication, it seems that viral proteins are made in the cytoplasmic ribosomes. The localization of vaccinia and poliovirus synthesis in cytoplasmic factory sites is probably necessary for vaccinia and polio to maintain adequate concentrations of the enzymes required for viral replication. The proteins necessary for the synthesis and assembly of nuclear viruses must also be made in the cell cytoplasm. Viral mRNA has therefore to leave the nucleus

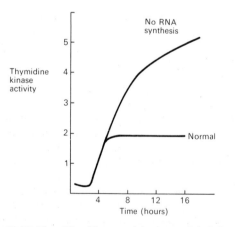

FIG. 13.12. Thymidine kinase activity in vaccinia-infected cells and in cells treated with an inhibitor of RNA synthesis. Normally this early enzyme activity increases and reaches a plateau, but if mRNA synthesis is inhibited within 2 hours after infection, then enzyme synthesis continues.

and the new viral proteins have to enter the nucleus before maturation of the virions can take place. Evidence in support of this mechanism has been obtained with herpesviruses using radioactive tracer techniques; although the proteins cannot be detected serologically in the cytoplasm soon after infection with herpes, adeno- and papova viruses, immunofluorescence demonstrates the presence of new viral antigens in the nucleus.

A rather more complex pattern is seen with the influenza viruses. The internal component, the ribonucleo-protein helical strand or RNP antigen, is first detected within the nucleus and then is found throughout the cell, in particular at the cell surface, the site at which virus maturation takes place. Two other components of the virion, neuraminidase and haemagglutinin, can be found initially only within the cytoplasm, often in a perinuclear position. Later, these components appear to be concentrated in the cytoplasmic membrane and are then incorporated into maturing virions.

Assembly and release of virions. Once a pool of viral nucleic acid has accumulated, increasing numbers of infective virions can be detected within cells. The complex T-even phages illustrate the manner in which assembly or maturation occurs. The first step is the condensation of viral DNA molecules into particles similar to phage heads. The mechanism of this condensation of a very large piece of DNA is not completely understood, but may occur by interaction of the DNA with internal head proteins known to be present in mature virions. Capsid subunits are then arranged around the DNA particles to form recognizable heads. Next, the tube-like structure present inside the sheath is attached to the head, often in association with the base plate. Once this stage has been reached, an uncontracted sheath is built around the tube, and finally the tail fibres are assembled from their subunits and attached to the base plate. This assembly process has some characteristics of crystallization, the initiation of each step requiring the completion of the previous step. By this stage of the replication cycle, a single bacterium may contain several thousand mature virions occupying almost the entire cell.

An essentially similar sequence occurs in the assembly of symmetrical animal viruses although the process varies from virus to virus. Herpesviruses and adenoviruses, for example, are assembled within the nuclei of infected cells. In ultrathin sections of infected cells examined in the electron microscope the earliest evidence of the assembly process is the detection of regular arrays of immature, small particles, which probably represent the DNA in association with an internal protein. Later, the particles acquire a definite hexagonal outline as the protein subunits are added to form the capsids. The symmetrical RNA viruses, e.g. polioviruses, are synthesized and assembled in membrane-associated sites in the cytoplasm. The complex poxviruses show some differences from simpler viruses in that a matrix, probably containing DNA, is enclosed initially within a primitive membrane. Differentiation takes place within the membrane, culminating in the development of the DNA containing nucleoid and the lateral bodies. At the same time, the membrane is modified and matures to show the surface structure associated with mature virions. This sequence fits with the observation that vaccinia virus structural proteins are made both as early and late proteins, and that some of the early proteins are apparently situated in the outer layers of the external membrane.

The envelopes of enveloped viruses are derived from host cell membranes, often as the virus is leaving the nucleus or the cell surface. Before virions begin to be enveloped the host cell membrane is modified by incorporation of virus-specific antigens. In herpes-infected cells, new glycoproteins are produced, and several of these are associated with cell membranes.

Electron microscopy of the cell after infection with herpesvirus reveals a thickened nuclear membrane with many convolutions. The nucleus at this stage contains particles of hexagonal outline with a diameter corresponding to the icosahedral capsid. These particles acquire a membrane by budding through the inner lamella of the nuclear membrane, as illustrated in Fig. 13.13B. Thus nuclear particles in thin section appear to have a core surrounded by a hexagonal shell with a diameter of 100 nm. In the cytoplasm, or usually within vesicles in the cytoplasm, the virions have a larger diameter and appear to be surrounded by two shells. The inner

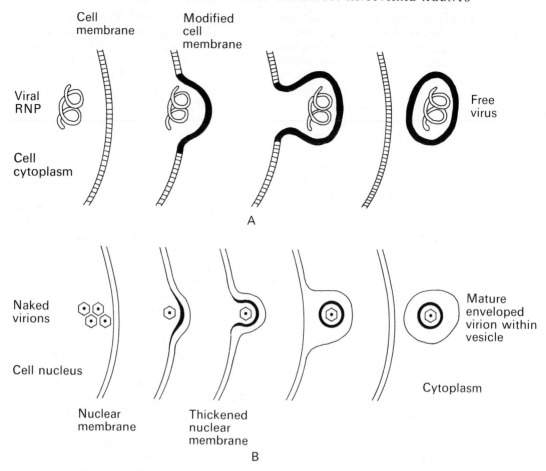

FIG. 13.13. Diagram of the envelopment and release of animal viruses.
  A. Orthomyxovirus or paramyxovirus ribonucleoprotein (RNP) located under cell membrane, in which viral components have been inserted. Virus then buds off from cell membrane, enclosing RNP.
  B. Herpesvirus DNA and capsids are assembled within the nucleus. Viral-specified components modify and cause thickening of the inner aspect of the nuclear membrane. The virus then buds through the membrane, thus being enveloped, and comes to lie within a cytoplasmic vesicle.

shell is the capsid, and the outer shell the envelope of modified host cell nuclear membrane.

The orthomyxo- and paramyxoviruses also acquire an outer envelope by a budding process; in these groups, however, the budding is from the surface of the cell and the envelope is derived from the modified cytoplasmic membrane (Fig. 13.13A). Envelopment occurs by a budding process in which the RNP component, after migrating from the nucleus, is surrounded by modified cell membrane, containing haemagglutinin and neuraminidase and released from the cell. The incorporation of viral antigens causes some thickening of the cell membrane, but perhaps the most striking change is the development of the property of haemadsorption. This ability to cause certain types of red blood cell to adhere to the cell surface is a useful property for the detection of virus-containing cells that do not always show a cytopathic effect after infection. The modification and use of host cell membranes by orthomyxo- and paramyxovirus implies that mature virus particles must contain host cell constituents in the viral envelope. This may be confirmed experimentally and indeed the lipid and carbohydrate composition of both the viral envelope and the host cell membrane can be shown to be similar. The viral neuraminidase may be important in the release of virus particles from the cell.

The budding process in orthomyxo- and paramyxovirus infected cells may continue over a period of time, in which the cell survives and many virions are produced. Some virions released by the budding method have been found to be capable of establishing a steady-state or non-cytocidal, productive infection; the cell survives and can divide, and at the same time virus is produced both from the parent and daughter cells. In such a culture, almost all cells are infected.

The alternative to the slow, prolonged release or leakage of these viruses is the rapid lysis of the infected cell, characteristic of the virulent T-even phages. As in the penetration stage, a bacterial virus has to overcome a very tough and rigid cell wall in comparison to the cell membrane encountered by animal viruses. To surmount this problem, the T-even phages probably rely on a muramidase. Increasing quantities of this enzyme can be detected late in the growth cycle and it attacks the cell wall from within. There follows a sudden disruption of the cell and the simultaneous release of the progeny virions. Poliovirus, like the phage, also has an early inhibitory effect on cell macromolecular synthesis and is released by bursting the cell. The gradual rundown of the cell functions may be severe enough to result in lysis of the cell. The process may be aided, however, by the release of lysosomal enzymes, which could attack and weaken the cell membrane from within.

Herpesvirus, which is assembled within the nucleus and enveloped at the inner layer of the nuclear membrane (Fig. 13.13B), may be transported across the cell cytoplasm in vesicles derived from the nuclear membrane ('reverse phagocytosis'). Other herpesviruses, e.g., varicella and cytomegaloviruses, may be cell-associated over a considerable period of time, and only low levels of released virus may be found in infected cell cultures.

Under optimal conditions several thousand virus particles may be produced by some animal viruses. It is notable, however, that only a small proportion of these are infective, as indicated by a high ratio of particles to infective virions. This is paralleled in ultra-thin sections by the absence of a core of nucleic acid from many particles. The lowest particle to infective virus ratios have been found with some of the picornaviruses, but these are still many times greater than the almost one to one ratios which can be obtained with many bacterial viruses.

DEFECTIVE VIRUSES

The term defective means that a virus cannot complete its replication cycle. Growth of such a virus may be possible with the assistance of another, or helper, virus. Defectiveness may be of varying degrees and may arise either from a lack of genetic information due to the small size of the virus, or as a result of a mutation in the genome of a normal virus. Such defective viruses may still be able to adsorb to and penetrate susceptible cells, and may also synthesize various virus-specified proteins and viral nucleic acid, but may be unable to complete the growth cycle; the exact point at which the cycle is interrupted depends on the site of the mutation in the viral genome. A lethal mutation in the genome causes an irreversible block in virus growth. However, mutants of both bacterial and animal viruses are known in which the results of the mutation are only lethal in certain conditions; these are termed conditional-lethal mutants. Temperature-sensitive mutants are one type of conditional-lethal mutant, in that the virus can grow well at a low temperature of incubation, 28° to 31°C, but if incubated at a higher temperature, 37°C, growth ceases. The phenomenon is thought to be due to changes in the secondary and tertiary structure of a protein, because of an amino acid substitution, with the result that the stability of the protein is much reduced at the higher temperature. Other types of mutant have been extensively studied especially with bacteriophages and will be discussed below.

The term *complementation* is used to describe the interaction between two viruses when the growth of a defective virus is aided by a helper virus which provides the gene function lacking in the defective virus. The progeny viruses of such a growth cycle, however, are identical to the parental infecting virions. This process may occur between conditional lethal mutants of the same virus, i.e. reciprocal complementation, or between one defective virus and another helper virus, i.e. non-reciprocal complementation. In some other situations a defective replication cycle may occur when a normal virus is inoculated into an unusual type of host cell. This form of host dependent defectiveness gives rise to *abortive* infection.

Adenovirus and its associated virus. Various strains of adenovirus have been shown to contain two types of symmetrical particle. One of these, 70 to 85 nm in diameter, corresponds in appearance to a mature adenovirus, whilst the other has a diameter of 20 nm. The smaller particle is referred to as the adeno-associated virus or AAV. In comparison with other DNA viruses, the AAV has sufficient DNA (3.5×10^6 daltons) to be independent. However, AAV replication has been detected only in cells that are simultaneously infected with an adenovirus. The helper adenovirus can be of any type, but the nature of the assistance required by the AAV is unknown.

SV40—adenovirus interactions. SV40, or simian virus 40, is a member of the papova group and grows well in simian tissues. In the laboratory, SV40 can produce cell transformation and tumours, and is therefore an oncogenic virus. The adenoviruses grow well in human cells, but are unable to grow in monkey cells unless SV40 virus is present simultaneously. Adenoviruses seem to be able to penetrate monkey cells but for completion of the cycle and the production of mature adenovirus virions, SV40 must be present. If the virions produced in such a mixed infection are examined, adenovirus capsid protein can be found to contain adenovirus DNA, SV40 DNA or DNA from both virus types. Some of these mixed particles were first detected after attempts to adapt human adenoviruses to monkey cells as a means of attenuating the viruses for use as vaccines. The populations of 'adapted' virus could be shown to contain not only the adenovirus particles but also some hybrid types. The dangers of such a process are obvious and should serve as an indication of the potential dangers of such an attenuation procedure.

Rous sarcoma virus and the Rous-associated viruses. Rous sarcoma virus (RSV) is an oncogenic RNA virus that can transform a range of cell types. A cell transformed by RSV is altered in its behaviour, and usually continues to produce RSV particles. In chicken cells, certain strains of RSV, notably the Bryan strain, seem to be unable to complete the replication cycle. The infected cells are transformed and behave as such, but no new virus is produced. These cells can be made to produce RSV if a helper virus called the Rous-associated-virus (RAV) is added; and there are fifty such helper viruses, all, like the Rous virus, members of the avian leukosis group. In fact, many stocks of Rous sarcoma virus contain RAV. The function provided by RAV is the synthesis of the outer coat of the virus. In the presence of a helper virus RAV_1, the RSV released from the cell will have a coat of antigenic type RAV_1. This means that the RSV genome is surrounded and enclosed by a RAV_1 coat. If the antigenic type of helper virus is changed to RAV_2 then the coat surrounding the RSV genome becomes antigenic type RAV_2.

Another strain of RSV, the Schmidt-Ruppin strain, is not defective in chicken cells, but is defective in mammalian cells. Transformation of the mammalian cell can be demonstrated, but no infective progeny virions are produced. This state is conditioned by the host cell and not by the virus. Transformed mammalian cells may be fused with chick cells, and as a result Rous virus may be detected. This fusion process or heterokaryon formation is induced by an ultraviolet-irradiated, inactivated paramyxovirus. Production of virus presumably occurs because the Rous virus genome present in the transformed cell gains access to the chicken cell, a permissive cell, and the replication cycle can be completed.

VIRUS GENETICS

The study of bacterial viruses has been of great importance in the development of genetics. Studies designed to map the location of genes in the viral genome are practicable because phages contain a single molecule of nucleic acid and a relatively small number of genes. Bacterial viruses have been studied in some detail, but the study of the genetics of animal viruses is not as far advanced, mainly due to the complexity of the animal cell compared with the bacterial cell.

Virus genetic studies are based on the use of a parent or wild-type virus and a variety of mutants. Two main types of mutant have been studied (1) plaque-type mutants, and (2) mutants that have a lethal effect only in certain restrictive conditions (conditional-lethal mutants).

1. *Plaque-type mutants.* These mutants were extensively used until the more useful conditional-lethal mutants were described. The major drawback of the plaque mutant is that only a small portion of the viral genome is concerned and hence no information can be gained about most of the genome. Mutants may be discovered quite readily if a large number of phage plaques are examined. Variation of size (minute) and appearance (turbid) may be used to distinguish plaques. Among the T2 and T4 phages, so-called rapid lysis mutants may be detected by the altered plaques they produce. Normally, during the development of a plaque, release of virus becomes asynchronous and results in the superinfection of some already infected cells; if this happens during the latent period, lysis inhibition will occur. The effect of this inhibition of lysis on the appearance of the plaque is the production of a halo around the central clear area. The halo is a zone formed by the normal lysis of some cells and the survival of lysis-inhibited cells. Rapid lysis mutants may be isolated which do not develop the halo around the plaque, but have a clear sharp edge due to a lack of lysis inhibition.

Another important type of plaque mutant is the host-range mutant which can grow only on a new mutant type of host cell. The host-cell variants can be selected out by growing the resistant bacterial cells from the rare colonies that survive challenge by the virus. Cultures of the resistant host bacteria can then be used to isolate phage mutants which can grow in these cells. Host-range mutants can infect host cells that are resistant to the parental wild-type phage, but can also infect cells susceptible to the wild-type phage. The host-range mutants can be readily identified by plating phage suspensions on mixed cultures of the susceptible and resistant host cells. Wild-type virus can grow on the susceptible host and produce diffuse turbid plaques due to the survival and growth of resistant cells. The host-range mutant, on the other hand, can grow in and lyse both types of cells and as a result a clear plaque is produced. As a further step, each of these phages may have the rapid lysis characteristic and, therefore, four combinations of plaque type are possible.

Animal viruses can produce plaques in monolayer cell cultures and plaque mutants have been identified in several groups of animal viruses.

2. *Conditional-lethal mutants.* Temperature-sensitive mutants are known for both bacterial and animal viruses. These mutants can be grown at 28° to 31°C, but growth ceases or is prevented if the incubation temperature is raised to 37°C. The other major class of conditional-lethal mutant is the suppressor-sensitive mutant, which can be detected only in cells with a 'suppressor' gene. This gene suppresses 'nonsense mutations' that may occur in the viral genome, thus allowing the virus to replicate. If no suppression occurs, the nonsense mutation is transcribed to mRNA, and protein synthesis is interrupted.

The so-called 'amber' mutants are of this type and have a mutation that results in premature termination of a peptide chain during translation of the viral mRNA. If a suppressor gene is present in the cell, peptide synthesis may continue as the cell gene inserts an amino acid instead of terminating the chain. The effect of the substitution will vary in that the resulting protein may be active, or may still be defective.

The 'ochre' mutants are of the same type, and different suppressors are required if viral mRNA translation is to be successful. Mutants of this type can occur at many different sites on the genome.

The probability that a defined mutation will occur during one replication cycle is called the mutation rate. This varies considerably and values of one in 10^4 to one in 10^8 have been found for spontaneous mutation rates. Mutations can also be produced by the intracellular or extracellular action of substances on the viral nucleic acid. The substance 5-bromouracil can be incorporated into DNA and produce false-base pairing during DNA replication, and hence mutations are more commonly found if the compound is present during the replication cycle. Nitrous acid is another substance that causes a chemical change in DNA, which results in false base-pairing during replication and hence mutation. The acridines are a class of chemical mutagens that act by becoming inserted into DNA, thus separating neighbouring bases, and causing mismatching of bases during replication.

With the definition and identification of these different types of mutant the working out of the genetic map of bacterial viruses became feasible. Early experiments with rapid lysis and host-range mutants of T-even phages showed that genetic recombination could occur during phage replication. When cells are infected with different parental viruses, recombination can be demonstrated in that a proportion of the progeny virions (recombinants) will possess properties derived from both parents. Recombinants arise from the pool of replicating viral DNA by the methods outlined in Chapter 7 for bacteria.

As more genetic markers became available, the genetic map of a phage could be constructed. This depends on the principle that in recombination studies the greater the distance between two markers, the greater the frequency of recombination. As more markers are added, a more detailed analysis is possible. The best studied viral genetic map is that of T4 phage. All the genes of T4 can be placed in a defined sequence, and located on a circular map, which seems to contradict the experimental observation that the DNA within T4 virions is not circular. This difficulty is overcome by the hypothesis that the DNA molecules in T4 are linear pieces of DNA on which the genes are located as if the DNA had been derived from a closed circle of DNA which was opened at different, randomly distributed points. These strands of DNA are said to be circularly disposed. Support for this idea has come from the detection of terminal redundancy in the strands of DNA recovered from virions. Short lengths of complementary bases can be found at opposite ends of each of the strands of the double-stranded DNA. If these projecting pieces come into contact, base pairing can occur, and a closed double-stranded circular form of DNA results. The circular genetic map is not typical of all phages, e.g. the coliphage lambda (λ) has a linear map.

In the T4 map, genes appear to be grouped according to function. Genes concerned with viral DNA replication are grouped together, as are those involved in the synthesis of head and sheath proteins. Another group is responsible for the production of tail fibres and host-range mutants map in this region.

Genetic studies among animal viruses are not so well developed. The genetic markers used in these studies cover a wide range. Some temperature-sensitive virus mutants are now known and other markers, such as plaque morphology in cell monolayers, pock production on the chorio-allantoic membrane, serological type, haemagglutinin and neuraminidase type and pathogenicity in animals, have been used. Recombination can be demonstrated, but at a lower frequency than with bacterial viruses, perhaps because the large volume of the animal cell reduces the chances of contact between nucleic acid molecules. Of the animal viruses so far studied, poliovirus is probably the best understood because of the small number of genes and the knowledge available of the normal growth cycle.

The importance of recombination in animal viruses may lie in the development of new strains of virus. Some viruses, e.g. influenza virus of man, show a great deal of genetic variation, and recombination may be important to this process. A knowledge of recombination may be of value not only in understanding virus variation but also in the development of virus vaccine strains.

LYSOGENY

The reproductive cycle already described regularly ends with the lysis of the infected cell and the release of the progeny virions. This is the lytic cycle of a virulent virus. Among bacteriophages another association between host cell and virus has been described; this is the phenomenon of *lysogeny*, in which infection with a *temperate* phage leads to a stable association, between the viral genome and the bacterial chromosome. In this state, lysogenic cells grow and divide in a normal fashion.

After infection of a bacterial cell with a temperate phage, two alternative interactions may occur (Fig. 13.14). In some cells a normal

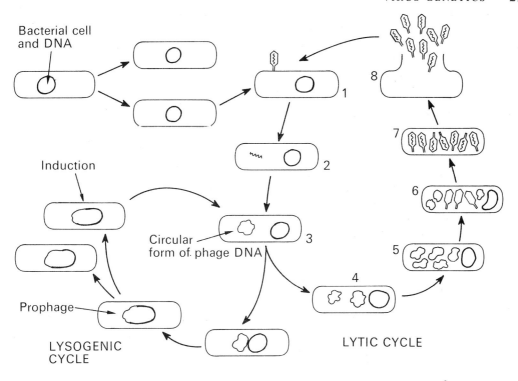

Bacterial cell and DNA

Induction

Circular form of phage DNA

Prophage

LYSOGENIC CYCLE

LYTIC CYCLE

Fig. 13.14. Growth cycles of a temperate phage. After phage adsorption and injection of nucleic acid (1) and (2) the DNA assumes the circular form (3). The DNA may then be inserted as the prophage into the host cell DNA and replicated with the host cell (lysogenic state), or may replicate (4) and (5), synthesize structural protein (6), mature (7) and be released by the disruption of the infected cell (8).

lytic cycle of replication occurs, culminating in the lysis of the host cell and the release of progeny virions. Alternatively, the phage DNA is inserted into the host DNA, where it exists in a stable, heritable, non-infectious form, known as the *prophage*. The prophage is replicated and segregated to the daughter cells during bacterial division. A cell that contains a prophage is unable to support a productive infection with the same virus; these cells are said to be immune to superinfection, and this phenomenon differs from resistance, in that the phage can adsorb to the bacteria and can inject its nucleic acid, but this does not replicate. The plaques produced by a temperate phage are turbid since only a proportion of infected cells experience a lytic cycle. Occasionally, virus replication does occur in a lysogenic cell and phage particles are released. This *induction* process can be enhanced by various factors, e.g. exposure of the bacteria

to ultraviolet irradiation and chemicals such as mitomycin C.

In lysogenic cells, bacterial conjugation experiments reveal that the prophage is associated with the bacterial chromosome, and can be mapped along with the bacterial genes. The location of the prophage of the coliphage λ (Fig. 13.15) is between the genes for galactose utilization (*gal*) and biotin synthesis (*bio*). Examination of cells carrying several different prophages shows that each phage has a characteristic locus on the bacterial chromosome.

By the use of standard phage genetic techniques with suppressor sensitive mutants, plaque type and other markers, a genetic map of the λ phage can be derived. During vegetative replication, the phage has a linear map, but the relative position of genes on the prophage or integrated map may be different from the vegetative map. The explanation of this altered

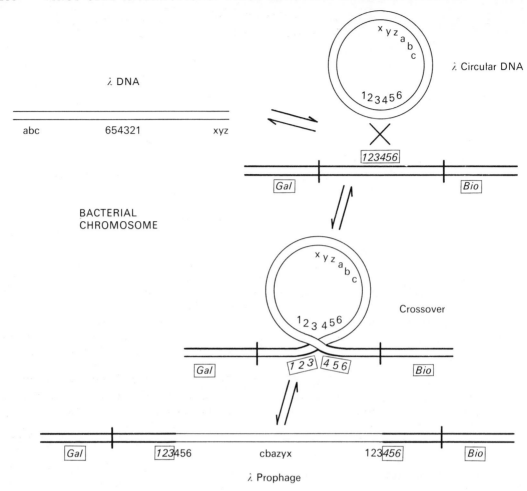

FIG. 13.15. Diagram of the insertion of the λ prophage into the bacterial chromosome. The λ DNA first assumes a circular form. The λ attachment site must then undergo a breakage and reunion crossover with the bacterial DNA at the insertion site. The induction process, culminating in the release of virus, occurs by a reversal of this mechanism. During induction, bacterial genes, e.g. gal, may be removed along with the λ prophage.

Gal = galactose locus; Bio = biotin locus of *Esch. coli.*

Numbers and letters on the λ DNA and bacterial DNA represent sites on the chromosome.

linkage pattern is that before integration the λ DNA assumes a circular form which can then be inserted by a single breakage and reunion step, as in genetic recombination to give a linear sequence within the bacterial chromosome. A viral enzyme, integrase, aids this insertion process. The λ DNA may assume the circular form due to the presence of short, complementary, single-stranded segments at each end of the molecule, which could be circularized by base-pairing between these sections.

Before insertion, λ DNA undergoes several replication cycles. Once inserted, the phage DNA replicates in association with the host cell DNA. The control or repression of most of the viral functions is due to the action of a repressor protein acting on a specific site or operon of the phage DNA to prevent transcription. A similar mechanism has been described in the regulation of the *lac* operon of *Esch. coli.* The presence of this repressor protein is the explanation of the phenomenon of superinfection immunity. The

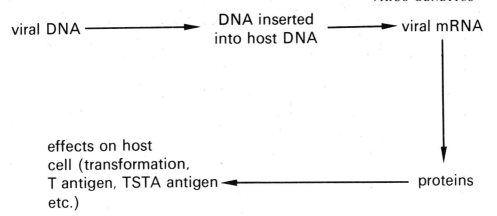

FIG. 13.16. Diagram of the association of an oncogenic DNA virus with a transformed cell.

repressor will act on a superinfecting virus entering a lysogenic cell, provided the prophage and the incoming phage are closely related. In the process of induction, ultraviolet light or alkylating agents act as inducing agents by either destroying or preventing the synthesis of the repressor protein or by forming an inducing substance.

The point on the circularized λ DNA at which attachment and insertion occurs is always the same, so this region must be brought into contact with a specific region of the bacterial DNA, perhaps by the action of the integrase enzyme. The induction process or release of the viral genome occurs as a reversal of the insertion mechanism.

The presence of a prophage within the bacterial chromosome may alter the properties and the behaviour of the host cell (lysogenic conversion). The state of lysogeny has many similarities with the latent infections seen with some animal viruses, especially the DNA tumour viruses.

Oncogenic Viruses

The behaviour and properties of the different groups of animal viruses (oncogenic viruses) that transform cells to malignancy is discussed in detail in Chapter 49. In order to compare the state of viral transformation with the lytic growth cycle and the lysogenic state, a brief account is given here. The transforming effect of tumour viruses on cells in culture leads to a change in behaviour; cells grow more rapidly and in a less controlled and organized fashion than normal cells and can cause tumours when inoculated into animals. There is loss of contact inhibition so that tumour cells or transformed cells can be seen in culture as clumps of randomly orientated, heaped up cells. They can continue to grow in culture and divide indefinitely, in contrast to untransformed cells which die off after a limited number of cell divisions.

Virus-transformed cells can be shown to possess new antigens with a specificity determined by the transforming virus. The production of new antigens on the surface of transformed cells may lead to their immunological rejection in the whole animal by mechanisms such as transplant rejection and cell-mediated immune responses.

Among the DNA viruses, some papovaviruses and adenoviruses produce tumours in the laboratory, but rarely in nature. Among the RNA viruses, members of the leukovirus group have been associated with tumours of animals, induced experimentally or occurring naturally.

Oncogenic DNA viruses. Polyoma and SV40 and some of the oncogenic adenoviruses have been studied in greatest detail. A common feature of these viruses is that no infectious virus can be detected after successful transformation of a cell (Fig. 13.16), although there is evidence that all or part of the viral genome is present. The DNA of polyoma virus has been found to be a circular double-stranded molecule, like λ phage. The transformation of a cell resulting from infection with polyoma or SV40 can be compared with the phenomenon of lysogenic conversion.

Transformed cells can be shown to possess two new types of virus-specific antigens, the nuclear T (tumour) antigens and the tumour-specific transplantation antigens (TSTA) located in the cytoplasmic membrane. These antigens can be detected by a variety of immunological techniques including immunofluorescence and complement fixation. The nuclear T antigens are identical with early proteins produced in the lytic cycle of infection by the same viruses. Indeed, transformation by the DNA viruses is a rare event, and just as a temperate phage may undergo a lytic cycle, so these animal viruses regularly undergo lytic cycles in the appropriate cell system.

After infection of a cell with a polyoma virus, the nuclear T antigens are produced, even in the presence of FUdR which will prevent viral DNA synthesis. Host-coded-DNA-synthesizing enzymes are then activated and DNA synthesis occurs in cells previously in a contact-inhibited state. Integration of the viral genome, or part of the viral genome, may then occur, with repression of most of the late viral functions so that no infectious virus is produced. Evidence for the persistence of polyoma genes has been derived from the immunological studies of T and TSTA antigens and from the detection of viral specific mRNA within transformed cells by molecular hybridization with viral DNA. Apparently not all of the viral genome is necessary for transformation as studies with SV40 virus treated with doses of ultraviolet irradiation sufficient to prevent the development of a lytic cycle show that this defective virus can still transform cells. However, in many instances all of the viral genome is present as has been demonstrated with SV40 transformed cells. If these cells are fused with grivet monkey cells, which support a lytic cycle of this virus, a proportion of the heterokaryons formed produce infectious SV40 virus.

Oncogenic RNA viruses (leukoviruses). These viruses differ from DNA tumour viruses in that they are commonly associated with tumour production in their natural hosts and also in that transformed cells regularly produce infectious virus. Most of the leukoviruses cause steady state, non-cytocidal infections in the appropriate cells. Rous sarcoma virus (RSV), a member of the fowl leukosis group, is the best studied of this group, and transformation by this virus has been shown not only in cultured chick cells, but also in mammalian cells.

Before transformation can occur there is a requirement for DNA synthesis, and if transformation is to be maintained mRNA transcription from DNA must continue (Fig. 13.17). These observations were confusing until the recent description of unusual enzymic activities within the virions of members of the leukovirus group. Purified virions have been shown to contain the enzymes RNA-dependent DNA polymerase ('reverse transcriptase'), DNA-dependent DNA polymerase, DNA nuclease and DNA ligase. This discovery suggests that the viral RNA genome may be copied to produce a DNA strand which may then be replicated and finally inserted into a host chromosome. In this manner the viral genome may persist as an integrated DNA copy, and the maintenance of the transformed state may depend on the transcription of the integrated component.

VIRAL INTERFERENCE AND INTERFERON

Double infection of cells does not always result in complementation or cooperation, more commonly *interference* occurs. With bacterial viruses previous viral infection may alter the cell surface so that it cannot adsorb other viruses (lysogenic conversion). Interference at the same level, i.e., the cell surface, may occur among the orthomyxo- and paramyxoviruses as a result of the destruction of receptor sites on the cell surfaces by the viral enzyme neuraminidase. In these circumstances, superinfection with a similar or related virus may be unsuccessful as a result of receptor destruction. Interference at an intracellular level also occurs and is more important with bacteria, e.g., after infection of a cell with a T-even phage, a rapid destruction of host DNA occurs, and the metabolic activities of the host cease. Superinfection by another, usually less virulent, phage may be completely inhibited, especially if the challenge virus relies on a host cell function for a step in the growth

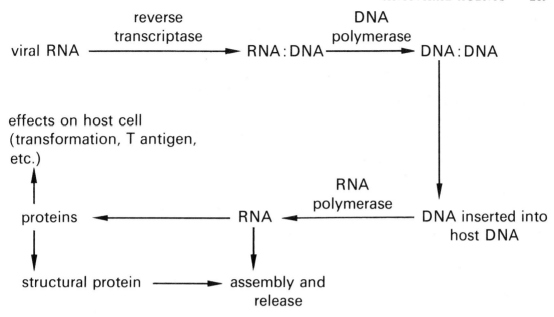

FIG. 13.17. Diagram of the association of an oncogenic RNA virus with a transformed cell.

cycle. The mechanism with viruses and eucaryotic cells depends on a unique substance, interferon.

Interferon. Among animal viruses, interference of one virus with the replication of another may be mediated by a protein called interferon which is produced by the cell after infection with the first virus. The ability to produce interferon seems to be a widespread property of vertebrate cells; both DNA and RNA viruses stimulate interferon, but there is considerable variation in inducer efficiency.

Interferon has been found to be a protein with a MW of approximately 30 000 daltons. As a result of its size, interferon is readily released from cells, and in the body can diffuse throughout the extracellular fluids. It is also a very stable protein, and extraction by treatment at pH 2·0 does not reduce its activity although it inactivates the inducing virus.

Interferon may be assayed by a plaque reduction test in monolayer cell cultures which are treated with interferon before challenge with a sensitive indicator virus. The end-point is the highest dilution of interferon that can reduce the virus plaque count to 50 per cent of the value in untreated controls.

In cell cultures, interferon is detected soon after infection with a virus, and its concentration increases and declines with the virus growth cycle. Inactivated viruses also induce synthesis of interferon; the replication of the virus is not essential for interferon production. Factors decreasing virus growth often increase interferon production, e.g., if infected cell cultures are incubated at higher temperatures than normal e.g. 40°C, virus growth may be diminished whilst interferon production may be enhanced.

In addition to avirulent or partially inactivated viruses, a number of other substances induce interferon synthesis; foreign nucleic acids and synthetic polynucleotides have this ability. In particular, double-stranded RNA and double-stranded polyribonucleotides are effective inducers, and these offer some prospect of using the antiviral properties of interferon in the control of human virus infections.

The mechanism of induction involves synthesis of cellular RNA and protein, i.e., it is sensitive to actinomycin D and puromycin. The incoming viral nucleic acid may therefore act as a derepressor of the cell DNA leading to synthesis of interferon (Fig. 13.18).

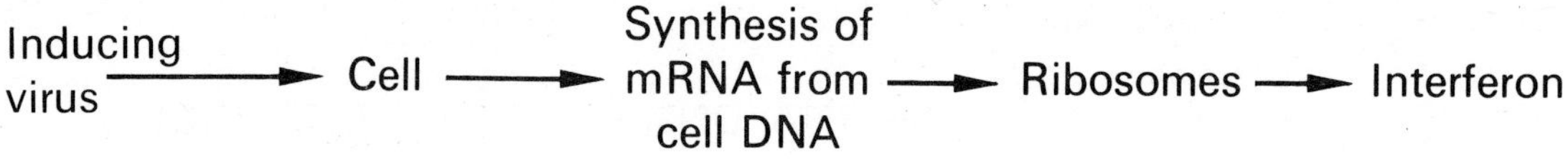

Inducing virus ⟶ Cell ⟶ Synthesis of mRNA from cell DNA ⟶ Ribosomes ⟶ Interferon

FIG. 13.18. Sequence of events leading to the synthesis of interferon.

Mode of action. Any explanation of the mode of action of interferon must account for its ability to inhibit the growth of a wide variety of DNA and RNA viruses. Another important property of interferon is the narrow species specificity: that is, interferon prepared in one species of cell in culture, has very little effect in another species. This property is relevant to the use of interferon in human infection when the substance has to be produced in human cells. The mechanism of action of interferon has been explored by adding it to cells for a period before the challenge or assay virus. If, during this lag period, the exposed cells are treated with actinomycin D and puromycin, the viral inhibiting effect of the interferon is not demonstrable so it seems that interferon itself is not the virus inhibitor but causes the cell to manufacture the proteins which have a direct effect on virus multiplication (Fig. 13.19). These proteins, called translation inhibiting proteins (TIP), are thought to prevent translation of viral mRNA. Interferon has no effect on cellular protein synthesis and must therefore be able to distinguish between viral and cell mRNA.

Inhibition of translation of the viral RNA or mRNA would account for the broad spectrum of activity; the need to induce the cell to manufacture TIPs might be related to the property of species specificity.

Interferon production by a cell already infected may not save the cell but due to its small size and ready release, interferon may reach other cells of a culture before the infecting virus and thus induce TIP synthesis and protect them. (See Chap. 14.)

VIRAL CHEMOTHERAPY

Viral chemotherapy is limited by the major difficulty of the very close relationship between virus and host cell. The virus synthesizes protein and nucleic acid utilizing ribosomes and the host cell's enzymes. Although compounds affecting these cell functions will also inhibit virus growth, their lack of selectivity renders them useless for the treatment of human virus infections. Thus, actinomycin D interrupts transcription of RNA from DNA, and will

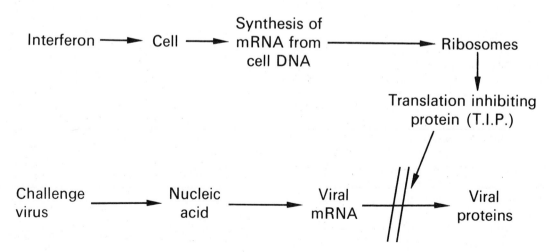

FIG. 13.19. Mode of action of interferon in preventing replication of a virus.

block viral and cellular transcription. The drug has proved of great value in the study of the virus growth cycle *in vitro*, but is too toxic for therapeutic use (cf. inhibitors of protein synthesis such as puromycin and parafluorophenylalanine).

With the recent knowledge of virus growth cycles the possibility exists of developing compounds to attack unique stages in virus replication, e.g. during (1) adsorption, penetration and uncoating and (2) macromolecular synthesis. Stage 1 might be blocked by removing or modifying the viral receptors. Alternatively, it might be possible to find a compound that could react with the viral capsid and either cause it to break up or so stabilize the capsid that the viral nucleic acid could not be released inside cells, even although the virus was still able to adsorb to and penetrate these cells. Stage 2 includes various virus specific steps in the synthesis of nucleic acid and protein. For example, the synthesis of viral RNA is known to depend on a viral specified enzyme in the poxviruses. RNA viruses replicate RNA on an RNA template; inhibition of this unique process should allow a selective effect on virus growth. Viral mRNA must differ in some way from cellular mRNA (see *Interferon*) and might be a suitable point of attack for an antiviral agent. Another possible approach might be to attack the infected cell so that only these cells were killed by a drug.

The application of a selective antiviral drug to the treatment of human infections may depend on other factors. The diagnosis of a virus infection may be difficult, and too late to allow the rational use of a drug. Thus many viral infections with a long incubation period may have no recognizable prodromal illness. By the time signs or symptoms of infection develop, virus may be disseminated throughout the body and may have caused considerable cell damage. Another difficulty may result from the successful development of highly specific compounds active against one type of virus or virus group. Administration of such a compound, which might have toxic side effects, would not be justified unless there was laboratory confirmation of the clinical diagnosis. At present, with a few exceptions, the laboratory diagnosis of a viral infection in its early stages takes some

time. Thus the development and application of antiviral agents might have to depend on improvements in diagnostic virology.

In the following section a number of compounds that are known to have a selective antiviral effect are described. Not all of them are of practical value in the treatment of viral infections of man, but are included to illustrate principles.

Isoquinolines. Viruses known to be sensitive *in vitro* are members of the orthomyxo- and paramyxovirus groups. The compounds were discovered to have an inhibitory effect on the enzyme neuraminidase and, as this is present on the surface of influenza and other viruses, these were tested for sensitivity to the drugs. The mechanism of inhibition does not appear to be directly on viral neuraminidase, but may involve interaction with the virus envelope to block the uncoating step.

Amantadine is the L-amino derivative of adamantane, a tricyclic saturated hydrocarbon. An inhibitory effect can be demonstrated against influenza A and C and rubella viruses *in vitro* apparently at the stage of penetration and uncoating. Administration of the drug to contacts of patients with influenza infections has been claimed to reduce the number of illnesses developing in the contacts. However, the neurological side effects may make this compound unsuitable for widespread use.

The substances mentioned above, acting in the early stages of virus growth, are most effective if they are administered to patients before exposure to virus. This prophylactic action might be applicable to certain groups of the population known to be at risk from a prevalent viral infection, e.g. influenza.

Drugs acting on viral macromolecular synthesis. The group of compounds related to Rifamycin have an inhibitory effect on transcription by DNA dependent RNA polymerase in the bacterial cell. In the light of knowledge of the 'uncoating' enzyme the effect of *Rifampicin* on the growth of vaccinia and other poxvirus has been investigated. Inhibition occurs but the exact stage in virus replication that is attacked may not be the early function of the virus-specific polymerase as immature forms of virus are synthesized within infected cells exposed to the drug.

The mode of synthesis and action of *interferon* have been discussed. A product of cells, it is non-toxic, and this, allied to its broad spectrum of activity, make it appear an ideal antiviral agent. Considerable difficulty has been encountered in the production and purification of sufficient quantities of human interferon for adequate testing in the treatment of infections. A more hopeful approach is to develop effective non-toxic interferon inducers. Synthetic double-stranded polyribonucleotides are effective inducers. Polyinosinic-polycytidilic acid (poly I:C) has been studied both *in vitro* and *in vivo*, and can be shown to ameliorate experimental infections in animals. However, endotoxin-like reactions have been noted.

The *thiosemicarbazones* are a group of compounds with antibacterial activity, especially for *Mycobacterium tuberculosis*. In addition, various derivatives have been shown to have an inhibitory effect on the replication of poxviruses. *N*-methylisatin-β-thiosemicarbazone or *methisazone* is the derivative which has been tested most extensively. The stage of replication at which methisazone acts is believed to be late in the growth cycle. As a result of its action, late viral proteins are not manufactured, perhaps due to an action on late viral mRNA to prevent translation. Methisazone can be shown to have a protective effect in mice infected with vaccinia virus, and it is one of the few compounds to have been extensively tested in man—both in the prevention and treatment of smallpox and vaccinia infections. The most striking effect was observed in a large trial in Madras when the drug was administered to contacts of smallpox patients. Two doses of 3 g of the drug were found to be effective in reducing both the number of infections and the case-mortality in contacts; it cannot, however, replace vaccination in the control of the disease in endemic areas. In non-endemic areas, the drug might be of value in the initial protection of contacts of an imported infection.

The value of methisazone in the treatment of clinical smallpox has not been established. The drug is said to have improved the condition of some patients suffering from some of the complications of vaccination, e.g. disseminated vaccinia, or vaccinia gangrenosa which may develop in patients with defective immune responses. A high incidence of vomiting from administration of the drug is a major disadvantage.

Some compounds act on the replication of viral nucleic acid; the earliest known antiviral substances were the compounds 2-(α hydroxybenzyl) benzimidazole (HBB) and guanidine. Both inhibit the growth of some members of the picornavirus group. At the time of discovery they were of special interest because of their activity against poliovirus. The exact mode of action is not clear, but a functioning viral RNA polymerase does not appear in treated infected cells. Drug-resistant strains of virus can be isolated very readily and if resistance is used as a marker in genetic studies, this character is found to be located in the same region of the genome as the genes for viral coat proteins. It is possible, therefore, that these compounds act via a coat protein to affect the secondary or tertiary structure of the viral polymerase. The modes of action of HBB and guanidine are not identical as cross-resistance between the two compounds is not observed.

The ease of isolation of drug-resistant strains of virus makes the successful application of these compounds impractical. Their discovery is of interest in that it is an indication that interruption of this stage of virus replication is possible. Derivatives of these compounds, which retain the selective antiviral effect but with a reduced tendency of the virus to develop drug resistance may be found.

The *halogenated deoxyuridines* also act at the stage of viral DNA synthesis. The halogen is substituted for a methyl group of uracil and the substituted compound is an analogue of thymidine. The substituted deoxyuridines were introduced for cancer chemotherapy to inhibit preferentially the higher rate of DNA synthesis in tumour cells: 5-fluoro 2'-deoxyuridine (FUdR), 5-bromo 2'-deoxyuridine (BUdR) and 5-iodo 2'-deoxyuridine (IUdR) or *idoxuridine* have all been shown to be effective in blocking the replication of viral DNA. Within cells, the enzyme thymidine kinase phosphorylates these compounds to produce the 5-monophosphate derivatives. The mode of action of FUdR differs from BUdR and IUdR in its inhibitory effect on the enzyme thymidylic synthetase, thus preventing the incorporation of thymidine into

DNA. As a result of this action, FUdR has been invaluable in the laboratory study of the virus-cell interaction, but it has not been used in the treatment of viral infections. Both BUdR and IUdR can be incorporated into DNA in place of thymidine, and the inhibitory effect may result from false transcription and the synthesis of non-functional proteins. The apparent selective action of these compounds on viral replication, at least in vaccinia and herpesvirus infections may depend on the activity of the enzyme thymidine kinase. Cells infected with either of these viruses show elevated enzymic activity since both viruses code for their own enzyme. In these circumstances, increased phosphorylation of BUdR and IUdR can be expected, and therefore the inhibitory effect on DNA synthesis will be greater in infected compared with uninfected cells. In addition, in the whole animal at any instant, many cells are not dividing and are not synthesizing DNA, and would be resistant to the inhibitory action of these chemicals.

As a result of their potential toxicity, use of these compounds has been restricted mainly to the treatment of superficial infections with vaccinia and herpes simplex virus. The cornea is one important site of herpetic infection, and IUdR or idoxuridine has been shown to be effective in this condition. Idoxuridine is said to produce a reduction in the discomfort and in the duration of the symptoms of skin and mucous membrane infections with herpes simplex virus. In this situation, however, penetration of the drug to the affected cells may be difficult to achieve due to its poor solubility. Other deriva-tives such as 5-methylaminodeoxyuridine and trifluorothymidine are under investigation and may be more effective. The systemic use of IUdR has been confined to a few serious infections with the herpes virus, especially encephalitis. Severe effects on the bone marrow and hepatic necrosis have been reported, and the real value of the drug in this condition has not been established.

A potential difficulty in the development of idoxuridine as an antiviral agent is the emergence of drug-resistant strains of herpes simplex virus.

The compound *cytosine arabinoside* has also been tested for antiviral activity. In this compound, arabinose is substituted for the normal sugar deoxyribose and the effect is to inhibit DNA synthesis by preventing the conversion of cytidilic acid to deoxycytidilic acid, but its use may be limited due to the low level of selective antiviral activity.

Viral chemotherapy is at a very early stage of development, and only a few effective drugs are available. The value of methisazone and idoxuridine is established, but perhaps the best prospects for future development are the use of compounds that can stimulate endogenous interferon production.

FURTHER READING

FENNER, F. (1968) *The Biology of Animal Viruses*, Vols. 1 and 2. New York: Academic Press.

HAYES, W. (1968) *Genetics of Bacteria and Their Viruses*, 2nd Edn. Oxford: Blackwell.

LURIA, S. E. & DARNELL, J. E. (1967) *General Virology*, 2nd Edn. New York: J. Wiley & Sons.

14. Virus Infections: Pathogenesis: Immunity

Pathogenicity is the ability that a virus has to infect an animal host. Although fever and clinical manifestations of disease frequently accompany the onset of infection there are many occasions when there are only trivial effects or the host reaction is clinically inapparent.

When a virus strain regularly produces severe clinical effects on its animal host it is said to be more *virulent* than other strains that lack this property. The term 'virulent' is best reserved for the damage by microorganisms on the whole animal host. For the destructive effects that viruses may have on cultivated cells it is best to use 'cytocidal' or 'cytolytic'. Cytocidal viruses are not always highly virulent for animals and, contrarily, non-cytocidal viruses, e.g. influenza viruses, can often have very striking clinical effects.

The initiation of viral infection depends on the survival of the extracellular virions in their natural environment and their successful transmission to their next susceptible host cells.

The events following entry of the virus depend to a great extent on the portal of entry of the virions and the circumstances of their transmission.

(a) Infection by the Respiratory Tract

Viruses of many different kinds are inhaled and often they are trapped in the layer of mucus that coats the surface of the ciliated epithelium lining the upper respiratory tract. Rhinoviruses, for instance, inhaled through the nose are engulfed in the mucus of the nasal passages and, provided they are not inactivated by specific antibody or inhibited by other protective mechanisms, enter and infect the ciliated columnar epithelial cells in that situation. As they multiply, the inflammation and irritation they set up is followed by the copious exudation of fluid that is the familiar rhinorrhoea of the common cold.

At a lower level a 'muco-ciliary blanket' similar to that of the nasal passages extends from beneath the larynx to cover the bronchial tree as far as the finer bronchioles. Viruses, e.g.

myxoviruses, and foreign particles alighting here are caught in the mucus and are swept upwards by the action of the cilia to be expectorated or swallowed. Some, however, manage to adhere to and enter the underlying ciliated epithelial cells; if they have not been inactivated by specific antibody or firmly combined to glycoprotein inhibitors in the mucus, they are able to enter the host and initiate infection. From the first small focus of multiplication increasing numbers of new virions involve neighbouring cells until considerable amounts of infective virus are continuously extruded into the tissue fluids in which they are propelled by ciliary action in currents that flow over large areas of the bronchial tree. An intense capillary congestion with inflammation and necrosis of the superficial cells follows and it is at this point that fever and clinical signs of influenza become obvious. Healing is usually rapid and complete but for a short time the viral damage leaves open a pathway for the entry of pathogenic bacteria such as *Haemophilus influenzae*, or pneumococci or *Staphylococcus aureus*, which may invade lung tissue and initiate the lesions of bronchopneumonia.

Distal to the finer bronchioles the mucociliary carpet is absent and here it is the macrophages that play a major role. They engulf inhaled particles and viruses and convey them to the local pulmonary lymph nodes and also to lymphatics and onwards into the blood stream. For example, the ectromelia virus under experimental conditions has been observed to invade lung tissue by this mechanism.

Although a great many pathogenic viruses can enter the respiratory tract and succeed in establishing foci of infection there are others, as for instance the arboviruses, that are unable to infect man by this route.

(b) Infection by the Alimentary Tract

There are many occasions when viruses are introduced through the mouth. Usually they enter in foodstuffs contaminated by infected human carriers but fomites of various kinds may also be involved.

As they are being swallowed the viruses encounter the host cells for the first time, usually the stratified epithelium lining the oral cavity or the lymphoid cells that are situated very close to the surface in the nasopharynx. There is very little evidence to indicate how the viruses initiate infection either in the oropharynx or lower down the alimentary tract.

Most viruses are destroyed before they reach the small intestine. Myxoviruses with their fragile bile sensitive envelopes and the acid-sensitive rhinoviruses are inactivated long before they can reach the jejunum. Only a few viruses are able to resist the digestive enzymes, mucus, acid and bile that they encounter after ingestion; of these the enteroviruses belonging to the picorna group and the hepatitis viruses are the most important because of their pathogenic effects. Adenoviruses, the only DNA viruses able to establish intestinal infection, are probably derived from primary lesions in the upper respiratory tract. Reoviruses also possess the ability to infect the gut as well as the respiratory tract.

Polioviruses are known to have an affinity for lymphoid cells and the early stages of invasion with this virus frequently occurs in the Peyer's patches throughout the small intestine although lymphoid tissue in the oropharynx may also be involved. The mechanisms of attachment and penetration of the polioviruses have been studied intensively by Holland (1964) who demonstrated host cell receptors that determine organ, tissue and host cell specificity for enteroviruses. The receptors are necessary for efficient infection because they provide the mechanism of absorption and cause a temperature-dependent alteration of viral capsid which is a prerequisite to the release of the RNA genome of the virus.

The access of enteroviruses to the columnar epithelial cells of the intestinal villi may be hindered or entirely prevented by mucus or antibodies produced locally by the lymphoid tissue. The latter are immune globulins of the dimer IgA class and are to be found at the cell surface or in faeces where they are known as copro-antibodies. After infection with attenuated live vaccines of the Sabin type much IgA antibody together with interferon is produced and the intestine becomes resistant to reinfection by polioviruses.

(c) Infection via the Conjunctiva and Through the Skin and Mucous Surfaces

The *conjunctiva* is often exposed to minute airborne droplets some of which may carry infective microorganisms which, if they find susceptible cells at hand, are able to set up a local infection. The majority of the droplets, however, are washed away by the tears and carried down the nasolachrymal ducts to situations in the upper nasal passages where the infective microorganisms may have a second opportunity to establish infection.

The eyes of an infant at parturition are particularly susceptible to contact infection by the microorganisms present in the mother's birth canal. The chlamydia of inclusion blenorrhoea may give rise to severe purulent conjunctivitis in children and trachoma results from an inflammatory lesion caused by a closely related organism which may be introduced by contact.

Adenoviruses may reach the eyes in airborne droplets or on contaminated fomites such as towels and there are records of their transmission in contaminated lotions used for irrigation in eye clinics. They may infect the surface epithelium and some serotypes, e.g. type 8, cause a severe keratoconjunctivitis. On one occasion a veterinary surgeon contracted fatal rabies by accidentally splashing his eyes while performing a necropsy.

The *skin* is often subjected to small superficial abrasions through which virus may gain access to susceptible cells in the deeper layers of the epidermis or in the dermis itself. Probably many primary infections with herpes simplex viruses are contracted by labial or genital skin contact when the virus in infected tissues is introduced to the new host through breaches in the surface epithelium. The human wart virus, a *papovavirus,* can penetrate in this way and after a long incubation period gives rise to proliferation of the epithelial cells at the point of entry with the formation of a local papilloma. Warts are often situated on the feet where they are specially liable to damage; in swimming baths blood from a wart, with the virus it contains, easily introduces the infection through skin abrasions to other bathers. Plantar warts occur frequently in schoolchildren and can be painful and troublesome. Another infection that is introduced superficially into the skin by direct contact is molluscum contagiosum. The cause is a poxvirus which produces local and intensely irritant papules.

In all these instances the viruses are introduced superficially and produce localized papular lesions. Spread is limited to the area at the site or sites of entry and there is no systemic spread of infection.

The subcutaneous tissues may be penetrated by one of the following means:

1. IMPLANTATION FOLLOWING INJURY is exemplified as the mode of viral transmission in rabies and herpes virus B infections of man and in pseudorabies in cattle.

In rabies human infection follows severe damage to the tissues by the bite of an animal whose saliva contains the virus. The passage of the virions along the neurones and the involvement of the central nervous system is discussed in Chapter 48.

Human infection with herpesvirus B takes the form of severe encephalitis and follows the bite of an infected monkey.

Pseudo-rabies has for its natural host the pig in which it causes only mild or inapparent infection although when it is transferred to cattle it involves the central nervous system in fatal encephalomyelitis. The pseudo-rabies virus probably enters the bovine animal through minute skin abrasions and is derived from nasal secretions of pigs kept in the same building. These latter two infections cause only minor effects in their natural hosts, but on obtaining access to abraded skin and nerve fibres in unusual host species they rapidly invade the central nervous system usually with fatal results.

2. TRANSMISSION BY INSECTS. When arthropods bite man their saliva is introduced into the subcutaneous tissues before they withdraw his blood. Because arthropods may attack many different species of mammals as well as man they often convey viruses from one animal in the viraemic phase of an illness to another susceptible host (Chap. 47). Arboviruses multiply in their vectors which may carry the infection for the rest of their lives and in many instances pass the virus on to their progeny through the egg and onwards in subsequent stages of reproduction. Thus arthropod-borne transmission is an effective way for viruses to cross species barriers and be transferred to new hosts that are particularly susceptible because they have had no previous exposure to the infection.

After injection into a new host arboviruses in the subcutaneous tissues are engulfed by macrophages and conveyed to the lymphatics and lymphoid tissue where they begin to multiply; later they reach the blood stream and are carried in the circulation to establish further foci of infection.

3. ARTIFICIAL INOCULATION occurs when hypodermic syringes contaminated with virus or any other contaminated instrument is used in breaching intact skin. The most notorious example of a disease transmitted in this way is serum hepatitis. The source of this infection is the blood of a human carrier who is often without any sign or symptom of disease. The increasing use of blood transfusion, the injection of blood products, and the introduction of the methods of renal dialysis have been accompanied by a greatly increased incidence of serum hepatitis (Chap. 46).

(d) Infection of the Foetus in Utero

So far the mechanisms of virus transmission that have been discussed all involve transference of infection from one individual to the next—a process sometimes called 'horizontal transmission'.

When infection is transferred from the mother to the foetus *in utero* the process is called 'vertical infection'. Usually this happens during the course of a viraemic illness in the pregnant woman when the virions can be transmitted to the foetus at any stage in its development; rubella virus is a good example.

SYSTEMIC SPREAD OF VIRUSES WITHIN THE BODY

When a virus has succeeded in gaining a foothold at its point of entry it is able to initiate its early cycles of reproduction and to involve neighbouring cells in a small focus of primary infection. Such foci are difficult to detect; many are situated in the lymphoid tissue of the oropharynx or the gastrointestinal tract but some in the respiratory tract are notable because disruption of the host cell membranes allows the cytoplasm to engulf several nuclei and to form 'syncytial masses' as in measles and RSV infection.

From the primary foci newly formed virions are extruded into the tissue fluids and are carried via the finer lymphatic channels to the local lymph nodes that drain the site of entry. Most of the virus is taken up by macrophages lining the sinuses of the lymph nodes and is digested and degraded but some may escape and multiply in the lymphatic tissues. From here the virus passes onwards in the lymph and finally is discharged through the thoracic duct into the blood stream. This is the phase of *primary viraemia* when there is little damage to the tissues and only minor prodromal symptoms of illness. The amount of virus in the blood stream is often small and may not be detected by blood culture methods.

Removal of virus from blood is effected by the platelets and lymphocytes and by the monocytes of the circulating blood, the process of phagocytosis inactivating many of the infective particles. Some however survive and may multiply in the cells that carry them to reach new susceptible host cells in distant situations. In this way they may be lodged in the lining cells of capillary endothelium where new foci of infection are established.

Most of the virions and infected cell debris in the phase of primary viraemia are cleared from the blood by macrophages, especially those that are fixed in linings of the extensive sinusoids in the spleen, liver and bone marrow. If, however, multiple foci of viral proliferation are established in these areas and in the capillaries, vast numbers of new virions are produced and released into the blood to constitute the phase of *secondary viraemia.*

So far it has been seen that viraemia is for the most part *cell associated,* with macrophages playing a key role in viral pathogenesis. It must also be remembered that erythrocytes may be involved in carrying viruses in the blood and that arbo, myxo and swine fever viruses are spread in the body during adhesion to the envelopes of red blood cells. It sometimes happens that clearance of virus from the blood is not complete and that virus remains free circulating in the plasma. *Plasma viraemias* are characteristic of serum hepatitis in man and of lymphocytic choriomeningitis in mice. A state of immune tolerance may permit the protracted persistence of infective virions in the blood stream.

When the primary phase of viraemia subsides the prodromal symptoms and fever decline and a temporary clinical improvement follows. But this lull soon ends if the phase of heavy secondary viraemia develops and many virions are discharged into the blood from infective multiple foci throughout the body. High fever is at once obvious and during the succeeding 48 hours the various target organs reveal obvious clinical involvement in the disease process.

The interval between the first entry of infective virus and the first onset of fever and clinical signs is the *incubation period* which may be measured in just a few hours as in the common cold or may be as long as three weeks in mumps or even several months as in serum hepatitis.

Target Organs

The *skin* is one of the principal targets for virus attack and rashes are characteristic of many acute viral infections. Virions in the blood invade the endothelium of the capillaries and venules of the dermis where they produce local lesions. A sustained local dilatation of sub-papillary dermal blood vessels produces a macule which, if followed by oedema and cellular infiltration of the area, becomes a papule. The epidermis over such lesions may be involved in desquamation or changes in pigmentation.

If the primary process of viral invasion is in the epidermis with an outpouring of a fluid exudate and an ingress of mononuclear cells the layers of the epidermis are split. As the process continues a vesicle is produced with keratin and the granulosa cells forming its roof and degenerating epithelial cells and a monocytic inflammatory exudate constituting the base. Secondary bacterial invasion may follow with the formation of a pustule which gradually dries and in the final stage a firm scab is formed. Some of the skin lesions of viral exanthemata are characterized by intracellular inclusions and the formation of multinucleate giant cells. The skin lesions in many exanthemata as for instance in measles, varicella and smallpox are so typical and so constant in their distribution that the clinician can often make his diagnosis without laboratory help (see Table 14.1).

Table 14.1. Generalized rashes of Viral Exanthemata

1. Maculopapular rashes	**Measles**
	Rubella
	Echovirus 4, 6, 9, 16
	Coxsackie A 9, 16, 23
	Some arboviruses of
	Groups A and B
2. Vesicular rashes	**Herpes simplex**
	Varicella
	Zoster
	Vaccinia
	Coxsackie
	Smallpox
3. Haemorrhagic rashes	Smallpox
	Measles
	Arboviruses,
	e.g. Dengue,
	Ckikengunga and
	several others

Heavy type indicates common infections

Rashes occur not only in the skin but the mucous membranes of the oropharynx. In this situation there is no dense covering of keratin to contain the fluid exudate within the vesicles which are more easily ruptured than those elsewhere. Thus virus is liberated early in oropharyngeal secretions which thereby often constitute the first and most important vehicle in the transmission of infection as in measles.

It has been suggested that the skin offers a peculiarly sensitive situation for viral growth because of its lower temperature. Some viruses are unable to multiply at temperatures much higher than that of body heat; the smallpox virus, for instance, has a ceiling temperature for growth at 38·5°C. It might be that with the wide general distribution of the smallpox virus the only situation in the body offering acceptably cool temperature conditions could be the skin. THE CENTRAL NERVOUS SYSTEM provides another important target for viruses which may reach it either by the blood stream or by entering damaged nerve trunks and passing centrally along the neurones or the tissue spaces between the nerve fibres. Although haematogenous spread is the principal route for infection of the nervous system, extraneural multiplication and a high degree of viraemia are essential prerequisites for the general invasion of nervous tissues.

The structure and constitution of the capillary walls in the central nervous system is so compact that the so-called 'blood–brain barrier' is formed and as long as it is intact no virions or macromolecules can pass through it. The capillary endothelium rests on a basement membrane which is very closely ensheathed by the cytoplasm of the pericapillary astrocytes. The extracellular spaces are very small and in electron micrographs are represented by gaps of the order of only 15 to 20 nm wide. The movement of metabolites from the blood to the brain is probably achieved only by a process of selective active transport across the pericapillary glia or during inflammatory reactions.

Penetration of the blood–brain barrier may, however, occur when it is damaged by trauma or some pathological process. A few viruses, e.g. enteroviruses, are able occasionally to infect the capillary endothelial cells and invade the pericapillary astrocytes. In this way they grow through the barrier. At first there is a limited spread of virions from cell to cell but, as the infection spreads through the brain parenchyma, neurones become involved in cytocidal processes in which cell necrosis, neuronophagia and perivascular infiltration with inflammatory cells give rise to the syndrome of encephalitis.

The coxsackie-B group of viruses multiply in the cells of the choroid plexus and from this site are disseminated generally through the tissues of the nervous system in the cerebrospinal fluid; cells of the meninges in particular are infected and a meningo-encephalitis with or without neuronal damage results.

Apart from physical damage, there are a number of other factors known to aid the localization of virions from the blood-stream in the brain tissue. Exercise, the injection subcutaneously of irritant substances and repeated sensory stimulation, e.g. pinching, are thought to cause reflex vaso-dilation in the related areas of the brain or spinal cord. It is well known that there is an increased risk of paralytic poliomyelitis after the injection of alum-containing vaccines, after tonsillectomy, and after severe exercise or the treatment of a fracture.

Another predisposing condition is pregnancy, especially in the first trimester, possibly because of hormonal influences.

Direct invasion of the central nervous system may happen when the virus contaminates damaged nerve trunks. The viruses pass centrally, usually along perineural or interneural tissue spaces. After the bite of a rabid dog the rabies virus enters the torn nerve fibres and slowly travels upwards to reach the brain. Polioviruses and herpesviruses are also able to enter the open endings of peripheral nerve fibres and to pass centrally to the brain where they may initiate generalized inflammatory lesions. In each case the damage done is limited to neurones.

Spread in the opposite direction occurs when latent varicella-zoster virus is reactivated in the dorsal root ganglion and passes peripherally along sensory nerves to reach the related skin area where the painful papulo-vesicular eruption of shingles is located.

The liver is another target organ for circulating virions. Normally the sinusoidal endothelial cells and the Küpffer cells form an intact lining which separates the hepatic parenchyma from the blood. However, infective virions of the hepatitis, some poxviruses, and probably the Epstein-Barr virus of infectious mononucleosis, have been shown by immune-fluorescence to be phagocytosed by the Küpffer cells where they multiply before penetration and generalized invasion of the substance of the liver.

Striated and cardiac muscle are involved in severe necrosis caused by coxsackie viruses which may also involve the pancreas and the brown fat.

HOST RESPONSES TO VIRAL INFECTIONS

Of the many defences that vertebrates possess to protect them against the effects of virus infection the most important and the best understood is their immunological response.

THE IMMUNE RESPONSE essentially has two features: in one there is an outpouring into the circulation of antibodies which are immunoglobulins specifically adapted to react with the invading virus, and in the other a cell-mediated resistance that conveys to the tissues the power to respond vigorously against the infection in a process known as delayed hypersensitivity.

ANTIBODY-MEDIATED IMMUNITY is associated with the production of a number of immunoglobulins to combat infecting viruses, of which the most important in viral infections are IgG, IgM and IgA (Chap. 10). During the viraemic phase great quantities of viral antigens are carried to the liver, spleen, lymph nodes and other tissues which are the main sites of production of immunoglobulins. There begins a copious production of circulating antibodies. A peak level of IgG is reached gradually but significant amounts of it may continue to be produced for many years. IgM is the antibody produced when the host encounters a virus for the first time; it appears very early after the onset of the infection, reaches its peak rapidly and declines quickly until at the end of a few months it is barely detectable. Both IgG and IgM are found in quantity not only in the blood but also in the tissue spaces. Their antiviral activities are due to their ability to neutralize the processes of viral attachment, penetration and uncoating.

IgA is produced locally by plasma cells in the mucous membranes of the respiratory and gastrointestinal tracts where, for example, it provides a defence against common cold viruses reaching the nasal mucosa, or against enteroviruses passing through the intestine. Although its major protective activity is local at the site of its production IgA is also transported in secretions such as the bronchial mucus, saliva and intestinal fluids in a dimeric complement-fixing form and it is also present in serum as a monomer or polymer. IgA probably plays a major role in affording a barrier to the systemic spread of viruses from localized surface areas. The monomer has a molecular weight of 160 000 million daltons, and does not cross the human placenta. It participates in many antibody reactions but does not fix complement.

CELL-MEDIATED IMMUNITY. Some children lack the power to produce virus neutralizing antibodies because they suffer from a congenital inability to synthesize adequate amounts of gammaglobulins (hypogammaglobulinaemia). These children, however, quite often recover quite normally from acute exanthemata like measles, chickenpox and mumps, and local viral lesions, as for example those following smallpox vaccination, heal in the usual fashion. They owe their resistance to a specifically provoked, slowly evolving, mixed cellular reaction in which lymphocytes and macrophages infiltrate the virus-sensitized tissues to produce an intense inflammatory reaction. It must be explained that sensitized lymphocytes and activated macrophages dispose cells that contain any viral antigens. This phenomenon, which requires 24 to 48 hours to develop, is known as the *delayed hypersensitivity reaction* and it is largely independent of circulating antibodies (see Chap. 10).

The accelerated reaction that follows the revaccination of immune individuals against smallpox is a typical example of delayed hypersensitivity to a virus. Similarly, intracutaneous inoculations of the mumps virus and the agents of psittacosis and lymphogranuloma venereum in patients previously infected by these microorganisms produce delayed inflammatory flares at the site of injection. These hypersensitive reactions provide positive evidence of previous infection and constitute the 'skin tests' that provide the clinician with evidence of considerable diagnostic value.

When both cell-mediated immunity and antibodies are lacking as occurs in the Swiss-type of hypogammaglobulinaemia the infants invariably die from infection early in life.

IMMUNE COMPLEXES AND DISEASE. All of the effects of immune reactions are not beneficial. Specific reactions between antibodies and their antigens may lead to the formation of immune complexes. The ratio of antibody to antigen determines the ability of the complex to damage the tissues. When antibody is in excess the complexes are insoluble and may be relatively harmless for they can be rapidly eliminated by the cells of the reticulo-endothelial system. Complexes in which the antigen is in excess are usually soluble and tend to remain in the circulation for a long time before being deposited in sites for which they have a special affinity.

Immune complexes are formed in many viral infections. In man they have been observed in rubella and, especially, during the course of serum hepatitis. In the latter disease small aggregates of particles of Australia antigen coated liberally with antibody have been found by electron microscopy in the circulating blood of fulminating cases—a situation in which there is an excess of (IgG) antibody (Almeida and Waterson, 1969). Larger aggregates of irregularly shaped spherical and tubular particles of Australia antigen have been found in conditions of antigenic excess (Chap. 46).

DURATION OF IMMUNITY. After some virus infections there follows a prolonged immunity that may last for life but in others it may last for only a few weeks. A prolonged immunity is characteristic of infections where there has been an extensive viraemic phase and where the virus concerned is antigenically stable and monospecific. In such infections as measles, mumps, varicella, smallpox and yellow fever, the immune state persists for many years and second attacks of these diseases are extremely rare. Because the illness follows two phases of viraemia, the secondary antibody response is early enough to prevent infection and to suppress the secondary viraemia.

Limited immunity of short duration occurs when there has been no phase of viraemia and when there are frequent variations in the antigenic structure of the virus. Influenza, the common cold and many other infections of the upper respiratory tract are followed by a short-lived immunity and attacks of these illnesses are frequently repeated. Sufferers from these infections are often encountering for the first time an antigenic type of the virus to which they have never before been exposed with the resultant stimulus that incites the production of the specific protective immunoglobulin IgA in their mucous membranes.

Non-Immunological Responses

In addition to specific immune responses directed at particular viruses there are many important general physiological defences.

PHAGOCYTOSIS. It has been seen that lymphocytes and macrophages play a particularly important part in limiting the dissemination of viruses throughout the body especially during the viraemic phases of infection. Macrophages circulating in the blood stream (monocytes and lymphocytes) ingest virus particles and carry virions to different parts of the body where foci of infection may be established but they may also produce enough interferon to neutralize any possible cellular damage.

Polymorphonuclear leucocytes seem to have no protective role to play against viruses and indeed are usually numerically depressed during severe viral infections. There is often a leuco-poenia with a relative lymphocytosis in acute viral infections and the inflammatory reaction at the site of cellular damage is characteristically monocytic with few if any polymorph cells.

INTERFERON. The nature of interferon and its production at a cellular level is discussed in Chapter 13. There is no doubt that this antiviral protein is produced in many tissues of intact animals as a result of the stimulus of different viruses or even inert substances. The interferon response is very rapid and is not specific for individual viruses. Interferon may play a role in the recovery from a first infection possibly because it appears significantly earlier than do circulating antibodies. When mice are given interferon intravenously or inoculated with a paramyxovirus known to stimulate interferon production, they survive the challenge of other-wise lethal doses of viruses.

In man the local instillation of interferon into the conjunctival sac has been shown to be beneficial in herpetic and vaccinial infections. The stimulation of the host to produce interferon for himself may offer better prospects for anti-viral therapy than the difficult tasks of produc-tion and purification of a host specific substance in quantities large enough and stable enough for use as an antiviral chemotherapeutic agent.

PYREXIA. In almost all overt infections at the end of the incubation period there is a febrile response which coincides with the wide distribu-tion of the virus. Body temperatures of 38° to 41°C. are often reached and these may well offer a protective mechanism that prevents the further multiplication of a heat-sensitive virus (e.g. smallpox, Chap. 40). On the other hand, fever, either naturally or artificially induced, may promote viral multiplication as in the activation of latent herpes simplex virions lying dormant in the tissues to produce a recurrence of 'fever blisters' at muco-cutaneous junctions.

Many other non-specific factors such as age, nutrition, race and hormonal status all influence the pathogenesis of microbial infection.

The Outcome of Viral Infections

So far the nature of the pathogenic mechanisms of viruses and the way that their host combats them have been considered. The interplay between these two forces may have many differ-ent effects. Sometimes the virus seems able to produce a *clinically* obvious illness in practically all the people it infects. This is true when fully susceptible persons are infected with measles, smallpox and varicella. But in others even though there is definite viral proliferation only a small proportion of those infected develop an illness whereas most show little or no untoward effects as in poliomyelitis. Such events are known as *inapparent* or *subclinical* infections. Whether the patient develops a severe or a mild illness or escapes altogether any observable effect of the infection, is determined by many interacting factors, of which the size of the infecting dose, the virulence of the virus, and the effectiveness of the immune and physiological responses are the most important.

LATENT INFECTIONS may be of very long duration and are inapparent. They occur when an equilibrium has been established between the virus and the host. The virus may persist in an occult form in the tissues indefinitely without causing damage. Its presence is only revealed when it is conveyed to a new susceptible host as occurs for instance in hepatitis, or when the equilibrium is upset by some factor that damages the host or favours the virus as in herpes simplex.

SLOW VIRAL INFECTIONS are characterized by progressive tissue damage continuing throughout a very long incubation period and are probably a sequel to acute infections. The interval between the first infection and the appearance of clinical signs of the disease may be as long as several years.

TOLERATED INFECTIONS with viruses occur when the virions become established early in intrauterine life before the embryo has devel-oped any immunological responses. In the absence of antibodies and when there is no cellular response the virus survives indefinitely in the tissues of a host who is 'immunologically tolerant'. The classical example of this pheno-menon is the intrauterine infection of mice with the benign lymphocytic choriomeningitis virus.

The embryo mice are infected and remain quite unharmed although the virus continues to multiply in their tissues and is excreted in their urine throughout their life. Similar situations exist in murine leukaemia and avian leucosis.

REFERENCES AND FURTHER READING

ALMEIDA, J. D. & WATERSON, A. P. (1969) Immune complexes in hepatitis. *Lancet*, **ii**, 983.

BANG, F. B. & LUTTRELL, C. N. (1961) Factors in the pathogenesis of virus diseases. *Advances in Virus Research*, **8**, 200.

FENNER, F. (1968) *The Biology of Animal Viruses*, Vol. 2, Chap. 12 to 15. New York: Academic Press.

LE BOUVIER, G. L. & McCOLLUM, R. W. (1970) Australia (hepatitis associated) antigen: physicochemical and immunological characteristics. *Advances in Virus Research*, **16**, 357.

MIMS, C. A. (1964) Aspects of the pathogenesis of virus diseases. *Bacteriological Review*, **28**, 30.

MIMS, C. A. (1966) Pathogenesis of rashes in virus diseases. *Bacteriological Review*, **30**, 739.

NATHANSON, N. & COLE, G. A. (1970) Immunosuppression and experimental virus infection of the nervous system. *Advances in Virus Research*, **16**, 397.

SMITH, H. & PEARCE, J. H. (1972) *Microbial Pathogenicity in Man and Animals*. (Chapters by R. Bablanian, p. 239; F. B. Borg, p. 415; and C. A. Mims, p. 333.) Cambridge University Press.

Symposium on Immune Complexes and Disease (1971) *Journal of Experimental Medicine*, **134**, No. 3, Part 2.

Volume 1 : Part 2
Bacterial Pathogens and Associated Diseases

15. Staphylococcus
Skin and Wound Infections: Abscess: Osteomyelitis

The genus *Staphylococcus* consists of cluster-forming Gram-positive cocci. It is important because it includes the common and versatile pathogenic species *Staphylococcus aureus* (syn. *Staph. pyogenes*). This staphylococcus is the cause of a wide range of different kinds of major and minor pyogenic infections, and also occurs harmlessly as a commensal parasite in the anterior nares and on moist areas of skin in 20 to 30 per cent of healthy persons ('carriers'). Other staphylococci, called *Staph. albus* (syn. *Staph. epidermidis*), are harmless commensals that grow on the whole surface of the skin and in the nostrils and mouth of all persons throughout their life, but they occasionally act as opportunistic pathogens in persons with defective antimicrobial defences, e.g. damaged heart valves or urinary tract anomalies. The staphylococci can survive and grow in high salt concentrations, e.g. in drying sweat and pickled meat, and produce lipases and esterases that enable them to utilize the lipids of sebaceous secretion as a source of carbon and energy. The *albus* variety is frequently found in acne lesions, though its role in acne is doubtful.

Definition of the Genus Staphylococcus

Gram-positive cocci that grow in irregular, grape-like clusters, are facultatively anaerobic, form acid from glucose under either aerobic or anaerobic conditions, produce catalase, and occur as parasites on the skin in man and other vertebrate animals.

Other genera of cluster-forming Gram-positive cocci are harmless saprophytes that live in soil, water and foodstuffs: *Micrococcus* differs from *Staphylococcus* in being strictly aerobic, *Sarcina* differs in forming cubical packets of eight cocci, and *Aerococcus* in not producing catalase. *Peptococcus* consists of strictly anaerobic cocci that live as harmless commensals in the throat, intestine and vagina.

DEFINITION OF THE TWO SPECIES OF STAPHYLOCOCCUS

Staphylococcus aureus: coagulase-positive, toxin-forming, pathogenic staphylococci. Most strains form golden-pigmented (aureus) colonies; some form white or cream coloured colonies.

Staphylococcus albus: coagulase-negative, non-toxin-forming and non-pathogenic staphylococci. Most strains form white (albus) colonies, but a few form pigmented ones (lemon, yellow, red).

STAPHYLOCOCCUS AUREUS

DESCRIPTION

Morphologically, these are Gram-positive cocci about 1 μm in diameter, mainly joined in grape-like clusters, but some cocci are single and some in pairs; non-sporing, non-motile and non-capsulate. After culture for 24 hours at 37°C on nutrient agar, milk agar or blood agar the colonies are circular, 2 to 3 mm in diameter, with a smooth, shiny surface, relatively opaque to transmitted light, and pigmented golden, yellow, orange or fawn, or, in a few strains, white or cream coloured. Milk agar containing 7 per cent NaCl or broth containing 10 per cent NaCl may be used as a selective medium for culture of staphylococci from materials such as faeces and food which contain many bacteria of other kinds.

COAGULASE. This is a soluble enzyme-like product of *Staph. aureus* that converts the fibrinogen in citrated human or rabbit plasma into fibrin aided by an activator in the plasma. *In vivo* it may contribute to pathogenicity by inactivating a bactericidal substance in normal serum or by protecting the cocci with a fibrin barrier against phagocytosis. Staphylo-coagulase occurs in two forms, viz. *soluble coagulase* which can be demonstrated by adding a drop of a young staphylococcal broth culture into a tube containing 0·5 ml citrated human or rabbit plasma diluted 1 in 10 (tube test); and *bound coagulase* (clumping factor) which is demonstrated when clumping of the staphylococci occurs within ten seconds of adding a trace of undiluted plasma to a saline suspension of the organism on a glass slide (slide test). Doubtful reactions with the slide test should be checked by the tube test.

OTHER VIRULENCE FACTORS. A number of its cell components and soluble toxins and nontoxic aggressins, including coagulase, contribute to the ability of *Staph. aureus* to overcome the body's defences and to invade, survive in, and colonize the tissues. Probably most important are the toxins that kill phagocytes and the cell-surface components that enable the cocci to resist killing by lysosomal enzymes after ingestion by polymorph leucocytes or macrophages. The cocci are highly resistant to intracellular killing unless they are sensitized before phagocytosis by exposure to serum factors, including heat-labile complement. Even then they sometimes outlive the phagocyte that has ingested them. The cell-wall components of the coccus include (1) mucopeptide, (2) a species-specific antigen, protein A, which is a precipitant of gamma-globulin, (3) alpha and beta ribitol teichoic acids, also antigens, and (4) one or more of over 30 different type-specific antigens. Which if any of these substances protect it against intra-phagocytic digestion is unknown. Rare strains of *Staph. aureus* also have an antiphagocytic carbohydrate capsule.

Most strains of *Staph. aureus* produce a soluble fibrinolysin (plasminogen activator) and a hyaluronidase ('spreading factor') but neither of these substances appears to play an important part in pathogenesis.

TOXINS. Exotoxins are secreted by the growing *Staph. aureus* cells and are demonstrable in bacteria-free filtrates of cultures. Toxins that probably play a part in the pathogenicity of the staphylococcus are α-toxin and the Panton-Valentine (PV) leucocidin.

Alpha-toxin has haemolytic, leucocidal (kills macrophages), cytotoxic, dermonecrotic and lethal effects. Its action on smooth muscle causes constriction of small veins and ischaemic necrosis of the affected tissue. It is an antigenic enzyme, which appears to act on cell membranes and is probably responsible for some of the

symptoms in fatal cases of staphylococcal septicaemia.

Panton-Valentine (PV) leucocidin is a nonhaemolytic toxin that kills polymorphs and macrophages with morphological changes but without lysis. It consists of two antigenic proteins, F and S, that act synergistically on the phospholipids in the leucocyte membrane.

Other staphylococcal toxins are *beta toxin,* a weak haemolytic toxin, which is found mainly in strains of animal origin and *delta-toxin* which is haemolytic, leucocidal (and leucolytic) and cytotoxic; delta-toxin appears to be a non-antigenic enzyme active on phospholipids and is neutralized by alpha and beta globulins in normal serum.

Enterotoxin is an intestinal toxin, formed by 30 to 50 per cent of strains of *Staph. aureus,* mostly in phage-group III. It is heat-stable and withstands exposure at 100°C for a few minutes, a treatment that will kill the staphylococci. When ingested in food, commonly cooked meats, in which the staphylococcus has been growing profusely, the enterotoxin causes nausea, vomiting and diarrhoea within 6 hours (staphylococcal food-poisoning). Five antigenic types of enterotoxin, A to E, are distinguishable in gel-diffusion precipitin tests, and the presence of one of these toxins may be demonstrated by a precipitin test made on an extract of the food.

PATHOGENESIS

Staph. aureus, which is present in the nose and on the skin of a variable proportion of healthy people, is an opportunistic pathogen in the sense that it causes infection most commonly in tissues and sites with lowered host-resistance, e.g. damaged skin and mucous membranes, or the haematoma in the cancellous tissue of a long bone, following injury, which predisposes to osteomyelitis. But the more pathogenic strains of staphylococci are also well endowed with enzymes (coagulase, lipase, esterase) and toxins to help establish and protect the organism in the host's tissues. The most common staphylococcal lesion, the boil, results from the invasion of hair follicles or sebaceous glands, aided by the lipase-esterase enzyme whilst coagulase, α-toxin and PV leucocidin combat host reactions and phagocytosis. Even after phagocytosis, intracellular destruction facilitated by complement may not be completed as happens with other pyogenic cocci, and this resistance may lead to chronic staphylococcal infection.

Staph. aureus is the cause of a wide variety of acute suppurative infections; some of these, e.g. boils, are almost exclusively due to it, but others, e.g. wound infections, may also be caused by other pyogenic bacteria.

1. Superficial infections: skin pustules, boils, carbuncles, impetigo, pemphigus neonatorum, sycosis barbae, paronychia, styes, blepharitis, and conjunctivitis: infections of accidental and surgical wounds, and burns.

2. Subcutaneous and submucous abscesses: e.g. whitlow of finger or palm of hand, and breast abscess.

3. Osteomyelitis, bronchopneumonia, particularly post-influenzal, and pyelonephritis.

4. Lymphangiitis, lymphadenitis, bacteriaemia, septicaemia, pyaemia, and acute bacterial endocarditis.

5. Staphylococcal food-poisoning, a common cause of vomiting and diarrhoea, and staphylococcal enterocolitis, a rare, generally fatal infection that follows abdominal surgery preceded or accompanied by the oral administration of broad-spectrum antibiotics to eliminate the normal flora of the alimentary tract.

The staphylococcus is capable of initiating an infection in apparently intact skin, but infection is facilitated if the skin is breached or damaged. Infections of deep tissues, such as osteomyelitis and pyelonephritis, are presumably blood-borne from a minor superficial lesion or a cryptogenic focus, e.g. in the upper respiratory tract.

Staph. aureus is a very common cause of infection in hospitals, and is most liable to infect newborn babies, surgical patients, old and malnourished persons, and patients with diabetes and other chronic diseases. In maternity hospitals it generally causes minor skin and conjunctival sepsis in 5 to 20 per cent of the newborn babies and more severe infections such as bullous impetigo (pemphigus neonatorum), bronchopneumonia and osteomyelitis or other deep seated lesions in a smaller proportion. Transfer of a virulent hospital strain of *Staph. aureus* from the nose or nasopharynx of the baby into the milk ducts of the nursing mother causes breast abscess in about 1 to 2 per cent of the mothers, developing usually 3 to 6 weeks after delivery. In surgical units *Staph. aureus* may cause sepsis in the operation wounds in 1 to 10 per cent of patients. Some of these infections take place in the theatre during the operation and others post-operatively in the ward.

IMMUNITY IN STAPHYLOCOCCAL INFECTIONS. Neutralizing antibodies are developed against the alpha-toxin, PV leucocidin and coagulase during the course of natural infections in man, and in men and animals given injections of staphylococcal vaccines and toxoids. There is some evidence that these antibodies may have a protective effect, but serotherapy and active immunization procedures have not been widely used. Most normal human sera contain small amounts of antibodies to alpha-toxin and PV leucocidin, but the amounts of these antibodies become greatly increased in severe or deep seated infections such as osteomyelitis and their levels may be measured for diagnostic purposes.

LABORATORY DIAGNOSIS

One or more of the following specimens may be collected for examination: (1) *pus* from abscesses, wounds, burns, etc., preferably in a screw-capped container, otherwise on a liberally soaked swab. (2) *sputum* from cases of lower respiratory tract infections, e.g. influenzal pneumonia, coughed up from the bronchi into a wide-mouthed jar; the specimen should not consist of saliva from the mouth; (3) *faeces* or *vomit* from patients with suspected food poisoning; 1 to 5 ml into a universal container; also convenient quantities of the *remains of foods* suspected of causing food-poisoning into separate containers; (4) *blood* from patients with suspected bacteriaemia, e.g. in osteomyelitis or endocarditis; 5 ml transferred aseptically into a blood-culture bottle containing 50 ml broth; (5) *urine* from patients with suspected cystitis, pyelonephritis or post-catheterization infection; a mid-stream specimen into a wide-mouthed jar or universal container; (6) *anterior nasal* and *perineal swabs* from suspected carriers; the swabs should first be moistened, if possible, with sterile water or broth, and the nasal swabs should be rubbed in turn over the anterior walls of both nostrils, which are covered by squamous epithelium.

The specimen is generally examined as follows: (1) An attempt is made to demonstrate the presence of *Staph. aureus* in it by (a) examination of a Gram-stained smear, except in the case of blood and swabs, (b) culture on a plate of nutrient, blood or milk agar and inspection for characteristic golden, cream-coloured or white colonies, and (c) performance of the coagulase test on a golden colony or, if there are no golden colonies, on a white one. (2) The sensitivity of the isolated strain of *Staph. aureus* to a selection of different antibiotics is tested by the disk diffusion method on a nutrient agar plate inoculated confluently from a colony. When the Gram-stained direct smear shows many Gram-positive cocci, sensitivity test disks may be used on the primary culture (Vol. II, Chap. 18). (3) The phage-type or serotype of the isolated strain may be determined if this information is required for epidemiological purposes.

Phage-typing

Strains of *Staph. aureus* may be differentiated into several hundred different 'phage-types' by observation of their pattern of susceptibility to lysis by a set of 24 different anti-*Staph. aureus* bacteriophages. A strain is tested by inoculating it confluently over a nutrient agar plate marked out in 24 squares and dropping the 24 phage preparations in specially measured dilutions (routine test dilutions) one on each square before the plate is incubated. The type of the strain is designated by the symbols of all the phages that lyse it with the production of a clear area in the film of growth. Thus a strain of type 3B/3C/55 is one that is lysed by phage 3B, phage 3C and phage 55 but not by any of the other phages.

Strains isolated from patients, carriers and fomites may by this means be precisely identified ('finger-printed') and their source and pattern of spread in an outbreak discovered. For example, a group of surgical wound infections may be traced to a surgeon who is a nasal carrier, or to a patient who is shedding staphylococci into the ward, by the demonstration that the strains from all the infected wounds belong to the same phage-type as the one isolated from the surgeon or the shedding patient.

A few of the many phage-types of *Staph. aureus*, e.g. 'type 80' (correctly, type 52/42B/42C/44A/80/81), have been found to be more virulent than the majority of types and more liable to cause cases and epidemics of sepsis in hospitals. Thus, in a period of 12 months as many as 100 to 200 phage-types of staphylococci may be isolated from patients and carriers in a maternity unit or a surgical ward, yet only 10 to 20 types may be found in cases of clinical infection and only 2 or 3 types, such as type 80, may be responsible for the large majority of the clinical infections.

The strains of *Staph. aureus* of different phage-types can be allocated to three main phage-groups, I, II and III, according to their susceptibility to three groups of related phages. Group I contains many hospital epidemic strains, e.g. those of types 80 and 52A/79. Group II contains many of the strains causing minor sepsis outside hospital and strains of types 71 and 3B/3C/55, most commonly causing impetigo and pemphigus neonatorum. Group III includes strains of animal origin, many of the antibiotic-resistant hospital strains (e.g. type 47/53/75/77) and most of the enterotoxin-producing strains. The strains of the three groups produce antigenically distinct forms of coagulase.

SEROTYPING. Strains of *Staph. aureus* can also be divided into a number of different types by a serological method which depends on their possessing different combinations of type-specific surface antigens that are demonstrable in slide agglutination tests with absorbed antisera. There are three main serotypes I to III, which correspond with the phage-groups I to III, and some minor types. Serotyping has been much less extensively used than phage-typing in epidemiological studies largely because of technical difficulties.

ANTIBIOTIC THERAPY OF
Staph. Aureus INFECTIONS

Sensitivity to Antibiotics

Strains of *Staph. aureus* isolated from different patients and carriers differ in their degree of sensitivity to particular antibiotics, and some strains are resistant to particular anti-staphylo-coccal antibiotics at the highest concentrations that can conveniently be achieved in the patient's tissues. At the present time (1973), most (e.g. 50 to 75 per cent) of the strains infecting patients and carriers *outside hospitals* are sensitive to penicillin (minimum inhibitory concentration of benzyl-penicillin = 0.03 $\mu g/$ml), ampicillin (MIC = $0.1\,\mu g/ml$), streptomycin, chloramphenicol, tetracycline, fucidin, erythro-mycin, novobiocin, and lincomycin, whereas most (e.g. 75 per cent) of those infecting patients and carriers *in hospitals* are resistant to penicillin (MIC benzyl-penicillin $> 1000\,\mu g/ml$) and many of these penicillin-resistant strains are also resistant to some of the other anti-staphylo-coccal antibiotics (multi-resistant strains). Patients under antibiotic treatment in hospital commonly become cross-infected with a multi-resistant 'hospital' staphylococcus and such strains are often highly virulent. Staphylococci are poorly susceptible to sulphonamides, except when the sulphonamide is used in combination with trimethoprim in the preparation cotri-moxazole (marketed as Septrin and Bactrim).

Resistance of staphylococci to penicillin depends on the inherent property of the penicillin-resistant strains to produce penicillin-ase, an enzyme that decomposes and inactivates benzyl-penicillin, phenoxymethyl (oral) peni-cillin and ampicillin. Most penicillin-resistant staphylococci are therefore sensitive to the modified penicillins that are insusceptible to penicillinase, e.g. methicillin (MIC = $2\,\mu g/ml$) and cloxacillin (MIC = $0.25\,\mu g/ml$), and to fucidin and the cephalosporins. Penicillin-sensi-tive strains of *Staph. aureus* never mutate to become penicillinase-producing, though sensi-tive strains can readily mutate into forms resistant to streptomycin, erythromycin, fucidin or novobiocin, and less readily into forms resistant to chloramphenicol or tetracycline. The multi-resistant hospital staphylococci have prob-ably arisen by a succession of mutations confer-ring resistance to these different drugs in strains that were originally penicillin-resistant. Resist-ance to the antibiotics other than penicillin and ampicillin is a true insusceptibility and is not due to the production of an antibiotic-destroying enzyme.

Penicillin-resistant strains of *Staph. aureus*

existed before the introduction of penicillin into medical use in 1942, but they were rare and comprised only a very small proportion ($<$ 1 per cent) of the strains isolated at that time. The property of penicillinase production may originally have evolved because the enzyme acted on some natural substrate chemically similar to penicillin or because it protected the cocci when growing in habitats contaminated with a penicillin-like antibiotic, e.g. in fungal skin lesions. After the medical use of penicillin had become general, there was a progressive, large increase in the prevalence of the penicillin-resistant staphylococci and this increase was more rapid in hospitals than in the general com-munity. In one London hospital, for instance, the proportion of strains isolated from septic infections in patients that were penicillin-resistant was 14 per cent in 1946, 38 per cent in 1947 and 59 per cent in 1948. In contrast, the proportion of resistant strains isolated from septic infections in outpatients of British hos-pitals only reached about 10 per cent by 1950 and 40 to 50 per cent in 1960. Proportionate increases in the percentage of resistant strains took place among those isolated from carriage sites in patients and healthy doctors and nurses in hospitals, and among those isolated from healthy carriers in the general community. The high prevalence of resistant strains in hospital staff is exemplified by the finding that in 1957 in an Edinburgh hospital staffed by about 900 doctors and nurses, 53 per cent of the staff were carriers of *Staph. aureus* and 90 per cent of these carriers harboured a strain of *Staph. aureus* that was penicillin-resistant.

Since most hospital patients with septic lesions were treated systemically with penicillin, it is understandable that penicillin-sensitive strains of *Staph. aureus* would tend to be elimin-ated both from their lesions and carriage sites, and that the lesions and carriage sites would thus become susceptible to replacement infec-tion with a penicillin-resistant strain from a hospital source. In one hospital it was observed that the nasal carriage rate, which was less than 20 per cent at the time of admission, rose to over 60 per cent after 8 to 9 days in the patients who were treated with penicillin, but remained lower ($<$ 40 per cent) in those not treated with an antibiotic.

The high carriage rate of resistant strains by healthy hospital staff must have had another explanation, since high rates were observed at a time when many of the carriers had had no previous therapy with penicillin. Hospital staff are, however, frequently exposed to airborne penicillin-containing dust produced from penicillin accidentally spilt in wards and pharmacies, and penicillin excreted by patients under therapy, and it has been demonstrated that staff may inhale sufficient amounts of this dust into their noses to eliminate penicillin-sensitive staphylococci and allow their replacement by penicillin-resistant ones.

Before 1960, when methicillin, the first of the penicillinase-resistant penicillins, was brought into use, about 1 per cent of strains of *Staph. aureus* were 'methicillin-resistant' and by 1970 in Britain their proportion had risen to about 5 per cent. These strains are tolerant of, and able to grow in the presence of, low therapeutic concentrations of methicillin, cloxacillin, benzyl-penicillin and ampicillin. They do not destroy methicillin and cloxacillin, but most of them are penicillinase-producing as well as being 'methicillin-resistant' and therefore inactivate benzyl-penicillin and ampicillin. The clinical significance of this resistance is uncertain since infections may be cured with a high dosage of methicillin.

CHOICE OF ANTIBIOTIC FOR THERAPY. Since different strains of *Staph. aureus* differ in sensitivity to different antibiotics, the choice of antibiotic for use in treatment of a patient should be based on the results of sensitivity tests made on a culture of the strain isolated from the patient. Pending receipt of the results, the treatment of severe infections suspected of being staphylococcal should be begun with the injection of methicillin or cloxacillin. If tests show that the infecting organism is penicillin-sensitive, the drug of choice for further treatment is benzyl penicillin, which is narrow-spectrum and bactericidal. If the strain is found to be penicillin-resistant, methicillin or cloxacillin should be continued. If the patient is hypersensitive to penicillin, one of the cephalosporins, vancomycin or gentamicin should be given by injection for severe infections, and fucidin or erythromycin in combination with novobiocin by mouth for less severe ones.

EPIDEMIOLOGY OF *Staph. Aureus* INFECTIONS

Sources of Infection

1. PATIENTS WITH LESIONS DISCHARGING STAPHYLOCOCCI INTO THE ENVIRONMENT. Especially large numbers of cocci are disseminated in pus and dried exudate discharged from large infected wounds and burns and secondarily infected skin lesions, e.g. psoriasis, eczema and dermatitis, and in sputum coughed from the lung of a patient with bronchopneumonia. Small discharging lesions, e.g. pustules and paronychiae, on the hands of doctors and nurses are a special danger to their patients.

2. HEALTHY CARRIERS. *Staph. aureus* grows harmlessly on the moist invaginated skin in the nostrils in 10 to 30 per cent of healthy persons and on that of the perineum in about 10 per cent. The cocci are spread from these sites into the environment by the hands, handkerchief, clothing and dust (consisting of skin squames and cloth fibres). Some carriers, called 'shedders', disseminate exceptionally large numbers of cocci comparable to the numbers disseminated by patients with large superficial lesions or lower respiratory tract infections.

During the first day or two of life the body surfaces of most babies become colonized by staphylococci acquired from their mother, nurse or environment. In babies born in hospital, the nose, umbilical stump and moist areas of skin are commonly colonized by *Staph. aureus,* often by a virulent multi-antibiotic-resistant strain. Nasal carriage in babies, as in older persons, is usually long-lasting. When a particular strain of *Staph. aureus* has colonized a carrier site in an individual, it tends to persist in that site for many months or several years, and to prevent colonization of the site by other strains, whether more or less virulent (bacterial interference). In babies who are nose carriers the occurrence of an intercurrent viral infection of the respiratory tract greatly increases the dissemination of staphylococci into the environment ('cloud babies'). Babies with skin infections or who are carriers of an 'epidemic' strain of staphylococcus may bring infection into the household from the hospital.

3. ANIMALS of domesticated and some wild

species may disseminate *Staph. aureus* from infected lesions or carriage sites and so cause infections in man, e.g. a dairy cow with staphylococcal infection of the udder may give infected milk which can cause staphylococcal food-poisoning.

Modes of Infection

The mode of acquisition of an infection may be either (1) *exogenous*, i.e. directly from a source in another person or animal; e.g. the operation wound of a patient may be infected from hand-carriage by a surgeon who sweats the organisms through glove punctures or by a nurse who is a nasal carrier; or (2) *endogenous*, i.e. from a source, either carriage site or minor lesion, elsewhere in the patient's own body; e.g. a boil may be caused by cocci transferred on the fingers from a carriage site in the nostrils to a hair follicle on the back of the neck, and a surgical wound may be infected post-operatively by contaminated fingers or by dust-borne staphylococci derived from the patient's nostrils or perineum.

The relative importance of exogenous and endogenous infection in the causation of surgical sepsis with *Staph. aureus* appears to vary from hospital to hospital. In some studies a much higher incidence of sepsis (e.g. 8 per cent) has been found in patients who were nasal or perineal carriers than in those who were not (e.g. 2 per cent), but in other studies the incidence has been similar in the carriers and non-carriers.

VIABILITY OUTSIDE THE BODY. Staphylococci do not grow outside the body except occasionally in moist nutrient materials such as meat, milk and dirty water. They are, however, very hardy and, though not spore-forming, may remain alive in a dormant state for up to several months when dried in pus, sputum, clothing or dust. They are fairly readily killed by heat, e.g. by moist heat at 65°C in 30 min, by exposure to light and by strong disinfectants.

Mechanisms of Transmission in Cross-infection

These include:

1. CONTACT. The readiest method of spread is thought to be direct contact (touching) with the contaminated hand or clothing of an infected person, e.g. with a hand on which there is a septic sore, or the hand of a nasal carrier who has picked his nose. Hundreds of staphylococci may pass in a drop of sweat exuded from the hand of a carrier surgeon through a puncture in his rubber glove or from his forearm through the moistened sleeve of his gown. Moderate numbers of staphylococci may be transmitted indirectly on the hands of non-carrier nurses who have contaminated their hands by touching infected patients or babies. Small numbers of staphylococci are likely to be spread by contact with objects, such as furniture, clothing, bedding, towels, hand-basins and baths, that have been contaminated by a patient or carrier. *Staph. aureus* is commonly present on such fomites. Newborn babies have been shown to become colonized with *Staph. aureus* by contact with infected shirts, napkins and blankets, though less frequently than by contact with infected hands.

2. AIR-BORNE DUST. Staphylococci carried on fragments of desquamated keratin, fibres of cloth and particles of powdered dried pus or sputum are readily shed into the air from the skin, handkerchief, clothing, bedding and surgical dressings of patients and carriers when these objects are disturbed or moved even slightly. For example, several thousand *Staph. aureus*-carrying particles may be shed into the air by a carrier shaking open his handkerchief, changing his clothing or making his bed; most (e.g. 90 per cent) of these particles will fall out of the air within 15 to 20 min, but a few will remain air-borne for up to 2 hours or more. *Staph. aureus*-carrying particles are likely to be present in considerable numbers in the air of occupied rooms and hospital wards during periods of activity such as bed-making, sweeping, dusting, etc. They may fall on to the body surfaces, surgical wounds or vehicles of infection such as surgical instruments, or they may be inhaled into the respiratory tract.

3. DROPLET-SPRAY AND AIR-BORNE DROPLET-NUCLEI, which are freely disseminated in speaking, coughing and sneezing by healthy nasal carriers and patients with broncho-pneumonia, are probably the *least important* of the different methods of spread, since relatively few of the droplets or droplet-nuclei contain *Staph. aureus*.

Transmission of Infection to Newborn Babies in Hospital

The circumstances that babies are born free from bacterial colonization and are highly susceptible to colonization with *Staph. aureus* have made it possible to compare the relative importance of different sources and mechanisms of transmission of *Staph. aureus* in the nurseries of maternity hospitals. Studies in which strains of *Staph. aureus* were distinguished by phage-typing suggest that it is usually a carrier nurse or a nurse with a septic lesion that introduces an epidemic strain into a nursery, that thereafter the colonized babies serve as the main source of that strain for other babies, and that the main means of transmission between the babies is by contact with the hands and clothing of the nurses that attend them. However, in a number of studies, measures taken to exclude the possibility of contact spread by nurses, e.g. disinfection or gloving of the hands, wearing of masks, and change of gown between babies, have failed appreciably to reduce the rate at which the babies became infected, and there is evidence that infection has been transmitted by air and by fomites. The practice of nursing the baby alongside its mother instead of in a communal nursery or the use of several small nurseries in which successive cohorts of babies are nursed has helped to reduce staphylococcal infection among neonates.

PREVENTION OF STAPHYLOCOCCAL INFECTION IN HOSPITAL

Prevention is very difficult. The measures that may be attempted include the following:

1. MEASURES AGAINST THE SOURCES OF INFECTION. (a) Patients with discharging lesions should be neutralized as sources of infection by the use of antibiotic therapy, occlusive dressings, barrier nursing and, where possible, isolation in single-bed rooms with exhaust ventilation to the outside. Particular attention should be paid to patients with large septic wounds or burns, large areas of infective dermatitis, staphylococcal pneumonia or any open infection with a known epidemic strain.

(b) Surgeons, nurses, anaesthetists and surgical orderlies who have an open infected lesion on any part of the body, even if this lesion is small, e.g. paronychia, a discharging pustule, or a patch of secondarily infected psoriasis, or who have a lesion of the hand or arm even if it is not discharging, should not attend patients until healing is complete. Covering the lesion with an occlusive dressing is not an adequate safeguard.

(c) Carriers among patients and staff may be detected by nasal and perineal swabbing and treated with twice-daily application of neomycin-chlorhexidine cream to the carriage site. Carriers are generally numerous among the hospital staff and they should not be removed from duty unless they are known to be carrying a strain of a phage-type that is currently causing an outbreak of clinical infection. Since bacteriological screening for carriers in a large staff is very laborious, it is usually not done unless there is a serious outbreak of sepsis.

2. MEASURES AGAINST SPREAD THROUGH THE ENVIRONMENT. Mostly these are measures that are generally applicable in the control of hospital infection. They include recognized aseptic and antiseptic procedures during operations; aseptic and antiseptic techniques applicable in the wards for post-operative patients and for the impedimenta of nursing care (baths, basins, weighing baskets, etc.) in infant nurseries; early recognition and isolation of any infected case and special protection of highly susceptible patients such as premature babies in special units or single rooms; and measures against the hazards of airborne infection from infected dust, etc. in operating theatres, wards, dressing stations and special units.

3. ANTIMICROBIAL PROPHYLAXIS. It is generally undesirable to give antibiotics to patients with the object of preventing their acquiring a staphylococcal infection. The antibiotic thus used will tend to eliminate the sensitive members of the body's commensal bacterial flora and, by removing competitors, facilitate infection with a hospital strain of *Staph. aureus* or another species that is resistant to the antibiotic. If it is decided to attempt prophylaxis, the *topical application* of a drug is preferable to systemic application, since it is possible to use the more toxic drugs, e.g. a mixture of polymyxin, neomycin and bacitracin, which

are not used for systemic therapy; or a chemical antiseptic e.g. hexachlorophene may be applied (Chap. 5). If systemic prophylaxis is required it is preferable to use a narrow-spectrum antibiotic such as cloxacillin rather than a broad-spectrum one.

4. BACTERIAL INTERFERENCE. This method for the control of staphylococcal infection in the newborn has been applied successfully in trials in several American hospitals but because of its hypothetical dangers is unlikely to come into general use. Its effectiveness, however, is of considerable interest because it demonstrates the marked ability of established commensal cocci to prevent the colonization of carriage sites by other, more virulent or antibiotic-resistant strains and thus to reduce the likelihood of endogenous septic infections. A strain of *Staph. aureus,* chosen for its low virulence, may readily be induced by the deliberate inoculation of bacteria from a culture to colonize the nasal and umbilical carriage sites in newborn babies who have not yet acquired a staphylococcal flora by natural infection. Colonization with the inoculated strain is only rarely achieved in older babies and adults already carrying another strain of *Staph. aureus* unless the resident strain is first eliminated by topical treatment with antibiotics. Carriage of *Staph. albus* has some protective effect against the inoculation of *Staph. aureus,* but the degree of interference is less than that between two different strains of *Staph. aureus.*

In the American trials, a special strain of *Staph. aureus* of low pathogenicity, no. 502A, was able to establish itself when applied to the nostrils and umbilicus in doses of 10^4 to 10^6 cocci in 95 per cent of babies without previously resident staphylococci but only in 55 per cent of those already colonized by *Staph. albus* and in 12 per cent of those carrying another type of *Staph. aureus.* The value of this 'prophylactic' procedure was tested in infant nurseries where epidemics of staphylococcal infection were occurring. Only 5 per cent of babies successfully colonized with the special strain, 502A, became carriers of the epidemic strain compared with 40 per cent of the uninoculated babies, and in a follow-up period only 9 of 96 inoculated babies developed septic infections compared with 26 of 45 babies who had acquired the epidemic strain

type 80/81 and 10 of 54 babies who had become carriers of other strains of *Staph. aureus.*

STAPHYLOCOCCUS ALBUS

Staph. albus is defined as consisting of the coagulase-negative staphylococci. It receives its name from the fact that most strains form white (albus) colonies. It differs from *Staph. aureus* in not forming toxins or other aggressive factors, so that it is devoid of primary pathogenicity. It is a constant, harmless commensal which grows on all areas of skin and in the nostrils, mouth, external ear and urethral meatus throughout life. By contact with the skin and by the shedding of skin squames large numbers of the cocci are disseminated on to clothing and fomites and into dust and air. For this reason the organism is a common accidental contaminant of clinical specimens and laboratory cultures, and in most cases its finding in such specimens may be regarded as being without any clinical significance.

Occasionally, however, *Staph. albus* acts as an opportunistic pathogen and causes infection in persons with defective resistance, e.g. cystitis in persons with urinary-tract abnormalities, septicaemia or endocarditis in patients after cardiac surgery, meningitis with bacteriaemia in patients fitted with ventriculo-venous cerebrospinal fluid shunts, and septicaemia in immunosuppressed and immunodefective patients. These cases are recognized by the finding of significantly large numbers of cocci (e.g. 10^5 per ml in urine, 5 per ml in blood) in repeated specimens and the infections should be treated with an antibiotic indicated by the results of sensitivity tests on the infecting strain.

OTHER GRAM-POSITIVE CLUSTER-FORMING COCCI

The distinguishing characters of the other Gram-positive cluster-forming cocci are given in Volume II, Chapter 18. They are harmless commensals and saprophytes that very rarely cause even opportunistic infections. One variety of *Micrococcus* (subgroup 3) has, however, been implicated as the cause of a number of urinary tract infections.

FURTHER READING

ELEK, S. D. (1959) *Staphylococcus pyogenes and its Relation to Disease*. Edinburgh: Livingstone.

MAIBACH, H. J. & HILDICK-SMITH, G. (1965) *Skin Bacteria and their Role in Infection*. New York: McGraw-Hill.

MUDD, S. (1970) In *Infectious Agents and Host Reactions*, Chap. 9. Edited by S. Mudd. Philadelphia, London, Toronto: Saunders.

WILLIAMS, R. E. O. (1959) Epidemic Staphylococci. *Lancet*, i, 190.

WILLIAMS, R. E. O., BLOWERS, R., GARROD, L. P. & SHOOTER, R. A. (1966) *Hospital Infection*. 2nd Edn. London: Lloyd-Luke.

WORLD HEALTH ORGANIZATION (1968) Staphylococcal and streptococcal infections. *World Health Organization Technical Report Series* no. 394, Geneva.

16. Streptococcus

Sore Throat: Scarlet Fever: Impetigo: Bacterial Endocarditis: Rheumatic Fever: Glomerulonephritis

Several species of Gram-positive cocci have their main habitat in the upper respiratory tract of man. They include the pneumococci and streptococci found mostly in the throat and the staphylococci predominantly present in the anterior nares. Within each of these groups, often recognizable by their characteristic cell arrangements in pairs, chains or clusters, there are commensals, pathogens and potential pathogens, the last of these affecting particularly tissues with lowered resistance, e.g. causing secondary bronchitis after a primary virus infection. Most streptococcal infections are caused by the pathogenic haemolytic streptococci of Lancefield's group A—*Streptococcus pyogenes* (see below) and the most common infective syndrome is an acutely inflamed throat with or without exudate (tonsillitis or pharyngitis) which requires both clinical and laboratory skills for its accurate diagnosis. Another typical streptococcal infection is scarlet fever—sore throat plus a generalized erythematous rash. Haemolytic streptococci also cause various suppurative conditions and certain skin infections, erysipelas and impetigo contagiosa. In addition, streptococcal sore throat may be followed by an attack of rheumatic fever whilst acute glomerulonephritis may be a sequela of sore throat or impetigo.

CLASSIFICATION OF STREPTOCOCCI

The streptococcus belongs to the family *Lactobacillaceae* along with the pneumococcus and the lactobacillus. The streptococci are Gram-positive, spherical or oval cells arranged in chains of varying length; each cell is approximately $1 \cdot 0$ μm in diameter, non-motile, non-sporing and may be capsulate. The majority are facultative anaerobes, but there are species that are anaerobic or microaerophilic.

The facultatively anaerobic streptococci may first be divided into those that produce a soluble haemolysin and those that do not. The first of these groups usually causes a clear zone of haemolysis on fresh blood agar—called beta (β) haemolysis; it includes most of the species associated with primary streptococcal infections in man and animals. These haemolytic streptococci may be subdivided into a number of broad groups determined by the chemical nature of the carbohydrate (or C antigen) contained in the body of the organism (Lancefield groups A, B, C, D etc.). Strains that belong to Lancefield group A (*Streptococcus pyogenes*) are responsible for over 90 per cent of human streptococcal infections; these group A strains may be further divided by specific agglutinating or precipitating sera into Griffith types according to their surface protein antigens (M, T and R). The M protein is the antigen of most importance and it exists in over 50 different antigenic forms, each of which is present in a different serotype of *Strept. pyogenes* (type 1, type 2, etc.). The determination of the serotype of strains of *Strept. pyogenes* isolated from patients and carriers plays a valuable part in the epidemiological investigation of outbreaks of infection in a way comparable to the use of phage-typing in the study of *Staph. aureus* infection. The extracellular toxins and enzymes produced by *Strept. pyogenes* and which may contribute to its pathogenicity are discussed later.

Facultatively anaerobic streptococci that do not produce soluble haemolysin may be divided into two broad categories according to their appearance when grown on blood agar. Those that cause a greenish pigmentation with a narrow zone of partial haemolysis are called alpha (α) haemolytic streptococci or *Streptococcus viridans*. Culturally, they have some resemblance to pneumococci but the two species may be differentiated by certain biochemical and biological tests (Vol. II, Chap. 19). Those without effect on the blood-containing medium are called non-haemolytic, or gamma (γ) streptococci and include the faecal streptococci (*Streptococcus faecalis*). Whilst most of the Lancefield group A streptococci produce beta-haemolysis, some variants are non-haemolytic. Conversely, a variant of *Strept. faecalis* (Lancefield group D) may be actively haemolytic on blood agar, although it does not produce a soluble haemolysin.

The strictly anaerobic streptococci (or peptostreptococci) have different biological and pathogenic characteristics from the aerobic streptococci.

CLINICAL INFECTIONS DUE TO
Strept. pyogenes

The most common and most typical infection caused by *Strept. pyogenes* is an acute sore throat called tonsillitis if the tonsils are maximally involved or pharyngitis if there is little or no tonsillar tissue in the fauces. There is acute inflammation often with oedema and exudate on the faucial tissues including the soft palate, accompanied by fever and usually an associated cervical adenitis. If the infecting streptococcus is capable of producing a considerable amount of an erythrogenic toxin and the host has not developed antibodies to this toxin, the sore throat may be accompanied by a generalized punctate erythema or rash and this syndrome is called *scarlet fever*. Local extension of the streptococcal infection from the throat may result in such complications as peritonsillar abscess (quinsy), sinusitis, otitis media, mastoiditis or meningitis.

Puerperal sepsis or child-bed fever is traditionally associated with infection with *Strept. pyogenes* although there are other causal agents. Besides local inflammation of uterine tissues, infection may spread to the adnexa (pelvic cellulitis or peritonitis) or may become generalized (septicaemia). Wounds, burns and chronic skin lesions (eczema, psoriasis) may become infected with *Strept. pyogenes*; these superficial infections may extend in the local tissues (cellulitis) or be carried by lymphatics to regional lymph glands (lymphadenitis) or get into the blood stream.

Strept. pyogenes may cause two types of skin infection—erysipelas and impetigo. The former infection is a spreading inflammation of the dermis seen most commonly on the face and neck and may be associated with antecedent streptococcal infection of nose, throat or ear. Repeated attacks may occur, which may be related to an allergy to the streptococcal toxins. Impetigo contagiosa, characterized by multiple vesiculo-pustular or ulcerated skin lesions usually on exposed parts of the body (legs, arms, face) and affecting mostly school and pre-school children, is nowadays uncommon in temperate climates but is prevalent in many warm-climate countries where it is a more likely precursor of acute glomerulonephritis than is streptococcal sore throat. Impetigo may also be caused by *Staphylococcus aureus*: the primary skin lesion may be bullous rather than vesicular (bullous impetigo or pemphigus neonatorum).

Scarlet Fever

Scarlet fever, a specific infectious disease, most often consists of a combination of streptococcal sore throat and a generalized erythema; occasionally the rash will accompany a streptococcal or staphylococcal wound infection (surgical scarlet fever). The rash is due to an erythrogenic toxin produced by the infecting organism in the primary lesion; only strains of *Strept. pyogenes* that have been infected with temperate bacteriophage, i.e. are lysogenic, can produce the erythrogenic toxin (cf. toxigenic diphtheria bacilli, Chap. 21). The toxin, suitably diluted, may be used to test susceptibility or immunity to scarlet fever by intradermal injection; a localized erythema appearing within 8 to 12 hours indicates susceptibility (positive Dick test). Conversely, serum from a convalescent case of scarlet fever or artificially prepared streptococcal antitoxin will, when injected intradermally, cause local blanching of a scarlatinal rash (Schultz-Charlton reaction) due to neutralization of the toxin.

In localized outbreaks of scarlet fever, as in a school, there are usually cases of sore throat without rash and many healthy throat carriers; serological examination of the streptococci will show that these children are infected with the same streptococcal type as those with scarlet fever. They have developed streptococcal anti-toxin which protects them against the rash (but not against the primary streptococcal infection), presumably because of previous infections by strains that produce small amounts of toxin. Laboratory studies have shown that there are many different serotypes of *Strept. pyogenes* but only one main erythrogenic toxin. An individual may therefore suffer from frequent attacks of streptococcal sore throat but only one attack of scarlet fever. Specific antibodies to the M protein, the virulence antigen of the infecting streptococcus, develop slowly after sore throat or other streptococcal illness and persist for a long time so that repeat attacks by the same streptococcus serotype are unlikely; but this specific antibody does not protect against infection with other serotypes.

Besides the acute inflammatory and septic lesions caused by *Strept. pyogenes*, there are two other syndromes, acute rheumatic fever and acute glomerulonephritis (q.v.) that may follow an antecedent streptococcal infection. These two diseases are usually regarded as allergic tissue manifestation affecting predominantly heart and joint tissues (rheumatic fever) or kidney tissue (glomerulonephritis).

PATHOGENESIS

The most common route of entry of *Strept. pyogenes* is by the upper respiratory tract where the primary infection is established, usually in the throat. As is customary with this and other pathogens, only a proportion of infected individuals develop a clinical syndrome such as tonsillitis, pharyngitis or scarlet fever. The others may have mild atypical infections or become symptomless carriers. The nose is much less frequently infected and the streptococci usually disappear much earlier from the nose than from the throat. After an acute attack of sore throat the convalescent patient may carry the infecting streptococci in the fauces for some weeks; a few of these convalescent carriers may continue to carry the streptococci in throat or nose for much longer periods (persistent or chronic carriers), more especially if there is diseased tonsillar tissue or nasal deformity. A nose carrier sheds far greater numbers of

streptococci (e.g. 100-fold) into the environment than does a throat carrier and consequently nasal carriers, often with an associated sinusitis, are more likely sources for the spread of infection than are throat carriers although numerically nose carriers are much less common. The saliva of both cases and carriers may become contaminated, sometimes heavily, with haemolytic streptococci and may be responsible for spreading infection.

Strept. pyogenes is well-endowed with secretory enzymes or 'toxins', including two forms of *haemolysin*, streptolysin-O which is oxygen-labile and streptolysin-S which is not (these are toxic to a variety of tissues); *streptokinase* which lyses fibrin; *hyaluronidase* which increases tissue permeability by hydrolysing the tissue cement, hyaluronic acid; *DNAase* and *leucocidin* which destroy leucocytes. One or more of these substances may help the streptococcus in its attack or defence against the host tissues but the invasiveness or virulence of *Strept. pyogenes* is related particularly to a surface antigen, the M-protein, which is present during the acute phase of infection but may be scanty or absent in the later convalescent phase when variant forms of the coccus are present. Two other surface proteins, T and R, do not play any part in virulence but are useful in identification of the infecting serotype. The M-protein is responsible for the virulence of *Strept. pyogenes* because it is the main anti-phagocytic factor of the coccus. Hyaluronic acid capsules are produced by the cocci when spreading in the blood and tissues and in the early hours of artificial culture, but they have only a weak antiphagocytic effect. Antibodies to M-protein are the antibodies mainly responsible for immunity to *Strept. pyogenes*. They act as opsonins, counteracting the anti-phagocytic action of the M-protein and they are effective only against the homologous serotype of streptococcus.

A characteristic feature of streptococcal infections, whether the portal of entry be the throat or the skin or the genital tract, is the spread or permeation of the inflammation through the tissues in contrast to the much more localized inflammatory lesion which is characteristic of staphylococcal infections. A classical example of the spreading lesion is erysipelas and it is tempting to suppose that this permeation of the infection through the skin is related to the production of hyaluronidase; but *Straphylococcus aureus* also produces hyaluronidase and rarely causes spreading infections in the skin.

LABORATORY DIAGNOSIS

Since sore throat, with or without inflammatory exudate, may be caused by different agents and consequently requires different treatments, the physician should, whenever possible, obtain a laboratory report on material taken from the throat and, if need be, from the blood. The differential diagnosis may rest between streptococcal or viral infection, diphtheria, Vincent's angina, thrush, infective mononucleosis (glandular fever) and such blood dyscrasias as agranulocytosis and leukaemia when the throat becomes 'dirty' because of the absence of the normal scavengers, the phagocytes.

In taking a throat swab, the doctor or nurse must have a good view of the fauces, which means a good light and in most young children, a tongue depressor; the child's hands and head may have to be held by an attendant. If there is likely to be a delay of more than a few hours between taking the throat swab and its arrival at the laboratory, the swab should be placed in a transport or holding medium, e.g. Pike semisolid agar (q.v.), or a serum-coated swab may be used. When search is being made for carriers, e.g. in an institutional outbreak of sore throat and/or scarlet fever, deep nasal as well as throat swabs must be taken. In many cases, and particularly in children over 3 years of age, a specimen of saliva expectorated into a wide-mouthed container is easier to obtain and gives a higher proportion of positive results than a throat swab in both convalescent and chronic carriers (Ross, 1971). It may be desirable in the differential diagnosis to collect a sample of blood for leucocyte count (total and differential), erythrocyte sedimentation rate, and antistreptolysin or other streptococcal antibody tests.

CHEMOTHERAPY

Strept. pyogenes is highly sensitive to a wide range of antibacterial drugs—penicillin, erythromycin, tetracyclines, sulphonamides, etc.—but strains resistant to sulphonamides and tetracyclines are fairly common. A penicillin preparation is the drug of choice; penicillin-resistant strains of *Strept. pyogenes* are unknown, so that antibiotic-sensitivity tests are unnecessary if *Strept. pyogenes* is identified as the infecting organism. In an acute infection, early dosage should be given parenterally, e.g. a combination of benzyl and procaine penicillin, or a long-acting penicillin, e.g. benzathine penicillin (Penidural), which obviates the need for continuing oral penicillin therapy for 7 to 10 days. This prolongation of treatment for some days after the clinical infection has subsided is required if the infecting streptococcus is to be eliminated from the throat and the risk of septic and allergic complications (rheumatic fever, glomerulonephritis) reduced to a minimum. Bacteriostatic drugs like sulphonamides or tetracyclines should not be used for this purpose.

Although 50 to 70 per cent of cases of acute sore throat are caused by pathogens other than *Strept. pyogenes*, e.g. rhino-, adeno-, myxo- and entero-viruses which are not sensitive to antibacterial drugs, it seems wise to initiate antibiotic therapy in all cases and decide on the continuation or not of drug therapy after the laboratory report on the throat swab is received.

EPIDEMIOLOGY

The severity of streptococcal infections has become steadily and markedly reduced in many countries in the past century. The strongest evidence in support of this statement comes from the mortality rates for scarlet fever which has long been a notifiable disease. Death rates in Britain from this once dreaded disease have fallen from approximately 1000 per million population in the decade 1860–69 to virtually zero at the present time. The remarkable reduction in the severity of scarlet fever was accompanied by declines in the incidence, and mortality, of other severe streptococcal infections such as septicaemia, puerperal sepsis and malignant endocarditis and was apparent before the chemotherapeutic era. This general amelioration was probably related to a steady improvement in nutrition and in social and environmental conditions compared with the abject poverty and gross overcrowding during and after the industrial revolution when the rapid transfer of *Strept. pyogenes* in a highly susceptible population probably led to an exaltation in the virulence of the pathogen. However, despite the great reduction in severity, it is doubtful if there has been a corresponding reduction in the incidence of the commonest streptococcal syndrome, sore throat. It is true that notifications of scarlet fever have declined markedly in recent years but the doctor is not likely to notify what is nowadays a mild infectious disease which can be effectively treated at home without upsetting the family with notification and household disinfection.

Sources and Modes of Spread

Streptococcal throat infections have their highest incidence in school children in the age range 5 to 8 years and are rare (or rarely detected) in children under 2 years. The attack rates among school children in temperate climates are probably around 10 to 20 per cent per annum and may be higher among troops in training or in other closed or semi-closed communities. Streptococcal throat infections, and in particular scarlet fever, are much less commonly recognized in tropical countries, but such complications as otitis media and rheumatic heart disease are common enough. Glomerulonephritis is prevalent in some tropical and semi-tropical countries but the antecedent infection is more likely to be streptococcal impetigo than sore throat.

If a throat carrier of *Strept. pyogenes* speaks, coughs or sneezes towards an exposed blood-agar plate within a radius of 1 to 2 feet from his mouth, very few of the expelled droplets will carry haemolytic streptococci. A nose carrier, on the other hand, sheds large numbers of streptococci which abundantly contaminate his clothing and his environment and can be readily recovered from floor dust, bedding, books and the like in his immediate vicinity, where they may remain alive for days, weeks or months if shielded from daylight. This environmental contamination suggested that dust and fomites were more likely vehicles for the spread of streptococcal infections than droplet spray, and this view was supported by the studies of Wright, Cruickshank and Gunn (1944) on the control of

secondary streptococcal complications among hospitalized cases of measles by dust-suppressive measures. However, later studies by American workers (see Wannamaker, 1954) showed that men in barracks were remarkably resistant to primary throat infection from dust or bedding heavily contaminated with streptococci. Instead, there was a direct relationship between the incidence of infection and the proximity of the contact (a radius of about 8 feet) to the infected patient so that early transfer of *moist* secretions from an acute case or heavy nasal carrier by direct contact or by contaminated fomites may be the main mode of spread of *primary* streptococcal infection in healthy subjects. Dried secretions in contaminated dust and the like may nevertheless commonly infect highly susceptible tissues such as burns, or the respiratory mucosa after a primary virus infection, e.g. measles, influenza or common cold.

Besides the acute case of sore throat and the nasal or saliva carrier, other dangerous sources of infection are patients with streptococcal otitis media, vulvo-vaginitis or infected skin lesions. Although the nose carrier is the most likely focus for the initiation of streptococcal infections the throat and/or saliva carrier is the more common and more persistent reservoir of *Strept. pyogenes*; some 5 to 10 per cent of children will be throat carriers at any one time and this proportion increases sharply at times and in places of greater prevalence of clinical infection. The throat carrier rate may be 2 to 3 times higher in children with tonsils than in those without, and acute streptococcal infections tend to be more common in the former group; but this is not an argument in favour of indiscriminate tonsillectomy.

CONTROL OF STREPTOCOCCAL INFECTIONS

The early treatment of patients with streptococcal sore throat or other streptococcal infections with a bactericidal drug, such as penicillin or erythromycin, will quickly reduce the numbers of streptococci in the lesion to nil or to small numbers. At the same time as treatment is begun, a swab from the lesion should be sent to the laboratory for bacteriological examination, since more than half of sore throats are non-bacterial in origin. In streptococcal sore throat complete elimination of the infecting organism can be obtained only if treatment is continued for 7 to 10 days with an oral penicillin or erythromycin, or by giving a single large injection of a long-acting penicillin, e.g. benzathine penicillin. However, this last drug is more likely to produce sensitizing reactions than are other penicillins given orally. Unfortunately, a large proportion of children with sore throats will not be seen by a doctor during the acute episode: such patients will disseminate the infecting organism in the community and be themselves liable to develop secondary septic or non-septic complications.

In outbreaks it is important to search as early as possible for the dangerous spreader, most commonly a nasal carrier, but it may be a child with suppurating otitis media or an infected skin lesion. Such individuals should be isolated and treated with antimicrobial drugs. Heavy nasal carriers are best treated with systemic rather than local therapy, as there is often an associated sinusitis. Treatment of these dangerous carriers is particularly important in children's wards, where young sick patients may develop serious secondary infections. In some hospitals admission swabs are taken to detect a dangerous carrier so that he may be temporarily isolated. Because gross environmental contamination quickly occurs in closed spaces, such as hospital wards, dormitories, and barracks, where there may be dangerous 'shedders' of haemolytic streptococci, bedding and floors should be washed and disinfected regularly and particularly after an outbreak of infection. In children's wards the communal use of toys, books, pencils, and the like should be prohibited. Dust control measures in hospitals or barracks, such as oiling of floors and blankets, present technical difficulties and are probably not of much value unless there are patients with highly susceptible tissues, e.g. burns or virus respiratory infections.

NON-SUPPURATIVE COMPLICATIONS OF STREPTOCOCCAL INFECTION

1. Rheumatic Fever

There is nowadays general agreement that an attack of acute rheumatic fever is related to an antecedent streptococcal throat infection occurring 1 to 5 weeks earlier. Support for this association is based on epidemiological, bacteriological, serological and therapeutic evidence.

Outbreaks of streptococcal sore throat in schools have been followed a few weeks later by a crop of cases of rheumatic fever; in army training camps in North America, 3 to 4 per cent of patients with proven streptococcal tonsillitis or scarlet fever have developed rheumatic fever; and in institutions for convalescent cases of rheumatic fever, outbreaks of streptococcal infection have been followed by a high incidence of rheumatic fever relapses. Sometimes the association is much less obvious. Among school children suffering from streptococcal sore throats, rheumatic fever is nowadays a rare sequela occurring in, perhaps, 1 in 500 to 1 in 1000 of such cases. However, rheumatic heart disease may be discovered in children with no clear history of antecedent sore throat or rheumatic fever; this finding occurs particularly in tropical countries where the rheumatic syndrome has its greatest incidence in young children (3 to 7 years old) in comparison with the later peak (8 to 12 years) in Britain, and even later in U.S.A.

Laboratory evidence for antecedent streptococcal infection is based on bacteriological and serological data. *Strept. pyogenes* has been isolated from the throats of 50 to 80 per cent of cases of rheumatic fever occurring a few weeks after an untreated primary sore throat; and the social class and age distribution of the rheumatic syndrome correlates well with the distribution of streptococcal carrier rates. The demonstration of raised or rising levels of streptococcal antibodies, e.g. antistreptolysin 0 and/or antistreptokinase, antihyaluronidase, anti-DNAase in 95 per cent of cases of rheumatic fever is perhaps the strongest evidence of the association with an earlier streptococcal infection. These antibodies are usually at higher levels and persist for longer periods in rheumatic disease than happens in uncomplicated streptococcal infections.

The supporting chemotherapeutic evidence comes mainly from the prophylactic value of prolonged therapy with penicillin or sulphonamides in patients who have already suffered from one or more attacks of rheumatic fever. Recurrent attacks are not uncommon (20 to 50 per cent) after a fresh streptococcal infection and these can be largely prevented by the long-term administration of an antistreptococcal drug, preferably one of the penicillins. Similarly, if the patient is under medical care, treatment of the primary streptococcal throat infection with penicillin for 7 to 10 days will eliminate the pathogen and minimize the risk of a subsequent attack of rheumatic fever.

In summary, there is conclusive evidence of the association between rheumatic fever and an antecedent streptococcal throat infection but not with primary streptococcal infections of other tissues. The streptococci are not present in the lesions in the heart and joints. No particular streptococcus serotypes are incriminated as happens with glomerulonephritis and it is for this reason that repeat throat infections with different serotypes occur and cause relapses of rheumatic fever; the evidence indicates that some antigenic component of *Strept. pyogenes,* cellular or extracellular, is involved, perhaps in association with cardiac tissue (muscle or valve) in establishing an allergic hypersensitivity which produces the syndrome of rheumatic fever. There can be little doubt that selected individuals are prone to develop the rheumatic syndrome and the patient with this rheumatic genotype, once he has suffered an initial attack of rheumatic fever, is particularly liable to recurrent attacks after further streptococcal sore throats. However, the significance of the hereditary predisposition in families is very difficult to disentangle from predisposing environmental factors. Of these factors, the most important is overcrowding in families and in communities which facilitates the spread of streptococcal infection. For example, the rates of rheumatic heart disease among school children in Scotland is lowest in the Northern and North-Eastern regions (28 to 46 per 100 000), intermediate in the Eastern and South-Eastern regions (75 to 95 per 100 000) and highest in the Western region (116 per 100 000) which corresponds with the degree of urbanization and overcrowding in these five regions. On the other hand, congenital heart disease, with much higher rates, shows little variation in the four more populous regions (Fig. 16.1). This factor of crowding is

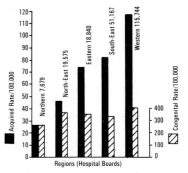

FIG. 16.1. Organic heart disease in Scotland, from the school medical inspection in 1964. Rate per 100 000 per region.

the main reason for the high prevalence of rheumatic heart disease in the cities of many developing countries. Another interesting but unexplained phenomenon is the increasing disparity in the deaths from rheumatic heart disease between men and women with advancing age. Although the primary rheumatic infection has similar morbidity and mortality rates in the two sexes, total deaths from rheumatic heart disease in Scotland have been in the ratio of 2:3 for males and females in the age-range 25 to 44 years, about 1:2 in the age-range 45 to 64 years and nearly 1:3 in those aged 65 years or older. The sex difference in the *death rates* has been maintained in the 45 to 64 years age group in recent years, but has gradually disappeared in the younger, 25 to 44 years age group (Fig. 16.2 and 16.3).

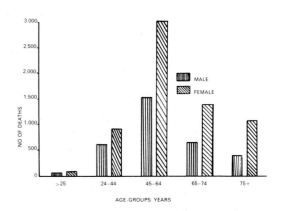

FIG. 16.2. Deaths in males and females from rheumatic heart disease, Scotland, 1958 to 1970.

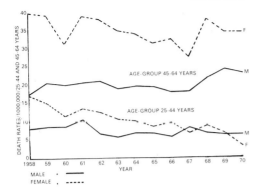

FIG. 16.3. Death rates in males and females from rheumatic heart disease, Scotland, 1958 to 1970.

2. Acute Glomerulonephritis

Acceptance of the association between acute glomerulonephritis and an antecedent streptococcal infection is based on similar evidence to that for rheumatic fever. The pathogenesis of this form of nephritis is possibly similar to that of the rheumatic syndrome; that is, an acquired tissue hypersensitivity or autoimmune disease with the kidney as the involved organ developing 1 to 4 weeks after a primary streptococcal infection. *Strept. pyogenes* is not found in the kidneys or urine. There are several distinctive features about this streptococcus-mediated disease: (a) it follows infection with a limited number of streptococcal 'nephritogenic' serotypes; (b) the primary infection may affect the skin and not the throat; in warm climate countries particularly, streptococcal impetigo or secondarily infected scabies is more likely to be the antecedent infection than a sore throat; and (c) second attacks are very rare. In throat infections, the infecting streptococcus is most commonly Griffith type 12, less often types 4 and 25; in impetigo, type 49 is most commonly incriminated, but types 2, 52, 55, 57 have also been involved; the M antigen may be masked by an associated T antigen of another type, e.g. T type 14 antigen may mask the M 49 antigen (Maxted *et al.,* 1967).

In temperate climates, the incidence of acute glomerulonephritis tends to be episodic dependent, presumably, on the occurrence of primary throat infections with nephritogenic streptococci. School children and young adults are most often affected; mild or atypical cases with transient albuminuria and haematuria are found during outbreaks in institutions or epidemic waves in a community. However, recognized nephritogenic types, e.g. type 12, may cause epidemic or sporadic throat infections without an associated nephritis. In tropical countries, the age of attack is earlier than in temperate climates with the peak around 3 to 4 years of age. Experimentally, Matheson and Reed (1959) were able to produce acute nephritis in rabbits and monkeys after intravenous injection of a culture filtrate of nephritogenic streptococcus type 12 or of a purified polypeptide fraction. Other workers have been less successful. Early penicillin therapy of the primary streptococcal infection seems to reduce the risk of subsequent kidney disease.

OTHER BETA-HAEMOLYTIC STREPTOCOCCI

Beta-haemolytic streptococci of groups other than group A are only occasionally incriminated as human pathogens; such strains belong almost invariably to groups C, G, B and D of the 18 Lancefield groups, labelled A to T.

Group C streptococci are predominantly animal parasites; 4 biochemical types are recognized and that designated *Strept. equisimilis* is the one most commonly associated with human disease, e.g. it has been found in cases of puerperal infection, and has also been isolated from cases of cellulitis, tonsillitis, wounds and scarlet fever.

The majority of group G strains have been found as commensals in the human oropharynx; its pathogenic role is restricted to occasional cases of puerperal infection and possibly pharyngitis; it has been responsible for epidemics of canine tonsillitis.

Colonies of group B on blood agar do not produce such marked β-haemolysis as do group A strains. Some strains give α-haemolysis or are non-haemolytic. It is encountered as a commensal in the human vagina and throat but is only rarely pathogenic to the human subject; it may cause pharyngitis and has been recorded in a few cases of puerperal infection and ulcerative endocarditis. As *Strept. agalactiae,* it is the most common cause of bovine mastitis.

Group D or *Strept. faecalis* (enterococcus) is discussed on p. 255.

STREPTOCOCCUS VIRIDANS: BACTERIAL ENDOCARDITIS

Streptococcus viridans, so-called because of the green pigmentation that surrounds colonies of the organism grown on blood agar and more distinctively on heated (chocolate) blood agar, is a normal commensal of the oropharynx. Morphologically it resembles *Strept. pyogenes* and has a tendency to occur in short chains when grown in a fluid medium. It is non-capsulate. On ordinary blood agar, colonies are small and convex and are surrounded by a zone of partial haemolysis (alpha-haemolysis) and green discoloration; there may be a thin outer rim of complete lysis, especially after overnight refrigeration. Because of the green pigmentation colonies of *Strept. viridans* resemble pneumococcal colonies but *Strept. viridans* is distinguishable from the pneumococcus by being non-capsulate, non-bile-soluble, resistant to optochin and non-virulent for the mouse. Biochemical reactions and antigenic characters are little used in identification or classification although several distinct serotypes have been recognized in strains isolated from the oropharynx and from cases of bacterial endocarditis. *Strept. viridans* is not a single defined species but is the name given to streptococci belonging to several species that produce alpha-haemolysis, e.g. *Strept. mitis, Strept. sanguis* and *Strept. salivarius.*

Pathogenicity

Strept. viridans is a constant and numerous commensal of the mouth, being present in most persons throughout life in numbers in the order of 10^9 per ml saliva. It has little intrinsic pathogenicity, but may act as an opportunistic pathogen and attack tissues with lowered resistance. It is one of the varieties of non-haemolytic streptococci which play a major role in the causation of dental caries (q.v.) and is a pathogen in periodontal infections. It is, however, its causative role in subacute bacterial

endocarditis that has given *Strept. viridans* an important place in medicine. This infection, which before the advent of penicillin was almost invariably fatal after a febrile course of 6 to 10 weeks, affects heart valves that have been damaged by antecedent rheumatic infection, syphilis and, in more recent years, arteriosclerosis or malignant disease, or are congenitally malformed; other congenital abnormalities such as ventricular septal defects and aortic stenosis also predispose to infection. When rheumatic fever was more common than it is nowadays, subacute bacterial endocarditis occurred most frequently among young adults; in recent years a much higher proportion of the cases occur in the age range 40 to 70 years and tend to run a more rapid course. In the earlier period, *Strept. viridans* was the causal organism in approximately 90 per cent of cases and there was a close association between periodontal sepsis and/or tooth extraction and the onset of bacterial endocarditis due to the bacteriaemia that generally is produced for 5 to 15 min after dental extractions. With the shift to the older age groups, the range of incriminated bacteria has widened and includes non-haemolytic and micro-aerophilic streptococci, *Strept. faecalis, Staphylococcus albus, Haemophilus influenzae,* bacteroides, and *Coxiella burnetii*, with presumably other primary foci than the oropharynx such as the respiratory and urinary tracts. In a proportion of cases (10 to 20 per cent), repeated blood cultures have failed to isolate any bacterium. Since *Staph. albus* from the skin is the commonest contaminant of blood cultures the finding of *Staph. albus* in a blood culture requires confirmation by further blood culture and its significance proved by the demonstration of specific antibody to the isolated staphylococcus.

Treatment

With the greater range of incriminated bacteria, the rational and optimal antimicrobial therapy of patients with bacterial endocarditis requires close collaboration between the bacteriologist and the physician. Although *Strept. viridans* is generally more resistant to penicillin than is *Strept. pyogenes,* a penicillin preparation is still the first drug of choice but with more resistant bacteria such as *Strept. faecalis* a combination of penicillin and streptomycin may be required or other drugs may be used according to the drug-sensitivities of the infecting organism. Treatment with adequate dosage must be continued for 4 to 6 weeks; even so, the case-fatality for patients under 40 years of age with *Strept. viridans* infections will vary from 20 to 30 per cent, and in the older age groups with underlying cardiac or other disease, the case mortality will be much higher (60 to 80 per cent). Any patient with recognized valvular disease of the heart or congenital cardiac abnormality who requires dental treatment should be given penicillin (100 000 units benzyl penicillin, plus 300 000 procaine penicillin) *one half to one hour and no earlier* before treatment and this prophylaxis against bacteriaemia should be continued for 24 to 48 hours. The pathogenesis and treatment of bacterial endocarditis was fully discussed in a recent R.C.P. Symposium (1970).

STREPTOCOCCUS FAECALIS (ENTEROCOCCUS)

This streptococcus which almost constantly inhabits the intestine of man and animals as a commensal is oval in shape and occurs in pairs (like spectacles) or short chains. Ordinarily, its colonies do not cause any change in blood agar but a variant causes a clear zone of haemolysis without producing soluble haemolysin, and the species is classified antigenically as Lancefield group D. *Strept. faecalis* grows on MacConkey's and other bile-salt lactose media (forming very small, pink colonies) and also in the presence of a high salt content (6·5 per cent). Characteristic features are its resistance to heat at 60°C for half an hour, fermentation of aesculin and of mannitol with gas formation.

At most, it is an opportunistic pathogen when it gains access to the urinary tract, either alone or more often in association with coliform organisms. It is also one of the less common streptococci in cases of subacute bacterial endocarditis. It has a high degree of resistance to many antimicrobial drugs.

STREPTOCOCCI AND DENTAL DISEASE

Certain alpha-haemolytic and non-haemolytic streptococci, e.g. *Strept. mutans*, *Strept. sanguis*, *Strept. mitis* and *Strept. faecalis*, are commonly found in large numbers in dental plaque, carious teeth and root abscesses and probably play an important part in initiating caries and periodontal disease.

Dental Caries

When fed on a sucrose-rich diet, rats and hamsters with a normal oral flora develop caries. Germ-free animals fed on the same diet remain free from caries, but readily develop it when they are later infected with a pure culture of *Strept. mutans* or *Strept. sanguis* and sometimes do so when infected with *Lactobacillus casei* or *L. acidophilus*.

In man, streptococci form about half the bacterial population of 'plaque', a soft whitish material that accumulates on the surfaces of the teeth if they are not regularly cleaned. *Strept. mutans* and *Strept. sanguis* are the principal bacteria in the plaque that forms on smooth surfaces and are the cause of *smooth-surface caries*. They convert dietary sucrose into dextran, an insoluble, inert, gelatinous polysaccharide which enables them to adhere to the dental surface. These streptococci, as well as the less numerous but more highly aciduric lactobacilli present in the plaque, ferment part of the sucrose and other dietary carbohydrates to form lactic acid. The acid is held locally by the diffusion-inhibiting dextran and protected from neutralization by the saliva. It dissolves the hydroxy-apatite (calcium phosphate/hydroxide) of the tooth enamel and dentine, allowing lactobacilli to invade the tubules of the dentine and continue the process. *Fissural caries,* which begins in crevices protected from mechanical scouring, is caused by a variety of streptococci and lactobacilli, including non-dextran-producers, without need for the production of a very gelatinous plaque.

Periodontal Disease

Plaque that forms in the angle around the crown of the tooth just above the margin of the gum, contains principally *Strept. mitis* and *Strept. faecalis*. When teeth are not brushed, this marginal plaque grows down into the gingival crevice where it induces a change of flora to one dominated by anaerobic Gram-negative cocci (veillonellae), bacilli, vibrios and spirochaetes and this change leads to the development of gingivitis and pyorrhoea.

ANAEROBIC STREPTOCOCCI

Streptococci that can grow only as obligate anaerobes have undoubted pathogenicity for man. *Peptostreptococcus putridus* is the best documented species.

They are Gram-positive cocci resembling facultatively anaerobic streptococci but frequently much smaller (0·5 μm or less) and exhibiting pleomorphism in artificial culture. After anaerobic incubation for 48 hours, colonies on blood agar are smooth, low-convex, approximately 1 to 2 mm in diameter; no alteration occurs in the medium. Cultures in meat broth are proteolytic and usually give off an exceptionally foul odour.

Attempts have been made to classify the anaerobic streptococci on their biochemical reactions; provided that a sulphur compound is present (e.g. 0·1 per cent sodium thioglycollate) in the medium, *Pepto. putridus* strains ferment glucose, maltose and fructose with abundant gas production.

Pathogenicity

The main normal habitats of the anaerobic streptococci are the vagina and the intestine. *Pepto. putridus* is incriminated in low-grade puerperal sepsis, probably as an endogenous infection precipitated by trauma and the presence of necrotic material; characteristically it produces a septic thrombophlebitis in the pelvic veins with metastatic abscesses in the lungs. It has also been isolated from brain abscess, infected wounds, e.g. post-operative synergistic bacterial gangrene, and anaerobic streptococcal myositis. Strains are sensitive to penicillin which should be used in large doses therapeutically for 1 to 2 weeks.

LABORATORY DIAGNOSIS. Strictly anaerobic methods are required if isolation is to be successful. Inoculation of blood agar plates and incubation for 48 hours in a McIntosh and Fildes' jar produces colonies as described above. For details of the classification and pathogenicity of anaerobic species other than *Pepto. putridus* the report by Thomas and Hare (1954) should be consulted.

REFERENCES AND FURTHER READING

MATHESON, B. H. & REED, R. W. (1959) Experimental nephritis due to type specific streptococci. *Journal of Infectious Diseases,* **104,** 213.

MAXTED, W. R., FRASER, C. A. M. & PARKER, M. T. (1967) *Streptococcus pyogenes* type 49: a nephritogenic streptococcus with a wide geographic distribution. *Lancet,* **1,** 641.

R.C.P. SYMPOSIUM (1971) *Bacterial Endocarditis. Proceedings of the National Symposium,* Royal College of Physicians, London.

ROSS, P. R. (1971) Beta-haemolytic streptococci in saliva. *Journal of Hygiene, Cambridge,* **69,** 347.

THOMAS, C. G. A. & HARE, R. (1954) The classification of anaerobic streptococci and their isolation in normal human beings and pathological processes. *Journal of Clinical Pathology,* **7,** 300.

WANNAKER, L. M. (1954) The epidemiology of streptococcal infections. In *Streptococcal Infections.* New York.

WORLD HEALTH ORGANIZATION (1966) Prevention of Rheumatic Fever. *Technical Report Series* No. 342, Geneva.

WORLD HEALTH ORGANIZATION (1968) Streptococcal and straphylococcal infections. *Technical Report Series* No. 394, Geneva.

WRIGHT, JOYCE, CRUICKSHANK, R. & GUNN, W. (1944) The control of dust-borne streptococcal infection in measles wards. *British Medical Journal,* **ii,** 611.

The pneumococci are primarily concerned with infections of the upper and lower respiratory tracts, but are carried in the throat by many healthy persons. They are the commonest primary pathogens in lobar, lobular and broncho-pneumonia, and bronchiolitis and are frequently associated as secondary pathogens, after primary virus infections of the respiratory tract, in acute and chronic catarrhs, sinusitis, bronchitis and otitis media. The pneumococci are, therefore, major contributors to a vast amount of morbidity and economic loss since respiratory infections are responsible for 30 to 40 per cent of the illnesses requiring medical attention and of sickness absenteeism in schools and industries. They are particularly frequent and severe at the extremes of life.

The pneumococci are also associated with such suppurative infections as empyema, meningitis, peritonitis and arthritis.

DESCRIPTION

The pneumococcus belongs to the family *Lactobacillaceae* and the generic name *Diplococcus pneumoniae* is commonly used although the term *Streptococcus pneumoniae* may be found in some textbooks. It is a Gram-positive coccus, about 1.0 μm in diameter, ovoid or lanceolate, occurring in pairs with the broader ends apposed (Plate 2.3). In infective material, the pneumococcus shows a well-defined capsule surrounding the diplococci but after artificial cultivation the capsules are less easily seen whilst the cocci are more rounded and may occur in short chains. It is an aerobe and facultative anaerobe but most strains prefer an atmosphere of 5 to 10 per cent CO_2 for primary culture. The addition of 0.1 per cent glucose or of 5 to 10 per cent blood or serum facilitates growth which is optimal at $37°C$. On a blood agar medium, the colonies are small and flat with, later, a raised rim (draughtsman); around the colony there is partial clearing of the blood (alpha-haemolysis)

with green coloration like that around colonies of *Strep. viridans*. The pneumococcus is distinguishable from the latter organism by being capsulate, uniformly turbid in broth culture, bile-soluble, sensitive to optochin and highly virulent for the mouse. The pneumococcus ferments various carbohydrates including, as a rule, inulin. It dies rather easily on repeated subculture which also leads to a change from the smooth (S) capsulate form to a rough (R) non-capsulate form with concomitant loss of virulence. R forms originate as spontaneous mutants from S forms and outgrow the parental S forms under the conditions of prolonged or repeated artificial culture. *In vivo*, R mutants are selectively eliminated by phagocytosis.

Antigenically, the pneumococci are divisible into some 80 serotypes, related to the specific chemical composition of the capsular polysaccharide substance. Identification of the serotype may be made by agglutination tests with suspensions of a pure culture or by the so-called capsule-swelling ('quellung') reaction, a phenomenon in which the pneumococcal capsule becomes sharply delineated but not swollen when it comes in contact with its specific antiserum. This test may be carried out on fresh infective material, e.g. sputum, or on a young culture or on mouse peritoneal exudate (see Vol. II, Chap. 20). Serotyping of pneumococci may have value in both the medical care and control of pneumococcal pneumonias.

PATHOGENESIS

It is important to distinguish two main categories of disease syndromes associated with the pneumococcus. One category includes lobar pneumonia and some suppurative infections, e.g. meningitis and peritonitis, which are mostly caused by a limited number of pneumococcus serotypes—1, 2, 5, 7, 12, 14—possessing infectious and invasive qualities that facilitate primary attack on healthy tissues. The other category includes secondary infections of upper and lower respiratory tracts, e.g. sinusitis, bronchitis, broncho-pneumonia, by opportunistic or potentially pathogenic pneumococci—types 4, 6, 10, 18, 19, 22, 23, etc.—already resident in the oro- or nasopharynx and ready to attack tissues of lowered resistance. Two pneumococcus types, 3 and 8, are probably intermediate in invasiveness but, because they are rich in capsular substance, they may produce very severe infections, particularly in elderly debilitated persons.

In lobar pneumonia, the highly virulent pneumococcus, once it has penetrated the bronchial mucosa, spreads diffusely through the hitherto healthy lung via the peribronchial tissues and lymphatics. In bronchitis and bronchopneumonia, on the other hand, the pneumococci, which are generally less virulent, spread along the mucosal surface of the bronchial tree, which is probably already damaged by a predisposing viral infection or other condition, and invade the lung tissues only to a short distance from the mucosa. The causal role of pneumococci, like that of *Haemophilus influenzae*, in chronic bronchitis and its acute exacerbations is probably facilitated by the excessive secretion of bronchial mucus in that syndrome which may be due primarily to tobacco smoking, atmospheric pollution, allergy or other as yet unknown causes.

Pneumococci are frequently inhaled into the upper and lower respiratory tracts but the usual outcome of such introductions is elimination of the organisms by phagocytosis and other normal defence mechanisms. In some persons the introduction leads to the establishment of symptomless carriage in the nasopharynx. It is possible that the introduction of a virulent type of pneumococcus sometimes causes nasopharyngitis, but whether pneumococci can act as primary pathogens in producing an exogenous clinical infection of the throat is uncertain. The available evidence suggests that pneumonia is seldom if ever caused by the direct inhalation of pneumococci from the environment into the lungs, i.e. by direct exogenous infection. Probably the infecting pneumococcus first becomes established in the nasopharynx and then some days or weeks later, if the carrier is subjected to a predisposing condition, it may spread to and infect the lung, the middle ear, a paranasal

sinus or the meninges. The conditions most commonly predisposing to pneumonia are probably virus infections, including the common cold, but chilling, excessive intake of alcohol and deep anaesthesia, conditions that predispose to aspiration of secretions from the throat into the lower respiratory tract, may also be effective.

Capsule as Virulence Factor

The main virulence factor of the pneumococcus is its capsular polysaccharide which, because of its highly acidic and hydrophilic properties, renders the pneumococci, when suspended in fluid, very difficult for phagocytes to trap and ingest. Non-capsulate mutant (R) forms of pneumococci lack this resistance to phagocytosis and are entirely non-virulent for experimental animals like the mouse and rabbit, and presumably also for man. Capsulate pneumococci, although resistant to phagocytosis when suspended in fluid, are nevertheless moderately susceptible to phagocytosis when lying on a surface, e.g. a bronchial or alveolar wall, or a deposit of fibrin, against which the phagocytes may trap them. Infection of the respiratory tract is therefore facilitated by conditions, such as primary virus infections, that cause an excessive secretion of mucus, since this mucus protects the pneumococci from 'surface' phagocytosis and allows their free growth. There is evidence suggesting that lobar pneumonia may be produced in the hitherto healthy lower respiratory tract of a throat carrier of pneumococcus when, in the course of a viral infection of the upper respiratory tract, nasopharyngeal secretion containing pneumococci is aspirated into the lower tract.

TOXINS. Pneumococcus is generally cited as an example of a pathogen combining high invasiveness with minimal toxigenicity. The failure to demonstrate its production of a significantly potent toxin has left in doubt the mechanism by which it causes death in cases of pneumonia and septicaemia. A weak oxygen-labile haemolysin (pneumolysin) and a weak oxygen-labile leucocidin with some general cytotoxic activity have been demonstrated in bacteria-free filtrates or centrifuged supernates of cultures, but their role is unknown.

Immunity

Since the antiphagocytic capsule is the principal virulence factor of the pneumococcus, the principal protective antibody is antibody specific for the capsular polysaccharide. This antibody exerts a strong opsonic effect so that the capsulate pneumococcus is easily phagocytosed. Production of anticapsular antibody in the course of infection is probably the main factor bringing about recovery, for example by 'crisis', that often takes place about the 7th or 8th day in untreated cases of lobar pneumonia. Since the anticapsular antibody is type-specific, the acquired immunity is specific for each of the 80 different types of pneumococcus, and a person recovered from pneumonia due to one type of pneumococcus may at any time suffer a second attack of pneumonia due to infection with a pneumococcus of a different type. In the period before sulphonamides and penicillin became available for the treatment of pneumococcal pneumonia, horse or rabbit antiserum was administered to patients with a beneficial and often life-saving effect; it was necessary for this purpose that the type of the pneumococcus infecting the patient should be determined and that antiserum specific for this type should be given. Similarly if vaccines are to be used effectively for active immunization against pneumococcal infection, they must contain a mixture of the capsular polysaccharides from all the more common types of pneumococcus likely to cause infection in the community (see p. 261).

Many persons who are not known to have suffered pneumococcal infection nevertheless possess antibodies to various types of the organism. They may have developed these antibodies either as a result of having carried the corresponding pneumococci for a long period (e.g. many months) in the nasopharynx or by ingestion of cross-reacting antigenic polysaccharides in vegetable foodstuffs. If prolonged throat carriage does lead to the production of protective antibodies, then the danger of endogenous infection being induced in a carrier through exposure to a precipitary factor, such as an upper respiratory-tract virus infection, must be limited to the early weeks after the start of carriage.

Pneumonia, which on the basis of clinical and radiological findings is divisible into lobar, segmental, lobular and broncho-pneumonia, is a disease syndrome of varied microbial aetiology. For these pneumonias and for other severe chest infections, e.g. bronchiolitis and croup in children, chronic bronchitis, primary atypical and interstitial pneumonias in adults, precise aetiological diagnosis is often essential for effective antimicrobial therapy and good medical care. Sputum that has been coughed up (not salivary secretion) or, when sputum is not available, a laryngeal swab should be transmitted to the laboratory as early and as quickly as possible with all relevant information including any history of anti-microbial therapy before admission. In addition, blood for culture and for the first of two serum specimens for virus antibodies and cold agglutinins should also be obtained on admission. Sputum is homogenized by shaking with water and glass beads in a mechanical shaker and inoculated on plates of blood agar and heated blood agar. It may also be injected intraperitoneally into a mouse when a search is to be made for scanty pneumococci. The inoculated plates are incubated for 18 hours at $37°C$ in an atmosphere of 5 to 10 per cent CO_2 and suspected colonies of bacterial pathogens—pneumococci, *H. influenzae*, staphylococci and β-haemolytic streptococci—are picked for further identification. The second serum specimen is taken after 2 to 3 weeks and the paired sera are tested for antibodies against influenza and parainfluenza viruses, the adenovirus group, psittacosis, Q fever, and cold agglutinins or antibodies to mycoplasma infection (Vol. II, Chap. 11).

In a series of 156 adult patients with pneumonia or severe bronchitis, admitted to an Edinburgh hospital, pneumococci were isolated from sputum and/or blood in 44 per cent; in 13 per cent of these cases there were associated *H. influenzae* which were also isolated as the main pathogen in another 10 per cent of cases. *Staphylococcus aureus* was the significant pathogen in 8 per cent. In 38·5 per cent of all patients, no bacterial pathogens were isolated; since a quarter of these cases were classified as lobar pneumonia in which the pneumococcus is much the commonest pathogen and since 39 per cent of all patients had antimicrobial drugs before admission, it was assumed that many of the pathogen-negative cases were in fact pneumococcal infections. Serological evidence of recent virus infection was found in 18 per cent of all cases (Bath *et al.,* 1964).

It has been argued that routine blood culture and pneumococcus serotyping are worthwhile procedures in adult cases of pneumonia because of their prognostic significance. Austrian (1970) reported a case-fatality of 18 per cent in a large series of bacteriaemic pneumococcal pneumonias; in type 3 pneumococcus infections, it was 48 per cent. In an Edinburgh series of 137 cases of pneumococcal pneumonia, 50 (36 per cent) were type 3 infections and 5 of these died (4 with positive blood culture): the overall case fatality was 7·3 per cent (Calder, McHardy and Schonell, 1970).

For the isolation of bacterial pathogens in lower respiratory tract infections of young children, a serum-coated laryngeal swab, plated on blood agar and certain selective media, gave satisfactory results in a London series of 191 hospitalized patients (mostly under 5 years of age) in whom pneumococci were the most common pathogens followed by *Staphylococcus aureus, H. influenzae, β*-haemolytic streptococci and coliform bacilli in that order of frequency (Morrison *et al.,* 1957). If there is likely to be delay in the swab reaching the laboratory, it should first be inoculated into a modified Pike medium and plated out after overnight incubation.

CHEMOTHERAPY

The pneumococcus is sensitive to a wide range of antimicrobial drugs including the penicillins, tetracyclines and sulphonamides. In the treatment of pneumonia in adults or children at home or in hospital, identification of the infecting pathogen may not be sought or is known only after chemotherapy has been started. In such circumstances, broad-spectrum bactericidal drugs like ampicillin or the combination of trimethoprim and sulphamethoxazole (cotrimoxazole), both of which can be given orally is likely to be effective. In severe infections, parenteral injections of combined penicillin and streptomycin may be preferred. If and when the

infecting pathogen has been identified and its drug sensitivity ascertained, a switch may have to be made to the appropriate antimicrobial drug. Tetracycline-resistant pneumococci are now not uncommon (Percival, Armstrong and Turner, 1969) and recently, penicillin-resistant pneumococci, developing sometimes in the course of treatment or chemoprophylaxis, have been encountered (Calder, unpublished; Hausman *et al.,* 1971). The treatment of chronic bronchitis is considered in Chapter 20.

EPIDEMIOLOGY

The number of deaths from pneumonia in England and Wales has been increasing in recent years (41 027 in 1968) and with bronchitis and influenza (total 78 335) these respiratory infections rank fourth to cardiovascular diseases, cancers and cerebrovascular diseases in the mortality table. The increase in deaths and in mortality rates from pneumonia probably reflects the greater longevity of the population and the weakening of resistance to infection in old age; seven-tenths of all pneumonia deaths occur in persons over 65 years of age. Young children are the other highly susceptible age group and account for one-tenth of all deaths from pneumonia. Although the death rate from pneumonia at all ages is almost equal in male and females, it is much higher for men than for women in the age group 55 to 64 years (71 versus 40 per 100 000) and this disparity is even greater for the death rates from bronchitis in the same age-group (217 versus 39). In the Morbidity Statistics for General Practice (Report, 1962) respiratory infections constituted one quarter of practitioner consultations, the age groups most affected being 0 to 5 years and 65 years or over. The highest consultation rates were in urban communities and the lowest in rural areas; and they were, of course, highest in the winter months. There was a steeply rising gradient from social class I to V of consultation rates for pneumonia and bronchitis among males aged 15 to 64 years and for bronchitis in children aged 0 to 5 years.

Source and Mode of Infection

Pneumococci of one or other type are found growing, apparently like commensals, in the nasopharynx of about 30 per cent of healthy persons examined on a single occasion, and in lesser numbers in the oral and nasal secretions of many of these throat carriers. The pneumococcus is relatively resistant to drying and other common environmental conditions and it therefore may readily be spread from the throat of one person to that of another by any of the routes generally applicable to respiratory-tract infections, e.g. by the distribution of dust derived from dried respiratory-tract secretion, which may become airborne and be inhaled, by contact with fingers and other articles soiled with secretion and possibly, by secretion droplet-spray and droplet-nuclei.

It is important to emphasize that most of the severe chest infections at the extremes of life are endogenous infections by opportunistic resident bacteria such as pneumococci, *H. influenzae* and staphylococci and that they develop when respiratory mucosal resistance is lowered by antecedent virus infections or from social and environmental causes. On the other hand, most cases of lobar pneumonia in older children and healthy adults are primarily exogenous infections derived from cases or carriers of the limited number of the more infectious and invasive pneumococcus types. Outbreaks of lobar pneumonia are rare but have occurred in army training camps and in heavy industries such as steel works. Because most of the younger patients with lobar pneumonia respond well to chemotherapy, they are nowadays often treated at home whereas older persons with severe respiratory infections are usually admitted to hospital. When detailed investigations including pneumococcus typing are made in these hospitalized cases, pneumococcus type 3 is found to be the most frequent pathogen and with type 8 accounts for over 50 per cent of the pneumococcal pneumonias (Calder, McHardy and Schonell, 1970); 30 to 40 years ago pneumococcus types 1 and 2 were the causal agents in the pneumonias of 50 to 70 per cent of the hospitalized patients, a large proportion of whom were 20 to 40 year-old adults.

CONTROL MEASURES

Chest infections take their heaviest toll at the extremes of life. In the old, a terminal pneumonia has been called 'the old man's friend', but much of the high morbidity and mortality from bronchitis and pneumonia in young children is preventable. The incidence of primary respiratory virus infections may be the same in all social classes but the secondary bacterial infections are mostly associated with poverty and overcrowding. What particular factor (or factors) in this social complex is important in precipitating severe secondary infection is still unknown but besides crowding, inadequate clothing and undue exposure to climatic changes may play a part. As yet, there are no prophylactic virus vaccines (apart from influenza vaccine) that can be used against the upper respiratory infections so that continuing efforts must be made to improve the social and environmental conditions which predispose to bronchitis and pneumonia in young children.

The prophylaxis of lobar pneumonia has been attempted by the use of combined vaccines of the prevalent pneumococcus types in circumstances where there is a high incidence of infection, e.g. among native labourers in the South African mines, where the results were disappointing, and in army camps, where more encouraging results have been obtained. In particular, a controlled trial during the second World War of a combined antigen of purified polysaccharides prepared from four of the main epidemic types (types 1, 2, 5 and 7) indicated that a high degree of protection could be obtained against infection with these types after a single injection of 0·06 mg of each of the polysaccharides (McLeod *et al.*, 1945). Recently, Austrian (1970) has advocated the use of prophylactic vaccines made from the purified polysaccharide antigens of the more common invasive pneumococcus types in the civilian community on the grounds that, in U.S.A., 75 per cent of bacteriaemic pneumococcal pneumonias are caused by 10 serotypes which are also responsible for 72 per cent of the deaths from these infections. In the Edinburgh series of 137 cases of pneumococcal pneumonias, 84 per cent were caused by 9 serotypes (1, 2, 3, 5, 7, 8, 10, 12, 14): from 19 of the 20 bacteriaemic cases, five (1, 2, 3, 5, 8) of these nine types were isolated, and in seven deaths, only types 3 and 1 were incriminated. Since influenza is a common precipitating factor in the pneumonias of elderly people, a case could perhaps be made for combined influenza virus and multiple pneumococcus polysaccharide vaccines for the protection of those at greatest risk from these respiratory infections.

REFERENCES

AUSTRIAN, R. (1970) The current status of pneumococcal disease and the potential utility of polyvalent pneumococcal vaccine. *International Conference on the Application of Vaccines against Viral, Rickettsial and Bacterial Diseases of Man.* Pan American Health Organization. World Health Organization, Washington, D.C.

BATH, J. C. J. L., BOISSARD, G. P. B., CALDER, M. A. & MOFFAT, M. A. J. (1964) Pneumonia in hospital practice in Edinburgh, 1960–62. *British Journal of Diseases of the Chest,* **58,** 1.

CALDER, MARGARET A., MCHARDY, V. U. & SCHONELL, M.E. (1970) Importance of pneumococcal typing in pneumonia. *Lancet,* **i,** 5.

HAUSMAN, D., GLASGOW, H., STURT, J., DEVITT, L. & DOUGLAS, R. (1971) Increased resistance to penicillin of pneumococci isolated from man. *New England Journal of Medicine,* **284,** 175.

H.M.S.O. REPORT (1962) Studies on medical and population subjects, No. 14. *Morbidity Statistics from General Practice.* Vol. iii. London: H.M.S.O.

MCLEOD, C. M., HODGES, R. G., HEIDELBERGER, M. & BERGHARD, W. G. (1945) Prevention of pneumonia by immunization with specific capsular polysaccharides. *Journal of Experimental Medicine,* **82,** 445.

MORRISON, BRENDA, BASS, D., DAVIS, J. A., HOBSON, D., MADSEN, T. I. & MASTERS, P. L. (1957) Acute lower respiratory infections in childhood. *Lancet,* **ii,** 1077.

PERCIVAL, A., ARMSTRONG, E. C. & TURNER, G. C. (1969) Increased incidence of tetracycline-resistant pneumococci in Liverpool in 1968. *Lancet,* **i,** 998.

18. Lactobacillus Dental Caries

Definition

The genus *Lactobacillus* consists of Gram-positive rod-shaped bacteria that are non-sporing, non-motile, either facultatively or strictly anaerobic, strongly acid-producing (acidogenic) by fermentation of carbohydrates, and exceptionally capable of survival and growth under acid conditions (aciduric).

The lactobacilli are common commensal parasites of vertebrate and invertebrate animals and also occur widely as saprophytes in fermenting animal and vegetable matter, e.g. souring milk, cheese and silage. Apart from a common involvement in dental caries and an extremely rare occurrence in subacute bacterial endocarditis, they are entirely harmless to man. There is, indeed, evidence that the lactobacillary flora of the intestine and vagina has a beneficent, protective effect in tending to inhibit colonization by potentially harmful organisms.

DESCRIPTION

The bacilli are fairly large, e.g. 1 to 5 μm × 1·0 μm, and, unlike the corynebacteria, commonly occur in pairs in-line and in short chains. Filamentous, club-shaped and swollen, ovoid forms occur in aged, involutionary cultures. Lactobacilli are non-sporing and, except for rare strains, non-motile and non-capsulate. Staining is Gram-positive and uniform in young cultures, but may be Gram-variable or granular in old ones.

Plates for primary isolation should be incubated for 2 to 4 days at 37°C under anaerobic conditions in a jar containing hydrogen or nitrogen plus 5 per cent carbon dioxide. Growth is poor on ordinary nutrient agar but is improved by the addition of glucose, whey, yeast extract or blood. A good non-selective medium is that of De Man, Rogosa and Sharpe (1960). Colonies after 48 hours are small, e.g. 0·5 mm, in diameter, and usually have an irregular edge and a granular surface.

Lactobacilli grow best at about pH 5·8 but can survive and grow slowly at pH values as low as 3·0 to 4·0. This exceptionally aciduric character is exploited in the use of acid media for the selective culture of lactobacilli from saliva, faeces and other materials containing a mixture of bacteria capable of outgrowing the lactobacilli on ordinary media. Hadley's tomato juice agar, pH 5·0, and the glucose-yeast extract-acetic acid agar of Rogosa, Mitchell and Wiseman (1951), pH 5·4, are good selective plating media.

All species grow at 37°C, but some, grouped as *low-temperature species,* can grow at 15°C though not at 45°C, and others, *high-temperature species,* can grow at 45°C though not at 15°C.

The lactobacilli have complex nutritional requirements and the different species differ in the range of amino acids and vitamins required. Certain species with requirements for particular growth factors are used in microbiological assays of these factors, e.g. *Lactobacillus leichmannii* in assays of cyanocobalomin (vitamin B 12).

Lactobacilli resemble streptococci in obtaining energy solely by the fermentation of carbohydrates, etc. They lack cytochromes and other enzymes necessary for aerobic respiration, and form neither catalase nor oxidase. In fermenting glucose and other sugars, *homofermentative* species form only lactic acid, whilst *heterofermentative* species form acetic acid, formic acid, ethanol, CO_2 and other products as well as lactic acid. The heterofermentative organisms may be recognized by the demonstration that CO_2 is produced from glucose but, because CO_2 is soluble in water, a special method is required to demonstrate the gas (Gibson and Abd-el-Malek, 1945). All species ferment glucose and most ferment lactose, maltose and sucrose. The species may be classified by their differing abilities to ferment particular substrates among these and other carbohydrates (Cowan and Steel, 1965).

Agglutination tests with antisera distinguish serotypes within individual species, but deep antigens extracted with acid and identified in precipitation tests with group antisera distinguish six groups corresponding to some of the main species: namely, the bulgaricus, casei, casei-helveticus, fermenti, lactis-brevis, and plantarum groups.

OCCURRENCE OF LACTOBACILLI

Alimentary Canal

Lactobacilli form a major part of the normal commensal flora of the mouth, stomach, small intestine and large intestine in man and most other warm-blooded animals, and are present in large numbers in the faeces. Within the first 2 to 3 days after birth the alimentary canal of the baby is colonized with lactobacilli, probably derived from its mother's vagina, mouth and intestine. A heavy colonization with bacilli numbering in the range 10^6 to 10^{10} per ml of fluid contents is maintained throughout life, except for periods when certain antibiotics are given by mouth. The numbers of lactobacilli are higher when the diet is rich in cereals and sugars than when it is deficient in these and rich in protein. A variety of species are present, the commonest usually being *Lacto. acidophilus*. In the mouth, the lactobacilli are usually outnumbered by commensal streptococci, neisseriae and veillonellae, and in the colon by anaerobic Gram-negative bacilli of the bacteroides and fusiformis groups, but elsewhere in the alimentary canal they are usually the most numerous commensal organisms (Smith, 1965).

Vagina

Lactobacilli constitute the predominant members of the commensal flora of the vagina during the periods of life when, under the influence of oestrogenic hormone, a large amount of glycogen is deposited in the cells of the multi-layered epithelium. In these periods, notably between puberty and the menopause, the vaginal secretion is highly acid, e.g. at pH 4·5, due to the presence of lactic acid formed from the glycogen. The breakdown of glycogen to lactic acid

may be brought about in part by vaginal-tissue enzymes, but probably mainly by the lactobacilli, some strains of which can attack glycogen directly whilst others may ferment glucose split from the glycogen by different bacteria or by the vaginal enzymes.

Cruickshank and Sharman (1934) have shown that large amounts of glycogen formed under the influence of maternal oestrin are present in the vaginal epithelium during the first week of life. The pH of the secretion, which is about 5·5 to 6·0 at birth, falls to 4·5 to 5·0 when, after 2 or 3 days, lactobacilli colonize and become the predominant commensals in the vagina. During the next month, the maternal oestrin is eliminated through the kidneys, glycogen disappears from the epithelium, the lactobacilli are largely replaced by a mixed flora of streptococci, staphylococci, diphtheroid bacteria, coliforms and vibrios, and the secretion becomes nearly neutral in reaction (pH 6·5 to 7·5). This condition continues until puberty when the glycogen is again deposited abundantly, lactobacilli recolonize the vagina and very largely displace the other bacteria, and the secretion again becomes highly acid (e.g. pH 4·5). During the early months of pregnancy the secretion may be less acid, but in the later months it is again highly acid. After the menopause, glycogen becomes scanty, the lactobacilli may be replaced by a mixed flora and the secretion then becomes less acid.

The high acidity due to the fermentation of glycogen is antagonistic to microorganisms other than the aciduric lactobacilli and yeasts (candida) and is probably responsible for the predominance of these organisms during the reproductive period of life. It is probably also protective against the acquisition of infections of or through the vagina. Thus, the susceptibility of pre-pubertal girls to gonococcal vulvovaginitis and pneumococcal peritonitis and the common occurrence of post-menopausal vaginitis may be due to the non-acid state of the vaginal secretion at these ages.

Dental Caries

Together with certain streptococci, the commensal lactobacilli of the mouth probably play an important part in the causation of dental caries.

These bacteria are thought to ferment dietary carbohydrates, such as sucrose, with the production of acid which dissolves the mineral component (calcium phosphate/hydroxide) of the enamel and dentine. The lactobacilli are more aciduric than the streptococci and other oral bacteria and can therefore survive and continue to ferment carbohydrate under more strongly acidic conditions, e.g. at pH 3·0 to 4·0. Their number in the saliva has been shown to be much higher, e.g. over 10^5 per ml, in the presence than in the absence of caries. Even in carious mouths, however, the lactobacilli are greatly outnumbered by the streptococci and form only 1 to 2 per cent of the salivary flora. They make up a larger proportion, e.g. 5 to 10 per cent, of the bacteria in the plaque on the surface of carious teeth and an even larger proportion, e.g. 50 to 100 per cent, of the bacteria invading carious dentine. The greater numbers of the streptococci in the plaque and the observation that germ-free rodents fed on a sugar-rich diet develop caries much more readily when infected with a pure culture of a dextran-producing streptococcus, such as *Strept. mutans,* than when infected with a lactobacillus suggest that the lactobacilli are less important than the streptococci in the *initial* stages of caries production. After the enamel has been eroded, however, lactobacilli such as *Lacto. casei* and *Lacto. fermenti* appear to be the organisms that most commonly take the lead in invading and decalcifying the dentine. For a review and references, see Scherp (1971).

Table 18.1

Type of fermentation	Temperature for growth	Species
Homofermentative	High	*Lacto. acidophilus* *Lacto. bulgaricus* *Lacto. helveticus* *Lacto. lactis* *Lacto. leichmannii* *Lacto. salivarius*
Homofermentative	Low	*Lacto. casei* *Lacto. plantarum*
Heterofermentative	High	*Lacto. fermenti*
Heterofermentative	Low	*Lacto. brevis*

'LACTOBACILLUS BIFIDUS'

This bacterium resembles other lactobacilli in being a non-sporing non-motile Gram-positive bacillus which strongly ferments sugars to lactic and acetic acids, is highly aciduric and strictly anaerobic, and occurs commonly as a numerous commensal inhabitant of the intestine. It is more liable than most lactobacilli to produce bizarre involution forms in fully grown and old cultures. It commonly shows Y-shaped, branching (bifid) forms, to which it owes its name, as well as swollen ovoids, filaments, club-shaped forms and forms with lateral buds. This pleomorphism, which is seen in faeces as well as in culture, resembles that resulting from defective synthesis of the mucopeptide 'rigid layer' of the bacterial cell wall.

Recent studies have suggested that the organism is not a true lactobacillus but is more closely related to the corynebacterium group. Thus, DNA analyses have shown that the true *Lactobacillus* species resemble each other, and also streptococci and pneumococci, in having a mole percentage of guanine plus cytosine (GC ratio) of 38 to 40, whereas *Lacto. bifidus* has a GC ratio of 56, which is close to that of the corynebacteria. It has been suggested that the organism should be called *Bifidobacterium bifidus*.

Lacto. bifidus is commonly the predominant intestinal commensal organism in breast-fed infants, of whose faecal flora it may form as much as 99 per cent associated with a highly acid reaction in the stools (pH 5·0 to 5·5). It is present less regularly and in smaller numbers in the mixed flora of the faeces of bottle-fed infants, in which *Lacto. acidophilus* is usually predominant, and in that of adults. The nutritional advantages of human milk and the greater freedom from infective gastroenteritis observed in breast-fed as compared with bottle-fed babies has been attributed to the effects of a nearly pure intestinal flora of *Lacto. bifidus*.

One strain of *Lacto. bifidus* has been shown to require for normal cell-wall formation and growth a supply of derivatives of *N*-acetyl-glucosamine which are present in human milk and which serve the bacillus as precursors for synthesis of the muramic acid component of the cell-wall mucopeptide. When cultured on a medium with a small content of α,β-methyl-N-acetyl-D-glucosaminide, the bacillus at first grows in the form of simple rods but later, when the glucosaminide is exhausted, forms branching, swollen and other abnormal forms (Glick *et al.*, 1960). The specific requirement of *Lacto. bifidus* for growth factors present in sufficient amount in human milk but not in cow's milk may be one reason why a predominant colonization by this organism is dependent on breast feeding.

REFERENCES

COWAN, S. T. & STEEL, K. J. (1965) *Manual for the Identification of Medical Bacteria*. p. 58. Cambridge University Press.

CRUICKSHANK, R. & SHARMAN, A. (1934) The biology of the vagina in the human subject, I, II and III. *Journal of Obstetrics and Gynaecology of the British Commonwealth*, **41**, 190, 208 and 369.

DE MAN, J. C., ROGOSA, M. & SHARPE, M. ELIZABETH (1960) A medium for the cultivation of lactobacilli. *Journal of Applied Bacteriology*, **23**, 130.

GIBSON, T. & ABD-EL-MALEK, Y. (1945) The formation of carbon dioxide by lactic acid bacteria and *Bacillus licheniformis* and a cultural method of detecting the process. *Journal of Dairy Research*, **14**, 35.

GLICK, M. C., SALL, T., ZILLIKEN, F. & MUDD, S. (1960) Morphological changes in *Lactobacillus bifidus* var. *pennsylvanicus* produced by a cell-wall precursor. *Biochimica et biophysica acta*, **37**, 361.

HADLEY, F. P. (1933) A quantitative method of estimating *Bacillus acidophilus* in saliva. *Journal of Dental Research*, **13**, 415.

ROGOSA, M., MITCHELL, JOYCE, A. & WISEMAN, R. F. (1951) A selective medium for the isolation and enumeration of oral and fecal lactobacilli. *Journal of Bacteriology*, **62**, 132.

SHERP, H. W. (1971) Dental caries: prospects for prevention. *Science*, **173**, 1199.

SMITH, H. W. (1965) Observations on the flora of the alimentary tract of animals and factors affecting its composition. *Journal of Pathology and Bacteriology*, **89**, 95.

19. Bordetella   Whooping-cough

The genus *Bordetella* belongs to the family Brucellaceae, small, ovoid to rod-shaped Gram-negative bacilli; two of its members, *Bord. pertussis* and *Bord.parapertussis*, cause one of the most frequent bacterial respiratory infections of childhood in communities not effectively protected by vaccination. The name whooping-cough is given to this infection because of the tendency for a paroxysm of coughing to end with a long inspiratory high-pitched note or whoop. The disease in its typical form is prolonged and debilitating and may affect 70 to 80 per cent of unprotected children with a high incidence and severity of attack in infants under 2 years of age.

Available bacteriological and serological methods of laboratory diagnosis fail to demonstrate bordetella infection in a substantial proportion of cases diagnosed clinically as whooping-cough. Probably most of the cases giving negative results are bordetella infections that are not demonstrated by the laboratory tests because the methods used are insufficiently sensitive or because the time or method of collection of the specimens is unsuitable. Some of the 'negative' cases, however, may be due to infection with other kinds of microorganisms and there is evidence suggesting that a clinical syndrome simulating whooping-cough may be caused by adenoviruses of types 1, 2 and 5 (Connor, 1970), some other respiratory viruses, and *Mycoplasma pneumoniae*.

DESCRIPTION

Bord.pertussis used to be classified with *Haemophilus* because a culture medium rich in blood was needed for its primary isolation. But the bordetellae are not dependent on nutritional factors in blood for growth and the other two members of the genus, *Bord.parapertussis* and *Bord.bronchiseptica* are less exacting in their growth requirements than *Bord.pertussis*.

Bord.pertussis is a small, Gram-negative coccobacillus uniform in size and shape in primary culture but definite bacillary forms occur on subculture and become more numerous in 'rough' cultures. The organism is non-motile and non-sporing; capsules are demonstrable in young cultures. In culture films, the organisms tend to form loose clumps with clearer spaces between, giving a 'thumbprint' distribution.

Bord.pertussis is an aerobe and grows best at 35° to 36°C. Catalase and a substance, e.g. albumin or charcoal, which will absorb toxic products (possibly unsaturated fatty acids) are essential for growth. For primary culture the special medium of Bordet and Gengou containing 33 per cent fresh blood or a modification of it should be employed. On this medium, which should be kept moist, growth occurs slowly and after two or three days or even longer there appear small raised greyish white colonies which are highly refractile to light, resembling a bisected pearl or a mercury drop. The colonies are cohesive and may be picked off entire for slide-agglutination. Penicillin (0·25 units per ml) is usually incorporated for the suppression of commensal bacteria and diamidine (M & B 938) may also be included to make the medium more selective (Vol. II, Chaps. 6 and 22).

Bord.pertussis differs from *Haemophilus influenzae* in its continued viability at low temperatures (0° to 10°C). It is killed by heat at 55°C for half an hour. It has no fermentative properties.

Recently isolated strains appear to be closely related in antigenic characters and react with the same agglutinating and complement-fixing antisera. There are, however, a number of surface agglutinating factors, numbered 1 to 6, of which 1 is common to all strains. Thus, agglutination with absorbed, single factor sera distinguishes three common serotypes, type 1,2, type 1,2,3, and type 1,3, according to their content of agglutinating factors 1, 2 and 3.

A number of other distinguishable antigenic fractions have been isolated from *Bord.pertussis*, e.g. haemagglutinin, protective antigen, histamine-sensitivity fraction, and endotoxin. It is difficult to assess the significance of these and other factors in the pathogenicity or toxicity of the organism (Pittman, 1970).

Bord.parapertussis is related antigenically to *Bord.pertussis* but produces a milder form of whooping-cough which is rare in Britain but common in some other European countries, e.g. Denmark and Czechoslovakia. It differs from *Bord.pertussis* in its more rapid growth so that the pearly colonies are well developed after two days' incubation on Bordet-Gengou medium. The underlying medium becomes greeny-black due to the production of a brown pigment. *Bord.parapertussis* actively produces catalase and on subculture grows readily on ordinary culture media. It can be specifically identified by agglutination with an absorbed antiserum.

term sequel. Convulsions and, more rarely, encephalopathy may occur as a feature of severe infections in young children and may be related to anoxaemia. An early leucopenia is soon followed by a leucocytosis (total white blood cells: 15 000 to 30 000 per cmm with 70 to 80 per cent lymphocytes) related to a lymphocyte-stimulating factor. A very high leucocytic count with a considerable proportion of polymorphonuclear cells indicates a secondary bacterial infection, e.g. bronchopneumonia.

Animal pathogenicity. Intranasal inoculation of *Bord.pertussis* cultures in mice anaesthetized with ether produces an interstitial pneumonia which may be fatal. Mice are also highly susceptible to intracerebral injection of virulent strains. A condition similar to clinical whooping-cough has been produced in monkeys and chimpanzees by introduction of pure cultures into the respiratory tract.

PATHOGENESIS

Whooping-cough is predominantly an infection of the respiratory mucosa, running a protracted course of four to eight weeks after an incubation period of 7 to 14 days. The bacilli can be demonstrated adhering to the cilia and luminal surface of the epithelium of the bronchioles, bronchi and trachea. They grow only on the surface of ciliated epithelium, without invading the mucosa more deeply; they cause damage to the cilia and consequently initiate the irritation that induces increased secretion of mucus and the stimulus for the paroxysmal coughing and bronchospasm. Some workers, however, believe that the syndrome may be related to the production of a neurotoxin by the bacillus. The organisms are expelled in droplets during coughing and in scanty viscid sputum, and are most readily demonstrable in the first two or three weeks of infection. Later, toxic damage may affect the submucosa and extend into lung tissue accompanied by peribronchiolar infiltration with lymphocytes and polymorphonuclear cells. Blocked bronchioles lead to areas of lung collapse and patches of emphysema. Secondary bronchopneumonia due to infection with pyogenic cocci may ensue and sometimes causes death, or bronchiectasis may develop as a long-

LABORATORY DIAGNOSIS

A specimen for bacteriological diagnosis can be obtained most conveniently by use of a pernasal swab. For this purpose, a fine pledget of cotton wool is mounted on a long, very flexible nichrome wire (21 SWG) and the swab is passed into the post-nasal space through the nose. The tip of the swab, moistened in nutrient broth, is directed along the floor of the nasal passage for about 2 inches and left *in situ* for a few seconds when it touches the posterior pharyngeal wall. An assistant should hold the child's head steady. The swab should be inoculated on to a plate of selective Bordet-Gengou medium within 2 to 3 hours. If there is likely to be a longer delay, the swab should be placed in Stuart's transport medium. The inoculated plate is incubated at 35° to 36°C for 3 days and, if negative, reincubated for 2 more days. An alternative procedure is the use of a 'cough plate' which is held about 4 inches in front of the child's mouth while the child is encouraged to direct 4 to 6 coughs on to the plate. Typical colonies are picked for slide-agglutination: detailed antigenic analysis for agglutinating factors is best done in a reference laboratory, although monospecific agglutinating antisera are available.

Because of the poor rate of isolation of *Bord. pertussis* by culture from patients with suspected whooping-cough, laboratory diagnosis has also been attempted (i) by immunofluorescent microscopical demonstration of *Bord.pertussis* in specimens of the patient's respiratory secretion and (ii) by demonstration of *Bord.pertussis* antibody in the patient's serum by agglutination, complement-fixation or immunofluorescence methods. In some series these methods have given more positive results than culture.

Serological diagnosis of whooping-cough may be attempted by the use of complement-fixation and agglutination tests on paired blood sera with the second specimen of blood taken as late as possible in convalescence because of the slow development of demonstrable antibodies. In a recent study in Scotland, these two tests were found to give comparable results with some bias in favour of the complement-fixation test which has also certain technical advantages (Scottish Report, 1970). The serological tests compared poorly with *Bord.pertussis* isolations in 73 infants under 6 months of age (19 per cent positive CFTs vs 42 per cent isolations) whereas serological tests gave much better results than isolations in ill children over one year of age (65 per cent vs 19 per cent respectively). Taking isolation and serological results together, evidence of *Bord.pertussis* infection was obtained in about 50 per cent of the hospitalized cases diagnosed clinically as whooping-cough.

Since the cultural method of diagnosis gives negative results in many cases in which the serological method gives positive results and the serological method gives negative results in many in which culture is positive, it is evident that each of these methods commonly fails to detect *Bord.pertussis* infection. For this reason, the obtaining of negative results with either or both methods should not be taken as excluding *Bord.pertussis* infection.

CHEMOTHERAPY

Bord.pertussis is sensitive to a wide range of antimicrobial drugs including the tetracyclines, chloramphenicol, erythromycin and ampicillin but is relatively resistant to benzyl penicillin. Unfortunately, whooping-cough is often not recognized clinically until the infection is well established by which time chemotherapy has little or no effect on its severity or duration. A controlled trial (M.R.C. Report, 1953) in which three groups of approximately 100 children under 5 years of age were given chloramphenicol, chlortetracycline or a placebo showed that the two antibiotics could reduce the number and severity of coughing paroxysms *only if given within the first ten days of infection*. Another recent trial with small numbers of children but including two additional drugs (ampicillin and erythromycin) gave similar results (Bass *et al.*, 1969). It is possible that a drug with a restricted antibacterial spectrum such as erythromycin could be used chemoprophylactically to protect young siblings of an older child who brings whooping-cough into the home. Penicillin is, of course, valuable for the treatment of secondary bronchopneumonia due to pyogenic cocci that are penicillin-sensitive.

EPIDEMIOLOGY

Source and Transmission of Infections

Patients with clinical whooping-cough appear to be the only significant sources of infection. Healthy carriers are probably rare but a few subclinical infections have been detected by culture in healthy home contacts of patients. The bacillus is not very resistant to drying or other environmental conditions and transmission probably takes place mainly by contact with fingers and other objects contaminated with sputum or saliva, or by direct spraying of the eyes, nose or mouth with cough droplets.

Incidence

Mortality from whooping-cough has declined dramatically over the past half century. Whereas this infection killed some 40 000 children in England and Wales in the decade 1921 to 1930, there were only 279 deaths in the 10 years 1959 to 1968; 216 or 77 per cent of these occurred in the first year of life and 171, or 4 out of 5 of these 216 deaths were in infants under 6 months of age. The recorded incidence of whooping-cough has been falling in the past two decades but notifications give a gross underestimate of total morbidity because of poor reporting.

However, the data indicate that the national use of pertussis vaccines has reduced the incidence of the disease because the epidemic waves, which used to have a biennial periodicity, now occur at 3 to 4 year intervals and with decreasing amplitude (Fig. 19.1): but the health administrator must be cautious about attributing the downward slope of the epidemic wave to the introduction of some new preventive measure like prophylactic vaccination.

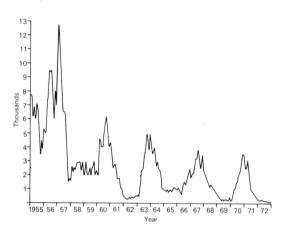

FIG. 19.1. Whooping-cough notifications: England and Wales: 1955–1972. (Pertussis vaccination of young children came into general use about 1957.)

Whooping-cough is essentially a disease of early childhood. There is little or no transfer of passive immunity from mother to offspring so that infections occur in early infancy and some 10 per cent of unprotected infants in urban areas develop whooping-cough in the first year of life. The attack rate is about the same for each of the next 4 years of life so that half the child population has been affected by the age of 5 years. Morbidity and mortality rates are rather higher in females than in males in contrast to most other specific childhood fevers. One attack does not necessarily confer long-lasting immunity and clinical infections, often unrecognized, may occur in adults, e.g. parents of affected children.

Transfer of infection requires fairly intimate contact. Thus, the secondary attack rate is 80 to 90 per cent among susceptible siblings (home exposures) but much lower for contacts outside

the home; in day and residential nurseries the infection may spread in a slow and smouldering fashion in contrast to the explosive outbreaks of measles. A child with whooping-cough is most infectious in the first 2 to 3 weeks after onset before any whoop develops; duration of convalescent carriage of the pathogen is probably shortened by early chemotherapy or previous vaccination.

CONTROL MEASURES

Whooping-cough due to *Bord.pertussis* can be controlled, if not wholly prevented, by prophylactic vaccination. After encouraging results reported by the Danes in the epidemics on the Faroe Islands and by Kendrick and Eldering in Grand Rapids, Michigan, a series of controlled trials of different vaccines was carried out in Britain during the 1950s under the sponsorship of the Medical Research Council. In all, some 50 000 children, mostly in the age range 6 months to 2 years, were involved and 25 different vaccines were tried. The main findings as summarized in the final Medical Research Council Report (1959) were:

The results of the trials clearly showed that it was possible by vaccination to produce a high degree of protection against the disease, as shown by the substantial reduction in the attack rate amongst home contacts, and, in those cases where vaccination failed to give complete protection, to reduce the severity and duration of the disease. The results also showed that the different vaccines employed varied a great deal in their protective action; the poorest gave an attack rate in home contacts of 87 per cent, and the most effective an attack rate of 4 per cent.

The protective efficacy of different vaccines was checked against a number of laboratory tests of which the mouse protection test was found to correlate best with the results of the field trials. But sometimes there was considerable divergence between the mouse test and the clinical results. In a recent reassessment, pertussis vaccines that had passed the laboratory test failed to give any significant protection to vaccinated children exposed to infected siblings (P.H.L.S. Report, 1969). Thus, the attack rate among fully vaccinated children under 5 years after exposure in the home to a bacteriologically proven case was 56 per cent and the corresponding rate for non-vaccinated children was 67 per cent. The poor protection in the vaccinated children was not apparently affected by the age of the child, the interval since vaccination or the absence of a booster dose. It was, however, noted that the serotype of the strains in the vaccines used in the late 1950s was type 1,2 whereas the infecting strains in the late sixties were predominantly type 1,3. Preston (1970) has attributed the inadequacy of these vaccines to the appearance of new antigenic variants but Pittman (1970) believes that the total amount of immunizing antigen is the critical factor in the prophylaxis of whooping-cough. Improved methods for testing the antigenic potency of pertussis vaccines and ensuring better protection have been proposed (Perkins, 1969; Preston, 1970), but despite improved modifications in British vaccine production since 1968, notifications of whooping-cough again reached a high level in 1970 to 1971 (see Fig. 19.1). Obviously, more determined efforts to improve antigenicity and reduce toxicity of pertussis vaccines are needed.

There is conflicting but mostly negative evidence about the protective value of seroprophylaxis with human immunoglobulin given to intimately exposed contacts.

Early recognition and isolation of an infected child in a day or residential nursery may help to limit the spread of infection to other children.

REFERENCES

BASS, J. W., KLENK, E. L., KOTHEIMER, J. B., LINNEMANN, C. C. & SMITH, M. H. D. (1969) Antimicrobial treatment of pertussis. *Journal of Pediatrics*, **75**, 768.

CONNOR, J. D. (1970) Evidence for an aetiologic role of adenoviral infection in pertussis syndrome. *New England Journal of Medicine*, **283**, 390.

M.R.C. REPORT (1953) Treatment of whooping-cough with antibiotics. *Lancet*, **i**, 1109.

M.R.C. REPORT (1959) Vaccination against whooping-cough. *British Medical Journal*, **i**, 994.

PERKINS, F. T. (1969) Vaccination against whooping-cough. *British Medical Journal*, **iv**, 429.

PITTMAN, M. (1970) In *Infectious Agents and Host Reactions*, p. 239. Edited by Stuart Mudd. Philadelphia and London: W. B. Saunders.

PRESTON, N. W. (1970) Technical problems in the laboratory diagnosis and prevention of whooping-cough. *Laboratory Practice*, **19**, No. 5.

P.H.L.S. REPORTS (1969, 1973) Efficacy of whooping-cough vaccines used in the United Kingdom before 1968. *British Medical Journal*, **iv**, 329; **i**, 259.

SCOTTISH REPORT (1970) Diagnosis of whooping-cough: comparison of serological tests with isolation of *Bordetella pertussis*. *British Medical Journal*, **iv**, 637.

20. Haemophilus
Respiratory Infections: Meningitis

Haemophilus influenzae was originally described as the causal organism of epidemic influenza and has been designated *haemophilic* in virtue of its inability to grow on culture medium without the addition of whole blood or certain growth-promoting substances, termed X and V, present in blood. These growth factors, however, are not restricted to blood, but are present also in certain vegetable tissues. The Koch-Weeks bacillus, isolated from cases of acute conjunctivitis, shows the same growth requirements as *Haemophilus influenzae*, and may appropriately be grouped with it. If the term *haemophilic* were used in a broad sense to designate organisms which require blood for their growth it would embrace a number of heterogeneous species, and the generic term *Haemophilus* is therefore restricted to those organisms which are dependent on one or both of the growth factors required by *Haemophilus influenzae*.

Haemophilus influenzae was first described by Pfeiffer in 1892 as the cause of influenza in the 1889 to 1892 pandemic because of its 'constant presence in the characteristic purulent sputum— in uncomplicated cases in absolutely pure culture and in almost incredible numbers'. In 1893, he was able to grow the bacillus on a blood-containing medium. Doubts about its causal relationship to influenza developed during and after the 1918–19 pandemic, mainly because other bacterial pathogens were being incriminated in the secondary influenzal pneumonias. Only in 1933, however, did doubt become certainty with the discovery of the influenza virus A by Smith, Andrewes and Laidlaw. The view that there may be a special relationship between the virus and the bacillus found support in Shope's studies of swine influenza but the modern concept is that *H.influenzae* is a secondary pathogen on respiratory mucosa that has become susceptible to bacterial attack after the primary influenza virus infection. It seems to play a similar role in chronic bronchitis. Later, the demonstration by Pittman that *H.influenzae* is

divisible into capsulate and non-capsulate strains and that the capsulate strains could be differentiated serologically into 6 types, labelled a to f, of which type b, in particular, was causally concerned as a primary pathogen in acute purulent meningitis and laryngo-epiglottitis (croup), helped to define the importance of this organism. The great majority (>95 per cent) of strains of *H.influenzae* found in the healthy or diseased respiratory tract are non-capsulate and generally are pathogenic only in a secondary role. The minority of capsulate strains which may colonize the throats of a few healthy carriers may act as primary pathogens in the respiratory tract and meninges.

CLASSIFICATION

H.influenzae is a small Gram-negative bacillus. It shows considerable pleomorphism from coccobacillary forms which predominate in young cultures and often as small clumps in sputum to filamentous forms in older cultures and in the spinal fluid of cases of purulent meningitis. *H.influenzae* needs good quality nutrient media for its growth but specifically it requires two nutritional factors, called X and V, which are present in blood. X factor, highly heat-resistant, is present in haemin and probably acts as a substrate in the synthesis of catalase, cytochromes, etc., which are required for the aerobic growth of the bacillus; V factor, which has been variously named co-enzyme I and II, di- and triphosphopyridine nucleotide (DPN and TPN) and nicotinamide adenine dinucleotide and its phosphate (NAD and NADP) is essential as a hydrogen receptor in the cell's metabolism and is destroyed by heating at 120°C for a few minutes. In ordinary blood agar, the V factor tends to be imprisoned in the intact red blood cells; in chocolate agar (containing blood heated to 80 to 90°C), the V factor is released so that this latter medium, or a transparent medium containing blood extracts (Levinthal agar, Fildes' peptic digest agar), gives the best growth of *H.influenzae*. V factor is also produced by certain bacteria and fungi: the staphylococcus can be used to demonstrate the dependence of *H.influenzae* on this growth factor by noting enlarged colonies of the bacillus around colonies of staphylococci in primary mixed cultures (satellitism) or by streaking a culture of staphylococcus across a plate inoculated with suspected *H.influenzae*. Capsulate strains are best demonstrated by their colonial features on a transparent medium like Levinthal agar on which the colonies are mucoid, rather opaque and when viewed obliquely with transmitted light, characteristically iridescent. Typing of capsulate strains can be done by slide agglutination or by the capsule swelling reaction with monospecific antisera to types a to f.

Other haemophili that conform generically in their nutritional requirements for X or V factors or both are (a) the Koch-Weeks bacillus (*H.aegyptius*), requiring both X and V factors and closely resembling *H.influenzae*; (b) *H.parainfluenzae*, requiring only V factor and occasionally associated with subacute bacterial endocarditis, besides being a commensal in the upper respiratory tract; (c) *H.haemolyticus*, also dependent on V factor and a commensal that may cause confusion in cultures of throat swabs because of its colonial and haemolytic resemblance to β-haemolytic streptococci; (d) *H. aphrophilus*, requiring X factor and CO_2; and (e) *H.ducreyii*, the causative organism of the venereal disease, chancroid or soft sore, with special nutritional requirements besides dependence on X factor. Clotted fresh rabbit blood is a good medium for its isolation.

PATHOGENESIS

H.influenzae is a very common commensal in the upper respiratory tract, mostly as the non-capsulate variety. From different surveys, mainly in urban communities, rates of 60 to 80 per cent have been obtained for carriage of non-capsulate strains in the throat or nasopharynx of young children and rates of 3 to 4 per cent for the carriage of capsulate strains, notably type b;

rather lower carrier rates (30 to 80 per cent) of non-capsulate strains were obtained in older children and adults; capsulate strains were rarely found in these older age-groups. Much higher carrier rates of capsulate haemophili may occur in semi-isolated communities of young children without overt disease (see Turk and May, 1967). These findings resemble those for the pneumococci, there being high throat carrier rates of types that are only potentially pathogenic and low carrier rates of the virulent invasive types.

The diseases with which the haemophilus genus is associated fall into two groups: (1) acute primary (exogenous) infections caused by capsulate haemophili, usually type b, and (2) acute and chronic secondary (endogenous) respiratory infections associated with non-capsulate haemophili.

1. Capsulate haemophili, particularly type b, may act as primary pathogens in producing nasopharyngitis (sore throat with fever), laryngo-epiglottitis (croup), acute bronchitis, pneumonia, otitis media, septicaemia, meningitis, septic arthritis and pericarditis. Age seems to be an important factor in the incidence of clinical infection with the capsulate haemophili; acute purulent meningitis occurs mostly in the age range 2 months to 3 years and laryngo-epiglottitis (a form of croup with greatly enlarged and inflamed epiglottis) mostly in the age-range 2 to 7 years. Both types of infection have an associated septicaemia or bacteriaemia and blood culture should be done when either is suspected. The route of infection of the meninges is probably from the nasopharynx via the blood. The restriction of these infections to infants and young children is probably related to the finding by Fothergill and Wright (1933) that bactericidal antibodies against a capsulate strain of haemophilus from a case of meningitis could not be demonstrated in blood samples from children between the ages of 2 months and 3 years but were more common in children between 3 and 10 years and constantly present in the blood of older children and adults. When type-b *H.influenzae* first infects a baby after it has lost protective maternal antibody at 2 to 3 months of age, it commonly causes naso-pharyngitis with fever and in some cases may spread to cause infection elsewhere in the

respiratory tract or invade the blood and cause meningitis or other metastatic infection. Subsequently these children are protected by the active production of specific type-b antibodies.

2. Non-capsulate haemophili have in the past two decades been frequently found in the sputum of cases of chronic bronchitis, particularly during acute exacerbations, and in cases of bronchiectasis. Difficulty in the demonstration of haemophili in sputum because of their irregular distribution has been overcome by homogenization of the specimen either by pretreatment with a mucolytic enzyme such as pancreatin or by shaking the specimen with sterile water and glass beads for 15 to 30 minutes. Although haemophili are not regarded as a primary etiological factor in the causation of chronic bronchitis, its importance as a secondary infecting agent has been demonstrated by the studies of May and others (Turk and May, 1967). Three points may be emphasized: (1) the more frequent association of haemophili with purulent than with mucoid sputum in cases of chronic bronchitis; (2) the clinical improvement with antimicrobial therapy that eliminates, temporarily, *H.influenzae*, and the association of clinical relapse with its return; and (3) the presence of high levels of species-specific antibody to *H.influenzae* in the blood of patients with chronic bronchitis, particularly those with purulent sputum, and the low level of such antibody in patients with asthma and in healthy subjects. Both *H.influenzae* and pneumococci are associated with acute exacerbations of chronic bronchitis, just as both are important agents in the causation of secondary bronchopneumonia.

In young children, particularly, non-capsulate haemophili are often found in pure culture in cases of paranasal sinusitis, and less commonly, in otitis media; in such cases, the haemophili are presumably secondary pathogens after a primary virus infection.

Laboratory Diagnosis

In cases of *H.influenzae* meningitis, an early and rapid laboratory diagnosis may be life-saving because infants with fulminating infections may die within 24 hours of onset. Conversely, cases may have been treated with antimicrobial drugs for some days before admission to hospital and the infection drags into a subacute phase. Smears of the centrifuged deposit of the cerebrospinal fluid from any case of purulent meningitis must be stained by Gram's method with dilute carbol-fuchsin as the counterstain for haemophili which stain poorly and also with methylene blue. Careful search of stained smears may be needed to demonstrate the pathogen, which is most likely to be meningococcus, *H.influenzae* (often in pleomorphic form) or pneumococcus. The urgency of a precise diagnosis lies in the need for the early administration of an appropriate antimicrobial drug, e.g. a sulphonamide plus penicillin for meningococcus, chloramphenicol (usually with streptomycin or sulphadiazine) or ampicillin for *H.influenzae* or coliform bacilli, and penicillin for pneumococcus or other Gram-positive coccal pathogens. When haemophilus meningitis is suspected, immediate verification may be obtained if type-b antiserum is available. Either a loopful of the antiserum may be mixed with the fresh deposit and the mixture examined microscopically for capsular swelling which demonstrates the haemophili more easily than a Gram-stained film; or the cerebrospinal fluid may be layered on top of the antiserum in a capillary tube when a white precipitate will appear at the interface.

The deposit should be plated on ordinary blood agar and on chocolate agar but it is emphasized that good quality nutrient agar base in the blood-containing medium is essential for the growth of *H.influenzae*. Where facilities are available, a few drops of the cerebrospinal fluid may be layered on the culture medium directly from the lumbar puncture needle. Capsulation and satellitism are best demonstrated by subculture to a transparent medium and serological typing may be done locally or at a reference laboratory. Blood culture is advisable in meningitis cases and is essential for the diagnosis of acute laryngo-epiglottitis since the haemophili are not easily demonstrable in cultures from the local lesion.

For the isolation of haemophili from the sputum of cases of chronic bronchitis or bronchiectasis, the specimen must first be homogenized, smears stained by Gram's method, and cultures made on blood agar and chocolate agar. Suspected haemophilus colonies may be confirmed by the application of disks containing X factor, V factor or both factors to different areas on a nutrient agar plate after it has been seeded from the colony. The laboratory procedures are similar for the culture of material from infections such as conjunctivitis, sinusitis and otitis media.

Haemophilus strains are sensitive to refrigeration and neither specimens nor cultures should be kept at 0–4°C.

CHEMOTHERAPY

H.influenzae is sensitive to a fairly wide range of antimicrobial drugs, including sulphonamides, penicillin, ampicillin, streptomycin, chloramphenicol, tetracyclines and erythromycin, in minimal inhibitory concentrations that range between 0·2 ug/ml to 1·0 µg/ml. For acute infections with capsulate haemophili and, in particular, meningitis and epiglottitis, chloramphenicol is probably the drug of choice because it diffuses readily from the blood into the cerebrospinal fluid and respiratory secretions and drug resistance to it is rare. It may have to be given initially by a parenteral route if the child is unconscious or vomiting. Ampicillin is a good alternative drug and may be preferred because of its low toxicity although this hazard is very rare with chloramphenicol given for 4 to 5 days only. In cases of haemophilus meningitis that do not respond quickly to chemotherapy with a single drug, streptomycin or sulphadiazine (or sulphadimidine) may be additionally prescribed.

The chemotherapy of chronic bronchitis is concerned with (a) control of the chronic infection, and (b) treatment of acute exacerbations. For the former, only cases with purulent sputum will respond and for them, ampicillin or trimethoprim — sulphamethoxazole (cotrimoxazole) may be preferred to tetracycline because of their two-step bactericidal activity. Opinions differ as to whether one of these drugs should be given continuously through the winter months or intermittently, as indicated by sputum purulence or clinical relapse. There is evidence of an increasing incidence of tetracycline-resistant pneumococci from cases of acute and chronic respiratory infections (Percival, Armstrong and Turner, 1969). For the acute exacerbation, in which haemophili or pneumococci or both may be implicated, treatment is urgent and parenteral injections of combined penicillin and streptomycin or of ampicillin for 5 to 7 days are indicated.

EPIDEMIOLOGY AND CONTROL MEASURES

Hospital data on haemophilus meningitis from a number of countries have indicated that the incidence has been increasing in the last few decades, particularly in North America and probably in Britain. Analyses of bacteriologically confirmed cases of purulent meningitis of all ages reported by the Public Health Laboratory Service over the 4 years 1967 to 1970 showed that meningococcal infections were most frequent (average 457 per annum) and that cases of haemophilus (average 338) were slightly ahead of cases of pneumococcal meningitis (294) although the relative proportions of meningitis cases due to these three pathogens varied in different areas. Haemophilus meningitis occurs predominantly in the age-range 2 months to 3 years, related, as already indicated, to the absence of protective antibody either derived transiently from the mother or acquired by latent infection in early childhood. Type-b haemophilus is the infecting strain in 98 per cent or more of the cases; there is little difference in sex incidence. Cases occur sporadically but groups of unrelated cases have been noted to appear synchronously and type-b haemophili are frequently found in the throats of family contacts. Fatality rates in series of cases treated with modern chemotherapy have ranged from 4 to 15 per cent; most deaths are due to fulminating infections; brain damage is a common sequel among cases treated late or inadequately.

There are no effective control measures against primary haemophilus infections although family contacts may be given a short course of an appropriate antibiotic. The possibility of using a protective vaccine prepared from type-b capsular antigen is being explored.

Clarification of the etiological factors in chronic bronchitis and other respiratory infections in which non-capsulate haemophili may be secondary pathogens make it obvious that control measures must be directed at cigarette smoking, atmospheric pollution, respiratory virus infections and other agents that lower the resistance of the respiratory mucosa to secondary bacterial infection.

REFERENCES

FOTHERGILL, L. D. & WRIGHT, J. (1933) Influenzal meningitis: relation of age incidence to bactericidal power of blood against causal organism. *Journal of Immunology*, **24**, 273.

PERCIVAL, A., ARMSTRONG, E. C. & TURNER, G. C. (1969) Increased incidence of tetracycline-resistant pneumococci in Liverpool in 1968. *Lancet*, **i**, 998.

TURK, D. C. & MAY, J. R. (1967) *Haemophilus influenzae: its Clinical Importance*, London: English University Press.

21. Corynebacterium; Erysipelothrix; Listeria

Diphtheria: Erysipeloid: Listeriosis

Diphtheria is today a rare infection in most developed countries that have carried out effective immunization programmes. The future doctor of these countries, which include Britain, may well ask: is it necessary to learn about a disease that I am unlikely to see in my medical practice? To this question the teacher could reply that (1) diphtheria still occurs in sporadic episodes in this country and unfamiliarity with its clinical and epidemiological features may be disastrous; (2) much of our knowledge about the pathogenesis and control of toxic infections has depended on early and continuing researches on diphtheria toxin and antitoxin; and (3) diphtheria is still prevalent in many Commonwealth countries and so concerns students who come to Britain for their medical education. It therefore seems prudent that the future doctor should learn something about this infection.

CORYNEBACTERIUM DIPHTHERIAE

Corynebacterium diphtheriae (literally, the club-shaped rod of the membrane) is the causative organism of diphtheria which is a localized inflammation of the throat with greyish white adherent exudate (sometimes called false membrane) and a generalized toxaemia due to the secretion and dissemination of a highly potent toxin, the characteristic feature of this *toxigenic* species. The corynebacteriaceae are a large family, consisting mostly of non-pathogenic diphtheroid bacilli, some of which are commensals in the oropharynx and on the skin of man but at least one pathogenic species *C.ulcerans* causes localized ulcerations in the throat. Certain other species of corynebacteria (*C.pyogenes, C.ovis*, etc.) cause acute or chronic suppurative lesions in various domestic animals. *Erysipelothrix* and *Listeria* which belong to the family Corynebacteriaceae, are primary pathogens in animals but sometimes cause infections in man.

DESCRIPTION

Morphologically, *C.diphtheriae* (or the Klebs-Loeffler bacillus) has a characteristic appearance when films from growth on suitable culture media are stained with selective dyes to show the volutin (metachromatic) granules, which are intracellular depots of polyphosphate. Because the bacilli on dividing snap and bend abruptly, they are seen as angled pairs or parallel rows (palisades) looking like Chinese lettering; the average size is $3 \cdot 0 \times 0 \cdot 3\ \mu$m but there is considerable pleomorphism with club-shaped, oval and globular forms appearing in older cultures. The rods are Gram-positive but are easily decolourized. When stained with polychrome methylene blue or a selective stain (Neisser, Albert-Laybourn) the volutin granules stain very darkly purple in contrast with the brown or green counterstain, and so give the rods a 'beaded' or 'barred' appearance. With short diphtheria bacilli, the granules are polar but they are absent in most short diphtheroids. *C.diphtheriae* is non-motile, non-sporing and non-capsulate.

Culturally, the corynebacteria are aerobes or facultative anaerobes, growing best at 37°C (range 20° to 40°C) on a blood or serum-containing medium. The earlier dependence on Loeffler's serum slopes for quick growth and characteristic morphology in selectively stained films has been supplemented by the use of more selective blood or serum tellurite media in Petri plates on which the diphtheria bacilli grow more slowly as greyish to black colonies. The shape, size and colour of these colonies enable the bacteriologist to take the first step in differentiating the toxigenic strains into three main biotypes, called *gravis, intermedius* and *mitis* because of a relationship with the clinical severity of the infection (severe, intermediate and mild, respectively).

Fermentation reactions are important in differentiating toxigenic strains from diphtheroids and from each other: the toxigenic (and some non-toxigenic) types produce acid from glucose and maltose, but not as a rule from sucrose or mannitol, which are usually fermented by non-toxigenic strains; only the *gravis* type ferments starch and glycogen. All types are non-proteolytic. Other characters, e.g. uniform turbidity or granularity in fluid medium and haemolysis of ox or rabbit blood, which are used in differentiating the biotypes, may not be stable and some strains do not fit into any of the three main types.

The demonstration of toxin-production is the final test in differentiating toxigenic from commensal corynebacteria. A test of toxigenicity is particularly needed with mitis-like strains and with cultures from sites other than the throat, e.g. nose, ear, conjunctiva. Throat cultures that can readily be identified as *gravis* or *intermedius* types are mostly toxigenic but 10 to 20 per cent of *mitis* strains isolated from 'sore throats' are non-toxigenic. Toxigenicity is demonstrated by the agar-gel precipitation (Elek) test or by intradermal injection in the guinea-pig. Toxigenicity is associated with lysogeny and can be induced in receptive non-toxigenic strains by diphtheria β-phages. Conversely, strains may be 'cured' of lysogeny and lose their toxigenicity when grown in culture containing anti-β-phage serum.

PATHOGENESIS

When diphtheria bacilli find a foothold on the faucial mucous membrane, they cause an inflammatory exudate and necrosis of the mucosal cells. The infection may spread into the postnasal cavity or into the larynx where it may cause respiratory obstruction requiring tracheostomy or intubation. The sero-cellular exudate clots and remains adherent to the fauces so that attempts to remove the thick greyish smelly 'membrane' leave a raw bleeding surface. The diphtheria bacilli do not as a rule penetrate deeply in the underlying tissues, or into the blood, but as they multiply they produce a very powerful toxin which diffuses through the body by the blood stream and has a special affinity for certain tissues such as heart muscle, adrenal tissue and nerve-endings. This potent poison affects cellular activity by interfering with protein synthesis by the ribosomes, probably by inactivating the enzyme transferase II (Gill *et al.*, 1969). The amount of toxin produced in clinical infections is greater with *gravis* and *intermedius* than with *mitis* strains, related, perhaps, to the greater invasiveness and more rapid multiplication of the two former types which are more likely to be found in the deeper oedematous tissues. Diphtheria toxin is produced most actively when the bacterial iron content is decreased although *gravis* strains can elaborate toxin in culture media containing iron levels approaching those of the tissues, an attribute which has been equated by some workers with its invasiveness.

Death is generally the result of heart failure, presumably due to the cardiotoxic effect of the toxin, or, in cases of laryngeal diphtheria, to asphyxiation due to obstruction of the gap between the vocal cords by the diphtheritic membrane. The survival value of toxin production to the pathogen presumably lies in the role of the toxin in assisting colonization of the throat by killing the cells of the pharyngeal mucosa and the polymorph leucocytes attempting to phagocytose the bacilli. Non-toxigenic strains are able to colonize the throats of some healthy persons but such strains are less common and apparently, less successful parasites than the toxigenic strains. The marked diminution in the healthy carriage rate of toxigenic diphtheria bacilli brought about by national programmes of artificial *antitoxic* immunization is further evidence suggesting a role for the toxin in facilitating colonization of the throat.

IMMUNITY AND THE SCHICK TEST

It is generally agreed that diphtheria toxin and its specific antitoxin are the main participants in the occurrence of, and protection against, diphtheria. A simple screening test to separate susceptible from immune individuals is the injection intradermally of a small amount (0·2 ml) of a suitably diluted and stabilized diphtheria toxin, usually on the volar aspect of the forearm (Schick test). A localized erythema (with some oedema) reaching its maximum size (1 to 3 cm) and intensity in 2 to 4 days is a positive reaction and indicates that there is little or no neutralizing antitoxin in the tissues; that is, the individual is susceptible to diphtheria. If there is no reaction, he is immune. A control test with heated toxin or purified toxoid, injected into the other arm, sometimes results in a small erythematous patch which fades quickly and is presumably due to tissue hypersensitivity to some non-toxic protein fraction; this pseudo-positive reaction usually occurs in older children and adults who have already a naturally or artificially acquired immunity to diphtheria (Barr, Stamm and Stevens, 1957). Similarly, a localized swelling may occur after the *subcutaneous* injection of a small amount of toxoid (Moloney test). These hypersensitive individuals should not be given injections of diphtheria toxoid since (a) they may have violent local and/or systemic reactions to the injections; (b) most are already immune; and (c) the Schick test itself will have stimulated more antitoxin production.

The reaction to the Schick test serves only as a rough guide to the amount of antitoxin in the blood; negative reactions are very unlikely if the level is less than 0·004 unit/ml but positive reactions may occur in individuals with values up to 0·01 unit/ml. Precise antitoxin measurements will obviously give better assessments of immunity and there is a good measure of agreement between the antitoxin titres and the degree of immunity. Thus, in the extensive studies by Hartley, Tulloch and their colleagues (M.R.C. Report, 1951) in Tyneside and Dundee, two-thirds of the children with diphtheria had on admission to hospital antitoxin levels between 0·001 and 0·01 unit/ml, whereas less than a quarter of the control normal children had these low levels. When diphtheria occurred in artificially immunized children—and it was usually infection with the invasive *gravis* type—the clinical syndrome was often that of a localized tonsillitis or pharyngitis without general toxaemia or complications.

In communities where diphtheria is endemic, natural immunization by subclinical infection is common, particularly after an epidemic wave of *gravis* infection as happened in Britain before World War II and in Europe during that period when there were some three million cases of diphtheria. In temperate climates this natural immunization is due to latent or atypical faucial infections and is accompanied by high throat-carrier rates. Under such circumstances of high endemicity and absence of artificial immunization, a large majority of the population (e.g. 90 per cent) become immune through contracting subclinical infection during childhood. In tropical countries latent diphtheritic infection of skin lesions probably plays a more important role (Marples, 1965; Bezjak and Farsey, 1970).

LABORATORY DIAGNOSIS

The primary diphtheritic lesion occurs most often in the throat, though sometimes in the nasal cavity or larynx. For laboratory diagnosis, the lesion is swabbed and the material inoculated on to selective culture media and blood agar as soon as possible. A direct smear should be made and stained by Gram's method, not for the diagnosis of diphtheria, but for the identification of coarse spirochaetes and fusiform bacilli present in cases of Vincent's angina and sometimes in infectious mononucleosis. The best selective medium is one containing whole blood (heated, laked or plain) plus approximately 0·04 per cent potassium tellurite which is markedly inhibitory to most microorganisms other than the corynebacteria. Since the tellurite also slows the growth of diphtheria bacilli, incubation should be continued for 24 to 48 hours before a negative report is given. In endemic areas where an early report may be helpful, a Loeffler serum slope which encourages quick growth and characteristic morphology should also be inoculated; an Albert-stained smear of the mixed growth on the slope after 12–18 hr is examined for bacilli with metachromatic granules.

The tellurite-containing medium, besides being selective, allows an early provisional identification of the infecting biotype from the colonial appearance, which may be prognostically valuable to the physician. The case-fatalities from diphtheria in a very large collected series were respectively 8·1, 7·2 and 2·6 per cent for *gravis*, *intermedius* and *mitis* infections;

haemorrhages and post-diphtheritic paralyses were much more common with the former two types than with *mitis* infections.

Further identification and virulence tests are necessary with diphtheria-like cultures from sites other than the throat; they consist in the main of fermentation reactions and the agar-gel precipitation or guinea-pig intradermal tests for toxigenicity.

CHEMOTHERAPY

The corynebacteria are sensitive to penicillin in the range 0·004 to 0·02 units/ml and to other antibiotics active against Gram-positive bacteria. The most useful of these is erythromycin which may be preferred to penicillin for eliminating diphtheria bacilli from the throat, particularly of persistent carriers. Antibiotic therapy can be a useful adjunct to, but not a substitute for, antitoxin in the treatment of clinical diphtheria since it helps to eliminate the organism but has no effect on preformed toxin. It is mandatory to give antitoxin as early as possible to any patient with *suspected* diphtheria since the fatality rate is directly related to the period of delay in giving antitoxin, rising from 0 to 20 per cent between days 0 and 5 of the infection: the average case fatality is 5 to 7 per cent.

EPIDEMIOLOGY

Source and Mode of Transmission

In communities where diphtheria is endemic healthy throat carriers are commonly present, e.g. 1 per cent of schoolchildren, and for every clinical case there may be up to 100 healthy carriers who may spread infection to susceptible persons. The bacillus is therefore maintained principally in the throats or noses of healthy carriers and the majority of clinical infections are probably contracted from carriers rather than patients. The nasal carrier is particularly dangerous because he sheds large numbers of bacilli. The diphtheria bacillus is relatively resistant to drying and other adverse environmental influences. It may survive for many weeks in dust and on dry fomites (toys, books, pencils, etc.) contaminated with nasal, oral or pharyngeal secretion. The dust in hospitals and institutions may become heavily infected with dried, pulverized secretions. The infection is probably spread by airborne infected dust, by contact with fingers, eating utensils and fomites contaminated with secretion and, possibly, by secretion droplets or droplet-nuclei. The source of infection in localized outbreaks is most often a nose carrier as in streptococcal infections, but other reservoirs should be looked for, e.g. children with diseased tonsils, discharging ears or skin lesions.

Incidence

Diphtheria is an infection confined to man although, very rarely, it may be transmitted by cow's milk contaminated from superficial teat lesions which, in turn, have been infected from a human source. Infection usually spreads directly from person to person and is facilitated by intimate and continuous contact as in the family, school, residential nursery or other institution. Children are susceptible from the age of 3 to 6 months when passive immunity derived from the mother via the placenta has disappeared. Incidence is highest among primary school children and then among toddlers: for example, in the city of Manchester in 1936–37 before national immunization in Britain, the proportion of clinical cases in the age groups 0 to 4, 5 to 14 and 15 or over years was respectively 22, 64 and 14 per cent. Outbreaks have occurred among teenagers and young adults in service training units. In the course of national immunization programmes directed at pre-school and school children there may be a shift in distribution of cases to older age groups.

In some tropical centres where latent skin infections may play an important part in the natural acquisition of immunity, faucial diphtheria is less common than in endemic temperate countries: it has its highest incidence in pre-school children and is reported mainly from the towns. In these circumstances, improvements in social and environmental conditions may lead to an increasing incidence of faucial infections as skin sepsis declines.

During national immunization programmes,

the carrier rate of virulent diphtheria bacilli diminishes *pari passu* with the fall in incidence of clinical infections so that carrier rates of 0·5 to 2·0 per 100 schoolchildren in the pre-immunization period are reduced to rates of 0·1 to 0·01 or less after 60 to 70 per cent of pre-school and schoolchildren have been immunized. Yet localized outbreaks, mostly in schools or in families, have occurred in London and other urban areas in Britain during the past two decades; *mitis* has been the most common infecting type and symptomless carriers have considerably outnumbered clinical cases. The possibility that localized outbreaks of diphtheria in non-endemic areas are due to the importation of infection either by immigrants or by British subjects returning from abroad must be kept in mind and investigated. A more precise epidemiological marker than the biotype might be useful for tracing possible sources of these outbreaks, e.g. serological typing (Robinson and Peeney, 1936; Hewitt, 1947), phage typing (Saragea and Marimesceu, 1966) or bacteriocin typing.

In recent years throat infections due to *C.ulcerans* have been reported in Britain; they accounted for half the corynebacterial clinical cases (25 out of 49) reported by the Public Health Laboratory Service in the years 1965 to 1969 (Pollock, personal communication); raw milk may be a vehicle; symptomless carriers are rare.

Prophylactic Immunization

The evidence in favour of a national immunization programme for the control of diphtheria in communities where the infection is endemic is now overwhelming. For example, in England and Wales where large-scale immunization was begun in 1941 the incidence of diphtheria has fallen from a pre-immunization level of around 55 000 cases annually with 2 780 deaths, to an average of 17 cases per annum for the five years 1964–68 and only 6 deaths in that period. In the intervening years, when both morbidity and mortality rates were falling steadily, the ratio of diphtheria in immunized and unimmunized members of the community was 1:4 and the mortality rate in the ratio of 1:25.

The choice of diphtheria prophylactic and the times at which injections are to be given will depend on local circumstances. An alum-adsorbed toxoid is the most effective antigen when used singly; two or three injections at 6 to 8 week intervals are best given in the second six months of infancy. However, it is usually more expedient to give combined antigens, e.g. diphtheria and tetanus toxoids (not alum-adsorbed) mixed with pertussis vaccine, when three doses should be given, beginning as early as the third month of life and at intervals of 6 to 8 weeks, and 4 to 6 months between first and second and second and third injections respectively (Chap. 58). A booster dose of diphtheria toxoid (combined with tetanus toxoid if the two antigens have been used together for primary immunization) is given at school entry. There is no need for further booster doses unless, in adult life, the individual is going to a country where diphtheria is still endemic, and then only after preliminary Schick testing.

The control of localized outbreaks of diphtheria in immunized communities requires close collaboration between the Medical Officer of Health or school medical officer, the bacteriologist and the local practitioners. All home and close school contacts must have swabs taken from both nose and throat or any other possible focus (discharging ear, skin lesion), preferably on two separate occasions; infected persons (cases and carriers) should be removed to the isolation hospital and given antibiotic therapy (preferably, erythromycin) as well as antitoxin where necessary; and the immunization histories of all home and school contacts are reviewed. Where a primary course or a boosting dose of prophylactic has been given within the previous two years, no further immunization is necessary. Those immunized more than two years previously should be given a boosting dose, either a small dose of alum-adsorbed toxoid or of toxoid-antitoxin floccules (TAF). Close contacts not previously immunized require urgent protection and this is best achieved by combined active/passive immunization; a dose of 500 units refined antitoxin is given in one site and 0·5 ml of alum-adsorbed toxoid in another site; the dose of toxoid is repeated 4 to 6 weeks later. In older children and adults it is advisable to do Schick tests before giving the prophylactic, which should be restricted to positive reactors without any pseudoreaction. These procedures are described in more detail by Taylor, Tomlinson and Davies (1962) following their experience with outbreaks of diphtheria in the London area.

OTHER CORYNEBACTERIA

There is a great variety of species within the genus *Corynebacterium*. At least one of these, *C.ulcerans*, is pathogenic for man and a number are animal-pathogens, e.g. *C.ovis* or the Preisz-Nocard bacillus, the causative organism of pseudotuberculosis in sheep and of a suppurative lymphadenitis in horses, *C.pyogenes*, associated with suppurative lesions in pigs and cattle, including bovine mastitis; *C.renale*, causing cystitis and pyelonephritis in cattle; *C.equi*, reported as a cause of pneumonia in foals and pseudotuberculous lesions in other animals, and *C.murium*, which causes chronic caseating lung lesions in the mouse. Non-pathogenic corynebacteria, some of which may be opportunistic pathogens, are usually called diphtheroids; they include *C.hofmannii*, a common commensal in the oropharynx, *C.xerosis*, often present on the conjunctivae but of dubious pathogenicity, and *C.acnes*, frequently found in acne lesions. Some of these diphtheroids are short and ovoid in shape with a tendency to show polar staining with methylene blue but devoid of volutin granules as demonstrated by selective stains; other diphtheroids which may be present in respiratory secretions or purulent discharges from infected wounds, middle ear, etc. resemble *C.diphtheriae* morphologically and in their staining reactions but usually ferment sucrose and are non-toxigenic.

C.ulcerans

This corynebacterium has been isolated from exudative or ulcerative throat lesions which clinically resemble diphtheria. It is a pleomorphic bacillus with club, coccoid and filamentous forms, particularly after 48 hours culture. Although Gram-positive, it stains irregularly and may be Gram-negative in older cultures. It resembles the *gravis* biotype of the diphtheria bacillus in its sugar reactions but also ferments

trehalose late and liquefies gelatin. There is a narrow zone of haemolysis round the colonies on blood-agar. *C.ulcerans* produces two distinct toxins—one immunologically identical with diphtheria toxin and the other similar to the toxin of *C.ovis*. Subcutaneous inoculation into a guinea-pig results in death with *post mortem* findings similar to those produced by *C.diphtheriae* but death may not be prevented by prophylactic diphtheria antitoxin. Intradermal inoculation causes a necrotic ulcerative lesion.

Epidemiologically, the throat infection may be derived from raw cow's milk or from contact with cattle. Contact carriers are uncommon but several cases may occur in a family from a common source such as milk. Any infected patient should be treated as though he were a case of diphtheria; erythromycin is regarded as the antimicrobial drug of choice.

ERYSIPELOTHRIX: LISTERIA

Erysipelothrix and *Listeria*, which are members of the family Corynebacteriaceae, have many similar biological characters and some workers would place them in the same species. They are common pathogens of both domestic and wild animals and birds and sometimes produce infection in man.

ERYSIPELOTHRIX RHUSIOPATHIAE (ERY. INSIDIOSA)

The causative organism of swine erysipelas and human erysipeloid.

Description

Morphologically, the organisms are slender, Gram-positive, non-motile, rod-shaped bacilli 1–2 μm by 0·2–0·4 μm, occurring singly and in chains. In culture media, longer and filamentous forms are observed. True branching has been described, and on this account the organism was once classified as an actinomycete. Growth occurs on ordinary media even at room temperature, though the optimum is about 37°C. The organism shows a tendency to be microaerophilic when first isolated, and in agar-shake cultures may grow best just below the surface, but is able to grow under both aerobic and anaerobic conditions. In gelatin-stab culture a line of growth occurs along the wire track with lateral spikes or disks radiating from the central growth. Surface colonies on plates are of two types: one is exceedingly minute and dewdrop-like, with a smooth surface; the other is larger and has a granular appearance. Various carbohydrates are fermented (without gas production), e.g. glucose and lactose; sucrose and mannitol are not fermented. Different groups of the organism have been recognized according to their antigenic characters.

ANIMAL PATHOGENICITY. Mice, rats, rabbits and pigeons are susceptible to inoculation. Mice and pigeons are specially susceptible, and usually die of an acute septicaemia within four or five days after experimental inoculation. Subcutaneous injection in rabbits produces a spreading inflammation and oedema with a fatal result. Experimental inoculation with cultures in swine reproduces the disease as it occurs naturally. The smooth-colony type of culture is the more pathogenic.

PATHOGENESIS. In pigs the bacilli can be observed in the characteristic diamond-shaped skin lesion, and in internal organs, e.g. lungs, spleen and kidney. In some cases there is a septicaemic condition and the organism is detectable in blood films, particularly in leucocytes. In the chronic form of the disease, in which a 'verrucose' endocarditis occurs, the bacilli may be confined to the cardiac lesions.

A similar organism, *Erysipelothrix muriseptica*, is responsible for epizootic septicaemia in mice. It is doubtful whether this organism constitutes a separate species.

Ery. rhusiopathiae may occur in apparently healthy pigs, and has been isolated from the tonsils, intestines and faeces. It has a wide distribution in other animals and in birds. It is also found, apparently as a commensal, on the skin and scales of many fish (particularly members of the perch family).

Human Infection

Cases of human infection with this organism are known as 'erysipeloid' and have a distinctive clinical picture. There is very severe pain and swelling of a finger or part of the hand with a dusky, greyish discoloration of the skin of the affected area. The condition is an occupational hazard for those who handle infected animals or fish; most recorded cases have been in abattoir workers, butchers, fishmongers, laboratory workers and veterinary surgeons.

LABORATORY DIAGNOSIS. According to Sneath *et al.* (1951) it is seldom possible to recover *Erysipelothrix rhusiopathiae* from swabs, and the most satisfactory method is to obtain a biopsy from the actively growing edge of the lesion and to incubate this for 48 hours in 1 per cent glucose broth, subculturing on to blood agar. An attempt should be made to cultivate the organism from the blood in acute cases. Inoculation of infective material may also be made in mice or pigeons. An agglutination test is applicable.

LISTERIA MONOCYTOGENES

This organism owes its specific name to the fact that infection by it in laboratory animals, e.g. rabbits and guinea-pigs, produces a monocytosis in the blood. The disease, listeriosis, is now recognized to have a world-wide distribution, affecting many species of wild and domestic animals (foxes, dogs, gerbils, chinchillas, etc.), birds and fishes as well as man. It is regarded as a zoonosis but transmission from animal to man is often difficult to demonstrate. In man, listeriosis manifests clinically as a meningo-encephalitis in older adults but a generalized infection (granulomatosis infantiseptica) may occur in neonates following a symptomless infection in the mother.

Description

Morphologically *Listeria monocytogenes* is a Gram-positive straight or slightly curved non-sporing rod, 2 to 3 μm by 0·5 μm, often in pairs at an acute angle. Sometimes elongated filaments may be observed, particularly in solid medium at room temperature. It is feebly motile at 37°C, but in young broth cultures at 25°C it is more active and exhibits up to four flagella. Young cultures of the organism are Gram-positive, but after 48 hours many are Gram-negative, and in older cultures they may be entirely Gram-negative.

Cultures can be obtained at 37°C under aerobic conditions on ordinary media, but growth is better on media containing liver extract, blood, serum or glucose. The colonies are at first very small and droplet-like; after a few days' growth they may attain a diameter of 2 mm, being smooth and transparent, though later they may be more opaque. Surface colonies on blood agar are surrounded by a narrow zone of complete haemolysis. Gelatin and Löffler's serum are not liquefied. In glucose, maltose and certain other common sugars acid is promptly produced without gas; lactose and sucrose, but not mannitol, are fermented slowly.

Listeria produces an exotoxin in the form of a haemolysin which probably plays little part in pathogenicity. Experimentally, the organism is pathogenic for rabbits, mice and guinea-pigs, but not for rats and pigeons. It gives rise to focal lesions on the chorio-allantoic membrane of chick embryos.

Listeria is susceptible *in vitro* to penicillin, streptomycin, the tetracyclines, chloramphenicol and erythromycin, but resistant to sulphonamides, bacitracin and polymyxin.

Human Infection

Cases of meningo-encephalitis in man are characterized by a suppurative meningitis with mostly a mononuclear or polymorphonuclear exudate in the CSF and a monocytosis.

An intra-uterine infection, characterized by extensive focal necrosis especially of liver and spleen, known as granulomatosis infantiseptica, first described by continental workers, causes a high mortality in the affected foetus or newborn child.

LABORATORY DIAGNOSIS. Isolation of the organism is made by culture of the blood or lesions in generalized infections in infants and of spinal fluid in cases of meningitis. The pathogen may be misdiagnosed as a contaminating diphtheroid. The cerebrospinal fluid in cases of meningitis is slightly turbid (300 to 20 000 cells/ml polymorphs and lymphocytes) and has a higher glucose content than might be expected; the diphtheroid-like bacilli may be seen in a stained film of the centrifuged deposit. White cell counts of the blood show a relative monocytosis.

EPIDEMIOLOGY. In recent years evidence has accumulated of the widespread distribution of listeriosis in man and animals, especially in certain European countries (Germany, Czechoslovakia, Denmark, Sweden) and in North America. Authenticated cases of listeria meningitis in England and Wales, as reported by the Public Health Laboratory Service, range around 20 per annum, a rate of 0·45 per million population. The infection occurs mostly in adults over 40 years of age and is more common in males than in females. Inapparent infections may occur at any age; in pregnant women it may be followed by abortion, usually in the 5th to 6th month, by perinatal death or by severe generalized infection in the neonate.

REFERENCES AND FURTHER READING

BARKSDALE, L., GARMISE, L. & HORIBATA, K. (1960) Virulence, toxinogenicity and lysogeny in *Corynebacterium diphtheriae*. *Annals of the New York Academy of Sciences*, **88**, 1093.

BARR, M., STAMM, W. P. & STEVENS, P. J. (1957) Immunity to diphtheria; evaluation of Schick test as preliminary to immunization. *British Medical Journal*, **i**, 1337.

BEZJAK, V. & FARSEY, S. J. (1970) *Corynebacterium diphtheriae* in skin lesions in Uganda children. *Bulletin of the World Health Organization*, **43**, 643.

GILL, D. M., PAPPENHEIMER, A. M. Jnr, BROWN, R. & KURMICK, J. T. (1969) Studies on the mode of action of diphtheria toxin. *Journal of Experimental Medicine*, **129**, 1.

HEWITT, L. F. (1947) Serological typing of *C. diphtheriae*. *British Journal of Experimental Pathology*, **28**, 338.

MARPLES, MARY J. (1965) *Ecology of Human Skin*. Illinois: C. J. Thomas.

M.R.C. REPORT (1950) A study of diphtheria in two areas of Great Britain. Medical Research Council Special Report Series No. 272.

ROBINSON, D. T. & PEENEY, A. L. P. (1936) The serological types amongst *gravis* strains of *C. diphtheriae* and their distribution. *Journal of Pathology and Bacteriology*, **43**, 403.

SARAGEA, ALICE & MAXIMESCU, P. (1966) Phage typing of *Corynebacterium diphtheriae*. *Bulletin of the World Health Organization*, **35**, 681.

SNEATH, P. H. A., ABBOTT, J. D. & CUNLIFFE, A. C. (1951) Bacteriology of erysipeloid. *British Medical J.*, **ii**, 1063.

TAYLOR, I., TOMLINSON, A. J. H. & DAVIES, J. R. (1962) Diphtheria control in the 1960's. *Royal Society of Health Journal*, **82**, 158.

THOMSON, D. (1966) Mass immunization in the control of infectious disease. *British Medical Journal*, **ii**, 427.

ZABRISKIE, J. B. (1970) Bacterial protein toxins. In *Microbial Toxins*, Vol. I, p. 213.

22. Mycobacterium Tuberculosis

Pulmonary Tuberculosis: Other Tuberculous Infections

The mycobacteria, or acid-fast bacilli, have distinctive biological characters differentiating them from most other microorganisms. They belong to the order Actinomycetales and therefore have some affinity with the pathogenic actinomycetes and nocardiae. Because of a waxy material in their cell walls, the mycobacteria are not easily stained but treatment with hot carbol fuchsin allows impregnation by the dye which is retained despite attempts to remove it with acid or alcohol. The mycobacteria are thus called 'acid-fast' organisms. Another characteristic feature is the very slow growth of the pathogenic mycobacteria or even failure to grow, e.g. *Mycobacterium leprae*, on artificial culture media.

Mycobacteria are widely distributed throughout the world and only a few species are pathogenic to man and other mammals, birds, reptiles, and fish. The pathogenic species that merit particular attention are the mammalian tubercle bacilli, namely *Myco. tuberculosis*, or the human type of tubercle bacillus, whose main host is man, and *Myco. bovis*, the bovine type of tubercle bacillus, which is pathogenic to man as well as to cattle, its main host, and other animals; *Myco. avium*, which is pathogenic to birds and some animals, e.g. pigs, but very rarely a cause of disease in man; mycobacteria causing skin ulcerations; certain opportunistic ('atypical' or 'anonymous') mycobacteria which are infrequently pathogenic; and *Myco. leprae*, the cause of leprosy, which today occurs mostly in tropical and subtropical countries.

Mycobacteria characteristically produce chronic granulomatous lesions, which, in the case of tuberculosis, break down by caseation. The most common site of infection is the lung (pulmonary tuberculosis) but glands, bones, joints, the brain and meninges, and other internal organs may be affected. Leprosy affects the skin, certain mucous membranes and peripheral nerves and occurs in either a mild tuberculoid form or the more severe lepromatous nodular disease; it is a very chronic infection.

MYCOBACTERIUM TUBERCULOSIS: MYCO. BOVIS

Occurrence

The two types of tubercle bacilli that ordinarily affect man are the human type, *Myco. tuberculosis*, and the bovine type, *Myco. bovis*. Man is the main host of the human type of bacillus and the bacillus is spread almost exclusively through patients with 'open' pulmonary tuberculosis who cough and spit out infected sputum. The human type of bacillus has also sometimes been found in natural infections of monkeys, dogs, cattle and pigs. The prime hosts of the bovine type of tubercle bacillus are cattle, but this organism also is a common cause of tuberculosis in many other mammals, including horses, pigs, cats and dogs. Man is also commonly infected with the bovine bacillus when there are ready opportunities for contact with infected animals or drinking of infected milk. Infection with the bovine bacillus is a zoonosis and this bacillus rarely spreads from man to man. There are no true healthy carriers of either the human type or the bovine type of tubercle bacillus.

DESCRIPTION

The human and bovine types of tubercle bacilli show certain differences in morphology, in cultural characters and in their pathogenicity for laboratory and domestic animals. In films of sputum the human strains may be slender and straight or slightly curved rods, 3 μm × 0·3 μm; and the bovine strains are straight and stubby. They may occur singly or in pairs often forming an obtuse angle, or in small bundles of parallel bacilli. The organisms are non-motile. They are non-sporing but possess considerable resistance to drying and some disinfectants.

Tubercle bacilli do not grow on unenriched culture media. Primary growths may be obtained on blood or serum media or preferably on a medium containing whole egg or egg-yolk, incubated aerobically at 37°C. Growth is slow and becomes visible by 10 to 14 days at the earliest or as late as 6 to 8 weeks after primary inoculation from the infected host.

Human strains grow more luxuriantly in culture (eugonic) than do bovine strains (dysgonic). The addition of a low percentage of glycerol to the medium encourages the growth of human strains, but has no such effect on the growth of bovine strains and may inhibit them. Sodium pyruvate enhances the growth of bovine strains and also of those strains of tubercle bacilli, both human and bovine, that have been damaged by chemotherapy and, as a result, grow feebly or not at all on standard media. A low concentration of an inhibitory dye, malachite green, is usually added to egg media to prevent growth of contaminants. Discrete colonies of the human type are raised, irregular in shape, with dry wrinkled or mamellated surface and of tough, tenacious consistency; the colour, at first creamy white, later becomes buff. By contrast, the bovine type grows as flat, white, smooth, moist colonies which 'break up' more readily when touched.

Tubercle bacilli will grow on top of a liquid medium as a wrinkled pellicle if the inoculum is carefully floated on the surface and the flask left undisturbed. Otherwise they will grow as floccules throughout the medium. These growth characters are due to the lipid, hydrophobic surface of the bacilli. However, a diffuse growth can be obtained by adding a wetting agent or detergent such as the polyoxyethylene sorbitan monooleate commercially known as 'Tween 80' to a medium containing casein hydrolysate, bovine serum albumin, asparagine and certain salts (Dubos medium). This medium can be solidified and used to give surface growth by incorporating agar.

Biochemical reactions are not ordinarily used in the identification or classification of tubercle bacilli. Antigenic analysis has shown that there are four main serological groups of mycobacteria: mammalian (human, bovine and murine), avian and reptilian tubercle bacilli, and saprophytic mycobacteria. The human and bovine types of tubercle bacilli appear to be identical in antigenic composition thus explaining their cross-reactions in tuberculin hypersensitivity tests and the successful use of a bovine bacillus (BCG) vaccine for immunization against human-type bacillus infections.

The thermal death time at 60°C is 15 to 20 minutes, an important point to remember in connection with the pasteurization of milk. The organism is relatively resistant to injurious chemical substances; it can survive in putrefying material, and in sputum may resist 5 per cent phenol for several hours. It is highly susceptible to sunlight and ultraviolet radiation, whilst ordinary daylight, even through glass, has a lethal effect. If protected from light, however, the tubercle bacillus may remain viable in moist sputum, or in dried and pulverized sputum for weeks or months.

Animal Pathogenicity

The guinea-pig is highly susceptible to experimental infection with both human and bovine types of tubercle bacilli. After subcutaneous injection of infective material, a local swelling appears within 10 days, the neighbouring lymph nodes become involved, and infection then spreads to other lymph nodes and tuberculous nodules appear in spleen and liver, less commonly in lungs and kidneys. Death occurs within 8 to 12 weeks. Two-thirds of the strains of human tubercle bacilli derived from patients in South India are less virulent for the guinea-pig than strains from British patients.

Mice are much less susceptible to experimental tuberculosis than are guinea-pigs but after intraperitoneal, intravenous or intracerebral inoculation they develop progressive or chronic lesions according to the dose and virulence of the strain. These experimentally infected mice are very useful for studying the effects of new antituberculosis drugs.

Myco. bovis is more virulent to cattle and other domestic animals than *Myco. tuberculosis*. In the ox it produces a fatal tuberculosis, whereas the human type of bacillus causes only a localized lesion which heals spontaneously.

The difference in virulence between the two types of bacillus can be elicited in rabbits by *intravenous* injections of a suspension in saline of 0·01 to 0·1 mg (dry weight) of a culture from solid medium. The bovine bacillus produces an acute generalized tuberculosis, and the animal usually dies within 3 to 6 weeks; the human bacillus produces a more limited infection and the animal either survives or dies only after several months, with lesions confined usually to the lungs and kidneys.

Strains that deviate in their characters from the standard human and bovine species may be met with. Thus, strains isolated from lupus vulgaris may be atypical in that their virulence for laboratory animals is attenuated. The greatly attenuated bovine strain BCG (Bacille Calmette-Guérin) which is used for prophylactic vaccination against tuberculosis and which may be isolated from post-vaccinal lesions, grows eugonically like a human strain but is, of course, avirulent for laboratory animals.

PATHOGENESIS

The tubercle bacillus does not appear to contain or produce any significant toxin and the injection of killed bacilli or extracts of bacilli does not produce an early toxic effect apart from the hypersensitivity reaction which develops only in persons or animals previously infected with the organism. The bacilli multiply slowly in the body (generation time 6 to 12 hours) and they have no noticeable ability to resist capture and ingestion by phagocytes. Their pathogenicity appears to depend on their being able to resist destruction by lysosomal enzymes when inside the phagocyte, and they proceed to multiply in the cytoplasm of the phagocytes, in particular in the macrophages which are particularly active in their ingestion. After intracellular growth has taken place, macrophages become laden with numerous bacilli, the macrophage dies and disintegrates, and the liberated bacilli continue to multiply extracellularly in the tissue fluids or, after ingestion by other phagocytes, again intracellularly.

The termination of infection in patients who recover spontaneously appears to depend on the development of cell-mediated immunity and a consequent production of activated macrophages which have a greatly increased ability to kill ingested bacilli.

The commonest form of primary infection with the tubercle bacillus is a pulmonary lesion known as the primary complex. This primary complex comprises two components, namely, a lesion at the subpleural site of infection, or primary (Ghon) focus, and lesions in the draining lymph nodes. The organisms, usually *Myco. tuberculosis* but rarely *Myco. bovis*, are inhaled in very small particles (not more than 5 μm in diameter) directly into the terminal bronchioles or the alveoli. The primary lesion presumably develops at the site of implantation of a *single* airborne particle bearing one or a few bacilli. It may occur in any part of the lungs, and may be difficult to locate because of its small size. From it, the organisms are carried by lymphatic drainage to the regional mediastinal lymph nodes in which there may be progressive enlargement and involvement, followed by caseation and later calcification. More generalized infection may follow spread of the organism either through the blood-stream or the bronchi, leading to miliary or bronchopneumonic tuberculosis, usually with lesions in other organs besides the lungs, e.g. in the brain and meninges (tuberculous meningitis), spleen, liver and kidneys. Primary infection may also occur via the intestine with involvement of the mesenteric lymph nodes or via the tonsils with secondary cervical adenitis; such alimentary tract infection results usually from ingestion of milk infected with *Myco. bovis* but sometimes from use of eating utensils or ingestion of food contaminated with *Myco. tuberculosis*. Again, the pattern of the primary complex with a minimal initial lesion and more obvious involvement of the draining lymph nodes is produced but these forms of primary tuberculosis have become much rarer now that most milk supplies are pasteurized and bovine tuberculosis is virtually eradicated from Britain. From studies during the Second World War about a quarter of the cases of cervical adenitis in children under ten years of age were at that time caused by the human type of bacillus and about three-quarters of the cases of meningeal and bone and joint tuberculosis were also due to the human type. The few isolates of *Myco. bovis* in recent years in Britain have been from adults; these bacilli may have originated by activation of a lesion produced in a primary infection many years previously in which the bacilli had remained alive though dormant. Intracutaneous BCG vaccination may produce a form of primary complex with local skin lesion and an associated axillary adenitis.

Although tuberculous meningitis occurs characteristically as an early extension of a primary lung infection in very young children, it may also develop as an apparently primary infection in older children and young adults. In such cases, as in many instances of renal and bone and joint tuberculosis, there has presumably been an early 'seeding' of tubercle bacilli, blood-borne from the primary lesion in the lung or elsewhere, which has lain latent until some factor has encouraged fresh activity. Sometimes, too, an active lesion in one area may help to reactivate a latent infection in another organ or tissue.

The post-primary (or adult) form of pulmonary infection is the most common form of clinical tuberculosis in which one or more lung lesions progress to caseation and cavitation and, involving the bronchial tree, create a case of open or infectious tuberculosis. This clinical lesion occurs characteristically in young adults and may sometimes be due to a fresh exogenous infection; in older people pulmonary tuberculosis is most likely to be a reactivation of an earlier healed primary or secondary lesion. Tuberculous ulcerations in the larynx and intestine, when they occur, are usually sequelae of pulmonary tuberculosis spread by infected sputum; similarly secondary infections of ureter, bladder, epididymis may follow renal tuberculosis.

Laboratory Diagnosis

Since tubercle bacilli do not occur as commensals in healthy persons, their demonstration in the tissues or secretions of a patient is proof of the existence of tuberculous disease. Since, moreover, commensal or saprophytic mycobacteria are rarely found in the respiratory tract, the finding of acid-fast bacilli in sputum is good presumptive evidence of the presence of pulmonary tuberculosis. Such a provisional diagnosis based on microscopical findings is of great value because the final identification of *Myco. tuberculosis* by culture or animal inoculation takes several weeks.

Tubercle bacilli are most numerous in lesions showing rapid caseation, e.g. adult-type pulmonary tuberculosis. In miliary tuberculosis they appear to be relatively scanty. In more chronic or closed lesions few tubercle bacilli are observed, and they may not be detectable microscopically though they are demonstrable by culture or animal inoculation, e.g. in the pus from a tuberculous abscess, the urine of renal tuberculosis or the gastric lavage from a child with hilar gland infection.

Sputum collected from patients with open pulmonary lesions is the specimen in which tubercle bacilli are most commonly demonstrated. It is important to ensure that the specimen does consist of purulent secretion coughed up from the bronchi and is not merely saliva spat from the mouth. Suitable specimens are best collected during a bout of coughing soon after the patient awakes in the morning.

To demonstrate tubercle bacilli by direct microscopy, a strongly acting dye with a mordant, e.g. carbol fuchsin, is required with the application of heat to facilitate impregnation; this is followed by decolourization with 20 per cent sulphuric acid and application of a counter-stain such as malachite green or methylene blue, as in the Ziehl-Neelsen modification of a method originally described by Ehrlich. The tubercle bacilli stain red and this may cause difficulty for colour-blind people. To obviate this hazard, a blue-green screen, or filter, may be placed in front of a high-intensity illuminant when the bacilli and debris appear black, whereas if the counterstain is malachite green the background of cells almost disappears, rendering the bacilli easily recognizable. The use of a 1/7 (3·6 mm) fluorite oil immersion lens which allows more rapid scanning of smears is recommended but even so a prolonged examination may be necessary in some smears where the bacilli are relatively scanty. A negative result does not exclude tuberculosis, since at least some 100 000 tubercle bacilli must be present in 1·0 ml sputum for the reasonably ready demonstration of a positive microscopic finding.

Fluorescence microscopy, after staining with auramine, may be substituted for ordinary microscopy with Ziehl-Neelsen stained films and has some advantage in speed when large numbers of sputum smears have to be examined.

In suspected cases of pulmonary tuberculosis with no obvious sputum, coughing may be induced by the use of two laryngeal swabs, the expectoration collected on one being used to prepare a film for microscopic examination and that on the other used for culture. Alternatively, stomach contents obtained by gastric lavage may be examined microscopically and should be cultured without undue delay because of the bactericidal effect of the acid gastric secretion.

Urine, pleural and *peritoneal fluids* are centrifuged, films are made from the deposit and stained by the Ziehl-Neelsen method. As tubercle bacilli are often scantily present in these fluids, the deposit from 50 to 100 ml should be used for both direct microscopic examination and for culture; or the cultural method recommended by Ives and McCormick (1956) may be used, i.e. 100 ml of pleural fluid is added directly to 100 ml of double strength Sula liquid medium.

With all urinary specimens it is essential to treat the film with ethyl alcohol (two minutes) after decolourization with acid in the Ziehl-Neelsen process, in order, if possible, to exclude the commensal smegma bacilli that may be present in the external genitalia and which are generally decolourized with alcohol. In examining urine it is advisable to obtain the sediment from three consecutive morning specimens or the deposit from a 24-hour collection because of intermittency of excretion.

Cerebrospinal fluid is allowed to stand in a stoppered tube for an hour or longer, when a 'spider-web' coagulum usually forms in the fluid. The clot is carefully transferred to a slide, the preparation is dried, fixed by heat and stained by the Ziehl-Neelsen method. In the absence of clotting the fluid is centrifuged, the deposit, usually small, is taken up in a pasteur pipette, dropped without spreading on a slide, allowed to dry slowly and then stained.

Direct microscopic examination is an insensitive screening method for demonstrating the presence of acid-fast bacilli which may or may not be *Myco. tuberculosis*. Because of this limitation and because cultures of tubercle bacilli are often required for accurate identification and for drug-sensitivity tests, suspected tuberculous material should always be cultured, usually on an egg-containing medium such as the Löwenstein-Jensen medium without starch and in test tubes that can be sealed, e.g. screw-cap containers, in order to preserve moisture during the prolonged incubation period of up to 6 to 8 weeks. Properly conducted culture may be expected to detect tubercle bacilli when present in numbers as low as 10 per ml of specimen. If the material is likely to be free from contaminants, e.g. cerebrospinal fluid or pus from a closed lesion, it is inoculated directly on to two tubes of Löwenstein-Jensen or similar medium on which small colonies may be seen within 10 to 14 days; the presence of the dye, malachite green, not only inhibits contaminants but also helps to show up the whitish or buff-coloured colonies. If the material, e.g. sputum, is likely to contain other organisms, e.g. pharyngeal commensals, it must first be treated with a homogenizing and anti-microbial agent such as 4 per cent NaOH, trisodium phosphate or a combination of a quaternary ammonium compound and a mucolytic agent. If this is not done, commensal bacteria which grow much more rapidly than the tubercle bacilli, suppress their growth. Tissues such as glands must be finely minced with scissors or homogenized in a blender before heavy inoculation. Growth that appears atypical must be further examined by tests which will differentiate *Myco. tuberculosis* or *Myco. bovis* from the 'atypical' or saprophytic mycobacteria.

Great care must be taken in the handling of tuberculous material, particularly liquid cultures or suspensions of cultures, and during manipulations the use of a separate room and a special hood is recommended (Memo, 1970).

Serological tests for production of specific antibodies in tuberculous infection have not proved to be of much diagnostic value. The complement-fixation test becomes positive in a high proportion of established cases but is usually negative in early or suspected cases. Middlebrook and Dubos (1948) described a haemagglutination test which depends on the agglutinating effect of patients' serum on sheep or group-O human red blood cells sensitized with an extract of tubercle bacilli. This test has received a good deal of study, but its practical value in the diagnosis of clinical tuberculosis is doubtful because of its lack of both specificity and sensitivity.

GUINEA-PIG INOCULATION. Where tubercle bacilli cannot be detected in specimens by microscopic examination, guinea-pig inoculation may be used in addition to direct cultivation, since it is as sensitive if not more sensitive a method of demonstrating small numbers of bacilli, and one or other or both of these procedures often yield positive results when microscopic examination is negative. With most materials, culture gives at least as high a proportion of positive results as guinea-pig inoculation and has the advantages that a positive finding can be reported earlier and the culture is immediately available for sensitivity tests. In suspected renal tuberculosis, on the other hand, guinea-pig inoculation of microscopically negative urinary deposits may be more often positive than culture.

The usual method of carrying out the guinea-pig inoculation test is to inject material subcutaneously in the flank or intramuscularly in the thigh of two guinea-pigs, one of which is killed and examined at necropsy at four weeks and the other at eight weeks.

CHEMOTHERAPY

Although the tubercle bacillus is sensitive to an increasing range of antimicrobial drugs, clinical experience has confirmed that effective 'first-line' chemotherapeutic substances in tuberculosis are, in order of potency, isonicotinic acid hydrazide (isoniazid), streptomycin, and para-amino-salicylic acid (PAS). The necessarily large dose of PAS nauseates some patients and it is now frequently replaced by the powerful, safe, and acceptable, antituberculosis drug, ethambutol. Because resistant mutants of the tubercle bacillus may appear within one to three months after commencing treatment with any *one* of these drugs, and cause failure of treatment, it is essential that (a) a combination of three, initially, and later two of these antimicrobial drugs be used from the onset of treatment in cases of tuberculosis in order to minimize this risk and (b) every effort must be made to culture and test the sensitivity of infecting strains as early as possible, since resistant mutants in a strain that is already resistant to one of a pair of drugs being used will soon emerge to the other. Alternatively, frequent microscopic examination of sputum may detect the emergence of resistant variants. Strains that are highly resistant to isoniazid usually show a decrease in virulence for the guinea-pig but not necessarily for man.

The drug-resistant mutant originates spontaneously at the rate of about 1 in 10^6 bacteria in the multiplying population of bacteria in the patient's body. It originates independently of the presence of the drug and probably in most cases is present before the start of treatment. It is only, however, after treatment with the drug has been given for one or two months that the mutant bacteria, by selective outgrowth, appear in demonstrable numbers.

Reserve drugs that may have to be used in patients whose infecting strain is resistant or develops resistance to two or three of the first-line drugs, or in those patients who become highly sensitized to one or more of these drugs, include ethambutol, rifampicin, pyrazinamide, prothionamide, cycloserine, capreomycin and thiacetazone. The first two are powerful anti-tuberculosis agents and remarkably free from side-effects. Pyrazinamide and prothionamide are effective but the former is hepatotoxic and the latter frequently causes nausea. *Myco. bovis* is naturally resistant to pyrazinamide. Cycloserine and capreomycin are relatively weak but they can be used to prevent the emergence of resistance to accompanying drugs. Cycloserine may cause severe depression, and capreomycin can damage the eighth nerve and the kidney. Thiacetazone is moderately effective but it is hepatotoxic and causes nausea. These side-effects are slight in some Asiatic and African races. In some developing countries, therefore, combined therapy with thiacetazone and isoniazid under careful supervision is administratively not too difficult, is usually curative, and is much less expensive than treatment with standard therapy. The physician prescribing any of these 'second-line' drugs must be aware of the cross-resistance of the tubercle bacillus to two or more of them and of the hazards of toxicity (see Citron, in Heaf and Rusby, 1968).

EPIDEMIOLOGY

In the 17th century tuberculosis, or the 'consumption', was aptly described by John Bunyan as 'the captain of all the men of death'. Today it is the most important infectious disease in the world because of its high global prevalence, its chronic debilitating character and its heavy attack rate on the wage-earning community. Recent estimates by the World Health Organization indicate a prevalence of some 15 million infectious cases of which 70 to 80 per cent are in developing countries; 2 to 3 million new cases occur and 1 to 2 million cases die every year. In technically advanced countries mortality from tuberculosis is much lower than in the less advanced, but in the past was very high. In Britain tuberculosis probably accounted for about 20 per cent of all deaths at the beginning of the 19th century, by 1870 it was responsible for about 15 per cent, in 1920 for 10 per cent, in 1950 for 5 per cent and in 1970 less than 0·5 per cent. Mortality rates have been falling steadily in most technically advanced countries with temporary set-backs during the first and second world wars but the decline in deaths has been accelerated since the widespread use of effective chemotherapy in the past two decades (Fig. 22.1).

Notification rates, where these are reliable, have shown a similar downward trend, lagging a few years behind the fall in mortality rates. In Britain, both mortality and morbidity rates are much higher for men than for women; about 60 per cent of all deaths from respiratory tuberculosis are in men over 55 years of age. The decline in notifications has been particularly evident in children under 5 years and in males aged 25 to 44 years; and yet there were nearly 12 000 notifications of new cases in 1970. Of 2 298 isolations of *Myco. tuberculosis* from infective cases reported by the Public Health Laboratory Service in the second half of 1970, two-thirds came from males of whom half were over 45 years of age; 81 per cent of isolates were from cases of pulmonary tuberculosis, 5 per cent from cases of urinary tuberculosis and 24 or 1 per

cent from cases of tuberculous meningitis. There were only 42 isolations of *Myco. bovis*, all from adults, in 1970 (*British Medical Journal*, 1971). It may be concluded from these data that clinical tuberculosis has become much less common among young children and young adults, ordinarily two of the most susceptible age-groups, and is nowadays more frequently seen as a disease of elderly men; but even among them, notifications are decreasing.

Sources and Spread

With the control of bovine tuberculosis, which in former years in Britain accounted for 5 to 10 per cent of all deaths from tuberculosis and about a quarter of the cases of childhood tuberculosis from drinking infected milk, infection is nowadays predominantly due to the human type of tubercle bacillus and is spread mostly from open cases of pulmonary tuberculosis. The organism is expectorated in large numbers in sputum and is expelled in smaller numbers in droplets during coughing and speaking. There have been instances of explosive outbreaks of tuberculosis in schoolchildren and others exposed to an infective teacher or singer. Since very small droplets that can be inhaled directly from the infective patient are much less likely to carry tubercle bacilli than are larger droplets or sputum, infection may occur more often indirectly from dried dust particles than directly from moist droplets or droplet nuclei. Tubercle bacilli survive slow drying for days or weeks if protected from the bactericidal daylight or sunlight. Sputum smeared on handkerchiefs, clothing, bed-clothes, furniture or floor is liable to become broken into a fine dust when it has become dried, and minute infected dust particles, including many less than 5 μm in diameter, may readily be stirred up into the air in the course of body movements. In comparative experiments, P. Chaussé (1914 and 1916) showed that guinea-pigs were much more readily infected by exposure to sputum-dust liberated by the shaking of a patient's soiled handkerchief than by exposure to the spray of numerous coughs.

The spread of infection from infected case to susceptible contacts by contaminated dust or fomites is probably facilitated in overcrowded,

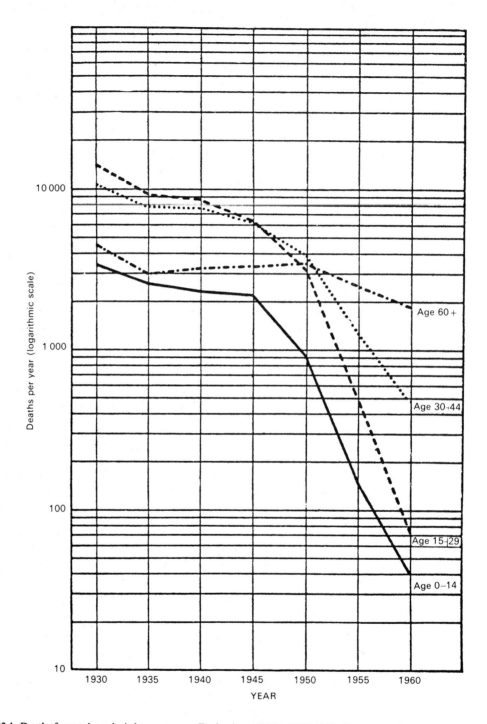

FIG. 22.1. Deaths from tuberculosis by age groups England and Wales 1930–1960. (Source, Registrar-General.)

badly lit rooms or buildings. Primary infection may occur at any age; if it occurs in early life (0 to 3 years) it is often associated with signs or symptoms of disease, e.g. hilar tuberculosis or the more serious systemic infections (tuberculous meningitis, miliary tuberculosis). At school age (5 to 15 years) infection usually occurs in an inapparent form, but in adolescents and young adults is again more likely to result in clinical disease.

Infection occurs earlier and is more likely to result in clinical disease among susceptibles who live in close contact with open cases than in subjects not so exposed, but many personal and environmental factors may contribute to overt tuberculosis, e.g. age (extreme susceptibility in early childhood and old age), malnutrition, other respiratory disease, hormonal dysfunction, pregnancy, stress, genetic constitution, etc.

Workers exposed to the inhalation of dusts containing silica have a high incidence of tuberculosis. Nurses, medical students, doctors and workers in pathology and bacteriology laboratories are more exposed and tend to have a higher than average rate of infection.

Tuberculin Test

The prevalence of tuberculous infection in contra-distinction to the clinical disease may be estimated by use of the tuberculin test which, when positive, indicates that the individual has at some time been infected by the tubercle bacillus without necessarily showing overt signs or symptoms of disease. A standardized tuberculin in the form of a purified protein derivative of *Myco. tuberculosis* (PPD/RT 23) with Tween 80 as a stabilizer is now available through the World Health Organization; the intracutaneous injection of a measured amount (usually 1 to 3 tuberculin units) allows comparison of the results obtained at different times and in different countries and is known as the Mantoux test. A positive test appears as a delayed hypersensitivity tissue reaction, manifesting as an area of oedema (or induration) with a wider erythematous zone; the diameter of the indurated area is measured after three days and the reading expressed in millimetres. In many warm climate countries where 'non-specific' tuberculin reactions, presumably related to infection with mycobacteria other than mammalian tubercle bacilli, are common, only reactions of 10 or more mm are likely to indicate previous tuberculous infection. The risk of misinterpreting tuberculin positive reactions in these communities may be minimized by dual tuberculin testing with the PPD-S (or human) tuberculin plus tuberculin prepared from a non-mammalian species, e.g. PPD-B (or Battey). In most countries with temperate or colder climates, nonspecific reactions are less common so that a positive test measuring 6 to 8 mm is suggestive of tuberculous infection.

An alternative method of testing for hypersensitivity makes use of a multiple puncture apparatus which pricks the skin through a film of stronger tuberculin (Heaf test). This method may also be used with undiluted BCG vaccine instead of tuberculin. The Heaf test is read as grades 1 to 4 according to the degree of reaction; grade 1 probably indicates a non-specific response. This test has the advantage of speed, acceptability and reproducibility but is not so easily standardized as the Mantoux test. (For technical details about tuberculin testing, see Heaf and Rusby, 1968.)

Tuberculin tests to measure prevalence of infection may be applied to children, say, at school entry (5 to 6 years) or at 10 to 13 years when in Britain it is used as the preliminary screening test before BCG vaccination. Comparison of the yearly findings of positive tuberculin tests among children aged 12–14 years and students has shown a steady downward trend in the prevalence of tuberculosis and the proportion of reactors in these age-groups in 1969 was 9·7 per cent. It has been suggested that the control of tuberculosis as a public health problem could be considered as being achieved when the prevalence of natural reactors among children aged 14 years has fallen to less than 1 per cent.

Other uses of the tuberculin test are (a) contact tracing of infectious cases of tuberculosis in the families and close relatives of young children who give positive reactions; (b) as an aid to the clinical diagnosis of suspected infection in young children; (c) as an indication of early clinical infection in older children who give strongly positive reactions (15 mm or more); these children require regular follow-up with X-ray examinations for 2 to 3 years; and (d) as a post-vaccination check on the efficacy of BCG vaccination.

CONTROL MEASURES

Tuberculosis is an infectious disease; it is also a social disease with its highest incidence among poor, malnourished and crowded communities. Control measures must therefore be directed at (a) reducing the load of infectious cases by case-finding and effective chemotherapy; (b) protecting the susceptible members by vaccination or, sometimes, by chemoprophylaxis and (c) improving personal, social and environmental conditions.

Case-finding and Chemotherapy

Reduction of the load of infection by 'case-getting' or case-finding followed by effective chemotherapy has played a major part in the dramatic reduction of mortality and morbidity from tuberculosis in sophisticated communities. Open cases of pulmonary tuberculosis become nearly non-infectious within a few weeks after the start of effective chemotherapy and remain so during maintenance of such therapy. Chest clinics to which suspected cases are referred by general practitioners have given the best returns in case-finding, with a current rate of 4 cases per 1 000 referrals in England and Wales. The organization of chest clinics, long since established in Britain, needs to be developed, perhaps in special units in health centres or polyclinics, in countries where a large proportion of the cases of pulmonary tuberculosis already have extensive disease before they are seen medically. In such countries, microscopic examination of sputum smears is the best and cheapest method of screening for infectious cases. Case-finding by mass miniature radiography is expensive and impracticable in most developing countries and should not be used until the load of infection has been reduced to reasonably low levels when it can help in detecting disease in older people and in special groups such as teachers, nurses and medical students, workers in certain industries, and staff in medical laboratories.

When an infectious case has been recognized, treatment with two or three of the first-line drugs must be initiated and maintained for at least one year and for two years in advanced cases in order to minimize the risk of relapse. Controlled trials of the treatment of infected cases in hospital or at home have shown that domiciliary treatment can be as effective as hospital treatment but some countries prefer to begin treatment with a spell of 2 to 3 months in hospital. The dangers of the development of drug-resistant strains of tubercle bacilli and of clinical relapses associated with ineffective chemotherapy have been illustrated by reports from many countries. In Britain, fortunately, surveys have shown that only 4 per cent of strains from untreated cases are resistant to one or more of the first-line drugs and 3 per cent are resistant to one drug only.

BCG Vaccination

Killed vaccines of the tubercle bacillus give little or no protection against tuberculosis. In 1921, two French workers, Calmette and Guérin, introduced a living vaccine prepared from a bovine strain that had been cultured for 239 subcultures on a bile-potato medium during the course of many years. This Bacille Calmette-Guérin (BCG) vaccine was at first given orally, but following Scandinavian practice is now given mostly by intradermal injection. Its value in the prophylaxis of tuberculosis has been much disputed, but in recent years controlled trials in different countries and with different communities and age-groups have demonstrated conclusively that BCG vaccination may give protection of the order of 80 per cent against clinical infection. Thus, in large-scale trials among school-leavers (14 to 15 years of age) in industrial areas in England, the incidence of clinical disease was reduced by approximately 80 per cent in the vaccinated groups during a follow-up period of 15 years (M.R.C. Reports 1963, 1972): (see Table 22.1). In a study among North American Indians (0 to 20 years old) a similar degree of protection persisted for some ten years after vaccination (Aronson et al., 1958).

These findings are in striking contrast to the poor results reported by Palmer and his colleagues from two controlled trials (a) in Puerto Rico where the protection rate was 31 per cent and (b) in Georgia and Alabama where it was only 14 per cent. Various factors have been

Table 22.1. *British M.R.C. Tuberculosis Vaccines Trial:* 1950–1971. Cases of tuberculosis starting within 15 years.

Section	Trial group	Number of participants	Cases of tuberculosis			Percentage protection
			Number starting within 15 years	Annual incidence per 1 000 participants*		
A	Children given BCG vaccine and those admitted concurrently with them	Negative unvaccinated	12 699	240	1·28	78·4
		Negative, BCG-vaccinated	13 598	56	0·28	
		Positive to 3TU	15 514	204	0·89	
		Positive only to 100TU	6 153	52	0·57	
B	Children given vole-bacillus-vaccine and those admitted concurrently with them	Negative unvaccinated	5 889	130	1·50	80·8
		Negative vole-bacillus-vaccinated	5 817	25	0·29	
		Positive to 3TU	8 783	118	0·91	
		Positive only to 100TU	3 068	32	0·70	

* After allowing for removals from population at risk, i.e. by death or by contracting tuberculosis.

blamed for these discrepant findings, such as malnutrition, variations in the protective potencies of the BCG vaccines, the strength of tuberculin used to distinguish susceptible from resistant individuals, and, in particular, the high level of non-specific hypersensitivity found in warm-climate countries (Table 22.2). A critical assessment of these factors has recently been made by Hart (1967) who, while admitting some protective effect from non-specific hypersensitivity, suggests that the low immunizing potency of the vaccines used in some of the American trials may have been the main contributor to the poor protection. Large-scale trials are at present being carried out in India in an attempt to solve these controversial problems.

Mycobacterium murium, the vole bacillus, causes tuberculosis in voles but is non-pathogenic to man. It has been used as a prophylactic vaccine and gives protection of the same order as that of BCG. However, it may give rise to local lupus-like reactions and its use has been discontinued.

CHEMOPROPHYLAXIS. Isoniazid, usually in a dose of 5 mg/kg body weight daily for one year, has been used for the chemoprophylaxis of tuberculosis in the U.S.A. where BCG vaccination has not been generally advocated. Best results have been obtained in young children with primary tuberculosis diagnosed by a positive tuberculin reaction (secondary chemoprophylaxis); these children have a relatively high risk of developing extrapulmonary complications; and with close child contacts of active cases of pulmonary tuberculosis who are at special risk of infection within the first year after recognition of the index case. However, the need to maintain treatment for a year among children who are not obviously sick must militate against the large-scale use of chemoprophylaxis in poor class communities where the need will be greatest.

Table 22.2. BCG vaccination: 6 trials (from *International Conference on the Application of Vaccines against Viral, Rickettsial and Bacterial Diseases of Man,* p. 463, W.H.O.).

Place	Age group (years)	Malnutrition	Tuberculin test dose	BCG activity	TB reduction (%)	Nonspecific hypersensitivity
Puerto Rico	1–18	±	low	? weak	31	+
Georgia and Alabama	5+	?–	low	? weak	14	++
Chicago	0–1	–	high	good	74	–
U.S.A. (Amerindian)	0–20	+	high	good	80	–
Britain	13–14	–	high	good	79	–
India	All ages	+	low	good	60	++

Hygienic Measures

Tuberculosis has its highest incidence in poor-class urban communities where overcrowding, poor housing and malnutrition are the main contributors. But even in such communities, the prevalence of infection, as indicated by the tuberculin test, is much higher in families where an adult (father, mother, grandparent) is an infectious case than in families without. Thus, the public must be taught that early recognition of pulmonary tuberculosis (persistent cough and spit, sometimes frank haemoptysis, fever and sweating) is advantageous both to the patient and to his family. Particular attention should be given to elderly, apparently bronchitic individuals. Avoidance of open coughing or spitting in the home, at the factory or in public transport has now become good social practice; good standards of household hygiene, lighting and ventilation will help to reduce the risks of family infection. Malnutrition is recognized as an important factor in reducing resistance to clinical disease. Persistent health education can help to direct attention to these hygienic and health measures but since social and environmental betterment takes time, most emphasis must be given to the more specific measures of case-finding, effective chemotherapy and prophylactic vaccination for the control of tuberculosis.

REFERENCES

ARONSON, A. D., ARONSON, C. F. & TAYLOR, H. C. (1958) A twenty-year appraisal of BCG vaccination in the control of tuberculosis. *Archives of Internal Medicine*, **101**, 881.

CHAUSSÉ, P. (1914, 1916) *Annales de l'Institut Pasteur*, **26**, 720, 771 and **30**, 613.

HART, P. D. (1967) Efficacy and applicability of mass BCG vaccination in tuberculosis control. *British Medical Journal*, **i**, 587.

HEAF, F. R. G. & RUSBY, N. L. (1968) *Recent Advances in Respiratory Tuberculosis*, 6th Edn. London: Churchill.

IVES, J. G. J. & MCCORMICK, W. (1956) A modification of Sula's method of cultivation of tubercle bacilli from pleural fluid. *Journal of Clinical Pathology*, **9**, 177.

MIDDLEBROOK, G. & DUBOS, R. J. (1948) Specific serum agglutination of erythrocytes sensitised with extracts of tubercle bacilli. *Journal of Experimental Medicine*, **68**, 521.

M.R.C. REPORT (1963) BCG and vole bacillus vaccines in the prevention of tuberculosis in adolescence and early adult life. *British Medical Journal*, **i**, 973.

M.R.C. REPORT (1972) BCG and vole bacillus vaccines in the prevention of tuberculosis in adolescence and early adult life. *Bulletin of the World Health Organization*, **46**, 371.

MEMO (1960/70) Precautions against tuberculosis infection in the diagnostic laboratory. Department of Health and Social Security, London.

23. Atypical Mycobacteria: Myco. Leprae

Chronic Respiratory Infections: Skin Ulcers: Leprosy

Acid-fast bacilli that are neither human nor bovine tubercle bacilli and which may be associated with disease in man have been provisionally named 'atypical' or 'anonymous' mycobacteria. They have attracted considerable attention in recent years because in those countries where the incidence of tuberculosis is declining, they have become relatively less rare. In Scotland they are still an exceptional cause of disease but in England and Wales the incidence appears to be just under 2 per cent among cases of tuberculosis. In some parts of the world they infect and sensitize large numbers of people and although their virulence is low, they occasionally cause disease that is clinically and radiologically indistinguishable from tuberculosis. The lungs are most frequently affected, generally the lungs of middle-aged men, especially if there has been antecedent pneumoconiosis, bronchitis or tuberculosis. They also infect the lymph nodes of the neck and in Britain they now appear to be the commonest cause of cervical lymphadenitis in children (Keay, 1969). They are resistant to most of the common antituberculosis drugs, and disease to which they give rise responds poorly to chemotherapy.

DESCRIPTION OF ATYPICAL MYCOBACTERIA

Atypical mycobacteria have been divided into four provisional groups (Runyon, 1959) according to the capacity of the cultures to become yellow on exposure to light (photochromogens, group I), or to produce an orange colour in the dark of the incubator (scotochromogens, group II), or to remain colourless (nonchromogens, group III), or to grow in three days (rapid growers, group IV). This grouping has proved valuable and is widely used. Further help in identification may be obtained from the bacterial morphology, colonial appearance, the effect on growth of incubating at low, medium, and high temperatures (say, 25°C, 37°C, 45°C); absence of niacin (nicotinic acid); catalase and arylsulphatase activity; susceptibility or resistance to, or effect on, certain chemicals; the pattern of sensitivity to antituberculosis drugs; their pathogenicity or lack of it for guinea-pigs, rabbits, chickens and mice; precipitation and agglutination reactions; bacteriophage typing; and lipid analysis. Some of these tests may be carried out in the hospital laboratory but the last three procedures are practicable only in certain reference centres.

The most important photochromogen is *Myco. kansasii*. The growth at first resembles *Myco. tuberculosis*, but when a young culture is exposed for an hour to light in the presence of air and then re-incubated it becomes canary yellow. *Myco. kansasii* infects the lungs of middle-aged men especially if there has been pre-existing disease. Consequently it is found in cities and industrial areas where the incidence of chronic bronchitis and lung damage due to air pollution is high. Women are seldom affected. There is little evidence that the organism is transmitted from man to man, and its source is unknown. It is the commonest pathogen among the opportunistic mycobacteria in Britain.

The scotochromogens are widely distributed in the environment and they occasionally contaminate cultures of tubercle bacilli. Some rather ill-defined strains—the scrofula scotochromogens—give rise to a mild cervical adenitis in children which simulates infection with the tubercle bacillus.

The nonchromogens, which produce no colour in the dark or after exposure to light, include *Myco. intracellulare*, formerly known as the Battey bacillus. It is so closely related to *Myco. avium* that some investigators regard them both as members of the same species. Infection with *Myco. intracellulare* occurs particularly in the South Eastern states of the U.S.A. and in

Western Australia, and in many warm climate countries. It is responsible for widespread, latent infection and tissue hypersensitivity which probably reduces the efficacy of BCG vaccination. It occasionally causes serious, progressive, pulmonary disease especially in middle-aged men whose lungs have already been damaged by air pollutants, and is, therefore, as a pathogen associated with urban and industrial life. Pulmonary disease due to *Myco. intracellulare* is refractory to chemotherapy. The source of the organism is obscure, but mycobacteria resembling or apparently identical with it have been isolated from soil. Human latent infections and tissue hypersensitivity may occur through contaminated skin lesions.

Myco. avium, another nonchromogen and the cause of tuberculosis in birds, may be endemic in flocks of poultry. Pigs that are closely associated with affected poultry may acquire an infection of the neck glands. Cattle may also be infected. Infection in man is rural rather than urban. The organism is an occasional cause of cervical adenitis in children. It may attack the damaged lungs of middle-aged men, and be the cause of a progressive, generalized infection with fatal outcome. Fortunately, these last two infections are rare as they respond poorly to chemotherapy.

A third nonchromogen is *Myco. xenopi* which was first isolated from a cutaneous lesion in the South African toad, *Xenopus laevis*. It occasionally causes chronic lung infection in man, and so far it has been identified in the South of England and in some European countries. *Myco. xenopi* is a thermophile, that is, it grows at 45°C as does *Myco. avium*; and it is moderately pathogenic for chickens. Because human infections have a coastal and estuarine distribution the mycobacterium may be derived from sea birds (Marks, 1969). It is susceptible to some of the antituberculosis drugs.

The rapid growers are usually saprophytes or commensals. They appear from time to time in pathological specimens and may be a source of confusion. *Myco. smegmatis* which is found in smegma (the sebum beneath the prepuce or around the clitoris and on the labia minora) may contaminate specimens of urine and may be seen as acid-fast rods in films of the deposits stained with the Ziehl-Neelsen stain. They usually do not resist decolourization with alcohol nor do they usually survive treatment with 4 per cent sodium hydroxide.

One rapid grower, *Myco. fortuitum*, is a pathogen of fish, amphibia and reptiles, and it may be recovered from water, soil and manure. In man it has been isolated from pustules and superficial abscesses, sometimes at the site of an injection. It has on rare occasions been the cause of lymphadenitis and pulmonary infections. It may harmlessly colonize the lungs of pneumoconiotics for a time without causing damage (Marks, 1969). When first isolated it should be cultured at 30°C, and it grows rapidly—within several days.

SKIN PATHOGENS

The skin may be infected by mammalian tubercle bacilli as in the lesions acquired by pathologists and butchers, or the ulceration of lips, external genitalia, or anus from tuberculosis of the associated organs; by attenuated mammalian tubercle bacilli in lupus vulgaris; by the artificially attenuated *Myco. bovis* of Calmette and Guérin from the site of a BCG vaccination; by *Myco. leprae*; and by *Myco. fortuitum* to produce a small abscess. Moreover, chronic skin ulcers may be colonized by commensal mycobacteria which can be isolated when appropriate methods are used.

There are two species of mycobacteria—*Myco. ulcerans* and *Myco. marinum*—which are exclusively skin pathogens. They remain strictly localized, multiplying only in the cool, superficial tissues, and they give rise to chronic skin ulcers. The regional lymph nodes are not enlarged and there is no systemic disturbance.

Myco. Ulcerans

Infection with *Myco. ulcerans* occurs in Victoria and Queensland, Australia, in Uganda (Buruli ulcer), the Congo, Nigeria, Malaya and Mexico; and foci of infection, generally near rivers and lakes, are probably widely distributed throughout the tropics. Although it is apparently a strictly human parasite, there is as yet no evidence of its spread from man to man; nor of carriage by insects although biting flies are prevalent in areas where infection with *Myco. ulcerans* is found. The organism may be introduced into the skin of an exposed part, usually an arm or leg, by some slight injury such as the prick of a thorn or an insect bite. In the course of a few weeks an area of induration develops which breaks down, and the ulceration spreads slowly under the skin and into the deeper tissues.

LABORATORY DIAGNOSIS. Smears from the spreading edge of the ulcer show the presence of masses of strongly acid- and alcohol-fast bacilli. Curettings treated for 15 minutes with 4 per cent sodium hydroxide yield on Löwenstein-Jensen medium at 32°C in the course of two months a poor growth of colourless, convex or flat colonies sometimes rough and not more than 3 mm across. Growth is never abundant and it does not develop either initially or on subculture at 37°C or 25°C. Films from the culture show that the bacilli are arranged in skeins or cords. The organism is non-pathogenic for guinea-pigs and rabbits, but inoculation of the foot pad of a mouse is followed by oedema progressing along the limb, and occasionally by ulceration.

Myco. Marinum

Myco. marinum (*balnei*) causes tuberculous disease in fish and amphibia, and these cold-blooded animals are the natural reservoir. *Myco. marinum* is not only a pathogen but can lead also a saprophytic existence in fresh or salt water lakes, swimming pools, and fish tanks. The organism infects man through an abrasion of the skin on the nose, fingers or toes, or over prominences such as the elbows, knees and ankles. A papule appears in the course of a week or so and breaks down into an indolent, circumscribed ulcer, the swimming-pool granuloma, which heals spontaneously in the course of a few weeks to a year. It may occur also on the hands of those who clean out fish tanks. The lesion is self-limiting so no treatment is required but cotrimoxazole is sometimes prescribed. The infection has been described in Europe and North America.

LABORATORY DIAGNOSIS. The bacilli are scanty and are scattered irregularly throughout the granulomatous lesion. They are acid-fast, long, beaded and banded rods rather larger than human tubercle bacilli. A homogenized snippet of skin may be used to inoculate Löwenstein-Jensen slopes, and cultures should be incubated at 30°C to 33°C. Growth will appear in about a fortnight. The colonies are round, convex, generally smooth and glistening, and yellowish; but after exposure to light followed by overnight incubation they become vividly golden. Subcultures grow in 3 days and become luxuriant. They grow less abundantly at 37°C. Films of the cultures show that the bacilli are not arranged in cords or skeins. *Myco. marinum* causes no disease in guinea-pigs but intradermal inoculation in the rabbit gives rise to a lesion like swimming pool granuloma in man. Inoculation into the foot pad of a mouse results after a few days in inflammation followed by breakdown and a discharge of pus. The lesion progresses much more rapidly than that following inoculation of *Myco. ulcerans*.

Notable differences between the two skin pathogens may be summarized as follows. *Myco. ulcerans* occurs in the tropics, the ulcer is progressive, the mycobacterium is abundant in the tissues, it grows poorly and slowly at 30°C to 33°C and not at higher or lower temperatures, and inoculation of the foot pad of the mouse causes slowly advancing oedema and ulceration. *Myco. marinum* occurs in temperate zones, the papule and ulcer develop quite quickly and are self-limiting, and the mycobacterium is scanty in the tissues. After subculture it grows in 3 days at 30°C to 33°C and also at 25°C and 37°C, growth becomes abundant and is bright yellow after exposure to light; inoculation of the foot pad of the mouse is followed by rapid onset of oedema and later discharge of pus.

Tests for Identification of Atypical Mycobacteria

In those regions where the incidence of primary resistance to antituberculosis drugs is low and 'atypical' mycobacteria acting as pathogens are a rarity, it is unnecessary to apply a series of tests for mycobacteria other than mammalian tubercle bacilli. It is sufficient to examine colonial and bacterial morphology and to confirm by testing for the presence of niacin that the strain is *Myco. tuberculosis*. *Myco. bovis* is niacin-negative, and it is occasionally resistant to PAS and always resistant to pyrazinamide. If the mycobacterium does not conform to the pattern for mammalian tubercle bacilli then certain other tests may be practicable and useful. Numerous tests have been proposed in the last 20 years to identify species and groups of mycobacteria. No single test has proved definitive, but the results of several may concur to give an unequivocal answer. The following may be helpful:

1. A fresh culture is exposed to bright light for an hour allowing access of oxygen by slackening the cap, and re-incubated overnight. If the culture becomes canary-yellow the strain is a photochromogen.

2. Subcultures are incubated at low, medium, and high temperatures (e.g. 25°C, 37°C and 45°C) and examined for growth daily for 5 days and thereafter at weekly intervals. At 25°C *Myco. fortuitum* and *Myco. marinum* grow in several days and *Myco. intracellulare* in about 3 weeks. At 45°C *Myco. avium* and *Myco. xenopi* grow in 3 weeks but other pathogenic mycobacteria do not do so.

3. Catalase activity is a rough guide. It is on the whole more active among the atypical mycobacteria than among the mammalian tubercle bacilli. It is further diminished in strains of the latter that are resistant to isoniazid.

4. Arylsulphatase activity may be used to distinguish between *Myco. avium* (negative) and *Myco. intracellulare* and *Myco. xenopi* (positive). It is helpful in identifying *Myco. fortuitum* which is highly active with a reduced quantity of the substrate, tripotassium phenolphthalein disulphate. It gives a strongly positive reaction in 3 days. [For technical details of these tests see Vol. II, Chap. 26.]

MYCOBACTERIUM LEPRAE

Leprosy is a disease of great antiquity: the leper has for centuries been a social outcast, partly because from biblical times he was regarded as 'unclean' and partly because his repulsive appearance and disabilities prevented him from being an acceptable member of the community. It is a very chronic disease affecting skin, mucous membranes and peripheral nerves and is manifest in two main clinical forms: lepromatous leprosy in which skin and mucous membrane lesions and granulomata cause much disfigurement, and tuberculoid or maculo-anaesthetic leprosy in which infiltration of nerves results in subcutaneous nodules, anaesthesias, and blanching of the skin, followed by trophic ulcers, burns and various deformities. The predilection of the bacillus for superficial tissues may be due to its preference for temperatures lower than 37°C.

DESCRIPTION

The leprosy bacillus, recognized inside cells from leprosy nodules in 1874 by Hansen, a Norwegian doctor, was the first bacterial pathogen to be described. Although Hansen maintained, against much opposition, that leprosy was contagious, the specific characters of the leprosy bacillus and its resemblance to the tubercle bacillus were not identified until some years after its discovery.

Morphologically, it is a straight or slightly curved slender bacillus, about the same size as the tubercle bacillus, with pointed, rounded or club-shaped ends; it is non-motile and non-sporing. With the Ziehl-Neelsen stain, it is less strongly acid-fast than the tubercle bacillus: the bacilli stain evenly in material from active lesions but usually show marked beading in smears from patients on effective chemotherapy: the proportion of solid staining to irregular staining bacilli is known as the 'morphological index'. The leprosy bacillus is Gram-positive, and can be stained fairly readily by Gram's method.

Many attempts have been made without success to cultivate this organism on artificial media and the cultures of acid-fast bacilli that have apparently been isolated from leprous lesions cannot be accepted as true leprosy bacilli. The leprosy bacillus, moreover, cannot be made to infect laboratory animals by conventional inoculation procedures, but much progress has been made in recent years in the cultivation of the leprosy bacillus in the footpad of the mouse. Infection has been initiated with strains from many countries, and since the bacilli survive well in wet-ice refrigeration, infective material may be sent by air to laboratories equipped to do the mouse foot-pad tests.

PATHOGENESIS

Leprosy is an infective granuloma, consisting of vascular fibrous tissue and many macrophages, packed with leprosy bacilli. Unlike the tuberculous lesion, the leproma does not necrose or caseate but frequently ulcerates with the discharge of infective exudate. In the *lepromatous* or *nodular* type, the granulomata form in the skin, mucous membranes and various organs (e.g. lungs, liver, spleen, testes): in the *tuberculoid* type, the granulation tissue infiltrates certain nerves and leads to motor and sensory paralysis, with characteristic trophic changes (e.g. anaesthetic skin areas—maculae). Bacilli are scanty in the tuberculoid lesions except during a reaction. Both types of the disease may occur in the same patient. Between these two polar types are the *indeterminate* cases, seldom bacteriologically positive and evolving to one or other type.

Experimental infection of the mouse foot-pad is helping in the study of the pathogenesis of leprosy and thymectomized irradiated mice provide a host that develops generalized infection including invasion of nerves, skin and other tissues. However, the very slow rate of division means that it may take 6 to 8 months for the leprosy bacilli to multiply 100 to 1 000 fold and the yields in the mouse foot-pad are limited to around 10^6 bacilli.

Laboratory Diagnosis

Films are made from any ulcerated nodule on the skin, or a non-ulcerated nodule may be punctured with a needle and squeezed till lymph exudes, from which films are made. Films may be prepared also from a scraping of tissue after a skin incision, particularly of the ear lobe, which may yield a positive result even when there is no obvious lesion: or a piece of skin (about 2 mm deep) overlying a nodule may be removed with curved scissors and smears prepared from the under-surface. Films should be made in all cases from scrapings or secretion from the nasal mucosa, as diagnostic information may be obtained in this way even when lesions are not present in the skin.

Films or sections are stained by the Ziehl-Neelsen method, substituting 5 per cent for 20 per cent sulphuric acid. The presence of the characteristic acid-fast bacilli, especially when they occur in large numbers inside cells, is diagnostic.

When the lungs are affected the bacilli may be demonstrated in the sputum and may be differentiated from the tubercle bacillus by differential Ziehl-Neelsen staining and by inoculation of a guinea-pig.

Infection of the mouse foot-pad which can be initiated with even a few leprosy bacilli, and is followed by the production of characteristic lesions, may be used to confirm a dubious diagnosis. This model is also useful in testing strains for drug resistance and in studying the antibacterial activity of new drugs. In clinical trials, the viability of the leprosy bacilli can be assessed more reliably by the mouse foot-pad test than by the morphological index (Rees and Weddell, 1970).

EPIDEMIOLOGY

The leprosy bacillus causes infections only in man and does not occur in healthy carriers. It is dependent for its maintenance on continued epidemic or endemic transmission through persons suffering from clinical leprosy.

In the middle ages, leprosy spread through Europe from its endemic centres in warm climate countries and persisted, particularly in Northern Europe, into the nineteenth century; there is still evidence of its former presence, e.g. in Norway and Scotland in the 'leper-slits' in the walls of churches and mansion houses where food was passed out to the leper in his wanderings as a licensed beggar. Leper houses (or spitals) were built for segregation of the lepers, and Liberton, a suburb of Edinburgh, is said to be derived from 'leper-town' where the sick congregated. Although there are still some 300 registered cases of leprosy in Britain, all of them acquired their infection elsewhere. Globally, it is estimated that there are some 10 million cases of leprosy, mostly in the tropical or subtropical belts of Africa, India, S.E. Asia, the Caribbean and Central and South America. In the past century, the disease has spread to Oceania and has heavily infected populations in the Hawaiian islands. New cases are being registered at the rate of 100 000 per annum in 75 countries but only a small proportion of all the cases are being treated or supervised.

Contrary to popular belief, the infectivity of the disease is low and requires long and close contact. The disease is most often acquired in childhood or early adult life and is most common among the lower social classes: males are more often affected than females. Infection is probably spread by direct contact through skin abrasions but may also be acquired by inhalation of infected dust via the nasal mucosa. Blood-sucking insects may possibly act as carriers. Patients with lepromatous lesions are much more infectious than tuberculoid cases. The incubation period is very variable (weeks to years) but is most commonly 2 to 4 years.

Because of its chronicity, crippling disabilities and social barriers, leprosy presents very large public health and economic problems in many developing countries.

CONTROL MEASURES

Lepromin: BCG Vaccination

Lepromin, as ordinarily used, is a boiled unstandardized extract of leprous tissue which, when injected intracutaneously, produces an area of nodular infiltration reaching its maximum in 3 to 5 weeks (Mitsuda reaction) in cases of tuberculoid leprosy and in a proportion of apparently healthy people. The reaction is usually negative in cases of lepromatous leprosy. Recently, efforts have been made to 'clean' and standardize lepromin by treatment in a tissue blender, washing, centrifugation, etc. in order to reduce the tissue content and homogenize the bacterial suspension. As a result, an antigen containing 160 million lepra bacilli per ml has been recommended as a 'standard' lepromin of which a 1 in 4 dilution containing 40 million bacilli would on intradermal inoculation be adequate to produce a nodule of 3 mm or more after 4 weeks as the criterion of positivity. A positive Mitsuda reaction indicates resistance to leprosy and the negative reaction in lepromatous cases may be related to a deficiency of cell-mediated immunity.

There is considerable overlap with positive tuberculin tests; for this and other reasons, controlled trials of BCG vaccines as a prophylactic against leprosy have been carried out in three regions—Uganda, Burma and New Guinea. The most promising results were obtained in Uganda against tuberculoid leprosy in children aged 0 to 15 years with a protection rate of 82 per cent among the vaccinated children over a period of 6 years. BCG vaccination gave some protection, particularly in the age range 10 to 29 years, in an aboriginal population in New Guinea with a high prevalence of tuberculoid leprosy and very little tuberculosis whereas a controlled trial among children in Burma where lepromatous leprosy is common gave negative results. Obviously, further evidence is needed before BCG vaccination can be recommended for routine prophylaxis against leprosy (W.H.O. Report, 1970).

Chemotherapy and Chemoprophylaxis

Oral administration of sulphones, in particular dapsone (4, 4'-diamino-diphenylsulphone, or DDS) has become the most practical chemotherapy for mass campaigns against leprosy. The recommended dosage, after tolerance to the drug has been established, has ranged from 6·0 to 10 mg per kg body weight per week over a period of 3 to 5 years or more, depending on the nature and extent of the infection. Smaller doses are recommended by some leprologists as being less likely to provoke severe lepra reactions or other secondary effects. The long-acting or repository sulphone, acedapsone (DADDS), or the riminophenazine, clofazimine (formerly known as B663 or lamprene), or other more bactericidal drugs are presently on trial.

Controlled trials in the long-term chemoprophylaxis of leprosy with dapsone among child contacts of infective cases have given encouraging results in India and the Philippines (W.H.O. Report, 1970).

Health education is an important element in any leprosy control programme, with the main objective of creating in the minds of the community, the patients and their families a reasoned attitude towards leprosy, which neither exaggerates the danger nor minimizes it.

REFERENCES AND FURTHER READING

KEAY, A. J. (1969) 'Atypical' mycobacterial lymphadenitis. *Tubercle, London*, Supplement, **50**, 85.

LESTER, W. (1966) Unclassified mycobacterial diseases. *Annual Review of Medicine*, **17**, 351.

MARKS, J. (1969) 'Opportunist' mycobacteria in England and Wales. *Tubercle, London*, Supplement, **50**, 78.

REES, R. J. W. & WEDDELL, A. G. M. (1970) Transmission of human leprosy to the mouse. *Bulletin of the World Health Organization*, **64**, 31.

RUNYON, E. H. (1959) Anonymous mycobacteria in pulmonary disease. *Medical Clinics of North America*, **43**, 273.

SELKON, J. B. (1969) 'Atypical' mycobacteria: a review. *Tubercle, London*, Supplement, **50**, 70.

W.H.O. REPORT (1970) Fourth report of expert committee on leprosy. *World Health Organization Technical Report Series*, no. 459.

24. Actinomyces: Nocardia

Actinomycosis: Mycetoma

Actinomycosis characteristically occurs as a chronic granulomatous infection in man and certain other animals and arises endogenously. In man the infecting species is *Actinomyces israelii* which occurs commensally in the buccal cavity. In bovines the infecting species is *Actinomyces bovis* and in dogs and cats the causal organism is *Actinomyces baudetii*. These three species of actinomyces are host-specific.

DESCRIPTION

Regardless of the species of the host, the causal organisms grow as colonies in the tissues and these eventually attain a size that allows them to be seen with the naked eye. Such colonies are commonly called sulphur granules since they show a yellow colouration during their development but in early lesions they are white and semitransparent. After developing the classical sulphur granule appearance they finally become dark brown or even black. When viewed in Gram-stained preparations after being crushed between two microscope slides the central filamentous mass is Gram-positive. There is commonly a surrounding zone of radiating clubs and these are Gram-negative; the clubs were once thought to be part of the organism but it is now considered that they represent lipoid material laid down by the host tissues in an endeavour to prevent further invasion by the filamentous growth.

When such preparations are stained by the Ziehl-Neelsen method, but with only 1 per cent in place of 20 per cent H_2SO_4 for decolourization, the peripheral clubs are acid-fast and the felted central mycelial mass is non-acid-fast. Club formation is less frequent in human than in animal lesions and is rarely if ever noted in films made from cultures; here the appearances are mainly of fragmented mycelium so that much of the material appears as bacillary or coccobacillary Gram-positive fragments.

The three species are similar in requiring anaerobic or microaerophilic conditions for growth *in vitro* although *Actino. bovis* is more tolerant of oxygen than the other two species. Growth is enhanced by increased concentrations of CO_2 and by use of media enriched with blood or serum and glucose. Colonies of *Actino. israelii* show considerable pleomorphism but surface growths always adhere firmly to the underlying medium whereas those of the other species do not. *Actino. bovis* colonies are smoother and softer in consistency than those of *Actino. israelii*; *Actino. baudetii* colonies are slow growing and require incubation for 4 to 5 days before showing as pin-head, dull white colonies.

If a shake tube culture is made in glucose agar, colonies grow optimally in a zone 10 to 20 mm below the surface where the CO_2 concentration is optimal and there is only a trace of free oxygen.

Strains show intraspecific antigenic homogeneity with no serological relationships among the three species.

CLINICAL INFECTION

Human actinomycosis still presents some puzzling features especially in that the infection, although endogenous, shows a much higher incidence in male agricultural workers than in any other occupational category: generally males are more frequently affected than females (3:1) and although no age group is exempt, the disease is most common between 20 to 29 years with the 10 to 19 year age group a close second; between them these two decades account for more than half the reported cases.

More than 65 per cent of lesions occur in the

cervico-oro-facial region and approximately 20 per cent are abdominal. Actinomycosis of lung, liver, kidney and skin also occur usually as blood-borne metastatic lesions. There is a tendency in human cases for secondary infection to occur, usually with pyogenic cocci.

At least two predisposing factors are recognized in human actinomycosis; namely, the presence of carious teeth and trauma; thus dental extraction may precipitate infection, and appendicectomy may be associated with the onset of abdominal actinomycosis. Similarly, external trauma, accidental or intentional, has also been noted to precede the onset of the disease.

LABORATORY DIAGNOSIS

The material submitted to the laboratory should be searched for sulphur granules which can be readily recognized and harvested by shaking the pus with water in a test tube; after standing for a few minutes the granules sediment and may be collected with a capillary pipette. A granule should then be crushed between two microscope slides and after fixation one of the films should be stained by Gram's method and the other by the modified Ziehl-Neelsen technique.

Granules to be used for inoculating blood agar plates or shake tubes of glucose agar should be washed several times in sterile saline before they are seeded. The microaerophilic nature of the resulting growth in the shake tube cultures (the largest colonies about $\frac{1}{2}$ in below the surface) combined with microscopic examination of stained films from colonies on blood agar to note the characteristic appearance is sufficient for diagnosis.

CHEMOTHERAPY

Treatment of actinomycosis before the introduction of penicillin was essentially surgical and surgery may still be required because the fibrotic granulomatous lesions are not readily penetrated by antibiotics. Penicillin remains the drug of choice and must be given in large doses for a long time, e.g. 0·5 to 1 mega units twice daily for two to three months. It is essential that patients apparently recovered from infection should be seen at regular intervals for a year or more since recurrence of infection is not uncommon.

CONTROL. Since the primary focus of infection is most often a carious tooth it is obvious that the incidence of actinomycosis would be greatly reduced if dental caries were prevented or adequately treated at the earliest possible stage.

NOCARDIA

Infection with *Nocardia* is rare in Britain. The majority of species in this genus are saprophytic but a few cause granulomatous and suppurative infections in men and animals. The most common human infection is mycetoma (madura foot), an infective granulomatous condition of the foot which occurs only in certain tropical and sub-tropical countries. Granules similar to those seen in actinomycosis can be found in the tissue lesions and pus.

The causal organism, e.g. *Nocardia madurae*, is a strict aerobe like other members of the genus; on culture colonies which are at first small, round and convex, later increase in size and become opaque and rosette-like; pigment production (yellow to pink) is very variable. It should be noted that *Noc. madurae* does not display acid-fastness. Mycetoma may also be caused by true fungi or *Madurella* (see Chap. 53).

Another species, *Nocardia asteroides*, is occasionally incriminated as the cause of pulmonary nocardial infection and secondary brain abscess or empyema. This species which is slightly acid-fast acquired its specific name from the star-shaped nature of its colonies after prolonged incubation.

25. Neisseria Meningitis: Gonorrhoea

The neisseriae are Gram-negative diplococci of which the pathogenic members, meningococcus and gonococcus, are characteristically found inside the polymorphonuclear pus cells of the inflammatory exudate. Although difficult to differentiate on morphological and cultural characters, these two pathogens are associated with entirely different diseases. *Neisseria meningitidis* is the cause of an acute purulent meningitis, variously called epidemic cerebrospinal meningitis, cerebrospinal fever or, because of a purpuric rash which is sometimes present, 'spotted fever'. It may also cause a subacute septicaemia with a petechial rash but without meningitis, particularly during epidemics of meningococcal meningitis. The term meningococcal infection is used to embrace these two syndromes. *Neisseria gonorrhoeae* is the cause of a sexually transmitted or venereal disease, gonorrhoea, a purulent infection of the mucous membrane of the urethra and also of the cervix uteri in the female; there may be rectal infection and secondary local and metastatic complications, e.g. epididymitis, salpingitis and arthritis may occur if the primary infection is not promptly treated. A purulent conjunctivitis of the newborn, ophthalmia neonatorum, and a vulvovaginitis in young girls also occur as primary gonococcal infections.

The non-pathogenic or potentially pathogenic members of the neisseria genus are common commensals of the upper respiratory tract, which is also the reservoir of the meningococcus. They include *N. catarrhalis*, *N. flava* and *N. sicca*.

Description

The two pathogenic neisseriae, *N. meningitidis* and *N. gonorrhoeae* are so similar in their morphological and cultural characters that they may be described together. They are Gram-negative oval cocci occurring in pairs with the apposed surfaces flat and even slightly concave (bean-shaped), and with the axes of the pair parallel, not in line as in the pneumococcus (Colourplate 1.2). In pus from inflammatory exudates, such as cerebrospinal fluid or urethral discharge, many diplococci are found in a small proportion of the polymorphonuclear cells; extracellular cocci also occur and there may be considerable variation in the size and intensity of staining of the cocci. In films from cultures, the diplococcal arrangement is less obvious and faintly staining involution forms are frequent in older cultures.

GROWTH REQUIREMENTS. Both the meningococcus and the gonococcus are exacting in their growth requirements due, perhaps, more to a susceptibility to inhibitory substances in the culture medium than to nutritional needs. The addition of lysed whole blood or ascitic fluid, or both, to nutrient agar will ensure good growth of colonies from infective material, provided incubation is done in a moist atmosphere containing 5 to 10 per cent CO_2, preferably at 35°C to 36°C. Growth is rather slow but on a good medium greyish glistening slightly convex colonies of 0·5 to 1·0 mm in diameter appear in 18 to 24 hours: aerobic incubation should, however, be continued for another 24 hours when the colonies are much larger disks (2 to 3 mm) with slightly roughened surfaces and a tendency to crenation of the margins, particularly in the gonococcus. Colonies of both pathogenic neisseriae react positively to the oxidase test (q.v.) and *quickly* develop a dark purplish colour; colonies of non-pathogenic neisseriae react more slowly.

To test for fermentative activities, subcultures are made on peptone serum agar slopes containing 1 per cent of the appropriate sugars plus an indicator: the meningococcus ferments glucose and maltose but not lactose or sucrose: the gonococcus ferments glucose only.

Gonococci are divisible into four biotypes (T1 to T4) related to colonial appearance, autoagglutinability and virulence as demonstrated by the induction of urethritis in human volunteers (Kellogg *et al.*, 1968). Types 1 and 2 have small (0·4 to 0·5 mm) glistening, convex, brown colonies, and are autoagglutinable and virulent; types 3 and 4 have large (1·0 to 2·0 mm) flat, unpigmented colonies and are avirulent. Virulence is probably associated with a surface antigen that is quickly lost on artificial culture.

The non-pathogenic neisseriae, which grow readily on ordinary, serum-free culture media, are either non-fermentative and non-pigmented, e.g. *N. catarrhalis*, or are pigmented and usually ferment glucose, maltose and sucrose, e.g. *N. flava* (see Vol. II, Chap. 26).

SEROLOGICAL CLASSIFICATION. Antigenically, the meningococci are divisible into four main serogroups now named A, B, C and D, a different terminology from some of the earlier classifications. Group A is in most countries the serogroup associated with epidemics of cerebrospinal meningitis, but in recent years group A has been supplanted by groups B and C as the main epidemic types, first among service personnel and now affecting civilian populations in the U.S.A. and Canada. A few new but still rare serogroups have been isolated, mainly from carriers but also from clinical cases, in Britain. The serogroup of a culture is usually determined by a slide agglutination test made with absorbed, group-specific antiserum. The addition of specific antiserum to a wet film containing meningococci in infective material or fresh culture will, in addition, demonstrate 'capsule-swelling', as with the pneumococcus.

The gonococci are antigenically more heterogeneous than the meningococci so that serogrouping has not proved practicable: they share certain somatic antigens with the meningococci and non-specific antibody tests with human sera may show cross-reactions with both neisseriae.

MENINGOCOCCAL INFECTION

PATHOGENESIS

The natural habitat of the meningococcus is the nasopharynx of man. Surveys of normal populations will demonstrate a carrier rate around 5 to 10 per cent. In communities in which outbreaks of cerebrospinal meningitis are occurring, the carrier rate of the epidemic strain may range from 20 per cent to 80 to 90 per cent and certain studies have shown that a sharp increase in the carrier rate of group A or other pathogenic groups of meningococci precedes the occurrence of clinical cases. However, this carrier:case ratio is variable in different outbreaks.

The route of spread of the meningococcus from the nasopharynx to the meninges is a controversial matter; the organism may either spread directly through the cribriform plate to the subarachnoid space by the perineural sheaths of the olfactory nerve; or, much more probably, it may be blood-borne. In favour of the latter route are the frequent positive blood cultures in the early stages of infection, the purpuric rash in many cases with the isolation of meningococci from the skin lesions, and the occurrence, particularly during epidemics, of meningococcal septicaemia with rash but no clinical meningitis.

It is important to realize that infection of the meninges is 'opportunistic' and irrelevant to the survival and spread of the meningococcal species. The bacterium spreads to other hosts from its site of carriage in the nasopharynx and never from the blood or meninges. In cases where the meningitis is fatal its production is disadvantageous to the causal strain of meningococcus by terminating its opportunities for dissemination from the nasopharynx.

The problem of main concern in pathogenesis is the occurrence of cerebrospinal meningitis among only a limited proportion of the population at risk. Recent studies have confirmed some early observations that the absence of bactericidal antibody in the blood is the factor most closely related to susceptibility to clinical infection. Evidence in support of this relationship is: (1) the age-distribution of meningococcal disease which has its highest incidence in infants and young children, from 3 months to 3 years of age, amongst whom humoral meningococcicidal antibodies are rarely found: the analogy with haemophilus meningitis is obvious; (2) the reciprocal relationship in the appearance of these bactericidal antibodies in older children and adults with the decreasing incidence of cerebrospinal meningitis, except when it occurs in outbreaks among adults brought together for special reasons, e.g. in service training centres and, in earlier days, in ships and jails; (3) prospective studies among military recruits which showed that whereas only 1 per cent of the total population at risk became clinically affected, 38·5 per cent of those lacking specific bactericidal antibody to meningococcus and who became infected with the epidemic group C strain developed meningococcal meningitis; and (4) patients convalescent from meningococcal infection develop typical immunoglobulins and bactericidal antibody to the infecting strains (Goldschneider, Gotschlich and Artenstein, 1969).

It is clear, nevertheless, from the relatively low incidence of meningitis in young children and the absence of meningitis in a large proportion of adults lacking specific antibody that in most persons the first infection of the nasopharynx with meningococcus leads to antibody production without the development of meningitis. Presumably non-specific defence mechanisms are generally successful in preventing infection of the blood and meninges.

LABORATORY DIAGNOSIS

Lumbar puncture should be done as soon as meningitis is suspected. In a case of meningococcal meningitis the spinal fluid is under pressure and is turbid in appearance due to the large number of pus cells present. In the early stages of infection the Gram-negative diplococci are present usually in considerable numbers in the purulent cerebrospinal fluid and can be recognized by microscopic examination of the centrifuged deposit. At a later stage they may be scanty and even apparently absent.

Films made from the sediment are stained by methylene blue and Gram's method (with Sandiford's counterstain). In the early untreated case, Gram-negative diplococci are seen, filling a limited number of the pus cells but also extracellularly; if the organisms are scanty, they may be more easily demonstrated in the smear stained with methylene blue. Cultures are made on blood or 'chocolate' (heated blood) agar and incubated for 18 to 24 hours in an atmosphere of 5 to 10 per cent CO_2. If Gram-stained films from the resulting growth show typical Gram-negative cocci, subcultures for biochemical tests are made by picking off single colonies on to sugar-containing serum agar slopes. The serological group may be identified by agglutination tests with the appropriate antisera.

For quick differential diagnosis, which is essential for early effective chemotherapy, microscopic examination is often sufficient. However, in the later stages of infection, or if sulphonamides have been administered, the organisms may be scanty or undetectable in the centrifuged deposit. In such cases a method sometimes successful is to add an equal volume of glucose broth to the cerebrospinal fluid, incubate the mixture for 18 hours, and subculture on blood agar; or the supernatant fluid, after centrifugation, may be layered on to the specific antiserum in a capillary tube, in search of a precipitin reaction. A retrospective diagnosis of meningococcal meningitis may be made by demonstrating the development of complement-fixing antibodies in the patient's blood serum.

In cases of suspected meningococcal septicaemia, and also in cases of meningitis, blood cultures should be carried out and subcultures made on blood agar every day for 4 to 7 days.

CHEMOTHERAPY

The meningococcus is ordinarily sensitive to the sulphonamides (80 to 90 per cent of strains) and to many other antimicrobial drugs. Because the sulphonamides diffuse readily into the cerebrospinal fluid, a sulphonamide compound, e.g. sulphadiazine given orally (or intravenously in comatose patients) is the best drug for proven cases of meningococcal meningitis except in areas where it is known that the meningococcus has become sulphonamide-resistant (MIC > 0·1 mg/ml). For these latter infections, benzyl penicillin or ampicillin parenterally should be used in addition to a sulphonamide; these drugs pass from the blood through inflamed, though not through normal, meninges into the cerebrospinal fluid. Otherwise chloramphenicol may be given orally since it diffuses even more readily into the cerebrospinal fluid. Prompt chemotherapy can be life saving and has reduced overall case-fatalities from a level of 20 to 40 per cent in untreated cases to 5 to 10 per cent. Fulminating infections, particularly in infants, sometimes with haemorrhagic involvement of the adrenals (Waterhouse-Friederichsen syndrome), may, despite treatment, end fatally within 24 hours of onset.

EPIDEMIOLOGY

The recorded number of meningococcal infections (mostly meningitis) in England and Wales fell from 1 390 in 1951 to 293 in 1967. From October 1968 all forms of 'acute meningitis' became statutorily notifiable in England and Wales and it is hoped that doctors will specify the infecting agent, where known, in the certificate of notification. Meanwhile it should be noted that the number of cases of meningococcal meningitis reported by the Public Health Laboratory Service has risen steadily from 358 in 1967 to 556 in 1970 (see *British Medical Journal*, 1971, **2**, 230). About two-thirds of the cases occur in the first five years of life and in this age group more than half the cases are in infants under 1 year of age. Incidence is considerably higher in males than in females. Because of the greater frequency and severity of meningococcal meningitis in early life, the death rate from this disease for the 5 years 1960–64 in England and Wales was around 70 per million in infants, 13 per million in 1 to 4-year-old children, 1·0 per million in the age range 5 to 14 years and less than 1 per million in adults.

The spring plateau of cerebrospinal meningitis that used to occur in Britain has now virtually disappeared and the infection occurs sporadically throughout the year. Widespread epidemics of infection with serogroup A, sweep through the dry belt of Africa below the Sahara, e.g. in Sudan and northern Nigeria, rising to a peak in the dry months, February to May, and ending abruptly with the onset of the rainy season. Whether crowding indoors during the hot, dusty weather or the effect of inhaled dust and dry air on the nasopharynx is responsible for the timing of these epidemics is unknown. Outbreaks have frequently occurred among young adult populations recently recruited to live together in semi-closed communities and what might have been limited epidemics in Britain were fanned into great conflagrations of cerebrospinal meningitis among troops in training in the early years of both world wars. In recent years, localized outbreaks have been a regular occurrence in some American Army base camps: the epidemic strains have been groups B or C, not group A. Intensive studies of the infection in these training centres have added much to our knowledge of the natural history of the disease. A high proportion of the recruits become meningococcus nasopharyngeal carriers and if the carrier strain is relatively avirulent, it induces bactericidal antibodies to virulent strains without causing clinical disease. On the other hand, clinical infection may occur in a high proportion of susceptible individuals who acquire the epidemic strain. The natural acquisition of immunity with increasing age from early childhood in civilian communities is therefore likely to be due to asymptomatic infection with avirulent strains.

Outbreaks of meningococcal meningitis require at least three factors: the presence in the population of a proportion of susceptible individuals who lack bactericidal antibodies to the current strains, a high transmission rate from person to person, and a virulent meningococcus. The first stage is the carrier epidemic which requires close personal contact although the large crowded barrack which seemed to be a dominant factor in the occurrence of outbreaks among troops in training in the first world war is not nowadays regarded as so important; nor is physical or emotional stress. The important factors that determine virulence and communicability of the meningococcus are still not understood.

Control Measures

In the control of outbreaks, mass chemoprophylaxis with sulphadiazine given orally, or inhaled like 'snuff' into the nose, for 2 to 3 days proved to be very effective in reducing carrier and case rates until the emergence of sulphonamide-resistant strains of meningococcus, initially in U.S.A. and more recently in Britain and other European countries. A satisfactory alternative drug for large scale chemoprophylaxis has not yet been found.

Since resistance to meningococcal meningitis is closely related to the possession of bactericidal antibodies, whether transiently derived from the mother or actively acquired by latent infection, the possibility of inducing immunity by vaccination has been explored from time to time and has now become reality with the separation from the epidemic serogroups A and C of high molecular specific polysaccharides which have been shown to be good immunizing agents. Vaccine trials with a group C polysaccharide vaccine in U.S. Army Training Centres have resulted in effective protection, not only against clinical infection, but also against the carrier state with the epidemic strain. However, the protection was group-specific and there were compensatory increases in both carrier rates and clinical disease with group B meningococci (Artenstein and Gold, 1970). Controlled vaccine trials in civilian communities are in train.

GONOCOCCAL INFECTION

PATHOGENESIS

The gonococcus is a strictly human parasite and all attempts to infect animals had failed until recently when chimpanzees have been experimentally infected. Its toxicity to mice on intraperitoneal injection of large amounts of culture is due to an endotoxin like that of the meningococcus. Unlike the meningococcus the gonococcus is not found in healthy carriers, but only in cases of acute or chronic infection; some cases of chronic infection are clinically inapparent, and such cases act as sources of infection. The initial infection generally affects the anterior urethra in men and the urethra and cervix uteri in women, but if untreated, the infection generally spreads more deeply into the genital tract and may become *chronic*. In acute urethritis the gonococcus infects the mucosa but does not ordinarily pass through it into the submucosal tissues. It is found in the urethral exudate on the surface of or within epithelial cells, within a proportion of polymorphonuclear leukocytes and also extracellularly.

In *men* the organism infects the urethra and produces a suppurative inflammation with purulent discharge. The cocci are present in large numbers in the discharge at an early stage, but later are scanty, sometimes with trivial discharges, and secondary infecting organisms, e.g. pyogenic cocci, coliform and diphtheroid bacilli may be present. Infection may extend along the mucous surfaces to the prostate, seminal vesicles and epididymis or may invade the peri-urethral tissue, producing an inflammatory reaction, peri-urethral abscess and subsequent stricture.

In *women* the urethra and cervix uteri are infected, but rarely the vaginal mucosa: discharge is often scanty. Infection may extend to the vestibular glands (bartholinitis), the endometrium (endometritis) and Fallopian tubes (salpingitis) and even the peritoneal cavity may be invaded.

Rectal infection (proctitis) occurs in both men and women. It is, of course, exogenously acquired by passive male homosexuals: in the female, it usually spreads to the anus from the genital infection.

Blood invasion may result from primary gonorrhoeal infections, and arthritis and tenosynovitis may occur as complications. Although the gonococcus has on occasion been cultivated from joint fluid in arthritis, the possibility of gonococcal arthritis being an allergic manifestation must be considered. A somewhat similar condition, Reiter's syndrome, characterized by urethritis, arthritis and conjunctivitis, is probably a sexually acquired infection of unknown aetiology. Secondary gonococcal conjunctivitis may be caused by transfer of infection from the urethra on the fingers. There have been recent reports of septic gonococcal dermatitis, usually associated with arthritis, arthralgia and fever. The skin lesions, varying from maculopapules to vesiculopustules are scanty, present mostly on the extremities or around joints and are more common in females than in males (Barr and Danielsson, 1971).

In female infants and children the gonococcus may produce a persistent vulvo-vaginitis with involvement sometimes of the rectum. Outbreaks of this infection used to occur in paediatric wards and children's institutions, but gonococcal vulvo-vaginitis is now rare, and associated mostly with sexual offences. In newborn infants, gonococcal ophthalmia (acute purulent conjunctivitis) may result from direct infection at birth when the mother has chronic gonorrhoea.

LABORATORY DIAGNOSIS

In *acute infections* thin evenly spread smears are made from the discharge. In *men*, specimens are taken from the urethral discharge; the meatus should be cleansed with sterile gauze soaked in saline solution, and specimens are taken either with a wire loop from within the meatus or drops of the discharge are taken directly on to slides. In *women* specimens are taken from the urethra and cervix uteri with a wire loop or swab and a vaginal speculum. Specimens may also be taken from the rectum and from the orifice of the greater vestibular gland.

Separate films are stained by methylene blue and Gram's method (with neutral red or Sandiford's stain as the counter-stain). In the acute stage, both in men and women, the occurrence of the *characteristic Gram-negative intracellular diplococci* is strongly suggestive of gonorrhoea. However, intracellular cocci may be scanty and pleomorphic, particularly if the patient has already received treatment; or only extracellular cocci are seen.

In *chronic infections*, the cocci may be relatively scanty in films and difficult to identify accurately among the secondary infecting organisms which may include Gram-negative commensal diplococci. In the male the 'morning drop' of secretion from the urethra should be examined, or films are made from a centrifuged urinary deposit or from any discharge after prostatic massage. In the female, secretion from the cervix uteri, and not vaginal discharge, should be examined. Any vaginal discharge should, however, be examined as a wet preparation for *Trichomonas vaginalis*.

Recently, fluorescent techniques for the identification of gonococci in smears have come into use but this 'on-the-spot' diagnosis must be confirmed by cultural and biochemical characters. Where there is a mixed infection, isolation of the organism may be technically difficult and a selective medium, e.g. that of Thayer and Martin (1966) or *Transgrow* containing trimethoprim should be used. Inoculation of material to be cultivated should, if possible, *be made directly from the patient on to a suitable medium pre-warmed to 37°C*, and the culture should be incubated at once, or at least within an hour or two, since the gonococcus may die quickly in an adverse environment.

When it is impracticable to make direct cultures, the specimen is taken with a charcoal-impregnated swab on a wooden applicator which is broken into a tube of Stuart's holding medium for transport to the laboratory.

Cultures are incubated at 35°C to 36°C for 1 to 2 days in an atmosphere of 5 to 10 per cent CO_2. In mixed cultures, e.g. from cases of chronic or symptomless infection in females, the oxidase reaction (q.v.) is useful in detecting colonies of the gonococcus, which *quickly* develop a purplish colour.

SEROLOGY. The complement-fixation test has been used with varying degrees of success, and is most useful for the diagnosis of chronic infection in females and for suspected gonococcal complications such as salpingitis and arthritis. Considerable care and experience are needed in the preparation of the gonococcal antigen to ensure maximum specificity without non-specific sensitivity. The degree of specificity of the test increases with increased positivity of the reaction but, with present procedures, both false-positive and false-negative reactions may be reported. Cross-reactions occur in patients with meningococcal infection and may be found in patients with chronic bronchitis and bronchiectasis related, perhaps, to antibody responses to commensal neisseriae. The test is, therefore, of doubtful value and not recommended for routine use.

CHEMOTHERAPY

The gonococcus is ordinarily sensitive to a wide range of antimicrobial drugs (e.g. MIC of penicillin = 0·005 units/ml) but a proportion of strains have developed resistance to those drugs which have been most commonly used in therapy, viz. the sulphonamides, penicillin and streptomycin. In many countries the proportion of strains highly resistant to sulphonamides increased from less than 10 per cent to 80 to 90 per cent between 1936 and 1946, by which time penicillin became generally available and replaced sulphonamide in the treatment of gonorrhoea. After use of sulphonamide had become infrequent, the prevalence of sulphonamide-resistant strains declined and these strains are now a small minority. Penicillin-resistant strains were not encountered until 1957 and although the incidence of penicillin-resistant strains has increased in the past decade to 10 to 20 per cent in some areas, the degree of penicillin-resistance is not very high (MIC = 0·1 to 1·0 units/ml) and infection may be susceptible to cure by treatment with high dosage. Crystalline penicillin (5 mega units) or procaine penicillin (1·2 to 2·4 mega units) is still the drug of first choice. The dose should be repeated on three successive days for women with chronic infection and for cases of proctitis. In patients that do not respond to such therapy, the additional use of probenecid (0·5 to 1 g) to delay renal excretion has given good results. Alternative drugs that have been used successfully are tetracyclines, spiromycin and kanamycin. The combination of trimethoprim and a sulphonamide, suggested by Garrod and Waterworth (1968) because of the *in-vitro* synergistic action of this combination, may indicate the usefulness of cotrimoxazole.

EPIDEMIOLOGY

Sources and Modes of Transmission

Patients with clinically apparent or chronic inapparent infection are the only sources, and the infection is transmitted from person to person almost exclusively by sexual contact, so that gonorrhoea is classified as a venereal disease. The reason why the gonococcus is mainly dependent on sexual contact for its transmission are firstly that its main portal of entry and exit from the body is through the urogenital tract and that the coccus is so exceptionally susceptible to killing by the conditions of the extracorporeal environment, e.g. drying, cold, exposure to air, absence of nutrients, that it can only very rarely survive transmission by means less direct than the immediate transfer from the urogenital tract of one person to that of another. There is evidence to suggest that occasionally it may survive rapid transfer of exudate on the fingers to the conjunctiva or on damp towels as in the spread of gonococcal vulvo-vaginitis in institutions.

Gonorrhoea has been increasing at an alarming rate in most countries of the world during the past decade. Its global incidence in 1970, estimated at 16 million new cases, makes it one of the commonest specific infectious diseases. In the U.S.A., where there were about 2 000 000 cases in 1970, giving a rate of 2 000 per 100 000 of population over 15 years of age; the present

prevalence is, therefore, regarded as being epidemic. In Britain, after a peak incidence immediately after the Second World War and relatively low levels in the early 1950s, probably as a result of effective chemotherapy, the annual returns from venereal diseases clinics in England and Wales have shown a steady increase since 1954 (17 536 cases) and had reached 53 525 cases in 1970 (see Fig. 25.1). This number does not include patients treated privately or in the Armed Forces. Concomitant with the increasing incidence, a larger proportion of the diagnosed cases (around 16 per cent) are occurring among teenagers with more girls than boys affected. The rate for girls under 16 years is about $4\frac{1}{2}$ times that for boys of the same age group. This sex ratio may be contrasted with that for adults which ranges from 3:1 to 4:1, males to females, due partly to the reservoir of promiscuous women and prostitutes and partly to the difficulties of recognition of infection in the female.

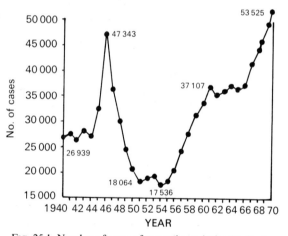

FIG. 25.1. Number of cases of gonorrhoea dealt with for the first time in England and Wales from 1940–70.

In recent years, a high proportion of the male cases (around 40 per cent) in England and Wales have been immigrants, mostly from the West Indies and Asia whereas less than 20 per cent of the female cases were born abroad.

The processes of modern life which have led to earlier maturity, greater mixing of the sexes, economic freedom for the young and increasing facilities for travel tend to lead to promiscuity.

Thus, factors that contribute to the mounting incidence of gonorrhoea are (a) an apparent increase in promiscuity, both heterosexual and homosexual, in a permissive society; (b) the easy availability of birth control methods and of effective chemotherapy for the infected; (c) difficulties in recognition (and therefore of treatment) in women and in passive male homosexuals; (d) greater population mobility within and between countries for cultural, commercial, touristic or military purposes; and (e) high infectiousness and short incubation which make the chain of infection difficult to break; to which may be added the development of drug resistance in the gonococcus which accentuates the need for accurate diagnosis, effective treatment and tests for cure.

CONTROL MEASURES

Control measures are aimed at the early recognition and effective treatment of clinical cases, tracing of infected contacts and bringing them in for treatment, use of physical and/or chemical barriers during intercourse, and health education. Treatment of venereal diseases in Britain is free and confidential at 'special clinics' (perhaps better renamed 'departments of genitourinary diseases') which are usually sited in the outpatient department of large general hospitals. These clinics·deal with a wide range of sexually transmitted and related conditions besides venereal diseases which affect only about one-quarter of all the patients who attend. Many of the clinics have attached social workers who help to tackle the problems of young people, unmarried mothers, unstable marriages, etc. A most important function of the clinics is contact tracing, which means seeking information from the patient about possible sources or recipients of infection and, hopefully, persuading them to attend the clinic for examination and treatment. There is, of course, no legal compulsion for prostitutes or promiscuous women to seek examination and treatment but most of those that are traced attend regularly. General practitioners may prefer to treat their own patients and if so, they, too, must endeavour to trace infected contacts. More health education is needed to warn the community that promiscuity carries a real risk of acquiring venereal diseases which, in women, may be easily missed and may be followed by serious sequelae. There is, for example, evidence of an increasing incidence of salpingitis which can lead to sterility.

Future developments may include greater emphasis on contact-tracing, better serological tests for the detection of symptomless infections in women, a combined birth control and antimicrobial substance to be applied locally, and the selective use of prophylactic vaccines.

REFERENCES

ARTENSTEIN, M. S. & GOLD, R. (1970) Current state of prophylaxis of meningococcal disease. *Military Medicine*, **135**, 735.

BARR, J. & DANIELSSON, D. (1971) Septic gonococcal dermatitis. *British Medical Journal*, i, 482.

GOLDSCHNEIDER, I., GOTSCHLICH, E. C. & ARTENSTEIN, M. S. (1969) Human immunity to the meningococcus. *Journal of Experimental Medicine*, **129**, 1307, 1327 and 1385.

KELLOGG, D. S. Jr., COHEN, E. B., NORINS, L. C., SCHROETER, A. L. & REISING, G. (1968) *Neisseria gonorrhoeae*: colonial variation and pathogenicity during 35 months *in vitro*. *Journal of Bacteriology*, **96**, 596.

THAYER, J. D. & MARTIN, J. E. (1966) Improved medium selective for culture of *N. gonorrhoeae* and *N. meningitidis*. *United States Public Health Report*, **81**, 559.

26. Salmonella: 1 Typhoid and Paratyphoid Fevers

The term *enteric fever* is frequently used in Britain to include typhoid and the paratyphoid fevers caused respectively by *Salmonella typhi* and *S. paratyphi A*, *B* or *C*: typhoid fever was confused with typhus fever until 1850 when Jenner, having examined 66 fatal cases of the two diseases both clinically and at post-mortem examination, clearly differentiated them before the causal agents of either had been discovered. Though the portal of entry and exit of the infecting bacilli is the intestinal tract, the enteric fevers are septicaemic infections with widespread involvement of tissues throughout the body.

Typhoid and the paratyphoid fevers are clinically similar and the assumption that cases of typhoid fever are invariably more severe is not always true. Also, the gross pathology of the enteric fevers is similar regardless of the causal organism and only bacteriological examination can differentiate between them. In Britain, typhoid fever is now relatively rare and the majority of recorded cases are imported from other countries. A significant endemic level of infection with *S. typhi* persists in the warm climate countries of Southern Europe. Outbreaks of infection due to *S. paratyphi B* outnumber other causes of enteric fever in Britain; *S. paratyphi A* infections are uncommon in this country but are frequently encountered in Eastern Europe, the Americas, India and the Middle East; *S. paratyphi C* as a cause of paratyphoid fever is largely restricted to Eastern Europe and Asia.

DESCRIPTION

The genus *Salmonella* to which the enteric fever pathogens belong comprises more than 1 000 serotypes and unlike other salmonellae, which are primarily parasites of animals other than man, *S. typhi* and its cousins, the three paratyphoid bacilli, are essentially parasites of man.

Morphologically members of the genus *Salmonella* are indistinguishable from each other or from other members of the family Enterobacteriaceae to which they belong: they are motile and non-capsulate. Culturally they are similar to most other enterobacteria except that on MacConkey or DCA medium they are lactose-non-fermenting after incubation for 18 to 24 hours; on such differential media their colonies are pale-coloured and similar to those of the other common pathogenic genus, *Shigella*.

Reference to Chapter 28 shows that differentiation of salmonellae from shigellae is a fairly straightforward matter; but to identify a member of the genus *Salmonella* and give it serotype status is time-consuming but necessary for epidemiological purposes. The particular isolate must first have its group status recognized by identifying its somatic (O) antigens and thereafter determining its serotype within the particular group by identifying the flagellar antigens which the isolate possesses. Strains of *S. typhi*, *S. paratyphi A* and *B* and *S. typhimurium* may be subdivided by phage-typing (see Vol. II, Chap. 29).

PATHOGENESIS

Natural infection in the enteric fevers is most often by ingestion followed by penetration through the mucous membrane of the small intestine; possibly the bacilli sometimes enter through the pharyngeal mucosa. From the results of observations on experimental salmonella infections it appears that the bacilli attach to the epithelial cells of the intestinal villi and induce their own intake into the cells by a process akin to phagocytosis. They pass through the cells and within 24 hours are found in the lamina propria and submucosa where they are rapidly phagocytosed by polymorphs and macrophages. The pathogenicity of the salmonellae appears to depend primarily on their ability to

314

remain alive and to multiply within the phago-cytes, which they may then kill and thus escape. From the submucosa of the small intestine the organisms pass via the lymphatics to the mesen-teric lymph nodes, whence after a period of multiplication they invade the bloodstream via the thoracic duct; the liver, gallbladder, spleen, kidney and bone-marrow become infected dur-ing this primary bacteriaemic phase in the first 7 to 10 days of the incubation period. After multiplication in these organs, bacilli pass into the blood, causing a secondary and heavier bacteriaemia, the onset of which approximately coincides with that of the pyrexia and other signs of clinical illness. From the gallbladder a fur-ther invasion of the intestine results, and lymphoid tissue—Peyer's patches and lymphoid follicles—is particularly involved in an inflam-matory reaction and infiltration with mono-nuclear cells, followed by necrosis, sloughing and the formation of characteristic typhoid ulcers. Haemorrhage of varying degree may occur and, less frequently, perforation through a necrotic Peyer's patch may complicate the illness. Fever and illness continue for 3 to 4 weeks.

As well as being present in the blood, *S. typhi* is present in large numbers in the infected organs, in the ulcers and is found in the intestinal con-tents and the faeces. As a consequence of its dissemination in the bloodstream, the bacillus may localize in the kidney and appear in the urine, sometimes producing a marked bacilluria. It may also infect other tissues and produce such occasional complications or sequelae of typhoid fever as acute suppurative periosteitis and osteitis, abscess of the kidney, acute chole-cystitis, bronchopneumonia, empyema and ul-cerative endocarditis.

In 2 to 5 per cent of convalescents, the typhoid bacillus persists in the body for over a year and many of these persons continue to be carriers for the remainder of their life. In such *chronic carriers*, the bacilli are most commonly present in the gallbladder, or rarely in the urinary tract, and are excreted in the faeces or urine. The long duration of the carrier state enables the bacillus to infect small, relatively isolated, communities or families as happened in the case of the cook called 'Typhoid Mary'.

Recent studies in induced typhoid fever among human volunteers have given new and valuable information about the pathogenesis of this disease. Using a pathogenic strain of *S. typhi*, well equipped with Vi, O and H antigens, Hornick and his colleagues (1970) found that a dose of 10^9 organisms was needed to induce clinical infection in most adults, whereas the ID50 was 10^7 organisms and the ID25 was 10^5 organisms. With the higher doses the incubation periods were shorter (5 to 7.5 days) than with the smaller ID25 (9 days) but the clinical fea-tures were not affected by dosage. Faecal excre-tion of typhoid bacilli was common in the first few days of incubation, then ceased and re-appeared about the end of the first week of fever, persisted for the next 3 weeks and then rapidly stopped. Faecal excretion of similar pattern occurred in a number of volunteers who did not become clinically ill; excretion was not affected by chloramphenicol therapy. Relapses after treatment with chloramphenicol occurred in 15 to 20 per cent of patients (in non-treated cases the relapse rate varies from 5 to 10 per cent).

Whilst the pathogenicity of salmonellae ap-pears primarily to depend upon the ability of the bacilli to survive and grow inside phagocytes (other than 'activated' macrophages) and on the toxicity of their lipopolysaccharide endotoxins, which is their O antigen, the typhoid and para-typhoid C bacilli have an additional aggressive factor in the possession of a microcapsule con-sisting of a glycolipid called the virulence (Vi) antigen. This Vi substance appears to protect the bacillus against the lytic action of antibody and complement and to impede phagocytosis to some extent. In the experimental studies of typhoid infection in human volunteers a dose of 10^7 organisms caused clinical infection more commonly (51 per cent) with a Vi-containing strain than with a non-Vi variant (26 per cent).

Volunteers rendered tolerant of the typhoid endotoxin by repeated intravenous injections were not more resistant to challenge than the controls despite high levels of O antibody. There was no evidence that humoral antibodies con-tributed to immunity against typhoid infection. Specific immunity appears to be cell-mediated; lymphocytes sensitized to the salmonella antigen and triggered by contact with the antigen acti-vate fixed and wandering macrophages so that the latter are enabled to kill phagocytosed bacilli.

CLINICAL INFECTION

Those who have had wide experience of the diagnosis and treatment of the enteric fevers in Britain and abroad are well aware that besides the 'classical case' there are numerous variations in the clinical picture owing to the variable virulence of the four causal organisms, possibly variation in infecting dose and in the 'resistance' of the patient. In Britain, paratyphoid B usually runs a milder course than typhoid fever often with initial diarrhoea and has a much lower case fatality.

Characteristically the history of a case of typhoid fever reveals exposure to infection 10 to 14 days before the onset of symptoms but this incubation period can be as short as 7 days or as long as three weeks; the onset is usually insidious and early symptoms are often vague and may be referable to tracts other than the bowel. A dry cough and epistaxis associated with anorexia, a dull continuous headache, abdominal tenderness and doughiness are among the most common symptoms; early in the illness many patients will complain of constipation. In the untreated case the temperature shows a stepladder rise over the first week of the illness, remains at 39·5°C to 40°C for 7 to 10 days and then falls by lysis during the third or fourth week. In the untreated cases, relapses occur in 5 to 10 per cent and although usually shorter and of milder character than the initial illness they can be severe and may end fatally.

When the infection is recognized early and appropriate antimicrobial treatment prescribed the illness loses its typical course and is much abbreviated with temperature falling to normal in 3 to 4 days. Differential diagnosis presents little problem when cases are being seen during an epidemic but in endemic areas alternative diagnoses include miliary tuberculosis, brucellosis and typhus fevers which have to be eliminated as well as other less common causes of pyrexia of uncertain origin (PUO), e.g. bacterial endocarditis and virus pneumonias associated with leucopenia.

LABORATORY DIAGNOSIS

Although the causal organisms may be recovered from the bloodstream throughout the illness, they are most commonly found during the first 7 to 10 days of the clinical illness and during relapses; 5 to 10 ml of blood obtained by venepuncture may be added to a blood culture bottle containing bile-salt broth. The technique of inoculation and the laboratory procedure are given in Vol. II, Chap. 29. Alternatively, clot culture may be performed; here 5 to 10 ml of venous blood are placed in a sterile universal container and the blood allowed to clot. The serum is then removed to perform a Widal test, the clotted blood digested with streptokinase or minced up with scissors and added to a bottle of bile-salt broth which is incubated and examined as in the blood culture technique; the advantages of clot-culture over blood cultures are that it may yield a higher percentage of positive results, it does not require a stock of special blood culture bottles to be maintained or to be taken to the patient and it allows a base-line titre of antibodies to be determined against which the results of further Widal tests can be judged.

Specimens of faeces and urine should be submitted for examination in an endeavour to isolate the causal organism but it must be remembered that the isolation of a salmonella strain from either of these specimens does not necessarily mean that the patient is suffering from a clinical infection—he may be a carrier. In the clinical case, stool cultures are usually positive from the second week and urine cultures from the third week of infection. In paratyphoid-B infections the clinical course is much shorter (7–10 days) than in typhoid; diarrhoea is usually early and stool cultures are often positive in the first week of the illness.

Faeces or urine (after centrifugation) are plated on DCA medium and are also inoculated into fluid enrichment media; e.g. tetrathionate or selenite broth; the broth culture is subcultured to a fresh plate of DCA medium after incubation at 37°C for 18 to 24 hours. Pale, lactose-non-fermenting colonies on the original DCA plate or on that inoculated from the enrichment broth are then tested for urease production (negative for salmonellae), motility (positive) and for their ability to utilize certain sugar substrates with gas production. With the exception of *S. typhi* itself, all members of the genus produce gas.

Colonies that give characteristic reactions are then identified by determining serologically their group (O) and type (H) antigens. *S. typhi* and *S. paratyphi C* possess an additional surface antigen, the Vi antigen, which may obscure agglutination with somatic antisera; identification of such organisms can be made with Vi antiserum or by removing the Vi antigen by boiling a suspension of the organisms before testing with O antisera.

Similarly, when attempting to determine the serotype within the O group to which the isolate belongs, the bacteriologist may be frustrated if the flagellar antigens are in a non-specific phase when they will react with several H antisera; on such occasions he attempts to harvest the minority population which have type-specific flagellar antigens by the technique known as the Craigie tube method. This entails growing the organisms in a medium containing non-specific flagellar antiserum which will immobilize organisms in the non-specific phase and only those which possess specific flagellar antigens will be free to move away from their non-specific partners and be collected for subcultivation and re-testing against the relevant type specific antisera.

Widal Test

Tests for specific antibodies (O and H) in the patient's serum can be performed but the interpretation of the results of such Widal tests are valid only if note is taken of certain findings which may otherwise cause false positive results. The level of 'enteric' antibodies in the healthy population must be known and may be variable; again, previous inoculation with TAB vaccine can give relatively high titres of specific antibodies as can previous clinical or latent infection, although only the H antibodies tend to persist at detectable levels. Not infrequently false-positive results in the Widal tests stem from the presence of non-specific antibodies such as fimbrial antibody. The usefulness of the Widal test is greatest when on testing a second specimen of the patient's serum 4 to 7 days after a first specimen a four-fold or greater rise in O and H antibody titres occurs.

In the search for typhoid carriers, either as part of the routine examination of food handlers or water-works employees or after an outbreak of typhoid fever, a useful screening test is to examine blood-serum specimens for specific antibodies; in particular, if the Vi antibody is present in a titre of 20 or higher, the individual may be a carrier and should have several stool examinations plus bile examination by duodenal aspiration, preferably in hospital. Typhoid patients may be similarly examined 6 months or more after discharge from hospital, if there was a significant titre of Vi antibody at the time of discharge.

CHEMOTHERAPY

Specific effective therapy in the enteric fevers only became available in 1948 with the introduction of chloramphenicol; before this good nursing care and the patient's own defence mechanisms were the main contributors to recovery. These factors are still important but the dramatic effect of chloramphenicol therapy, first noted during a trial of the drug against scrub typhus in Malaya, has greatly improved prognosis. Huckstep (1962) reported a fatality rate of only 5·4 per cent in a series of 240 cases in Africa when without the use of chloramphenicol the expected rate may well have been 30 to 50 per cent. This low case fatality included patients with complications, e.g. intestinal perforation and haemorrhage. Chloramphenicol therapy, as already noted, has usually been accompanied by a higher relapse rate although some authors claim to prevent this increase in relapses by varying the dosage and duration of chloramphenicol therapy and/or using TAB vaccine therapeutically. More recently the chemotherapeutic value of trimethoprim combined with sulphamethoxazole (Cotrimoxazole) has been assessed in typhoid fever and if the early promising results are confirmed in large scale clinical trials then another valuable antimicrobial agent will be available for treatment.

EPIDEMIOLOGY

The typhoid and paratyphoid bacilli are essentially human parasites and are acquired almost exclusively from human sources, namely patients and carriers. They thereby contrast with the salmonellae that cause food-poisoning in man, which are primarily parasites of other species of animals.

The commonest cause of enteric fever in Britain nowadays is *S. paratyphi B*. The ratio of cases of paratyphoid B to typhoid fever in Britain is now around 3:1, 3045 and 1133 corrected notifications respectively being made for England and Wales in the decade 1957–66.

Sources and Modes of Spread

The typhoid and paratyphoid bacilli are spread from the faeces (or urine) of a patient or carrier to other persons by the 'faecal–oral routes', namely, (1) water-borne, (2) food-borne and (3) by contact with hands, eating utensils and other fomites.

The infecting dose in paratyphoid fever is probably much larger than for typhoid so that multiplication in some suitable substrate, e.g. milk, cream, artificial cream, etc. often precedes ingestion and infection. Because of this the peak incidence of paratyphoid fever in Britain tends to be in mid-summer as with salmonella food-poisoning rather than in the autumn when typhoid fever was most prevalent. The source may be a mild missed case, or a chronic carrier. The risk of paratyphoid outbreaks from imported frozen egg and dried egg albumen (not uncommon some years ago) has been largely obviated by pasteurization procedures of bulk supplies before or after importation.

Water is rarely incriminated as the immediate vehicle of infection. However, a recent outbreak of paratyphoid B due to phage-type Taunton and affecting mostly schoolchildren in four villages, was almost certainly water-borne: a number of cows on a nearby farm were also infected, presumably from the contaminated water supply (Report, 1971).

Infection due to *S. typhi* is usually imported by visitors to this country or by holidaymakers returning from areas where typhoid fever is still endemic.

The sources of infection are usually chronic carriers and classically the vehicle of spread from such sources is water; the proof for such a statement is exemplified by the fact that typhoid fever was quite common in Britain until the water supplies were subjected not only to filtration but subsequently to chemical treatment, usually chlorination, so that water being distributed to householders and other users contained a small residual quantity of chlorine. Nonetheless precautions should be taken by laboratory tests against the risk of employing typhoid carriers who may be involved in water undertakings or food processing. The risks from eating raw shellfish, e.g. oysters and mussels, that may have fed in contaminated river estuaries or sea shores must be kept in mind.

Spectacular epidemics, such as that in Aberdeen in 1964, have resulted from importation of canned food contaminated at source abroad. In these outbreaks, sewage contaminated river water has been used in the cooling process after sterilization of the canned food and has been sucked into the can through unsealed joints. Such contaminated cans are unlikely to be 'blown' from gas formation as *S. typhi* is anaerogenic.

PHAGE-TYPING. Great assistance may be obtained and sources of infection delineated by the application of the phage-typing method for identifying different strains of the salmonella serotype. *S. typhi* is divisible into about 80 different phage-types, *S. paratyphi A* into at least 10 and *S. paratyphi B* into 45. In general, it may be expected that all patients infected from a common source will yield salmonella strains of the same phage-type. If the suspected source is a carrier the isolation of a culture of the epidemic phage-type from this carrier is usually confirmatory evidence of his role as the source of infection.

CONTROL MEASURES

A rapid reduction in the incidence of typhoid fever in Britain followed the provision of safe water supplies accompanied in time by adequate means for the proper disposal of human excreta, e.g. by a water-carriage system; in communities thus safeguarded patients with enteric fever returning from an endemically infected country rarely give rise to secondary cases. Obviously people employed in water-works, dairy farms and the food industry should be closely supervised and ideally they should be screened serologically and bacteriologically before being so employed and at intervals thereafter. Bacteriological sampling of imported foods such as tinned meats is another preventive measure which is now generally practised. Chronic carriers must be advised and if necessary restricted as to their employment, and the Medical Officer of Health is required to maintain an Enteric Register for his community which lists all known chronic carriers.

Prophylactic vaccination is commonly practised in countries with a high endemic level of typhoid fever. TAB vaccine, which is most often used, consists of a mixture of cultures of *S. typhi*, *S. paratyphi A* and *S. paratyphi B*, killed by heating at about 60°C and preserved in 0·5 per cent phenol.

Controlled vaccine trials have shown that *S. typhi* vaccines, acetone-killed and preserved in the dry state, can give a very high degree of protection in endemic areas, e.g. in Guyana, Yugoslavia and Poland, that the protection is maintained at a high level for 5 to 7 years and that a single dose of typhoid vaccine given to children in hyper-endemic areas apparently gives as good protection as two doses (Ashcroft *et al.*, 1967). Phenolized vaccines are less effective. The triple TAB vaccines should be avoided because the paratyphoid A and B components are either not needed or in the doses ordinarily used give no protection. In non-endemic areas typhoid vaccine should be given to people particularly at risk, e.g. troops or visitors going to a country where the disease is endemic, laboratory workers handling specimens or live cultures and people living in the same house as a chronic carrier.

Prolonged treatment (1 to 3 months) with ampicillin has resulted in cure of chronic gall-bladder carriers (Christie, 1964; Simon and Miller, 1966). If antibiotic therapy fails, cholecystectomy is highly effective. Urinary typhoid carriers are much rarer, although perhaps more dangerous, than faecal carriers; here the carrier usually has some abnormality in the urinary tract and may be cured by surgical intervention.

REFERENCES AND FURTHER READING

ASHCROFT, A. T., SINGH, B., NICHOLSON, C. C., RITCHIE, J. M., SOBRYAN, E. & WILLIAMS, F. (1967) A seven-year field trial of two typhoid vaccines in Guyana. *Lancet*, ii, 1056.

CHRISTIE, A. B. (1964) Treatment of typhoid carriers with ampicillin. *British Medical Journal*, i, 1609.

HORNICK, R. B., GREISMAN, S. E., WOODWARD, T. E., DUPONT, H. L., DAWKINS, A. T. & SNYDER, M. J. (1970) Typhoid fever: pathogenesis and immunologic control. *New England Journal of Medicine*, **283**, 686 and 739.

HUCKSTEP, R. L. (1962) *Typhoid Fever and Other Salmonella Infections*. Edinburgh: Livingstone.

SIMON, H. J. & MILLER, R. C. (1966) Ampicillin in the treatment of chronic typhoid carriers. *New England Journal of Medicine*, **274**, 807.

REPORT (1971) *On the State of the Public Health*. Annual Report of the Chief Medical Officer, Department of Health and Social Security for the year 1970.

27. Salmonella: 2 Bacterial Food-poisoning

Food-poisoning can result from the ingestion of various materials including inherently poisonous substances but this chapter deals only with bacterial food-poisoning and not with the accidental or deliberate ingestion of poisonous substances that have been mixed with articles of food or drink. The term bacterial food-poisoning is conveniently restricted to cases or epidemics of acute gastro-enteritis that are caused by the ingestion of food contaminated with bacteria or their products. Bacterial food-poisoning does not encompass specific gastro-intestinal infections such as bacillary dysentery, the enteric fevers or cholera. Botulism which is the most spectacular of all illnesses resulting from the ingestion of foodstuffs contaminated with bacteria or their products should also be considered separately since the essential symptomatology of botulism is associated with the central nervous system and not with the gastro-intestinal tract.

Bacterial food-poisoning may follow the ingestion of food or drink containing preformed toxins, e.g. from *Staphylococcus aureus* and *Clostridium welchii* and this, *toxic-type* food-poisoning, is dealt with in Chapters 15 and 35. Bacterial food-poisoning is more commonly caused by ingestion of foods contaminated with any of the numerous serotypes of the genus *Salmonella*. This *infective type* of food-poisoning requires multiplication of the salmonellae in the food before ingestion and multiplication in the intestine so that infective, or salmonella, food-poisoning contrasts with toxic food-poisoning in having a longer incubation period followed by a pyrexial illness with diarrhoea and vomiting of several days duration and in some instances a systemic infection.

DESCRIPTION

Members of the genus *Salmonella* responsible for cases of food-poisoning cannot be differentiated microscopically, culturally or biochemically from the enteric fever bacilli, particularly the paratyphoid bacilli; only by serological techniques can the types be differentiated from these and from each other (Vol. II, Chap. 29). There are over 1 000 different salmonella serotypes of which the most common as causes of food-poisoning in Britain are currently *S. typhimurium*, *S. heidelberg*, *S. enteritidis*, *S. newport*, *S. infantis* and *S. thompson*. In contradistinction to the typhoid and paratyphoid bacilli which are primarily parasites of man in which they cause the septicaemic disease called enteric fever, the numerous serotypes of salmonellae that cause food-poisoning are primarily parasites of other animal species. They cause septicaemic typhoid-like infections in their natural animal host, but only, apart from rare exceptions, localized gastro-enteritis in man. The fact that man is not a natural host of the food-poisoning salmonellae is probably the reason both why human infections are not septicaemic or, except rarely, serious, and why the dose of bacilli required to cause the infection is very high, so high as to be obtainable only through eating food in which the salmonellae have grown profusely; the infective dose in food-poisoning may be 10^8 bacilli or greater.

Clinical Features

Although in common with toxic types of food-poisoning, salmonellosis shares the symptoms of vomiting, abdominal pain and diarrhoea, the last of these is usually the main presenting symptom but its severity varies from the very slight, i.e. passage of one or two loose stools which may be disregarded by the patient, to a violent diarrhoea which leaves the patient severely prostrated. Abdominal pain of a griping nature occurs early but is not usually severe and similarly vomiting if it occurs is not severe. Pyrexia is common and evidence of the severity of the infection, e.g. headache, general body pain and shivering, is often obvious. Rarely, the infection becomes septicaemic, particularly with certain salmonella serotypes, e.g. *S. dublin*.

Laboratory Diagnosis

Specimens of faeces, vomit and any suspected foodstuffs must be sent to the laboratory and the procedures for isolation and identification of any suspect colonies are identical with those for the enteric fever pathogens. If the salmonella isolated is one of the common food-poisoning serotypes, e.g. *S. typhimurium* or *S. enteritidis*, it may be subjected to phage-typing, so that the phage-type of the isolates from patients may be matched with those from the infected food and from a suspected animal source.

Chemotherapy

The majority of patients afflicted with salmonella food-poisoning suffer a relatively mild infection so that specific treatment is rarely necessary; however, patients debilitated by other diseases or the young or very old may, if they suffer severe diarrhoea, become rapidly dehydrated and then restoration of electrolytes and fluid balance by intravenous therapy becomes essential.

Specific antimicrobial therapy if judged by the results of *in vitro* tests should be very efficient in salmonella food-poisoning and certainly specific drugs seem to be widely used for such cases. However, controlled trials have shown that antibiotics do not shorten the duration of the diarrhoea, do not eliminate the causal organisms and have no influence on the carrier rate. Thus the practitioner, although he may have a feeling of futility in being unable to offer specific treatment, should refrain from exhibiting what are in cases of salmonella food-poisoning, useless and potentially harmful drugs.

EPIDEMIOLOGY

The incidence of bacterial food-poisoning is highest in the summer months, probably associated with the higher temperatures which encourage bacterial multiplication: all consumers of infected food are at risk but infection is often most severe in elderly persons.

Sources and Spread

The carcases or products, e.g. cooked meats, eggs or milk of naturally infected domestic animals are the commonest sources of food-poisoning infection. Flesh may be infected when an ill, septicaemic animal is slaughtered. More commonly, uninfected meat or carcases may be infected in the abattoir, packing station or butcher's shop with infected intestinal contents from a 'carrier' animal killed at the same time as healthy animals (abattoir and shop cross-infection). Poultry, particularly hens, ducks and turkeys are the most significant reservoirs of food-poisoning salmonellae in Britain. Duck eggs are particularly suspect since infection occurs in the oviduct before the egg is shelled. However, hen eggs may become contaminated with salmonellae through the air pores in the blunt end of the shell if they are laid in contact with soil contaminated with infected hen faeces. Pigs, cattle and, in some Commonwealth countries, lambs and calves, also act as sources of infection so that much of man's foodstuffs can be contaminated at source or during its preparation and manipulation by man. Rats and mice are commonly infected with food-poisoning salmonellae and if they gain access to human foodstuffs may contaminate it with their faeces. Food-poisoning may also be caused by food contaminated by a human case or carrier.

Thus, even if the foodstuff is *ab initio* free of salmonellae the chance of contamination from 'the hoof to the home' is high and the more sophisticated the manipulation of the food the greater the chance of contamination. For example, one duck egg containing salmonellae, if eaten by an individual, probably will not give rise to infection; on the other hand, if such an egg is pooled with others free of salmonellae, as in preparing a custard or trifle for communal consumption, then conditions of temperature and time may readily allow multiplication of the salmonellae with a potential of an epidemic amongst those who eat the contaminated food.

Likewise, a clean carcase can be contaminated at the abattoir via instruments or by hanging alongside an infected carcase in the chilling hall or during transportation to the wholesale and retail butchers' premises. Again, the aggregation of pigs in holding pens greatly increases the occurrence of cross-infection before slaughter. Infection in pigs is most often due to the feeding of swill containing infected animal matter or to contaminated and usually imported feeding stuff, e.g. bone, fish and meat meals.

S. typhimurium has remained at the top of the league table of organisms causing salmonella food-poisoning for several decades—not only in Britain but in the rest of Europe and in America and this fact reflects its nature as a primary pathogen in a wide variety of animals which are eventually consumed by man, or which may contaminate food in his environment (rodents, cats, dogs).

Numerous studies in different countries have demonstrated a close correspondence between the types of salmonellae prevalent in animals (particularly pigs and poultry) and the types that cause infection in man. However, sometimes certain serotypes are frequently incriminated in food-poisoning outbreaks but are rarely found in animals, e.g. in recent years in Britain *S. heidelberg*, *S. brandenburg* and *S. panama* (Soyha and Field, 1970).

Infection of food with salmonellae is not in itself sufficient to cause food-poisoning. It is necessary that the infected food is moist and stored long enough under conditions allowing heavy growth of the bacteria, e.g. for 24 hr in a warm area of a kitchen, or several days in a cool larder, and that the food should not, before eating, be subjected to thorough cooking, which would kill the non-sporing bacilli (susceptible to 60°C in 10 minutes). Although cooking of liquid foods easily renders them safe, heating of solid foods often fails to do so because of the poor rate of penetration of heat. Thus, a cold or chilled joint of meat, a poultry carcase or a large meat pie may be heated in an oven until the surface is well cooked, whilst the central part is still insufficiently heated to destroy vegetative bacteria.

Food-poisoning incidents occur most dramatically as explosive outbreaks among members of a community sharing communal meals, e.g. in factories, hospitals, schools or after some celebration feast. Localized incidents may affect a single family or a single person. In all three categories salmonella infections are the most common and in Britain account for over 90 per cent of food-poisoning incidents in which the causal agent has been identified.

Salmonellosis may also occur as a nosocomial infection spreading from case to case, particularly *among young children in a hospital or nursery*, and with a relatively small infecting dose.

Control Measures

The principles for the prevention of salmonella food-poisoning can be readily enunciated, viz., the raising of animals free from infection, the elimination of contamination by rodents at all levels of food-production, the prevention of contamination by human handlers at the wholesale, retail and hotel levels; yet the barriers of economic husbandry, out-of-date premises and perhaps most important of all, the need for continuing education of food handlers at all levels of production make implementation of these principles difficult.

In an endeavour to reduce the incidence of food-poisoning—whether due to salmonellae or other bacteria—two basic precepts must be observed; firstly, raw foodstuffs, which are potentially contaminated, must never have contact, either direct or indirect, with cooked foods. Secondly, if a foodstuff is, or thought to be, contaminated with salmonellae, it should be treated or held under temperature conditions which prevent the organism from growing, i.e. either under refrigeration or at sufficiently high temperatures (and then consumed immediately) so that at the least the inoculum ingested by any one individual is minimal.

Too often when an outbreak of salmonella food-poisoning has been investigated it is found that the incriminated food had been cooked some hours or perhaps a day or two before and then left at room temperature before being reheated immediately before serving; this procedure ensures that salmonellae which survived the initial cooking or gained access to the cooked food had an excellent milieu and ideal temperatures at which to multiply in the interval before being warmed up for consumption.

As in most other endeavours to control the spread of infection the human element is the weakest link in the chain so that health education, particularly of food handlers, is a continuing requirement.

REFERENCE

SOJKA, W. J. & FIELD, H. I. (1970) Salmonellosis in England and Wales 1958–1967. *Veterinary Bulletin*, **40**, 515.

28. Shigella Bacillary Dysentery

Dysentery, or the bloody flux of biblical times, is a clinical entity, characterized by the frequent passage of blood-stained mucopurulent stools. Aetiologically, it is divisible into two main categories—amoebic and bacillary dysentery; both forms are endemic in most warm climate countries. Bacillary dysentery, caused by members of the genus *Shigella*, is also prevalent in many countries with temperate climates, but over the past half century there has been a steady and remarkable change in the relative frequency of the different shigella species in Britain and other European countries; infections due to *Sh. dysenteriae* (Shiga bacillus) have virtually disappeared and the Sonne dysentery bacillus has largely supplanted the Flexner types, particularly in the north-western countries of Europe, with an associated lessening in the severity of the disease. Today in Britain, most shigella infections, caused by the Sonne type, are relatively mild; only in the very young and the old or debilitated are typical dysenteries sometimes seen. If, as has been said, the prevalence of dysentery reflects the hygienic standards of a country or a community, it is disturbing that the recorded incidence of Sonne dysentery in England and Wales mounted in waves of increasing size in the post-war years, reaching a peak of 49 009 notifications in 1956.

DESCRIPTION

The genus *Shigella* is one of several genera in the large family Enterobacteriaceae; a distinctive character is that its members very rarely parasitize forms of life other than man and, possibly, primates. Microscopically, shigellae are Gram-negative bacilli very similar to other enterobacteria; but they are non-motile and non-capsulate. Culturally they are similar to most other enterobacteria except that on MacConkey or DCA medium they are lactose-non-fermenting after incubation for 18 to 24 hours; thus on such differential media colonies are 'pale' and similar to those of the other common pathogenic genus, *Salmonella*.

By simple tests shigellae can be differentiated from salmonellae since the latter almost invariably produce gas as well as acid when grown in sugar solutions and are motile; only a few serotypes of *Shigella* produce small volumes of gas and one serotype of salmonella, *S. typhi*, is anaerogenic. Tests for indole production will reveal that members of the genus *Salmonella* are persistently negative whereas some species of *Shigella* have this ability; conversely H_2S production is common in salmonellae but does not occur in shigellae. Thus a pale (lactose-non-fermenting colony) from a DCA plate can be speedily recognized as probably belonging to one or other genus by testing its fermentative ability on a narrow range of substrates and by noting whether or not the isolate is motile, and whether or not it produces indole or H_2S.

Within the genus *Shigella* there are four groups; A, B, C and D which are named respectively *Sh. dysenteriae*, *Sh. flexneri*, *Sh. boydii* and *Sh. sonnei*; one of these, *Sh. dysenteriae*, is unique in being mannitol-non-fermenting; another group, D or *Sh. sonnei*, is a late lactose fermenter, i.e. colonies growing on MacConkey or DCA media for more than 24 hours acquire a pink colouration. Identification of a shigella isolate is made with group specific antisera; members of group A (*Sh. dysenteriae*) can be subdivided into 10 specific serotypes, *Sh. flexneri* into 6 serotypes and *Sh. boydii* into 15 serotypes. On the other hand, members of group D (*Sh. sonnei*) are serologically homogeneous and for epidemiological purposes a useful marker is the ability of such strains to produce different colicines, which allows subdivision into 17 types.

PATHOGENESIS AND CLINICAL FEATURES

Infection occurs by ingestion; it is probable that the infecting dose is much smaller than for salmonellae (except *S. typhi*). After reaching the large intestine the shigella bacilli appear to attach themselves to the luminal ('brush') border of the epithelial cells of the villi in the mucosa of the large intestine and induce these cells to ingest them. They then multiply within the epithelial cells and spread laterally into adjacent cells; some spread into and multiply in the lamina propria. The infected epithelial cells are killed and the lamina propria and submucosa develop an inflammatory reaction, with capillary thrombosis. Patches of necrotic epithelium are sloughed and ulcers form. The cellular response is predominantly by polymorphonuclear leucocytes and these are readily noted on microscopic examination of the dejecta. Dysentery bacilli rarely invade other tissues and bacteriaemia has only occasionally been reported (Savage, 1972).

The severity of the clinical illness, bacillary dysentery, is to some extent associated with the particular species involved; infection with *Sh. dysenteriae* is usually associated with a severe illness in which there is a sudden onset of abdominal pain, tenesmus, pyrexia, prostration and sometimes convulsions; the stools lose their usual faecal character, are small and frequent, and are composed mainly of fresh blood, pus and mucus. The special virulence of *Sh. dysenteriae* is due to its forming a potent exotoxin that has a fluid transuding action on the intestinal mucosa (enterotoxin) in addition to the lipopolysaccharide endotoxin formed by all shigella species. Because of the neurological effects resulting from vascular endothelial damage produced by this toxin when injected intravenously, it has formerly been described as a 'neurotoxin'. At the other end of the clinical spectrum of bacillary dysentery, the illness associated with *Sh. sonnei*, in an otherwise healthy person, may be confined to the passage of a few loose stools with vague abdominal discomfort and the patient often continues at school or work.

The illness caused by members of *Sh. flexneri* and *Sh. boydii* groups is usually more severe than Sonne dysentery and may be as prostrating as that caused by *Sh. dysenteriae*. Death from bacillary dysentery is uncommon; it occurs mostly at the extremes of life or in individuals who are usually suffering from some other disease or debilitating condition.

LABORATORY DIAGNOSIS

A specimen of faeces is preferable to a rectal swab; rectal swabs do not allow adequate macroscopic and microscopic examination of the stool and unless properly taken, and bearing obvious traces of faeces, may be no more than a swab of the perianal skin. Again, because of drying of the swab, pathogenic species die off more rapidly on it than in specimens of faeces. An added advantage in submitting faecal specimens is that the onus of collecting and delivering the specimen can be placed on the patient or a relative. When faecal specimens are likely to be in transit to the laboratory for one or more days it is wise to add the specimen to a container with fluid preservative (e.g. glycerol saline) to ensure survival of pathogens.

Microscopic examination of fresh unstained films of faeces should be undertaken to eliminate the presence of protozoa or their cysts and also to note the character of the cellular exudate.

Before inoculation on to culture media the specimen should, if necessary, be emulsified in sterile physiological saline; mucus, if present in the specimen, may be used as the inoculum.

The material is plated on DCA medium and a tube of selenite enrichment broth should also be inoculated; the latter is subcultured to a fresh plate of DCA medium after incubation at 37°C for 18 to 24 hours. Pale lactose-non-fermenting colonies from DCA are subjected to tests for urease production (negative for shigellae), motility (negative) and for ability to utilize certain sugar substrates. Colonies that give the characteristic reactions must have their identity confirmed by serological investigation with group specific sera and then with type specific antisera if the strain belongs to group A, B or C. With isolates belonging to group D colicine typing may be performed.

Tests for specific antibodies in the patient's serum are of little value since in an endemic area the patient's serum rarely shows any increased level of specific antibody compared with sera from healthy people.

CHEMOTHERAPY

Sulphonamides, both soluble and insoluble, singly or in combination, were originally used with great success in treating cases of bacillary dysentery, e.g. in North Africa in World War II. The marked and fairly rapid development of resistance as judged by *in vitro* tests has mirrored the decreasing clinical usefulness of this group of antimicrobial drugs.

More recently, reports from numerous centres emphasize that dysentery bacilli are efficient at acquiring resistance through resistance transfer factors (see Chap. 7) to antibiotics which at one time may have been effective in assisting clinical cure. In Sonne ·dysentery it is more prudent to treat the mild case of bacillary dysentery with a non-specific agent, e.g. kaolin, because in most cases such therapy gives rapid symptomatic relief with cessation of diarrhoea.

Specific antibiotic therapy should not be given until laboratory investigation shows that the antibiotic selected by the clinician is active against the patient's strain *in vitro*; even then certain antibiotics may prolong the period during which loose stools are excreted and, at the bacteriological level, population studies show that clearance of the pathogen may not occur significantly earlier than when non-specific treatment has been given.

EPIDEMIOLOGY

On very rare occasions epidemics of bacillary dysentery have been traced to captive monkeys, but for practical purposes, human cases and carriers are the only important sources of infection. Spread is by the faecal–oral route.

The infection in Britain nowadays is caused mainly by *Sh. sonnei* although in certain communities, e.g. Glasgow and Liverpool, a significant proportion of cases are caused by *Sh. flexneri* serotypes which are rarely isolated elsewhere in the country except in some mental hospitals.

Sources and Spread

Usually bacillary dysentery is spread from hand to mouth, i.e. the case or carrier, after contaminating his hands while cleansing himself at toilet, touches and thus contaminates door handles, washbasin taps, hand-towels, etc., which, when handled by another individual, allows transference of dysentery bacilli to this recipient's hands and thence to his mouth. Such spread is facilitated by separating the washbasin from the w.c. compartment so that the handle of the intervening door acts as a vehicle of infection. The carrier may also handle and thus infect food that is eaten, or eating utensils that are used, by another person who is thereby infected. Dysentery bacilli are also liberated into the air in an aerosol when an infected loose stool is flushed from the toilet and after settling on the surfaces of toilet seats, furniture, etc. may survive for several days in a moist atmosphere.

An important feature of the epidemiology of bacillary dysentery in Britain and other countries with good environmental sanitation is that the main patient group involved is school-age children and particularly primary school children; here inadequate toilet facilities at school undoubtedly play a part. The seasonal distribution of bacillary dysentery in Britain is bimodal with the highest incidence in spring and a second peak in October/November. Incidence is at its lowest during the summer months, i.e. when schoolchildren are on holiday and during the period of the year when domestic insects have their flight season; thus insect vectors play no part in transmission. However, in communities without satisfactory methods of sewage disposal insects can gain access to infected human excreta and transfer dysentery bacilli mechanically to foodstuffs; foods may also be contaminated directly by human cases or carriers. Occasional epidemics of bacillary dysentery can be traced to water supplies when chlorination of the supply has not been instituted or has been defective. Such water-borne epidemics are usually spectacular in the large number of people simultaneously infected and in the speed with which they can be terminated when the water supply is adequately treated. In U.S.A. labour camps, the incidence of bacillary dysentery has been lower in households with water available in the home than in households with stand-pipe or other less accessible supplies.

Control Measures

The mild and often fleeting nature of the clinical illness associated with *Sh. sonnei* infection means that frequently the case of bacillary dysentery remains ambulant and follows his daily labour and leisure pursuits; hence he remains in circulation as a disperser of the causal organism. The pressure on toilet facilities, particularly in schools, allows hand to mouth spread of the bacilli. The provision of washbasins in the same compartment as the toilet pedestal would allow some reduction in spread especially if flushing mechanisms and washbasin taps could be operated by foot instead of by hand. Adequate toilet facilities must be made available at schools, and hand drying, at home or in communal toilets, should be by individual towels and not by roller or other communally used articles. There is no evidence that prophylactic use of antimicrobial agents protects individuals in semi-closed communities, e.g. in day or residential nurseries; similarly, isolation in hospital does not appear to reduce the incidence of the infection since cities where hospitalization is still commonly practised have no more favourable experience than those in which hospital isolation is undertaken rarely and then only for social reasons.

The incidence of bacillary dysentery in a community can be taken as an index of the personal hygiene of the population and if toilet areas were properly designed and equipped and people washed their hands thoroughly after being at stool a reduction in incidence should follow.

In hyper-endemic areas in Yugoslavia, some success has been obtained in controlled trials with live oral Flexner and Sonne shigella vaccines given to troops in training or to young children (Mel *et al.*, 1971). However, frequent dosage and the sero-specificity of protection makes this prophylactic measure difficult to implement on a large scale in civilian communities.

REFERENCES

MEL, D., GANGAROSA, E. J., RADOVANOVIČ, M. L., ARSIČ, B. L. & LITVENJENKO, S. (1971) Studies on vaccination against bacillary dysentery. 6. Protection of children by oral immunisation with streptomycin-dependent *Shigella* strains. *Bulletin World Health Organisation*, **45**, 457.

SAVAGE, D. C. (1972) In *Microbial Pathogenicity in Man and Animals*, p. 25. Edited by H. Smith and J. H. Pierce. Cambridge University Press.

29. Escherichia Coli: Klebsiella: Proteus: Providencia
Gastro-enteritis: Urinary Tract Infections

Strains of *Escherichia coli* and related coliform bacteria predominate among the aerobic commensal flora present in the gut of men and animals and are also widely distributed in the environment. All persons have a rich flora of *Esch. coli* in the lower ileum and in the colon. It is acquired in the first few days after birth, when the child ingests bacilli derived from its mother or attendant. *Esch. coli* is incriminated as a pathogen outside the gut and particularly in the urinary tract and in wounds where the infection may be endogenous from the patient's own intestine or acquired from an exogenous source. Some antigenically identifiable strains with special enterotoxic characteristics also cause gastro-enteritis, particularly in infants.

Some species of coliform bacteria such as *Klebsiella aerogenes* and *Citrobacter freundii* commonly grow in the soil, vegetation, natural waters and other environments outside the body. *Esch. coli*, on the other hand, appears to grow only as a parasite of man and animals, mainly in the intestine. Being excreted in very large numbers in faeces, it comes to contaminate the environment, including the soil, very widely and the bacilli may survive without growth for several days to a few weeks outside the body. When *Esch. coli* is found in a water supply, it is considered to indicate that the supply has recently been subjected to contamination with human or animal faeces.

Description

Esch. coli is a Gram-negative, motile, non-sporing bacillus, morphologically identical with salmonellae and on ordinary culture media their colonies are also very similar; however, on MacConkey's medium *Esch. coli* strains yield rose-pink colonies since they ferment the lactose in the medium. They grow poorly if at all on the more selective DCA or SS media. The species can be differentiated from others within the enterobacteria by biochemical reactions but as always in the Enterobacteriaceae, a minority of strains are atypical and difficult to allocate to any one genus or group (see Table 29.1).

Antigenic schemas for the genus are based on the presence of various O, H and K antigens and most interest centres on strains bearing the K types of antigen—a group of antigens designated L, A or B on the basis of differing physical characteristics. These K antigens occur as envelopes or capsules and like other surface antigens they may prevent somatic agglutination of living strains by the homologous O-antisera. When abundant, the K antigen appears

Table 29.1

Group or genus	Usual features						
	Gas from glucose	Motility	Indole	Gelatin liq.	V.-P.	M.-R.	Citrate
Escherichia	+	+	+	−	−	+	−
Alkalescens-Dispar	−	−	+	−	−	+	−
Citrobacter	+	+	−	−	−	+	+
Klebsiella	+	−	−	−	+	−	+
Cloaca	+	+	−	+	+	−	+
Hafnia*	+	+	−	−	+	−	+

* Results when tests are performed at 20°C.

to act as a virulence factor, impeding phago-cytosis and protecting the bacillus from killing by the action of antibody and complement. Its role may be similar to that of the Vi antigen in *S. typhi* (Glynn, 1972).

Identification studies of faecal isolates in healthy persons show that the types of *Esch. coli* present are not only multiple at any one examina-tion in an individual but that repeated examina-tions over a period of time reveal changes in the main serotypes; one or two 'dynastic' types persist over relatively long periods of time whereas other serotypes are quite transient. Commensal strains isolated from faeces are distributed over many O-groups; relatively few of these possess K-antigens of which only about 50 per cent are of the L variety.

PATHOGENESIS

Esch. coli, as a pathogen, is associated with two main clinical syndromes; (1) acute gastro-enteritis in infants up to 2 years of age and rarely, in adults with possibly some lowered resistance, and (2) infections of the urinary tract, particu-larly in married women but also in girls and in elderly men with prostatic enlargement. *Esch. coli* may also be the causal organism in appen-dicular abscess, peritonitis, cholecystitis, wound infections, etc.

Gastro-enteritis

The enteropathogenic strains of *Esch. coli* seem to belong to a limited number of O-serotypes with an associated B-type K antigen. At present about a dozen O-serotypes have been incrimina-ted, of which the more common and most widely distributed are O26, B6; O55, B5; O111, B4 and less frequently O119, B14; O126, B16; O86, B7; O127, B8; O128, B12. Outbreaks of acute gastro-enteritis occur in infant nurseries and in day nurseries and paediatric units with a high proportion of babies under 18 months of age. More widespread outbreaks may occur in the general community as happened in Aberdeen and other cities in the post-war years and are usually associated with only one or two of the enteropathogenic serotypes. On the other hand, among infants with gastro-enteritis admitted sporadically to hospital, recognized types of enteropathogenic *Esch. coli* may not be isolated from more than 10 to 30 per cent of the cases. However, it seems likely that other entero-pathogenic serotypes of *Esch. coli* than those already incriminated may be found to be causally related to acute gastro-enteritis both in infants and in older persons.

The pathophysiology of infantile gastro-enteritis associated with enteropathogenic *Esch. coli* is characterized by massive fluid loss from the gut, causing acute dehydration, acidosis and hypovolaemic shock. At post-mortem examina-tion, there is little or no inflammatory reaction in the intestinal mucosa which is pale and oedematous: there may be some associated toxic and fatty changes in the liver. These largely negative findings closely resemble those which characterize cholera in older children and adults and the infantile syndrome has been fittingly called 'cholera infantum'.

The pathogenesis of infantile gastro-enteritis seems to be related to the production of an enterotoxin similar in action to the cholera enterotoxin. Laboratory experiments with whole cultures, lysates and filtrates of enteropathogenic strains of *Esch. coli*, injected into isolated loops of rabbit, mouse or piglet intestine result in a rapid outpouring of an isotonic fluid, which may be activated by enzymic disturbances of the intestinal secretions as in cholera. The reason for the restriction in activity of the entero-pathogenic *Esch. coli* serotypes to infants is not known but could be related to the absence of any acquired local immunity to the enterotoxin of these *Esch. coli* strains. Such strains are rarely found in the intestinal commensal flora of adults and older children so that their main source in outbreaks is likely to be other infants with diarrhoea.

In addition to the cholera-like action without apparent damage to mucosal cells, there is evi-dence, particularly in experimental animals, that certain strains of *Esch. coli* may be locally in-vasive like the shigellae or may penetrate more deeply like the salmonellae. *Esch. coli* may, therefore, in its pathogenicity pattern in the gut, be the prototype of other defined intestinal pathogens.

Urinary Tract Infections

The importance of coliform bacilli in urinary tract infections has long been known and the relationship of urinary retention and stasis in pregnancy and in elderly males in predisposing to infection has been emphasized. Recently, the interpretation of finding coliform bacilli in urinary specimens has been clarified by making quantitative counts per ml on *freshly voided urine*. Kass (1955) by relating bacterial counts to clinical history in pregnant women, developed the concept of 'significant bacteriuria', by which is meant that counts of 100 000 or more bacteria per ml indicated multiplication of the organisms in the urinary tract whereas lower counts were usually associated with contaminants from the urethra or external genitalia. Various workers, examining large series of pregnant women, have found that 5 to 8 per cent have significant bacteriuria. Coliform bacilli (*Escherichia, Klebsiella* and *Proteus*) have been most commonly incriminated. The incidence of significant bacteriuria in schoolgirls and nuns is around 1·0 per cent.

The main factors predisposing to bacteriuria in married women are pregnancy and sexual intercourse. The hormonal effects in reducing the tone of the ureteric musculature in pregnancy aided, perhaps, by mechanical pressure from the gravid uterus leads to urinary stasis and so encourages bacterial growth in urine which is an excellent culture medium. However, Sleigh and his colleagues (1964) found an 8 per cent incidence of significant bacteriuria in married but completely infertile women, and they suggested that sexual intercourse was an important predisposing factor. The detection of a symptomless significant bacteriuria in early pregnancy may be followed by clinical signs of urinary infection in a considerable proportion (30 to 40 per cent) of women so that suppression of the bacteriuria in early pregnancy by appropriate chemotherapy should reduce the risk of symptomatic cystitis, pyelitis or pyelonephritis later in pregnancy and in the puerperium. It has been claimed that the incidence of prematurity, perinatal deaths and small birth size is also related to significant bacteriuria. Various screening tests for the detection of this condition in early pregnancy have been devised and are further discussed in Chap. 55.

Esch. coli is the most common coliform species present in the urine of pregnant women with significant bacteriuria and only a limited number of the 145 O-serotypes seem to be commonly involved—e.g. types O1, O2, O4, O6 and O75. Over 90 per cent of urinary specimens in such cases contain only one serotype. Early relapses of infection after temporary cure is most often with the original infecting type but later recurrences are frequently due to another O-serotype (Ganguli, 1970). High antibody titres to the infecting type may be present in women with persistent bacteriuria and this finding may indicate infection of the upper urinary tract and tissues (pyelonephritis) rather than lower urinary tract infection (cystitis).

There is evidence that strains of *Esch. coli* rich in K-antigen are more liable than K-poor strains to infect the kidneys, whereas the proportion of strains causing cystitis that are K-rich is no greater than that of strains found in the faeces (Glynn, 1972).

LABORATORY DIAGNOSIS

It must be emphasized that in their morphology, cultural appearances and biochemical activities enteropathogenic strains of *Esch. coli* do not differ from strains that are commensal in the gut or strains isolated from non-enteric pathological material: therefore, antigenic analysis must be undertaken when isolates are obtained from suspect cases of gastrointestinal infection. Such isolates of *Esch. coli* on blood agar or MacConkey's medium which has been seeded with faecal material from cases of gastro-enteritis must be examined serologically to determine whether an enteropathogenic strain belonging to certain O-groups and possessing a B-antigen is present; this is the only method of detecting such strains and at least ten colonies must be tested from each diagnostic plate, firstly with polyvalent antisera and if agglutination occurs, further tests are made with individual type-specific antisera which comprised the polyvalent serum.

Specimens from non-enteric infections, e.g. urine, pus, etc., are stained by Gram's method and *Esch. coli* will show as Gram-negative rods identical to other members of the

Enterobacteriaceae. Here again, the material is plated on to blood agar and MacConkey's medium and if more detailed identification of characteristic lactose-fermenting colonies on the latter medium is required, resort must be made to biochemical and serological tests, although these steps are rarely necessary unless epidemiological studies are being undertaken.

It is emphasized that urinary specimens must be sent to the laboratory as soon as possible after the specimen has been collected. In women, preliminary cleansing of the external genitalia is usually recommended and in all cases, a midstream specimen is best. Special arrangements may have to be made for the early collection of urinary specimens submitted by general practitioners, or special containers packed with ice, may be used. Methods for quantitative counts are described in Vol. II, Chap. 31.

Chemotherapy

In cases of infantile gastro-enteritis caused by enteropathogenic strains of *Esch. coli*, there is a wide spectrum of clinical severity of the illness from the mild or missed case to the fulminating fatal case. The essential treatment of severely ill dehydrated infants is rehydration and restoration of the electrolyte balance. Antibiotics have little part to play in the treatment of the acute stage in severe cases of gastro-enteritis because they cannot act fast enough to stop further fluid loss in a dehydrated child and may, by causing vomiting, add to dehydration. However, appropriate chemotherapy given in the early stages of a mild case may prevent further deterioration.

Perhaps the most significant decision as to whether to treat babies with antibiotics after correction of fluid and electrolyte loss depends on whether the infant is returning to his own home or to a residential nursery; in the former case it is unlikely that another susceptible infant will be there and he does not therefore require antimicrobial therapy. However, when the baby is to be discharged to an institution it is wise to give specific treatment in an endeavour to eradicate the enteropathogenic strain.

Epidemiology

Outbreaks of gastro-enteritis occur most commonly in institutions and affect either newborn babies in a maternity nursery or infants up to 18 months of age in paediatric wards or other residential institutions.

The infection occurs much more frequently in artificially fed babies than in wholly breast fed babies, which focuses attention on the milk feed and feeding bottles as the most likely vehicles of infection, indirectly from a case or from a carrier involved in the preparation of the feed. But dust and communal articles like brooms and weighing baskets may help to disseminate the infecting organism in an institution.

Infantile enteritis is prevalent in most developing countries and occurs most often in infants during or shortly after weaning (sometimes called weanling diarrhoea). Besides poor standards of personal and household hygiene, the most important predisposing factor is malnutrition which enhances both the susceptibility to, and the severity of, infantile gastro-enteritis. However, only a proportion of such cases can be attributed to infection with *Esch. coli*: other intestinal pathogens, known and unknown, are major contributors.

Control Measures

Since outbreaks of gastro-enteritis may result in high fatality rates in maternity nurseries and institutions caring for young children, every precaution must be taken to prevent the introduction of infection, particularly by infants coming from another institution. This may require some system of preliminary quarantine and bacteriological screening of the new admissions. If infection becomes established, drastic measures for its control may be needed, including temporary closure of a ward, nursery or institution.

Generally, the prevention of infantile gastro-enteritis demands that bottled milk feeds served to infants must be sterile and in hospital this is best effected by terminal heat sterilization of the fully prepared feed in the feeding bottle. In the home mothers should be encouraged to use domestic pressure cookers for the same purpose and to observe high standards of personal hygiene in preparing the feed but, of course, this kind of advice is very difficult to implement in conditions of poverty and poor environment. Undoubtedly, the most effective preventive measure is breast feeding (without supplements) for the first 6 to 9 months of life and every effort must be made to encourage mothers, particularly in the developing countries, to appreciate that 'breast is best' for their babies.

For the control of urinary tract infections special arrangements should be made for the screening of specimens of urine for significant bacteriuria at antenatal and diabetic clinics.

KLEBSIELLA

Most strains of *Klebsiella* are saprophytic and are found in many parts of the environment particularly in natural waters. *Klebsiella* species are sometimes detected as commensals in the human and animal intestine. They display an opportunistic pathogenic ability in the respiratory tract, the urinary system or as the cause of surface infections, particularly when there is some lowered tissue resistance or other predisposing factors, and are associated with both endemic and epidemic infections in hospitals.

Description

Klebsiella species have the general features of the other members of the enterobacteria but are never motile; they are capsulate both in natural environments and as human pathogens. *In vitro* they usually produce large capsules and an abundance of loose extracellular slime so that colonies are normally very mucoid. Most strains ferment lactose and so give pink colonies when grown on MacConkey's medium.

The capsular (K) antigen and the mucoid (M) slime antigen in any one strain are identical but the almost constant presence of these antigens masks the underlying somatic (O) antigens so that capsular, and not O antisera, are utilized in typing procedures; the 'capsule swelling' reaction resembles that used in serotyping of pneumococci and more than 70 serotypes of *Klebsiella* have been recognized.

Species

The six species described below may be distinguished by their biochemical reactions. Some authors, however, recognize only three species and include *Kl. aerogenes*, *Kl. pneumoniae*, *Kl. edwardsii* and *Kl. atlantae* in one species named *Kl. pneumoniae*. More than one species are represented in certain of the capsule serotypes of *Klebsiella* (Cowan et al., 1960).

Klebsiella aerogenes. This species occurs mostly in environmental sources such as soil, vegetation and water but may be found in the human intestine, particularly in hospitalized patients. Hospital acquired intestinal strains are frequently multidrug resistant and apparently well adapted to cause endogenous infections, e.g. in the urinary tract, or to be transmitted to other hospital patients. Types 8, 9 and 10 have been identified in urinary tract infections, but the prevalent serotypes in hospital vary in time and place. Seventy-two serotypes are known.

Klebsiella pneumoniae (serotype 3), or Friedländer's bacillus, is a rare cause of bacterial pneumonia (less than 1 per cent of cases in Britain), but its significance lies in the high case mortality (more than 50 per cent) in such cases. *Kl. edwardsii* (types 1 and 2) and *Kl. atlantae* (type 1) also rarely cause respiratory infections, including pneumonia.

Respiratory infections with klebsiellae are not uncommon in warm climate countries where they vary considerably in severity. Klebsiella types 1 to 6 are those most often derived from patients with respiratory infections, but other serotypes are also identified with respiratory disease.

Klebsiella rhinoscleromatis strains mostly belong to serotype 3 and can be differentiated from *Kl. pneumoniae* biochemically. This klebsiella is the cause of rhinoscleroma, a chronic granulomatous condition prevalent in South-Eastern Europe. Lesions occur in the mucous membranes of the nose, throat and mouth, and the bacilli are sited intracellularly in the lesions.

Klebsiella ozaenae is associated with ozaena and other respiratory tract infections and belongs to serotypes 3, 4, 5 and 6. The main distinguishing biochemical reactions of the more common pathogenic klebsiella are listed in Table 29.2.

Table 29.2

Species (and serotype)	Gas from glucose	Acid from lactose	Acid from dulcitol	V.-P.	M.-R.	Citrate
Kl. aerogenes (1–72)	+	+	+ or −	+	−	+
Kl. pneumoniae (3)	+	+	+	−	+	+
Kl. edwardsii (1, 2)	−	(+)	−	+	+ or −	+ or −
Kl. atlantae (1)	+	(+)	−	+ or −	+	+
Kl. ozaenae (3, 4, 5, 6)	+ or −	(+)	−	−	+	+ or −
Kl. rhinoscleromatis (3)	−	−	−	−	+	−

(+) = positive at 7 days.

PROTEUS

Description

Members of the genus *Proteus* occur widely in man, animals and in the environment and can be readily recovered from sewage, soil, garden vegetables and many other materials. The organism is a Gram-negative, actively motile, non-capsulate, rather pleomorphic, coliform bacillus.

Reflecting the wide parasitic and saprophytic distribution is the ease with which *Proteus* species can be grown *in vitro*. On media such as nutrient agar or blood agar, incubated aerobically discrete colonies are rarely seen; instead the growth spreads or swarms over the surface of the medium, usually in successive waves with flat sheets of thin growth alternating with rings of thick growth. Swarming is due to vigorous motility although its cause is not clearly established and it can be inhibited by various means, e.g. by incorporating certain chemicals in or on the surface of the medium or by increasing the concentration of agar in the medium.

Proteus species form pale colonies and do not swarm on MacConkey's and DCA media. They are distinctive in decomposing urea rapidly in the urease test and this feature differentiates them from other enterobacteria. Four biotypes within the genus (*Pr. vulgaris*, *Pr. mirabilis*, *Pr. morganii* and *Pr. rettgeri*) can be recognized by their ability or inability to utilize mannitol, maltose and citrate and whether or not they liquefy gelatin or produce indole. All strains can transform phenylalanine to phenyl-pyruvic acid, a characteristic which they share only with the genus *Providencia* within the family Enterobacteriaceae.

Clinical Infection

Strains isolated from the faeces of healthy human beings and also those from pathological specimens usually belong to the biotype *Proteus mirabilis*. There is still doubt as to the specific relationship of *Proteus morganii* to the syndrome known as summer diarrhoea in infants. *Proteus* strains are often found as concomitants of shigellae and make their appearances in the stools of patients recovering from bacillary dysentery. They are found either alone or often associated with pyogenic cocci in some cases of chronic otitis and also occur as secondary invaders in wounds, bedsores and the like where the infection is often endogenous. *Proteus* species are also incriminated in urinary tract infections and although infection may again be endogenous, the possibility of infection being introduced from an exogenous source during diagnostic or therapeutic instrumentation must not be forgotten. The urease activity of proteus probably is an important factor determining its pathogenicity in the urinary tract. The organisms rapidly form ammonia from the urea in the urine, which becomes very alkaline. In the tissues of an infected kidney the ammonia may promote infection by inactivating the fourth component of complement, whilst in the pelvis and bladder the alkalinity may cause deposition of phosphate stones which promote infection by increasing the retention of residual urine.

Laboratory Diagnosis

The spreading nature and fishy odour of the growth on blood agar or nutrient agar combined with the appearance of pale colonies on MacConkey or DCA media are sufficient for identification in routine diagnostic work but tests for urease activity and the phenylpyruvic acid reaction may also be done. If necessary the biotype may be established and similarly antigenic analysis within the biotype may be made since each biotype comprises numerous somatic antigen groups; these can be further subdivided into serotypes on the basis of flagellar antigens; seroanalysis, however, is rarely performed.

The swarming nature of proteus on ordinary media will cover the colonies of any other bacterial species that may be present in the culture so that the subcultivation, identification and determination of the antibiograms of the other species will be delayed; methods for preventing the spreading growth have already been mentioned.

CHEMOTHERAPY. Treatment of proteus infections should whenever possible be guided by the results of *in vitro* sensitivity tests since strains vary markedly so that the sensitivity of any one strain is difficult to forecast. Kanamycin and neomycin are most likely to be successful; the former is less toxic. As in infections with other species, infections of the urinary tract with proteus may be associated with structural or pathological abnormalities; these impede eradication of infection or, if the primary infecting strain is eliminated, promote its replacement with other species.

PROVIDENCIA

These Gram-negative motile bacilli are closely allied to the genus *Proteus* and indeed were formerly termed *Proteus inconstans*. They share the ability of proteus to deaminate phenylalanine although they rarely produce urease, and never exhibit swarming. They produce pale colonies on DCA and MacConkey's medium and are motile so that they might be confused with salmonellae by the unwary. However, even if urease and phenylalanine deaminase tests are not done, the observation that the organism produces indole prevents such confusion.

Providence species occur in normal faeces and have also been isolated from epidemics and sporadic cases of diarrhoea in man but it is at present difficult to assess their importance in relation to diarrhoeal disease. They also occur in infections of the urinary tract where there is no doubt as to their significance. Some laboratories do not seem to identify *Providencia* strains perhaps because their distinguishing characters are not sufficiently recognized.

REFERENCES

COWAN, S. T., STEEL, K. J., SHAW, C. & DUGUID, J. P. (1960) A classification of the klebsiella group. *Journal of General Microbiology*, **23**, 601.

GANGULI, L. (1970) Serological grouping of Escherichia coli in bacteriuria of pregnancy. *Journal of Medical Microbiology*, **3**, 201.

GLYNN, A. A. (1972) In *Microbial Pathogenicity in Man and Animals*, p. 75. Edited by H. Smith and J. H. Pearce. Cambridge University Press.

KASS, E. H. (1955) Symposium on newer aspects of antibiotics: chemotherapeutic and antibiotic drugs in the management of infections of urinary tract. *American Journal of Medicine*, **18**, 764.

SLEIGH, J. D., ROBERTSON, J. G. & ISDALE, M. H. (1964) Asymptomatic bacteriuria in pregnancy. *Journal of Obstetrics and Gynaecology of the British Commonwealth*, **71**, 74.

30. Vibrio: Spirillum   Cholera: Rat-bite Fever

A series of six pandemics of cholera, originating in the Bengal basin, ravaged the world in the nineteenth and early twentieth century, so that cholera, like plague, became a disease of fear. Characterized by the sudden onset of intense vomiting and diarrhoea with rapid dehydration and hypovolaemic shock, many patients died within 2 days of onset and case fatality rates of 20 to 30 per cent were recorded. Cholera today, if treated early and efficiently, can be shorn of its terrors and the patient can be quickly restored to health without complications. Unfortunately, after a few decades when cholera was being increasingly contained within the endemic foci and surrounding areas in India and Bangladesh, there has occurred a seventh pandemic due to

the El Tor biotype of the cholera vibrio; this originated in 1961 in Indonesia, spread to the Far East (Philippines, Hong Kong, probably the Chinese mainland, Taiwan, Korea, etc.) and then swept back through Indo-China, Malaysia, Thailand, Burma to India, West Pakistan, the Middle East and southern U.S.S.R. Since then (1970–71), the pandemic has invaded Africa where already some 22 countries have been affected (Fig. 30.1). The El Tor biotype (see below), originally isolated from pilgrims at the quarantine station of that name and for long regarded as of doubtful pathogenicity, supplanted the classical biotype of cholera vibrio in India and spread into Indian states previously free from the infection. But in spite of the ever

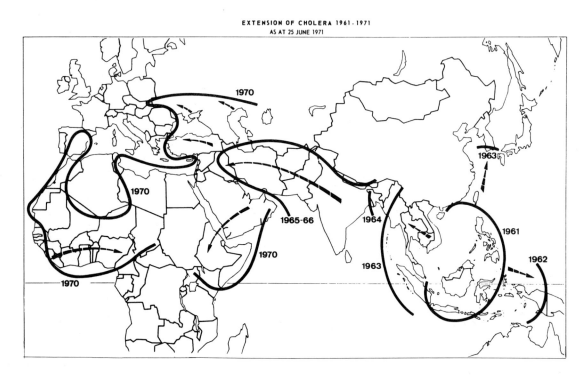

FIG. 30.1. Extension of cholera 1961 to 1971, as at June 1971.

increasing geographic distribution of cholera since 1961, there has been until the outbreaks in refugee camps in India, a marked decrease in its reported incidence which indicates that the El Tor vibrio is highly infective but less virulent than the classical strain; that is, the ratio of infection to clinical disease is high (see Fig. 30.2). There may be an analogy here with the Sonne and Flexner types of shigella infection in that Shiga and Flexner infections have been largely supplanted by Sonne dysentery in many countries with temperate climates.

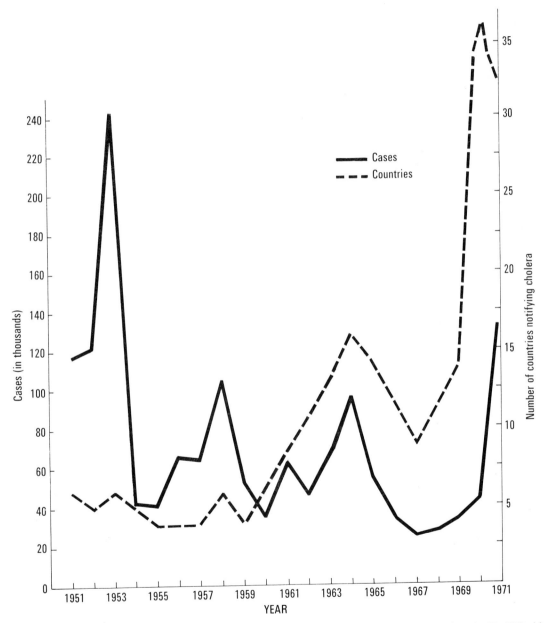

FIG. 30.2. Incidence of cholera and number of countries notifying cases, 1951 to 1971 (figures according to the *World Health Statistics Report*, provisional figures for 1971).

DESCRIPTION

The vibrios are allocated to the family Spirillaceae and are characterized as Gram-negative motile rods, usually curved (the comma bacillus), with a single polar flagellum. They are non-sporing, non-capsulated, facultative anaerobes, fermenting glucose without gas, hydrogen sulphide negative, and with enzyme activities on certain amino-acids (lysine+, ornithine+, arginine− for vibrios) which serve to distinguish them from two closely related genera, *Aeromonas* and *Plesiomonas*. Indeed, it has been suggested that these three genera should be grouped in a new family Vibrionaceae. Only two vibrios, the classical and El Tor biotypes of *Vibrio cholerae*, are associated with the cholera syndrome but other vibrios may be causally related to diarrhoeal disease. Reference is made in Vol. II to *Vibrio parahaemolyticus* which causes a form of acute food-poisoning in Japan, S.E. Asia, U.S.A. and possibly elsewhere. Many non-pathogenic vibrios are found in nature, mostly in water and in fish. All vibrios, being motile, have O and H antigens; the cholera vibrios can be differentiated from other vibrios on the basis of a somatic antigen, O1 which is specific to the classical and El Tor biotypes of *V. cholerae* so that other vibrios that lack this antigen are sometimes called non-agglutinating (NAG) or non-cholera vibrios (NCV). The two pathogenic biotypes may each be divided into two serological subtypes, called *Inaba* and *Ogawa*, based on the presence of a subsidiary O antigen. The El Tor biotype was first differentiated from the classical biotype by its production of haemolysin; other distinctive characters are its resistance to one of the four cholera phages (group IV) which Mukerjee has used to subdivide the classical vibrios, resistance to polymyxin B (50 units) and haemagglutination of chicken or sheep red cells. However, the haemolytic test may give variable results and most of the recently isolated El Tor strains are non-haemolytic; differentiation should therefore be based on reliable tests such as resistance to group IV phage at routine test dilution, resistance to polymyxin B and direct haemagglutination of chicken or sheep red blood cells.

Clinical Infection

Cholera is typically characterized by the sudden onset of effortless vomiting and profuse watery diarrhoea. Vomiting is a common feature but the rapid dehydration and hypovolaemic shock which may cause death in 12 to 24 hours are related mainly to the profuse 'rice water' stools —watery, colourless with flecks of mucus and distinctive sweet, fishy odour—which contain little protein (<0·1 per cent) and are very different from the mucopurulent blood-stained stools of classical dysentery. Anuria develops, muscle cramps occur and the patient quickly becomes weak and lethargic with loss of skin turgor, low blood pressure and absent or thready pulse. But there are all grades of severity and the milder cases of cholera, which are more common in El Tor infections, cannot be distinguished clinically from non-vibrio diarrhoeas. Symptomless infections are common.

PATHOGENESIS; PATHOPHYSIOLOGY

The sequence of events leading to cholera are basically simple and confined to the gut. The cholera vibrios are ingested in drink or food and, in the natural infection, the dosage must often be very small; after passing the acid barrier of the stomach juices, the organisms begin to multiply in the alkaline medium of the small intestine. As they multiply, they produce a potent exotoxin, called *enterotoxin*, which stimulates a persistent outpouring of isotonic fluid by the gut mucosal cells. The toxin is thought to react with a receptor in the membrane of the intestinal epithelial cell, then to activate adenylcyclase in the membrane and thereby raise the intracellular level of cyclic adenosine monophosphate (CAMP) which induces increased secretion of water and electrolytes into the intestinal lumen (Craig, 1972). There is no convincing evidence of any inflammatory reaction involving increased capillary permeability. Obviously a number of factors, some still unknown, must contribute to the occurrence of clinical cholera in any infected person; for example, cholera strains vary in toxigenicity, and variations in host resistance probably explain the infrequency of more than one case in a family.

Much new knowledge about the pathogenesis of cholera has come from experimental studies in animals, e.g. baby rabbits (10 to 14 days old) in which a syndrome resembling cholera can be produced, localized infection in isolated intestinal loops (rabbit, fowl, etc.) characterized by outpouring of isotonic fluid, and experimental cholera in dogs after neutralization of the stomach acids.

It is now generally accepted that there is no inflammatory denudation of the bowel mucosa in cholera and no invasion of the intestinal wall, deeper tissues or blood although the gall bladder may become a reservoir. The pathophysiological changes are directly related to the massive loss of isotonic fluid with excess of sodium bicarbonate and potassium through the gut, leading to hypovolaemic shock, acidosis and haemoconcentration with a consequent sharp rise in plasma proteins. Delay in rehydration may result in renal failure due to acute tubular necrosis; hypokalaemia from excess loss of potassium is likely to occur in children.

Immunity

More than one attack of clinical cholera is rare but reinfections are not uncommon in endemic areas where evidence from serological surveys indicates that from infancy to adulthood an increasing proportion of the population have vibriocidal antibodies, presumably related to repeated exposure and the occurrence of symptomless or mild infections; this phenomenon has been called 'salting' of the population. After a clinical attack, specific antibodies (agglutinins, vibriocidal antibodies) are demonstrable in the blood within a few days, reaching a peak in 7 to 14 days and thereafter declining to low levels after about 3 months. The antibody responses are poorer in pre-school than in schoolchildren or adults. The vibriocidal antibody titre correlates well with resistance to infection so that in endemic areas the incidence of clinical cholera falls progressively with age; two-thirds of the cases may be children under 15 years of age.

Despite the important part played by enterotoxin in the pathogenesis of cholera, the role of antitoxin in protection against the infection has not yet been elucidated.

LABORATORY DIAGNOSIS

In the acute stage of cholera, vibrios are abundantly present in the watery stool (10^7 to 10^9/ml) which is best collected with a no. 24 to 26 rubber catheter into a test-tube or screw-capped container; or a rectal swab may be used. Collection from a bedpan should be avoided because of the risk of contamination or the presence of antiseptic. In the examination of contacts and possible carriers, the rectal swab is most convenient, or the specimen may be collected from a stool passed on to clean paper or a large leaf. If there is likely to be delay in examination of the faecal specimen, a transport medium such as salt sea water or its equivalent (Venkatraman-Ramakrishnan fluid) or alkaline taurocholate tellurite liquid medium may be used; or strips of thick blotting paper may be soaked in the stool and wrapped in plastic or other impervious material to prevent leakage or evaporation.

Where there is urgency in making the bacteriological diagnosis of a case, a vibrio-immobilization test with dark field microscopy using two drops of the fresh fluid specimen on a glass slide or two drops of a young peptone water culture may be used. After the remarkable motility of the vibrios (like a cloud of gnats) has been seen, a drop of either Inaba or Ogawa antiserum is added to the bacterial suspension and specific immobilization can be demonstrated in 60 to 80 per cent of acute cases of cholera.

In the early stages of infection, the stool is plated directly on to one or more selective solid media. From bile salt agar typical bluish grey colonies can be picked off, with or without the use of a stereo-plate microscope, after overnight incubation or as early as 5 to 6 hours. Precise identification of biotype and serotype depends on further biological, serological and phage-sensitivity tests (see Vol. II, Chap. 32). Serological examination of paired serum samples taken within 48 hours of onset and after 7 to 10 days will usually show a significant rise of agglutinating and vibriocidal antibodies and may be used to check the reliability of bacteriological diagnosis; serological micro-techniques using very small amounts of the reagents give satisfactory results so that finger-prick specimens of blood are adequate.

In epidemiological investigations for the detection of contact or convalescent carriers when the number of vibrios in the stool may vary from 10^2 to 10^5 per g, inoculation of a large sample (2 to 3 g) of stool into 50 to 100 ml alkaline peptone water will give best results although moistened rectal swabs have often to be used for convenience. More than one subculture after 6 hours incubation in alkaline peptone water or other enrichment medium may be necessary when the vibrios are scanty. Induced purging sometimes reveals a hidden carrier of El Tor vibrios and duodenal incubation has helped in detecting persistent carriers of El Tor vibrios after clinical infection.

CHEMOTHERAPY

The first and essential requirement in the treatment of cholera is rehydration but chemotherapy plays a useful supporting role. The cholera vibrios are sensitive to the tetracyclines, chloramphenicol, streptomycin, furazolidone and other chemotherapeutic drugs active against most Gram-negative organisms. In practice, dosage with 2 g daily of tetracycline or furazolidone (in divided doses) for 2 to 3 days quickly eliminates the vibrios from the stools and sharply reduces the duration of the diarrhoea and associated loss of fluid.

EPIDEMIOLOGY

Man is the only natural host of the cholera vibrio and the spread of infection is from person to person with contaminated water or certain foods such as uncooked seafoods (shrimps, etc.) or vegetables as the most common vehicles. Cholera is characteristically an infection of crowded poor class communities living in low lying areas and it tends to persist in such communities which share communal water supplies such as 'tanks', ponds, canals or rivers for bathing, washing of linen and household uses. Outbreaks occur either as explosive epidemics, usually in non-endemic areas, or as protracted epidemic waves in endemic areas. The seasonal incidence is fairly consistent in different endemic regions but the climatic conditions during epidemic waves may be distinctive for each region.

For example, in Bangladesh the cholera season (November to February) follows the monsoon rains and ends with the onset of the hot, dry months; across the Bengal delta the main epidemic wave in Calcutta (May to July) rises to its peak in the hot, dry season and ends with the onset of the monsoon but extends inland to neighbouring states during the rainy season. In endemic areas, clinical infection is most common among the 'unsalted' pre-school children although it is rare in infancy. In explosive outbreaks, often associated with fairs, festivals and pilgrimages, or in non-endemic areas, adults are more commonly affected. In rural India infection spreads along lines of human communication from village to village just as it does on the global scale.

Spread is probably facilitated by the high ratio of symptomless carriers to clinical cases, varying from 10:1 to 100:1 depending on living conditions as well as on biotype. Symptomless carriers occur much more frequently in El Tor than in classical cholera infections. Although the clinical disease is similar after infection with one or other of the two biotypes, the epidemiological features may be distinctive, related to the high infectivity, low virulence and greater hardiness of the El Tor biotype which facilitates more direct person-to-person spread (e.g. by fomites and feeding utensils) than is the case with the classical biotype, for which water is the most likely vehicle. The symptomless carrier probably plays an important part in spreading El Tor infection into new communities.

In non-epidemic periods in endemic areas, carriers or mild missed cases are essential links in maintaining the reservoir of infection since the vibrios do not multiply or survive for long on possible vehicles such as water, food, fruit, vegetables. After an acute attack of cholera, the vibrios may be excreted for a few weeks in convalescence although more persistent El Tor carriers have been reported. Maintenance of the reservoir of infection seems to depend on the chain infected case → water → infected case plus more direct person-to-person spread with the resistant El Tor biotype. Detection of human reservoirs may be attempted by the bacteriological examination of sewage, e.g. collected night soil as has been done in Hong Kong or bucket latrines as in Calcutta.

Phage-typing has not yet contributed much information about the epidemiology of cholera, mainly because only types 1 and 3 of the five phage-types of classical *V. cholerae* are commonly found and because there is some instability among the provisional six El Tor phage-types.

CONTROL MEASURES

It seems unlikely that cholera can be controlled in the endemic areas until good water supplies are installed in individual houses, better provision is made for sewage disposal, and the necessity or habit in certain countries of using communal water in ponds, canals and rivers for washing of bodies and linen as well as for household use can be abolished. A most disturbing feature of the seventh pandemic is that the number of affected countries in Asia and Africa has been rising steadily in the past decade and in India the infection is more widespread than it has been for many years. A number of European countries have also been invaded. This wide geographic dissemination is wholly due to the El Tor biotype which, because of its greater hardiness and higher infectivity/virulence ratio than the classical biotype, is likely to establish endemic foci in many crowded centres in African and Asian countries with poor standard of environmental sanitation and household hygiene. It is noteworthy that Japan has resisted invasion despite several introductions of cholera and it seems unlikely that cholera will become endemic in countries with good environmental sanitation and high public health standards.

A number of controlled trials in different countries to test the efficacy of prophylactic vaccination has shown that with the presently available killed whole cell vaccines, protection of about half of the inoculated community lasts for only 3 to 6 months. In an endemic area, one dose of vaccine is more effective when given to the 'salted' schoolchildren than are two doses given at 4 to 6 weeks' interval to the highly susceptible pre-school children (Feeley, 1970). Controlled trials with monovalent antigens (Inaba and Ogawa) have indicated that protection is specifically against the infecting serotype. Mass immunization of schoolchildren with one dose of vaccine at the beginning of the *epidemic* period in endemic areas might be practicable and help to control the spread of infection. Mass immunization of pilgrims on their way to Mecca and of those attending religious festivals, and perifocal inoculations during a localized outbreak, e.g. in a refugee camp, may also be useful prophylactic measures. However, it has been concluded that cholera vaccination as a general public health measure is ineffective in preventing the introduction of cholera into a community, in containing its spread or in reducing mortality where adequate treatment facilities are available (Mosley, 1970). The possible usefulness of cholera toxoid, whole cell vaccine plus toxoid, purified antigens with or without adjuvant, and live attenuated oral vaccines are presently under consideration.

Meanwhile, there is evidence that in some areas where cholera is now endemic, e.g. the Philippines, improved sanitation in the shape of readily available water supplies and/or cheap privy construction will reduce the incidence of cholera and presumably other diarrhoeal diseases, and will, in the long term, be economically preferable to repeated mass vaccination.

Control of incipient outbreaks in non-endemic areas requires prompt recognition of suspected clinical cases and quick laboratory confirmation so that early treatment and suitable preventive measures, e.g. chemoprophylaxis among close contacts, are put in train. Unfortunately such facilities are not usually available in developing countries but W.H.O. has been active in fostering training courses and laboratory services in countries where the risks of importation seem greatest. A rational use of the International Health Regulations, which aim at combining a maximum of safety with a minimum of interference in international traffic and trade instead of unnecessarily restrictive quarantine and trade measures against countries reporting cholera, would help to minimize economic and political upheavals. Health administrators must know, and make it known, that cholera, if promptly recognized, is certainly curable if not yet preventable. Measures against the importation of cholera to European countries are discussed in a memorandum 'Cholera Control in the European Region' issued by the European Regional Office of

World Health Organization (Copenhagen, 1971).

SPIRILLUM MINUS

A causative organism of rat-bite fever, this organism, though often described as a spirochaete, conforms in its biological characters to those of a spirillum and the name *Spirillum minus* is generally used. A similar clinical syndrome is caused by *Streptobacillus moniliformis*.

Description

Spirillum minus is a short spiral organism about 2 to 5 μm in length and relatively broad, with regular short coils numbering one for each micron of the length of the organism. Longer forms up to 10 μm may also be observed. This organism is very actively motile, showing darting movements like those of a vibrio. Movement is due to terminal flagella, which are variable in number—from one to seven at each pole. In moving, the organism itself remains rigid and shows no undulation. It can be demonstrated easily by dark-ground illumination in fresh preparations. It is most readily stained by a Romanowsky stain (e.g. Leishman's), but can also be stained by ordinary aniline dyes. The organism has probably never been cultivated successfully.

The clinical syndrome is characterized by a relapsing febrile illness with a local inflammatory lesion, enlargement of regional lymph glands and a macular skin eruption, all these lesions fluctuating in parallel with the temperature. This form of rat-bite fever occurs mainly in Japan and the Far East.

Laboratory Diagnosis

In rat-bite fever the spirillum may be demonstrated in the local lesion, the regional lymph glands and even in the blood, either by direct microscopical methods or by animal inoculation. If the spirillum cannot be detected microscopically in the local lesion, or if the original bite-wound has healed, an enlarged lymphatic gland may be punctured by means of a hypodermic syringe; 'gland juice' is aspirated and investigated by direct methods or animal inoculation. Guinea-pigs, white rats and mice are susceptible to infection; the spirilla appear in the peripheral blood and can be detected by dark-ground illumination. Guinea-pigs develop a progressive disease and die from the infection. The intraperitoneal inoculation of human infective material in mice is followed by no sign of disease; spirilla appear in the blood after 5 to 14 days, but always in very small numbers.

Spirillum minus occurs naturally in wild rats and certain other wild rodents, producing a blood infection. Conditions similar to rat-bite fever have also been reported following the bites of cats and ferrets.

Spirillum minus infections respond to treatment with the tetracyclines and penicillin.

REFERENCES AND FURTHER READING

CRAIG, J. P. (1972) The enterotoxic enteropathies. In *Microbial Pathogenicity in Men and Animals*, p. 129. Edited by H. Smith and J. H. Pearce. Cambridge University Press.

MOSLEY, W. H. (1970) In *World Health Organization Public Health Papers*, no. 40, p. 23. Geneva.

FEELEY, J. C. (1970) In *World Health Organization Public Health Papers*, no. 40, p. 87. Geneva.

The genus *Pseudomonas* comprises more than 140 species, but only one of these is pathogenic to man, i.e. *Pseudomonas pyocyanea* (*Ps. aeruginosa*). The others are essentially saprophytic and occur widely in nature. Some species have been given specific rank on the most flimsy evidence, frequently according to the source from which they have been isolated, e.g. *Ps. tomato*. Although Baginski recognized the pathogenic nature of *Ps. pyocyanea* in 1908, and in particular its ability to infect newborn babies, it is only in the last two decades that the wider significance of *Ps. pyocyanea* in human infections has attracted attention, especially as a nosocomial (hospital acquired) infection.

Classical strains of *Ps. pyocyanea* may be isolated from a wide variety of environmental sources, e.g. earth, sewage and water, and undoubtedly these potential pathogens are competent and hardy saprophytes. The ability of the strain to persist and multiply in wet places and on wet equipment in hospital wards, bathrooms and kitchens is of particular importance. Its isolation from many ordinary and exotic plants and animals, e.g. the arctic fox, and from both warm and cold blooded species underlines the ability of *Ps. pyocyanea* to thrive parasitically in a wide variety of circumstances. The organism is also found in the faeces and on the skin of a proportion of healthy persons, in whom it appears to grow as a commensal.

The remarkable adaptation of *Ps. pyocyanea* may be emphasized by noting that it has entered the space age at the same time as man since it has been isolated from jet fuels and incriminated as a cause of corrosion of the linings of fuel tanks.

DESCRIPTION

Ps. pyocyanea is Gram-negative, bacillary in shape, usually motile by virtue of one or more polar flagella, non-sporing and non-capsulate. It is a strict aerobe and grows on a wide variety of laboratory media. The majority of isolates produce pigments when grown *in vitro* and classically the colony is greenish-blue due to production of pyocyanin and fluorescin, pigments which diffuse rapidly into the surrounding medium. Some strains produce pyorubrin which endows the colony with a reddish-brown appearance and a minority of strains, perhaps 10 to 15 per cent, do not produce obvious pigment although they do so when grown on special media. Individual colonies of *Ps. pyocyanea* are large, low convex with an irregular surface and edge which is translucent in comparison with the pigmented centre.

Unlike some other Gram-negative bacilli, *Ps. pyocyanea* is not very active biochemically and of the substrates normally employed in diagnostic bacteriology only glucose is utilized. However, all strains give a positive oxidase reaction when tested in the same way as the neisseriae; although a few other Gram-negative bacilli are also oxidase-positive, none reacts as swiftly as *Ps. pyocyanea* which gives a positive reaction within 30 seconds. Thus the oxidase test is diagnostic for strains that do not produce pigments.

For epidemiological purposes both serological and bacteriophage-sensitivity techniques have been used to differentiate *Ps. aeroginosa* into 'types' but neither method is as readily applicable nor as internationally acceptable as *pyocine typing* which depends on the production of pyocines (bacteriocines) by the strain under investigation. Pyocine production is demonstrated by the various patterns of inhibition given by the strain under test against a standard set of eight indicator strains. Some 37 pyocine types of *Ps. pyocyanea* have so far been recognized (Gillies and Govan, 1966; Govan and Gillies, 1969).

CLINICAL INFECTIONS

Infections caused by *Ps. pyocyanea* are not unknown in the open community where the organism usually gives rise to mild superficial infections, e.g. otitis externa; such infections are often chronic although not disabling. In hospital practice pseudomonas infections are much more common. In a recent survey the incidence of clinical pseudomonas infection in the open community was 1·25 per 10 000 of the population as compared with 269 per 10 000 patients in one hospital serving the same community. Fortunately, even in hospital-acquired cases the infection is usually localized, as in urinary tract infections, infected bedsores, infected burns and eye infections. In patients debilitated either by reason of age or concomitant infection and in patients receiving immunosuppressive agents or corticosteroids, pseudomonas infections frequently become generalized and the organism may be isolated from blood cultures and, *post mortem* from all tissues and tracts of the body.

Laboratory Diagnosis

The isolation of *Ps. pyocyanea* is a straightforward procedure. Specimens, e.g. sputum, urinary deposits, swabs from ulcers or burns etc., are plated on to blood agar; blood culture specimens are treated in the usual manner and specimens of faeces are, in addition, inoculated on to a plate of DCA medium. Resultant colonies are usually easily identified and in cases of doubt an oxidase test may be performed. Pyocine typing of the isolate (q.v. Vol. II, Chap. 33) is undertaken for epidemiological purposes. Tests for antibodies in the patient's serum have no place in diagnostic procedures at present.

Chemotherapy

In vitro tests of sensitivity must be undertaken as a guide to intelligent antimicrobial therapy. The fact that *Ps. pyocyanea* is naturally resistant to most of the commonly employed antimicrobial agents adds to the dilemma created by its emergence as a human pathogen; the only agents to which strains are regularly sensitive are gentamicin, carbenicillin and polymyxin. Other agents to which some strains may be sensitive

are streptomycin, neomycin and kanamycin but varying degrees of cross-resistance between these agents have been reported.

Ps. pyocyanea is resistant to, and may multiply in, 'in-use' dilutions of certain of the disinfectants commonly used in hospital, e.g. cetrimide and chloroxylenol.

Epidemiology

The hospital-acquired nature of infections with *Ps. pyocyanea* has already been noted and whilst some patients suffer endogenous infection, particularly of the urinary tract, it is probable that the vast majority of infections are acquired from exogenous sources. Healthy carriers of *Ps. pyocyanea* usually harbour strains in the bowel but carrier surveys of healthy individuals in the open community reveal a low carrier rate. Contrarily, such surveys conducted in patients in hospital show that acquisition of *Ps. pyocyanea* is very rapid and up to 28 per cent of patients have been shown to be excreting strains within two days of admission and 38 per cent to be parasitized at some time or other during their stay in hospital.

Baginski's statement, made more than 60 years ago, that '*Ps. pyocyanea* is one of the commonest enemies of infancy' has been frequently confirmed in recent times. Epidemics of pseudomonas infection in newborn and young infants in maternity units and paediatric wards are not uncommon. The ability of *Ps. pyocyanea* to survive, and occasionally to flourish, in many supposedly antiseptic or disinfectant solutions explained the method of spread in some of these episodes. For example, in a large maternity unit pseudomonas infections had been sporadic over a period of two years when suddenly 71 cases of infection occurred among the infants in the space of five weeks. All these babies were artificially fed and no breast-fed infant was affected. Naturally therefore the milk kitchen came under suspicion and although the bulk milk supply was sterile, as were the feeding bottles which had been autoclaved before filling, *Ps. pyocyanea* was recovered from milk feeds immediately prior to being used. Investigation showed that once the milk had been introduced into the bottle the top was occluded with a rubber bung which was kept in place while the feeds were stored. After use these bungs were washed and stored in a solution of antiseptic. The epidemic strain of *Ps. pyocyanea* was isolated from the stored bungs. The introduction of terminal heat sterilization of the fully prepared and teated milk feeds terminated the epidemic.

Burned patients are another category peculiarly at risk from this opportunistic pathogen and the presence of *Ps. pyocyanea* in ward air and dust in such instances is easily demonstrated, suggesting that infection is dust-borne. After such a ward has been vacated *Ps. pyocyanea* may be isolated from many situations, e.g. underneath skirting boards, in the traps of sinks, baths and drains, and from minute pieces of eschar from discharged patients. Patients with pseudomonas infection of chronic skin lesions, e.g. psoriasis, similarly cause heavy contamination of the hospital environment.

Contact spread has also been demonstrated and may take place directly or indirectly. Patients requiring tracheostomy with artificial ventilation are especially susceptible to infection with *Ps. pyocyanea* and pulmonary infection in such instances not infrequently is a prelude to septicaemia. It is very difficult to clean modern respirators and there is little doubt that such apparatus may cause spread from one case to another.

The remarkable viability of *Ps. pyocyanea* and its opportunistic ability has been frequently seen in recent years in cases undergoing ophthalmic surgery when instillation of a supposedly sterile medicament, which, however, contained *Ps. pyocyanea*, was made into the patient's eye; the resulting infection not infrequently ended with loss of sight.

Control Measures

Once *Ps. pyocyanea* has gained access to the hospital environment it is notoriously difficult to eradicate. Three guide-lines to control of infection are offered in the knowledge that it is not always easy to follow them.

1. When a patient comes into the high-risk category in being susceptible to infection with *Ps. pyocyanea*, e.g. a patient being evaluated for renal transplant, he should not be admitted to a ward where cases of pseudomonas infection are present but should be investigated or treated in strict isolation.

2. A patient infected with *Ps. pyocyanea* should, if at all possible, be isolated until the infection has been eradicated. Otherwise he will remain as a disperser of his organism to other patients with whom he shares a communal ward environment.

3. A general requirement, applying not only to the control of pseudomonas infections but to all hospital-acquired infections, is that all instruments and apparatus, dressings, etc., must be not only clean but sterile. Antimicrobial and other therapeutic substances and solutions must also be free from bacteria; a particular danger exists when multi-dose containers, e.g. for eye-droppers, are used to treat several individuals over a period. Initially the preparation may be sterile but contamination can easily occur between uses and since *Ps. pyocyanea* can multiply readily at room temperature in many medicaments, contamination of such containers may allow growth with the consequent danger on application to damaged tissues.

LOEFFLERELLA

Only two species within the genus *Loefflerella* have any significance in human medicine and both are essentially parasitic on animals; man is only occasionally infected. *Loefflerella mallei* causes an infection called glanders in horses and its incidence nowadays is restricted to Asia. It is a Gram-negative, slender bacillus, non-motile and non-sporing which stains irregularly, giving a beaded appearance. It is an aerobe and facultative anaerobe with a wide temperature range and grows on ordinary media, although for primary isolation it is advantageous to adjust the pH of the media to a slightly acid reaction (pH 6·6). Young colonies are semi-transparent, whitish and often mucoid; older colonies become opaque and ochre in colour.

Guinea-pigs are remarkably susceptible to inoculation of cultures and the Straus reaction can be demonstrated if an inoculation is made intraperitoneally into a male guinea-pig; the tunica vaginalis is rapidly invaded by the bacilli and swelling of the testis is obvious. The infected animals die within a few days of inoculation and generalized lesions can be seen at necropsy.

Glanders in the natural host gives a profuse catarrhal discharge from the nose, and the nasal septum shows nodule formation; later in the disease the nodules break down with the production of irregular ulcers. When infection occurs in superficial lymph vessels and nodes, following infection through the skin, e.g. via abrasions caused by a rubbing harness, the clinical term farcy is used to describe the infection. The lymph vessels show irregular thickening, become corded and are termed 'farcy pipes'.

Man may become infected via skin abrasions or wounds which come in contact with the discharges of a sick horse.

The other species within the genus, *Loefflerella pseudomallei*, causes melioidosis which is a glanders-like infection occurring epizootically among rodents in Asia, e.g. India, Malaysia and Indonesia. *Loeff. pseudomallei* resembles *Loeff. mallei* but is motile by virtue of a tuft of polar flagella. It grows well in and liquefies gelatin at 20°C. It is oxidase-positive, grows on MacConkey's medium and does not produce H_2S. Although a Straus reaction can be elicited with cultures the species is serologically distinct from *Loeff. mallei*.

Rats are probably the most important source of infection for man. Although the disease has been transmitted experimentally by the rat flea it is more likely that infection is transmitted by foodstuffs that have been contaminated with rats' excreta. In man the disease usually develops as an acute pulmonary infection followed by bacteriaemia, the formation of multiple abscesses and death after an illness that may last for weeks or months.

Recently, *Loeff. mallei* has been classified as *Acinetobacter mallei* because it resembles other *Acinetobacter* species in its non-motility and failure to ferment any carbohydrate. *Loeff. pseudomallei* has been classified as *Pseudomonas pseudomallei* because it resembles *Pseudomonas* species in having polar flagella and giving a positive oxidase reaction.

REFERENCES

GILLIES, R. R. & GOVAN, J. R. W. (1966) Typing of *Pseudomonas pyocyanea* by pyocine production. *Journal of Pathology and Bacteriology*, **91**, 339.

GOVAN, J. R. W. & GILLIES, R. R. (1969) Further studies in the pyocine typing of *Pseudomonas pyocyanea. Journal of Medical Microbiology*, **2**, 17.

32. Anthrax Bacillus

Malignant Pustule: Woolsorter's Disease

Anthrax is a disease primarily of animals caused by infection with *Bacillus anthracis*. Man is infected accidentally by contact with infected animal products. It is a disease of world-wide distribution, important and interesting for a number of reasons. It is the disease in which Koch (1877) first showed that the organism could be isolated from the blood of infected animals, could be seen to divide and to produce heat resistant spores. Furthermore, he demonstrated that pure cultures reproduced the disease in animals. Koch's work on anthrax led to the development of the present day methods of isolation and identification of bacteria and to the 'Koch postulates' (see Chap. 1). Pasteur showed that animals could be actively immunized by infecting them with cultures of *B. anthracis* that had been attenuated by growth at 42 to 43°C. Anthrax is a disease in which the infection is transmitted by the spore of the bacillus and the source of the spores is usually bacilli shed in large numbers from the nose, mouth and anus of animals in the terminal stages of the infection. The disease is therefore unusual in that the infection is spread only from a dying or dead host. The pathogenesis was not understood until the 1950s, at which time the exotoxin produced by the bacillus was demonstrated and subsequently a protective vaccine for man was produced from it.

B. anthracis belongs to the genus *Bacillus* whose members are large straight Gram-positive rods, occurring in chains, growing aerobically and forming heat-resistant spores. Most of these organisms exist as saprophytes in soil, water, air and on vegetation—e.g. *Bacillus cereus* and *Bacillus subtilis*. *B. anthracis* is the only pathogen of the group for man, though very occasionally *B. cereus* has been implicated in food infections.

BACILLUS ANTHRACIS

DESCRIPTION

B. anthracis is a non-motile, straight, sporing bacillus, rectangular in shape and 4 to 8 μm by 1 to 1·5 μm, i.e. just smaller in length than the diameter of a red blood corpuscle. The spore is oval, refractile, central in position and of the same diameter as the bacillus. The organism is a strongly Gram-positive aerobe and facultative anaerobe with a temperature range for growth of 12° to 45°C (optimum 35°C); it grows on all ordinary media as typical colonies with a wavy margin and small projections, the so-called 'medusa head' appearance.

Spores are never found in the tissues but appear when the organism is shed or grown on artificial media; they stain only with special spore-staining procedures. The spores are resistant to chemical disinfectants and heat; e.g. the spores of many strains will resist dry heat at 140°C for one to three hours and boiling or steam at 100°C for 5 to 10 minutes. However, autoclaving at 121°C (15 lbs/in²) destroys them in 15 minutes. The spores are relatively resistant to chemical agents with the exception of 1 in 1 000 mercuric chloride and 4 per cent potassium permanganate which destroy them in 30 minutes and 15 minutes respectively.

PATHOGENESIS

Experimental Infection

All mammals are susceptible, though to a varying degree. Birds of prey (vultures) which have fed on infected carcases excrete the spores in their faeces but seldom die. Guinea-pigs and mice are highly susceptible to experimental inoculation. If a guinea-pig is injected subcutaneously with pathological material containing the bacilli, or with pure cultures, the animal dies, usually within two to three days, showing a marked inflammatory lesion at the site of inoculation and extensive gelatinous oedema in the subcutaneous tissues. Large numbers of the bacilli are present in the local lesion, and are also profusely present in the heart-blood and in the capillaries of the internal organs. They are specially numerous in the spleen, which is enlarged and soft, giving rise to the description 'splenic fever' in the ox and the German name for the organism—Milzbrandbazillus (spleen-destroying bacillus).

Experimentally the production of anthrax in monkeys and guinea-pigs by inhalation of contaminated aerosols has also been studied. Spores deposited on the alveolar walls are taken up by phagocytes and carried to the tracheo-bronchial glands which become inflamed and enlarged. Infection spreads via the lymphatics to the general circulation. The LD50 is about 20 000 organisms if the particle size of the aerosols is less than 5 μm since the smaller particles are more likely to penetrate in the air-stream to the alveolar walls, but is much higher if the particles are larger.

The pathogenesis of anthrax was obscure for many years. No lethal exo- or endotoxins could be found in artificial cultures of the organism and it was believed that death was due to the massive terminal septicaemia; the bacilli were thought to block the capillaries and exhaust the tissues of essential nutrients and oxygen. It is now recognized that the virulence of *B. anthracis* is determined by at least two unconnected factors—an extracellular toxin and the capsular polypeptide (Smith, 1960). The toxin was first detected in the sterile plasma of guinea-pigs dying of anthrax, but it has now been produced *in vitro* and consists of at least three components which act synergistically (Stanley and Smith, 1961). These three components have been designated factor I (chelating agent), factor II (protein) and factor III (protein) and a mixture of them 'anthrax toxic complex'. The main effect of the toxic complex is to increase vascular permeability and it is generally agreed that death is due to this complex (Smith and Stoner, 1967),

although changes in the circulation dynamics, renal changes and alterations of carbohydrate metabolism play a part in the processes leading to death.

The capsular polypeptide is composed of D-glutamic acid and this substance is found only in virulent strains. The capsule appears to function by inhibiting opsonization and phagocytosis. It is of interest that extracts of human tissue differ in their ability to decapsulate the bacillus, e.g. extracts of lymph nodes are very active and extracts of thyroid and skin are very inactive (Zanev *et al.*, 1968).

Clinical Infections

The anthrax bacillus produces an epizootic disease in herbivorous animals, particularly among sheep and cattle. Although the condition is usually septicaemic in nature, subacute and chronic disease also occurs in animals as do localizing pustules which are analogous to the malignant pustule in man. In animals the portal of entry is the mouth and intestinal tract, the spores being ingested with coarse vegetation which probably predisposes to trauma of the mucosa. Infection may also take place by the inhalation of dust-containing spores into the respiratory tract or by the entry of spores through abraded skin.

The spores germinate and the vegetative cells produce toxin leading to the formation of gelatinous oedema and haemorrhage. In the susceptible animals the bacilli resist phagocytosis and reach the lymphatics and thence the bloodstream. Before death the bacilli multiply freely in the blood and tissues. In the resistant animal there is a more profuse leucocyte response with phagocytosis and decapsulation of the organism.

In man, infection is acquired from animal sources, usually through damaged skin or mucous membranes, or more rarely by inhalation of spores into the lungs. Infection occurs most commonly through the skin in persons such as farmers and veterinary surgeons handling infected animals, or among dock workers, factory workers and farmers from handling carcases and hides, animal hair and bristles, shaving-brushes, feeding-stuffs, bone-meal, and other bone products. The resulting lesion is cutaneous anthrax, sometimes described as a *malignant pustule*. The lesion starts as a papule and becomes a blister within 12 to 48 hours and then a pustule with an increasing area of inflammation depending upon the resistance of the host. Coagulation necrosis of the centre results in the formation of a dark-coloured *eschar* which is later surrounded by a ring of vesicles containing serous or sero-sanguineous fluid; outside this is an area of oedema and induration which may become very extensive. The degree of oedema varies and may be quite small with a large malignant pustule or very extensive with a tiny local lesion. The degree of oedema and toxicity is important, the prognosis being poor in patients with severe toxic signs and widespread oedema and in those developing septicaemia.

Infection may result from inhalation of spores carried in dust or filaments of wool from infected animals, as in the wool factories—'wool-sorter's disease'. The organisms settle in the lower part of the trachea or in a large bronchus, and an intense inflammatory lesion results, with haemorrhage, oedema, spread to the thoracic lymph nodes, involvement of the lungs, and effusion into the pericardial and pleural cavities; the organisms are present in considerable numbers in the lesions; septicaemia or haemorrhagic meningitis may supervene.

Infection may occur by the intestinal route, but this is relatively uncommon except in primitive societies eating infected animals which have been found dead. The outbreaks may carry a high fatality rate.

LABORATORY DIAGNOSIS

Malignant Pustule

A swab is taken from one of the vesicles or the fluid is collected into a capillary tube which is then sealed at both ends and dispatched to the laboratory. Films are also made from the fluid at the time of collection. These films are stained by Gram's method: the finding of bacilli morphologically like *B. anthracis* is suggestive of anthrax.

Cultures are made from the fluid or swab on a nutrient agar plate. The typical medusa head colonies are obtained after overnight incubation: the presence of *B. anthracis* is shown by Gram staining of films from the colonies when some spores will be seen in long tangled chains of large Gram-positive bacilli. Confirmation that the organism is *B. anthracis* is provided by animal inoculation. When the animal dies the post-mortem appearances are characteristic and bacilli can be demonstrated in the heart blood and spleen in large numbers. In smears stained by polychrome methylene blue, the bacilli are blue and are surrounded by a purplish-red granular staining which is the disrupted capsular material (McFadyean's reaction). This appearance is given only by *B. anthracis*.

The methods for isolation of *B. anthracis* from heavily contaminated material, e.g. hair and wool, and the details of a precipitin test (Ascoli reaction) with tissue extracts of suspected animal deaths from anthrax are described in Vol. II, Chap. 34.

The spores of *B. anthracis* are not affected by the antibiotics in the concentrations used in the selective culture media and are able to become vegetative cells and grow on the media. The colonies which grow have usually to be identified as *B. anthracis* by virulence tests.

CHEMOTHERAPY

Most antibiotics to which the anthrax bacillus is sensitive in *in vitro* tests have been used successfully in the treatment of anthrax in man, e.g. penicillin and streptomycin. The case fatality in cutaneous anthrax since the introduction of antibiotics has fallen from 20 per cent to 5 per cent. Chemotherapeutic agents have no effect upon the toxins already produced; therefore it is important to institute therapy as soon as possible.

The serum of artificially immunized animals, e.g. Sclavo's serum, which was used in the treatment of human anthrax in the pre-antibiotic era, is not now ordinarily given.

In animals, treatment is not often possible as most cases are not diagnosed till moribund or dead. Penicillin in large doses should be given possibly combined with immune serum.

EPIDEMIOLOGY

Anthrax is a zoonosis: a disease of animals transmissible secondarily to man. The annual incidence of human anthrax throughout the world is not known accurately due to a large number of cases not being notified, but probably is between 20 000 and 100 000 cases, mostly in rural areas.

In the terminal stages of the septicaemic disease in animals the bacilli are present in very large numbers in faeces, urine and saliva and these contaminate the ground and pasture. Contamination of the soil and pasture may also result from the exudates from dead animals. The vegetative cells sporulate rapidly after being shed and the spores may remain viable for many years.

When anthrax infection becomes established in livestock in a district, a relatively permanent enzootic focus of infection is created because of the prolonged viability of the spores in soil. Heavy contamination of the soil exists in many parts of the world, particularly Asia, Southern Europe and Africa.

In the United Kingdom, the disease is sporadic amongst cattle and is commonest in the winter months when it can be traced usually to imported feeding stuffs that have been contaminated with anthrax spores, especially bone-meal imported from areas where animal anthrax is common, e.g. the Indian continent (Jamieson and Green, 1955). In the report of the Committee on Anthrax (1959) 18 out of 21 samples of bone-meal from India and Pakistan were contaminated with anthrax spores and experience since then confirms this finding.

In countries where the disease is relatively rare in animals, industrial anthrax from contamination with imported materials is the commonest form of infection in man. In general, the infectivity of the anthrax bacillus for man is not of a high order and when a case of anthrax occurs in an industrial establishment, spores of the bacillus are often widely distributed and in large numbers in the environment. In 1958 Liverpool Docks handled over 6 000 tons of dry hides and when discharged from the ships, one-quarter of the hides were contaminated with anthrax spores (Semple and Hobday, 1959). Yet, anthrax is very rare amongst the hide handlers, only six cases having been recognized in five years. Cutaneous anthrax is by far the commonest human lesion. Cases have been described among nurserymen and amateur gardeners distributing infected bone-meal into bags or spreading this infected material on rosebeds (Green and Jamieson, 1958). In the 17 years up to 1960, 109 cases of human anthrax were reported in New York State and in all but two instances the patient suffered from malignant pustule (Miller, 1961). Pulmonary anthrax, common in Great Britain and Germany as woolsorter's disease in the nineteenth century, is now rare and the 1957 outbreak in New Hampshire is claimed to be the first in the twentieth century (Brachman et al., 1960). In this small epidemic there were 5 cases (4 fatal) of inhalation anthrax during a 10-week period in a mill processing imported goat hair. During handling there was an excessive amount of dust and the air contained large numbers of anthrax spores.

PROPHYLAXIS AND CONTROL

In outbreaks of animal anthrax, affected animals must be promptly diagnosed and isolated. Carcases must be buried deeply in quicklime or cremated to limit sporulation of the organism from the tissues and spread to pasturage and other animals. The limitation of the import of animal hides and hair to a single port (Liverpool), where facilities for mechanical handling and disinfection ('Duckering') are available, has done most to reduce the danger of anthrax in the United Kingdom (see Anthrax Order, 1938).

The eradication of anthrax in animals can be assisted by active immunization procedures and numerous vaccines have been used. Historically live attenuated bacilli were first used by Pasteur in 1881 in his famous experiment at Pouilly-le-Fort. The attenuation of the bacilli was achieved by growth at 42 to 43°C. Theoretically vaccines of bacilli should be effective since the bacilli are important in the disease.

Live spore vaccines have been employed extensively in the immunization of animals (e.g. the Sterne strain) with considerable success. The spore vaccine is directed against the commonest form of the organism to cause infection and vaccines that stimulate mechanisms for removing spores entering the body should be effective. Protection for one year is produced by a single injection of these vaccines. Spore vaccines are not considered safe for man.

Alum-precipitated toxoid is very safe and has been used to immunize people liable to be exposed to anthrax infection. In the United Kingdom an alum precipitated toxoid (Darlow *et al.*, 1956) is available through the P.H.L.S. laboratories at Colindale, Liverpool and Bradford. It is given in three doses (0·5 ml each) intramuscularly at successive intervals of six weeks and six months with a reinforcing dose yearly. No serious side effects have been reported following its use.

BACILLI BIOLOGICALLY ALLIED TO BACILLUS ANTHRACIS

These organisms are saprophytes and represent a large number of different species. They are found in soil, water, dust and air. Being ubiquitous, they are frequent contaminants of culture media in the laboratory, and therefore important to bacteriological workers.

The species are differentiated by a number of criteria, one being the size of the bacillus. There are two groups, the large-celled, e.g. *B. megaterium*, *B. cereus*, and the small-celled, e.g. *B. subtilis*, *B. stearothermophilus* (see Wilson and Miles, 1964).

The following species are of special interest either in connection with antibiotics or in tests of the effectiveness of sterilization procedures.

B. subtilis. Some strains produce an extracellular penicillinase. The enzyme concerned is an adaptive one and is produced in appreciable amounts only when the organism is grown in the presence of penicillin.

B. subtilis var. globigii is used as a test organism for the efficiency of ethylene oxide sterilization. The spores of *B. pumilis* are used to test the efficiency of ionizing radiation methods of sterilization.

The spores of *B. stearothermophilus* have been used extensively for testing the efficiency of autoclaves. The bacilli are thermophilic and grow between 55° to 60°C; the spores are highly heat resistant and are killed only if heated at 121°C in an autoclave for at least 12 minutes. *B. polymyxa* is important as a source of the antibiotic polymyxin or aerosporin.

REFERENCES

BRACHMAN, P. S., PLOTKIN, S. A., BUMFORD, F. H. & ATCHISON, M. M. (1960) An epidemic of inhalation anthrax: The first in the twentieth century. II. Epidemiology. *American Journal of Hygiene*, **72**, 6.

DARLOW, H. M., BELTON, F. C. & HENDERSON, D. W. (1956) The use of anthrax antigen to immunize man and monkey. *Lancet*, **ii**, 476.

GREEN, D. M. & JAMIESON, W. M. (1958) Anthrax and bonemeal fertilizer. *Lancet*, **ii**, 153.

JAMIESON, W. M. & GREEN, D. M. (1955) Anthrax and bonemeal fertilizer. *Lancet*, **i**, 560.

MILLER, J. K. (1961) Human anthrax in New York State. *New York State Journal of Medicine*, **61**, 2046.

H.M.S.O. REPORT (1959) *Report of the Committee of Inquiry on Anthrax*, Cmnd. 846. London: H.M.S.O.

SEMPLE, A. B. & HOBDAY, T. L. (1959) Control of anthrax. *Lancet*, **ii**, 507.

SMITH, H. (1960) Studies on organisms grown *in vivo* to reveal the bases of microbial pathogenicity. *Annals of the New York Academy of Science*, **88**, 1213.

SMITH, H. & STONER, H. B. (1967) Anthrax toxin complex. *Federation Proceedings*, **26**, 1554.

STANLEY, J. L. & SMITH, H. (1961) Purification of Factor I and recognition of a third factor of the anthrax toxin. *Journal of General Microbiology*, **26**, 49.

WILSON, G. S. & MILES, A. A. (1964) *Principles of Bacteriology and Immunity*, 5th Edn. London: Edward Arnold, Ltd.

ZANEV, N., BARDAROV, S. & TOMOV, A. (1968) Uber die wirkung von Extrakten menschlicher organe auf die kapsel des milzbrandbazillus. *Zeitschrift für Bakteriologie*, **207**, 466.

33. Brucella Brucellosis

The genus *Brucella* consists of a group of Gram-negative bacilli that are essentially pathogens of animals, mainly the domestic animals, goats, cattle, sheep and pigs. Infection in pregnant animals, particularly cows, leads to abortion and involvement of the mammary glands may cause the brucella organisms to be excreted in the milk for many months or even years. Human infections arise through contact with infected animals or their discharges, through the handling of infected carcases or through consumption of infected milk or milk products. Brucellosis is a typical zoonosis and infection does not spread from man to man. The infection may remain latent or subclinical or it may give rise to a variety of symptoms of varying intensity. Fever, chills, sweating, malaise, weakness and various aches and pains predominate. Acute brucellosis in its more severe form sometimes causes the characteristic intermittent waves or undulations of temperature that gave the name 'undulant fever' to describe the human disease, a term that can be misleading, since many brucella infections do not manifest this symptom.

DESCRIPTION

Brucella organisms are Gram-negative bacilli that are mostly so short as to appear more like cocci (coccobacilli) about 0·4 μm in diameter. Some more definite bacillary forms may also be observed. They occur singly and in groups and are non-motile, non-capsulate and non-sporing.

Brucellae are aerobic. However, *Br. abortus* when first cultured is unable to grow without the addition of 5 to 10 per cent carbon dioxide to the atmosphere. All strains grow best in a medium enriched with animal serum and glucose. Their optimum temperature is 37°C. The colonies take several days to appear and are normally smooth, moist, transparent and glistening, about 1 mm in diameter.

Brucella organisms may survive in the soil and in manure for many weeks and remain viable in dried foetal material for even longer periods. They have been isolated from butter, cheese and ice-cream prepared from infected milk (fresh goats' milk cheese is a potent source of *Br. melitensis* infection). The organisms may survive in carcase meat, pork and ham and may remain viable after refrigeration for several weeks and after pickling. They are killed in 10 minutes by a temperature of 60°C and infected milk is rendered safe by pasteurization. The brucellae are very sensitive to direct sunlight, and moderately sensitive to acid so that they tend to die out in sour milk and in cheese that has undergone lactic acid fermentation for some time; they are likely to be destroyed by the acid secretions of the stomach.

CLASSIFICATION

There are three main species of *Brucella* that differ in their choice of animal host, in certain cultural and biological characteristics and in the amount of the two main antigens that are common to all three species. They are *Brucella melitensis* which infects goats and sheep, *Br. abortus* which infects cattle and *Br. suis* which infects pigs. The host-parasite relationship is not absolutely specific and both man and domestic animals are susceptible to all three species. Within the species, strains that differ in some respects from the normal prototypes occur and are considered to be biotypes. There are at least nine biotypes of *Br. abortus*, three of *Br. melitensis* and four of *Br. suis*.

A number of other *Brucella* species have been named although some authorities prefer to regard them as biotypes of one or other of the main species. They are *Br. ovis* which is mainly responsible for a testicular infection of rams in various parts of the world including Australia and New Zealand; *Br. rangiferi tarandi* that has been isolated from reindeer (*Rangifer tarandi*) in the U.S.S.R. and from caribou (*Rangifer arcticus*) in Canada and Alaska where it is responsible for outbreaks of human brucellosis among Eskimos, presumably through their contact with the animals that constitute their main source of meat; *Br. canis*, a strain found to be the cause of a number of outbreaks of canine abortion among beagles in breeding kennels in the U.S.A. Other breeds of dog appear to be resistant but cases of human brucellosis have occurred among laboratory workers handling cultures of this strain; and *Br. neotomae*, a rodent strain isolated from the desert wood rat in Utah, U.S.A.

Differential Tests for Brucella Species

The three main species of *Brucella* differ in certain characteristics that form the basis of their conventional classification. These are (1) the need for added carbon dioxide for growth; (2) the amount of hydrogen sulphide produced during growth; (3) sensitivity to the dyes, basic fuchsin and thionin; (4) urease activity; and (5) agglutination by monospecific antisera (see Table 33.1). Techniques for these differentiating tests are fully described in Vol. II, Chap. 35.

IDENTIFICATION OF BIOTYPES. Brucellae having the biochemical characteristics of one species and the serological characteristics of another frequently occur and are regarded as biotypes of one or other of the three main species. They are identified by certain oxidative metabolic tests—and by their susceptibility to phage.

Variation

Whilst typical virulent brucellae of the three main species yield colonies that are smooth and transparent, their growth on laboratory media results in mutation to a rough type of colony formation with a corresponding loss in virulence. Mucoid variants may also appear. The organisms also change antigenically, losing their somatic (O) antigen and are no longer readily agglutinated by homologous sera. It has been suggested that the susceptibility or resistance of an individual may be determined by the presence or absence of a factor in his serum which suppresses the rough variants, thus favouring the multiplication of the more virulent smooth types. Resistant individuals do not have this factor and the smooth to rough (avirulent) mutation readily occurs. The two species, *Br. ovis* the cause of sheep disease and *Br. canis* isolated from beagles, only occur in the rough form and have no relationship with smooth forms of any of the three main *Brucella* species.

PATHOGENESIS

Each of the three main species is pathogenic to man. The incubation period is variable, usually about 10 to 30 days, but sometimes symptoms are delayed for several months. The organisms enter the body through abraded skin surfaces, through the mucous membranes of the alimentary and respiratory tracts and sometimes through the conjunctiva, and reach the bloodstream by way of the regional lymphatics. The

Table 33.1. Some differentiating biological and biochemical characters of the three main brucellae

	CO_2 requirement	H_2S production (days)					Basic fuchsin 1:25 000	Thionin 1:50 000	Methyl violet 1:50 000	Urease activity demonstrable within (minutes)	Abortus	Melitensis
		1	2	3	4	5						
Br. melitensis	−	− (or slight)					+	+	+	variable	−	+
Br. abortus	+	+	+	+	−	−	+	−	+	120 or more	+	−
Br. suis (American strains)	−	++	++	++	+	+	−	+	−	15–30	+	−
Danish strains of *Br. suis* are similar to the American strains but do not produce H_2S											+	−

Growth in presence of — spanning Basic fuchsin, Thionin, Methyl violet columns; Serological — spanning Monospecific serum Abortus Melitensis.

infection may persist for some time without causing any clinical manifestations, or it may give rise to classical undulant fever although this syndrome occurs more frequently with *Br. melitensis* than with *Br. suis* and *Br. abortus* infections. Infection by all three species, however, may give rise to a variety of symptoms and, without the fluctuating temperature to act as a guide line, clinical diagnosis may be difficult. The organisms subsequently localize in various parts of the reticulo-endothelial system, liver, spleen, bone, etc. with the formation of granulomatous lesions resulting in a variety of complications that may involve any part of the body. Surviving organisms within these granulomata may cause relapses of the acute disease or a chronic hypersensitive condition may develop associated with a long continued illness with vague symptoms of malaise, low-grade fever, lassitude, insomnia, irritability and swelling of joints. This type of chronic brucellosis may follow an acute attack or develop insidiously over a number of years without previous acute manifestations.

LABORATORY DIAGNOSIS

Blood cultures should be carried out repeatedly on all clinically suspected patients but are not likely to be positive in more than 30 to 50 per cent of cases. *Br. melitensis* and *Br. suis* are more readily isolated from the blood than is *Br. abortus*. It is not necessary to limit the tests to the febrile phase and at least 10 ml of blood should be withdrawn as the organisms may be relatively scanty. Blood cultures should be carried out in duplicate in glucose-serum broth, one of each pair being incubated in 10 per cent carbon dioxide. Subcultures on to solid media are made every few days and characteristic colonies looked for. The blood cultures should be retained for as long as six weeks before they are discarded as negative. *Br. melitensis* may sometimes be isolated from the urine.

Serological Tests

A positive agglutination reaction may be detected 7 to 10 days after onset of clinical infection.

In the acute stage of the disease the serum agglutinating antibodies increase to give titres of well over 1 000 before beginning to fall again. Since prozones may occur in the agglutination test with high-titre sera, it is advisable to make a range of serum dilutions sufficiently high (e.g. to over 1 000) in order to avoid false-negative readings. Both agglutinating and complement-fixing antibodies are present in the acute stage, the former being mainly associated with the high molecular weight immunoglobulin fraction of the serum (IgM) and the latter with the low molecular weight (IgG) immunoglobulin.

As the disease progresses from the acute to the chronic form and the organisms become localized intracellularly in various parts of the body, the IgM antibodies decrease, so that the agglutination titre falls to a low level and may finally be absent even when the patient is still ill. The absence of agglutination therefore does not rule out the possibility of infection. As long as infection continues, IgG antibodies are present in the serum and these may be detected by complement-fixation tests (Kerr *et al.*, 1966).

Another method of detecting non-agglutinating (IgG) brucella antibodies is by using an anti-human globulin serum as in the Coombs test (Wilson and Merrifield, 1951). This results in the agglutination of the brucella suspension already sensitized by the non-agglutinating antibodies in the patient's serum.

It should be noted that because of previous inapparent or latent infections the sera from a proportion (about 1 to 2 per cent) of the normal population agglutinate brucellae in low dilutions. The percentage is higher in rural than in urban communities. In latent or chronic infection the complement-fixation test is likely to be positive whereas in past infection it is negative. Agglutinins for brucella organisms may be present in the serum of persons who have been immunized against cholera and of those who have antibodies to *Francisella tularensis*. After recovery from brucellosis the complement-fixing antibody level falls slowly sometimes taking many months to reach low levels.

Reference to the table on page 353 may help in interpreting the results of the three main diagnostic tests.

The brucellin skin test, giving a delayed hypersensitivity reaction like tuberculin, is sometimes used in the diagnosis of brucellosis but its

Table 32.2

Type of brucellosis	Agglutination test	Complement-fixation test	Anti-human globulin test
Acute	positive	positive	. . .
Chronic	weak or negative	positive	positive
Past infection	weak or negative	negative	weak or negative

interpretation is difficult because in communities frequently exposed to infection, e.g. in farming areas, there may be a high incidence of positive skin reactions as a result of latent infection (P.H.L.S. Report, 1972).

CHEMOTHERAPY

Brucella infections respond to a combination of streptomycin and tetracycline. Intensive treatment in the acute stage of the disease is advisable to prevent the infection from progressing to the chronic form which is less likely to respond to treatment. The effectiveness of therapy should be checked by testing a series of serum specimens for antibody titre during and after the course of treatment.

EPIDEMIOLOGY

Br. melitensis infections were the first to be studied. They still persist in Southern France and other Mediterranean countries where the disease is sometimes called Mediterranean fever or Malta fever. The causative organism was first isolated in 1886 from the spleens of fatal cases by David Bruce, an army doctor serving with the British army stationed on the island of Malta. He described it as a coccus. At that time the disease had a high incidence among the army and navy personnel and also among the island's civilian population. The name 'Brucella' was subsequently given in honour of Bruce who established it as the cause of Mediterranean fever by transmitting the infection to monkeys. Twenty years later Zammit, a Maltese bacteriologist, showed that the organism was carried by goats and was being transmitted to man in goats' milk. After Zammit's discovery, the Mediterranean Fever Commission, a body formed to study the problem as it affected the British service men, recommended the prohibition of goats' milk and goats' milk products; when this restriction was put into effect there followed a spectacular fall in the number of cases among the services personnel from 916 cases with 23 deaths in 1905 to 21 cases with 1 death in 1907, whereas among the civilian population, who continued to drink goats' milk, the corresponding figures were 663 cases with 88 deaths in 1905 and 714 cases with 78 deaths in 1907.

Br. abortus infects cattle in many parts of the world. The disease occurs mainly in farming communities and tends to be an occupational disease affecting farmers and veterinary surgeons. In Great Britain *Br. abortus* is the only species responsible for human brucellosis. Five of the nine biotypes of *Br. abortus*, viz. biotypes 1, 2, 3, 4 and 9 have been isolated from dairy herds in various parts of the country. In spite of widespread vaccination of cattle, which has reduced the incidence of bovine abortion, the infection still remains endemic in cattle and milk is still a major source of human infection. A milk ring test (MRT) to detect the presence of brucella agglutinins is used as a screening test for infection in dairy cattle (Hamilton and Hardy, 1950). Although the organism is present in a high proportion of samples of unpasteurized market milk, the incidence of overt cases of human brucellosis due to the consumption of milk is relatively low; but antibodies indicating subclinical or unrecognized infection are present in about 30 per cent of the population in rural areas in some parts of the country. Surveys have shown that dairy farmers and veterinary surgeons who come into close contact with infected cattle are at greater risk of acquiring infection than their wives and families, even though they all drink raw milk. A history of close contact with cattle in a patient with a chronic febrile illness of uncertain diagnosis (PUO) should raise a suspicion of brucellosis.

However, it should be borne in mind that persons who are no longer infected but who are repeatedly exposed to infection may maintain high IgG levels in their sera due to secondary stimulation of that antibody (McDevitt, 1970; Coghlan and Longmore, 1973).

Human brucellosis due to *Br. suis* is almost entirely an occupational disease arising from contact with infected pigs or pig meat. It has been reported mainly from the U.S.A. where it accounts for more than 50 per cent of the human cases of brucellosis and occurs mainly among meat packers, especially those who handle raw meat shortly after slaughter.

There is evidence that in some European countries hares and other rodents act as reservoirs of *Br. suis* infection of livestock. Dogs may sometimes spread brucella infection in herds of sheep and cattle by transporting infected foetal material derived from aborted animals from one area to another.

Horses are susceptible to the three species of *Brucella* and human infections have been derived either from the consumption of mares' milk or through contact with horses suffering from suppurative lesions of brucella origin.

PREVENTION AND CONTROL

Vaccination

Vaccination of cattle between six and eight months of age protects them from abortion due to invasion of the uterus during the first and subsequent pregnancies. However, protection against infection is not fully achieved.

A living attenuated strain of *Br. abortus*, similar to the one used to immunize cattle, has been used in certain parts of the world to protect workers who are at a high occupational risk and is said to be effective. However, because of undesirable side-effects and the possibility that hypersensitivity to brucella protein may develop, vaccination of man is not recommended (W.H.O., 1964).

Pasteurization

Pasteurization of milk eliminates the risk of brucella infection arising as a result of the consumption of infected milk or milk products. However there remains the possibility of infection due to contact with infected cattle or their tissues so that veterinarians and farmers are particularly at risk.

Eradication of Brucellosis

Prevention of brucellosis in man and domestic animals depends on the eradication of the infection from animals by a policy of testing the animals and slaughtering positive reactors. Some countries have already eradicated brucella infection from cattle. The State-Federal Brucellosis Eradication Programme of the U.S.A. has resulted in the herds of nineteen States being 'Certified Brucellosis-free', and all except four States have 'Modified Certified Brucellosis' status. This achievement has resulted in a spectacular fall in the incidence of human brucellosis, from 6 321 cases (4·4 cases per 100 000 population) in 1947 to 231 (0·11 per 100 000 population) in 1969. In 1969, 70 per cent of the human cases reported in the U.S.A. were in persons working in meat processing plants and the majority were due to *Br. suis*, derived from infected pigs. A similar eradication scheme for the control of brucellosis of swine is now under way in Britain. In Northern Ireland a scheme for the eradication of brucellosis in cattle, begun in 1959, was made compulsory in 1963, and over 90 per cent of herds are now free of the infection. A similar scheme for the rest of Britain has been introduced; compulsory eradication of brucellosis in cattle in certain selected areas has begun, and some areas have already been declared free of infection.

REFERENCES AND FURTHER READING

COGHLAN, J. D. & LONGMORE, H. J. A. (1973) The significance of brucella antibodies in a rural area of South West Scotland. *The Practitioner*. (In press.)

HAMILTON, A. V. & HARDY, A. V. (1950) The brucella ring test. Its potential value in the control of brucellosis. *American Journal of Public Health*, **40**, 321.

KERR, W. R., COGHLAN, J. D., PAYNE, D. J. H. & ROBERTSON, L. (1966) The laboratory diagnosis of chronic brucellosis. *Lancet*, **ii**, 1181.

McDEVITT, D. G. (1970) The relevance of the anti-human globulin (Coombs) test and the complement-fixation test in the diagnosis of brucellosis. *Journal of Hygiene, Cambridge*, **68**, 173.

P.H.L.S. REPORT (1972) Appraisal of the Brucellin skin test.

Report of a working party on brucellosis. *Lancet*, **i**, 676.

SPINK, W. W. (1956) *The Nature of Brucellosis*. University of Minnesota Press.

WILSON, M. M. & MERRIFIELD, E. V. O. (1951) The anti-globulin (Coombs) test in brucellosis. *Lancet*, **ii**, 913.

WORLD HEALTH ORGANIZATION (1964) Expert committee on brucellosis. *World Health Organization Technical Report Series*, no. 289.

34. Yersinia: Pasteurella: Francisella
(Pasteurella Group) Plague: Mesenteric Adenitis: Tularaemia

The Pasteurella group consists of a number of small, Gram-negative bacilli with similar characteristic morphological and cultural features. These organisms are essentially animal parasites that under certain conditions are transmitted to man, sometimes directly and sometimes through intermediary insect vectors, viz: certain species of fleas and ticks. The pasteurella infections are, therefore, zoonoses. Each species of Pasteurella gives rise to its own particular disease manifestations. The four species implicated in human infections are commonly known as *Pasteurella pestis, P. pseudotuberculosis, P. multocida* (sometimes called *P. septica*) and *P. tularensis*. However, as a result of improved knowledge, the group has recently been classified into three separate genera, viz: *Yersinia* (*pestis, pseudotuberculosis* and *enterocolitica*), *Pasteurella* (*multocida*) and *Francisella* (*tularensis*) (Mair, 1969).

The most notable of the pasteurella organisms is *Y. pestis*, the cause of plague in rats and man. *Y. pseudotuberculosis* is a parasite of guinea-pigs and other rodents, causing a fatal disease in those animals and sometimes, though rarely, a severe, typhoid-like illness in persons who come into contact with infected animals. It is also one of the causes of acute mesenteric lymphadenitis in children and of erythema nodosum sometimes associated with this disease. *P. multocida* is responsible for 'haemorrhagic septicaemia' in a wide range of animals and birds. It has been known as an important cause of animal disease since the time of Louis Pasteur who isolated it from chickens suffering from 'fowl cholera' and used it to develop an effective attenuated vaccine. But only in recent years has it been recognized as causing various forms of infection in man, in particular, superficial and deep-seated septic infections following dog and cat bites. *F. tularensis* is the cause of tularaemia, a plague-like illness of squirrels and other rodents in North America and some European countries including Scandinavia. The infection is transmitted directly from animal to animal or from animal to man but may also be spread by ticks, or through polluted drinking water. Human tularaemia manifests itself as a prolonged febrile illness sometimes with local ulcerative lesions and glandular involvement. Laboratory infection is readily acquired.

YERSINIA PESTIS
(*Past. pestis*)

DESCRIPTION

Yersinia pestis is a small ovoid Gram-negative bacillus, 1·5 μm by 0·7 μm, showing pleomorphism, i.e. extreme variation in size and shape, under certain conditions of culture. True capsules are formed in living tissues but are less readily seen in culture. When stained with methylene blue the stain is taken up more densely at both ends—bipolar staining. The organisms are non-motile and non-sporing. Growth occurs aerobically and anaerobically but *Y. pestis* is somewhat sensitive to oxygen and small inocula may not grow readily on ordinary culture media incubated aerobically. The optimum temperature for growth is 27°C which is unusual for parasitic organisms. Unlike the other members of the genus, *Y. pestis* grows poorly at 37°C.

The plague bacillus is essentially a parasite of rodents. In certain parts of the world burrowing animals such as gerbilles and voles act as chronic carriers and provide a continuing reservoir of infection that may be transmitted by fleas to more susceptible animals of the same species and to other species of rodent such as bandicoots, marmots and squirrels. These animals suffer from outbreaks of plague, and fleas from them may attack man and give rise to sporadic cases of human plague. This form of plague in man occurs in rural areas as a result of endemic infection in wild rodents and is referred to as 'wild plague' (previously known as sylvatic plague). It tends to affect such persons as farmers and trappers who are likely to come into contact with infected animals. More serious for man is the spread of infection to rats especially the species of black rat known as *Rattus rattus* that flourishes in and around human habitation. This constitutes the most important source of infection for man and outbreaks of human plague following epizootics in rats (domestic plague) have in the past sometimes developed into pandemics.

History of Plague

Human plague was introduced into Europe from Asia in the 13th century when infected black rats with their flea colonies spread westwards by land and sea with the returning crusaders. This led to the great pandemic known as the Black Death. During the years 1347 to 1348 about a quarter of the population of Europe succumbed to the plague. For two centuries after this pandemic had subsided the infection remained enzootic in

the rats in Europe and continued to give rise to outbreaks of human plague until in 1665 there occurred the last major epidemic in England, the Great Plague. Plague disappeared spectacularly from Europe during the 17th and 18th centuries. This may have been due to the natural spread of the brown (sewer) rat (*Rattus norvegicus*) from Asia into Europe so that it largely displaced the black rat except around the sea ports where shipping continued to re-introduce the black rat from abroad. *R. norvegicus*, although highly susceptible to plague does not frequent human dwellings to the same extent as *R. rattus* and its fleas are therefore less likely to attack man directly. Improvements in standards of housebuilding, leading to the more general exclusion of rats from homes, may also have played an important part in the elimination of plague from Europe. The decline in the incidence of human plague was interrupted by a major outbreak in Hong Kong in 1894, that led to a new pandemic, the main centres of the disease being North and West India where, during 1904, over one million persons are known to have died of plague. Plague-infected rats were carried by

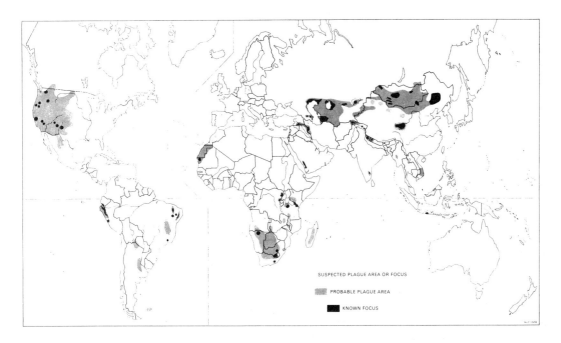

SUSPECTED PLAGUE AREA OR FOCUS

PROBABLE PLAGUE AREA

KNOWN FOCUS

Fig. 34.1. Known and probable foci and areas of plague, 1969.

ships to most of the major sea ports of the world whence they subsequently spread the infection to the indigenous rodent population of the countries concerned.

The plague bacillus was first described in 1894 by Yersin at the time of the Hong Kong outbreak. During the following years of the pandemic a great deal of experimental and investigational work was carried out by a number of Governmental Plague Commissions including the British Plague Commission that investigated the Bombay outbreak. These studies resulted in a much greater understanding of the nature of the disease, the mode of spread and ways in which it may be controlled.

In recent years urban plague has become a rarity and rural bubonic plague is limited to sporadic outbreaks in endemic areas. However, as long as plague exists in rodents in many areas of the world a constant surveillance has to be maintained to prevent its spread to more populated areas especially those where living conditions are still below standard and where rats and their ectoparasites can flourish. The incidence of plague in endemic areas such as India was greatly reduced following the widespread use of DDT in the control of malaria.

PATHOGENESIS OF HUMAN PLAGUE

The virulence of the plague bacillus is related to certain factors that protect it from phagocytosis, the main one being the capsular (envelope) antigen. Two somatic antigens V and W when present also play a part in enabling the organism to resist phagocytosis in the absence of a visible capsule (Burrows and Bacon, 1956). Aggressive factors that enhance spreading and increase capillary permeability have been demonstrated in extracts of tissues of experimentally infected animals. No exotoxin has been identified but suspensions of dead plague bacilli and extracts of them produce local necrotic lesions and general toxaemia when inoculated into laboratory animals. This protein endotoxin appears to act on the peripheral vascular system and causes injury to the liver and kidneys.

There are two severe forms of human plague,

viz. bubonic plague and pneumonic plague. In *bubonic plague* the lymph nodes draining the area of the flea bite become infected. The adenitis results in painful swellings or buboes in the inguinal, axillary or cervical regions depending on the site of the bite. From these primary buboes the plague bacilli may spread through the body. In the absence of antibiotic therapy there is a case fatality of 25 to 50 per cent. Occasionally it is no more than a localized infection (pestis minor).

In *pneumonic plague* there is a severe haemorrhagic bronchopneumonia, the sputum contains numerous plague bacilli, septicaemia develops and in the absence of antibiotic therapy the outcome is invariably fatal. *Septicaemic plague* may also occur primarily as well as a complication of bubonic or pneumonic plague.

LABORATORY DIAGNOSIS

Plague is confirmed by demonstrating the plague bacillus in fluid from buboes in the case of bubonic plague, in the sputum in pneumonic plague and by blood culture when generalized infection is suspected.

The bubo is punctured with a hypodermic syringe and some of the exudate withdrawn. A film is made and stained with methylene blue. The characteristic bacilli showing bipolar staining can be confirmed as *Y. pestis* by culturing some of the exudate on blood agar to obtain a pure culture for further investigation, and by inoculating the material on to the nasal mucosa of guinea-pigs or white rats.

Similarly in pneumonic plague sputum is examined microscopically, culturally and by animal inoculation. In septicaemic plague the bacilli may be demonstrated in blood culture or from smears of spleen tissue at *post mortem* examination. Identification of characteristic colonies is made by various cultural and biochemical tests and by demonstrating the ability of the bacilli to form chains in broth culture and 'stalactite' growth from oil drops layered on the surface of fluid medium.

Chemotherapy should be started without waiting for confirmation of the diagnosis. Tetracycline in large doses is the drug of choice for both bubonic and pneumonic plague (W.H.O. Report, 1970).

Epidemiology of Bubonic Plague

Bubonic plague is a zoonosis. The plague bacilli are transmitted from animal to animal and from animal to man by fleas, notably *Xenopsylla cheopis*, one of the ectoparasites of rats. It has been shown experimentally that fleas, lice or ticks are essential for the spread of infection among rodents. Transmission from rats to man is dependent on fleas. In cool humid weather fleas multiply and plague spreads readily among susceptible rats. Hot, dry weather, on the other hand, tends to limit spread of the infection. Its ability to spread rapidly and exponentially in a population of rats depends on the animals having a high *flea index*, or mean number of fleas per rat (e.g. index of 2 or more), since an infected rat is unlikely to pass on the infection to a larger number of other rats than the number of its fleas.

In the sick animal, an intense septicaemia develops and when a flea feeds on the blood of such an animal, plague bacilli are sucked into the midgut where they multiply to such an extent that they block the proventriculus. On the death of the animal the flea seeks an alternative host which may be another rodent or man. Because the 'blocked' flea is unable to suck readily, some of the infected blood of the previous host is regurgitated and injected into the bite wound of the new victim. 'Unblocked' infected fleas may also pass on infection, but less readily than 'blocked' ones. When the weather changes to hot, dry conditions, the fleas tend to die. This may happen at the time when the epizootic among the rats has reached a stage where the number of susceptible animals has greatly decreased through death or developing immunity. Those two factors contribute to the termination of the rat epizootic and thus, also of the human epidemic. The renewal of an epizootic and epidemic in the following or later years depends on the growth of a fresh population of young susceptible rats and their heavy infestation with fleas. The infection may be introduced into this fresh population from an old, surviving 'carrier' rat with intermittent bacteriaemia or from infected wild rodents.

Epidemiology of Pneumonic Plague

In some patients contracting bubonic plague from a rat or sylvatic rodent (e.g. tarbagan in Eastern Siberia) the bacteriaemia may lead to infection of the lungs and the development of severe bronchopneumonia. The sputum from these pneumonic patients contains plague bacilli and under certain circumstances the infection may spread epidemically, from man to man, by the respiratory route. Epidemics of pneumonic plague have occurred particularly in colder regions such as North China where conditions have been favourable to airborne transmission of infection within dwelling houses. Whether the bacilli are transmitted in respiratory droplet-nuclei or sputum-dust is unknown.

Control Measures

Plague prevention consists essentially in measures to control both wild and domestic rodent population in towns and villages. The construction of dwelling houses to a standard that facilitates the exclusion of rats from them is of primary importance. Rat-proofing of buildings especially warehouses in dock areas, the fumigation of ships or the building of ships in which rats can no longer establish themselves have succeeded in preventing the spread of plague from one country to another. Periodic surveys in areas where wild plague is endemic are advocated to determine the prevalence of rodents and fleas and the degree of infection among wild and domestic rodent hosts in order that, where necessary, control measures can be put into effect. When an epidemic is in progress, control is most quickly achieved by the eradication of fleas from the rats by the liberal application of insecticide to rat runs.

Vaccination

Y. pestis contains many antigens, somatic, heat-stable antigens and a heat-labile capsular antigen. The effectiveness of plague vaccine is not well established but is thought to depend to a large extent on the presence of the capsular protein. Both live vaccine, prepared from avirulent strains of *Y. pestis* and vaccine from inactivated virulent cultures are available but immunity resulting from their use is of short duration and revaccination is necessary after some months.

YERSINIA PSEUDOTUBERCULOSIS
(*P. pseudotuberculosis*)

Description

This is a small, ovoid Gram-negative bacillus which is slightly acid-fast. It is closely related to *Y. pestis* but differs from it in being motile. Motility, however, is observed only in cultures grown at ambient temperature (22°C). It may also be differentiated from *Y. pestis* by its ability to produce a rapid colour change in urea medium due to the production of urease. These differential tests are important when the organisms are isolated from rats that may be infected with plague bacilli; unlike other members of the pasteurella group, both *Y. pseudotuberculosis* and *Y. pestis* are capable of growing on MacConkey's medium.

ANTIGENIC CHARACTERS. There are five serological types of *Y. pseudotuberculosis* (types 1 to 5) based on type-specific, thermostable, somatic antigens and thermolabile flagellar antigens. There are also a number of sub-types. A group somatic antigen is shared by all five types and also by *Y. pestis*. There is an antigenic relationship between type 2 and group B salmonellae and between type 4 and salmonellae of groups D and H. Identification of a particular strain of *Y. pseudotuberculosis* is determined by slide agglutination tests using single-factor O-agglutinating antisera prepared in rabbits (Mair *et al.*, 1960).

Pathogenicity

In guinea-pigs infection by *Y. pseudotuberculosis* causes a disease characterized by multiple nodules rather like those of tuberculosis in the liver, spleen and lungs. Human infections have, on rare occasions, resulted in a severe typhoid-like illness with fever, purpura and enlargement of the liver and spleen which is usually fatal. A more frequent result of human infection, however, is mesenteric lymphadenitis simulating acute or subacute appendicitis that affects mainly male schoolchildren aged 5 to 15 years. It is also a cause of erythema nodosum.

Laboratory Diagnosis

Y. pseudotuberculosis infection is confirmed by isolating the organism from the blood or mesenteric glands, particularly the ileocaecal glands, or by demonstrating specific antibodies in the patient's serum either by slide or tube agglutination carried out during the acute phase of the illness. The agglutinins decline rapidly and reach a low level within 3 to 5 months.

TREATMENT. Little has been reported on the subject of treatment since most cases of mesenteric adenitis usually make an uneventful recovery. *In vitro* tests have shown that broad-spectrum antibiotics would be the drugs of choice, were these deemed necessary.

Epidemiology

It has not been possible to show a relationship between human infections and animal contact but the occurrence of the organism in epizootic form in guinea-pigs and turkeys and the sporadic outbreaks in many other animal and bird species suggest that human infections are derived from animal sources.

PASTEURELLA MULTOCIDA
(*P. septica*)

Strains of this organism have been generally named in the past according to the animal from which they were isolated (*P. boviseptica*, *P. oviseptica*, *P. aviseptica*, etc.) but they are now regarded as members of the same species, *P. multocida*, that differ in their parasitic adaptations to particular hosts.

Description

Like the other members of the pasteurella group they are small, oval, Gram-negative bacilli that exhibit bipolar staining when treated with methylene blue. They are capsulate and nonmotile; they grow under aerobic and anaerobic conditions on blood agar but do not grow on MacConkey's medium.

Table 34.1. To show differentiating characters among the main pathogens in the pasteurella group

Species	Growth on bile salt medium	Motility at 18–22°C	Motility at 37°C	Acid from maltose	Indole production	Urease activity
Y. pestis	+	–	–	+	–	–
Y. pseudotuberculosis	+	+	–	+	–	+
P. multocida	–	–	–	–	+	–
Y. enterocolitica	+	+	–	+ (late)	–	+

ANTIGENIC CHARACTERS. Attempts to group strains from different sources on the basis of their antigenicity have proved unreliable, probably due to antigenic variation that occurs readily with this species. Four groups have been defined but not all strains conform to the grouping and there is no relationship between serological group and animal source.

Pathogenicity

Pasteurella multocida is extremely virulent to many species of birds and animals causing haemorrhagic septicaemia which is usually fatal. However, the organisms may be carried by apparently normal cattle, sheep, swine, dogs, cats and rats. Reports of human pasteurella infections are comparatively rare. Just as normal animals may act as carriers, the organisms may sometimes be present as commensals in the respiratory tract and nasal sinuses of persons associated with animals. Clinical manifestations in man usually take one of three forms (1) a local abscess following an animal bite with cellulitis, adenitis, abscess formation and sometimes osteomyelitis; (2) meningitis following head injury; (3) infections of the respiratory system such as pleurisy, pneumonia, empyema, bronchitis, bronchiectasis and nasal sinusitis in which, although not always the direct cause, *P. multocida* probably contributes to the course, severity and duration of the illness. Cases of appendicitis from which *P. multocida* was isolated in pure culture from the pus have also been reported. It appears that the organism becomes pathogenic to man only after trauma resulting from animal bites, operation, cranial fracture, and the like.

Laboratory Diagnosis

Identification is confirmed by isolating the organism on blood agar from swabs of dog or cat bite wounds, from cerebrospinal fluid in cases of meningitis and from the infective secretions in suppurative conditions of the respiratory system, followed by certain cultural and biochemical tests (see Table 34.1).

Agglutinating antibodies against the infecting organism may be detected in the patient's serum.
TREATMENT. *P. multocida* is moderately sensitive *in vitro* to penicillin, sensitive to sulphonamides, tetracycline and to streptomycin. Therapy may have to be continued for up to 8 weeks in cases of osteomyelitis following animal bites.

Epidemiology

Infection following animal bites is a direct one, the organism passing directly to man in the animals' saliva. In those cases described under (2) and (3) above, the organisms, although no doubt derived from animals in the first place, may have existed as commensal in the upper respiratory passages until conditions were favourable to their spread and establishment at the site of infection.

FRANCISELLA TULARENSIS
(*P. tularensis*)

This organism is now classified in a separate genus, *Francisella*, and is called *Francisella tularensis*.

Like other members of the pasteurella group, this is a small Gram-negative, encapsulated, coccobacillus. It is 0·7 μm by 0·2 μm when first isolated but larger, up to 1·5 μm long, when in culture. It has a marked tendency to pleomorphism in artificial culture. *F. tularensis* cannot be cultured on ordinary media but requires the addition to fluid media of pure egg yolk or pieces of sterile rabbit spleen or of cysteine and glucose to human blood agar.

Pathogenicity

F. tularensis produces a disease (tularaemia) in wild rodents with lesions reminiscent of those found in plague-infected animals. The organisms are found in large numbers within the cells of the liver and spleen, suggesting that it may multiply as an intracellular parasite. Infection in man may result in a prolonged febrile illness (typhoidal) with glandular lesions and ulcers of the skin, but the clinical manifestations may be mild or influenzal, as described in water-borne outbreaks in Europe.

Laboratory Diagnosis

Human infections are usually diagnosed by inoculation of laboratory animals, e.g. guinea-pigs or mice, with exudates from the glands or ulcers (and isolation of *F. tularensis* from infected tissues, e.g. spleen, on glucose cysteine blood agar). The patient's serum should be tested for agglutinating antibodies. It should be noted that the serum of persons infected with *Brucella* species may agglutinate *F. tularensis*.

Epidemiology

The disease has a world wide distribution and has been reported from several European countries. The infection, which is a typical zoonosis and which is largely tick-borne among its natural hosts (lagomorphs and rodents) is transmitted to man during the handling of infected animals, e.g. rabbits and hares; or laboratory cultures (it is highly infective for laboratory workers). Tularaemia is sometimes water-borne as a result of pollution of water with the excreta of infected rodents such as water rats.

YERSINIA ENTEROCOLITICA

In the last few years a group of organisms resembling *Y. pseudotuberculosis* has been isolated from diarrhoeal and other diseases of man. This group has been named *Yersinia enterocolitica*. These organisms have also been isolated from a wide range of wild and domestic animals. Although no epidemiological connection has been established, it is likely that human infections are directly or indirectly derived from animal sources and may be contracted through the ingestion of contaminated food.

Like *Y. pseudotuberculosis*, for which it may have been mistaken in the past, *Yersinia enterocolitica* is motile when grown at 22°C, but the two species differ from one another in some biochemical respects. Although the pathogenicity of the organism has not been finally established, there is evidence to suggest a relationship between its presence and the symptoms of disease. It has been isolated from patients with acute terminal ileitis, mesenteric adenitis, appendicitis and erythema nodosum, as well as from those with mild and severe gastroenteritis. Human infections have been reported mainly from Sweden and Belgium where they have been most looked for, but also from other European countries including Britain and from other parts of the world, e.g. Central Africa; they are probably much more common and widespread than is presently realized.

REFERENCES

Burrows, T. W. & Bacon, S. A. (1956) The basis of virulence in *Pasteurella pestis*, an antigen determining virulence. *British Journal of Experimental Pathology*, **37**, 481.

Mair, N. S. (1969) The laboratory diagnosis of infections with *Pasteurella pseudotuberculosis*. In *Recent Advances in Clinical Pathology*, 4th Edn, Chap. 3.

Mair, N. S., Mair, H. J., Stirk, E. M. & Corson, J. G. (1960) Three cases of acute mesenteric lymphodentis due to *Pasteurella pseudotuberculosis*. *Journal of Clinical Pathology*, **13**, 432.

World Health Organization (1970) Expert committee on plague, 4th report. *World Health Organization Technical Report Series*, no. 447.

35. Bacteroides: Donovania: Streptobacillus

Suppurative Thrombophlebitis: Granuloma Venereum: Rat-bite Fever

Bacteroides Group

The Bacteroidaceae are a rather heterogeneous family of strictly anaerobic non-sporing Gram-negative bacteria that have been variously sub-classified, particularly on a morphological basis; some workers recognize at least three genera— *Bacteroides, Fusobacterium* and *Sphaerophorus*. As some spindle-shaped forms are produced by members not included in *Fusobacterium*, and as many members of the Bacteroidaceae are highly pleomorphic with rather variable biochemical activities in currently available tests, it seems advisable to avoid a detailed subdivision at present, but rather to refer to the *Bacteroides-Fusiformis* group as a whole, embraced by the label *Bacteroides*.

These organisms are extremely abundant as commensals in the lower intestinal tract of man where they may exceed 10^{10} viable bacteria per gram of gut content and greatly outnumber coliform organisms and enterococci there (Table 35.1). They also abound in the mouth and oro-pharynx and may be present in the lower genito-urinary tract in the female. In the ali-mentary tract they probably play an important role in excluding other invaders, partly by their production of butyric and acetic acids, but they are themselves potentially pathogenic; they appear to be held in check under normal conditions despite their very large numbers and they are not highly invasive. When various circumstances alter the host's local or general resistance, however, the *Bacteroides* group has much potential for harm and human infections with this group of organisms are commoner than is generally appreciated.

Clinical Infections

Although these infections may arise in the absence of an obvious predisposing cause, they are commonly associated with such precipitating factors as bowel surgery, neoplastic disease, diverticulitis, diabetes, gingivitis and dental conditions, immunosuppressive or cytotoxic therapy or steroid therapy, alcoholism, drug addiction and other debilitating states. The bacteria may simply contribute to a localized infection, but occasionally and typically they enter the bloodstream and cause more widespread trouble, sometimes localizing in a remote site such as the brain. After surgical operations, a local bacteroides infection may produce sloughing of the edges of the incision or there may be sinus formation. Localized bacteroides infections are often associated with a foul odour.

Occasionally, appendicitis or peritonitis may be caused by *Bacteroides spp*. Early involvement of regional veins is typical of bacteroides infections and septicaemia or pyaemia may follow a suppurative thrombophlebitis. Post-operatively, a bacteriogenic shock syndrome may be precipitated; this insidious complication can kill a patient if it is not quickly recognized and treated intensively. Bacteroides bacteriaemia may be the initial stage in such a condition, but an initially unsuspected bacteriaemia is sometimes

Table 35.1. The bacterial flora of faeces of English subjects[*]

Bacterial group	Mean $\log_{10}$ no. per g[**]
Bacteroides spp.	9·8
Bifidobacteria	9·8
Clostridia	c. 5·0
Veillonella spp.	4·2
Lactobacilli	6·5
Bacillus spp.	3·7
Enterobacteria	c. 7·9
Streptococcus spp.	7·1
Enterococci	5·8
Total anaerobes	10·1
Total aerobes	8·0

[*] From Hill *et al.* (1971).
[**] Mean $\log_{10}$ no. of viable organisms per gram of faeces.

associated with an infective endocarditis. Although this is not a common form of endocarditis, it calls for special treatment and must not be missed.

A large and important group of bacteroides infections occur following abortion and less frequently after normal childbirth in which the presenting sign is puerperal fever due to suppuration in the genital tract. The infection is often a mixed one with bacteroides organisms, anaerobic cocci and coliform bacteria, but it may be a pure bacteroides infection. Another important group of cases suffer from bacteroides empyema with or without lung abscess. Brain abscess caused by bacteroides, alone or in association with anaerobic cocci, is a difficult clinical challenge. The association of fusiform bacilli with borreliae in Vincent's infections of the oropharynx is well recognized (Chap. 38). Ulceration of the throat, sometimes after tonsillectomy, and purulent gingivitis after dental extractions, are also manifestations of the infection. Localized lesions in the skin and subcutaneous tissues may be found in workers who are obliged to handle infected animals. Bacteroides organisms can be isolated from specimens of urine, but their possible pathogenic role in the urinary tract is not yet defined.

Some strains of bacteroides organisms can be shown to deconjugate the bile acid conjugates secreted in bile; for example, sodium taurocholate is decomposed to cholic acid and taurine and the activity of the conjugate is lost. This is of note to clinicians interested in the possibility that the overgrowth of such strains at various points in the intestine may be related to malabsorption syndromes. It has also been postulated that intestinal bacteria may be able to produce carcinogens from dietary fats or from bile steroids and the bacteroides organisms are linked with this hypothesis (Hill et al., 1971).

DESCRIPTION OF SUB-GROUPS

The group can be sub-classified according to various morphological, cultural and biochemical characteristics. Rapid presumptive identification can be based on the results of tests of sensitivity to various antibiotics (Sutter and Finegold, 1971).

The bacteroides organisms that predominate in the human gut are exemplified by *B. fragilis*; they differ in their appearance and characteristics from those generally isolated from the mouth and exemplified by *B. necrophorus*. A third miscellaneous group contains organisms with special characteristics that distinguish them from the *fragilis-necrophorus* groups. This provisional classification is set out as follows:

1. *Bacteroides fragilis.* This is a delicate rod (2 to 3 μm by 0.4 to 0.8 μm) often showing irregular staining and moderate pleomorphism. It is a normal commensal of the gut and is the Gram-negative anaerobic bacterium most frequently isolated from clinical material. It is typically resistant to penicillin.

2. *Bacteroides necrophorus* is a fairly large and sometimes markedly pleomorphic organism. Characteristically, it is filamentous with a central bar that stains less deeply than the rest of the organism, but many other forms are seen ranging from elongated slender filaments to small Gram-negative bacilli. It is typically sensitive to penicillin. Synonyms are *Sphaerophorus necrophorus* or *Fusiformis necrophorus*.

3. Miscellaneous species include the following:

Bacteroides melaninogenicus typically produces a black pigment (colloidal ferrous sulphide) in cultures on blood agar. This is not an invariable or specific property as other *Bacteroides spp.* can do so if certain factors are provided (Tracy, 1969).

Bacteroides corrodens. Colonies of these strains characteristically produce pitting on nutrient agar or blood agar. The taxonomy of this fairly homogeneous group is debated as many of the strains are not strictly anaerobic (Hill, Snell and Lapage, 1970; Jackson et al., 1971).

The above sub-grouping will almost certainly require re-appraisal in view of current clinical interest in and experience with the Gram-negative anaerobes. There may be a good case for the retention of the genus *Fusobacterium* as it is at present difficult to include this unreservedly in the *necrophorus* group; one member merits particular mention:

Fusobacterium fusiforme (Fusiformis fusiformis) is a concomitant of *Borrelia vincentii* in Vincent's angina and in other necrotic inflammatory conditions such as gingivitis and stomatitis. Characteristically the organism is a large spindle-shaped or cigar-shaped bacillus and it often has a central area that stains less deeply.

Antibiotic Sensitivities of the Bacteroides Organisms

Although *B. necrophorus* is typically sensitive, most strains of *B. fragilis* are relatively resistant to the penicillins. There is evidence that an increasing number are becoming resistant to the tetracyclines, but they are generally sensitive to chloramphenicol.

Erythromycin and lincomycin are probably the drugs of choice in the treatment of bacteroides infections. The organisms are usually sensitive, but there are technical problems associated with sensitivity testing. Clinical results with 7-chloro-lincomycin have been particularly promising, though a bactericidal effect is not invariable. The group varies in its sensitivity to trimethoprim-sulphamethoxazole, but many strains are sensitive. They are often sensitive to fucidin. Metronidazole (Flagyl), a drug used until now primarily as an antiprotozoal agent, is markedly bactericidal to bacteroides organisms *in vitro*.

Bacteroides organisms are generally relatively resistant to the aminoglycosides and especially resistant to neomycin and to streptomycin. They are often resistant to vancomycin and they tend to develop resistance to rifampin.

DONOVANIA AND STREPTOBACILLUS

The systematic positions of the following two organisms are doubtful. Only in their pleomorphic character, their Gram-negative staining and their potential pathogenicity for man have they any features in common with the *Bacteroides* group. They are aerobes and have no known relationships to bacteroides organisms or to each other.

STREPTOBACILLUS MONILIFORMIS

This organism occurs as a normal inhabitant in the nasopharynx of wild and laboratory rats and is the cause of a spontaneous disease of mice characterized by multiple arthritis often involving the joints of the feet and leading to swellings of the feet and legs. It is also the cause of a proportion of cases of 'rat-bite fever' in man particularly in the Americas. Although the organism is usually introduced through a bite, this history cannot always be obtained. The infection seems sometimes to be acquired by the ingestion of contaminated food: for example a group of cases in U.S.A., characterized by fever, multiple arthritis and an erythematous eruption (Haverhill Fever), was shown to be associated with the organism which was swallowed in contaminated milk.

Description

The organism is an aerobic Gram-negative pleomorphic bacterium, occurring as short rod-shaped forms (1 to 3 μm by 0·3 to 0·4 μm) or as elongated filaments that are either undivided or consist of chained bacilli. They may show characteristic fusiform, oval or spherical enlargements sometimes projecting laterally from the filaments. The organism is non-capsulate and non-motile.

Growth can be obtained if there is a high proportion of blood, serum or ascitic fluid in the medium. Löffler's serum serves well for cultivation. The colonies are small (1 mm). Viability in culture is feeble and cultures die in 2 to 4 days. On solid media, after 2 to 3 days' incubation, raised granular colonies 1 to 5 mm in diameter develop. Adjacent to these, and best seen with the plate microscope, a variable number of minute colonies 0·1 to 0·2 mm in diameter may be seen; they grow into the depths of the medium and can only be transferred by excising a small portion of the agar. These small colonies breed true on subculture and constitute the 'L forms' or 'L phase' of the organism's growth; they consist mainly of very small coccoid or coccobacillary elements but larger and bizarre forms may be present.

'L' organisms are extremely resistant to penicillin, although the streptobacilli are very sensitive to this antibiotic. However, both forms have identical fermentative properties and one antigen is common to them. L forms lack an antigen present in the streptobacillus and they have little or no virulence for laboratory animals. It is now generally accepted that the L forms are variants of *Streptobacillus moniliformis* in which there is a defective mechanism of cell wall formation. It should be noted that L phase variation occurs spontaneously to a greater or lesser extent with all strains of *Streptobacillus moniliformis*. In other bacteria where L phase dissociation is recognized, abnormal cultural conditions are required to induce the production of L-type colonies.

Mice are susceptible to experimental inoculation and develop either a rapidly fatal generalized infection without focal lesions or a more slowly progressive disease with swelling of the feet and multiple inflammatory lesions of joints. LABORATORY DIAGNOSIS. The organism has been isolated by blood culture, and from joint fluid in patients with arthritis. In fluid culture, colonies of the organism take the form of 'fluff balls' situated on the surface of the sedimented blood cells.

It should be noted that another type of rat-bite fever (Soduku) is caused by *Spirillum minus* (see Chap. 30) and clinically may be indistinguishable from that caused by *Streptobacillus moniliformis*.

DONOVANIA GRANULOMATIS

This organism, whose biological relationships are still doubtful, is responsible for a chronic granulomatous disease ('granuloma venereum') observed in tropical and subtropical countries. The initial lesion is on the genitalia. In the mononuclear cells of the lesions the organism is seen as a small Gram-negative pleomorphic bacillus (1 to 2 μm in length). It may show polar staining and appears to be capsulate. Extracellular forms are also observed. The organism has proved difficult to cultivate on the usual bacteriological media, but cultures have been readily obtained in the yolk sac of the chick embryo; after adaptation, growth can be obtained on enriched artificial media. Laboratory animals are not susceptible to inoculation, but the disease has been reproduced in man by inoculating yolk sac cultures. The organism is not filterable. Sterilized cultures produce an allergic skin reaction in infected persons, and give a complement-fixation reaction with patient's serum. A capsular material has also been found to fix complement with sera from patients with the disease. The organism has morphological resemblances to *Klebsiella* and cross-reacts serologically with *Klebsiella rhinoscleromatis*.

It should be noted that this infection is quite different from lymphogranuloma inguinale with which it should not be confused (see Chap. 50).

REFERENCES

HILL, L. R., SNELL, J. J. S. & LAPAGE, S. P. (1970) Identification and characterisation of *Bacteroides corrodens*. *Journal of Medical Microbiology*, **3**, 483.

HILL, M. J., DRASAR, B. S., ARIES, V., CROWTHER, V. S., HAWKSWORTH, G. & WILLIAMS, R. E. O. (1971) Bacteria and aetiology of cancer of large bowel. *Lancet*, **i**, 95.

JACKSON, F. L., GOODMAN, Y. E., BELL, F. R., WONG, P. C. & WHITEHOUSE, R. L. S. (1971) Taxonomic status of facultative and strictly anaerobic 'corroding bacilli' that have been classified as *Bacteroides corrodens*. *Journal of Medical Microbiology*, **4**, 171.

SUTTER, V. L. & FINEGOLD, S. M. (1971) Antibiotic disc susceptibility tests for rapid presumptive identification of Gram-negative anaerobic bacilli. *Applied Microbiology*, **21**, 13.

TRACY, O. (1969) Pigment production in Bacteroides. *Journal of Medical Microbiology*, **2**, 309.

36. Clostridium: I: Cl. welchii and other Clostridia

Gas Gangrene: Food-poisoning

The genus *Clostridium* comprises the Gram positive spore-bearing anaerobic bacilli. Most species of this genus are saprophytes that normally grow in soil, water and decomposing plant and animal matter; they play an important part in the process of putrefaction. Some, e.g. *Clostridium welchii* and *Cl. sporogenes*, are commensal inhabitants of the animal and human intestine, and just before or immediately after the death of their host, rapidly invade the blood and tissues and play a major part, along with aerobic bacteria such as *Proteus*, in putrefying and decomposing the corpse. A few species are opportunistic pathogens and can produce disease; these include *Cl. welchii, Cl. septicum* and *Cl. oedematiens*, the causes of gas gangrene and other infections; *Cl. tetani*, the cause of tetanus; and *Cl. botulinum*, the cause of botulism. With only a few exceptions, the bacteria producing powerful exotoxins belong to this genus. *Cl. welchii* is also known as *Cl. perfringens*; and *Cl. oedematiens* as *Cl. novyi*.

The bacilli are typically large, straight or slightly curved rods with slightly rounded ends. Pleomorphism is common and a pure culture may contain many forms, including filaments, citron bodies, spindle-shaped (clostridium is a little spindle) and club forms. Some members of this group tend to lose their Gram-positive reaction early in culture, especially in broth culture, and may then appear Gram-negative. All produce spores and these enable the organisms to survive under adverse conditions, for example in soil and dust and on skin. *Cl. welchii* and the type species *Cl. butyricum* are the only capsulate members. Almost all members of the genus are motile, but *Cl. welchii* is an important exception.

The clostridia are biochemically active, frequently possessing both saccharolytic (carbohydrate-decomposing) and proteolytic (protein-decomposing) properties. *Cl. welchii, Cl. septicum, Cl. tertium* and *Cl. fallax* are examples of predominantly saccharolytic clostridia. *Cl.*

sporogenes, Cl. histolyticum and *Cl. tetani* are proteolytic or predominantly so. There is, however, no hard and fast line of demarcation between the two groups. Thus, *Cl. welchii* has slight proteolytic activity, and *Cl. sporogenes* has some saccharolytic properties.

A few clostridia can grow in the presence of trace amounts of air and some actually grow slowly under normal atmospheric conditions, but most species are obligate anaerobes. The spores of the true anaerobes do not germinate and growth does not normally proceed unless a suitably low redox potential (Eh) is obtained. In general, this usually involves the exclusion or removal of oxygen and the presence of reducing agents. The requirement for anaerobic conditions, the capacity to sporulate and the ability to produce potent toxins and aggressins are evident in the mechanisms of pathogenicity associated with the pathogenic clostridia. Recent evidence indicates that, although spores of clostridia are involved in their ability to withstand exposure to severely adverse conditions, vegetative cells can be recovered from inocula that have been at least transiently exposed to the air (Collee, Rutter and Watt, 1971) and vegetative forms can be recovered from soil (Garcia and Mackay, 1969). Thus, the transmissibility of gas-gangrene organisms from soil to wounds may not necessarily depend solely on spores, but it is likely that spores are often involved.

CLOSTRIDIUM WELCHII

(Cl. perfringens)

DESCRIPTION

Cl. welchii is the organism most commonly associated with gas gangrene. There are five types designated A to E and distinguished by the various combinations of toxins they produce. The classical *Cl. welchii* of gas gangrene belongs to type A, and a subgroup within type A is typically associated with *Cl. welchii* food poisoning in man. The other types are more commonly associated with diseases in animals and they are not discussed here.

The organism is a relatively large stout Gram-positive bacillus, about 4–6 μm by 1 μm, with stubby rounded ends, occurring singly or in pairs, and always capsulate when seen in the tissues. It is non-motile. Spores are formed under natural conditions, for example in the bowel, but only under special conditions in laboratory media.

Cl. welchii is an anaerobe, but it is not strictly demanding and may grow under microaerophilic conditions. It grows rapidly in cooked meat broth at 37°C and even more rapidly at temperatures up to 45°C. *Cl. welchii* is essentially saccharolytic and is only mildly proteolytic. However, it has various enzymes that enable it to break down cell membranes and connective tissue materials including collagen in animal tissues. On horse blood agar the colonies are large, round, smooth and usually regular with a variable zone of complete haemolysis and sometimes with a wider zone of incomplete haemolysis or darkening. In litmus milk medium this actively saccharolytic organism produces an acid clot that is disrupted by gas production; this is the mechanism of the typical 'stormy clot' reaction.

VIABILITY. *Cl. welchii* spores resist the action of the routinely used antiseptics and disinfectants. The spores of classical type-A strains of *Cl. welchii* are only moderately heat-resistant and will not survive boiling for more than a few minutes. The spores of so-called 'typical food-poisoning strains' and certain type-C strains are markedly heat-resistant and may survive boiling for at least 30 minutes and generally for several hours.

TOXINS

The types of *Cl. welchii* differ in the combinations of various toxic and enzymic factors that they produce. Several of these factors have haemolytic, lethal or necrotizing properties and others have enzymic activity against biological substrates (see below).

Table 36.1 shows that the various types of *Cl. welchii* can be differentiated on the basis of their production of the four major lethal toxins. Type-A strains produce alpha toxin; type-B strains typically produce alpha, beta and epsilon toxins; type-C strains produce alpha and beta toxins; type-D strains produce alpha and epsilon toxins; and type-E strains produce alpha and iota toxins.

Neutralization tests may be performed by intracutaneous or intravenous administration of mixtures of toxin and antitoxin to guinea-pigs or mice respectively. Epsilon and iota toxins do not occur in fully active form in cultures and

Table 36.1. The major lethal toxins and minor lethal or non-lethal factors produced by the various types of *Cl. welchii* (after Brooks, Sterne and Warrack, 1957)

Type	Occurrence	Major lethal toxins				Minor lethal or non-lethal factors							
		α	β	ε	ι	γ	δ	η	θ	κ	λ	μ	ν
A	Gas gangrene												
	Puerperal infection: Septicaemia	+++	−	−	−	−	−	(+)	+−	+−	−	+−	+−
	Food-poisoning	+++	−	−	−	−	−	−	(+)	+−	−	+−	++
B	Lamb dysentery	+++	+++	++	−	++	(+)	−	++	−	+++	+++	++
C	'Struck' in sheep	+++	+++	−	−	++	+++	−	+++	+++	−	−	+−
	Enteritis in other animals	+++	+++	−	−	?	−	−	+++	+++	−	−	+−
	Enteritis necroticans in man	+++	++	−	−	++	−	−	−	−	−	−	+++
D	Enterotoxaemia of sheep and pulpy kidney disease	+++	−	+++	−	−	−	−	++	++	++	+−	+−
E	Doubtful pathogen of sheep and cattle	+++	−	−	+++	−	−	−	++	++	++	(+)	+−

+++ = produced by all strains.   ++ = produced by most strains.   +− = produced by some strains.
(+) = produced by very few strains.

these prototoxins require to be activated by trypsinization of samples of the culture filtrates prior to neutralization tests.

Alpha Toxin

Alpha toxin is produced by all types of *Cl. welchii* but notably by type-A strains. This is the most important of the lethal toxins of the organism and is generally considered to be the main cause of the profound toxaemia associated with gas gangrene in man (but see p. 370). The alpha toxin is lethal for laboratory animals and it is necrotizing on intradermal inoculation. It is relatively heat stable, being only 50 per cent inactivated after five minutes at 100°C. The toxin is an enzyme—phospholipase (lecithinase C). In the presence of free Ca^{2+} or Mg^{2+} ions it can split lipoprotein complexes in serum or egg-yolk preparations with resulting opalescence. The reaction can be inhibited by specific antitoxin.

The phospholipase also attacks constituents of the membranes of red blood cells of various animals, and the alpha toxin is thereby haemolytic for the red cells of most species except the horse and the goat. The clear zones of haemolysis typically seen around colonies of classical type-A strains of *Cl. welchii* grown on horse blood agar are produced by the theta toxin and not by the alpha toxin. With the red cells of the sheep in particular the alpha toxin provides an example of a 'hot-cold' lysin. The alpha toxin similarly damages the membranes of other types of tissue cells and is thus a general cytotoxin.

NAGLER'S REACTION. Several clostridia and other bacterial species are able to produce opalescence in both human serum and egg-yolk media, due to the production of phospholipases that cause visible precipitates in these media. The reaction was first demonstrated with the alpha toxin of *Cl. welchii* and is specifically neutralized by *Cl. welchii* alpha antitoxin (but the serologically related phospholipase of *Cl. bifermentans* is also inhibited). This reaction has been utilized for the rapid detection of *Cl. welchii* in direct plate culture, and allows a serologically controlled identification of the organisms to be made within 20 hours of inoculating the plate from the wound exudate (Hayward, 1943). Further developments of this type of medium have included the incorporation of neomycin sulphate to inhibit aerobic spore-forming and coliform bacteria (Lowbury and Lilly, 1955).

Beta toxin. Types B and C produce this toxin, which is lethal and necrotizing.

Epsilon toxin is produced by type-B and D strains as a prototoxin which is thereafter activated by proteolytic enzymes. It is lethal and necrotizing. Filtrates may be trypsinized before assay.

Iota toxin. Only type-E strains produce this toxin, which is also lethal and necrotizing and, like epsilon toxin, is formed as a prototoxin which is then activated by proteolytic enzymes.

Theta toxin is an oxygen-labile haemolysin that is antigenically related to streptolysin O; it is a lethal toxin and a general cytolytic toxin. It is produced by most strains of *Cl. welchii*, types A–E, but is not produced by typical food-poisoning strains or by strains associated with enteritis necroticans in man. It lyses the red cells of the horse, ox, sheep and rabbit, but is virtually inactive against mouse erythrocytes. Many animal sera inhibit theta toxin and, although this may be due to contained antibodies, it is known that tissue lipids and cholesterol inactivate it.

Gamma toxin is a minor lethal toxin.

Delta toxin is lethal. It is also haemolytic for the red cells of even-toed ungulates (sheep, goats, pigs, cattle).

Eta toxin is said to be an insignificant lethal toxin.

Kappa toxin is a collagenase which attacks native collagen as well as hide powder and gelatin.

Lambda toxin is a proteinase and gelatinase. It will decompose hide powder, but it does not attack native collagen.

Mu toxin is a hyaluronidase.

Nu toxin is a deoxyribonuclease.

Cl. welchii thus produces a wide range of potentially toxic or aggressin-like substances. In addition, cultures of this organism have been shown to possess other enzymic properties. Enzymes are produced, particularly by some type-B strains, that destroy blood-group substances. The organism also renders red blood cells inagglutinable by the myxoviruses (Chap. 43), by destroying virus receptors at the red cell surface. This is due to a receptor-destroying enzyme (neuraminidase) similar to that of *Vibrio cholerae*. *Cl. welchii* renders red blood cells panagglutinable by exposing their T antigens so that they lose their specificity and react with any of the ABO antisera. A diffusible haemagglutinin elaborated by *Cl. welchii* causes agglutination of the red blood cells of man and most animals. It is produced by some strains after prolonged artificial subculture, but it is not produced by freshly isolated strains (Collee, 1961, 1965). Virulent strains of *Cl. welchii* are said to produce an aggressin that has been named 'bursting factor', but this agent has not yet been adequately characterized. The organism also produces a deconjugase enzyme that releases free bile acid from bile salt.

Animal Pathogenicity

Virulence for animals varies greatly with different strains. Some are markedly pathogenic to guinea-pigs by subcutaneous or intramuscular injection of 1 ml of a 24-hour, toxin-containing culture in cooked-meat broth into the thigh, and the animal may die within 24 hours. A control animal may be protected by a prior injection of *Cl. welchii* antitoxin, e.g. 300–500 units. At necropsy, a spreading inflammatory oedema with gelatinous exudate and gas production is noted in the subcutaneous tissue; necrosis occurs in the underlying muscles which are sodden, friable and pink. The products of growth of the bacillus increase its aggressiveness and, as toxin production occurs during early growth, young cultures should be used. The pathogenicity of a strain may be further enhanced by incorporating an equal amount of a sterile 5 per cent solution of calcium chloride in the inoculum immediately before injection. Pigeons are exceedingly susceptible to experimental inoculation of *Cl. welchii*.

The ill effects of *Cl. welchii* gas gangrene are closely related to toxic mechanisms. Evans (1945) produced indirect evidence that the virulence of *Cl. welchii* is primarily related to the production of alpha toxin, but it is debatable whether the toxic products of *Cl. welchii* that are recognized in in-vitro studies are the sole agents involved. Bullen (1970) has questioned whether the classical exotoxins have a primary role. There is no doubt that *Cl. welchii* is of relatively low infectivity. Nevertheless, it is potentially highly toxigenic and, once established in devitalized tissue, it is fiercely invasive; the organism grows rapidly into surrounding tissue and extends along tissue planes, and the patient rapidly becomes toxaemic and profoundly shocked. Van Heyningen (1955) postulated the development of a 'muscle toxin', i.e. a toxic product resulting from muscle decomposition *in vivo*; and Collee (1965) suggested that the organism's neuraminidase could alter host tissue to expose deep T antigens and precipitate a shock mechanism or allow other toxins access to otherwise protected sites.

Occurrence

Cl. welchii occurs normally in the large intestine of healthy man and animals. It is possible that post-gastrectomy diarrhoea is associated in some cases with abnormal growth of *Cl. welchii* in the proximal small intestine (Duncan *et al.*, 1954). The organism can be recovered from human faeces and its spores are ubiquitous in soil, dust and air; they are regularly present on human skin, especially in the region of the perineum, buttocks and thighs. The organism may pass from the bowel to the blood stream in a moribund patient and, multiplying in internal organs after death, produces the small gas cavities sometimes noted (e.g. in the liver) at necropsy. Lowbury and Lilly (1955) showed that *Cl. welchii* could be isolated from the air of operating theatres. Thus, when gas gangrene occurs after surgical intervention, such as amputation, pinning of a hip fracture or general abdominal surgery, the surgeon may be apt to blame environmental factors such as poor theatre facilities or an inadequate ventilating system, but it is likely that many of these cases arise as a result of endogenous infection (see Bittner *et al.*, 1970).

CLOSTRIDIUM SEPTICUM

(*Vibrion septique*)

Description

This Gram-positive bacillus varies considerably in its appearance. It is generally about 4–6 μm by 0·6 μm, but shorter forms, long forms, and very long filaments also occur. Spores are readily formed and, as they develop, various shapes arise ranging from swollen Gram-positive 'citron-bodies' to obviously sporing forms in which the oval spores may be central or subterminal and are clearly bulging. Older Gram-negative cells may be seen.

The organism is actively motile with numerous peritrichous flagella. It is one of the less exacting anaerobes and grows well at 37°C on ordinary media. It is saccharolytic and glucose promotes growth.

Surface colonies are irregular, transparent, droplet-like, later becoming greyish and opaque, with projecting radiations that are coarser than those of *Cl. tetani*. On horse blood agar, haemolysis is observed. If the surface of the medium is not relatively dry, the culture spreads across it.

ANTIGENIC CHARACTERS. Combinations of two somatic antigens (1, 2) and five H-antigens (a–e) distinguish six groups. There is considerable antigenic cross-relationship with *Cl. chauvoei* which shares a common spore antigen.

An exotoxin with lethal, necrotizing and haemolytic properties, the alpha toxin, can be demonstrated in cultures, and a specific antitoxin can be produced. The beta toxin is a deoxyribonuclease, the gamma toxin is a hyaluronidase, and the delta toxin is an oxygen-labile haemolysin. A fibrinolysin has also been reported. Dafaalla and Soltys (1951) considered that a haemagglutinin produced by *Cl. septicum* is cell-bound, but Gadalla and Collee (1967) considered that it was essentially soluble.

ANIMAL PATHOGENICITY. Intramuscular injection of cultures in laboratory animals produces a spreading inflammatory oedema, with slight gas formation in the tissues. The organisms invade the blood and the animal dies within a day or two. Smears from the liver show long filamentous forms and also citron bodies.

Epidemiology

The primary habitat of *Cl. septicum* is either the soil or the animal intestine. Areas with large numbers of spores appear to be associated with a higher incidence of *Cl. septicum* infections in man and animals than less heavily infected areas. It has been assumed that the spore is the primary agent of infection, but recent evidence indicates that vegetative forms of the organism may be abundant in the soil, and this finding merits further investigation.

Cl. septicum is responsible for braxy in sheep and for malignant oedema following wound infection in cattle and sheep.

CLOSTRIDIUM OEDEMATIENS
(*Clostridium novyi*)

This Gram-positive bacillus resembles *Cl. welchii* in morphology, but is larger and more pleomorphic and it is a much more strict anaerobe, being readily inactivated when its vegetative cell is exposed to air. It possesses peritrichous flagella, but its motility is inhibited in the presence of oxygen. The spores are oval, central or subterminal. The organism occurs widely in soil and is associated with disease in man and animals. The *Cl. oedematiens* species includes four types—A, B, C and D—distinguished on the basis of the permutations of the toxins and other soluble antigens they produce. Only type-A strains are of medical interest as they cause some cases of gas gangrene in man.

Cl. oedematiens gas gangrene is associated with profound toxaemia. Culture filtrates are highly toxic and possess at least four active substances (α, β, δ and ε toxins) that account for the various haemolytic, necrotizing, lethal, phospholipase and lipase activities of this organism.

The species as a whole is of considerable veterinary importance, and it is also of wide biological interest as a model for the study of anaerobiosis. Type-B strains are stricter anaerobes than type-A strains, and type-D strains are said to be among the most demanding anaerobes that are grown. Type-D strains do not grow readily on the surface of anaerobically incubated solid medium unless the medium is freshly poured and supplemented with a special reduced system (see Collee, Rutter and Watt, 1971; Watt, 1972).

Other Gas-Gangrene Clostridia

There are many other pathogenic clostridia that may be associated with gas gangrene on occasion. When these pathogens are isolated from infected wounds, they are usually in combination with various facultatively anaerobic pyogenic organisms, and sometimes several clostridia are involved. Pathogenic clostridia that are encountered in this way from time to time include organisms of the *Cl. bifermentans–Cl. sordellii* group and *Cl. histolyticum* which is a less strictly anaerobic member of the genus.

CLOSTRIDIUM SPOROGENES

This Gram-positive motile bacillus is very widely distributed in nature, e.g. in soil and in the intestines of animals, and is generally regarded as a harmless saprophyte. It is about 6–8 μm by 0·8 μm and Gram-negative forms are frequent in older cultures. Its oval, central or subterminal spores may be highly resistant and the organism is frequently encountered in mixed cultures in the laboratory, even after preliminary heating of these cultures to select heat-resistant pathogens. Its spores may survive boiling for periods of from 15 minutes up to 6 hours. *Cl. sporogenes* is frequently isolated from wound exudates in association with accepted pathogens. Whilst its presence may accelerate an established anaerobic infection by enhancing local conditions, it does not by itself cause gas gangrene and cannot be regarded as a pathogen in its own right.

GAS GANGRENE

Several different species of clostridia are associated with rapidly spreading oedema, myositis, necrosis, gangrene of the tissues, and gas production, occurring as a complication of wound infection in man. The patient's general condition deteriorates rapidly and severe shock develops. The main source of the organisms is animal and human excreta. Gas gangrene was prevalent among the armies in Europe during the war of 1914–18 and much less frequently in the war of 1939–45. Data obtained in the two wars indicate that of the three principal pathogens, *Cl. welchii* occurred most frequently (in about 60 per cent of all cases) in gas gangrene, whilst *Cl. oedematiens* and *Cl. septicum* occurred, respectively, in about 20–40 per cent, and 10–20 per cent of cases. Other clostridia, such as *Cl. bifermentans*, *Cl. sordellii*, and *Cl. histolyticum* occurred much less frequently. *Cl. welchii* occurs widely in soil and dust and on the skin, and it is readily cultured and identified in the laboratory, whereas *Cl. oedematiens* is a much more demanding organism. These facts should be borne in mind in relation to the above data.

The infection usually results from the contamination of a wound with soil (particularly that of manured and cultivated land), dirty clothing, street dust, etc., but may also be derived from the skin, especially in areas of the body that may be contaminated with intestinal organisms. Impairment of the normal blood supply of tissue with a consequent reduction in oxygen tension, e.g. by the crushing or severing of arteries, and the presence of devitalized or dead tissue, blood clot, foreign bodies or coincident pyogenic infection, are factors that promote the occurrence of gas gangrene in a wound. The predisposing factors later discussed in detail with regard to tetanus (Chap. 37) are equally applicable in the case of gas gangrene. The spores and vegetative bacilli cannot initiate infection in healthy tissues, presumably because the Eh of the tissues is too high for their growth and they are unable to avoid destruction by phagocytosis. Once infection has been initiated in a focus of devitalized anaerobic tissue in a wound, the clostridial toxins are produced. These spread into adjacent viable tissue, particularly muscle, kill it and render it anaerobic and suitable for colonization by the bacilli. Growth of the bacilli in the newly colonized tissue produces more toxin, which diffuses onwards into fresh tissue, killing it and leading to yet further spread of the bacilli. The infection extends along tissue planes. Thus the infection spreads until the whole of a muscle group or segment of a limb is involved. The surgical management of wounds should be prompt and adequate in the first instance; it is particularly important that devitalized tissue and debris are removed.

In puerperal infections, and especially in cases of septic abortion, the organisms may gain access from faeces-contaminated perineal skin to necrotic or devitalized tissues in the uterus or adnexa and set up a dangerous pelvic infection or invade the blood stream to produce intravascular haemolysis and anuria. *Cl. welchii* may also be involved in infections occurring as a result of extension of the organism from the alimentary tract, as in cases of appendicitis or intestinal obstruction.

If a preparation of adrenalin used for injection is contaminated with clostridial spores, the combination of an infective focus with the local ischaemia that follows the injection may be catastrophic. Gas gangrene is well recognized as a complication of surgical operations on the lower limb or hip area of patients in whom the blood supply may be inadequate and this is discussed below.

Other less severe forms of clostridial infection may occur without the typical toxaemia, such wounds having a foul odour and showing evidence of gas formation. Moreover, potentially pathogenic anaerobes may be cultivated from a wound that never shows any signs of gas gangrene. MacLennan (1943) has classified anaerobic infections on clinical grounds and he recognizes (a) simple contamination of a wound with clostridia; (b) anaerobic cellulitis, in which muscle is not involved; and (c) anaerobic myositis, which includes clostridial gas gangrene but may also be caused by anaerobic streptococci.

LABORATORY DIAGNOSIS

The bacteriological diagnosis of gas gangrene is usually combined with a general bacteriological examination of the infected wound with which this condition is associated. Clinical clues include crepitus in the adjacent tissues and signs of toxaemia or developing shock. Prompt diagnosis and intensive surgical and antimicrobial treatment greatly influence the patient's chance of survival.

If there are sloughs or necrotic tissue present in the wound, small pieces should be placed in a sterile screw-capped bottle and used for microscopic examination and culture. Specimens of exudate should be taken from the wound, particularly from the deeper tissues and from parts where the infection seems to be most pronounced. Films are made in the usual way and stained by Gram's method. If gas gangrene is present, Gram-positive bacilli may predominate, although *Cl. oedematiens* may appear to be relatively scanty in the wound exudate, even in an active infection. Thick, rectangular, Gram-positive bacilli suggest the presence of *Cl. welchii*, *Cl. fallax* or *Cl. bifermentans*; 'citron bodies' and boat or leaf-shaped pleomorphic bacilli with irregular staining may indicate *Cl. septicum*; slender bacilli with round terminal spores suggest *Cl. tetani* or *Cl. tetanomorphum*; *Cl. oedematiens* occurs in the form of large bacilli with oval subterminal spores. The laboratory diagnosis of gas gangrene is detailed elsewhere (Vol. II).

Direct microscopic examination of tissue smears stained with specific antisera conjugated to different fluorescent dyes and illuminated by ultraviolet light allows prompt recognition of *Cl. oedematiens* and prompt differentiation between *Cl. septicum* and *Cl. chauvoei* which are closely related (Batty and Walker, 1963).

TREATMENT OF GAS GANGRENE

Chemotherapy

Much work on the antibiotic sensitivities of numerous clostridia isolated from wounds suggested that the order of activity of the common antibiotics is, in general, tetracyclines > penicillin > chloramphenicol (Garrod, 1958). However, many factors must be considered in the antibiotic treatment of clostridial infections in addition to *in vitro* proof of antibiotic sensitivity (MacLennan, 1962). Penicillin has been widely used and may be administered together with a tetracycline. There is no evidence of antagonism, but some of the clostridia may now be resistant to tetracycline. The treatment of gas gangrene with penicillin (5 to 20 M units daily) and other measures has been reviewed by Bittner *et al.* (1970).

Hyperbaric Oxygen

Enthusiastic claims are made for the efficacy of hyperbaric oxygen therapy in gas gangrene (see Boerema, Brummelkamp and Meijne, 1964). Patients are placed in a special pressurized chamber in which they breathe oxygen at 2–3 atmospheres pressure absolute for periods of 1–2 hours twice daily on several successive days. Hyperbaric oxygen therapy involves special equipment and, as oxygen is potentially toxic, it requires special experience and careful monitoring. Nevertheless, this form of treatment is likely to gain more widespread recognition; when it is used by experienced operators the anaerobic extension of gas gangrene may be halted and the need for major surgical intervention avoided in some cases.

PROPHYLAXIS OF GAS GANGRENE

The prevention of gas gangrene should be considered separately in relation to planned surgical wounds and to accidental wounds. In the former case, it should be recognized that *Cl. welchii* is normally present in large numbers in human faeces and that its spores occur on the skin, especially in the areas of the buttocks and thighs. As clostridial spores are markedly resistant to most antimicrobial chemicals, they are likely to survive normal pre-operative skin preparation and a proportion of the spore population persists in the area of the planned incision. The numbers can be reduced by more prolonged skin preparation involving the sustained application of povidone-iodine for a day or two before operation and this procedure has a place in orthopaedic surgery. When the factors of inevitable skin contamination and likely survival of spores are combined with circumstances that predispose to devitalization of tissue and reduced oxygen tension, a patient is seriously vulnerable to the development of post-operative gas gangrene. These circumstances arise if an elderly patient or a patient with vascular insufficiency is subjected to major operative surgery involving the hip or lower limb. In such cases, there are strong arguments for insisting that penicillin should be given immediately pre-operatively (i.e. within a few hours) and for 5 to 7 days thereafter to guard against the possible germination and outgrowth of clostridial spores (British Medical Journal, 1969; Parker, 1969).

The prevention of gas gangrene in accidentally sustained wounds must take account of the endogenous factors noted above and the exogenous factors that relate to the general occurrence of clostridial spores and vegetative forms in soil, their contamination of clothing, and the increased risk of anaerobic infection developing when foreign bodies such as soil, clothing, metal (bullet, shrapnel) and skin are driven into an area of devitalized tissue. Prompt and adequate surgery is of paramount importance. This principle is recognized in military circles, but delays in surgical treatment in civil practice are inevitable when major disasters such as earthquakes or large explosions occur. *Prophylactic* administration of benzyl penicillin (500 000 units each of potassium and procaine penicillin, repeated at intervals of six hours) in cases of serious, contaminated wounds, has largely replaced the prophylactic use of gas gangrene antisera. The use of an antibiotic in this manner must never preclude prompt and adequate wound toilet.

Specific Prophylaxis

A polyvalent serum is available for prophylactic use and for treatment of cases in which the causal organism has not been determined. The prophylactic dose, given intramuscularly (or in urgent cases intravenously), is 10 000 international units *Cl. welchii* antitoxin, 5 000 units *Cl. septicum* antitoxin and 10 000 units *Cl. oedematiens* antitoxin. The therapeutic dose, given intravenously, should be at least three times the prophylactic dose, and the administration should be repeated as necessary. Monovalent sera are also available for the treatment of cases after the causal organism has been identified. Reactions to antitoxin administered intravenously may be severe and precautions should be taken.

CL. WELCHII FOOD-POISONING

Strains of *Cl. welchii*, conforming in most respects to type-A but producing non-haemolytic or feebly haemolytic colonies on horse-blood agar, are associated with a mild form of food-poisoning (Hobbs *et al.*, 1953). The mechanism of *Cl. welchii* food-poisoning is not fully understood, but it probably depends upon the ability of the food-poisoning strains to produce an enterotoxic exotoxin. An enterotoxic effect can be demonstrated in studies in which bacteria-free culture filtrates are injected into ligated intestinal loops in animals (Hauschild, Niils and Dorward, 1968). Ingestion of large numbers of the viable organisms in contaminated food appears to be necessary for the production of the typical disease in man (Dische and Elek, 1957) and it seems that production and release of the enterotoxin is related to sporulation of the organisms in the gut. Typical symptoms are abdominal cramps beginning about 8 to 12 hours after ingestion, followed by diarrhoea. Fever and vomiting are not typically encountered. The condition is usually transient and symptoms normally subside within 24 to 48 hours. Spores of so-called 'typical food-poisoning strains' are markedly heat-resistant, surviving boiling for several hours. Non-haemolytic strains of *Cl. welchii* occur frequently in human faeces (Collee, Knowlden and Hobbs, 1961), but carrier rates for 'typical food-poisoning strains', i.e. non-haemolytic on horse-blood agar and producing spores that resist boiling in cooked-meat broth for one hour, range from 2·2 per cent in the general population to 20 to 30 per cent in hospital personnel and patients. Food-poisoning strains of *Cl. welchii* are widely distributed, occurring in the faeces of healthy men and animals. The vehicle of infection is usually a pre-cooked meat food that has been allowed to stand at a temperature conducive to the multiplication of *Cl. welchii*. Whilst the heat-resistance of spores of food-poisoning strains ensures their survival in cooked foods and presumably accounts for the association of these potentially heat-resistant strains with most of the reported outbreaks of *Cl. welchii* food-poisoning, similar trouble can be caused by classical heat-sensitive β-haemolytic strains which may gain access to food during the cooling period under conditions suitable for their subsequent multiplication (McKillop, 1959). The essential property that enables some strains of *Cl. welchii* to cause food-poisoning is presumably the ability to produce enterotoxin, and although this ability is most commonly expressed by heat-resistant and non-haemolytic strains, it is clearly present in heat-sensitive, haemolytic ones.

such strains from *food* by selective heating is rarely successful because spores of *Cl. welchii* are not normally abundant in food. The vegetative organisms are often abundant and can be recovered by selective culture methods. The serological type of a typical food-poisoning strain is determined by slide agglutination tests (Hobbs' types)[1]. Untypable strains are not infrequently encountered.

It should be noted that the methods in current use for the detection of typical food-poisoning strains of *Cl. welchii* automatically exclude heat-sensitive strains. If large numbers of classical strains of β-haemolytic *Cl. welchii* are isolated from suspected food by quantitative methods, this finding should not be dismissed solely because the organism does not conform to the criteria of typical food-poisoning strains. It is now well recognized that heat-sensitive classical *Cl. welchii* and strains of intermediate heat resistance can cause food poisoning. On the other hand, the isolation of large numbers of classical β-haemolytic strains of *Cl. welchii* from *faeces* is *per se* of no significance as regards *Cl. welchii* food-poisoning. Warrack (1963) made a plea for more general typing of *Cl. welchii*, particularly in investigations of food-poisoning caused by this organism.

A sub-group of *Cl. welchii* type-C has been reported as the cause of a condition occurring in Germany affecting man and named *enteritis necroticans*. The spores of these strains, originally referred to as *Cl. welchii* type-F, are markedly heat-resistant. There is evidence to suggest that type-C strains of *Cl. welchii* are also involved in a disease called 'pig-bel' that affects New Guinea natives and is associated with pork feasts.

LABORATORY DIAGNOSIS

Bacteriological diagnosis involves the isolation of similar strains from faeces of patients and from those at risk and from the suspected food. Isolation of *Cl. welchii* from *faeces* is facilitated by their being present in spore form and a selective heating procedure is usually employed that is based on the known heat resistance of spores of typical food-poisoning strains. Isolation of

REFERENCES

BATTY, I. & WALKER, P. D. (1963) Differentiation of *Clostridium septicum* and *Clostridium chauvoei* by the use of fluorescent labelled antibodies. *Journal of Pathology and Bacteriology*, **85**, 517.

BITTNER, J., RACOVITA, C., CRIVDA, S. & ARDELEANU, J.

[1] Dr Betty C. Hobbs, Director, Food Hygiene Laboratory, Central Public Health Laboratory, Colindale Avenue, London.

(1970) Combined therapy in post-operative gas gangrene. *Journal of Medical Microbiology*, **3**, 325.

BOEREMA, I., BRUMMELKAMP, W. H. & MEIJNE, N. G. (1964) Clinical application of hyperbaric oxygen. *Proceedings of the 1st International Congress*. Amsterdam and Barking: Elsevier.

BRITISH MEDICAL JOURNAL (1969) (Leading Article) Post-operative gas gangrene. *British Medical Journal*, **iii**, 665.

BROOKS, M. E., STERNE, M. & WARRACK, G. H. (1957) A re-assessment of the criteria used for type differentiation of *Cl. perfringens*. *Journal of Pathology and Bacteriology*, **74**, 185.

BULLEN, J. J. (1970) In *Microbial Toxins*, Vol. 1, p. 233, edited by S. J. Ajl, S. Kadis and T. C. Montie. New York and London: Academic Press.

COLLEE, J. G. (1961) The nature and properties of the haemagglutinin of *Clostridium welchii*. *Journal of Pathology and Bacteriology*, **81**, 297.

COLLEE, J. G. (1965) The relationship of the haemagglutinin of *Clostridium welchii* to the neuraminidase and other soluble products of the organism. *Journal of Pathology and Bacteriology*, **90**, 13.

COLLEE, J. G., KNOWLDEN, J. A. & HOBBS, B. C. (1961) Studies on the growth, sporulation and carriage of *Clostridium welchii* with special reference to food poisoning strains. *Journal of Applied Bacteriology*, **24**, 326.

COLLEE, J. G., RUTTER, J. M. & WATT, B. (1971) The significantly viable particle; a study of the subculture of an exacting sporing anaerobe. *Journal of Medical Microbiology*, **4**, 271.

DAFAALLA, E. N. & SOLTYS, M. A. (1951) Studies on agglutination of red cells by clostridia. I. *Cl. septique*. *British Journal of Experimental Pathology*, **32**, 510.

DISCHE, F. E. & ELEK, S. D. (1957) Experimental food-poisoning by *Clostridium welchii*. *Lancet*, **ii**, 71.

DUNCAN, I. B. R., GOUDIE, J. G., MACKIE, L. M. & HOWIE, J. W. (1954) Some effects of partial gastrectomy on the intestinal flora. *Journal of Pathology and Bacteriology*, **67**, 282.

EVANS, D. G. (1945) The *in vitro* production of α-toxin, haemolysin and hyaluronidase by strains of *Cl. welchii*

type A, and the relationship of *in vitro* properties to virulence for guinea-pigs. *Journal of Pathology and Bacteriology*, **57**, 75.

GADALLA, M. S. A. & COLLEE, J. G. (1967) The nature and properties of the haemagglutinin of *Clostridium septicum*. *Journal of Pathology and Bacteriology*, **93**, 255.

GARCIA, M. M. & MACKAY, K. A. (1969) On the growth and survival of *Clostridium septicum* in soil. *Journal of Applied Bacteriology*, **32**, 362.

GARROD, L. P. (1958) The chemoprophylaxis of gas gangrene. *Journal of the Royal Army Medical Corps*, **104**, 209.

HAUSCHILD, A. H. W., NIILS, L. & DORWARD, W. J. (1968) *Clostridium perfringens* type A infection of ligated intestinal loops in lambs. *Applied Microbiology*, **16**, 1235.

HAYWARD, N. J. (1943) The rapid identification of *Cl. welchii* by Nagler tests in plate cultures. *Journal of Pathology and Bacteriology*, **55**, 285.

VAN HEYNINGEN, W. E. (1955) In *Mechanisms of Microbial Pathogenicity*, p. 17. 5th Symposium of the Society of General Microbiology, Cambridge.

HOBBS, B. C., SMITH, M. E., OAKLEY, C. L., WARRACK, G. H. & CRUICKSHANK, J. C. (1953) *Clostridium welchii* food-poisoning. *Journal of Hygiene (London)*, **51**, 75.

LOWBURY, E. J. L. & LILLY, H. A. (1955) A selective plate medium for *Cl. welchii*. *Journal of Pathology and Bacteriology*, **70**, 105.

MCKILLOP, E. J. (1959) Bacterial contamination of hospital food, with special reference to *Cl. welchii* food-poisoning. *Journal of Hygiene (London)*, **57**, 31.

PARKER, M. T. (1969) Postoperative clostridial infections in Britain. *British Medical Journal*, **iii**, 671.

MACLENNAN, J. D. (1943) Anaerobic infections of war wounds in the Middle East. *Lancet*, **ii**, 63, 94, 123.

MACLENNAN, J. D. (1962) The histotoxic clostridial infections of man. *Bacteriological Reviews*, **26**, 177.

WARRACK, G. H. (1963) Some observations on the typing of *Clostridium perfringens*. *Bulletin. Office international des épizooties*, **59**, 1393.

WATT, B. (1972) The recovery of clinically important anaerobes on solid media. *Journal of Medical Microbiology*, **5**, 211.

37. Clostridium : II : Cl. tetani : Cl. botulinum

Tetanus and Botulism

Tetanus occurs in man and animals when a wound is infected with *Clostridium tetani* under conditions that allow the organism to multiply and produce toxin. Absorption of the toxin to the central nervous system leads to hyperexcitability of voluntary musculature and the disease is characterized by increased muscle tonus and exaggerated muscular responses to trivial stimuli. Trismus occurs when the muscles of the jaw are affected and, as this is quite frequently an early sign of tetanus in man, the disease is sometimes called lockjaw.

CLOSTRIDIUM TETANI

DESCRIPTION

This is the causative organism of tetanus in man and animals. It is generally seen as a straight, slender, rod-shaped organism, 2 to 5 μm by 0·4 to 0·5 μm with rounded ends, but longer filaments may occur. *Cl. tetani* is motile and has numerous peritrichous flagella. It is a classical spore-former; the fully developed spore is terminal and spherical, two to four times the diameter of the bacillus, producing the 'drumstick' appearance that is a striking morphological feature of the organism. It is Gram-positive, but there is considerable variation and Gram-negative forms are usually encountered, especially in material from wounds and in broth cultures that are not intentionally examined at an early stage.

The tetanus bacillus is an obligatory anaerobe. It is readily grown in cooked-meat medium or in Fildes' peptic blood broth. On solid media, surface colonies of the normal motile type of tetanus bacillus are characterized by their very delicate branching projections.

The spores may be highly resistant to adverse conditions, but the degree of resistance varies; sporing forms of many strains are killed by exposure to boiling water for a few minutes whereas rarer more resistant strains may resist boiling for up to three hours. They may resist dry heat at 150°C for one hour, and 5 per cent phenol or 0·1 per cent mercuric chloride for up to two weeks or more. Iodine 1 per cent in watery solution and hydrogen peroxide (10 volumes) are said to kill the spores within a few hours.

Antigenically, ten types are distinguishable by agglutination tests involving flagellar (H) antigens. Type VI consists of non-flagellate strains. All types produce the same neurotoxin, and toxigenic and non-toxigenic strains may belong to the same type.

Toxin

The exotoxin, of which the neurotoxic component *tetanospasmin* is the essential pathogenic constituent, develops in broth cultures after 5 to 14 days' growth at 35°C, the optimum time varying with the strain. Toxin yields from *Cl. tetani* cultures vary from strain to strain and also depend upon the culture medium used. *Tetanolysin* is another toxic constituent and causes lysis of red blood corpuscles. It is oxygen-labile and related to streptolysin-O and the theta toxin of *Cl. welchii*. *Tetanospasmin* has been separated as a pure crystalline protein with an estimated lethal dose for the mouse of 0·0000001 mg. Tetanus toxin is thus an extremely powerful poison, second in potency only to the exotoxin of *Cl. botulinum*. When tetanus toxin is injected into guinea-pigs or mice, the animals die within a day or two with the typical signs of tetanus, the tetanic spasms usually starting in the muscles related to the site of injection ('local tetanus'). The toxin reaches the central nervous system by passing along the motor nerves, being absorbed probably by the motor end-plates and spreading up the spaces between the nerve fibres. Toxin adsorbed by motor nerves present in or near the infected wound passes first to the part of the brain stem or spinal cord containing the motor neurones of these nerves and causes 'local tetanus'; then, by local spread up the spinal cord produces 'ascending tetanus'. Toxin that is absorbed by motor nerves from the general musculature of the body after blood-borne distribution from the wound reaches the CNS first in the brain stem since the motor nerves from this centre are short, and then spreads downwards, so causing lockjaw followed by 'descending tetanus' (Kryzhanovskyi, 1967). Tetanus toxin has the effect of causing over-action of the motor cells in the anterior horn of the spinal cord and may then diffuse to involve the whole central nervous system. The toxin appears to act by interfering with the normal inhibition of motor impulses exercised by the upper motor neurone over the lower, producing an increase in tonus and tonic spasms. This affords an explanation of the clinical manifestations of tetanus, but the actual mode of action of tetanus toxin is not known. Whereas the toxin of *Cl. botulinum* produces visceral symptoms and signs, tetanus toxin does not appear to do so directly (Wright, 1955). Dysphagia and urinary retention observed in clinical tetanus can be attributed to paralysis of associated skeletal muscles. Certain strains of *Cl. tetani* produce a factor that enhances the lethal action of tetanospasmin for rabbits and this factor may facilitate access of the toxin to its susceptible cell substrate, which is a ganglioside in nervous tissue. Consideration of the specific affinity of the toxins of *Cl. tetani* and *Cl. botulinum* for nervous tissue, the relatively small amount of these toxins required to produce death, and the lag period between intoxication and its manifestation, has given rise to the theory that both of these toxins may act through interference with vital enzyme systems. A blocking effect on the normal mechanism of release of acetyl choline at certain nerve ends with a resultant inhibition of transmission and loss of a control system has been postulated, but the different symptomatology of tetanus and botulism has not been explained.

Occurrence

The tetanus bacillus occurs in the intestine of man and animals, but there is considerable variation in the frequency with which it is reported to have been isolated from their faeces. Tenbroeck and Bauer (1922) isolated *Cl. tetani*

from 34·7 per cent of stools from 78 individuals in Peking. Kerrin (1929) examined more than 300 human stools in Scotland and none yielded *Cl. tetani*. The wide divergence in these figures may be partly related to the different ways of life of the communities investigated. The use of human faeces (night-soil) as fertilizer in the fields of China, most of whose population lives in intimate contact with the soil, will play a part in the re-distribution of the bacillus. A warm climate may allow enrichment of *Cl. tetani* in the soil although it is still uncertain whether this organism flourishes as a saprophyte in the soil, as it seems to be derived primarily from the animal intestine. It is especially prevalent in manured soil, and, for this reason, a wound through skin that may be contaminated with soil or manure deserves special attention. Whether derived from the soil or the faeces, however, tetanus spores occur very widely; they are commonly present in street dust and may be present in the dust and plaster in hospitals and houses, on clothing and on articles of common use.

PATHOGENESIS

Tetanus is usually the result of contamination of a wound with *Cl. tetani* spores. The source of the infection may be soil, dirty clothing or dust. Spores of *Cl. tetani* and other anaerobes may be embedded in surgical catgut (prepared from sheep's intestine), and this has been the source of infection in some post-operative cases of tetanus. The sterility of surgical catgut is now rigorously controlled in Britain.

If washed spores alone are injected into an animal they fail to germinate, are phagocytosed and do not give rise to tetanus. It has been shown that the germination of spores of *Cl. tetani* is dependent on the reduced oxygen tension occurring in devitalized tissue and non-viable material in the wound. Infection, when it occurs, remains strictly localized in the wound and the tetanic condition is due to the effects of a potent diffusible exotoxin on the nervous system. Unlike the toxins of the gas-gangrene bacilli, tetanus toxin does not cause death of tissue adjacent to the infected wound and so does not bring about spread of the infection from its initial focus. Certain conditions favour the germination of the spores and the multiplication of the organisms in the tissues: e.g. lacerated wounds in which tissue is deprived of its blood supply by crushing or severing of arteries; deep puncture wounds; wounds accompanied by compression injury; necrotic tissue and effused blood; wounds contaminated with soil, the ionized calcium salts and silicic acid in which cause tissue necrosis; wounds containing foreign bodies such as pieces of clothing and shrapnel; infection by other organisms, such as pyogenic cocci and *Cl. welchii*. Thus, in war casualties, infection tends to occur when there are deep lacerated wounds caused by shrapnel which may carry in fragments of muddy clothing and particles of earth. Spores are then introduced under most favourable conditions for the development of the organism. Similar wounds may be sustained in civil life, notably as a result of accidents on the roads and on farms or after gunshot injuries. However, cases of tetanus have been reported, especially in children, in which the infection was apparently associated with a superficial abrasion, a contaminated splinter or a minor thorn-prick. In some cases the site of infection is assumed to be in the external auditory meatus (from which it is fairly easy to recover *Cl. tetani* if dust-borne spores are in the environment); thus, *otogenic tetanus* may be attributed to over-zealous 'cleansing' of the meatus with a stick. In other patients, the site of infection remains undiscovered and these are referred to as cases of *cryptogenic tetanus*. *Cl. tetani* infection may also occur in the uterus, as in cases of septic abortion. *Tetanus neonatorum* follows infection of the umbilical wound of newborn infants. Cases of post-operative tetanus have been attributed to imperfectly sterilized catgut, dressings or glove-powder, and some cases of post-operative tetanus have been attributed to dust-borne infection of the wound at operation.

Laboratory Diagnosis

Films may be made from the wound exudate and stained by Gram's method; the appearance of 'drum-stick' bacilli is suggestive but not conclusive evidence of the presence of *Cl. tetani* as other organisms with terminal spores, which are morphologically indistinguishable from *Cl. tetani*, may be present. Moreover, it is often impossible to detect the tetanus bacilli in wounds by microscopic examination.

Direct plating of unheated material on blood agar incubated anaerobically is often the best method of detecting *Cl. tetani*. Tetanus may be produced in mice by subcutaneous injection of an anaerobic fluid culture prepared from the wound. Control mice are protected with tetanus antitoxin. Material from the wound or from a sporing subculture may also be heated at various temperatures or for various times to exclude non-sporing organisms and then seeded on to a slope of nutrient medium. The advancing edge of a spreading filament of *Cl. tetani* may then be subcultured in due course.

Epidemiology

Tetanus ranks among the major infections that kill man. Bytchenko (1967) noted that no area in the world is free from the disease but, as it is not transmitted from case to case, it is not seen as an epidemic and there is much under-reporting. More than 38 000 deaths from tetanus were notified annually between 1956 and 1960 and, with allowance for incomplete notification, particularly in developing countries where the disease is most common, Bytchenko calculated that deaths from tetanus on a global scale probably exceeded 160 000 annually during the decade 1951–60.

The incidence of tetanus varies enormously from country to country. Areas of high incidence are inversely related to socioeconomic development, especially with reference to standards of living and preventive medicine in its widest sense. There is a direct relationship with fertile soil and a warm climate; thus, people in the agricultural areas of developing tropical countries are exposed to severe challenges (poor hygiene, lack of shoes, neglect of wounds, inadequate immunization) and suffer from a high incidence of tetanus (see Table 37.1).

In addition, certain local customs predispose to the occurrence of tetanus; for example, treatment of the umbilical cord stump with primitive applications that include animal dung greatly

Table 37.1. The reported mortality from tetanus in various countries (Rubbo, 1966).

High incidence area	Mortality per 100 000 population	Low incidence area	Mortality per 100 000 population
Haiti	46·2	Italy	0·90
Malaya	31·4	France	0·78
Panama	17·7	Japan	0·63
Nigeria	14·6	New Zealand	0·45
Philippines	9·0	Switzerland	0·35
Mexico	6·7	Australia	0·33
Venezuela	6·7	West Germany	0·30
Fiji	4·6	United States	0·13
Kenya	4·6	Finland	0·09
Thailand	4·3	England	0·05
Ceylon	4·0	Canada	0·03

increase the risk of neonatal tetanus which is common in such areas, sometimes affecting more than 80 per 1 000 live births, and with a very high case fatality. Veronesi (1967) noted that neonatal tetanus accounted for 25 per cent of all neonatal deaths in the Congo.

Attack rates are also high in young males up to 20 years old, during their accident-prone years, but girls may be significantly affected where ear-piercing is a local practice. Data from India (Suri, 1967) confirm that tetanus affects significant numbers of people in all age-groups from 0 to 50, including women of childbearing age in whom tetanus after abortion is not uncommon.

In general, with the exception of neonatal tetanus, fatality rates range from 15 to 50 per cent but the case fatality can be greatly reduced by modern methods of treatment in a specialist centre. Unfortunately, such help is available for only a small proportion of patients.

PREVENTION AND CONTROL

Prompt and adequate wound toilet and proper surgical débridement of wounds are of paramount importance in the prevention of tetanus as there is an increased risk that tetanus spores may germinate in a wound if there is delay in cleansing or if sepsis develops. Clean superficial wounds that receive prompt attention may not require specific protection against tetanus and it is unreasonable to insist that every small prick or abrasion requires protection with antibiotic or antitoxin. Moreover, some surgeons consider

that patients receiving thorough and prompt surgical treatment of their wounds, plus antibiotic therapy until healing is advanced, do not require tetanus antitoxin in addition, especially if there is a low incidence of tetanus in the area. It is wise to recommend specific prophylaxis in the case of deep wounds, puncture or stab wounds, ragged lacerations, wounds associated with bruising and devitalized tissue, wounds already septic, and animal bite wounds. The need for passive immunization with tetanus antitoxin is avoided if the patient is known to be properly immunized.

Active Immunization

Most authorities consider that all persons should be actively immunized against tetanus in infancy and their immunity maintained by booster doses of toxoid at intervals of five to ten years. This is of particular value in the case of allergic patients for whom serum prophylaxis in the event of wounding carries an increased risk of complications.

Tetanus toxoid is a preparation of refined toxin that has been rendered non-toxic by treatment with formaldehyde ('formol toxoid'). It is a good antigen and the soluble toxoid is made more effective in modern preparations by adsorption on to an aluminium hydroxide carrier ('adsorbed toxoid'). Tetanus toxoid is one of the components of the diphtheria-pertussis-tetanus triple vaccine given in childhood, and adsorbed toxoid by itself is used specifically for active immunization against tetanus.

A course of three 0·5 ml doses of tetanus

toxoid (preferably the adsorbed toxoid preparation) with intervals of 6 to 12 weeks between the first two, and 6 to 12 months between the second and third injections, is of proven value in the prevention of tetanus. A reinforcing (booster) dose of 0·5 ml toxoid may thereafter be given at intervals of five to ten years to maintain immunity; but if toxoid is given too frequently, there is a risk of sensitization.

A careful record should be kept of all prophylactic injections given, and information should include the batch numbers of the preparations used and the nature of any reactions observed. It is especially important that a record card should be given to the patient or his guardian.

The risk of developing tetanus is primarily related to the local incidence of tetanus and to the immune status of the individual. Whilst some degree of latent immunity is conferred even after only one injection of toxoid, for practical purposes it is wise to differentiate clearly between those likely to have a definite immunity and those who may not be immune. A patient may be regarded as *immune* for six months after the first two injections, or for 5 to 10 years after three injections (or a booster injection) of a planned course of adsorbed tetanus toxoid. Tetanus antitoxin should not be given to immune patients, but their active immunity may be enhanced when necessary by giving 0·5 ml of tetanus toxoid intramuscularly at the time of injury.

A patient is considered *non-immune* if he has never had an injection of tetanus toxoid or if he has had only one such injection. If more than six months have elapsed after a course of two injections, or more than 5 to 10 years after a full primary course of three injections (or a booster injection) of tetanus toxoid, he may be regarded as non-immune; recent evidence suggests that these time limits may be extended. He is non-immune if more than 1 to 2 weeks have elapsed since a previous injection of tetanus antitoxin. He should be considered non-immune if there is any doubt about his immunization history.

Passive Immunization with Antitoxin

Tetanus antitoxin, often called antitetanus serum or ATS, can be obtained by immunizing horses with toxoid. This serum is of value in the prophylaxis of tetanus, if given immediately after wounding. Its use as a curative agent after the development of tetanus is less effective than the corresponding antitoxin treatment of diphtheria.

The usual prophylactic dose of antitoxin is 1 500 International Units given by intramuscular or subcutaneous injection as soon as possible after injury. The dose is not reduced for a child. The injection may be repeated at weekly intervals as long as the risk of tetanus persists. Larger initial doses, e.g. 3 000 to 10 000 units, may be given when the wound is severe. Antitoxin is never given intravenously as a *prophylactic* measure.

The administration of equine antitoxin may be associated with untoward reactions and the incidence of unpleasant side-effects may be as high as 8 to 10 per cent of those that receive this heterologous serum. These include relatively trivial local reactions with erythema and urticaria; serum sickness which may be of the accelerated or delayed types; neuritic sequelae with varying degrees of loss of function; and anaphylactic shock that may occur immediately after the injection or may be delayed for 1 to 2 hours: but fatal anaphylaxis is rare (perhaps 1 death in about 100 000 recipients of equine antitoxin).

Some surgeons working in areas in which tetanus is a rare disease have virtually abandoned the use of equine antitoxin. Nevertheless, it should be categorically stated that there is good evidence to justify the administration of tetanus antitoxin to a wounded patient when the circumstances of the wound and the patient's non-immune state warrant it—especially if the wound is sustained in a high-incidence area. The risk of tetanus is greatly increased when there is delay in dealing with the wound and if sepsis develops. All of these predisposing factors are regularly encountered in many developing countries and it is disturbing that equine antitoxin is being prematurely discarded before there are supplies of human antitoxin to take its place; thus, patients at severe risk are in danger of being denied proper prophylaxis. The recommendations given in Table 37.2 must be considered carefully in this context. Even in Britain, human antitoxin is not generally available and it will be necessary to use equine antitoxin for some time to come. If antitoxin is given promptly as a prophylactic, and if proper surgical attention is given, protection is usually but not invariably afforded. In some non-immune patients, antitoxin may be contra-indicated or it may not be considered a sufficient protection. In such cases, the prophylactic use of an antibiotic is reasonable (see Table 37.2).

Antitoxins have been produced in the cow and the sheep in attempts to produce preparations associated with fewer side effects. These bovine and ovine antitetanus sera are available, but their protective efficacy is only assumed at present.

THE USE OF HUMAN ANTI-TETANUS GLOBULIN (ATG). The obvious way to avoid the main problems associated with heterologous sera is to develop adequate supplies of homologous antitoxin from human sources. In Britain, supplies of refined human antitetanus globulin are at present released for special prophylactic use or for treatment. This homologous antitoxin is not rapidly removed and a single dose of 250 units suffices for prophylaxis. In *treatment*, however, there is evidence to support the use of relatively large doses (see Adams, Laurence and Smith, 1969).

COMBINED ACTIVE–PASSIVE IMMUNIZATION. It is desirable that patients receiving passive protection with antitoxin after injury should also be actively immunized against tetanus with toxoid, because, apart from involving the risk of anaphylaxis, a second dose of antitoxin tends to be more rapidly eliminated than the initial dose and the passive protection afforded on the second occasion is reduced. Purified tetanus toxoid adsorbed on aluminium hydroxide is a powerful antigen released over a period of days and the use of this preparation of toxoid overcomes previous objections to the concurrent administration of tetanus antitoxin for immediate passive protection and tetanus toxoid for active immunization. Thus, an injured non-immune patient may receive from separate syringes, 1 500 units of equine tetanus antitoxin or 250 units of homologous ATG intramuscularly in one arm and 0·5 ml of the *adsorbed* toxoid preparation in the other. Active immunization is therefore started at an opportune moment and the patient is advised to have

a second injection of 0·5 ml of adsorbed toxoid 6 to 12 weeks later.

ANTIBIOTIC PROTECTION. Although the prophylactic administration of antibiotics to all cases of open wounds is not recommended, there is justification for the prophylactic administration of an antibiotic such as penicillin to a patient with a previous history of a severe immediate reaction to horse serum, in which case equine antitoxin is withheld. In the case of a deep contaminated wound or an open wound associated with much devitalized tissue, antibiotic protection should be given in addition to antitoxin because pyogenic infection is likely to occur in such wounds and this favours the development of tetanus. Penicillin may be given at the time of injury and dosage maintained (either by repeated administration or by the use of a long acting preparation such as benzathine penicillin) until healing is established. As in gas gangrene, this additional safeguard cannot take the place of prompt and adequate surgical wound toilet and it can be criticized on the grounds that strains of *Cl. tetani* vary in their sensitivity to penicillin, that access of antibiotic to the infected area may be impaired, and that penicillinase-producing organisms may also be present. Nevertheless, the prompt administration of antibiotics can prevent the development of tetanus in animals challenged with spores of *Cl. tetani*. There is good evidence that the combination of a prolonged course of antibiotic plus active immunization with adsorbed toxoid at the time of injury may prevent tetanus spores germinating until active immunity has developed (Smith, 1964).

Table 37.2, slightly amended from that proposed originally by Rubbo (1966), illustrates a realistic approach to the integration of antibiotic prophylaxis with the other measures discussed above.

Treatment

In the *treatment* of established tetanus, antitoxin is of proven value (Brown *et al.*, 1960). Reliance is frequently placed on the intravenous injection of a large initial dose of antitoxin (30 000 to 200 000 units) followed by intramuscular injections; results of current investigations suggest that an initial dose of 50 000 units, given wholly or partly intravenously, gives as good results as those obtained when 200 000 units of antitoxin are injected as the initial dose (see Laurence and Webster, 1963). When intravenous antitoxin is prescribed, it should be preceded by a subcutaneous test dose, followed by an intramuscular test dose, at half-hour intervals (see below). The antitoxin should be diluted, warmed to room temperature and injected very slowly into the recumbent patient. All of the precautions listed below should be observed. Intrathecal administration of antitoxin may cause dangerous reactions.

Encouraging results have been obtained with human antitetanus serum in the treatment of tetanus, but better results may be at least partly attributable to increasing skill in the general management of tetanus cases (Ellis, 1963).

PRECAUTIONS TO BE OBSERVED WHEN GIVING ANTITOXIN. In view of the risk of anaphylactic reactions following injections of antitoxin, routine precautions should be taken before antitoxin is administered. Information should be obtained from the patient regarding previous serum injections and any history of

asthma, infantile eczema, urticaria or other allergic condition elicited. In the absence of any of these contra-indications the full dose of antitoxin may be injected forthwith, but a sterile syringe and needle with adrenalin (1 ml of 1 in 1 000 solution) should be at hand. The patient should be kept warm before and after treatment and he should be under observation for at least 30 minutes after the injection.

If the patient has had a previous injection of serum, but gives no history of allergy, a subcutaneous trial dose of 0·2 ml antitoxin should be given, and a full dose of antitoxin may be given if no general reactions have occurred within 30 minutes. If the patient gives a history of allergy, the initial trial dose should be 0·2 ml of a 1 in 10 dilution of antitoxin subcutaneously. If no general symptoms develop within 30 minutes, this may be followed by 0·2 ml of undiluted antitoxin subcutaneously. The full dose may be given if there are no general reactions after a further 30 minutes.

CHEMOTHERAPY. A course of systemic penicillin or tetracycline therapy should be given in cases of established tetanus. There may be some

Table 37.2. A scheme for tetanus prophylaxis after injury (amended from Rubbo, 1966).

Wound (after surgical cleaning and topical disinfection)	Immune status*	Low-incidence area	High-incidence area
Cleaned (soil, manure or devitalized tissue removed) within 6 hours	Immune	No treatment	Toxoid × 1
	Partially immune	Toxoid† × 1	Toxoid × 1
	Non-immune	Toxoid × 3	Toxoid × 3
Contaminated (traces of soil, manure or devitalized tissue not removed)	Immune	Toxoid × 1	Toxoid × 1
	Partially immune	Toxoid × 1	Toxoid × 1, +ATS, +antibiotics§
	Non-immune	Toxoid × 3, +ATG‡	Toxoid × 3, +ATS, +antibiotics
Infected (signs of clinical infection)	Immune	Toxoid × 1, +antibiotics	Toxoid × 1, +antibiotics
	Partially immune	Toxoid × 1, +antibiotics	Toxoid × 1, +ATS, +antibiotics
	Non-immune	Toxoid × 3, +ATG, +antibiotics	Toxoid × 3, +ATS, +antibiotics

* Defined as follows: *Immune*—Patient has had complete course of three injections of toxoid some time in the past.
Partially immune—Patient has had two injections of toxoid some time in the past.
Non-immune—Patient has had one or no previous injections of toxoid, or the matter is in doubt.
† Toxoid recommended is 'aluminium phosphate adsorbed' containing 5 limit-flocculation units per 0·5 ml given by intramuscular injection; ×3 = full course of 3 injections (see p. 380).
‡ Dose of ATG 250 units, ATS 1 500–3 000 units, each given by intramuscular injection. (ATG = homologous antitetanus globulin; ATS = equine antitoxin).
§ Antibiotic treatment consists of long-acting penicillin given by intramuscular injection or oral tetracyclines providing cover 'until healing is established'.

justification for the local instillation of antibiotic into the wounded area after adequate
débridement. Antibiotics may also be required
to control complications such as pneumonia.

CLOSTRIDIUM BOTULINUM

Botulism is a severe, usually fatal form of food
poisoning characterized by pronounced toxic
effects, mainly on the parasympathetic system,
that include oculomotor and pharyngeal paralyses and aphonia. It is not a common disease in
Britain, only four incidents having been recorded since the Loch Maree tragedy in 1922 when
eight victims died after eating duck paste infected with *Cl. botulinum*. Six main types of *Cl.
botulinum* have been differentiated on the basis
of their antigenically distinct toxins designated
A, B, C, D, E and F. Types A, B and E are those
most frequently associated with botulism in the
human subject, but types C, D and F have also
caused disease in man.

DESCRIPTION

Cl. botulinum is a strictly anaerobic Gram-
positive bacillus (about 5 μm by 1 μm). It is
motile and has peritrichous flagella. Its spores
are oval and subterminal. It is a widely distributed saprophytic organism. Its natural habitat is
soil, even virgin and forest soil, and it may be
found on vegetables, fruits, leaves, and in
mouldy hay, silage, animal manure, and sea
mud. The temperature for optimum growth is
about 35°C, but some strains have been shown
to grow and to produce toxin at temperatures
as low as 1 to 5°C.

The widespread occurrence of *Cl. botulinum*,
the organism's ability to produce a very potent
neurotoxin (see below) in food, and the resistance of its spores to deleterious influences combine to make it a formidable pathogen. Spores
of some strains of *Cl. botulinum* withstand moist
heat at 100°C for several hours. They are destroyed by moist heat at 120°C usually within 5
minutes. Spores of type-E strains are usually
much less heat-resistant. Insufficient heating in
the process of preserving foods is an important
factor in the causation of botulism, and great
care is taken in canning factories to ensure that
sufficient heating is achieved in all parts of the
can contents.

Toxin

In culture media and in contaminated foods,
Cl. botulinum can produce a powerful exotoxin
that is responsible for the pathogenic effects in
the disease. It appears to interfere with the
mechanism of acetylcholine release from the
endings of the motor nerves of the parasympathetic system. This toxin is destroyed when
exposed to a temperature of 80°C for 30 to 40
minutes.

The toxin of type A has been isolated as a
pure crystalline protein and quantitatively is
probably the most potent toxic substance in
nature, the estimated lethal dose for mice being
0·000000033 mg; in other words, 1 g would kill
30 000 million mice. In spite of its potency, the
action of the toxin is slow and victims or experimental animals may die many days after receiving
a lethal dose; the incubation period (which may
be a misnomer for a process of intoxication) is
usually 12 to 36 hours. The different types of the
bacillus produce toxins that are immunologically different and neutralizable only by the
appropriate antitoxin; thus, antitoxin produced
against toxin A does not neutralize toxin B, and
vice versa. Type A toxin is resistant to inactivation by proteolytic enzymes: type E toxin can
be activated by limited proteolytic action.

Antitoxin is prepared by immunizing animals
with toxoid preparations, and it is used therapeutically. In general, a bivalent serum containing antitoxins to the A and B types of toxin
has been employed for prophylaxis and treatment; its efficacy in the treatment of established
botulism is doubtful. Antitoxin to Type E
botulism should now be added as a routine.

PATHOGENESIS

Human cases of botulism have been found to
originate from a considerable variety of preserved foods, e.g. ham, sausage, home canned
meats and vegetables, etc. Type E strains typically occur in fish and marine products but
strains of other types may also have a sea source.
Foods responsible for botulism may not exhibit

signs of spoilage. The intoxication follows absorption from the intestine of toxin preformed by the bacilli in the food, but there may also be some formation of toxin by the organism after ingestion. The toxin primarily affects the cholinergic system and seems to block the release of acetylcholine at the presynaptic level. The early clinical symptoms may suggest a coronary thrombosis. The neurotoxic signs and symptoms follow — vertigo, oculomotor and pharyngeal palsies with diplopia and dysphagia, difficulty in speech and in breathing. Death due to respiratory failure occurs a few days after onset of symptoms.

The bacillus may sometimes be demonstrated in the stomach contents and faeces of victims, and *post-mortem* in the intestinal contents and in the liver and spleen. It can also be isolated from the food responsible for the outbreak.

Rare cases of wound infection by *Cl. botulinum*, resulting in the characteristic signs and symptoms of botulism, have been recorded.

Laboratory animals are susceptible to experimental inoculation and feeding with cultures (see Vol. II). Sporadic outbreaks of botulism have been reported in mink in America, Scandinavia and England.

LABORATORY DIAGNOSIS

As botulism is essentially a food intoxication, the suspected food should be examined bacteriologically. It may occasionally be possible to demonstrate the presence of toxin in the patient's blood or in post-mortem specimens of blood or liver by direct animal inoculation.

Gram-stained films of the food may first be examined for sporing bacilli. The food is then macerated in sterile salt solution and a filtered extract injected, in a series of toxin-antitoxin neutralization and protection tests with suitable control preparations, intraperitoneally into guinea-pigs or mice.

Cl. botulinum may be isolated in pure culture from the food by anaerobic culture of samples that have been heated at 65 to 80°C for various times to eliminate non-sporing bacteria. Subsequent identification of *Cl. botulinum* is based upon its biological characters and its toxigenicity; in addition, immunofluorescence staining may be used if conjugated antisera are available.

Prophylaxis

Home-canning of foodstuffs should be avoided and home preservation of meat and vegetables, especially beans, peas and root vegetables, is not advisable. Acid fruits may be bottled safely in the home, heating at 100°C, since a low pH is inhibitory to the development of *Cl. botulinum*. A prophylactic dose of antitoxin (10 ml) should be given intramuscularly to all asymptomatic persons who have eaten food suspected of causing botulism. Active immunity in man can be produced by the injection of three doses of mixed toxoid at two-month intervals, but the very small incidence of the disease under normal conditions does not justify this procedure. Similar immunization of animals against the predominant type may be economically worth while and has been carried out in Australia on a small scale.

REFERENCES

ADAMS, E. B., LAURENCE, D. R. & SMITH, J. W. G. (1969) *Tetanus*. Oxford and Edinburgh: Blackwell Scientific Publications.

BROWN, A., MOHAMED, S. D., MONTGOMERY, R. D., ARMITAGE, P. & LAURENCE, D. R. (1960) Value of a large dose of antitoxin in clinical tetanus. *Lancet*, **ii**, 227.

BYTCHENKO, B. (1967) Tetanus as a world problem. In *Principles on Tetanus*, p. 21, edited by L. Eckmann. Bern and Stuttgart: Hans Huber.

ELLIS, M. (1963) Human antitetanus serum in the treatment of tetanus. *British Medical Journal*, **i**, 1123.

KERRIN, J. C. (1929) The distribution of *B. tetani* in the intestines of animals. *British Journal of Experimental Pathology*, **10**, 370.

KRYZHANOVSKYI, G. N. (1967) The neural pathway of toxin. In *Principles on Tetanus*, p. 155, edited by L. Eckmann. Bern and Stuttgart: Hans Huber.

LAURENCE, D. R. & WEBSTER, R. A. (1963) Pathologic physiology, pharmacology and therapeutics of tetanus. *Clinical Pharmacology and Therapeutics*, **4**, 36.

RUBBO, S. D. (1966) New approaches to tetanus prophylaxis. *Lancet*, **ii**, 449.

SURI, J. C. (1967) The problem of tetanus in India. In *Principles on Tetanus*, p. 61, edited by L. Eckmann. Bern and Stuttgart: Hans Huber.

TENBROECK, C. & BAUER, J. H. (1922) The tetanus bacillus as an intestinal saprophyte in man. *Journal of Experimental Medicine*, **36**, 261.

VERONESI, R. (1967) Epidemiology of tetanus. In *Principles on Tetanus*, p. 43, edited by L. Eckmann. Bern and Stuttgart: Hans Huber.

WRIGHT, G. P. (1955) In *Mechanisms of Microbial Pathogenicity*, p. 78, edited by J. W. Howie and A. J. O'Hea. Cambridge University Press.

38. Treponema : Borrelia

Syphilis : Yaws : Relapsing Fever : Vincent's Angina

SPIROCHAETES

Spirochaetes are constructed in a far more complicated manner than ordinary bacteria. They are slender spiral cells that have an intrinsic active undulating motility although they lack flagella. They may consist of regularly spaced tight coils or loose irregular spirals of varying amplitude. Some propel themselves with rapid lashing movements, others by slow twisting and bending. They differ in length from 4 to 14 μm and in thickness from 0·1 to 0·6 μm. Larger spirochaetes can easily be seen in stained films but the very thin ones are barely detectable by this means and are best demonstrated by dark field microscopy in wet preparations.

The protoplasmic core of these spiral cells is enclosed within a cell wall and an inner cytoplasmic membrane; between these two layers there are overlapping sets of fine fibrils which are anchored by knobs at the two poles of the organism. The number of fibrils varies according to the genus from a single pair to six or more pairs. It is probable that the spiral shape of the organisms depends on the tension in the fibrils for if they have been ruptured the coiled appearance is lost and the cell straightens out. The serpentine movement of spirochaetes may also depend on the integrity of the fibres.

Spirochaetes belong to the order Spirochaetales which is divided into two families Spirochaetaceae and Treponemataceae. The former are free-living saprophytes and are not associated with disease. The latter consist of several genera that are pathogenic for man and animals; they include *Treponema, Borrelia* and *Leptospira.*

TREPONEMA PALLIDUM

This spirochaete is the causative organism of syphilis, a notorious venereal disease that has persecuted mankind since it was first recognized in epidemic form in Europe in the fifteenth century. *Tr. pallidum* is a slender flexuous helix 6 to 14 μm long. Its width is 0·13 μm in dried, electron-microscope preparations, but is about 0·2 μm in the wet, living state, when it is just great enough for resolution with the light microscope. It has 6 to 12 coils that are remarkably evenly disposed at 1·0 μm intervals and its two ends are tapered. Because of its weak refractility and slender thickness, about the limit of resolution by the light microscope, it is best observed in wet living preparations with the dark ground microscope. In dried preparations it needs to be thickened by silver impregnation methods to become visible. It is actively but rather lazily motile and there are three movements that propel it: slow undulation, corkscrew-like rotation, and a sluggish backwards and forwards motion. Occasionally the organisms can be seen to divide by binary fission. As the spirochaete slowly moves across the dark field of the microscope it often displays a characteristic tendency to bend at right angles near its midpoint. These features are best observed in exudates taken freshly from the patient and they enable the physician to make an immediate and reliable diagnosis on the spot. Experience is needed to identify most non-pathogenic commensal spirochaetes but generally they lack the regular spacing of the spiral coils at 1 μm intervals and their lashing rapid motility easily distinguishes them from *Tr. pallidum.* When dark field microscopy is not available the organism can be detected in wet films of the exudate mixed with India ink.

Tr. pallidum cannot be stained by simple aniline dyes or by Gram's method. In films stained by Giemsa's prolonged method for 24 hours the organism appears as a delicate pink thread in contrast to the deep purple colour of coarser spirochaetes.

Under the electron microscope the protoplasmic core of *Tr. pallidum* is seen to be enveloped by a cell wall inside which it is contained by the cytoplasmic membrane. Between

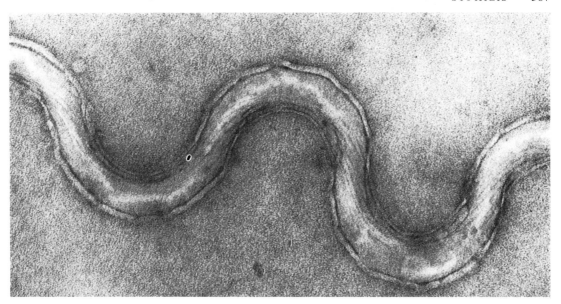

PLATE 38.1. *Treponema pallidum*. Part of an intact spirochaete. The outer cell wall is clearly defined but is covered by a slimy layer of irregular thickness. The four fibrils twisted around the spirochaete are clearly seen. (Stained by PTA. ×76 500.)

these two layers lie a number of axial filaments. It is frequently possible to see that two of the filaments are anchored by the insertion of their terminal knobs into the tapering tip at one end of the spirochaetal cytoplasm (Plates 38.1 and 38.2). A second pair are similarly anchored into the other tip of the spirochaete. Each pair is twisted spirally around the organism, those from one end overlapping those from the other for most of the length of the organism. Thus when a cross-section is made in the middle of a spirochaete the microtome knife transects four filaments.

ANIMAL PATHOGENICITY. All attempts to cultivate *Tr. pallidum* in artificial culture media, chick embryos or tissue cultures have failed and it is conceded that the organism cannot as yet be cultivated on artificial media. It is, however, possible to propagate the spirochaetes by inoculating living treponemes from pathological lesions into the testes, scrotum, skin, or eye of the rabbit. The experimental disease in the rabbit resembles the early course of the natural disease in man. A primary lesion rich in spirochaetes develops but the later manifestations in the rabbit differ from human tertiary syphilis in that a large number of the organisms persist in the tissues without the development of any progressive disease. The Nichol's strain used in the TPI test has been kept for many years (>25 years) by rabbit to rabbit intra-testicular passage since its first isolation from the brain of a fatal case of general paralysis of the insane (GPI).

Treponemes from rabbit 'syphilomas' of the testis preserved in the proper suspending fluids under anaerobic conditions remain actively motile for from four to seven days at 25°C or for two days at 37°C. Frozen in a medium containing 15 per cent glycerol at −65°C they remain viable for years and provide a reliable source of antigens for immunological tests.

Drying rapidly kills the spirochaetes as does exposure to heat at 41·5 to 42°C. They do not survive at 0 to 4°C for more than one or two days. They are rapidly immobilized by trivalent arsenicals, bismuth and mercurials. Minute concentrations of penicillin kill them, though rather slowly.

ANTIGENIC STRUCTURE. The pattern of the immune response to syphilitic infection includes at least three distinct antibodies but the antigens that evoke them are not well understood. The best known response is a non-specific complement fixation reaction, known as the

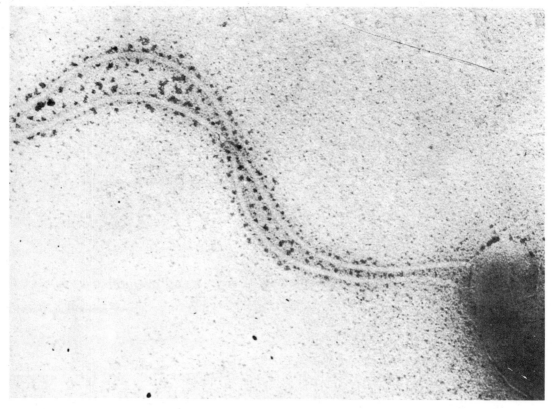

PLATE 38.2. *Treponema pallidum*. The tip of a spirochaete after 30 minutes tryptic digestion. Two fibrils remain inserted at the tip of the digested spirochaete but stream away from it. (Stained by PTA. ×60 800.)

Wassermann reaction in which an antibody reacts with a lipid hapten that can be extracted by alcohol from beef heart and other healthy tissues. This hapten is known as cardiolipin and has been identified as diphosphatidylglycerol; when mixed with lecithin and cholesterol it reacts with the Wassermann antibody not only in complement fixation tests but also in precipitation (or flocculation) reactions. This basic principle is employed in a number of serologic tests for syphilis (Standard Tests for Syphilis, STS) including the Wassermann, VDRL, Kahn, Hinton and Kleine tests, all of which detect the same antibody. For many years this lipoidophil antibody, which is contained in the IgM and IgG fractions, has been known as a 'reagin' but it is not to be confused with the reagin occurring in atopic disease, a globulin which belongs to the IgE class.

It is not known whether cardiolipin is contained in *Tr. pallidum* itself or whether it is released as a hapten from tissues damaged by infection. Since positive STS occur in other conditions than syphilis ('biological false positives') it seems that there may be a variety of disease processes presumably liberating antigenic materials which can generate anti-cardiolipin antibodies. Although the STS provide useful and sensitive screening methods they obviously are not sufficiently specific for complete diagnostic reliability.

The second antigen is contained solely within the treponemes themselves where it can be demonstrated by specific immune fluorescence (Fluorescent Treponemal Antibody or FTA test) and by the fact that when exposed to specifically protective antisera the spirochaetes lose their active mobility and are immobilized (Treponema pallidum Immobilization or TPI test). Both these phenomena are used for specific confirmation of syphilis in sera that react positively with cardiolipin antigens. False positive reactions are not known to occur in these *Tr. pallidum* antibody tests.

A third antigen is known to be present in both *Tr. pallidum* and also in the non-pathogenic Reiter's treponeme that grows in artificial culture media. This treponemal group antigen is shared by other treponemes and can be detected by complement fixation tests with antisera to the individual spirochaete strains. The Reiter complement fixation test is a valuable screening test often added to the STS but it is not as specific as the *Tr. pallidum* antibody tests.

PATHOGENESIS

Most cases of syphilis are contracted during sexual intercourse. The treponemes are present in superficial genital lesions and pass from one partner to the other through intact mucous membranes or through minor skin abrasions. Occasionally the source of the infection is extra-genital and in a small percentage of cases the primary lesion is found around the mouth. More rarely infection has been reported in lesions on the hands of medical or nursing staff after investigating or treating cases of syphilis.

An important reason why, in developed communities, syphilis is almost exclusively spread by sexual intercourse, i.e. why it is a venereal disease, is the extreme delicacy of *Tr. pallidum*. This organism dies very rapidly when outside the body, e.g. almost instantly when dried or within an hour when kept moist. Thus under normal conditions of social life there is scarcely any possibility for it to be spread by forms of indirect contact with fomites, clothing etc.

When the spirochaete has penetrated its new host it begins to multiply at the site of its entrance (its generation time is less than 5 hours) and during the next 10 to 90 days the initial sore of primary syphilis appears. It is a focus of inflammatory tissue infiltrated with lymphocytes and monocytes and is first noticed as a small red papule. The lesion is usually solitary and gradually enlarges; the centre breaks down to form a superficial ulcer about 1 or 2 cm in diameter. The base of the ulcer is indurated and the lesion

is referred to as a 'hard chancre' or as the 'primary sore'. It is the classical lesion of primary syphilis and in the male is often situated on the prepuce or the corona of the penis and in the female on the labia, the vaginal wall, or the cervix of the uterus.

There are very large numbers of treponemes in the primary sore and in the serum that exudes from it. In the early days of infection the spirochaetes invade the local lymph nodes where they cause an adenitis which in the male is in the inguinal region; and in the female is within the pelvis. The affected nodes have a firm rubbery consistency on palpation: from them the spirochaetes are soon conveyed to the blood stream in large numbers.

This generalization of the infection throughout the body continues for 2 to 12 weeks after clinical infection. Towards the end of this time in an untreated case the primary chancre begins to subside spontaneously and leaves only a small scar.

The secondary stage of syphilis accompanies the invasion of the blood stream by the spirochaetes and the most striking manifestations are widespread roseolar or papular rashes. Snail-track ulcers (mucous patches) in the oropharynx, and condylomata of the anus and the vulva, are other prominent lesions. Less commonly choreoretinitis, periostitis and meningitis may develop.

All the lesions of secondary syphilis, especially those involving mucous membranes on exposed surfaces, discharge very large numbers of treponemes. Like the primary chancre they constitute large reservoirs of infection and they present a hazard to medical personnel who investigate and treat cases of syphilis.

In distribution and duration the various lesions of secondary syphilis are extremely variable. Sometimes they are quite trivial and transient but more usually they are slow to heal and distress the patient for long periods. Secondary syphilitic lesions may remain infective for as long as four or five years but once healed the patient is no longer dangerous to others.

The mechanism that destroys the vast numbers of spirochaetes in the blood and tissues during secondary syphilis is quite unknown. It is unlikely to be phagocytosis, as happens in leptospirosis, because the treponemes seem able to resist engulfment by leucocytes. Probably the organisms are destroyed by a lytic process involving complement and specific antibody.

After the decline of the secondary stage of syphilis there is a period of quiescence known as 'latent syphilis'. During this period foci of infection may remain dormant and undetected in the tissues. In only about 50 per cent of untreated cases does the cure become permanent. The late manifestations of syphilis appear in the remainder and take the form of chronic granulomata known as 'gummata'. It may be as long as 10 to 20 years after initial infection before these lesions are detected. Damage to the cardiovascular system with destruction of elastic tissue and the formation of aneurysms in large arteries, as well as gummata in the brain, bone, skin and internal organs, are some of the principal pathological effects. In the central nervous system tabes dorsalis characterized by a chronic progressive destruction of nerve fibres in the spinal column is one important effect, as also is meningovascular syphilis where continuing damage to brain cells results in general paralysis of the insane. The lesions of tertiary syphilis contain very few spirochaetes and the extensive tissue damage that occurs is possibly the result of a delayed hypersensitive reaction to the products of the persisting treponemes.

Tr. pallidum can cross the placental barrier and a syphilitic mother, especially in the secondary stage, may transmit the infection to her foetus. The lesions of congenital syphilis are essentially similar to those already described but when the infection is massive the child may be still-born or survive only a short time. The most important defects in late congenital syphilis are mental deficiency, chronic meningitis, blindness and deafness.

LABORATORY DIAGNOSIS

Syphilitic Exudates

In primary and secondary lesions it is possible to find and identify *Tr. pallidum* by dark field microscopy. The method establishes the diagnosis quickly and with certainty but it is in some respects insensitive because in early lesions spirochaetes are rather scanty. In the usual conventional cover-slip preparation each oil immersion field contains 10^{-6} ml of the exudate. If the observer is to see one spirochaete in each field it follows that the specimen would require to have 10^6 organisms per ml. Thus negative findings can be misleading and prolonged and repeated searches are often necessary to detect the treponemes.

A fluorescent antibody test on acetone-fixed films of exudates is probably more sensitive than the conventional dark field method.

Antibody Tests

A specimen of 5 to 10 ml of clotted blood is needed; it should be placed in a sterile dry container without any preservative. If a TPI test is requested information *must* be provided about recent antibiotic treatment because traces of penicillin or other antibiotic in the blood interfere with the test. Specimens from babies should be taken by heel stab; cord blood from the newborn is not satisfactory.

TESTS FOR LIPOIDOPHIL ANTIBODY (STS). These tests, made with cardiolipin antigen, are usually the first investigations carried out to confirm the diagnosis of syphilis. A rapid slide flocculation test, such as the Venereal Disease Research Laboratory (VDRL) test, is often used for screening, although some prefer the Kahn test. A second test such as the Wassermann test is carried out quantitatively so that, besides confirming previous tests, it also provides a base line in assessing the effect of treatment.

Although these tests are very sensitive they are not immunologically specific and weak false positive reactions are frequently encountered. There are many microbial infections and pathological lesions that may liberate lipid antigens in the tissues with the consequent formation of lipoidophil antibodies and the occurrence of biological false positive reactions. Healthy blood donors, pregnant women and people who have been vaccinated against smallpox or suffer from various infections (e.g. leprosy, typhus, etc.), have all been observed as reacting positively but usually weakly to these tests.

In primary syphilis the Wassermann antibody is usually detectable about one week after the appearance of the primary chancre. In the secondary stage virtually all cases give positive findings with high titres. At first IgM and IgG antibodies can be demonstrated but in the latent infection and in late syphilis IgG usually, though not always, predominates. About 10 to 20 per cent of late cases give negative STS. Under treatment these tests become negative and remain so if the disease has been cured.

TESTS FOR TREPONEMAL ANTIBODIES. If the tests are positive when there is no clinical evidence to suggest syphilis they must be repeated and if they remain positive, verification by more specific tests such as the FTA or TPI tests for *Tr. pallidum* antibody or the RPCFT for treponemal group antibody will be required before a diagnosis of syphilis can be made with any certainty.

Treponemal group antibody. The RPCFT is technically simple and is often used as a screening test in parallel with the Wassermann test. Its value is that it detects treponemal group antibodies that arise both in syphilis and other treponemal infections. It is less sensitive than the anticardiolipin tests in early untreated syphilis but is more sensitive than these tests in latent or late syphilis. After treatment it becomes negative more slowly than the STS. Although the test has a high degree of specificity, false positive reactions do occur in about 1.0 per cent of healthy blood donors with negative STS.

Tr. pallidum antibody. When both the RPCFT and STS are positive the likelihood of syphilitic infection is very high and when both are negative the probability is low. In long-standing cases however both tests may be negative. If the clinical evidence is incompatible with the serological findings or if there is any conflict between the results of the various tests verification with more highly specific antitreponemal tests is essential. Of these, the most reliable is the *Treponema Pallidum Immobilization test* (TPI) in which the patient's serum is incubated with living virulent treponemes (Nichols strain) in the presence of complement. When specific antibody is present the spirochaetes are immobilized and killed. These antibodies appear later in the disease than the non-specific reagin so that the TPI test is not useful in the diagnosis of early syphilis; its main value lies in its ability to distinguish true from false positive STS and in the help it provides in the investigation of patients suspected of having latent or late syphilis.

Because the test is technically difficult and expensive it is reserved for use, usually in a reference laboratory, when the verification of the results of the other tests has become a necessity. Once this antibody has appeared the test remains positive for many years.

The *Absorbed Fluorescent Treponemal Antibody Test* (FTA ABS) is another highly specific reaction that is used as a verification procedure. It is technically easier to carry out than the TPI test and is highly sensitive at all stages of syphilis; it is particularly valuable in early primary untreated infections when 85 per cent or more cases react positively. Very occasionally the FTA ABS test gives false positive findings when the TPI test is negative; this may occur with sera containing abnormal globulins or the rheumatoid factor.

Of the classes of immunoglobulins that take part in the TPI and FTA ABS the most important is IgG though IgM is detectable in early syphilis.

An *indirect haemagglutination test* for the serodiagnosis of syphilis has been developed by Rathlev (1967). Formolized tanned sheep erythrocytes are conjugated with the antigens of a lysate of the Nichol's strain of *Tr. pallidum*. It is claimed that the test is simple to carry out and the results of the reaction between antibody and the coated cells give clear-cut and reproducible results. The specificity is said to be similar to that of the TPI test and the sensitivity comparable to that of FTA tests.

Cerebrospinal Fluid

For the investigation of a case of neurosyphilis 5 ml of cerebrospinal fluid taken in two moieties into dry containers are needed. The fluid in the second container (which must be labelled as such) is less likely to be contaminated by blood and the cells in it should be counted as soon as possible because even a delay of one hour is enough to permit them to disintegrate.

The investigations include all those routinely used in other infections of the nervous system together with the Lange gold curve, the Wassermann test and if required the TPI test. The cell count and the protein content give most information about the activity of the disease process and are the first to return to normal as the activity of the infection subsides. The Wasser-mann and Lange curve tests are the last to revert to normal.

Because antibodies do not normally traverse the blood-brain barrier positive Wassermann and TPI tests in the cerebrospinal fluid indicate only the activity of the infection in the nerve tissues with the local formation of immune globulins.

CHEMOTHERAPY

Penicillin is lethal to treponemes in a concentration of 0·003 unit per ml and is the drug of choice. In early syphilis the penicillin blood levels need to be maintained for two weeks and in late syphilis 4 to 6 weeks are needed. Other antibiotics are occasionally used. A prolonged follow-up is required to be sure of the effectiveness of the treatment.

EPIDEMIOLOGY

During the second world war the incidence of all venereal diseases rose to high levels and by 1947 in England and Wales the number of new clinical, infectious cases of primary and secondary syphilis had reached a peak of 23 878. When penicillin came into general use the number of new cases declined rapidly and during the years from 1964 onwards has remained at levels between 1 732 and 2 118. In recent years there has been little tendency for the incidence of syphilis to increase in Britain although that of gonorrhoea has risen steeply to surpass the peak of its war-time levels. The number of patients with gonorrhoea attending clinics is now 40 times greater than the number attending with syphilis, probably because gonorrhoea in women is often a symptomless infection and transmission of infection can occur very frequently without its source being traced. The primary chancre of early syphilis is obvious in the male, although less easily detected in the female; the male:female ratio is 4·3:1. Syphilis has occasionally been transmitted in transfusions of fresh blood: storage of collected blood at 0 to 4°C kills the spirochaetes within 1 to 2 days. Primary syphilis in the male is now found most frequently in homosexuals.

Non-venereal Syphilis

Although syphilis is a venereal disease, conditions with closely similar clinical manifestations occur in circumstances when it seems scarcely possible that infection was transmitted during sexual intercourse. Poor hygiene and the shared use of drinking and eating vessels apparently permit the rapid transmission of the delicate treponemes from person to person particularly by the mouth.

One such condition is *Bejel*, which is found in Bedouin Arabs in Syria and Iraq. Bejel occurs predominantly in young children who show mucous patches and other lesions of secondary syphilis without, as a rule, having any primary lesion. The infection is transmitted by close personal contact or by contaminated drinking vessels or other utensils. In some cases the child has been infected from a primary chancre on the nipple of the nursing mother. Meningovascular lesions may occur as late manifestations but involvement of the central nervous system is rare.

Closely similar diseases which are sometimes referred to as *endemic syphilis* have been reported in Bosnia, West Africa, Southern Rhodesia and in India. Except for the mode of transmission and the epidemiological findings endemic syphilis does not differ essentially from venereal syphilis and the laboratory diagnosis and treatment of both diseases is the same.

TREPONEMA PERTENUE

This spirochaete is the cause of *yaws* (*framboesia*), a chronic disease which is virtually limited to scantily clothed communities living in humid tropical areas in Africa, Asia and Central and South America. The primary lesion, which is practically always extra-genital, takes the form of a painless yellowish-red papule which slowly erodes and becomes an ulcerated discharging granuloma. This 'mother yaw' is followed six weeks to three months later by generalized secondary superficial more exuberant lesions situated on the limbs, neck and at muco-cutaneous junctions on the face and genitalia. The later manifestations of yaws include destructive lesions of bone in about 15 per cent of cases, but cardiovascular and neurological complications are rare. Treponemata abound in the exudates from the lesion and the infection is transmitted by direct personal contact, the spirochaetes entering the new host through small skin abrasions. Frequent skin-to-skin contacts between scantily clothed persons, and contact with freshly contaminated floor mats, permit sufficient opportunities for the delicate treponemes to be transmitted by non-venereal mechanisms. Flies may play a part as vectors of infection and the small gnat, *Hippolates pallipes* has been observed to feed on the open lesions; *Tr. pertenue* persists in the proventriculus of the insect for upwards of seven hours and is regurgitated when the fly feeds again.

Tr. pertenue is indistinguishable from *Tr. pallidum* in morphology, motility, staining properties, ability to provoke anti-cardiolipin and treponemal antibodies, and in its susceptibility to arsenical drugs and antibiotics. Thus the diagnostic procedures and treatment are the same as those used in syphilis. A long-acting penicillin is the drug of choice and a dramatic response follows its use. There is cross-immunity between yaws and syphilis and venereal syphilis is therefore generally absent from communities in which pre-adolescent children become infected with yaws.

TREPONEMA CARATEUM
(*Tr. Herrejoni*)

This spirochaete is the cause of *pinta*, a disease of dark-skinned races in Central and South America, the West Indies and in some of the Pacific islands. The primary lesion, which is extragenital and non-ulcerating, appears as an erythematous, scaly patch about one centimetre in diameter assuming later a psoriatic or licheniform appearance. About five months later secondary lesions of a similar nature appear and in time become characteristically depigmented and hyperkeratotic. Progressive hyperpigmentation of some areas follows to give a third stage of the illness characterized by multicoloured lesions. Involvement of the cardiovascular and central nervous systems occurs late in the disease. *Tr. carateum* can be demonstrated in the skin lesions and in the lymph nodes. Transmission is

non-venereal and usually occurs by direct contact. Like yaws, pinta may be spread by the gnat *Hippolates pallipes*.

Tr. carateum is morphologically indistinguishable from *Tr. pallidum* which it resembles closely in other respects. Immunologically, however, there may be some difference because patients with pinta can contract syphilis and syphilitic subjects have been successfully infected experimentally with pinta. The methods for the laboratory diagnosis and treatment of pinta are similar to those used for yaws and syphilis.

NON-PATHOGENIC TREPONEMATA

Treponema calligyrum (or *gracile*) is a commensal spirochaete that occurs in the normal secretions of the genitals and morphologically resembles *Tr. pallidum*. Its differentiation from the latter is therefore of practical importance in the diagnosis of syphilis. It is not usually found if care has been taken to collect only serum from below the surface of the chancre. It is thicker than *Tr. pallidum* and its spirals are shallower; by the dark-ground illumination method it appears 'glistening', whereas *Tr. pallidum* is 'dead-white'.

Treponema genitalis, which is very similar to *Tr. pallidum*, has also been described as a commensal on the genital mucosa.

Treponema microdentium flourishes in carious teeth, and may be found in the secretion between the teeth. It closely resembles *Tr. pallidum* in morphology, but is shorter (3–6 μm), has shallower coils and is more easily stained by the ordinary methods. *Treponema mucosum* is similar to *Tr. microdentium*, but produces a mucin-like substance. *Treponema macrodentium* occurs in the mouth; it is larger, thicker and more actively motile than *Tr. pallidum* and has less regular coils, usually two to eight in number.

BORRELIAE

These are large, motile, refractile spirochaetes about 10 to 30 μm long and 0·3 to 0·7 μm wide. They have irregular wide and open coils and are easily stained by the ordinary methods; they are

Gram-negative. When examined by electron microscopy borreliae are seen to have multiple fibrils (six or more) attached at each of the two poles and twisted around the body of the spirochaete (Plate 38.3) where they are situated between the cell wall and the cytoplasmic membrane. These spirochaetes are usually highly motile with lashing and rotating movements.

Some borreliae occur as commensals on the mucous membranes of healthy persons. Their presence there sometimes introduces diagnostic difficulties if the individual develops ulceration of the buccal mucous membranes or lesions in the anal or genital regions. However, the morphological characters of borreliae under the dark field microscope are so characteristic that they should easily serve to distinguish borreliae from *Tr. pallidum*.

BORRELIA RECURRENTIS: BORR. DUTTONII

At least two species of borreliae are known as causes of relapsing fever. *Borrelia recurrentis* (*obermeieri*) is the infecting organism of European Relapsing Fever which is transmitted from person to person by the body louse *Pediculus humanus var. corporis*. *Borrelia duttonii* is the cause of West African Relapsing Fever and is transmitted by ticks such as *Ornithodorus moubata* between animals and from animals to man.

These spirochaetes both have the general characters of the genus *Borrelia* and are coarse actively motile spiral organisms that are propelled by lashing, twisting and rotatory movements. Although morphologically almost identical they do represent distinct species. They are about 10 to 20 μm long and 0·3 to 0·5 μm wide. There are five to eight spiral coils spaced at regular intervals of about 2 μm.

These borreliae can be cultivated with difficulty in artificial culture media heavily enriched with serum from various species, but for primary isolation it is usually preferable to inoculate infective material intraperitoneally into mice or young rats.

Pathogenicity

The onset of relapsing fever occurs after an incubation period of three or four days and is sudden, with chills and high fever. This initial febrile episode lasts for three to five days during which time spirochaetes abound in the blood. Then the fever subsides and the patient, although weak, is much improved. During this period the spirochaetes are not found in the blood. After 4 to 10 days the fever returns and during the ensuing relapse the spirochaetes once more circulate in the blood. Ensuing febrile attacks may number between 3 and 10 but they become progressively less severe.

Fatal cases of relapsing fever have necrotic foci containing large numbers of spirochaetes in the liver and spleen and there are haemorrhages in the gastro-intestinal tract and in the kidneys. The brain and meninges may also be involved.

The phenomenon of successive regular relapses is related to the appearance of antibodies that are able to agglutinate or lyse the circulating spirochaetes and thereby terminate the bout of fever. Although these antibodies have the ability to destroy the infecting strain, they are ineffective against new antigenically distinct mutants, a succession of which arise spontaneously in the infecting population of spirochaetes. Each time an immunological variant emerges there is a relapse of the fever until the host has had time to develop new antibodies. The relapsing fever spirochaetes share with the sleeping sickness trypanosomes a high mutability in respect of their surface antigens and thus, by escaping in turn from each of a number of antibody responses, prolong the total period of their presence in large numbers in the blood and thereby increase their opportunity for transmission by blood-sucking insects.

PLATE 38.3. *Borrelia duttonii*. A spirochaete after 30 minutes tryptic digestion. The cell may be approaching binary fission. At the tip (usually just short of it) of the spirochaete 8 or 9 fibrils are inserted by terminal knobs but are freed from the restraint of the cell wall which has been digested away. The fibrils stream away from the spirochaete body retaining the curves of the spiral coils. At the very centre of the spirochaete are inserted the fibrils formed for two daughter cells; they too are displaced laterally. (Stained by PTA. ×10950.)

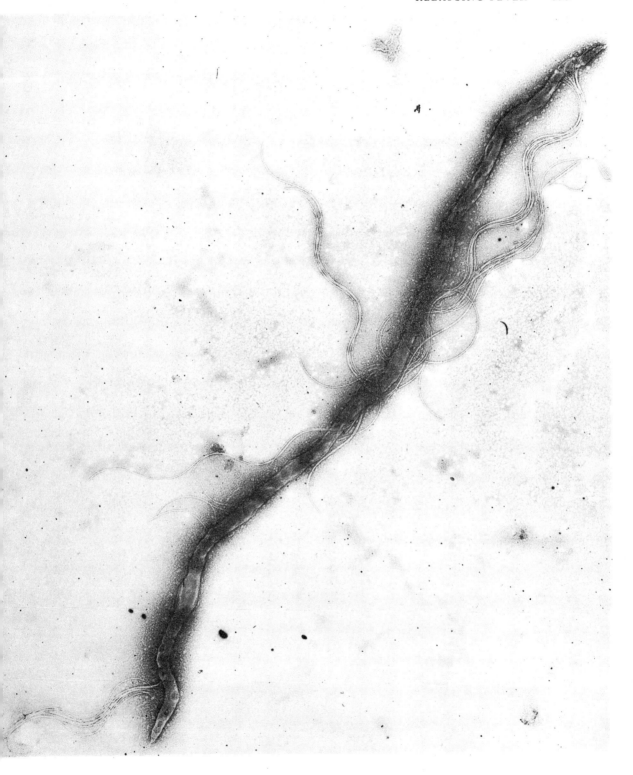

Laboratory Diagnosis

The spirochaetes can usually be found without difficulty in the blood during the pyrexial phases but seldom in the apyrexial intervals. Thick or thin films are made as in malaria diagnosis and stained by Leishman's method. Some workers prefer to stain the films with dilute carbol fuchsin.

If a drop of blood is mounted on a slide under a cover-slip and examined with the oil-immersion lens, the spirochaetes may be detected in the unstained condition and show active movement. A more satisfactory method of demonstrating them, however, is by dark-ground or phase-contrast illumination.

If spirochaetes are not detectable, intra-peritoneal inoculation of white mice with 1·0 to 2·0 ml blood may reveal the infection, the organisms appearing in considerable numbers within about 48 hours in the blood of the animals. A drop of blood from the tail of the inoculated animal is examined daily for a considerable period. An inoculum of 0·2 ml of blood into the chorio-allantoic sac of the chick embryo may also be used.

Lice taken from a case can be examined for spirochaetes by keeping them in a test-tube for a day, then placing them in drops of distilled water on slides and piercing them with a needle so that the haemocele fluid becomes mixed with the water, which is then examined microscopically by dark-ground illumination. The spirochaetes can also be demonstrated in ticks by examining stained films from the stomach contents.

TREATMENT. Penicillin, tetracyclines and chloramphenicol are all effective in the treatment of these infections.

Epidemiology

TICK-BORNE RELAPSING FEVER. Although rodents form the principal reservoirs for *Borr. duttonii* other mammals including pigs, porcupines, opossums and armadillos also harbour organisms of this species. The infection is a zoonosis.

The principal vector in North and South America, Central and South Africa and in Palestine and Iran is the tick. For 24 hours after being ingested the spirochaetes (*Borr. duttonii*) remain in the creature's stomach; then after disappearing for an interval of 6 to 8 days they can be demonstrated in the body cavity and in all the tick's tissues. They persist indefinitely throughout the life of the tick and are transferred through the ova to succeeding generations of ticks. Thus the infective reservoir is formed by both the population of infected ticks as well as by the mammalian hosts and the spirochaetes are able to survive in either for very long periods. There are many areas where infected ticks abound and the infection is transmitted by them from animal to animal or from animal to man. Human cases occur endemically usually as a result of a tick bite or from crushing the body of the tick between the fingers. Tick-borne relapsing fever as a zoonosis does not occur in epidemic form.

LOUSE-BORNE RELAPSING FEVER. In North Africa, Asia and Europe *Borr. recurrentis* is transmitted epidemically from man to man by the body louse. The infection occurs as a result of rubbing crushed lice into skin abrasions. There is no transovarial transmission of the spirochaetes. Numerous epidemics of louse-borne relapsing fever have been recorded and arise in verminous communities in crowded and insanitary conditions in the same fashion as epidemics of louse-borne typhus fever.

Prevention depends on the control of ticks and lice in their ecological environment and on the direction of human communities to avoid contact with these vectors.

BORRELIA VINCENTII

Together with large barred fusiform bacilli of the bacteroides group (*Fusobacterium fusiforme*) *Borr. vincentii* is found in large numbers in the exudates of ulcerative gingivo-stomatitis and ulcerative oropharyngitis (Vincent's angina).

Borr. vincentii is longer and coarser than the treponemes, being 17 to 18 μm long and 0·2 to 0·6 μm thick. There are three to eight loose coils of very variable size and the organism is actively motile. It is stained readily with weak carbol fuchsin and is Gram-negative. It is only cultivated with difficulty and requires an enriched medium and anaerobic conditions.

Pathogenesis

Borr. vincentii and the concomitant fusiform bacillus form a symbiotic combination that is found in small numbers inhabiting the healthy gum, but the numbers may increase enormously when the resistance of the local tissues is reduced. Thus infection with these organisms is superimposed when the superficial tissue is damaged by trauma, deficiencies of vitamins such as ascorbic acid or niacin, or infection with the viruses of herpes simplex and infectious mononucleosis. The infection is often seen as a complication, in granulocytopenia and leukaemia. Occasionally infective emboli containing Vincent's organisms are discharged into the circulation and are conveyed to the lungs where they initiate the formation of pulmonary abscesses.

Laboratory Diagnosis

Smears are made directly from the ulcerative lesions or from swabs and are stained with dilute carbol-fuchsin. A clinical diagnosis of Vincent's infection would be confirmed when very large numbers of both the spirochaetes and the typically barred fusiform bacilli are seen together with the many pus cells that indicate the presence of an active inflammatory process. Cultural procedures are not satisfactory for diagnosis of the infection but may be indicated when other pathogenic organisms such as haemolytic streptococci or diphtheria bacilli may also be present.

CHEMOTHERAPY. Vincent's organisms are highly sensitive to penicillin which is the drug of choice. The organisms are also sensitive to tetracyclines.

Epidemiology

The infection is usually endogenous and its source the patient's own mouth. The disease is thus not ordinarily contagious but sporadic. Epidemics of the infection have, however, been reported in children and young adults. During the First World War the condition was so common in soldiers that it was known as 'Trench Mouth'. Poor nutrition and poor dental hygiene are factors which are thought to facilitate infection and the transmission of a virus (e.g. herpes simplex) in a susceptible population may also play a part.

REFERENCES

RATHLEV, U. (1967) Haemagglutination test utilizing pathogenic *Treponema pallidum* for sero-diagnosis of syphilis. *British Journal of Venereal Diseases*, **43**, 181.

WILKINSON, A. E. (1970) The positive Wassermann reaction: investigation and interpretation. *British Journal of Hospital Medicine*, **4**, 47.

39. Leptospira   Leptospirosis

Throughout the world there exists a group of spiral microorganisms that are characterized by their slender appearance, numerous coils, hooked ends and active motility. They constitute the genus *Leptospira*. Many different types of these organisms exist, some are saprophytic and harmless to man and animals, whilst others are parasitic and potential pathogens. The parasitic leptospires are normally carried in the kidneys of rodents and other small mammals but in some parts of the world domestic animals, e.g. dogs, pigs, goats, cattle and other vertebrates, wading birds, snakes, frogs and tortoises have all been found to be infected although most of them probably play a minor role as carrier hosts. The organisms apparently cause no harm to their normal hosts, but if they are transmitted accidentally to other animals or to human beings, they may give rise to clinical infection, leptospirosis, with disease manifestations that vary from the relatively mild to extremely severe. The most virulent types may cause spirochaetal jaundice known as Weil's disease after the German physician who described the syndrome in 1886.

CLASSIFICATION AND DESCRIPTION

The various types of leptospires are indistinguishable morphologically and their differences in pathogenicity, geographical distribution and animal-host predilection are not sufficiently constant to form the basis for a classification into species. Certain biological tests, e.g. the ability of the saprophytes to grow in simple media without the addition of serum which is normally essential for parasitic strains, show that there may be fundamental differences between the saprophytic and parasitic strains, but the distinction is still not fully understood; strains with the biological characters of saprophytic leptospires have been isolated from cases of leptospirosis of which they have apparently been the cause. For the present, therefore, the genus is considered to have only one species named *Leptospira interrogans*. It consists of two broadly based complexes; one, containing mainly saprophytic strains, is known as *biflexa*; the other complex of parasitic and pathogenic strains is known as *interrogans*. Within each of these two complexes, serological tests have revealed many antigenic variations and on this basis the leptospires are classified as serotypes; certain serotypes with some antigens in common form serogroups. Within the interrogans complex there are 16 serogroups comprising over 100 different serotypes that have been isolated from man and animals (W.H.O. Report, 1967).

Leptospires are spiral organisms, 6 to 20 μm long, and 0·1 μm broad. They usually have hooked ends. The coils are very numerous and so closely set together that they are difficult to distinguish except in the living state by dark-ground microscopy or by electron microscopy. The active motility is mainly rotary with the organism spinning rapidly on its long axis, but it also glides rapidly across the field with either end foremost, occasionally forming secondary spirals and then straightening again into the rigid form that is so characteristic of the group.

The organisms stain poorly with the usual bacterial stains, but they may be demonstrated by the silver impregnation methods of Levaditi and Fontana and in such preparations the primary coils can no longer be seen.

Electron microscopy reveals two axostyles, one originating at either end of the organism and the two overlapping one another slightly in the middle. The cytoplasm is wound around the axostyles and the whole is contained within a clearly defined cell wall (Plates 39.1, 39.2).

Leptospires are readily cultured in fluid media but the parasitic members require the addition of animal serum, or a substitute provided by a fraction of bovine serum albumin. Phospholipids are important nutrient substances for leptospires and it is probable that the requirement for serum depends on its content of phospholipids (Ellinghausen and McCulloch, 1965). Leptospires

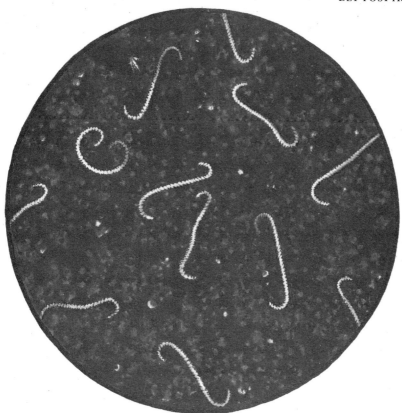

PLATE 39.1. Culture of living Leptospira ictero-haemorrhagiae in Fletcher's medium showing the different shapes which the leptospira commonly assumes during life. Note the very fine coils and the characteristic hooked ends. The brownish granular material of the background is Fletcher's medium. (Dark-ground illumination, ×1 500.) (From original painting by Dr Cranston Low, in Low and Dodds, *Atlas of Bacteriology*, 1947. Edinburgh: Livingstone.)

grow best at temperatures between 28°C and 32°C but for their primary isolation from animal tissues incubation at 37°C may be advantageous. Growth is slow, especially in primary culture and may not be obvious until 2 or 3 weeks after inoculation.

PATHOGENESIS

The clinical manifestations of human leptospirosis vary considerably in form and intensity. On the one hand there may be a mild influenza-like illness, sometimes with meningitis and usually with some degree of renal involvement as evidenced by albuminuria, whilst at the other extreme there may be a severe or fatal disease characterized by jaundice and haemorrhages— Weil's disease. Any of the pathogenic serotypes may cause the mild 'benign' form of leptospirosis, but the severe form is usually due to serotype *icterohaemorrhagiae*. In some parts of the world other serotypes, e.g. *andamana*, *australis*, *bataviae* and *pyrogenes* may also cause spirochactal jaundice.

Leptospires excreted in the urine of infected animals enter the human body through the skin, especially if this is cut or abraded, or through the mucous membranes of the nose, mouth or eyes after immersion in contaminated water. They probably multiply in the blood stream and circulate to all parts of the body, affecting any organ, e.g. liver, kidneys, lungs, meninges, etc., which accounts for the variety of signs and symptoms that characterize the disease. As antibodies

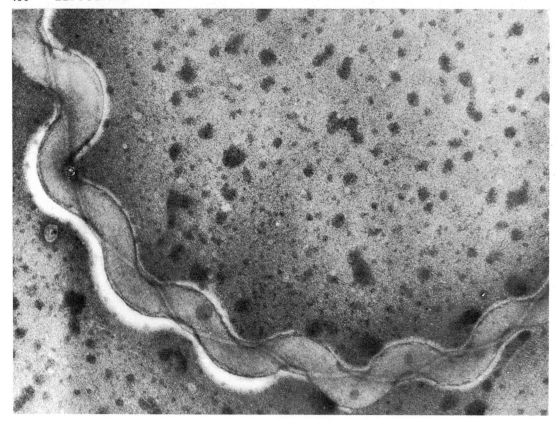

PLATE 39.2. An intact leptospira. The appearances seem to indicate that there are two axostyles, one of which passes over and under, while the other goes under and over the coils of the cytoplasmic cylinder. (×62 250.)

develop the organisms disappear from the blood and tissues, except from within the kidney cortex where they colonize the lumen of the convoluted tubules and remain during convalescence for several weeks.

LABORATORY DIAGNOSIS

Because of the variability in the clinical manifestations of infection and the frequent absence of jaundice, leptospirosis should always be considered in cases of undiagnosed pyrexia (PUO), especially when the patient could have been exposed to infection through the nature or place of his work or in some other way. After an incubation period of 5 to 12 days, there is a phase of leptospiraemia with later a phase of leptospiruria. Antibodies are detectable from the end of the first week onwards. The following points should be borne in mind when attempting a laboratory diagnosis.

1. The diagnosis is fully confirmed if leptospires are isolated in blood culture. Two or three drops of the patient's blood should be added to each of a number of small screw-capped bottles containing 3 ml of a suitable liquid medium. Successful isolation provides an opportunity for identification of the serotype responsible for the infection. However, leptospires are present in the peripheral blood during the first week of the disease only, rarely after the eighth day, so that by the time leptospirosis is suspected as a possible diagnosis, it may no longer be possible to obtain a positive blood culture. Peritoneal inoculation of guinea-pigs or golden hamsters with whole blood during the first few days of the illness followed some days later by cardiac

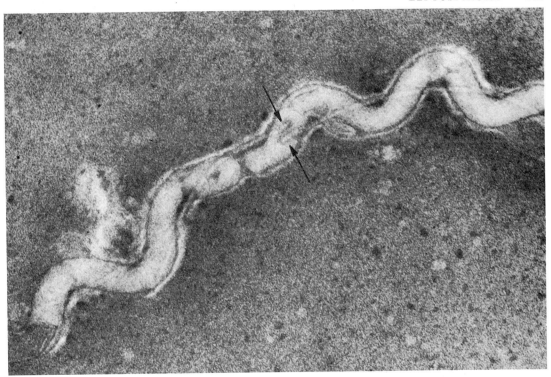

PLATE 39.3. A dividing leptospira. The cytoplasm has separated into two parts and the cell wall is just beginning to form a transverse septum. Two axostyles are clearly visible, both being inserted close to each other in the tip of the lower spirochaete. (× 60 000.)

puncture and culture of a few drops of the animal blood is an alternative method of isolating the organism. This is of particular value if a canicola infection is suspected.

Leptospires occasionally may be seen by dark-ground microscopic examination of the patient's blood, but care must be taken in their recognition because filamentous artefacts, called myelin bodies, which are derived from the red blood cells, may simulate them.

2. Leptospires may be present in the urine during the second week of illness and continue to be excreted intermittently for 4 to 6 weeks. They are most likely to be seen during the second and third weeks by dark-ground microscopic examination of the centrifuged urinary sediment. Direct culture of urine is not usually successful because of the presence of contaminating organisms, but positive isolates may be obtained by intraperitoneal inoculation of freshly voided urine into laboratory animals followed by culture of heart blood 4 to 5 days later. Because leptospires are very sensitive to acid urine and may be lysed by antibodies present in the urine, the urine should be examined for leptospires immediately after being voided.

3. For identification of the serotype of a newly isolated strain use is made of agglutination and agglutinin-absorption tests with a homologous antiserum prepared by immunizing a rabbit with a living culture of the unknown strain. The results should be compared with those obtained in parallel tests made with standard strains and their antisera. This is a specialized and time-consuming technique, and is best carried out in one of the WHO/FAO Leptospirosis Reference Laboratories to which all new isolates should be sent for identification.

4. Specific antibodies are detectable towards the end of the first week of the illness and increase

during the second to fourth weeks, after which they begin to decline. Residual amounts of *agglutinating* antibody may remain for many years after the infection has occurred. It is advisable to examine a specimen of the patient's serum during the early days of the illness and at 4 to 5 day intervals thereafter in order to demonstrate a rise in the antibody titre which is diagnostic of current infection. Several different serological tests are employed to demonstrate the presence of specific antibodies in the patient's serum. The microscopic agglutination test has been used extensively in the past. Since this test is serotype-specific, separate tests have to be set up against each serotype likely to be responsible for the case under investigation, or pools of different serotypes may first be used as screening tests to cover infection by all possible types. Alternatively, a rapid macroscopic slide agglutination test may be used. In the early stages of infection cross-reactions between the various serotypes used as antigens may be misleading, but subsequent tests usually result in the highest agglutinating titre being obtained against the specific infecting organism or a closely related serotype used to represent it in the test.

Other serological tests, that differ from the agglutination test in being genus-specific, have the advantage of being able in a single test to detect in human sera antibodies resulting from leptospiral infection due to any of the serotypes. Of these, the complement-fixation test has recently been widely used. The genus-specific antigen is prepared from a biflexa strain, viz. serotype *patoc.*, with the addition of antigens of several representative pathogenic serotypes. Since the complement-fixing antibodies tend to decline more rapidly than agglutinating antibodies, this test is suitable only for the diagnosis of current infection. The sensitized erythrocyte lysis (SEL) test, which does not require complement titration, may be used as an alternative. Immuno-fluorescence techniques may also be helpful, particularly the indirect method, to demonstrate specific antibody in the patient's serum.

CHEMOTHERAPY

Leptospirosis may respond to treatment with penicillin, streptomycin or tetracycline, pro-

vided these drugs are administered in large enough doses *early* in the infection. When there is impairment of kidney function, as sometimes happens in Weil's disease, it may be necessary to resort to renal dialysis to counteract the uraemia which is the main cause of death in fatal cases of leptospirosis.

EPIDEMIOLOGY

Leptospirosis is a zoonosis. Generally speaking, each leptospiral serotype has its own particular animal host. This is usually a rodent species, although sometimes domestic animals, e.g. dogs and pigs, appear to act as the natural reservoirs. Serotype *icterohaemorrhagiae* is carried normally by the brown rat (*Rattus norvegicus*); serotype *hebdomadis*, the cause of 'seven-day fever' of field workers in countries in the Far East, is carried by the field mouse, *Microtus montebelloi*; whereas serotype *canicola*, the cause of a benign form of leptospirosis, canicola fever, is carried mainly by dogs and pigs, no rodent host having yet been found. In localities where there is an abundant food supply, allowing many different animal species to exist together, as in the rice fields or sugar cane plantations of warm climate countries, one type of leptospire may be carried by a number of different animal species. Rarely, an individual animal may harbour more than one leptospiral serotype. The infected animal may be diseased but commonly acts as a chronic healthy carrier. Man, when infected, is an unnatural, or 'end' host, and does not, ordinarily, transmit the organism to other human or animal hosts.

Leptospires are exceptional among pathogenic microorganisms in being adapted to a mode of parasitic life dependent on transmission in the host's *urine*. The organisms localize in the kidneys of their normal hosts, colonizing the lumina of the convoluted tubules and a proportion of them are washed out in the urine, thereby contaminating the environment. Unlike the saprophytic types, pathogenic leptospires probably do not multiply to any extent outside the animal body, and they seldom survive for more than a few hours if the pH of the water or soil is more acid than 6·8. They also die quickly in salt or brackish water, in polluted water and in sewage, and very rapidly if they become dried. However, if the external conditions are favourable, e.g. in neutral water, slime, mud or moist earth, they may survive for a number of days and sufficiently long to be transmitted to other animals, including man, that may come in contact with them. They enter the body through cuts and abrasions of the skin and mucous membranes. Domestic animals, cattle, pigs and horses become infected through grazing in fields or from fodder contaminated with rodent urine. The infection may then be transmitted from animal to animal in herd epizootics. Man becomes infected from the rodents or domestic animals mainly through contact with water, soil or vegetation contaminated with the animals' urine. Workers in certain occupations are particularly likely to be exposed to infection, so that the disease is to a large extent an occupational hazard. Agricultural workers, miners working in damp coal mines, sewer workers and fish handlers are particularly liable to infection with the serotype *icterohaemorrhagiae*, since the conditions under which they work frequently encourage infestation with rats and moist conditions allow the leptospires to survive for a considerable time outside the animal body.

Because his work takes him into the natural environment of rats and mice, and because he commonly handles damp vegetation and soil which may be contaminated with their urine, the agricultural worker is particularly liable to contract leptospirosis. In some countries these workers go bare-footed in the fields, as in the rice fields and sugar plantations of warm climate countries. The leptospires in the rodent urine that contaminates the soil and vegetation readily penetrate the skin through cuts and abrasions of the feet and legs. In Great Britain, although the greater degree of mechanization on the farm tends to limit this mode of transmission, the majority of cases still occur among agricultural workers (Fig. 39.1).

A serotype known as *canicola* is the cause of 'canicola fever' of man, which often presents as a mild meningitis. It is a common infection of dogs and in them may give rise to a clinically recognizable nephritis, or the infection may be so mild as to escape notice. It has been observed that in a household with a dog (or dogs) the person most liable to infection is the one who tends

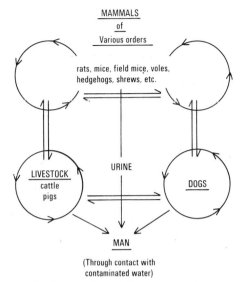

WILD VERTEBRATES

Portals of entry: damaged skin, eyes, nose, mouth.

FIG. 39.1. Transmission of leptospirosis from the main reservoir hosts to man and domestic animals. (Modified from a diagram by Turner, 1967.)

a sick puppy or cleans up its excreta. In spite of widespread infection in dogs, however, (reduced in recent years by the use of vaccine), human cases from this source have been comparatively few. A number of cases have occurred among workers in pig farms; it appears that the infection, after it is introduced into a herd of pigs, may be maintained there for many years, thereby providing a constant source of infection for those who tend the pigs (Coghlan and Norval, 1960).

Leptospiral infection may follow bathing or total immersion in stagnant ponds, canals or rivers polluted by rodents or other animal carriers, e.g. cattle or pigs, and in these cases the organisms probably penetrate the mucous membranes of the eyes and nasopharynx.

Prevention

Because leptospiral infections are derived from contact with infected urine from rodents and other animals, agricultural workers and other persons engaged in occupations that expose them to this type of contamination should protect their skin by wearing suitable gloves and boots when working in the fields, mines or sewers, or when digging ditches, harvesting sugar cane and rice, cleaning out pig-pens, cow-sheds or kennels, etc. Buildings that house animals or act as work places should be proofed against rats and the floors and work benches maintained in a good state of cleanliness and repair. They should be regularly washed down with sodium hypo-chlorite solution so that leptospires, if present, will not remain alive. Families or others who seek recreation in the country by bathing and paddling in country ponds or canals that may be fouled by rodents or domestic animals should be warned of the risks of acquiring leptospiral infection, especially through cuts or abrasions in the skin.

Prophylactic vaccination of certain groups of workers, with leptospiral strains known to be present in the locality, has been successfully carried out in parts of the world where the risk of infection is high e.g. among the rice field and sugar cane workers.

REFERENCES AND FURTHER READING

Coghlan, J. D. & Norval, J. (1960) Canicola fever in man from contact with infected pigs: further observations. *British Medical Journal*, **ii**, 1711.

Ellinghausen, H. C. & McCullogh, W. G. (1965) Nutrition of *Leptospira pomona* and growth of 13 other serotypes. Fractionation of oleic albumin complex and a medium of bovine albumin and polysorbate 80. *American Journal of Veterinary Research*, **26**, 45.

Turner, L. H. (1967, 1968, 1970) Leptospirosis; I, II, III. *Transactions of the Royal Society of Tropical Medicine and Hygiene*, **61**, 842; **62**, 880; **64**, 623.

World Health Organization (1967) Joint WHO/FAO expert committee on zoonoses. 3rd report. *World Health Organization Technical Report Series*, no. 378.

Volume 1 : Part 3
Pathogenic Viruses and Associated Diseases

40. Poxviruses
Smallpox: Vaccinia: Molluscum Contagiosum

The characteristic feature of the diseases caused by the pox group of viruses is the formation of papules, vesicles and pustules in the skin; generalized manifestations of illness may be very severe or entirely absent. In man these viruses cause smallpox, alastrim, vaccinia and molluscum contagiosum. In animals they give rise to cow-pox, swine-pox, monkey-pox (ectromelia) and to similar diseases in all domestic animals except the dog and cat. Myxomatosis in rabbits is the result of infection with a poxvirus. Avian poxviruses cause fowl-pox and similar infections in turkeys, pigeons, canaries and a wide variety of other birds. In avian-pox diseases the lesions tend to be proliferative rather than pustular with the formation of multiple tumour-like masses.

Poxviruses are within the size range 200 by 300 nm to 264 by 332 nm and are large enough to be visible with the light microscope. Most have a predilection for infecting epithelial cells, in which they produce characteristic eosinophilic intracytoplasmic inclusions. Many poxviruses can be cultivated on the chorio-allantoic membrane of chick embryo, where they give rise to pock-like lesions which are easily recognized with the naked eye. Under natural conditions, however, most of these viruses are restricted to a single host, although notable exceptions are the cow-pox and vaccinia viruses which can infect man, cattle and a number of other animals. Many animal pock-producing viruses are closely related antigenically to each other, but are distinct from the avian poxviruses.

THE VIRUSES OF SMALLPOX AND VACCINIA

DESCRIPTION

The appearances of the particles of these two viruses are virtually identical. By optical microscopy they are seen as small spheres 200 to 300 nm in diameter. They can be stained by aniline dyes as in Gutstein's or Paschen's methods but not by the Castaneda technique, which is used to demonstrate rickettsiae or chlamydiae. When dried films are stained negatively with phosphotungstic acid and examined under the electron microscope they are seen as brick-shaped particles with a dense central area covered by a multilayered membrane. The brick shape is probably an artefact because virions seen in ultra-thin sections of infected tissues are oval, measure 250 to 300 by 200 nm in diameter. The internal structure is complex and no precise symmetry can be detected. In the centre of the particle is an electron-dense disk-like structure —a 'nucleoid'—with a biconcave outline due to

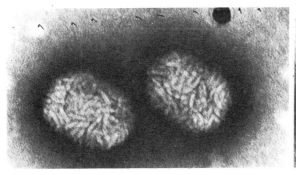
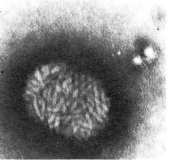

PLATE 40.1. Electromicrograph of vaccinia virus particles. Phosphotungstic acid, ×90 000.

the presence of two 'lateral bodies' adjacent to either side. This nucleoid is surrounded by a zone that has the appearance of a palisade of closely neighbouring hollow tubular structures which are spaced at regular intervals of 4·5 nm. The outer membrane covering the virion conforms to the surface of the palisade and has an irregular mulberry-like surface. Within this membrane is a meshwork of lipoprotein threads looping over the surface to form an interwoven lattice (Westwood et al., 1964).

The vaccinia virus contains approximately 5 per cent DNA, 2 per cent lipid and 2 per cent phospholipid; the remainder is protein. The core of the virion contains the viral DNA together with protein. The DNA is double-stranded and possibly circular; its molecular weight is 160 million daltons and its guanine and citosine content of 36 per cent is exceptionally low (see Table 12.4).

The protein complement of the vaccinia virus is extremely complex and at least 17 components have been identified by diffusion against antiserum in polyacrylamide gels (Joklik, 1966). A number of enzymes have also been identified within the viral cores; these include a DNA-dependent RNA polymerase, a phosphohydrolase, adenosine triphosphatase and ribonuclease activities.

Antigenic Structure

It is very difficult to distinguish the three viruses of variola major, alastrim and vaccinia by serological methods because they all share major common protein antigens. Purified suspensions of variola and vaccinia viruses can be shown to contain two antigens; one, the LS antigen, dissociates from the elementary bodies on standing at refrigerator temperature; the other, the nucleoprotein (NP) antigen, is associated with the virus particles themselves. The LS antigen is a loose combination of the L (labile) and S (stable) components in an elongated protein molecule which is known to have a molecular weight of $240\,000 \times 10^6$ daltons. The L component is inactivated by heat at 60°C, but the S component is stable at 90°C or above. Antibodies to the LS antigen precipitate and also fix complement with their homologous antigens,

but they do not protect an animal from the effects of the vaccinia virus nor do they neutralize the virus in laboratory tests. The NP antigen can be extracted from elementary bodies with dilute alkali; it is known to contain 6·0 per cent deoxyribonucleic acid and is a serologically specific component of the vaccinia virus. A soluble protective antigen shared by the vaccinia and rabbitpox viruses has been described by Appleyard, Zwartouw and Westwood (1964); it combines with the neutralizing antibody in hyperimmune sera and has a molecular weight of 100 000 to 200 000 daltons. It is developed during the early stages of the reproductive cycle of the virus, is smaller than the virus itself but is too large to be dialysable. The relationship of this protective, or 'serum blocking' antigen to the NP antigen, the haemagglutinin or other antigens detected by agar-gel precipitation tests is not yet decided.

Haemagglutination

Preparations of the vaccinia and variola viruses do not agglutinate the red blood cells of mammals, but erythrocytes from about 60 per cent of domestic fowls are sensitive to the virus. The haemagglutinin is smaller than the virus particle and can be separated from it by centrifugation; it is 65 nm in diameter and is mainly composed of lipoprotein. There is no loss of infectivity when the haemagglutinin is removed from virus preparations. The haemagglutinin is heat-stable and is distinct from the virus particles and from the LS and NP antigens. Antibodies to the haemagglutinin are developed soon after smallpox and after vaccination; they are not related to either neutralizing or LS antibodies.

Host Range

The host range of the smallpox virus is limited to the primates; apart from man, monkeys are the only animals susceptible to natural infection. Other animals are only slightly susceptible, and of these the rabbit was once used in Paul's test for the smallpox virus which was inoculated into the scarified cornea and produced a keratitis. Intracytoplasmic inclusions (Guarnieri bodies) in epithelial cells are characteristic of infection with variola and vaccinia viruses; they are round or oval, eosinophilic and there may be one or more in any one infected cell. The vaccinia virus has a much wider host range than the variola virus; calves, rabbits and sheep are all used regularly for the propagation of the virus for vaccine lymph, and monkeys, mice, rats, hamsters and guinea-pigs may also be infected, though they are rather less susceptible.

Both viruses grow well on the chorio-allantoic membrane of the ten-day-old chick embryo, each producing its own characteristic pocks. The variola virus gives rise to white circular plaques of epithelial hyperplasia which are visible to the naked eye 48 hours after inoculation and reach 1 to 2 mm in diameter in 72 hours; these lesions are uniform in size and often lie near the blood vessels of the membrane. The virus of alastrim grows less vigorously in the chick embryo than the variola major virus and is more sensitive to increases of temperature (Dumbell, Bedson and Rossier, 1961).

Vaccinia virus pocks are generally much larger and more variable in size than those of the variola virus; after incubation for 72 hours the majority are 4 to 5 mm in diameter with a definite yellowish colouration. Small seedling pocks beside the larger pocks of vaccinia are characteristic. The poxviruses can be differentiated by the maximum temperature of incubation at which they are able to produce pocks on the allantoic membrane of 12-day chick embryos. Bedson and Dumbell (1961) estimated these 'ceiling temperatures' for alastrim as 37·5°C, variola major 38·5°C, ectromelia and monkeypox 39°C, cow-pox 40°C and rabbit-pox and vaccinia 40·5 to 41°C; there was no correlation between these temperatures and the thermal stabilities of the viruses at 55°C *in vitro*. A useful distinguishing character is that variola virus will multiply and produce pocks at 38·25°C, whereas alastrim virus will not multiply or produce any lesions at this temperature. In general the higher the ceiling temperature of a virus the greater is its virulence for the chick embryo.

GROWTH IN CULTURED CELLS. Vaccinia virus grows readily in many types of tissue cultures; minced tissue suspensions of the Maitland type, explants in plasma clot of chick embryo and rabbit kidney tissues are all highly susceptible. In monolayer cultures of trypsinized human or monkey kidney, or in human amnion of HeLa cells the vaccinia virus produces a marked cytopathic effect within 48 hours of inoculation. In vaccine production bovine embryonic cells have been used successfully for virus propagation. Sometimes the cell damage seems to be due not to living virus but to some toxic action brought about by the synthesis of virus-induced proteins. In suitably prepared monolayer cultures of monkey kidney or other cells the virus gives rise to plaques visible to the naked eye.

The variola virus also grows in various types of tissue cultures but its lesions are smaller and develop more slowly.

The molecular biology of the process of the vaccinia virus growth cycle was described in Chapter 13. Multiplication is essentially intracytoplasmic and after the virion has been attached to the host cell and engulfed it is uncoated and the viral DNA is released. The process of the synthesis of the components and their assembly to form mature virion occupies about six hours. The virus is usually released by the disintegration of the host cell.

Viability

Variola virus is very stable and survives in exudates from patients for many months; living virus has been recovered from crusts kept at room temperature for over a year. It can be preserved in sealed ampoules at 4°C for many years and indefinitely by freeze drying. Vaccinia virus in calf lymph stored in the dark at −10°C retains its activity for at least three months. Between 0° and 10°C vaccine lymph retains its potency for at least 14 days, but at temperatures above 10°C its activity may be lost after seven days. Freeze-dried vaccine kept under an atmosphere of nitrogen at 37° and 45°C maintains its activity for two years and at 4°C indefinitely. The virus is destroyed by moist heat at 60°C in 10 minutes, but in the dry state can resist 100°C for 5 to 10 minutes. Both viruses withstand 1·0 per cent phenol at 4°C for several weeks, but are killed by it within 24 hours at 37°C. Ultra-violet light, X-rays and gamma rays are rapidly lethal; 0·01 per cent potassium permanganate and 50 per cent ethyl or methyl alcohol and acetone kill the virus within one hour. As does a pH value of 3.

SMALLPOX

Because the incidence of smallpox is diminishing rapidly, doctors outside the main endemic foci may never see the disease but it is important for them to be aware of it and to be suspicious of its occurrence in feverish patients who have travelled from abroad during the preceding two weeks. Mild infections with barely detectable skin lesions may occur in people who have been vaccinated several years previously.

Sometimes the disease is confused with chickenpox which in its severe form with a confluent rash may resemble variola just as chickenpox may resemble variola in the partially immune subject or have some of the features of variola minor. Doubtful cases should be referred without delay to the Public Health expert and suitable specimens should be sent immediately to the laboratory.

PATHOGENESIS. Smallpox virus enters the body through the upper respiratory tract; it first infects the mucosal cells and soon afterwards is thought to reach the regional lymph nodes. At this stage the patient is not infectious and it is improbable that there is an open lesion in the respiratory mucosa. A transient viraemia may follow with the infection of reticuloendothelial cells throughout the whole body; multiplication of the virus in these cells leads to a second and more intense viraemia which heralds the onset of the clinical illness. The virus can be isolated from the blood in a proportion of cases of smallpox, but the phase of viraemia is short-lived except in fulminant cases, and by the end of the second day of the fever the virus can no longer be detected in the blood. During the first 3 to 4 days of the fever the virus multiplies in the epithelial cells of the skin; focal lesions are formed which give rise to the rash, and in 2 to 3 days macules appear in typical centrifugal distribution and progress to papular, vesicular and pustular stages. Because of its low 'ceiling' temperature for growth, the virus after the onset of fever probably is able to grow only in the cooler tissues, particularly in the skin. Smears made from the early papular lesions show very large

numbers of virions and in the later stages crusts from the pustules still contain living virus.

Classical smallpox (variola major) has a case fatality which varies from 5 to 10 per cent in previously vaccinated patients to 10 to 50 per cent in unvaccinated cases. In fulminating and haemorrhagic cases the case fatality is over 90 per cent. Variola minor (alastrim) is much less severe than variola major at all stages of the illness, the rash is less profuse, the fever of shorter duration and the fatality rate is below 1 per cent. Variola minor may be indistinguishable from a mild case of variola major in a well vaccinated person. In other vaccinated contacts the infection may give rise only to fever and symptoms similar to those of the pre-eruptive phase without progressing further, a condition known as *variola sine eruptione*.

LABORATORY DIAGNOSIS

Often there is great urgency in confirming the clinical diagnosis of smallpox. The collection of the necessary specimens at each stage of the disease is described elsewhere (Vol. II, Chap. 10) and also in the Ministry of Health Memorandum (1972).

MICROSCOPY. The method of choice is the examination by electron microscope of skin exudates stained negatively with phosphotungstic acid (Christie *et al.*, 1961). The smallpox virus is easily recognized from its characteristic morphology and it is readily distinguished from the enveloped icosahedrons of the chickenpox virus. The investigation can be completed within two hours of the arrival of the specimen in the laboratory.

If access to an electron microscope is not possible smears from early lesions can be stained by Gutstein's alkaline methyl violet or by Nicolaus' method and large numbers of virions can be seen by the oil immersion objective of the light microscope. They are about 300 nm in diameter and can be demonstrated in some 60 per cent of cases of smallpox. Smears taken from pustules are unsatisfactory because they contain so much cellular debris and leucocytic granules that the virions cannot be recognized. Smears may also be examined by the indirect immunofluorescence technique (Murray, 1963). Smears

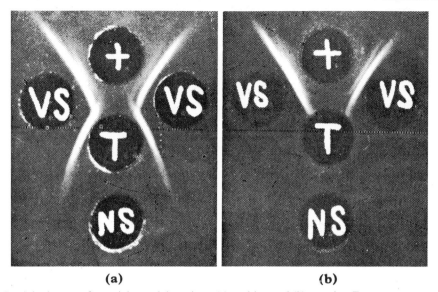

(a) **(b)**

PLATE 40.2. Precipitation tests for variola-vaccinia antigen. (a) positive, and (b) negative. T = test extract; + = positive control extract of variola crusts; VS = antivaccinal rabbit serum (undiluted and 1/2); NS = normal rabbit serum. (By courtesy of Bedson, S., Downie, A. W., MacCallum, H. O. and Stuart Harris, G. H. (1967) *Viral and Rickettsial Diseases of Man.* London: Arnold.)

made from chickenpox vesicles contain only sparse numbers of virions but multinucleate giant cells are quite often present and are characteristic of varicella.

SEROLOGY. Serological methods are valuable for the rapid detection of viral antigens in exudates from the skin lesions. Agar gel diffusion and immuno-electro-osmophoresis tests are useful and the materials need to be set up against high titre antivaccinial and anti-varicella-zoster sera. The results can be read with certainty after only a few hours (Dumbell and Nizamiddin, 1959). The complement-fixation test is very sensitive in detecting the variola virus antigens and is positive in over 90 per cent of smallpox cases (Downie and Kempe, 1969). This test, like the precipitation agar gel test and the microscopic techniques, does not distinguish between variola and vaccinia viruses. The complement fixation test has the disadvantage that skin exudates, heavily contaminated with bacteria, may confer anticomplementary properties on antigens made from them.

CULTIVATION. The virus can be isolated from the skin lesions or from the blood in the pre-eruptive phase of the illness. A suspension of vesicle fluid or ground-up crusts or serum from the blood is inoculated on to the chorio-allantoic membrane of 10- to 12-day-old chick embryos; after 48 hours small white pocks are present and by 72 hours they are 2 mm in diameter and identifiable as specific smallpox lesions. This procedure detects the virus in over 90 per cent of smallpox cases and serves to distinguish the virus of variola from that of vaccinia. All the methods, microscopy, serology and culture, must be used together so that the tests may serve to check each other. The combined use of these tests also helps to overcome the occasional difficulties which may arise from anticomplementary activity by the crust-suspension or the appearance of non-specific lesions on the chorio-allantoic membrane. The results of the tests provide a very sensitive indication of the presence of the variola virus and give reliable confirmation or exclusion of the clinical diagnosis.

ANTIBODY TESTS. Antibodies in patients' sera may be titrated by their power to neutralize the capacity of the vaccinia virus to form pocks on the chorio-allantois (Boulter, 1957). Another method employs complement fixation with an antigen prepared from vaccinial lesions in the rabbits' skin. Antibodies do not usually appear in the serum in smallpox until the eighth day of the disease, and the test is seldom of diagnostic value. As 30 to 40 per cent of persons vaccinated within 8 to 12 months give a positive result in neutralization tests, this method is only of limited value. Precipitation in agar gel against vaccinial or viral antigen is positive in most smallpox patients and negative in nearly all vaccinated persons.

Vaccination may provide a useful diagnostic procedure because less than 10 per cent of cases can be successfully vaccinated on the first day of the rash in smallpox, and none after the sixth day.

EPIDEMIOLOGY

The origin of infection in smallpox is a patient suffering from the disease. Infected particles may be inhaled directly by the susceptible contact. The virus may also be transmitted indirectly by clothing, bed-linen, utensils or dust, and there have been many occasions when workers in hospital laundries have contracted the infection from contaminated bed-linen. Patients are not infective during the incubation period of the disease, but from the time of the first appearance of the rash until all crusts disappear they may be a source of the virus. The period of greatest infectivity is the 3rd to the 10th day of the illness. The clinical picture of variola may be considerably modified by previous vaccination and persons who develop only minor symptoms of the disease may provide a dangerous source of infection.

In 1972, smallpox was endemic only in Bangladesh, India, Nepal, Pakistan and parts of Africa, a remarkable reduction since 1967 when smallpox was endemic in no less than 30 countries. In Britain the disease is no longer endemic and outbreaks, when they have occurred, have been traced to importation of the infection from abroad. The rapidity of modern methods of transport has greatly increased the risk of importation. Although smallpox is a highly infectious disease it has not as great an epidemic potential as measles or chickenpox. When the disease has been introduced from abroad into Britain, extensive epidemics have not occurred and spread has usually been limited to close contacts of cases. A full description of the epidemiology and clinical aspects of smallpox is given by Dixon (1962).

The age distribution of smallpox varies in different countries. In non-endemic areas and where compulsory vaccination is practised cases occur mostly in adults. But in highly endemic areas such as parts of India and Africa (and in England in the 18th century) the main incidence is amongst children.

CONTROL MEASURES

When a case of smallpox is diagnosed the patient must be removed to a hospital or unit specially reserved for variola cases and, after admission, strict isolation precautions must be observed. The patient's clothing, bedding, personal possessions and his house should be disinfected with steam or formaldehyde vapour. All persons who could possibly have been in contact with the patient or his possessions during the feverish phase of his illness must be traced, vaccinated and placed under supervision for 16 days. The source of the infection must be sought and the chain of contacts followed back to the first notified case. In such an investigation the results of laboratory tests may often be of great value in the diagnosis of doubtful and of missed cases.

Close contacts of smallpox patients should be vaccinated as soon as possible, but this measure may be effective only if used within 2 to 3 days of exposure. Immunoglobulin prepared from the serum of recently vaccinated persons in a dose of 1·0 g probably affords some protection and it may be used to supplement vaccination of previously unvaccinated close contacts (Pierce et al., 1958).

Strikingly successful results from the prophylactic oral use of the drug N-methylistatin B-thiosemicarbazone (also known as 'Marboran' or 'Methisazone') have been reported by Bauer et al. (1963). It is valuable for unvaccinated family contacts and people who have been heavily exposed to known cases. The drug is used in doses of 2 to 3 g given on successive days; it may be associated with some nausea and general malaise.

Vaccination

The practice of vaccination stems from 1798, when Jenner inoculated a boy on the arm with exudate obtained from a cow-pox lesion on the hand of a dairy-maid. When two months later this boy was exposed to experimental scarification of the variola virus no illness resulted and there was no local lesion. This simple and safe measure for protection against so serious an illness was soon taken into general use all over Europe. At first arm-to-arm variolation was practised, but this was later replaced by the inoculation of vaccinia lymph obtained from the skin of calves infected with the virus. The strains of vaccinia at present used in the production of 'vaccine lymph' are avirulent mutants of obscure parentage.

Vaccine lymph is usually obtained by inoculating the shaved skin of a calf or a sheep with pustular material from the skin of a rabbit similarly inoculated. After 5 to 7 days, the contents of the skin vesicles are harvested, homogenized and finally suspended in 50 per cent glycerol. The bacterial content is further reduced by the addition of 0·4 per cent phenol. The seed virus is maintained by the alternate inoculation of calves and rabbits, a procedure which is thought to hold its virulence at a constant level.

The potency of smallpox vaccines as glycerinated lymph declines at temperatures above 10°C and may be entirely lost after seven days. To overcome this difficulty and to facilitate transport over long distances in hot climates, Collier (1955) devised an improved method of preservation in which the lymph is suspended in 5 per cent bacteriological peptone in distilled water, adjusted to pH 7·4, and freeze dried. Vaccines prepared by this method are especially useful in tropical countries and have been shown to retain full potency, in that they gave 100 per cent successful vaccination rates after storage for periods of 32 and 64 weeks at both 37°C and 45°C (Cockburn *et al.*, 1957).

EGG VACCINES. Smallpox vaccine can also be prepared by cultivating the vaccinia virus on the chorio-allantois of chick embryos, a procedure which has the considerable advantage that it can be done under sterile conditions. Because the virus tends to lose some of its immunizing potency on repeated subculture in the egg, the seed virus used is obtained from calf lymph. Tests of potency and sterility are similar to those required for calf lymph. Although the efficiency of egg vaccines has not yet been assessed in extensive controlled trials, they appear to offer considerable promise. In Sweden an egg vaccine is used for public vaccination and 95 to 97 per cent of successful 'takes' on primary vaccination has been claimed (Dostal, 1962).

TISSUE CULTURE VACCINE. Bovine and chick embryonic tissues have been used for the propagation of the vaccinia virus for smallpox vaccine production (Kaplan and Micklem, 1961). The stability and potency of these vaccines are still in the process of development. In a comparative trial of a vaccine prepared from vaccinia virus propagated in chick embryo fibroblasts with the conventional vaccine, Shaw and Kaplan (1964) reported that the tissue culture vaccine produced fewer successful primary takes and fewer successful re-vaccinations. The vesicles and the size of the lesion with this tissue culture vaccine were smaller than with the conventional vaccine.

Technique of Vaccination

The multiple-pressure method is recommended. The skin is first cleansed with soap and water and allowed to dry. A drop of lymph is then

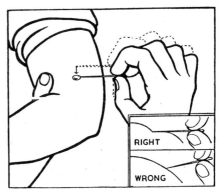

FIG. 40.1. The multiple pressure method of vaccination against smallpox. Notice the up and down motion of the needle and the angle at which it should be held. (Reproduced by permission of the Controller Of Her Majesty's Stationery Office from *Memo on Vaccination against Smallpox*. Ministry of Health (1948). London: H.M. Stationery Office.)

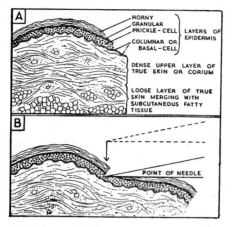

FIG. 40.2. The multiple pressure method of vaccination against smallpox. Diagram of a section of the skin of the arm. The motion of the needle and its final position penetrating only as far as the basal cell layer. (Reproduced by permission of the Controller Of Her Majesty's Stationery Office from *Memo on Vaccination against Smallpox*. Ministry of Health (1948). London: H.M. Stationery Office.)

placed at the site of inoculation and with the side of a Hagedorn needle held parallel to the skin, multiple 'pressures' are made to the skin through the lymph (Figs. 40.1 and 40.2). In this way the inoculum is forced into the deeper layers of the epidermis. The area inoculated may only be one-eighth of an inch in diameter. The number of 'pressures' varies from 10 to 30, e.g. 30 for primary vaccination of infants, 10 for primary vaccination of children of school-age. This procedure involves less risk of septic infection and less severe reactions than may occur with the scarification method. The method also has the advantage that it gives a higher success rate than the scratch method in persons previously vaccinated. A two-pronged instrument instead of the Hagedorn needle is now being widely used in W.H.O. campaigns.

Alternatively a single scratch a quarter of an inch in length may be made through the drop of lymph. Care should be taken to avoid any bleeding. The lymph should be allowed to dry *in situ* and no dressing is required until four to five days after vaccination.

In a person lacking immunity a papule forms at the site of inoculation in 3 to 4 days and this becomes vesicular in 5 to 6 days; in 8 to 10 days the vesicle becomes pustular with a zone of surrounding inflammation; finally the pustule heals with the formation of a crust which is desquamated about the 21st day, leaving a depressed scar. In persons who have been recently vaccinated and possess a satisfactory immunity, there may be no reaction, or a papule may appear more rapidly than in the non-immune subject and resolve without the development of a vesicle. Such reaction which is probably a hypersensitivity response cannot be accepted as indicating an effective immunity. In those who have been previously vaccinated but have lost most of their original degree of immunity, an accelerated 'vaccinoid' reaction is noted: a papule appears quickly, becoming vesicular and pustular more quickly than in the completely non-immune person.

Before a vaccination can be regarded as successful it is essential that the stage of vesiculation should have been reached. Primary vaccination of children in non-endemic areas is best done in the second year of life. There is a rather greater risk of generalized vaccinia and of neurological complications after vaccination in infancy (0 to 1 years) than in children 1 to 4 years old. Re-vaccination in non-endemic countries may be done at regular intervals of 5 to 7 years, for example on entering school and again on leaving, as well as in circumstances when there is a risk of exposure to smallpox. A certificate on a special internationally accepted form showing vaccination in the previous three years is required for entry into many countries.

Vaccination provides a powerful defence against the risk of contracting smallpox and gives a high degree of protection against the risk of death if the disease is contracted. Immunity can be demonstrated 8 to 9 days after vaccination and antibodies reach their peak within 2 to 3 weeks. Protection lasts for a variable period, in general 5 to 7 years pass before re-vaccination is necessary. Experience has shown that case fatality in smallpox is 5 or 10 times greater in unvaccinated than in vaccinated persons.

Complications of Vaccination

Associated with primary smallpox vaccination there is a definite and measurable risk. This varies in degree in different countries and with the extent of the practice of vaccination. In

England and Wales in 1971 there were 50 cases of secondary vaccinial infection; in 28 the virus had been disseminated from a deliberate vaccination and in 22 the virus had been introduced by accident. The risk of complications is much greater than that of contracting smallpox in the community at large and since July 1971, routine childhood vaccination has been discontinued in the United Kingdom.

Postvaccinial encephalitis is the most severe of the complications. Within a fortnight of being vaccinated for the first time the signs of an acute encephalomyelitis may supervene. The incidence of this condition is very low and varies from 1 in 8 000 to 1 in 70 000 vaccinations; the case fatality is up to 40 per cent. Young children in the first year of life and teenage adolescents are the age groups principally affected, and it is advisable to avoid vaccinating at these ages unless there is some very strong indication that protection against smallpox is immediately necessary. Clinically, the symptoms of encephalitis are accompanied by a flaccid paralysis which later becomes spastic. Histologically the characteristic lesion is that of demyelinization and perivascular infiltrations with mononuclear cells. A disease with very similar clinical and histological features has been recorded following variola, measles, varicella and vaccination against rabies.

The aetiology of post-vaccinial encephalitis is quite unknown and the virus has not been demonstrated in the lesions. A possible explanation is that the reaction is an auto-immune phenomenon.

Generalized vaccinia is a rare complication in which the vaccinia virus circulates in the blood. Discrete vaccinial lesions occur in crops over the surface of the body and there is a severe illness with a case fatality of 30 to 40 per cent. The incidence of generalized vaccinia is about 1 in 100 000 vaccinations.

Eczema vaccinatum occurs in people, especially in children, who suffer from eczema either as a complication of primary vaccination or from contact with a recently vaccinated person. Umbilicated vesicles and pustules appear on the eczematous lesions and spread over the healthy skin to give rise to a serious illness with a high fatality rate. As the immune response sets in, the fever subsides, the lesions begin to heal and in favourable cases recovery slowly follows. This illness resembles eczema herpeticum (Kaposi's varicelliform eruption), the cause of which is the herpes simplex virus.

Children who suffer from eczema or chronic skin diseases should not be vaccinated or if it is absolutely essential, they should be given anti-vaccinial immunoglobulin or methisazone at the time of vaccination.

Vaccinia gangrenosa is a very rare complication that is associated with abnormalities of the immune response. It is characterized by areas of deep ulceration and necrosis that extend gradually from the site of the primary vaccination to involve large areas of skin and subcutaneous tissue. The lack of an inflammatory reaction at the edge of the lesions indicates a failure of the delayed hypersensitivity response. The condition may respond to treatment with immunoglobulin but children with this illness usually deteriorate and die within 4 to 5 months.

ABORTION. Because the vaccinia virus may enter the circulation it is able to set up an intrauterine infection of the foetus and bring about abortion but this complication is rare. However pregnancy is a contraindication to vaccination unless there is some urgent reason for immunization against smallpox.

MOLLUSCUM CONTAGIOSUM

The lesions of this mild disease are small copper-coloured warty papules on the trunk, buttocks, arms and face. It is spread by direct contact or by contaminated fomites. In the epithelial cells very large inclusion bodies, mainly acidophilic in their staining reaction, can be observed. The inclusions may reach 20 to 30 μm in diameter and crowd the host cell nucleus to one side, eventually filling the whole cell. When material from the lesions is crushed, some of the inclusions are burst open and from them large numbers of elementary bodies escape. These virus particles have the size, internal structure and morphology of the vaccinia virus. The infection has been transmitted with filtrates to human subjects. The virus produces a cytopathic effect in tissue cultures of human cells but does not multiply readily.

A number of pox infections that primarily affect mammals other than man are occasionally transmitted to man.

Cow-pox

In cow-pox the eruption appears on the animal's teats as small papules which later give rise to vesicles and pustules. The cows themselves are not seriously affected and no generalized symptoms occur. Friction during the milking process often causes the lesions to break and raw tender areas are formed. Crusting follows and the dried scabs fall off in about ten days, leaving an unscarred surface. This disease was first described by Jenner, who realized that the infection could be transferred to the hands of milkers with vesicle formation. In man the lesions may occur in the interdigital clefts, or the back of the hands and also on the fore-arms and face. The lesions resemble those that follow primary vaccination, although they may be more indurated and the vesicle fluid is often blood-stained.

Poxvirus bovis is in size, morphology and resistance to heat and chemical agents identical with the vaccinia virus. It can be distinguished from vaccinia virus by the characteristic red haemorrhagic pocks to which it gives rise on the chorio-allantoic membrane of the chick embryo. The intracytoplasmic inclusions of the cow-pox virus are much larger than the Guarnieri bodies of vaccinia and have a denser matrix; they have also a tendency to distort the shape of the host cell. Serological studies indicate that there is a quantitative difference in the minor antigenic components of the two viruses.

Milkers' Nodes

A pox-like disease that to some extent resembles cow-pox. The lesions on the human skin are firm hemispherical red papules and are derived from the cow's udders. The incubation period in man is five days. Attempts to transmit the infection to laboratory animals have failed.

Contagious Pustular Dermatitis of Sheep (ORF)

The manifestations of this disease are pustules on the lips and round the mouth and on the mucosa of the mouth, the cornea, the feet and legs and other parts of the sheep's body. The infection is transmissible experimentally to lambs by inoculation of the skin with filtrates from the pustules. Human infections with the

Table 40.1. Classification of poxviruses.

Subgroup	Description	Special characters
A	Viruses closely related to variola Variola, alastrim, vaccinia, cow-pox, rabbit-pox, monkey-pox, ectromelia, camel-pox	Morphologically similar. Ether resistant. All closely related antigenically
B	Viruses related to orf Orf (contagious pustular dermatitis of sheep) Milkers' nodes (para vaccinia)	Morphologically similar (entwined pattern), moderately ether resistant
C	Viruses of ungulates Goat-pox, sheep-pox, lumpy skin disease of cattle	Some are partly ether sensitive
D	Avian pox viruses Fowl-pox, pigeon-pox and other bird poxes	Large virions contained in matrix of intracytoplasmic inclusion. Ether resistant, often transmitted by insects
E	Viruses related to myxoma Rabbit myxoma, rabbit fibroma, squirrel fibroma, hare fibroma	Ether sensitive, usually mechanically transferred by insects
F	Unclassified pox viruses Molluscum contagiosum Swine-pox, tanapox, yaba virus, horse-pox	These viruses cannot be placed in subgroups A–E

virus are sometimes seen as granulomata on the hands of those who handle diseased animals, their skins, or their carcases. The causative virus has the same size and morphology as the vaccinia virus, but little is yet known of its other characters. It has not been cultivated in the chick embryo but has been grown successfully in tissue cultures of human amnion. The only susceptible natural host at present available is the lamb. The disease in sheep has been controlled under field conditions by means of a living vaccine consisting of finely ground fully virulent scabs suspended in a 1 per cent concentration of glycerolsaline.

Tanapox

A disease characterized by a localized skin lesion in children. It was first found in Kenya associated with multiple skin lesions in the monkey. It is a poxvirus that is distinct from vaccinia; it will not grow in eggs but it can be cultivated in tissue cultures of cells from monkeys or other primates. It is probably a disease of monkeys and may be transmitted by arthropods (Downie et al., 1971).

Other Animal Pox Diseases

Brief description of other animal pox diseases, e.g. sheep-pox, swine-pox, ectromelia of mice and myxomatosis in rabbits and of some avian-pox infections are given in the 11th edition of this book (p. 378). Attention is particularly directed to the classical studies on the ecology of myxomatosis by Fenner and Ratcliffe (1965). A pox disease with tumour-like swellings on the hands and feet of monkeys has been recently described in West Africa and named *YABA*. The virus resembles vaccinia but has no haemagglutinin and no antigenic relationship with vaccinia virus (Olsen and John, 1970).

REFERENCES AND FURTHER READING

APPLEYARD, G., ZWARTOUW, H. T. & WESTWOOD, J. C. N. (1964) A protective antigen from the pox viruses. *British Journal of Experimental Pathology*, **45**, 150.

BAUER, D. J., ST. VINCENT, L., KEMPE, A. C. & DOWNIE, A. W. (1963) Prophylactic treatment of smallpox contacts with N-methylization β-thiosemicarbazone. *Lancet*, **ii**, 494.

BEDSON, H. S. & DUMBELL, K. R. (1961) The effect of temperature on the growth of pox viruses in the chick embryo. *Journal of Hygiene (London)*, **59**, 457.

BEDSON, H. S. & DUMBELL, K. R. (1967) Smallpox and vaccinia. *British Medical Bulletin*, **23**, 119.

BOULTER, E. A. (1957) The titration of vaccinial neutralizing antibody on chorio-allantoic membranes. *Journal of Hygiene (Cambridge)*, **55**, 502.

CHRISTIE, W. G., DONNELLY, J. D., FOTHERGILL, R., KER, F. L., MILLAR, E. L. M., FLEWETT, T. H., BEDSON, H. S. & CRUICKSHANK, J. G. (1966) Variola minor: A preliminary report from the Birmingham hospital region. *Lancet*, **i**, 1311.

COCKBURN, W. C., CROSS, R. M., DOWNIE, A. W., DUMBELL, K. R., KAPLAN, C., McCLEAN, D. & PAYNE, A. M-M. (1957) Laboratory and vaccination studies with dried smallpox vaccines. *Bulletin of the World Health Organization*, **16**, 63.

COLLIER, L. H. (1955) The development of a stable smallpox vaccine. *Journal of Hygiene (London)*, **53**, 76.

DIXON, C. W. (1962) *Smallpox*. London: Churchill.

DOSTAL, V. (1962) Advances in the production of smallpox vaccine. *Progress in Medical Virology*, **4**, 259.

DUMBELL, K. R., BEDSON, H. S. & ROSSIER, E. (1961) The laboratory differentiation between variola major and variola minor. *Bulletin of the World Health Organization*, **25**, 73.

DUMBELL, K. R. & NIZAMUDDIN (1959) An agar-gel precipitation test for the laboratory diagnosis of smallpox. *Lancet*, **i**, 916.

DOWNIE, A. W. & KEMPE, H. D. (1969) Poxviruses. In *Diagnostic Procedures for Viral and Rickettsial Infections*. Chap. 7, 4th Edn. Edited by E. H. Lennette and N. J. Smith. American Public Health Association Inc.

DOWNIE, A. W. (1970) Smallpox. In *Infectious Agents and Host Reactions*. Edited by Stuart Mudd. London: Saunders.

DOWNIE, A. W., TAYLOR ROBINSON, C. H., COUNT, A. E., NICHOLSON, G. S., MANSON-BAHR, P. E. G. & MATHEWS, T. C. H. (1971) *British Medical Journal*, **i**, 263.

FENNER, F. & RATCLIFFE, F. N. (1965) *Myxomatosis*. Cambridge University Press.

JENNER, E. (1798) An enquiry into the causes and effects of the variolae vaccinae, a disease discovered in some of the western counties of England, particularly Gloucestershire and known by the name of the Cow Pox. Reprinted in *Milestones in Microbiology*. Edited by T. D. Brock (1961). London: Prentice-Hall.

JOKLIK, W. K. (1968) The poxviruses. *Annual Review of Microbiology*, **22**, 359.

MEDICAL MEMORANDUM (1972) Department of Health and Social Security, Scottish Home and Health Department. *Diagnosis of smallpox*. Edinburgh: H.M.S.O.

MURRAY, H. G. S. (1963) The diagnosis of smallpox by immunofluorescence. *Lancet*, **i**, 847.

OLSEN, R. G. & JOHN (1970) *Journal of Virology*, **5**, 212.

PIERCE, E. R., MELVILLE, F. S., DOWNIE, A. W. & DUCK-WORTH, M. J. (1958) Anti-vaccinial gamma-globulin in smallpox prophylaxis.

SHAW, A. & KAPLAN, C. (1964) A field trial of tissue culture smallpox vaccine. *Monthly Bulletin of the Ministry of Health and Public Laboratory Service*, **23**, 2.

WESTWOOD, J. C. N., HARRIS, W. J., ZWARTOUW, H. T., TITMUSS, D. H. J. & APPLEYARD, G. (1964) Studies on the structure of vaccinia virus. *Journal of General Microbiology*, **34**, 67.

WORLD HEALTH ORGANIZATION (1959) Requirements for smallpox vaccines. (Requirements for biological substances No. 5.) *World Health Organization Technical Report Series* No. 180.

WOODSON, B. (1968) Recent progress in poxvirus research. *Bacteriological Reviews*, **32**, 127.

41. Herpesviruses

Herpes Simplex: Chickenpox-zoster:
Cytomegalovirus Infections:
Infectious Mononucleosis: Burkitt's Lymphoma

The herpesviruses are a large group of viruses infecting many animal species and sharing a number of properties although no group antigen is known.

Herpes simplex virus infection of man is widespread, as are chickenpox and zoster due to the varicella-zoster virus. Both of these cause vesicular skin eruptions, but can also involve nervous tissue. The Epstein-Barr virus and the cytomegaloviruses have been associated with the infectious mononucleosis syndrome and as with herpes simplex and varicella-zoster may establish a lifelong association after primary infection. Recurrent or reactivated forms of infection may be seen with some members of the group.

Herpesviruses are responsible for a number of infections of considerable economic importance in domestic animals. Infection with *Herpesvirus suis* is known as pseudorabies or Aujeszky's disease, and affects cattle, sheep and pigs. Equine rhinopneumonitis or equine abortion and avian infectious laryngo-tracheitis are also caused by members of the group. Of considerable interest is Marek's disease of chickens or neurolymphomatosis, an important cause of mortality in the poultry industry. The nature of the disease is discussed in Chapter 49.

DESCRIPTION

The viruses are all icosahedral in structure, with a capsid consisting of 162 hollow hexagonal and pentagonal capsomeres. The diameter of the capsid is between 70 and 100 nm, and mature particles are enclosed within a lipoprotein envelope with an overall diameter of 120 to 150 nm. The virions contain double-stranded DNA with a molecular weight in the range 70 to 100 million units. The DNA of different viruses varies in its content of the bases guanine and cytosine; the highest values are recorded for herpes simplex virus strains. All herpesviruses are relatively thermolabile.

With the exception of the Epstein-Barr virus, members of the group can be cultivated in cell culture, and all produce giant cells and Cowdry type A intranuclear inclusions in infected cultures. The typical inclusion is seen as a central eosinophilic body surrounded by a halo lying within a nucleus with a dense rim of marginated host cell chromatin.

The replication of the viral DNA and assembly of virions takes place within the nucleus of infected cells. The virus can code for many proteins and up to 42 virus specified polypeptides have been detected in cells infected with herpes simplex virus. Complete virions have been shown to contain 27 major proteins. The virus capsid proteins, and an arginine rich internal polypeptide, migrate from the cytoplasm into the nucleus where the viral DNA is enclosed within capsids. Viral glycoproteins are incorporated into cell membranes and much thickening and reduplication of the nuclear membrane can be visualized in the electron microscope. The viral envelope is usually acquired from the inner layer of the nuclear membrane as the virus buds out from the nucleus.

Herpesviruses vary markedly in the extent to which cell free virus is produced in cell cultures. Even the closely related type 1 and 2 herpes simplex viruses differ in this respect in that type 1 strains are more effectively released from cells. Cell free virus is difficult to prepare with varicella-zoster and the cytomegaloviruses. The Epstein-Barr virus has been grown only in cells derived from Burkitt lymphoma tumours or cultures of peripheral leukocytes.

Herpes simplex virus, herpesvirus B, varicella-zoster virus, the cytomegaloviruses and the Epstein-Barr virus with their associated diseases are discussed in this chapter.

419

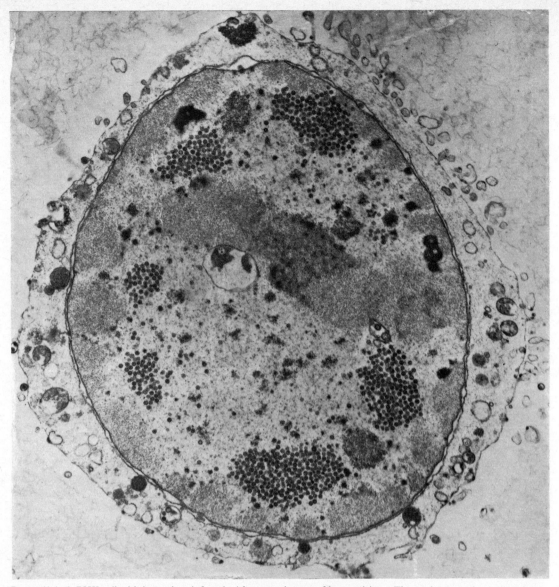

PLATE 41.1. A BHK cell with its nucleus infected with many clusters of herpesvirions. The nuclear membrane has characteristically been split into at least two layers and is greatly thickened. Some of the virions have moved into the cytoplasm and are free but within the cytoplasm. (× 9 300.)

HERPES SIMPLEX VIRUS (HERPESVIRUS HOMINIS)

The virus of herpes simplex has been studied for many years; despite this, many questions remain unanswered concerning the association between herpes simplex virus and man. The virus is widespread and as with other members of the group, infection may take several forms ranging from an acute illness to a lifelong latent or chronic state.

DESCRIPTION

The virus has the general structure and chemical composition as already described. In contrast to

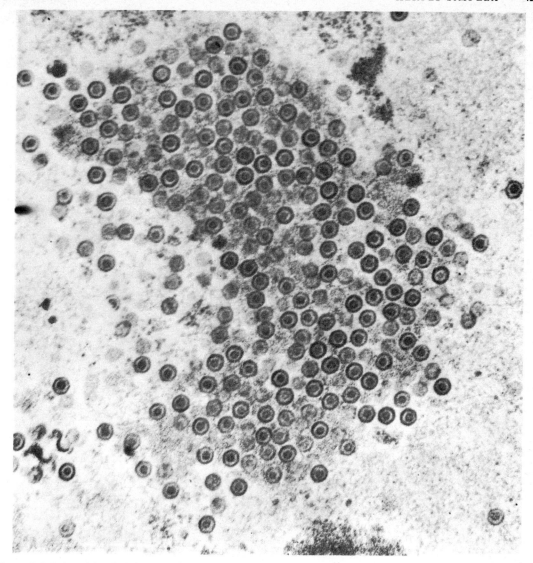

PLATE 41.2. Enlarged detail of Plate 41.1. A cluster of virus particles in the cell nucleus, some fully mature and others not fully developed. (× 60 000.)

other members of the group, herpes simplex virus can be grown in cells from a wide variety of species and can infect a variety of animals. The rabbit was the first species used for this purpose; it may be infected experimentally by several routes as may guinea-pigs and mice; the animals show a range of effects from localized skin lesions to meningoencephalitis. Herpes simplex virus also grows on the chorio-allantoic membrane of the developing chick embryo.

After 2 to 3 days' incubation lesions or pocks develop on the membrane; these represent foci of viral infection. There are two types of herpes simplex virus and they can be distinguished by the size of pock which they produce. Type 1 strains give rise to small white pocks which are almost always less than 0·75 mm even after 7 days' incubation and only involve the superficial epithelial cells; type 2 strains produce pocks greater than 1·00 mm and often as large

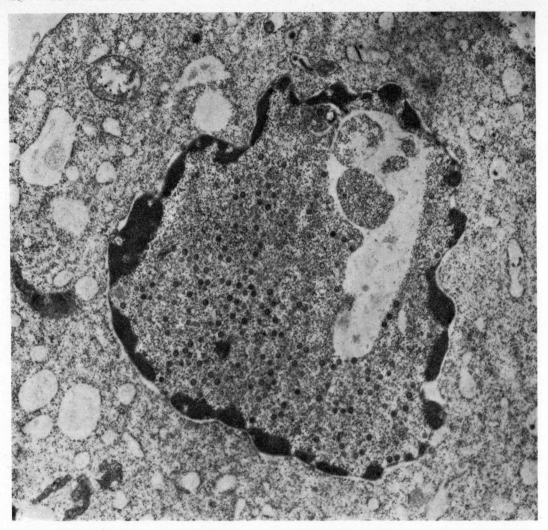

PLATE 41.3. A BHK cell infected with the herpes simplex virus. The nucleus contains many herpesvirus particles. The nuclear chromatin is condensed peripherally beneath the nuclear membrane. Only a few virions can be seen in the cytoplasm. Lead citrate. × 16 000.

as 2·0 mm after 7 days' growth. The large pocks are necrotic, and the virus spreads to sub-epithelial layers of the membrane. However, herpes simplex virus may be grown most conveniently in cultures of fibroblast and epithelial cells. Primary rabbit kidney and baby hamster kidney cells are most susceptible to the virus, although human amnion, human embryo, HeLa and HEp-2 cells can all support its growth. Growth is rapid and within 24 hours a cytopathic effect (CPE) may be visible, presenting as rounded, ballooned cells in foci which expand and eventually involve the entire cell sheet. Some virus strains may give rise to fusion of infected cells—syncytial formation, and the type of CPE may be used to identify virus strains. Virus is released from infected cells into the culture fluid, however, virus may spread directly from cell to cell despite the presence of specific antiviral antibody in the culture medium. Infected cells may show Cowdry type A inclusion bodies within the nucleus.

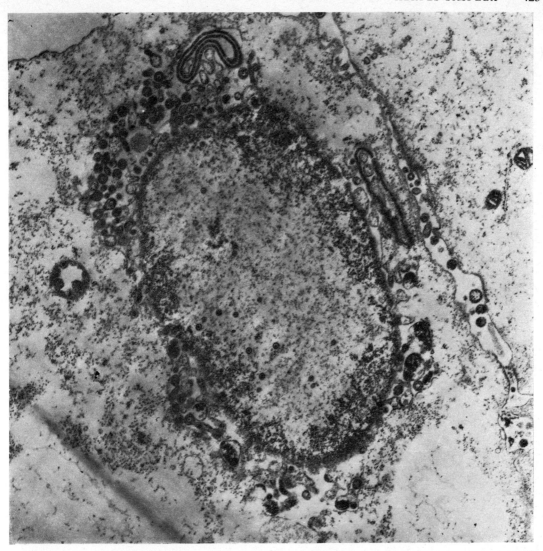

PLATE 41.4. The nucleus of a BHK cell with some of its cytoplasm. This is a later stage of the reproductive cycle of the herpesvirus. Notice that the mature herpesvirions have mostly moved peripherally and lie for the greater extent outside the nuclear membrane in the cytoplasm, where they are associated with thickened and folded regions of the nuclear membrane. Lead citrate. × 16 000.

Although type 1 and 2 strains share some antigens they can be separated into two types by neutralization tests.

Both type 1 and 2 viruses mature within the nucleus, but type 2 strains produce filaments or microtubules of unknown composition. Cell cultures infected with type 2 strains give poorer yields of virus than cultures inoculated with type 1 viruses. They also differ in their heat stability; type 2 strains are inactivated more rapidly than type 1 strains, at any temperature from 4° to 37°C. The two types are associated with different sites of infection in patients (see below); type 1 strains are associated with the mouth, the eye and the central nervous system and skin infections above the waist, whilst type 2 strains are associated with genital and associated sites of infection.

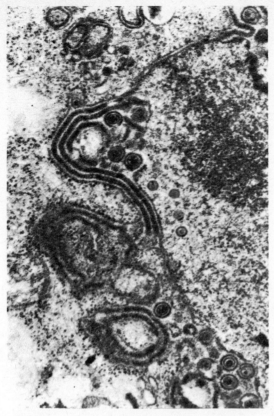

PLATE 41.5. The edge of the nucleus of a BHK cell infected with the herpesvirus. Some virions are seen within the nucleus and are associated with the altered cellular membrane. Lead citrate. × 32 000.

PATHOGENESIS AND CLINICAL FEATURES

The typical lesion produced by herpes simplex virus is the vesicle. An initial proliferation of epithelial cells is followed by degeneration and vesicle formation. The base of the vesicle contains giant cells and many of the nuclei of these cells contain the eosinophilic (Cowdry type A) inclusion body. The roof of the vesicle breaks down and an ulcer is formed; on the skin, the ulcer crusts over and heals. Primary herpetic infection usually involves the mucous membrane of the mouth, but may include the mucutaneous junction of the lips, the skin of the face, nose or any other site including the eye and genital tract. It may also involve the CNS, as meningitis, encephalitis or meningo-encephalitis. After primary infection, the virus probably remains in the host in a latent state or as a chronic infection and, over a period of many years, may reappear as a reactivated or recurrent infection. In a rare form of the disease in the newborn, almost all organs of the body show evidence of infection.

The age at which primary infection occurs depends on environmental factors. Classically, the infection presents as an acute febrile stomatitis in young, pre-school children. Vesicular lesions which rapidly ulcerate can be found in the front part of the mouth and on the mucous membrane of the tongue and cheek. Ulceration of the gums may occur and the condition may be described as an acute ulcerative gingivostomatitis. Vesicles may also develop on the lips and skin of the chin, or even on the fingers as the virus is spread in saliva. Cervical lymphadenopathy is usually present, and the child is miserable for a period of 7 to 10 days before the lesions heal. However, the majority of primary infections are unrecognized; the child may show only a low fever and the most likely diagnosis is 'teething'. Herpetic stomatitis also occurs in older children and young adults. If laboratory studies are performed, the virus may be recovered from the saliva or oral lesions and antibody to herpes simplex virus develops. Almost all oral strains of virus are type 1.

Recurrent or reactivated infection occurs at any of the sites listed above, except that recurrences within the mouth are rare. By far the commonest form of recurrent infection is the fever blister or cold sore (herpes febrilis). This is located most frequently on or around the lips (herpes labialis) or the anterior nares or cheek (herpes facialis) but may involve any skin or mucous membrane surface including the eye. There is also some evidence that recurrent infection of the central nervous system can occur. Reactivation of the virus may be achieved by a variety of stimuli such as sunlight, menstruation and, most commonly, fever, especially that associated with malaria, meningococcal and respiratory tract infections. Allergic reactions and stress have also been implicated. The mechanism is not completely understood. One explanation is that during primary infection in the mouth, the virus may ascend sensory nerve fibres to the sensory ganglion; in the nerve cells a latent non-cytolytic infection results and from this site the virus may descend along the nerve to affect the area of skin supplied by the nerve. In this way, recurrences on the face tend to be at one site in any individual. On other parts of the body a similar mechanism may operate. It is possible that the virus remains latent in skin or mucous membrane cells, but attempts to demonstrate virus within skin cells at a site subject to recurrent infection have failed. The development of recurrences after surgical interference in branches of the trigeminal nerve for intractable neuralgia supports the idea that the virus may be associated with the sensory ganglion. In this behaviour herpes simplex virus resembles the varicella-zoster virus. The exact form of the association between latent virus and cell is unknown, as are the factors which control the reappearance of the virus. There is evidence that in some sites, e.g., the mouth, the eye and genital tract, a chronic low grade infection may be present in which virus is shed in small amounts over prolonged periods. Reinfection could then occur at a related site, e.g., the lips, cornea or vulva and signs and symptoms develop. A puzzling feature of all recurrent infections is that antibody to herpes simplex virus is present in the patient's serum before and after the recurrence and usually no change in antibody titre can be demonstrated. It is likely that cell-mediated immune mechanisms play an important part in the control of recurrent infections. Immuno-suppressed patients, as for organ transplantation, may suffer a severe form of reactivated infection which does not heal readily.

SKIN INFECTION. In addition to the usual localization of herpetic lesions around the lips and face, nurses, doctors and dentists may contract a herpetic whitlow of the fingers, or a traumatic herpes may follow accidental pricking of the skin with a contaminated needle or other instrument. A severe form of cutaneous herpes may occur in children with eczema and this *eczema herpeticum* is recognized as one form of the Kaposi varicelliform eruption. Virus strains isolated from skin lesions above the waist are usually type 1; strains from some hand and most thigh, buttock and perineal infections are due to type 2.

EYE INFECTION. Involvement of the eye can arise during a childhood primary infection or may result from the transfer of virus from a cold sore via the fingers. Clinically, the patient suffers from a kerato-conjunctivitis associated with corneal ulceration and the production of branching dendritic ulcers; recurrences are frequent and may lead to permanent corneal scarring and impairment of vision. Recurrences may be related to a chronic infection of the lacrimal gland leading to the shedding of small numbers of virus particles in the tears and reinoculation onto the cornea. All eye infections are due to type 1 virus.

CENTRAL NERVOUS SYSTEM. Virus has been isolated from the blood during primary herpetic stomatitis in children and this may be the route whereby virus reaches the brain and meninges. Herpes simplex meningitis or encephalitis may develop, either as a localized necrotizing type or as a diffuse form with widespread involvement of the brain. Herpetic encephalitis has a poor prognosis and if the patient survives, considerable mental defect may remain. In some cases CNS infection may be due to reactivation of a latent infection. With the exception of virus strains isolated from the newborn, most CNS infections are caused by type 1 virus.

GENITAL TRACT. Both types of herpes simplex virus can infect the genital tract, although the usual association is with type 2 strains. At first the lesions are vesicular but they quickly rupture to produce raw ulcerated areas. In the male, the glans and shaft of the penis are the most frequent sites of infection, while in the female the labia and vagina (vulvovaginitis) or cervix, may be involved. Penile herpes and vulvovaginitis may be encountered in young children—usually in association with infection elsewhere, as in the mouth. In the sexually active age group, however, genital herpes behaves as a venereal disease, the spread of which is aided by the frequent recurrences. The main reservoir of the virus is probably the cervix where a chronic infection can be established leading to reinfection of the vagina and the labia. One serious result of genital infection in the female is that the virus may be transferred to a newborn infant during birth. If the maternal infection is recent the baby may be unprotected by maternal antibody and may die with a generalized infection. Type 2 virus is usually recovered from these infants. A further possible late effect of cervical infection is the development of carcinoma of the cervix (see below).

LABORATORY DIAGNOSIS

Direct demonstration of typical herpes virions is possible in the electron microscope. Vesicle fluid is a suitable specimen for examination, although brain biopsy material has also been examined in this way, but it is impossible to distinguish between herpes simplex virus and varicella-zoster virus by this method. Immuno-fluorescent staining of herpes specific antigens can also be used to detect the presence of the virus.

Virus isolation may be attempted from vesicle fluid or scrapings from the base of lesions. Infections of the CNS are difficult to diagnose, because virus may be demonstrable only in brain tissue. Many types of cell culture are susceptible, and rounding and ballooning of cells is usually evident within 24 to 48 hours. Virus is identified by neutralization with type specific antiserum. The appearance of the CPE may also be useful in typing the virus since type 2 strains tend to produce syncytia even on first isolation. The virus can be isolated on the chorio-allantoic membrane of chick embryos; the size of the pock, especially after prolonged incubation, may indicate the type of virus. The type of virus can be established by neutralization or immuno-fluorescent tests.

Complement fixation and neutralization tests are useful in diagnosing primary infections when a significant change in antibody titre can be expected. However, serological studies may be inconclusive in recurrent infections as changes in antibody titre are seldom demonstrable.

TREATMENT. Herpetic infections are among the few viral infections against which specific chemotherapy may be of value. The herpes-viruses are all susceptible to the inhibitory effect of 5-iododeoxyuridine (Idoxuridine) and herpetic infections of the eye in particular can be treated by the local application of this drug (Chap. 13). Treatment may reduce the severity and duration of symptoms although the relapse rate in recurrent ocular infection is apparently unaltered, perhaps because the lacrimal gland is the seat of infection. Treatment of skin infections has been attempted, but has not been completely successful, probably because the compound dissolves poorly in water so that it may be difficult to achieve effective concentrations at the site of infection. The acute tenderness of some genital lesions may be eased by the application of iodoxuridine as an ointment.

Systemic therapy with iodoxuridine has been tried in patients with herpetic encephalitis with uncertain results.

EPIDEMIOLOGY

Herpes simplex virus is probably transferred by direct contact, and the spread of infection can be followed among young children, especially in overcrowded conditions with low standards of hygiene. In this way most children acquire infection within the first few years of life. Outbreaks have been recorded, especially in nurseries and children's homes. Spread of infection may not occur so readily among children in better social conditions. As a result, primary infection may be delayed and may then develop in young adults.

A frequent source of infection in the family is a parent, or close acquaintance with a recurrent infection. Virus is plentiful in vesicle fluid, and may also be present in saliva so that eating and drinking utensils can be an important vehicle for both young children and adults. Genital infection, usually with type 2 strains of virus, is a venereal disease. Recurrent infections may occur at any age, but are probably most frequent in the young adult age-group. Recurrences of herpes labialis show a winter seasonal incidence due to reactivation during respiratory tract infections. Serological surveys indicate that more than 75 per cent of the population over the age of 30 years has been infected.

An association between genital infection with herpes simplex virus type 2 and the development of cervical carcinoma has recently attracted much attention. In America, studies among predominantly Negro populations have established that cervical smears with evidence of herpetic infection have a much higher incidence of cervical anaplasia than would be expected in the overall population. Herpes simplex virus antigens have been demonstrated in biopsy material from cervical carcinomas and in some cultures of cervical tumour cells. Further circumstantial evidence was obtained from serological surveys which showed that American, again predominantly Negro, women with cervical carcinoma had a higher frequency of antibodies to herpes simplex type 2 than controls matched for age and race. It has been suggested therefore that cervical herpetic infection, perhaps at some critical early age, e.g., during the first pregnancy, may lead to changes which manifest first as cervical dysplasia and carcinoma some years later.

However, not all serological surveys have confirmed these findings. If the control groups are matched more closely with the carcinoma patients with regard to a number of factors such as age at first pregnancy, then the differences between the carcinoma and control groups decrease. Indeed, no association with antibody to type 2 has been reported in some surveys among patients in areas other than America. The exact relationship, if any, of genital herpetic infection and carcinoma of the cervix, therefore, needs further investigation.

In support of an oncogenic role of the virus, transformation of hamster embryo cells has been reported after exposure to ultra-violet irradiated and chemically inactivated herpes simplex virus.

Herpesvirus Simiae (B Virus)

This virus is related antigenically to herpes simplex virus, but normally infects asiatic monkeys, e.g., rhesus and cynomolgus types. It causes a mild vesicular infection of the tongue and lips analogous to primary herpetic stomatitis in man. The infection rate in monkeys increases markedly if they are kept in crowded conditions. The importance of the virus to man is that he may acquire infection from a bite or after handling infected animals or in the laboratory from infected monkey cell cultures. Within 10 to 20 days local inflammation at the primary site of entry, usually the skin, is succeeded by an ascending myelitis or an acute encephalomyelitis. Very few individuals have survived this severe infection, and then usually with serious residual brain damage.

The virus can be isolated and identified in a wide range of cell cultures. Control of the disease may be attempted by avoiding overcrowding of captive monkeys and thus minimizing the spread of the virus.

VARICELLA-ZOSTER

Infection with varicella-zoster (V-Z) virus takes two forms. Primary infection, or chickenpox, presents as a generalized skin eruption with typical vesicular lesions, and occurs most often in children, whereas zoster, or shingles, is a localized vesicular eruption confined to one or a few dermatomes, and affects adults.

Description

The viruses isolated from patients with varicella or zoster are identical by all biological and serological tests applied; they have the general structure and composition of the herpesviruses. Virus replication takes place in the nucleus of an infected epidermal cell and histological examination of infected tissues may reveal typical Cowdry type A intranuclear inclusions and multinucleate giant cells identical with those of herpes simplex virus. The usual experimental animals and egg tissues are not susceptible to the virus and isolation was reported originally in human embryonic cell cultures. Human amnion and embryonic lung cultures are now most frequently employed for the detection of the virus, but it can grow and produce cytopathic effects in various kinds of human and monkey tissue culture. In most cell cultures cell-free virus may be difficult to detect and infection spreads through the cell sheet by direct transfer of virus to adjacent cells to produce focal lesions, consisting of rounded cells and multinucleate giant cells. Serial propagation of virus therefore usually requires passage of infected intact cells. Preservation of virus infectivity is best achieved by methods which preserve the intact cell. However, in vesicle fluid from clinical lesions, virus is cell-free and may remain viable for many years at $-65°C$.

PATHOGENESIS AND CLINICAL FEATURES

Varicella is a disease predominantly of children, characterized by a vesicular skin eruption. The earliest manifestation is a maculo-papular rash that progresses in a few hours to the vesicular stage. The vesicles characteristically are surrounded by a red rim; the lesions then rupture and crust, or may become secondarily infected and pustular before healing. The rash of chickenpox is centripetal in distribution in that the vesicles are most frequent on the trunk followed by the neck and proximal areas of the limbs. Successive crops of vesicles appear over 2 to 5 days, and as a result, at any one time will have lesions at various stages of development on the same area of skin.

In severity, varicella may vary from a mild disease with only a few scattered skin lesions, to a severe febrile illness with a widespread skin rash particularly in adults. Patients with leukaemia, or some other malignant diseases, may show an atypical generalized form of the disease with a haemorrhagic eruption. Cortisone therapy for various conditions, or immunosuppressive treatment, may predispose to this severe form of the disease, with a possible fatal outcome. In such cases, focal lesions consisting of cells with inclusions and multinucleate giant cells may be found in most organs of the body.

In a significant proportion of adult patients with varicella a primary atypical pneumonia follows the appearance of the rash. Involvement of the central nervous system is uncommon and may present as an acute cerebellar ataxia; it has a good prognosis, in contrast to the rare form associated with perivascular round cell infiltration, haemorrhage and demyelinization.

Zoster is a localized disease, usually unilateral, and confined to one or more dermatomes. The disease is seen predominantly in adults of whom 2 per cent may experience the infection, the incidence increasing markedly with age. Prodromal pain in the area supplied by a sensory nerve is a common feature and occurs before the skin lesions develop: these are identical to those of chickenpox, except in their distribution. The most frequently affected dermatomes correspond to the distribution of the rash in chickenpox in that the thorax, abdomen and face are the commonest sites. Involvement of the ophthalmic branch of the trigeminal nerve can cause severe corneal ulceration. In a few instances, paralysis of muscles occurs by extension of the lesions in the spinal cord to the motor nerve cells of the same or neighbouring segments. Encephalitis may also develop during the course of zoster, characterized by signs of meningeal irritation. Symptoms suggesting systemic involvement—fever and generalization of the skin lesions—occur in a small proportion of patients (5 to 10 per cent). Healing of the lesions takes place in 1 to 3 weeks, although painful sensations may persist in the affected area for some time—postherpetic neuralgia.

Round cell infiltration and focal haemorrhages occur in the posterior root ganglion of the affected area and are succeeded by nerve cell destruction and later fibrosis. Degenerative changes in the sensory nerve and in the posterior columns of the spinal cord can be demonstrated. Involvement of the CNS may be reflected in a marked increase of cells in the CSF.

LABORATORY DIAGNOSIS

On occasion it may be important to distinguish rapidly between varicella and smallpox. A number of laboratory techniques to distinguish these viruses are now available and are described in Vol. II, Chapters 10 and 11.

Examination of vesicle fluid, or scrapings from the base of lesions, in the electron-microscope may reveal typical herpesvirus particles. Light microscopy of the lesion scrapings may show Cowdry type A inclusions and multinucleate giant cells. Neither of these methods can distinguish between V-Z virus and herpes simplex virus.

V-Z virus can be grown in human embryonic cell cultures, and produces a focal cytopathic effect which expands slowly through the cell sheet. Unlike herpes simplex virus it will not produce pocks on the CAM of chick embryos. Vesicle fluid will usually give a positive result when tested by gel precipitation with a known positive zoster convalescent serum.

Serological studies with paired sera can be undertaken with a complement-fixing antigen prepared from infected cell cultures. This test may be used in primary infections, i.e. chicken-pox, when serological conversion occurs. In zoster the CF titres in serum are usually high by the time the eruption appears. Some degree of antigenic overlap exists between V-Z virus and herpes simplex virus.

EPIDEMIOLOGY

The upper respiratory tract is believed to be the usual route of entry for varicella virus, which is shed from ruptured vesicles or lesions in the oropharynx. Chickenpox may also be contracted after exposure to a patient with zoster. On the other hand, zoster rarely follows exposure to chickenpox, which is commonest in early child-hood; second attacks of varicella are very rare. It seems most likely that zoster is a localized reactivation of the latent virus acquired during varicella—the virus having persisted over very long periods despite the presence of circulating antibody. During an attack of zoster, antibody levels rise rapidly, indicative of a recurrent infection, but the virus is still not eliminated from the host as second attacks of zoster do occur. Zoster frequently complicates malignant disease, especially leukaemia, or treatment with steroids, immunosuppressive drugs or radio-therapy.

CYTOMEGALOVIRUS

The human cytomegaloviruses (CMV) belong to a large group of highly species-specific viruses, most of which have an affinity for salivary glands and kidney. The name is derived from the swollen appearance of infected cells (40 μm diameter) whose nucleus contains a large acidophilic inclusion body. Serological studies indicate that infection with cytomegaloviruses is widespread in man.

DESCRIPTION

The cytomegaloviruses have the same structure and composition as other members of the herpes group. They can be grown only in tissues of human origin, and preferably in fibroblast cells:

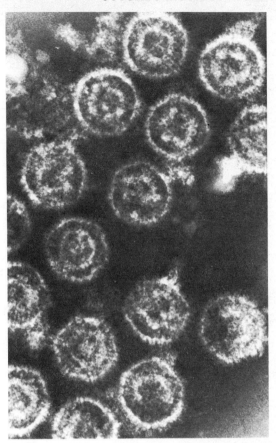

PLATE 41.6. Cytomegalovirus, salivary gland virus. In this group of virions from cultured cells, none have envelopes and most show a 50 nm core. This may illustrate the internal make-up of the capsid or may be only a staining artefact. (From Madeley, 1972 *Virus Morphology*. Churchill Living-stone.)

yields of virus are low, at least on first isolation, and growth of the virus may be detected by the presence of slowly expanding foci of enlarged cells. Subculture is best achieved by transfer of infected cells, since cell-free virus is difficult to produce, and the virus is sensitive to freezing and thawing. Serological differences can be shown between virus isolates but so far no definitive antigenic typing has been proposed.

CLINICAL FEATURES

A number of clinical syndromes have been associated with CMV although the majority of infections are unrecognized. As with other members of the group, a long-lasting association between host and virus can occur. In congenital infections, the earliest form to be recognized, the virus causes a severe and often fatal illness known as cytomegalic inclusion disease of the newborn. The characteristic histopathology is readily recognized in most organs, especially the kidney. The infant shows enlargement of liver and spleen, jaundice, thrombocytopaenic purpura and haemolytic anaemia. Among survivors mental retardation associated with microcephaly and cerebral calcification is usually evident, accompanied by chorioretinitis. Some children, infected in utero or from the cervix uteri during birth, do not show symptoms but may continue to excrete virus in the urine over a period of years despite the presence of circulating antibody.

Acquired infection is more frequent in families in poor home conditions and in institutions. Children carrying the virus excrete large quantities in their urine and saliva, but the exact route of entry of CMV is not clear. The association of CMV with adolescent mononucleosis suggests that like infectious mononucleosis, CMV may be spread in saliva during kissing, or by inhalation. Most infections are asymptomatic, but hepatitis and pneumonitis have been recognized. Indeed, liver involvement appears to be a common manifestation of infection and on occasion may be severe enough to cause jaundice. Haemolytic anaemia may also occur, and myocarditis, pericarditis and polyneuritis have been recorded. Chronic infections can occur in children and are associated with persistent hepatosplenomegaly.

CMV MONONUCLEOSIS

This syndrome has been recognized as occurring naturally but more especially a few weeks after the transfusion of whole fresh blood. Haematologically the findings suggest infectious mononucleosis with increased numbers of atypical mononuclear cells, although neither pharyngitis nor lymphadenopathy are prominent features. Tests for heterophile antibody (Paul-Bunnell) are negative, but serological tests indicate CMV infection. The post-perfusion syndrome occurs most often after open heart surgery when large volumes of blood are used. The source of the virus appears to be the leukocytes of a latently infected donor. An occult viraemia is readily demonstrated in many patients with acquired CMV infection or even in apparently normal individuals, by isolation of the virus from white cells.

Evidence of disseminated CMV infection can be obtained in children or adults with malignant disease, such as leukaemia, and in patients treated with immunosuppressive agents for organ transplantation, but its relationship to illness or death of the patient is difficult to establish. Pneumonitis is often a feature and may be associated with the protozoan parasites, toxoplasma and pneumocystis.

LABORATORY DIAGNOSIS

The earliest method available for diagnosis was the histological examination of necropsy or biopsy material. Most organs of children dying from cytomegalic inclusion disease characteristically contain large swollen cells with intranuclear inclusion bodies—'Owl-eye' cells. Similar cells with inclusions can also be demonstrated in the centrifuged deposit from the urine of affected children. These cells can sometimes be found in the salivary glands of children dying from other diseases.

The virus can be isolated from the urine, saliva, liver and other organs by inoculation of human embryonic fibroblasts cultures. Observation of inoculated cultures over a period ranging from 1 to 6 weeks may reveal foci of rounded cells. This CPE spreads slowly but may involve the entire cell sheet and characteristic inclusion bodies can be demonstrated.

Serological tests are available, using a complement-fixing antigen prepared from infected cell cultures: four-fold or greater changes in serum titre can be interpreted to indicate current or recent infection with the virus.

EPIDEMIOLOGY

Infection with CMV may be acquired in a variety of ways. Transmission can occur in utero, or an infant may be infected during birth from an infected cervix uteri. Children who acquire infection before or during delivery may excrete virus over a long period of time in urine and saliva, despite the production of both IgM and IgG antibodies, so that immunological tolerance to CMV does not develop.

The high incidence of inapparent infections in the population is indicated by the presence of CMV antibody in 50 to 80 per cent of adults. The mode of spread of the virus is not known, although saliva and urine appear to be the most likely sources.

INFECTIOUS MONONUCLEOSIS (GLANDULAR FEVER)

Infectious mononucleosis is an acute febrile illness seen most frequently in young adults who present with fever, pharyngitis and lymphadenopathy (glandular fever). General malaise precedes the onset of fever with headache and sore throat. In about three-quarters of patients, the pharynx and tonsillar areas are inflamed, and a white or grey exudate is frequently present. Small petechiae develop on the palate in about half the patients. Most show enlargement of the cervical lymph nodes; axillary and other lymph nodes may also be involved.

Splenomegaly is common and hepatomegaly associated with a mild degree of jaundice may develop in some patients. A morbilliform rash on the trunk is an uncommon finding (5 per cent) and meningitis occurs in 1 per cent of patients. Recovery usually takes place in 1 to 2 weeks, but occasionally symptoms may persist for weeks or months. Second attacks of the disease are rare, suggesting that only one serological type of virus is involved.

LABORATORY DIAGNOSIS

Within a few days of the onset of the infection, a blood count shows a decreased number of circulating polymorphs. Very soon, there is a significant increase in the number of circulating mononuclear cells to 10 000–50 000 cells per ml. In a blood film, characteristic 'glandular fever cells' can be recognized. These cells are lymphoblastic in type and are large atypical lymphocytes.

The kidney-shaped nucleus of such a cell contains a latticework of chromatin, and is enclosed within a vacuolated densely staining basophilic cytoplasm.

Evidence of liver involvement is usually obtained if liver function tests, such as enzyme and flocculation tests, are performed.

The standard diagnostic test for glandular fever is the Paul-Bunnell test for heterophile agglutinin, an IgM antibody that agglutinates sheep red blood cells. The antibody appears very soon after the onset of the illness and usually disappears within 1 to 2 months. False positive results may occur, but these can be detected by absorption procedures (see Vol. II, Chap. 11). Antibody titres of 10 or more are of diagnostic significance if the full test, complete with absorption, is performed. About 75 per cent of patients with a typical clinical presentation, and showing abnormal mononuclear cells in the peripheral blood, have a positive Paul-Bunnell test. Some young children with negative Paul-Bunnell tests, may be genuine cases of infectious mononucleosis, and some may be due to cytomegalovirus infection or some as yet unknown cause.

EPSTEIN-BARR VIRUS

This virus was first detected in cell lines derived from Burkitt's lymphoma, a disease seen almost entirely in central Africa. The epidemiological features of this tumour suggested that an insect vector might be involved in the transmission of the aetiological agent, perhaps a virus (see below). Cells can be grown from the tumours, and in a proportion of these cells Epstein and Barr detected a virus with the characteristic appearance and size of a herpesvirus, now called the Epstein-Barr virus or EBV. Although the exact nature of the association of EBV with Burkitt's tumour is still uncertain, strong evidence has been accumulated to establish a close link between EBV and infectious mononucleosis.

EBV can be maintained by serial cultivation of chronically infected carrier cultures. Normal human lymphocytes are incapable of indefinite propagation, but after mixing with irradiated EBV carrier cells, blast transformation of the cells occurs; they can then be shown to contain

EBV by electron-microscope examination and EBV antigens by immunofluorescence. Attempts to transfer the virus to other cell types have been unsuccessful due in part, perhaps, to the difficulty of producing cell-free virus.

The virus was originally demonstrated in Burkitt cells, but it has since been found in lymphoblasts from patients with infectious mononucleosis and even from normal individuals. The virus, when purified, has been shown to contain DNA with a molecular weight of 100 by 10^6 daltons.

EBV antigens can be detected in infected cell cultures by precipitation in agar gel with an immune serum, but immunofluorescent examination has been most useful in detecting intracellular virion antigens in fixed cell preparations, whilst new cell membrane antigens are demonstrable in unfixed cell preparations.

ASSOCIATION OF EBV
WITH MONONUCLEOSIS

The discovery that EBV is a cause of infectious mononucleosis is recent, and depends in part on the observation of accidental infections in laboratory technicians working with cultured Burkitt lymphoma cells.

The present evidence for the association of infectious mononucleosis and EBV can be summarized as follows. Cultures of peripheral leukocytes from patients with infectious mononucleosis regularly develop into cell lines that can be shown to contain EBV. Similar cultures from uninfected individuals do not grow into cell lines. Cultures from patients with a history of infection, or with antibody to EBV, yield intermediate results. A high success rate in establishing leukocyte cultures has been obtained using lymph node cells from antibody-positive patients. These results do not establish that EBV is the cause of infectious mononucleosis but show that EBV stimulates the growth of lymphoid cells and may be carried over a considerable period by healthy antibody-positive individuals.

Serological studies have provided good evidence of the association between EBV and infectious mononucleosis. Antibodies to the viral capsid and membrane antigens can be detected in the sera of patients in the acute stage of the illness. In addition, patients with well established histories of infectious mononucleosis have antibody to EBV but at a lower titre than patients with current infections. Again, sera collected before an attack of mononucleosis do not contain EBV antibody and this develops during the illness; individuals who have antibody to EBV are protected against infectious mononucleosis. Diagnostic changes in titre are difficult to detect, as the incubation period of infectious mononucleosis is long and by the time a patient seeks medical advice antibodies have developed and will persist, although at a reduced level, for many years. Under these circumstances, the shorter lasting heterophile antibody test (Paul-Bunnell) has remained a useful laboratory aid.

Experimental transmission of EBV has not been reported, but evidence has been obtained that blood transfusion can occasionally transfer infection.

EPIDEMIOLOGY OF
MONONUCLEOSIS

Infectious mononucleosis has an incubation period of 3 to 6 weeks and is most common in young adults aged 15 to 25 years. A less severe illness with a shorter incubation period is seen in children. Subclinical infections are common and occur most frequently in children; the age at which they acquire antibody to EBV is dependent on environmental conditions so that in areas where housing and hygienic conditions are poor, the virus spreads readily. As a result infectious mononucleosis is rarely seen in young adults from this background. The prevalence of antibody to EBV among adults may range from 40 to 95 per cent depending on country and environment.

The virus may be spread by saliva and in young adults and children, kissing and close personal contact are probably responsible. The disease is not highly infectious, and cases usually occur sporadically, although outbreaks in educational institutions and military camps have been documented.

Antibody develops after primary infection in a child or an adult and the EBV probably remains in the lymphoid cells of the host for life apparently without effect as there is no evidence that reactivation occurs as with other herpes-viruses.

Association of EB Virus and Burkitt's Lymphoma

The fact that EBV was first detected in cells derived from a malignant lymphoma (Burkitt's lymphoma) has led to intensive investigation of the possibility that EBV is the cause of this tumour. On the basis of the clinical picture, it was soon apparent that the tumour was found only in certain warm, moist parts of Africa and New Guinea. These early observations suggested that an insect-borne agent, perhaps a virus, might be concerned in the aetiology of this tumour. Routine virus isolation procedures yielded little information, but examination of cultured tumour cells led to the detection of EBV. The role of EBV in the causation of the tumour is not clear. In the areas of Africa where the tumour occurs, infection with the virus, as shown by the prevalence of EBV antibody, is widespread, but the tumour is rare. Subsequent studies have shown that EBV infection is world-wide, although lymphomas of the Burkitt type are rarely found in other parts of the world.

The known ability of EBV to form a long-lasting association with lymphoid cells suggested that the EBV could be present as a passenger virus in the tumour. The evidence for the close association of EBV with Burkitt lymphoma can be summarized thus: (1) patients with Burkitt's lymphoma have high titres of antibody to EBV: (2) there is good evidence that EBV is always associated with cell lines derived from Burkitt tumours. Although virus is demonstrable in only a small percentage of cultured cells, virus-specific antigens can be detected by immunofluorescence and complement fixation. In addition, cell lines which do not produce recognizable virus can be shown to contain EB virus DNA: (3) EBV can transform and alter the behaviour of normal leukocytes in culture in a manner analogous to certain animal tumour viruses. None of these observations prove that EBV is the causative agent of Burkitt's lymphoma, although the virus may act in conjunction with other factors to produce the clinical tumours. The geographical distribution of the tumour implied that an insect vector might be important and it has now been suggested that hyper- or holo-endemic malaria could be significant in the tumour aetiology. Even the combination of malaria and EBV cannot be the whole explanation, since if this were so, a much higher incidence of tumours should be found. It is possible that infection with EBV occurring at a certain age or stage of development of malaria could be important in the causation of the tumour. Elucidation of this problem may depend on the results of extensive prospective surveys in Africa.

High titres of EBV antibody in the sera of patients suffering from Hodgkin's disease and chronic lymphatic leukaemia have been reported, but the nature of the association between the virus and these lymphoproliferative diseases is unknown. Indeed, high antibody titres to EBV have been recorded in several non-malignant conditions, e.g. sarcoidosis, systemic lupus erythematosis and lepromatous leprosy, but the role of the virus, if any, in these conditions is not understood.

REFERENCES AND FURTHER READING

BIGGS, P. M., de-THE, J. & PAYNE, L. N. (Eds) (1972) *Oncogenesis and Herpesviruses.* Lyon: International Agency for Research on Cancer.

DUDGEON, J. A. (1970) In *Modern Trends in Medical Virology*, Chap 6, Vol. II. Edited by R. B. Heath and A. P. Waterson. London: Butterworths.

NAHMIAS, A. J., NAIB, Z. M. & JOSEY, W. E. (1971) In *Perspectives in Virology*, Vol. III. Edited by M. Pollard. New York: Academic Press.

WELLER, T. H. (1965) In *Viral and Rickettsial Infections*, 4th Edn. Edited by G. C. Horsfall and I. Tamm. London: Pitman Medical.

WELLER, T. H. (1971) The cytomegaloviruses. *New England Journal of Medicine*, **285**, 203.

42. Adenoviruses

Pharyngeal Infections: Respiratory Infections: Conjunctival Infections

Adenoviruses derive their name from the fact that they were first found in adenoid tissue removed at surgical operation. They are able to live in a latent or masked form in lymphoid tissue without any apparent harm to the individual. In other situations, however, they are responsible for a wide range of infections of the respiratory tract and the conjunctivae. Their role in infections of the intestine is still not clearly understood. Much attention has been focused on this group of viruses because they can induce malignant transformation in rodent cells *in vitro* and produce cancer when inoculated into the live baby hamster.

DESCRIPTION

The adenovirion is 65 to 80 nm in diameter, has an icosahedral form and is unenveloped. Its protein capsid is made up of 252 capsomeres within which is a dense deoxyribonucleoprotein core 30 nm in diameter. The 240 capsomeres that make the triangular facets and part of their edges are hollow and spherical or polygonal structures 7 to 8 nm in diameter. They each touch six neighbours and are called hexons. The remaining 12 capsomeres are situated at the apices of the icosahedron and since they have only five neighbours are known as pentons; in structure they are more complex, with a base 7 nm in diameter and a fibre with a terminal swelling. The fibres, which protrude from each of the 12 apices of the capsid, vary in length in different serotypes.

Deoxyribonucleic acid constitutes 11·3 to 13·5 per cent of the contents of the virion. It is double-stranded, non-circular and about 11 to 13 microns long; its molecular weight is 20 to 25 by 10^6 daltons.

The remaining 86·5 to 88·7 per cent of the virion is protein and there are nine different polypeptides. Three of these, each with its own characteristic molecular weight, are individually associated with the hexon, the penton base and the fibre. Three others, which are rich in arginine, are associated with the core DNA, and two more are involved in capsid-associated structures. The remaining polypeptide is completely heat labile and is probably an aggregate or break-down product.

Under natural conditions adenoviruses have been associated with infections of monkeys, bovines, swine, sheep, mice and birds, and each possesses its own particular characters. One adenovirus is the cause of Rubarth's disease—infectious canine hepatitis, and others cause fox encephalitis and canine laryngo-tracheitis.

HAEMAGGLUTININ. All adenoviruses have the ability to agglutinate the red blood cells of a number of animals. Rat, mouse and monkey erythrocytes are those most commonly clumped. The virions' organ of attachment is the penton fibre, but the nature of the receptor is not yet characterized.

Three groups of adenoviruses can be distinguished according to their power to agglutinate rhesus or rat erythrocytes.

Group I. Rhesus cells agglutinated, but not rat cells.

Types: 3, 7, 11, 14, 16, 20, 21, 25 and 28.

Group II. Rat cells agglutinated, but rhesus cells only to a low titre.

Types: 8, 9, 10, 13, 15, 17, 19, 22, 23, 24, 26, 27, 29 and 30.

Group III. Rat cells partially agglutinated, but not rhesus cells.

Types: 1, 2, 3, 4, 5, 6, 12, 18 and 30.

ANTIGENIC CHARACTERS. There are 33 established serotypes that affect human beings. These serotypes are distinguished by virus neutralization and haemagglutination inhibition tests. Within types 3 and 7 some antigenic heterogenicity has been described. The type specific antigenic component in neutralization tests resides in the hexon. All the antigenic types share at least two major antigens; one in the

434

hexon polypeptide, and the other in the penton base. For this reason they cross-react almost completely in complement fixation tests; a useful means of identification of the group is thereby provided which often suffices in medical work where the numerical serotyping is not always essential.

Growth in Cultured Cells

Adenoviruses grow well in continuous human cell-lines such as HeLa, Hep 2 or KB. Epithelioid cells are more susceptible than fibroblasts and primary human-kidney cells are especially sensitive. The human strains may multiply in the cells derived from non-human hosts but there is a marked tendency to abortive cycles of replication.

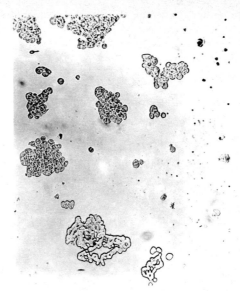

PLATE 42.2. HeLa cells. Cytopathic effect. Clustering. Seven days Adenovirus infection.

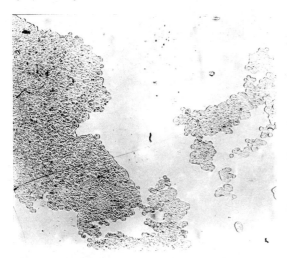

PLATE 42.1. HeLa cells. Cytopathic effect. Clustering. 48 h Adenovirus infection.

These viruses grow slowly and a definite cytopathic effect may take 2 to 4 weeks to become obvious. The changes develop over a period of several days and are irreversible. The infected cells are rounded off, granular, and refractile, and may be clustered together looking like bunches of grapes. They swell to about twice their size and with the increase of their metabolic activities the pH of the culture medium falls. Fixed and stained preparations reveal highly characteristic intranuclear Feulgen-positive inclusions which are easily seen by optical microscopy; in ultra-thin sections under the electron microscope they are seen to be composed of vast numbers of virions in crystalline array.

Virions attach to their receptors on susceptible cells and are rapidly engulfed; loss of infectivity follows with the shedding of the capsid. Thereafter the events that follow resemble essentially the reproductive cycle of any DNA virus (Chap. 13). There is, however, one special feature in that the viral DNA is replicated in the nucleus where the final stages of the assembly of the virion are completed. The capsid proteins are synthesized on cytoplasmic polyribosomes before rapid transfer to the nucleus. The virions are released by extrusion through the nuclear membrane.

PATHOGENESIS

Adenoviruses are stable and remain viable after 7 days at 36°C, 14 days at room temperature and 70 days at 4°C. They are completely inactivated by exposure to heat for two and a half to five minutes at 56°C. They resist lipid solvents and are stable within the pH range from 6 to 9·5 although above pH 10 or below pH 3 they lose infectivity. Human serotypes vary in their sensitivity to ultraviolet light and nitrous acid. Although human strains do not produce clinical disease in laboratory animals, certain types produce malignant tumours in baby hamsters. The oncogenic properties and the capacity of adenoviruses to transform rat and hamster cells growing *in vitro* have been used to form four subgroups. Subgroup A (types 12, 18, 31) has high and subgroup B (3, 7, 14, 16, 12) low oncogenic activity. Both transform cells *in vitro*. Subgroup C (types 1, 2, 5 and 6) and subgroup D (types 9, 10, 13, 15, 17, 19) are unable to induce tumours in animals but can transform rat and hamster cells *in vitro*. The last two subgroups can be distinguished from each other by T antigen specificity (see Chap. 13).

In man, infection with adenoviruses results in catarrhal inflammation of the mucous membranes of the eye and the respiratory tract, sometimes with enlargement of the regional lymph nodes. Adenoviruses have been recovered from enlarged mesenteric lymph glands removed at operation from cases of suspected appendicitis, from infants with intussusception and also from glands pressing on bronchi in bronchiectasis in children.

Types 1, 2, 5 and 6 are for the most part associated with mild, sporadic illnesses and are the common types found latent in the often enlarged tonsils and adenoids of children. Types 3, 4, 7, 14 and 21 are more frequently found in association with small epidemics of acute respiratory disease in closed communities.

Clinical Features

Acute pharyngitis is probably the most frequent manifestation of adenovirus infection. About half the cases are febrile and coryzal.

PHARYNGOCONJUNCTIVAL FEVER. The triad of fever, pharyngitis and conjunctivitis lasting for about one week is characteristic of infections with types 3, 7a and 14. This syndrome is encountered more frequently in the summer months, when it may spread rapidly amongst the members of a family and be associated with outbreaks in schools, day-nurseries or holiday camps.

ACUTE RESPIRATORY DISEASE (ARD) is a feverish coryza which, unlike virus influenza, has a gradual onset. Headache, sore throat and cough are common but not severe. This illness seldom has clear-cut characters in civilian practice, and the diagnosis is usually only made when epidemics occur in such communities as large military camps.

PNEUMONIA. The illness resembles primary atypical pneumonia. In children, type 7a is a frequent cause of the condition and in adults it occurs as a complication of ARD due to types 4 and 7.

ACUTE FOLLICULAR CONJUNCTIVITIS occurs principally in adults. The disease begins with a unilateral non-purulent inflammation of the conjunctiva with enlargement of the submucous lymphoid follicles and swelling of the pre-aruicular lymph node. Fever and systemic effects are usually absent. After a few days the other eye shows a similar involvement and the condition usually clears up within a week. Types 3 and 7a have been isolated from these cases.

EPIDEMIC KERATO-CONJUNCTIVITIS. This condition is due to infection with the single adenovirus, type 8. Factory workers are principally involved, especially those whose trade exposes them to the risk of small corneal abrasions from dust or metal particles such as are disseminated in arc welding and riveting, e.g. among shipyard workers. The acute phase of the infection may last for several weeks and healing is slow. Type-8 virus can easily be spread by contaminated towels to other members of a patient's family. Epidemics have been recorded where the virus was spread amongst patients in an ophthalmic clinic by means of solutions and instruments.

Table 42.1

Disease	Associated adenovirus type
Acute respiratory disease	**4**, **7**, 3, 14
Acute febrile pharyngitis	**1**, **2**, **3**, **5**
Pharyngoconjunctival fever	**3**, **7a**, 1, 2, 5, 6, 14
Virus pneumonia:	
(a) in infants	**7a**, 1, 3
(b) in adults	**4**, **7**, 3
Acute follicular conjunctivitis	**3**, **7a**, 1, 2, 5, 6, 14
Epidemic kerato-conjunctivitis	**8**, 3, 7a, 9

The most common types are given in heavy figures.

LABORATORY DIAGNOSIS

Virus isolation is carried out by inoculation into monolayer tissue cultures of human cells, preferably HeLa, HEp2 or primary cultures of human amnion in which adenoviruses produce a characteristic cytopathic effect. Because cellular changes take so long to develop (1 to 4 weeks) one blind passage is advisable. Isolates may be identified as members of the adenovirus group by their capacity to fix complement with a known positive human or rabbit antiserum. The type may be determined in neutralization or haemagglutination inhibition tests with type-specific rabbit antisera, but these time consuming techniques are mostly limited to research and epidemiological studies.

SEROLOGICAL TESTS. Infection with any one type of adenovirus stimulates the production of complement-fixing antibodies to the group soluble antigen. A rising titre with paired sera provides a simple and practical test for the detection of infections with the adenovirus group although it does not identify the type of the infecting strain. Complement fixing antibodies often rise from very low levels to a titre of 128.

Titres of type-specific antibodies to the adenoviruses may be measured in neutralization tests against serotypes in HeLa cell tissue cultures.

Immunity

The immunity that follows an adenovirus infection is long lasting and second attacks with the same serotype are rare. Neutralizing antibodies to one or more serotypes are present in more than 50 per cent of children over the age of 6 to 11 months. The incidence increases markedly with the age of the individual and between 6 and 34 years the majority of persons have neutralizing antibodies to more than three types. In the 6 to 15 years age group, antibodies to types-1 and 2 are particularly common and are found in 56 and 72 per cent respectively. Antibodies to types 3 and 4 are less prevalent at this age.

Complement-fixing antibodies are also commonly present and children who are born without them usually develop them by the age of six months. After natural infection these group complement-fixing antibodies persist for a variable period, perhaps for as long as seven years, but their presence or absence does not guarantee immunity against infection amongst people exposed to new adenoviruses when they move to a different environment.

Epidemiology

Adenoviruses are widespread in the continents of Europe and North America. In respiratory disease the viruses may be spread by the inhalation of infected particles and possibly through contamination of the conjunctiva and oropharynx by infected fingers or droplet-spray. The seasonal incidence is maximal in the winter, but pharyngoconjunctival fever occurs mostly in the summer months, and types 3 and 7a viruses are probably spread in swimming-bath water. In addition to being present in the exudates of the oropharynx and the eye, adenoviruses have been recovered from faeces and from mesenteric lymph nodes. Adenoviruses types from 9 to 28, excluding types 14 and 21, have been recovered almost exclusively from the intestinal tract, but the significance of their presence in the intestine is still in doubt.

Prophylaxis

Because there has been no urgent need for them adenovirus vaccines have never been recommended for general use. They have, however, been used effectively in preventing epidemics in communities of military recruits. Originally the vaccines contained types 3, 4 and 7 adenoviruses grown in monkey kidney cells and inactivated by formaldehyde, but their use had to be stopped when it was realized that there was frequent contamination with papova SV40-adenovirus hybrids that had oncogenic potentialities.

Two adenovirus vaccines designed to overcome this difficulty are under trial. One is made from the purified protein of the capsid antigen and avoids the possibility of contamination of genetic material from other viruses. The other contains live virus known to be uncontaminated; it is given orally in a coated capsule which dissolves and liberates the virus in the intestine. A subclinical infection follows and confers a high degree of resistance to wild strains. The vaccine virus has no tendency to spread from the vaccinated person to his contacts.

Adeno-associated Viruses (Adeno-satellite Viruses)

These are very small deoxyriboviruses belonging

to the *parvovirus* group. They are defective viruses and are unable to multiply unless the adenovirus is multiplying at the same time. The two viruses grow together in the cells of the human throat providing an example of complementation (Chap. 13).

Adeno-associated viruses are 18 to 22 nm in diameter and are naked icosahedral particles probably with 32 capsomeres. Their DNA is single-stranded and has a molecular weight of 1·2 to 1·8 million daltons. They multiply in the nucleus, and are heat stable and ether resistant. There are four antigenic types of adeno-associated viruses—types 1, 2 and 3 naturally infect man and type 4 infects monkeys. They are not related antigenically to the adenoviruses.

Adeno-SV40 Hybrids

Human adenoviruses will not multiply in monkey cells unless they are accompanied by a simian adenovirus. As the two viruses cohabit and multiply within the host cell, exchanges in part or in whole, of their capsids and genomes give rise to a projeny of many different hybrids. These genetic combinations may be of considerable importance in vaccine production and in the potential for oncogenesis (see Chaps 13 and 49).

FURTHER READING

GINSBERG, H. S. (1970) The biochemical basis of adenovirus cytopathology. In *Infectious Agents and Host Reactions*, Chap. 20. Edited by S. Mudd. London: Saunders.

HOGGAN, M. D. (1970) Adenovirus associated viruses. *Progress in Medical Virology*, **12**, 211.

SCHLESINGER, R. W. (1969) Adenoviruses: the nature of the virion and of controlling factors in productive or abortive infection and tumorigenesis. *Advances in Virus Research*, **14**, 1.

43. Orthomyxoviruses (Influenza viruses Types A, B and C) Influenza

The myxoviruses received their name from the special affinity they have for mucus. After the first isolations of the influenza viruses A and B were made in 1933 by Smith, Andrewes and Laidlaw and in 1934 by Francis respectively, the way was opened for the rapid development of medical virology as a laboratory science. Amongst the many advances made was the discovery of more myxoviruses as the causes of a variety of diseases of man and animals. The three that cause true influenza in man, types A, B and C, have been grouped together under the approved name of orthomyxoviruses (Wildy, 1971; Andrewes and Pereira, 1972).

Other myxoviruses differ in several respects. They cause mumps, measles and respiratory diseases in man as well as a variety of diseases in birds and mammals. They have been designated as paramyxoviruses (see Table 43.1 and Chap. 44).

DESCRIPTION

The virions are spherical, 80 to 120 nm in diameter, or may be filamentous up to several microns in length. They have a helical nucleocapsid with a core of single-stranded RNA (molecular weight 5 million daltons) probably in six separate pieces to which the protein capso-meres are attached (see Chap. 12). This ribonucleoprotein is usually wound tightly to form a rounded mass and corresponds to the 'S' or 'Soluble antigen'. It is covered by an envelope that contains lipids from the plasma membrane of the cell in which it replicated. From the envelope there project spikes that are 10 nm long and are triangular in cross section. These spikes, or haemagglutinins, are protein molecules of viral origin and are chemically linked to the host cell carbohydrate in the envelope (Plate 43.1). Between the spikes there are mushroom-shaped protrusions composed of neuraminidase. Both these proteins are of viral origin and are quite different from the proteins of the host cells.

The haemagglutinin combines specifically with glycoprotein receptors present on the surface of erythrocytes of various avian and mammalian species fastening them to each other in agglutinated masses. The enzyme neuraminidase, at its critical temperature, can split this virus-cell link and the virus is liberated unharmed. The glycoprotein receptors are, however, destroyed and the erythrocytes are no longer agglutinatable by the virus.

Host Range and Antigenic Composition

Although human influenza viruses of type A were the first to be isolated, other subtypes of

Table 43.1. Comparison of orthomyxoviruses and paramyxoviruses.

	Orthomyxoviruses	Paramyxoviruses
Particle size	80–120 nm	150–220 nm
Diameter of nucleocapsid	6 nm	18 nm
Filaments	+	−
Haemolysis	−	+
Site of formation of ribonucleoprotein	Nucleus	Cytoplasm
Antigenic stability	Frequent variations	Stable
Genetic recombination	Common	None
DNA-dependent RNA synthesis needed for multiplication	+	−
Actinomycin-D inhibition	+	−

439

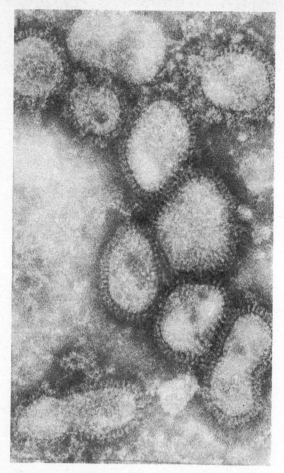

PLATE 43.1. Influenza A/NWS virus (HONI). All the main characters of orthomyxovirus are seen. Size 80 × 120 nm. Filaments larger. Note the fringes of haemagglutinin spikes on the surface of the virions. (By courtesy of Dr C. R. Madeley and Churchill Livingstone.)

this virus have been recovered from pigs, horses and a variety of avian species. All these strains of type A share the same common ribonucleoprotein antigen (the S antigen) while the strains of type B share a different one. Influenza C is distinct from both A and B.

The protein antigens on the viral surface are the haemagglutinins and neuraminidases already mentioned. In the case of type A virus there are at least 18 of these antigenic components which are shared in varying proportions by the viruses isolated in successive years (Webster and Laver, 1972). These changes in antigenic configurations usually show only minor differences from the structures of the strains of preceding years and the process has been described as one of 'antigenic drift'. However, especially in type A strains, a major interruption of these progressive changes can occur at long intervals varying from 10 to 30 years. This is a discontinuous variation and what is virtually a new virus emerges. The community possesses no immunological resistance to this novel infection which can rapidly spread to set up a pandemic. Variations of lesser degree are sometimes able to initiate smaller epidemics in very susceptible communities (Pereira, 1969).

It has become necessary to design a system of nomenclature to compare the nature of the virus strains as they mutate year by year and the following system was devised by the World Health Organization (1971). Strain designation of the types A, B and C contains the following details:

(1) Description of the ribonucleoprotein of the S antigen (A, B or C); (2) Host origin. If the isolation was made from man this is not indicated but it is stated for strains isolated from non-human hosts, e.g. swine, horse, duck, chicken, quail, tern, etc.; (3) Geographical origin; (4) Strain number; (5) Year of isolation.

In addition, for the influenza type A viruses, the character of the haemagglutinin subtype (H) is indicated, e.g.

Human H0, H1, H2, H3; Equine Heq1, Heq2; Swine Hsw1; Avian Hav1; etc.

Similarly, the neuraminidase subtype (N) is indicated:

Human N1, N2; Equine Neq1, Neq2; Avian N1.

The following are some examples of the full designation of type A strains: A/Hong Kong/1/68 (H3, N2); A/Turkey/Wisconsin/1/66 (Hav5, N2); A/Swine/Taiwan/1/70 (H3, N2).

CULTIVATION. For initial isolation the most suitable cells are primary kidney cells from either the monkey or the human embryo. Embryonic chick cells and those from various species of mammals are susceptible, but the rate of growth and the cytopathic effects vary with different strains. If continuous cell lines are used the cycle of viral multiplication is often abortive and in the past confusion arose from this difficulty.

Virions attach to the surface of the host cells

by means of their haemagglutinins. Entry of the virus follows the fusion of the viral lipid membrane with that of the cell wall and the nucleocapsid is released directly into the cytoplasm. The events of the ensuing few hours are not fully understood, but they follow the general pattern described for animal riboviruses in Chapter 13 (see Barry and Mahy, 1970).

Briefly, viral ribonucleoprotein (RNP) is first detectable by immunofluorescence in the nucleus of the cell while haemagglutinin is found only in cytoplasm. Migration of RNP from the nucleus occurs only after the synthesis of another protein and while this is proceeding the haemagglutinin and neuraminidase become incorporated in the plasma membrane of the cell rendering it capable of haemadsorption. There follows a budding process whereby virions are slowly released from the cell surface into the tissue fluids by the action of their own neuraminidase. The host cell does not seem to be damaged by the process.

VIABILITY. The influenza virus withstands slow drying at room temperature on articles such as blankets and glass; it has been demonstrated in dust after an interval as long as two weeks. When contained in allantoic fluid, or in infected tissues immersed in glycerol saline it will survive for several weeks at refrigerator temperature. It can be preserved for long periods at −70°C and remains viable indefinitely after freeze drying.

Exposure to heat for 30 minutes at 56°C is sufficient to inactivate most strains; the few which survive this treatment are killed by exposure for 90 minutes at the same temperature. These viruses are also inactivated by 20 per cent ether in the cold, phenol, formaldehyde in a concentration of 1 in 12 000, salts of heavy metals, detergents, soaps and many other chemicals. Iodine in the form of vapour or as a solution is particularly effective. Propylene glycol vapour is active against the virus present in airborne droplets.

TOXICITY. Influenza virus elementary bodies are toxic to such laboratory animals as mice and rabbits. After the intravenous inoculation of highly purified virus preparations the animals may die in 18 to 48 hours with gastro-intestinal haemorrhages and necrotic lesions in the spleen and liver. Immunized animals do not suffer these effects when given intravenous inoculations of the virus.

Clinical Features

'Influenza' is a vague term applied to a great number of mild conditions, but infection with the human viruses of types A and B are characterized by a brisk illness of sudden onset with high fever and muscular pains. The patient is often prostrated and there may be suffusion of the conjunctivae and an irritating cough, though usually without much catarrh. The illness usually lasts for 2 to 5 days but milder and abortive forms are quite common. Type C causes only mild effects or inapparent infections.

Pathogenesis

The virus is inhaled and reaches the mucous membrane of the nose, throat, trachea and finer bronchi. This occurs naturally in man and also experimentally in the ferret and the mouse. Characteristically, there is a necrosis of the ciliated epithelial surfaces and occasionally cells of the alveolar walls in the lungs may be affected (see Chap. 14). It is extremely rare for there to be any viraemic phase. The disease is rarely fatal, but some cases are complicated by bronchopneumonia when virus damaged tissues are invaded by such organisms as *Staphylococcus aureus*, pneumococci, *H. influenzae* or haemolytic streptococci. The formation of multiple abscesses with severe damage to the lung tissue is especially associated with staphylococcal invasion and a fulminating pneumonia is the cause of many influenzal deaths especially in the elderly.

LABORATORY DIAGNOSIS

Saline throat washings or carefully taken throat swabs should be placed in a suitable transport medium. If they cannot be examined immediately in the laboratory they should be preserved without delay in the deep frozen state.

The virus can be isolated by inoculating the material into the amniotic cavity of 13-day-old chick embryos. After incubation for 2 to 3 days at 33°C the virus is detectable in the amniotic fluid by the direct haemagglutination of human or guinea-pig erythrocytes. The viruses also grow well in human embryonic or monkey kidney cell cultures, but with minimal cytopathic effects; their presence is detected by haemagglutination or haemadsorption. Further identification is carried out in haemagglutination inhibition or neutralization tests with specific reference antisera. An additional criterion for strain differentiation is provided by the inhibition of neuraminidase activity by specific antisera. Immunofluorescence provides a specific and rapid method for the detection of the virus directly in the cells of respiratory secretions and in infected cell cultures (Hers, van der Kuyp and Masurel, 1968).

Serological confirmation of the diagnosis is obtained when a fourfold or greater rise of antibody titre can be demonstrated to any one type of virus. Complement-fixation reactions using the S antigens of the viruses distinguishes A from B and C infections. Differentiation of antibodies to different strains within the types is made by means of haemagglutination-inhibition, neutralization or strain-specific complement fixation tests.

Immunity

After an attack of influenza the ensuing immunity persists for a year or more and confers resistance to the virus strains concerned. It is related to the amount of neutralizing antibody (IgA) in the mucous secretions of the respiratory tract as well as to the titre of serum antibodies. When an individual experiences a second or third attack of influenza his humoral antibody response is determined by his previous experience of myxovirus infections. Usually the infecting strain shares antigens with earlier strains and provokes an anamnestic antibody response to them. Thus in any individual his dominant antibodies are mainly directed against the first strain that infected him early in life. If he encounters a strain that is totally unrelated to viruses he has previously experienced he is, of course, completely susceptible.

Treatment

There are hopes that recent trials of 1-amantadine hydrochloride and isoquinoline compounds will lead to the development of drugs that will be useful in prophylactic measures or in the chemotherapy of influenza. Findings to date indicate that L-amantadine hydrochloride is useful because it can block the entry of influenza virus A2 into cells and if given very early after exposure to the virus is able to prevent viral replication (Galbraith et al., 1971).

EPIDEMIOLOGY

Influenza is a short illness and the patients are only infectious for a few days, but subclinical infection is frequent and plays an important role in the dissemination of the virus in the community. Infections with both A and B virus types occur characteristically in epidemics but virus B outbreaks may be more localized, e.g. in schools. Virus A, unlike Virus B, is so subject to major antigenic changes that it causes occasional worldwide pandemics such as those of 1889–1890, 1918–1919 and 1957–1958. The first influenza virus A was isolated in 1933 and is designated as A0, a new sub-type A1 appeared in 1946–1947 and remained dominant until 1957 when the A2 or Asian sub-type arose to create a new pandemic. This strain had a new haemagglutinin and a different neuraminidase. Between the pandemics smaller epidemics are scattered in various different locations at intervals of two or three years.

The antigenic structure of type B virus is less liable to marked variation and although epidemics do occur at 3 to 6 year intervals they never reach pandemic proportions and their extent is usually limited to small communities.

The periodicity of outbreaks of influenza is characteristic, but the epidemiological picture between the major incidents becomes blurred by the existence of infections with other viruses such as the parainfluenza and adenoviruses (Hope-Simpson and Higgins, 1969). Epidemics of virus influenza are associated with attack rates as high as 20 to 40 per cent and a rapid spread over an irregularly defined region. Cold weather in the early spring and increased overcrowding are factors that facilitate the spread of the virus. In major epidemics it has been possible to trace the virus as it moves from point to point along travel routes and to map the advance of the epidemic geographically from country to country. The highest incidence of influenza is in the age group 5 to 15 years: and schools may be the reservoir from which infection spreads into the community. There follows a sharp decline in the 15 to 20 age group, but there is a rise between the ages of 20 and 30. Thereafter in older generations there is a downward trend to a low level.

Influenza virus type C does not cause epidemics and gives rise only to mild or inapparent infections.

PROPHYLAXIS

Because influenza has a very short incubation period and a high attack rate there is seldom time enough for the introduction of conventional control measures such as isolation and quarantine. The best that can be done to protect against infection is to use a suitable vaccine and to immunize especially those particularly at risk such as the very old, the very young and the debilitated. It is wise also to offer vaccination to key personnel and to the members of medical and nursing staffs.

The vaccine most commonly used is a purified and concentrated suspension of influenza viruses A and B grown in the chick embryo and inactivated with formaldehyde. A standard dose is inoculated subcutaneously and a booster dose is given after an interval of 4 to 8 weeks. Thereafter, annually each autumn, a single dose should be given (Tyrell, 1969). The vaccine viruses must be those currently circulating in the community, which means that the vaccines must be continually brought up to date. Thus in 1972 the vaccine in general use contained A2/Hong Kong/1/68 (H3, N2) and B/Tai/4/62. But in future years new strains will inevitably supersede them.

Influenza vaccines containing recently isolated strains are difficult to prepare in adequate amounts. Again, antigenic potency and infectivity may be reduced in continual egg passage of the viruses or if retained the incidence of reactions may be too great for large scale use of the vaccine. Controlled trials of influenza virus vaccines indicate that a moderate degree of protection (50 to 80 per cent) is attainable.

Live vaccines are in general more effective than killed vaccines and there have been many attempts to develop live influenza vaccines. They are introduced intranasally and by their multiplication stimulate the local production of antibodies of the IgA class. Circulating antibodies of the IgM and IgG classes are not raised to the same extent as when inactivated virus vaccines are injected. However, live virus vaccines do protect against the challenge of reinfection with the same strain although a disadvantage with some vaccines has been that too many reactions were produced for their use to be recommended on a large scale (Beare et al., 1968, a and b).

Attenuation of the virulence of virus strains has now been achieved quickly and effectively by recombination techniques whereby the desirable antigenic properties of a virulent strain can be transferred to another strain known to be of low virulence (Beare and Hall, 1971). This would seem to offer an effective means of producing 'tailor-made' live influenza vaccines to a required specification.

REFERENCES AND FURTHER READING

ANDREWES, C. H. & PEREIRA, H. G. (1972) *Viruses of Vertebrates*, 3rd Edn. London: Ballière Tindall.

BARRY, R. D. & MAHY, B. W. J. (1970) *The Biology of Large RNA Viruses*. London: Academic Press.

BEARE, A. S., BYNOE, M. L. & TYRRELL, D. A. J. (1968a) Investigation into the attenuation of influenza viruses by serial passage. *British Medical Journal*, ii, 482.

BEARE, A. S., HOBSON, D., REED, S. & TYRRELL, D. A. J. (1968b) A comparison of live and killed influenza-virus vaccines. *Lancet*, i, 418.

BEARE, A. S. & HALL, T. S. (1971) Recombinant influenza-A viruses as live vaccines for man. *Lancet*, ii, 1271.

GALBRAITH, A. W., OXFORD, J. S., SCHILD, G. C., POATTER, C. W. & WATSON, G. I. (1971) Therapeutic effect of 1-adamantanamine hydrochloride in naturally occurring influenza A/2 Hong Kong infection. *Lancet*, ii, 113.

HERS, J. F.PH., VAN DER KUYPH, L. & MASUREL, M. (1968) Rapid diagnosis of influenza. *Lancet*, i, 510.

HOPE-SIMPSON, R. E. & HIGGINS, P. G. (1969) A respiratory virus study in Great Britain. Review and evaluation. *Progress in Medical Virology*, 11, 354.

HOYLE, L. (1968) The influenza viruses. *Virology Monographs*, Vol. 4. Vienna: Springer-Verlag.

PEREIRA, H. G. (1969) Influenza. Antigenic spectrum. *Progress in Medical Virology*, 11, 46.

TYRRELL, D. A. J. (1969) Vaccination against respiratory viruses. *British Medical Bulletin*, **5**, 165.

WEBSTER, R. G. & LAVER, W. G. (1972) Antigenic variation in influenza virus. Biology and chemistry. *Progress in Medical Virology*, **13**, 271.

WILDY, P. (1971) Classification and nomenclature of viruses. *Monographs in Virology*, Vol. 5. Basel: Karger.

WORLD HEALTH ORGANIZATION (1971) A revised system of nomenclature for influenza virus. *Bulletin of the World Health Organization*, **45**, 119.

At one time paramyxoviruses and orthomyxoviruses were classified in a single group—*the myxoviruses*. However, it has now been realized that there are marked differences amongst these viruses and they have now been placed in two separate groups (see Table 43.1).

Although the paramyxoviruses resemble the orthomyxoviruses in morphology and symmetry, they are as a rule larger and more pleomorphic.

Included in the group are the parainfluenza viruses types 1 to 4 which are frequently recovered from patients suffering from a variety of respiratory illness, as well as the mumps virus and the Newcastle disease virus which is associated with severe infections of avian species.

The measles and respiratory syncytial viruses have also been placed in this group on the grounds of morphological similarity. However, this is clearly only a provisional classification because neither of these two viruses possesses a neuraminidase nor do they bear any antigenic relationships to any other paramyxoviruses.

Description

Electron-microscopy of negatively stained parainfluenza virions shows that they vary in diameter from 80 to 350 nm. Occasionally there are filamentous forms and giant forms up to 800 nm in diameter. The nucleocapsid is composed of helical coils of nucleoprotein some 18 nm in diameter forming a mass of about 100 to 200 nm in diameter; this is loosely enveloped by a lipoprotein membrane 10 to 13 nm thick, which is covered by projections 12 to 14 nm long and 2 to 4 nm wide. This virion is easily deformed by external forces and may assume many bizarre shapes.

Within the virion the genome is carried in a continuous thread 1 μm long of single-stranded RNA the molecular weight of which is 7 million daltons. Attached to each coil of the nucleic acid are some 15 protein capsomeres so that the diameter of the nucleocapsid of the paramyxovirion is longer and thicker than that of the orthomyxovirion. The virion contains some 70 per cent of protein, 20 to 40 per cent lipid, 6 per cent carbohydrate with approximately 0·9 per cent RNA. Analysis of the proteins shows that they contain three or more major and several minor polypeptides. An RNA-dependent RNA polymerase has been detected in the Newcastle virus.

The physico-chemical properties of the paramyxoviruses resemble very closely those of the orthomyxoviruses. All the paramyxoviruses possess haemagglutinins and most strains agglutinate chicken, guinea-pig and human erythrocytes. In tissue cultures, virus replication is easily detected by haemadsorption. The viruses also possess a neuraminidase which destroys the receptor sites on the surface of the erythrocytes. In addition, the virions have a haemolytic activity and are able to fuse mammalian cells in suspension and in monolayers.

All these viruses grow well in tissue cultures and usually cause a mild cytopathic effect with multiple acidophilic intracytoplasmic inclusions, syncytial formation and haemadsorption. Primary cultures of human or simian kidney cells or diploid strains of human fetal cells are suitable for isolation procedures. Only a few strains, e.g. the Sendai strain of parainfluenza 2 virus grows well in the chick embryo; other strains only do so after prolonged adaptation.

Virus multiplication is essentially intracytoplasmic. Paramyxoviruses differ from orthomyxoviruses fundamentally in that their replication cycle cannot be interrupted by actinomycin D, an antibiotic known to inhibit selectively the DNA-directed synthesis of RNA (see Chap. 13).

ANTIGENIC STRUCTURE. The parainfluenza, mumps and Newcastle viruses are all antigenically stable and are related to each other by virtue of sharing a group antigen. The measles virus is distinct but shares antigenic determinants with the canine distemper and rinderpest viruses of cattle. The respiratory syncytial virus is quite unrelated to any of the foregoing viruses.

PARAINFLUENZA VIRUSES

MYXOVIRUS PARAINFLUENZA 1. This group includes the haemadsorption virus type 2, or HA2 virus (Chanock *et al.*, 1958) and the Sendai virus which is also known as the Japanese haemagglutinating virus. The HA2 virus has been isolated frequently from cases of croup in young children, minor respiratory illness, bronchitis, and bronchopneumonia. The Sendai virus was originally isolated in mice from cases of pneumonitis in new-born children but its endemicity in stocks of laboratory mice makes it difficult to assess the significance of this finding. The Sendai virus is closely related antigenically to the HA2 virus, but differs from it in that it multiplies readily in the allantoic membranes of the chick embryo. The Sendai virus has never been isolated in Great Britain.

MYXOVIRUS PARAINFLUENZA 2, or the croup associated (CA) virus, has been isolated from patients with minor respiratory illnesses and bronchopneumonia and from cases of croup. It may not, however, be as commonly associated with croup as the parainfluenza 1 virus. This virus has no cytopathic effect on tissue cultures but is detected by its agglutination of chick (and to a lesser extent of human group O) erythrocytes. Adsorption and agglutination occur at 4°C and the virus elutes rapidly at 37°C. Antigenically this virus is related to the mumps virus but not to other myxoviruses. It is probably identical with an indigenous monkey myxovirus known as SV5; as many as 30 per cent of some batches of uninoculated monkey kidney tissue cultures have been found to carry the SV5 virus.

MYXOVIRUS PARAINFLUENZA 3 or haemadsorption type I (HA1) is associated, like the foregoing parainfluenza viruses, with respiratory illnesses and with croup and bronchopneumonia. It has also been found in the nasal secretions of cattle in transit and suffering from a respiratory illness known as 'shipping fever'. Unlike other parainfluenza viruses, parainfluenza 3 may produce a cytopathic effect seen as giant cell plaques in tissue cultures of human amnion cells growing under an agar overlay.

MYXOVIRUS PARAINFLUENZA 4 (M-25 strain) has recently been isolated from cases of mild respiratory illness. It has no cytopathic effect, does not grow in eggs, and is recognized by the use of the haemadsorption method in infected monkey kidney cells.

Laboratory Diagnosis

Primary isolation of parainfluenza viruses in the chick embryo may be difficult or impossible and tissue culture methods are preferred. Throat swabs or sputum are best preserved at 3 to 4°C. The viruses are very labile, and the specimens should not be frozen or incubated. Cultures of human kidney give the best result and should be inoculated without delay. Cultures of monkey kidney cells are also useful and primary human amnion, HeLa, or HEp2 cells are all satisfactory. The cytopathic effect produced is often minimal and may be absent; the viruses are detected by haemadsorption or

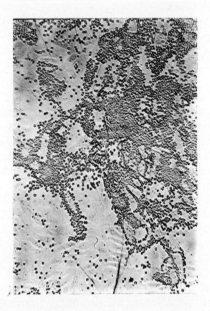

PLATE 44.1. Monolayer of monkey kidney cells infected with paramyxovirus. Extensive haemadsorption.

haemagglutination. Serologically the diagnosis is confirmed by the observation of rising titres of antibodies in paired sera using neutralization, complement-fixation, or haemadsorption or haemagglutination inhibition tests. Because of the antigenic sharing between these viruses and the mumps virus the results of these serological tests may be difficult to interpret. Parallel tests should always be carried out with the mumps S and V antigens for comparison.

RESPIRATORY SYNCYTIAL VIRUS

The respiratory syncytial virus was originally isolated from a cold-like illness in a colony of captive chimpanzees and was known for a time as the chimpanzees coryza associated (CCA) virus. It was however soon realized that it was also associated with human infection especially in young children.

DESCRIPTION

The virions are 90 to 120 nm in diameter and resemble other paramyxoviruses morphologically. There is a central coiled filament enclosed by an outer membrane. Since 5-fluoro-uracil inhibits the growth of the virus it probably has RNA as its nucleic acid. There has been no report of neuraminidase, haemagglutinin or haemolytic activity by the virus.

The virus does not grow in the chick embryo and it has no effect on mice, guinea-pigs, or rabbits. It grows rather slowly in continuous lines of human cancer cells such as HEp2, KB, HeLa, and also the Chang liver cells, but not so readily in primary kidney tissue cultures. One satisfactory method for the cultivation of the virus is to use monolayers of HEp2 cells grown in medium 199 with 10 per cent calf serum added; when ready for inoculation the monolayers are gently washed with medium 199 to rinse away the calf serum; for a maintenance medium during virus growth medium 199 is supplemented with 5 per cent chicken serum. The sodium bicarbonate content is increased by adding 4 per cent of the stock 1·4 per cent sodium bicarbonate solution; incubation is at 36°C.

The virus grows in the cytoplasm of the host cells where it may produce small eosinophilic inclusions. It produces an obvious cytopathic effect which becomes apparent 3 to 7 days after inoculation with the occurrence of giant cells and syncytia. Infectivity titres are usually low and are seldom above 10^5. Plaques are formed in HEp2 monolayers.

VIABILITY. The virus survives quick freezing at $-70°C$ but at higher temperatures its infectivity may rapidly be lost. Specimens such as throat swabs should not be refrigerated but should be treated with antibiotics and introduced into suitable tissue cultures with a minimal delay. The virus is destroyed at pH 3·0.

ANTIGENIC CHARACTERS. A complement fixing antigen is produced and is contained in a particle smaller than the virion itself. Complement-fixation and neutralizing tests can be used for diagnostic purposes.

Pathogenesis and Clinical Features

The virus causes colds and minor upper respiratory tract infections with cough in adults but in children, especially in infants aged 6 to 12 months, the lower respiratory tract is often involved and bronchitis, bronchiolitis and bronchopneumonia occur (Holzel et al., 1963). Young children aged 1 to 2 years may suffer from croup, 'virus pneumonia' or from mild cold-like illnesses.

Respiratory syncytical virus infections are essentially localized infections of the respiratory tract; protection from them is conferred mainly by the local production of IgA. Since this globulin does not pass the placenta, maternal antibodies have no value and it is only the IgA that is produced by the baby itself following infection that controls the events following re-exposure.

Epidemiology

Infection with the respiratory syncytial virus appears to be common in the population of this country; 66 per cent of all persons over the age of five years possess both complement fixing and neutralizing antibodies in the serum; and over the age of 15 years, 93 per cent have neutralizing antibodies. The lowest incidence of antibodies is in the age group six months to one year. Young children under the age of seven months seem to show a relatively poor serological response after infection; some 20 per cent develop a rising titre of complement fixing antibodies and 45 per cent neutralizing antibodies. It is a characteristic of this virus that it causes localized foci of infection which may be limited to one particular area or community. Infection occurs for brief periods in the winter months with long intervals between the outbreaks.

MUMPS VIRUS

Mumps is an acute contagious disease whose most constant and characteristic feature is a large painful swelling of one or both parotid glands. The disease is one of great antiquity and was one of the first infections to be recognized, for it was accurately described by Hippocrates in the fifth century B.C. The name is derived from the mumbling speech which is the result of the pain on moving the jaws. Usually there is a constitutional reaction and not infrequently other glands, e.g. the testes, pancreas as well as the parotids are involved.

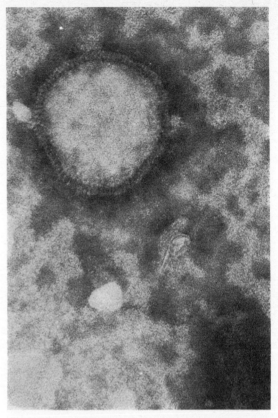

PLATE 44.2. A single mumps virion. (By courtesy of Dr C. R. Madeley and Churchill Livingstone.)

DESCRIPTION

The size of the elementary bodies of *myxovirus parotitidis* varies from 80 to 240 nm in diameter. Filaments have not been described. Morphologically it resembles the other paramyxoviruses and its envelope contains a haemagglutinin, a haemolysin and a neuraminidase.

The virus grows rather slowly in the amniotic and allantoic cavities of the chick embryo: 6 to 8 day old embryos are used and should be incubated for five days at 35°C. After two or three amniotic passages, most strains can be transferred to the allantoic cavity where they adapt themselves and grow very readily. A few strains, however, remain incapable of being transferred in this way. Primary cultures of human embryonic or monkey kidney are useful for primary isolation. Incubation is at 35°C and the best technique to detect the virus is haemadsorption.

The mumps virus agglutinates fowl, human and other red blood cells, fixes complement in the presence of specific antibody, and elicits a delayed allergic reaction in the skin of persons who have previously been infected. Like the Newcastle virus it causes the lysis of erythrocytes. Infective particles can be concentrated by ultra-centrifugation at 20 000 rev/min. Particles of the complement-fixing antigen require prolonged centrifugation at higher speeds.

VIABILITY. Infectivity is rapidly lost at room temperature. The virus is well preserved in skimmed milk at −50°C or −70°C or by freeze drying. The haemagglutinin, haemolysin and infective properties are destroyed by heat at 56°C for 20 minutes but the complement-fixing and allergic skin antigens withstand 65°C for an hour. Exposure to 0·2 per cent formaldehyde at 4°C for 24 hours and intense ultraviolet light irradiation for 0·28 seconds destroy the infectivity of the virus without impairing the haemagglutinin or complement-fixing antigens. Ether treatment at 4°C completely destroys infectivity. The virus is most stable between pH 5·8 and pH 8·0.

ANTIGENIC CHARACTERS. The mumps virus is a single antigenic entity distinct from other myxoviruses; it is not subject to variation and there are no obvious differences between strains. There are two components of the virus which are capable of fixing complement, the V or viral antigen and the S or soluble antigen. The V antigen is associated with the virus particle itself and the S antigen, which is analogous to the soluble antigen of the influenza virus, is a smaller particle extracted from infected cells in the early stages of infection.

PATHOGENESIS

The incubation period of mumps is 18 to 21 days. The common manifestations are fever with unilateral or bilateral parotitis. The virus is excreted in the saliva for about three days after the onset and transmission is by the inhalation of infected particles or by fomites contaminated with saliva. Patients are thought to be infectious for about three days before the onset and to remain so for about six days thereafter. In young children convalescence is uneventful and recovery is complete in about ten days. In about 30 per cent of cases infected with the virus the disease is inapparent. When the virus has been inhaled it multiplies locally in the oropharynx during the incubation period and after an interval reaches the bloodstream to be disseminated to distant organs. Although the virus may reach the parotid and submaxillary glands by direct spread from the mouth, infection of the testes, central nervous system, pancreas, thyroid gland, ovary, and breasts, is almost certainly bloodborne.

In males over the age of 13 years mumps may be complicated by orchitis which appears some 4 to 7 days after the onset of parotitis. Up to 20 per cent of patients are affected. In almost every case of mumps there seems to be some involvement of the central nervous system with an increase in the lymphocytes in the cerebrospinal fluid. Occasionally the condition proceeds to a frank meningoencephalitis which presents 4 to 7 days after the onset of parotitis; in these cases the mumps virus can be isolated from the cerebrospinal fluid. Sometimes mumps meningoencephalitis may occur without any sign of involvement of the salivary glands and is indistinguishable clinically from aseptic meningitis caused by other viruses such as those of the ECHO and Coxsackie groups. In many cases submaxillary gland involvement is encountered, but pancreatitis, oophoritis, and thyroiditis are rare complications. Mastitis may occur in up to 15 per cent of females infected.

LABORATORY DIAGNOSIS

Virus isolation is carried out by inoculating saliva or cerebrospinal fluid into fertile eggs. Saliva can conveniently be collected by placing dental cotton-wool rolls over the openings of the parotid ducts and leaving them in the mouth for about 20 minutes. The rolls are then removed and placed in screw-capped vials containing Hanks balanced salt solution with added antibiotics. The containers should be transported to the laboratory frozen at $-70°C$ in insulated boxes containing solid carbon dioxide. On arrival at the laboratory, the saliva is expressed from the rolls, added to the transport fluid and clarified in the centrifuge at 2000 rev/min for ten minutes. The supernatant is inoculated into the amniotic cavity of eight 11-day-old chick embryos; the eggs are then incubated for five days at 35°C. The primary isolation of the virus is sometimes a matter of difficulty because saliva may have toxic properties for the chick embryo, and because only a small proportion of inoculated eggs show evidence of infection. Alternatively, human or monkey kidney cells may be used (see above). The virus may be detected in the amniotic fluid by the haemagglutination of fowl red blood cells and its final identification is established serologically with specific antiserum in complement-fixation or haemagglutination inhibition tests.

SEROLOGICAL TESTS. Antibody rises can be detected in paired acute and convalescent sera. The complement-fixation test using both soluble and viral antigens is recommended. Antibodies to the S antigen develop early and are present in significant amounts within two or three days of the onset of the infection and they may reach their peak titre before the appearance of antibody to the V antigen. Antibodies to the V antigen appear on the eighth or ninth day of the disease, reach their maximum by the end of a month and thereafter decline very slowly. Subsequently, the anti-S antibodies disappear relatively rapidly and are seldom detectable nine months later. Antibodies to the V antigen persist for several years at very low, barely detectable levels. The haemagglutination-inhibiting antibody is similar in its duration to the anti-V antibody. The skin test for mumps is of little practical value in the diagnosis because the hypersensitive state is not developed until 3 to 4 weeks after onset of illness.

Epidemiology

Mumps is world-wide in its distribution, and the only reservoir of infection is man. The disease is predominantly one of children aged 5 to 15 years, but adults who have escaped infection in childhood are often attacked. The disease is probably transmitted by the same mechanisms as those in respiratory tract infections. Epidemics of mumps are not uncommon in young soldiers in army camps and the disease has been a common cause of invalidism among troops in wartime. Although mumps is one of the common diseases of childhood, it is not, apparently, as highly infectious as measles. Amongst adults the history of a clinical mumps infection is obtained in about 60 per cent of people but inapparent infections may increase the proportion of those infected.

Prophylaxis

Gamma globulin *prepared from mumps convalescent serum* may be of value in conferring passive immunity to exposed persons and if given immediately after the onset of parotitis reduces the incidence of orchitis. Gamma globulin from normal adults contains only traces of specific antibody and has no protective value.

Vaccines prepared from egg-grown strains inactivated by formalin or ultra-violet light have been used with some success in controlling mumps in army camps and in adults exposed to infection. Although antibody formation is stimulated by the vaccine, booster doses are needed after 6 to 9 months to maintain the antibody level. A living attenuated egg-adapted strain of mumps has also been used and is sprayed into the mouth; antibody production occurs at a low titre in about 90 per cent of the recipients. This vaccine is without side-effects and confers some protection on subsequent challenge. No clinical case of mumps has been reported as a result of the use of the live vaccine, and this method has been widely used in the U.S.S.R. for control of the infection.

MEASLES

Measles is probably the most infectious of the common fevers. The clinical diagnosis of the disease is seldom a difficult matter because a characteristic macular rash develops after a prodromal period of fever with catarrhal symptoms, conjunctivitis and the appearance of Koplik's spots on the buccal mucosa. The incubation period is 10 to 14 days and the rash often appears on the fourteenth day after exposure.

Description

The diameter of the virus in filtration experiments is 10 nm. The central core is composed of helices 16 nm in diameter with subunits arranged with a 4·5 nm periodicity. The virion is covered by an outer membrane on which there are radially disposed projections. The nucleic acid of the virus is RNA. In these respects the measles virus resembles the parainfluenza and respiratory syncytial viruses. However, it has no neuraminidase.

The virus can be isolated from the blood or throat washings of a patient during the first 24 hours after the onset of fever. For this purpose primary cultures of human amnion or chorion cells or a continuous line of amnion cells provide the most suitable tissue culture cells. Monkey kidney cells are less satisfactory.

Once established in tissue cultures, the measles virus will grow in a wide range of primate tissue cultures. Human kidney obtained at operation or at necropsy, and human embryonic lung or kidney all provide highly susceptible cells. The virus also grows in continuous lines of cells derived from human normal tissues such as heart, kidney, amnion and bone marrow, as well as in lines of carcinoma cells such as HeLa, KB and Hep2. In monolayers of monkey kidney cells and of some strains of HeLa cells small plaques are produced.

The cytopathic effect of the measles virus is characteristic, with the formation of large multinucleate giant cells or syncytial masses in which many vacuoles give a lacework appearance. After continued passage of the virus in human amnion cells the nature of the cytopathic effect alters, and in addition to giant cells, increasing numbers of refractile stellate cells appear. Variation of the constituents of the culture medium may modify the cytopathic lesions. With glutamine deficiency, for example, more giant cells are formed, but when the glutamine is restored the number of giant cells is diminished, the appearance of the cytopathic effect is delayed, and the virus yield is increased. The most constant feature of cells infected with measles virus is the late appearance of Cowdry type A eosinophilic intranuclear inclusions. Multiple intra-cytoplasmic inclusions also occur. Grown in monolayers of *patas* monkey kidney cells the virus produces countable microplaques. ANIMAL PATHOGENICITY. Measles can be reproduced in rhesus monkeys by the parenteral inoculation of blood or catarrhal secretions from patients or infected tissue culture fluids. The disease is usually mild and about one-third of the inoculated animals develop fever, conjunctivitis and a macular rash. Many monkeys imported for experimental use carry a virus, the Monkey-Intra-Nuclear Inclusion Agent (MINIA), which is indistinguishable from the measles virus. This infection is usually inapparent and is only manifest soon after the animals are captured. These circumstances make the majority of monkeys unreliable as experimental animals for measles research and the presence of MINIA in cultures of their kidney cells may give rise to considerable difficulties. Few mammals other than monkeys have been infected successfully with the measles virus. Some strains of the virus have been adapted to the amniotic cavity or chorioallantoic membrane of the chick embryo after their primary isolation in tissue culture.

VIABILITY. The virus survives over two weeks at 4°C or 22°C, and for many months in the frozen state in the temperature range $-15°$ to $-79°C$. Freeze drying preserves the virus well, though with some loss of infectivity. Formaldehyde in a concentration of 0·025 per cent at 37°C for four days brings about complete loss of infectivity without alteration of the complement-fixing activity. The virus is ether sensitive. Below pH 4·5 the virus is inactivated but it is stable within the range pH 5 to 9 for three hours at 0°C.

HAEMAGGLUTINATION. Concentrated preparations of the measles virus agglutinate rhesus monkey red blood cells at 37°C. The haemagglutinin does not elute spontaneously and is not related to the neuraminidase of the myxoviruses. Haemagglutination-inhibition may be used as a method for the estimation of serum antibodies. ANTIGENIC CHARACTERS. Measles virus strains are uniform antigenically. A complement-fixing antigen is present in infected tissue culture fluids; it can be separated from elementary bodies by centrifugation and has a particle size of 7 to 13 nm.

The measles virus is related antigenically to the virus of canine distemper. It is neutralized specifically by the serum of ferrets recovered from distemper, but not by normal ferret serum. Conversely, ferrets immunized by the measles virus are partially protected when challenged with distemper virus. There is also close relationship with the rinderpest virus.

Pathogenesis

Young children in the prodromal phase, when the catarrhal symptoms are prominent, are the main source of the measles virus. They discharge infected particles which are inhaled by the new victim and the virus reaches the respiratory tract, where it grows silently for some days in lymphoid tissue. When multiplication has continued to the point when many infected cells break open, the virus floods into the circulation and causes the prodromal illness. During the following two or three days the virus is localized in the skin and there produces the rash. This viraemia is quenched when antibodies appear in the blood.

Multinucleate giant cells (Warthin-Finkeldy cells) similar to those occurring in tissue cultures can be found in the organs of persons who have died during an attack of measles. It is probable that the giant cells begin to be formed about seven days before the appearance of the rash.

Laboratory Diagnosis

The simplest diagnostic method is to stain smears of the nasal secretions by Giemsa's method and to search for the typical giant cells. The virus can be isolated from throat swabs or washings taken during the 48 hours before and after the onset of the rash. It has also been recovered from the blood and urine in the prodromal period. After antibiotic treatment the materials are inoculated into grown monolayers of monkey kidney or human kidney cells. The cytopathic effect and giant cell formation may begin to appear after 48 to 72 hours but not infrequently are not detected for as long as 10 to 16 days. Subsequently the virus may be propagated in primary human amnion or HEp2 cells with greater yields.

Serum antibodies appear a few days after the onset of the rash, reach a peak about ten days later and decline slowly thereafter, but a detectable level remains indefinitely. Antibodies are most conveniently estimated by the complement-fixation method but neutralization and haemagglutination-inhibition techniques may also be employed.

Epidemiology

Measles is endemic throughout most countries of the world. The disease has a characteristic tendency to epidemicity every second year so that in Great Britain and North America there are 'measles years', usually commencing in the autumn which alternate with years in which a limited number of cases occur.

Measles is most infectious in the two or three days before the appearance of the rash; thereafter infectivity rapidly wanes and is lost after a few days. Transmission can occur by droplet nuclei as well as the orthodox modes of spread of respiratory infections.

The greatest incidence in measles is in the age group 1 to 5 years, and by the age of 20 years 90 per cent of persons have had an attack of the disease. After the first six months of life passively acquired maternal immunity disappears and susceptibility is practically universal. Although measles is usually benign it may cause severe or even fatal illnesses in young children or in elderly people. Secondary invasion with such pathogenic bacteria as haemolytic streptococci, staphylococci and *H. influenzae* cause the complications of bronchopneumonia, diarrhoea and otitis media and these bacterial complications are mainly responsible for the high case fatality from measles in some tropical countries. Another serious complication of measles is encephalomyelitis developing 2 to 6 days after the rash; the features of this condition may resemble those of aseptic meningitis but there is an average case fatality of 15 per cent. In Britain, encephalitis occurs in about 1 in 1 000 cases of measles, is commoner in girls than boys, and is more frequent in the 5 to 9 years age-group than in younger children (Miller, 1964).

When measles is introduced into an area where previously it was not endemic, a sweeping epidemic of great severity follows amongst a virgin population of highly susceptible persons. In these circumstances there is a high incidence of complications and the case fatality is increased. Epidemics of this type have occurred in isolated communities, especially on islands; one particularly severe outbreak occurred in Greenland in 1951. When the infection was first introduced into the Fiji Islands in 1875, it carried off 20 to 25 per cent of the entire population.

PROPHYLAXIS

Measles is so infectious and susceptibility to it so high that there is no point in isolating cases to control the spread of the infection in the population. Hospital patients with measles, however, should be isolated to protect them from the risk of cross-infection from patients ill with other diseases.

Passive immunity can be conferred on contacts by the subcutaneous inoculation of human immunoglobulin. The protective effect is complete if an adequate dose is given within five days of exposure; after this time the disease may not be prevented, but its severity is usually modified and the risk of complications reduced. Immunoglobulin prepared from pooled normal adult sera is effective in a dose of 15 mg per pound body weight.

VACCINES. Two types have been subjected to controlled trials. The first contains virus grown in tissue culture and inactivated by formalin; even after a series of three subcutaneous inoculations its antigenic potency is not sufficient to give full protection. The second type contains the living *Edmonston* strain which has been greatly attenuated by Schwartz. It is given at about the age of 12 to 18 months, after the complete disappearance of maternal antibody. Protective antibodies follow after a single injection in 95 per cent of recipients. The antibody levels that are produced are rather lower than those that follow natural infection, but the immunity conferred is long-lived. Low grade fever and modified rash occur in 5 to 10 per cent of inoculated children but these reactions are not regarded as contraindications to vaccination. However, vaccine should not be given to children who have any form of immunological incompetence or who are suffering from malignant disease.

The Measles, Canine Distemper, Rinderpest Triad

These three viruses are grouped together because of similarities in a number of their properties. Morphologically they have the helical symmetry and general appearances of the parainfluenza viruses. In their pathogenicity they are characterized by a sharp generalized illness with a viraemic phase and the complications of bronchopneumonia and encephalitis. There is a considerable volume of evidence to show that the three viruses share some common antigenic material in varying proportions. The canine distemper and rinderpest viruses were fully described in the eleventh edition of this book (pages 413–415).

REFERENCES AND REVIEWS

CANTELL, K. (1961) Mumps virus. *Advances in Virus Research*, **8**, 123.

CHANOCK, R. M., PARROTT, R. H., JOHNSON, K. M., KAPIKIAN, A. Z. & BELL, J. A. (1963) Myxoviruses: parainfluenza. *American Review of Respiratory Diseases*, **88**, 153.

HILLEMAN, M. R. (1963) Respiratory syncytial virus. *American Review of Respiratory Diseases*, Supplement **88**, 189.

MILLER, D. L. (1964) Frequency of complications in measles, 1963. *British Medical Journal*, ii, 75.

WATERSON, A. P. (1965) Measles virus. *Archiv für die gesamte Virusforschung*, **16**, 57.

44(b). Miscellaneous Viruses: Rubella, Corona, Arena Viruses

Rubella: Common Cold: Lymphocytic Choriomeningitis

The viruses in this section do not fall easily into any precise virus classification either because there is not yet sufficient information about them or because they may belong to groups so far undefined. In particular the rubella virus cannot yet be classified although it has a number of the characters of togaviruses. New taxa have been named coronaviruses associated with the common cold and arenaviruses that include the lymphocytic choriomeningitis virus.

RUBELLA VIRUS

Rubella or 'German Measles' is a common and mild infectious disease characterized by fever, a generalized macular rash and enlargement of the suboccipital, post-auricular and cervical lymph nodes.

DESCRIPTION

The virions are 50 to 70 nm in diameter: they have an electron-dense core about 30 nm in diameter covered by a pleomorphic triple-layered envelope about 8 nm thick. The virus is composed of a single piece of single-stranded RNA of a MW of about 3×10^6 daltons. The virus is inactivated by heat for 1 hour at 56°C and is stable at -65°C. It is sensitive to ether, chloroform and desoxycholate.

Haemagglutination by the virus is well observed in one-day-old chick erythrocytes and at a lower titre in goose and sheep red blood cells. CULTIVATION. In primary cultures of human thyroid tissue and in the cells of a transformed rabbit kidney cell, RK13, the virus regularly produces a definite cytopathic effect with focal changes and intracytoplasmic inclusions. In primary human amnion and in embryonic-skin-muscle cultures the cytopathic effect is less regular. In primary cultures of kidney cells from vervet and patas monkeys and in the HeLa and Chang liver cell lines the virus grows without cytopathic effect. The presence of the virus, in the absence of any cytopathic effect, can be detected by its *interference* (see Chap. 13) with growth of a challenge dose of a virus such as ECHO 2 or 9, Coxsackie A9, or Sindbis. There are no confirmed reports of the growth of the rubella virus in the chick embryo.

ANTIGENICITY. Like the measles and variola viruses, rubella is monotypic and there is no tendency to latent infection.

Pathogenesis

The only reservoir of infection is the human case from whom the virus is transmitted in naso-pharyngeal secretions borne in the air or dust. The virus is inhaled and multiplies in the mucosa of the upper respiratory tract. After an incubation period, usually 16 to 18 days, there is a viraemic phase with fever and the localization of the virus in lymph nodes and skin lesions. Complications are uncommon but arthralgia, arthritis, and paraesthesiae may occur, particularly in adults.

RUBELLA IN PREGNANCY

During the viraemic phase of the illness the virus is able to cross the placental barrier in a pregnant woman and multiply in the differentiating cells of the embryo. Infection of the embryo happens most frequently during the first month of pregnancy, but progressively less often in the second, third and fourth months. The effect on the embryo is the production of congenital abnormalities of which deafness is the most frequent, and then, in order of incidence, congenital heart disease, e.g. persistent ductus arteriosus and ventricular septal defects, chorio-retinitis and cataract, mental defects, micro-cephaly, etc. The rubella virus has often been recovered from the tissues of malformed foetuses removed at hysterotomy from mothers who had suffered from rubella early in pregnancy. There is no agreement on the assessment of the chances of an abnormal child being born to a woman who contracts rubella during pregnancy. In Britain and in Sweden 14 per cent of children born after rubella in the first trimester of pregnancy showed malformation of one or more kinds: about 30 per cent of these infants had some hearing loss, 20 per cent chorio-retinitis, and 18 per cent congenital heart disorders. Hill *et al.* (1958) estimated that the incidence of birth defects was 50 per cent if rubella was contracted during the first month of pregnancy, 25 per cent in the second month, 17 per cent in the third, 11 per cent in the fourth, and 6 per cent in the fifth, but thereafter the risk disappeared. The incidence of prematurity and stillbirths is also increased in women who contract rubella during the first trimester of pregnancy. The children of mothers exposed to but not contracting clinical rubella during pregnancy show no increased frequency of malformations.

It has been postulated that the teratogenic effects of rubella virus on the embryo is because it is relatively noncytocidal and thus allows infected cells to go on dividing, but at a diminished rate; and since spread occurs between contiguous cells, the virus is not affected by maternal antibody. This hypothesis is supported by the finding that, *in vitro*, fetal tissue cells infected with rubella virus multiply more slowly than noninfected cells.

Laboratory Diagnosis

Rubella virus is most easily isolated from throat swabs taken during the acute phase of the illness, but it can be recovered in the phase of viraemia from the blood, and also from leucocytes, the bone-marrow, the cerebrospinal fluid, the eye lens, or from almost any organ. Cell cultures that are susceptible include continuous cell lines such as RK13, BHK21 or SIRC where a variable degree of cytopathic effect or haemadsorption may occur. The virus may also be detected in these infected cells by immunofluorescence and it is obvious that virus replication occurs exclusively within the cell cytoplasm.

Serological evidence of rubella infection in the past is particularly important to the doctor caring for a pregnant woman who may have been exposed to infection. In these circumstances paired specimens of sera are required, the first collected as soon after exposure as possible, and the second 1 to 2 weeks later. The serological method of choice is the haemagglutination-inhibition test.

Congenital Rubella Syndrome

When a baby is born with congenital defects which could be related to rubella in the mother in early pregnancy, evidence of rubella infection in the infant may be obtained by examinations for excretion of rubella virus in the urine and other secretions. The question arises whether the offspring, infected early in utero, has acquired an immunological tolerance to the virus and antibody studies both on the fetus and on the infant for some months after birth have given the answer. IgM antibodies which are not transferable from mother to offspring begin to appear in the fetal tissues in the second trimester of pregnancy and steadily increase to reach maximum titres in the fourth to the sixth month after birth: IgG antibodies, present in fetal tissues and presumably derived from the mother, decline and disappear within 2 to 3 months of birth, but this is followed by a gradual rise of infant-manufactured IgG antibodies which reach a plateau in the first to the second year of life. There is therefore no evidence to support a hypothesis of immunological tolerance to rubella virus and such serological findings confirm a diagnosis of congenital rubella infection even in the absence of obvious neonatal defects.

The normal titres of rubella-specific globulins can be assessed precisely by the observation of the IgM, IgA and IgG antibody levels by serum-fractionation methods using immunodiffusion in agarose Biogel 5 m. Besides confirmation of the congenital rubella syndrome, there are a number of situations where the development or demonstration of these specific immunoglobulins are particularly useful:

1. When there has been a definite or suspected risk of exposure of a pregnant woman during the first two trimesters of her pregnancy. During these months a rising titre of IgM antibody as estimated in haemagglutination inhibition tests

gives a definite indication of a current infection.

2. After immunization it is important for newly-weds and pre-pubertal girls to know whether they have acquired a reliable measure of resistance to rubella as shown by the antibody titres.

EPIDEMIOLOGY

Rubella virus is demonstrable in the naso-pharynx of cases for several days both before and after the appearance of the rash. Infection is acquired by inhalation of infective material and perhaps by more direct contact, e.g. within the family and among young adults. Rubella is not so highly infectious as measles and the age of attack is later, mainly in schoolchildren and extending into adolescence and early adult life. The disease is endemic throughout the world but slowly spreading epidemic waves occur at inter-vals of 5 to 8 years in some countries. Because of its mildness, rubella is frequently missed or misdiagnosed: antibody studies have shown that in some industrialized countries with temperate climates, e.g. Britain and the United States, around 80 per cent of older schoolchildren have already been infected. The level is lower (50 to 60 per cent) in some warm climate countries, e.g. the West Indies, thereby increasing the risk of infection in pregnancy. One attack of the disease confers lasting immunity.

PROPHYLAXIS

No measures need to be taken to prevent the spread of this relatively mild infection amongst children and, indeed, deliberate exposure of young girls to the risk of infection has been advocated so that they may acquire an immunity before they reach the age of marriage. In preg-nant women exposed to infection normal immunoglobulin is of doubtful value in prevent-ing the clinical disease.

Active immunization against rubella can be conferred by a single subcutaneous (or intra-nasal) inoculation of a live attenuated vaccine. The vaccines available are the Cendehill vaccine which was developed in Belgium by passage in primary cultures of rabbit kidney cells; and the RA 27/33 virus vaccine which is grown in the WI 38 line of human embryonic cells. The Cendehill vaccine has been licensed for use in many different countries and, because it has been more attenuated than most other virus strains, only rarely produces arthritis in adults or reactions in children.

Multiplication of vaccine viruses in the reci-pient is usually symptomless though occasionally there may arise a mild transient fever with or without a rash, lymphadenopathy, or a minor degree of arthralgia or transient arthritis. As the vaccine virus multiplies in the tissues a few of the virions are discharged but they do not spread to infect susceptible contacts.

After successful vaccination rubella anti-bodies develop in about 95 per cent of the recipients and reach titres 4 to 8 fold higher than those attained in natural infection. These levels are maintained for several years.

The vaccine is best used at about the age of puberty in girls (11 to 13 years) and this is the recommended policy in Britain; however, some would advocate that all children be inoculated in the first two years of life in an attempt to eradicate the infection.

The vaccine must *not* be given to sero-negative pregnant women nor to anyone who might conceive during the following few weeks. Vacci-nation is relatively safe if it is done as soon as possible after the delivery of a first baby, but if it is postponed for even a short period, it may put early second pregnancies at risk.

When women are given this vaccine, they should understand that they must avoid be-coming pregnant during the succeeding eight weeks.

CORONAVIRUSES

Coronavirus is the generic name used for a con-siderable number of respiratory viruses of man; it also includes the virus of avian infectious bronchitis, the mouse hepatitus virus and the haemagglutinating encephelomyelitis virus of pigs.

DESCRIPTION

The virions are pleomorphic and 80 to 160 nm in diameter; they are covered by a fringe of petal-shaped projections, each about 20 nm long. Their resemblance to a crown has led to the use of the generic name of *coronavirus*. At first these viruses seem to be very similar to myxoviruses but on closer scrutiny, the internal nucleocapsid has been difficult to define and the petal-shaped protrusions from the envelope have their own special shape and are spaced much more widely apart than the haemagglutinin spikes of myxoviruses. Coronaviruses contain single-stranded RNA and are ether-sensitive. Human coronaviruses haemagglutinate the red blood cells of man and the vervet monkey at 4°C. Erythrocytes of the chicken, rat and mouse are agglutinated at room temperature or at 37°C. Neuraminic acid receptors are not involved in this process. There is a considerable amount of antigenic sharing by the human and murine coronaviruses.

CULTIVATION. When these viruses are first isolated they are propagated only with some difficulty. The most successful host-cell system is that of tracheal organ cultures, but primary human embryonic kidney cell cultures and human diploid cell strains are also susceptible and the presence of the virus is revealed by its cytopathic effect. Viral replication occurs in the cytoplasm and it is not affected by DNA inhibitors.

Pathogenicity

In man the coronaviruses give rise to acute upper respiratory tract infections, the majority of which are indistinguishable from the common cold. Infection of the lower respiratory tract is rare.

Laboratory Diagnosis

The viruses can be isolated from nasopharyngeal swabs in human embryonic ciliated tracheal endothelium organ cultures or in human diploid embryonic fibroblasts. Serologically a retrospective diagnosis can be made by demonstrating a significant rise of antibody in paired samples of sera using the complement-fixation technique.

ARENAVIRUSES

This group of viruses seem to contain RNA. The particles are round, oval or pleomorphic and vary in diameter from 50 to 80 nm. They are covered by an envelope with a structure of closely spaced projections. The interior of the particles seems to be granular and this characteristic has given these viruses their name which is taken from their resemblance to grains of sand. All strains share a group specific antigen.

The type species of this virus genus is the benign lymphocytic choriomeningitis virus but many other viruses, some of which were previously classified as arboviruses, have recently been included in this group.

LYMPHOCYTIC CHORIOMENINGITIS

Benign lymphocytic choriomeningitis is primarily an enzootic disease of wild mice. The virus is excreted in the urine and faeces and is transmissible in contaminated dust to man in whom it may rarely cause an influenza-like fever or a meningitis.

Description

The virions are 40 to 60 nm in diameter. They are well preserved by freeze-drying or storage at −70°C. In whole infected tissue stored in 50 per cent glycerol at 4°C the virus survives for several years: it is inactivated by 10 per cent ether overnight, 0·5 per cent formalin, and 0·01 per cent merthiolate: it is unstable at pH values below 7.

The virus grows on the chorio-allantoic membrane of 11 to 12 day-old chick embryos without pock production or any obvious effect on the embryo. Tissue culture cells of the chick, mouse, calves and monkey support the growth of the virus, but a cytopathic effect may not be obvious until the virus has been adapted by several passages.

When inoculated intracerebrally into healthy mice a severe encephalitis results in which the animals show marked muscular spasms and convulsions. In the guinea-pig the disease takes the form of generalized systemic infection. Rabbits are not susceptible.

Pathogenesis

In man the most obvious clinical picture is that of aseptic meningitis but the infection may be inapparent or show itself as a severe influenzal illness or as an 'atypical pneumonia'.

The lymphocytic choriomeningitis virus is essentially an inhabitant of mice and in these animals exists in a latent form which is transmitted by the mother to her young *in utero*. The virus is excreted by the mice in urine, faeces and nasal secretions. Most human infections are contracted from material contaminated by mice, and the most likely route of infection is thought to be through the respiratory mucosa.

Laboratory Diagnosis

The cerebrospinal fluid shows a marked cellular response; 200 to 1 000 cells per mm^3 are present and 90 per cent are lymphocytes. The protein is raised to 60 to 100 mg per 100 ml, but normal values are found for the chloride and sugar estimations; these findings help to distinguish lymphocytic choriomeningitis from tuberculous meningitis. The virus may be isolated from the cerebrospinal fluid by intracerebral inoculation of adult mice. Virus identification is carried out by neutralization tests or complement-fixation reactions with specific antisera.

Serological tests may give a retrospective diagnosis if virus isolation tests have not been carried out. Complement-fixing antibodies appear by the fourteenth day, but are slow to reach a peak. Three samples of serum are usually required to establish the existence of a rising titre of antibodies; the first should be taken as soon as possible after the onset of the illness, the second 14 days later and the third after an interval of 4 to 5 weeks.

There are no specific measures to control infection with this virus. Extermination of mice will usually eradicate the disease. Those whose work as laboratory assistants or rodent exterminators obliges them to come into contact with mice must take precautions to avoid inhaling infective material.

REFERENCES AND REVIEWS

BRADBURNE, A. F. & TYRRELL, D. A. J. (1971) Coronaviruses in man. *Progress in Medical Virology*, **13**, 373.

HILL, A. B., DOLL, R., GALLOWAY, T. M. & HUGHES, J. P. W. (1958) Virus diseases in pregnancy and congenital defects. *British Journal of Preventive and Social Medicine*, **12**, 1.

McDONALD, J. C. (1963) Gamma globulin for prevention of rubella in pregnancy. *British Medical Journal*, **ii**, 416.

SCHIFF, G. M. & SEVER, J. L. (1966) Rubella: recent laboratory and clinical advances. *Progress in Medical Virology*, **8**, 30.

WILSNACK, R. E. (1966) Viruses in laboratory rodents. *National Institute of Cancer Monographs*, **20**, 77.

45. Picornaviruses

(a) ENTEROVIRUSES:
Poliomyelitis: Aseptic Meningitis: Epidemic Myalgia
(b) RHINOVIRUSES:
Common Cold

Although the polioviruses were first isolated in monkeys and the original coxsackievirus in mice, the characterization of the picornaviruses and the isolation of many of them was possible only after the introduction of tissue culture methods.

As the name picornavirus suggests, these viruses are pico (small, 27 nm) RNA (RNA-containing) viruses and a-number of their principal features are shown in Table 45.1.

The polioviruses, coxsackieviruses and echoviruses are described as enteroviruses because they are all found in the intestines and excreted in the faeces. These three groups of viruses have a number of features in common: (1) they all replicate in the intestinal tract; (2) they commonly cause asymptomatic immunizing infections which protect against future infection; (3) they can give rise to a viraemia; (4) they occasionally cause infection of the central nervous system; (5) they are commoner in children than adults; (6) they cause infections usually in the summer and autumn.

The rhinoviruses are found in the upper respiratory tract and cause the common cold.

POLIOVIRUS

DESCRIPTION

The poliovirus is 27 nm in diameter. The virion is in the form of an icosahedron with 32 protein capsomeres enclosing an RNA core which constitutes 25 to 30 per cent of the particle.

Two outstanding characteristics of the virus are its affinity for nervous tissue and its narrow animal host range. The only animals readily susceptible are the primates, though it has been possible to adapt some strains to grow in small rodents and chick embryos. Cynomolgus and rhesus monkeys can be infected by the oral route and develop paralysis; in chimpanzees the infection is often asymptomatic. Under the influence of cortisone, monkeys become more

Table 45.1. Principal Features of Picornaviruses*

Group	Stability at pH 3–5	Important sites of infection in man	Method of isolation	Effect on	
				Monkey CNS	Suckling mice
Poliovirus	stable	Alimentary tract, CNS	MK, HA HEK	*paralysis*	none
Echovirus	stable	Alimentary tract, CNS, skin	MK, HA HEK, W1–38	rarely paralysis	none
Coxsackievirus	stable	Alimentary tract, CNS, muscles	group A = SM, group B = SM, MK, HA	rarely paralysis	*group A—myositis group B—encephalitis, necrosis of brown fat*
Rhinovirus	unstable	Upper respiratory tract	HEK W1–38, OC	none	none

*All the viruses are icosahedral and contain RNA.
MK = Monkey kidney tissue culture.
HA = Human amnion tissue culture.
HEK = Human embryo kidney.

W1–38 = Human diploid fibroblasts.
OC   = Organ culture, i.e. human embryo respiratory epithelium.
SM   = Suckling mice.

459

susceptible to small parenteral doses of the virus. The animals develop a viraemia which is suppressed when antibodies appear, and later they excrete the virus in their faeces. Polioviruses are most easily isolated and cultivated *in vitro* in tissue cultures of monkey kidney, primary human amnion or HeLa cells, in the last of which their cytopathic effect becomes rapidly apparent. They can be grown in a wide variety of human cells in tissue culture explants, e.g. embryonic skin, muscle, kidney, tonsil, prepuce, testis and uterus; monkey testis or lung can also be used.

Viability

The poliovirus is one of the most stable viruses. In aqueous suspensions of human faeces at 4°C it survives for many months, and in pieces of spinal cord in 50 per cent glycerol in normal saline it remains viable for periods of eight years or more. It can be preserved for many months or years at $-20°$ or $-70°C$. Unlike most other viruses its infectivity is not well preserved by freeze drying. In human stools the virus may remain infective at room temperature for as short a time as one day or for as long as several weeks, depending on the amount of virus present, the pH, the amount of faecal moisture and other environmental conditions. The virus is readily killed by moist heat at 50° to 55°C, but milk, cream and ice-cream exert a protective effect so that the virus in these foodstuffs may survive exposure to heat at 60°C. It is destroyed by the holding process of pasteurization of milk at 62°C, but the safety margin is not sufficient for certain inactivation and the flash method at 72°C is preferred.

In infected human spinal cord the virus is rapidly inactivated at pH values below 2 or over 11; it survives for ten days at 4°C in 1 per cent phenol, 18 hours at 4°C in 20 per cent ether and 0·1 per cent sodium deoxycholate. Inactivation of poliovirus in tissue culture fluids is complete after seven days exposure to 0·025 per cent formaldehyde at 37°C, but its antigenicity is retained so that it can be used as an immunizing agent. The most active disinfectants are oxidizing agents such as potassium permanganate and hypochlorites. In the absence of organic matter free chlorine in a strength of 0·05 parts per million will inactivate the virus, but higher concentrations than this are needed to disinfect swimming-bath water or materials contaminated by faeces.

Antigenic Characters

Three immunological types of the virus have been identified by neutralization tests carried out in the monkey or in tissue cultures. The prototype strains are; type 1, the Brunhilde and Mahoney strains; type 2, which includes the rodent adapted strains, the Lansing and MEF1 strains; and type 3, the Leon and Saukett strains. The three types are antigenically distinct, but overlapping in neutralization tests is not infrequent. Type 1 is the common epidemic type, type 2 is usually associated with endemic infections, and type 3 occasionally causes epidemics. The size, chemical and physical properties, and the resistance of the three types are all identical.

Virus Multiplication

Although the multiplication of poliovirus in cells is described here, the principles enunciated apply to the other picornaviruses also. The description applies to cells in culture and the same processes do not necessarily occur in the tissues of an infected person or animal.

The virion attaches to the cell by a specific cellular receptor which reacts with the protein capsid. The presence or absence of these specific receptors determines whether the cell is susceptible to infection by the virus or not. Once the virus particle is attached to the cellular receptor it is taken into the cell by pinocytosis. Inside the cell the virus is 'uncoated' and the viral RNA is released from the protein capsid. During this phase, the 'eclipse phase', the viral components cannot be demonstrated. The viral RNA acts probably as messenger RNA and gives rise to the formation of protein enzymes concerned with the production of viral RNA and the proteins of the capsid. The viral RNA consists of about 6000 nucleotides capable of producing genetic information to code for about 2000 aminoacids or 10 to 15 proteins. The synthesis of viral RNA and viral proteins occurs in the cytoplasm of the infected cell, probably near the nucleus, i.e. juxtanuclear.

When cells are infected with poliovirus, the

synthesis of cellular RNA and protein ceases and the lethal effects of the virus on cells is related to this effect. The end result of the replication is the appearance of the cytopathic effect which coincides with the release of infectious virus particles into the medium due to the shedding of the peripheral cytoplasm of the infected cell.

PATHOGENESIS

The only natural source of the virus is man; the virus is spread from person to person, and no intermediate host is known. The human reservoir of infection consists of persons who excrete the virus in their faeces and perhaps, less commonly, in their oropharyngeal secretions. Most of those infected have no paralytic mani-

festations of the infection and suffer no illness. The virus they excrete enters the new host by ingestion or inhalation.

In paralytic poliomyelitis, the virus can be found in the faeces for a few days preceding the onset of acute symptoms and is present in over 80 per cent of cases in the stool during the first 14 days. After three weeks some 50 per cent of patients still excrete the virus and at 5 to 6 weeks, 25 per cent. Only a few cases continue to excrete the virus after the twelfth week. No permanent carriers are known. The virus can be isolated from the oropharynx of many cases for a few days before and after the onset of the illness.

On entering the body of a new host the virus probably first invades the lymphoid tissues in the upper respiratory tract or the Peyer's patches of the small intestine and the associated mesenteric lymph nodes. During the next seven days

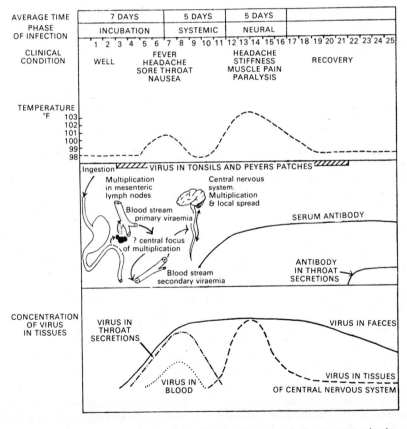

FIG. 45.1. A diagram to show the correlation between the clinical and pathological events occurring in a paralytic case of poliomyelitis.

large amounts of virus are produced locally in these extraneural sites until there is a spill-over into the lymphatics and invasion of the blood stream. In cases that die of an overwhelming infection within a short time from the onset, the Peyer's patches and the mesenteric lymph nodes are found to be greatly swollen and inflamed and to contain large amounts of virus (see Fig. 45.1).

The viraemic phase marks the end of the incubation period and is manifest in the patient by fever and generalized toxic symptoms; it is followed by a period of about 48 hours of relative well-being (the disease is biphasic) while the virus is invading nerve tissue and then, in serious cases, the signs of paralysis appear. Viraemia has been proved to occur after experimental infection of monkeys and has been demonstrated on several occasions in man. It is probable that the process can be arrested at various stages so that the virus may multiply in the intestine without ever reaching the blood stream, or once in the blood stream, the virus may be overcome by the patient's natural defence mechanisms before it can reach nerve cells. Even if the virus destroys nerve cells, it is only when certain critical areas are involved that paralysis results. In this way it is possible to explain abortive and non-paralytic forms of poliomyelitis. However, it is not yet known whether viraemia is a constant feature of the disease and no adequate explanation has yet been offered of the manner whereby the virus enters the nerve cells in paralytic poliomyelitis.

CLINICAL FEATURES

There are three types of poliovirus infection: (1) Asymptomatic infection or a mild transient 'influenza-like' illness; this infection is accompanied by excretion of the virus in the faeces for a limited time and an immunological response which protects against infection with the same strain in the future: (2) Infections with evidence of involvement of the central nervous system, so-called 'virus meningitis'; these patients, like those in (1), excrete virus and are protected against further attack, but they have a clinical illness characterized by meningitis without paralysis: (3) Paralytic poliomyelitis in which the patient develops paralysis during the course of the illness; this is the most dramatic form of the infection but is very uncommon, occurring in only about 1 in 1 000 of poliovirus infections. The paralysis may be spinal, bulbar, or bulbospinal depending on which anterior horn cells have been affected.

Factors Predisposing to Clinical Infection

A number of factors are known to shorten the incubation period, enhance the severity of the infection, and promote the localization of the virus in the central nervous system, thus predisposing to paralysis. Muscular activity during the preparalytic phase of the illness leads to paralysis of the limbs used. Pregnant women are more susceptible than non-pregnant women. Poliomyelitis occurring near full term is apt to be severe and may assume the bulbar form. Tonsillectomy carries an increased risk of bulbar poliomyelitis, and this risk persists for several months or even years after the operation. It is established that infants are less likely to develop paralysis than older children, but the peak incidence of clinical disease is still in the 1 to 3 year-olds; in recent epidemics over 60 per cent of fatal cases have been in patients over 15 years old in whom the infection tends to be more severe.

Paralytic poliomyelitis may also occur in children who have received immunizing injections of alum-containing diphtheria toxoid, particularly when combined with pertussis antigens, probably associated with the irritant properties of the adjuvant. A similar effect has followed the use of penicillin, arsenicals and heavy metals in mass campaigns against yaws. Paralysis occurs in the limb that receives the inoculation and its incidence is approximately 1 in 37 000 injections. There is much doubt about the manner in which the paralysis is precipitated; the irritant inoculum in the muscles may render the anterior horn cells of the corresponding segment of the cord more susceptible to virus invasion or it may provide a site for a focal proliferation of the virus circulating in the blood.

In paralytic poliomyelitis it sometimes happens that the patient has a double infection and that both the poliomyelitis virus and a coxsackievirus can be recovered from the faeces. Viruses of coxsackie group A occur with significantly greater frequency than those of group B in paralytic poliomyelitis. The frequency of the association of the poliomyelitis and coxsackie-viruses belonging to group A has been sufficient to suggest that infection with the latter predisposes to paralysis.

LABORATORY DIAGNOSIS

VIRUS ISOLATION. The virus may be recovered from faeces or from throat swabs taken early in the disease. Two such specimens should be collected on successive days as early as possible in the course of the disease. A 10 per cent faecal suspension is made in a balanced salt solution containing 100 units of penicillin and 100 μg of streptomycin per ml and is then centrifuged to remove coarse particles. Throat swabs are treated in a similar fashion. The material is then used to inoculate monkey kidney, human amnion, HeLa, HEp2 or other cell cultures. If the virus is replicating, a cytopathic effect is usually seen in the cells within 48 hours. Identification of the virus type is carried out by a neutralization test in which a measured dose of virus (approximately 100 $TCID_{50}$) is exposed to the action of standard type-specific antisera. In fatal cases specimens obtained at necropsy should include the cervical and lumbar enlargements of the spinal cord, the medulla, mesenteric lymph nodes and portions of small intestine and colon with their contents. After being homogenized, these tissues are treated in the same way as faeces. All types of infected material may be preserved in the refrigerator at 4°C, but better results are obtained when storage is at $-40°C$. Tissues should be placed in 50 per cent glycerol saline before storage.

Any poliovirus isolated from a patient may be either a 'wild' virulent virus or an attenuated vaccine strain. The only certain way to distinguish between these two possibilities is to carry out virulence tests in the monkey, but with attenuated strains of polioviruses types 1 and 2 there are certain genetic, *in vitro*, 'marker' characters which are sufficiently stable to be helpful.

SEROLOGICAL TESTS. Paired samples of serum are required; the first must be taken as soon as possible after the onset of the disease and the second after an interval of three to four weeks. Neutralization tests are usually employed with all the three virus types. If the first sample has been taken sufficiently early it is often possible to show a significant rise of antibodies to the infecting virus type in the second specimen, but in practice this may not always be achieved because of the insidious nature of the onset. Antibody tends to rise rapidly, and titres of 1 000 or higher are usual by the end of the third week of the disease. In type 1 infection some type 2 antibody may develop as well. Complement-fixation and flocculation tests are not generally used for routine diagnostic work.

EPIDEMIOLOGY

Since the wide use of poliovaccines in the 1960s in Western Europe, the North American continent and Australia, poliomyelitis, which used to be an endemic disease in these countries, has virtually disappeared and cases of infection in these areas have usually acquired the disease in countries where the disease is still endemic, such as the tropics. In the tropics the disease occurs uniformly throughout the whole year without any tendency to seasonal variation.

Prior to the use of poliovaccines, the disease was endemic with periodic epidemics, usually in the late summer in Europe, America and Australia. Where standards of hygiene were high the spread of the virus was impeded and individuals or whole communities escaped infection for many years. In this way, a situation arose in which a large proportion of the population had no immunity and when a poliovirus was introduced into such a community an epidemic could develop rapidly. The introduction of a strain of higher virulence may also be a factor in epidemic spread. It is difficult to know which of these factors was more important when in Britain in 1947 the incidence of poliomyelitis rose from the usual figure of 4 per 100 000 to 18 per 100 000 of the population.

Sources and Spread

Poliomyelitis is often contracted during a period of quite close proximity to an infected person so that family contacts are more likely to become infected than, say, school contacts. The virus may be inhaled in infected particles or ingested and may be frequently transferred by the hands of persons who are excreting the virus or by those who have touched contaminated fomites.

Faeces provide a rich and persistent source of the virus; it has been calculated that one gram of stool may contain several million infective doses of the virus. When poliovirus infection is prevalent, sewage in urban populations contains the virus throughout the summer and early winter months. Water supplies may occasionally be contaminated by sewage, and in rural areas this may be a means by which infection is spread. There is little evidence, however, that the virus can survive the purification processes used for a piped water supply, and urban water-borne epidemics have not been described. Faecal pollution of swimming-baths has been thought to spread the infection, but there is little direct evidence on this point and with adequate chlorination the risk is small. Flies may carry the virus to food on their feet or by regurgitation after feeding on exposed faeces or sewage.

Immunity is permanent to the virus type causing the infection. Although the three virus types are antigenically distinct there is some evidence to suggest that prior infection with type 2 virus may confer a measure of resistance to the paralytic disease caused by type 1.

Virus neutralizing antibodies are formed early during the disease (often before the seventh day) and persist for several decades. Complement-fixing antibodies are of much shorter duration.

Due to the intestinal infection by the virus there is a considerable amount of secretory IgA produced locally in the intestine.

Prophylaxis and Control

Since it has proved impractical to prevent the widespread dissemination of the virus and because it is impossible to recognize the trivial infections that the poliomyelitis viruses cause, it became obvious that the disease can be controlled only by raising the immunity of the population to a high level. Active immunization against poliovirus infection can be produced by

the use of:
  (a) inactivated poliovaccines (Salk) or
  (b) live attenuated poliovaccines (Sabin).

INACTIVATED POLIOVACCINES. The vaccine contains strains of the three types of virus, grown in monkey kidney cell culture, and inactivated by exposure to formaldehyde. The batches of vaccine are tested for the presence of residual live poliovirus and must be free from bacteria, fungi, mycoplasmas and viruses such as virus B and SV40, a simian virus which is oncogenic in hamsters. Inactivated poliovaccines have been produced in a number of countries, e.g. U.S.A., Sweden, and Britain. These vaccines have been used extensively and many millions of people have received them without ill effect; they cause no local or general reactions and have been proved to lower significantly the incidence of paralytic poliomyelitis. The British schedule of inoculation is that two doses of 1·0 ml of the vaccine are given intramuscularly at an interval of three weeks. Two booster doses are required, one 6 to 9 months after the second dose and the last a year or two later.

The inactivated poliovirus vaccine may be used simultaneously with the triple vaccine against diphtheria, pertussis and tetanus or it may be combined with it in a quadruple vaccine (Butler *et al.*, 1962). The latter has *not* been recommended for general use in Britain.

LIVE ATTENUATED POLIOVACCINES. These are now used extensively in many countries including Britain. The virus strains used in these vaccines are attenuated and lack all power to produce paralysis even when injected directly into the brain or spinal cord of monkeys. They were obtained by cultivating wild but relatively avirulent polioviruses in monolayer cultures of monkey kidney cells in which plaques were produced. By selection of a single plaque, pure clones of viruses were obtained and passaged until neurovirulence was lost. The strains most commonly used were developed by Sabin (1959).

Live attenuated vaccines have the great advantage over killed vaccines that they are given orally and are therefore much easier to administer; large numbers of persons can be immunized by feeding the vaccine during a very short space of time. In addition, this vaccine is much more economical in use than the inactivated vaccine because it is much simpler to prepare and the virus dose required is approximately one ten-thousandth part of the virus content of a single inoculation of the inactivated vaccine.

The immunity that follows feeding the attenuated viruses is effective in over 90 per cent of the subjects and the antibody response is as good as that induced by inactivated vaccines. The duration of immunity follows the same general pattern as that produced by the use of inactivated vaccines. In addition to evoking the production of humoral antibodies the growth of the vaccine strains in the gut creates a state of local resistance whereby the subsequent establishment of polioviruses in the intestine is prevented.

Administration of the attenuated strains in Great Britain is carried out by feeding a trivalent oral vaccine on three separate occasions spaced at 6 to 8 week intervals between the first and second dose and 4 to 6 months between the second and third dose (see Chap. 58). Children and adults receive the vaccine on a lump of sugar or in syrup (BP). The dose is 0·15 ml (3 drops) and contains all three of the Sabin strains. In infants the vaccine may be dropped directly into the mouth. An alternative schedule recommended by Sabin employs monovalent vaccines which are given in similar doses in the order of types 1, 3, and 2 at intervals of at least four and preferably six weeks.

Attenuated vaccines have the advantage that they can be administered very easily and quickly in mass vaccination campaigns. When used in this way in the face of a commencing epidemic they have been successful in halting the spread of infection, as in Singapore (1958–59), in Hull (1961) when type 2 strain was used, and in Dundee in 1962 when trivalent vaccine was employed. One disadvantage of the use of live vaccine is that the presence of another enterovirus in the community at the time of giving vaccine may prevent, by interference, the vaccine virus colonizing the alimentary tract and thereby interferes with the immune response. This hazard is likely to occur in crowded communities in warm-climate countries.

There is little doubt that a few cases of paralytic poliomyelitis have been closely associated with the use of the live vaccine. These few cases of paralysis have been discovered during surveillance programmes in various countries, and have occurred within 60 days of vaccination.

Most of these cases of paralytic poliomyelitis have been type 3 infections and the risk is about one in one million vaccinated individuals for type 3. The risk of paralytic poliomyelitis from types 1 and 2 live vaccine strains is much less. In view of the problem of the type 3 strain not being sufficiently attenuated, new strains of type 3 are being investigated and it is hoped a more stable strain will be discovered.

Passive immunity can be conferred by injecting gammaglobulin. To afford protection gammaglobulin must be used before or as soon as possible after exposure to the infection, i.e. when possible, before the risk has occurred. As it is in short supply and of rather doubtful value, gammaglobulin is reserved for special occasions; it is used for pregnant women after exposure, for children after tonsillectomy at epidemic periods, and for laboratory workers accidentally contaminated with the virus. It should *not* be used for family contacts of a recognized case.

ECHOVIRUSES

When tissue cultures began to be used for the isolation of polioviruses from stools, both in cases of poliomyelitis and illnesses stimulating nonparalytic poliomyelitis, it was found that many other viruses also could be recovered from the intestinal tract. These viruses can only be isolated in tissue cultures, optimally in those from monkey kidneys. Originally they were called 'orphan' viruses because they seemed to be unrelated to known diseases, and since they were present in faeces they were named 'enteric, cytopathogenic, human, orphan', i.e. echoviruses.

DESCRIPTION

The echoviruses are in general similar to the polioviruses in size, stability and resistance. They contain at least 25 to 30 per cent RNA. They survive long periods at 4°C, are not inactivated at 37°C, and are stable from pH 3 to pH 11. In general, they are killed by heat at 65°C for 30 minutes, survive well at −70°C, but lose much of their activity on freeze-drying. Continuous cell lines, e.g. HeLa, are not suitable for attempts at echovirus isolation, as the cytopathic effect may be absent or very slow to appear.

CULTIVATION. Most strains grow well in epithelial cells from the kidneys of rhesus or cynomolgus monkeys and also in human amnion, human embryonic kidney cells, and human diploid cells. Some types can be adapted to HeLa and HEp2 cells.

When echoviruses are seeded in dilute inocula on to the surface of a sheet of tissue culture cells, each single infective particle sets up an area of cell lysis or a plaque which is easily recognized. Some types produce large circular plaques with clearly defined edges and a diameter after a week's growth of 1 cm. Other types produce irregularly shaped plaques which develop slowly and seldom reach 0·5 cm in diameter (Hsiung, 1962).

The sequence of events in virus multiplication is similar to that of the other picornaviruses, taking poliovirus as a model.

Echoviruses are pathogenic for rhesus and cynomolgus monkeys; types 2, 3, 4, 7, 9, 13, 14, 16, and 18 induce a febrile illness with viraemia and an antigenic response (Wenner, 1962). Echo 9, especially after repeated passage in tissue culture, produces a fatal paralysis in mice resembling that caused by the type A coxsackieviruses.

Haemagglutination of human group-O erythrocytes is caused by types 3, 6, 7, 11, 12, 13, 19, 20, 21, 24, 29, and 30. These strains react with a receptor on human group-O cells which is distinct from that of the myxoviruses. The haemagglutinin is not separable from the virus particle.

ANTIGENIC CHARACTERS. Thirty-three distinct antigenic types have so far been distinguished by neutralization tests in tissue cultures. Cross reactions occur between types 1, 8, 12, and 13 in neutralization tests. Antigenic variation is known to occur in types 4, 6, and 9, and may be a common occurrence under natural conditions. The specificity of strains may be altered by cultivation in the presence of heterologous antiserum.

Clinical Features

Echovirus infections are preceded by a short incubation period, usually of 3 to 5 days, and may take the form of a simple fever, aseptic meningitis, diarrhoeal diseases or respiratory illnesses. A rubelliform rash may complicate these disease patterns or may occur as the sole manifestation of infection.

PATHOGENESIS

The sources of infection are human cases or carriers excreting echoviruses in their faeces or oropharyngeal secretions. When the viruses enter the body they multiply in epithelial cells in either the intestine or the respiratory tract. Some types, e.g. 6, 9, 11, 16, and 18, are able to penetrate the epithelial barrier of the gut to reach the blood stream and multiply in secondary target organs. The viraemic phase may begin five days before the beginning of the illness and continue until 24 hours after the onset. All except six of the serotypes have been recovered from the cerebrospinal fluid in cases of aseptic meningitis, the exceptions being 22, 24, 26, 29, 32, and 33. Echo 9 appears to be able to invade nervous tissue and infection with it is sometimes accompanied by mild transient paralysis. Recovery from echovirus infections is almost invariably rapid and complete; the number of human fatalities which can be ascribed with certainty to these viruses is exceedingly small.

Echoviruses are not infrequently found in the stools of healthy young children, but the significance of this finding is not yet clear. There is little evidence to suggest that they are intestinal commensals and it is more probable that they are carried for undefined periods after mild or inapparent infections.

LABORATORY DIAGNOSIS

Echoviruses are readily isolated from throat swabs, stools or cerebrospinal fluid; they are present in 80 per cent of cases in the faeces for two weeks after the onset. The procedure for isolation is that described for poliomyelitis and involves inoculation into monolayers of monkey kidney tissues. Human amnion cells, human embryo kidney cells and human diploid cells can be used, but HeLa cells are unsuitable. Strains are identified by testing first against pools of known antisera and then by neutralization with a single type specific antiserum (Hambling, Davis and Macrae, 1963). Infections with more than one echovirus type can sometimes be revealed by the different types of plaques produced in monolayer cultures. Serological tests are burdensome, and unless there is some indication of the prevailing type, it is impractical to set up the many neutralization tests required.

IMMUNITY. Type-specific circulating antibodies develop as a result of echovirus infection. Neutralizing antibodies appear within a fortnight after infection of the intestine. The antibodies usually persist for a number of years. Haemagglutination-inhibiting and complement-fixing antibodies appear a few days later than the neutralizing antibodies, and also disappear sooner.

EPIDEMIOLOGY

Echoviruses occur in all parts of the world. They are found more frequently in children than in adults and are more prevalent in the summer and autumn months in temperate climates. The method of spread of the viruses is the same as that of the polioviruses and they are widely and rapidly disseminated when hygiene and sanitation are poor. In closed communities of children and in schools, the viruses are transmitted easily so that a very high proportion of individuals are infected and excrete the virus.

Most of the echovirus types have been associated with sporadic cases of aseptic meningitis or one of the other disease patterns already mentioned. In the eruptive fevers caused by types 9 and 16 the aetiological relationship between the rash and the infective agent is well established. A number of types, notably 4, 6, 9, 16, 20, 28, and 30, have considerable epidemic potentialities and the clinical features are very varied. As examples, echovirus 9 epidemics have been common in Europe and North America and have taken the form of large outbreaks of a disease typically characterized by a biphasic fever, a sore throat, and exanthem in the form of macular or maculopapular rash on the face, neck and chest, and less commonly, on the lower trunk and extremities. A minority of patients show clinical signs of meningitis but many without distinct clinical signs have a pleocytosis in the cerebrospinal fluid.

Echovirus 16 epidemics have been called 'Boston Fever' after the city where the illness was first reported. Clinically, the infection starts with a sharp fever, abdominal pains and a mild sore throat. Commonly in children there appears, 24 to 48 hours after defervescence, a pink, discrete macular or maculopapular rash mostly on the face, chest and back. Aseptic meningitis is uncommon. Echoviruses 4, 6, and 30 epidemics have been associated with considerable outbreaks of aseptic meningitis in children and adults.

Echovirus 18 has been recovered from the faeces of many infants in an outbreak of diarrhoea. The children had no rash and no involvement of the central nervous system or meningeal reaction. Echovirus 20 was recovered from the throats of children suffering from cold-like illnesses and respiratory tract infections.

Other Enteroviruses

Echo-like viruses have been frequently isolated from animals. Monkeys appear to carry them asymptomatically and their presence is frequently detected by a cytopathic effect observed in uninoculated monkey kidney tissue culture cells. Often the cells show marked vacuolation and the viruses responsible have been known as 'foamy agents'. There are at least 25 enteric cytopathogenic monkey orphan (ECMO) viruses. Similar agents have been recovered from bovines (ECBO viruses) and from swine (ECSO viruses). Further investigation is required into the relationship of these animal viruses to human enteric viruses and the possibility of their transfer from one host to another.

NON-BACTERIAL GASTROENTERITIS

(WINTER VOMITING DISEASE)

It has been recognized for a considerable time that outbreaks of vomiting and diarrhoea occur in which no known bacterial agent can be isolated. The disease was first described in the U.S.A. by Zahorsky in 1929 and was called by him 'winter vomiting disease'. A similar disease has been described in Britain in families and in closed communities and is sometimes called 'epidemic vomiting'. The clinical features of the illness last 24 to 48 hours and include vomiting, diarrhoea, low grade fever and abdominal cramps. Cases seldom reach hospital.

Evidence has been obtained in some outbreaks that, when given by mouth a filtrate of faeces can induce the disease in volunteers. In Britain, Clarke *et al.* (1972) have demonstrated this transmission in volunteers and have shown that the agent responsible is less than 50 nm in diameter and ether stable. The agent does not replicate in a variety of types of cell cultures. In the U.S.A., Dolin *et al.* (1972) have described an agent—the Norwalk agent—that is capable of causing this illness in human volunteers; they induced the disease through three serial passages. The Norwalk agent has a diameter of less than 36 nm and is ether and acid stable. Preliminary experiments suggest that this agent replicates in fetal intestinal organ cultures but not in cell cultures. The agent appears to be host specific for man and to confer a short-term immunity. Until methods are available for cul-

tivating this and other similar agents, it will not be possible to characterize the agents fully nor to determine how widespread non-bacterial gastroenteritis is nor the degree of immunity following infection.

COXSACKIEVIRUSES

The third group of the enterovirus family contains the 30 coxsackieviruses which cause such diverse illnesses as aseptic meningitis, epidemic myalgia or pleurodynia, herpangina and neonatal myocarditis. The group was named coxsackieviruses by Daldorf after the place where a member of the group was first isolated. In their properties and in their reactions to chemical and physical agents, coxsackieviruses do not differ materially from other enteroviruses.

DESCRIPTION

The most outstanding characteristic of the coxsackieviruses is their pathogenicity for newborn mice and hamsters. During the first 48 hours of life these animals are fully susceptible

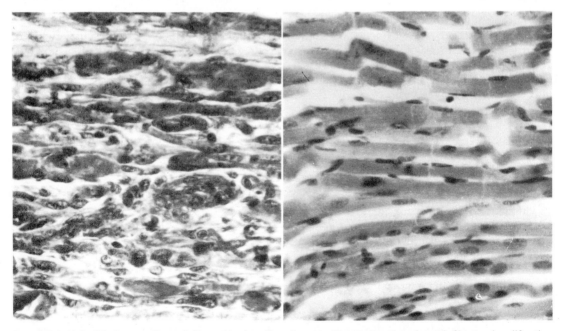

PLATE 45.1. (a) Suckling mouse. Group A Coxsackie virus, Ontario strain. Note destruction of muscle fibres and proliferation of sarcolemma. (b) Normal muscle in suckling mouse for comparison. (From Rhodes and Van Rooyens, *Textbook of Virology*, Baltimore: Williams and Wilkins.)

to infection; thereafter they acquire a natural resistance and after the age of five days they can no longer be infected. By definition coxsackieviruses are unable to infect adult mice. Two broad groups of the viruses have been made according to the histological nature and the situation of the lesions they produce in mice.

Group-A viruses, of which there are 24, cause lesions in only one tissue, a widespread severe myositis involving skeletal muscles throughout the whole body. The principal muscles to be involved are those of the hind limbs, and in life the mice appear to have a flaccid paralysis. Usually the signs of infection appear 4 or 5 days after inoculation and progress until the animal dies 4 or 5 days later.

Group-B viruses, of which there are six, cause widespread lesions in many organs. The myositis produced is characterized by focal lesions and gives rise to tremors, incoordination and a paralysis resembling the spastic type. The viruses also cause areas of necrosis in the brown fat lobules, especially those in the interscapular and cervical pads of brown fat. They also cause meningoencephalitis and pancreatitis. The incubation period of group B infections in mice is prolonged and symptoms may not be obvious until the tenth day after inoculation. Inoculated mice must be kept under observation for three weeks.

HAEMAGGLUTINATION. Types A20, A21, A24, and B1, B3, B5, agglutinate human group O-cells and type A7 will agglutinate fowl cells which are sensitive to the vaccinia haemagglutinin.

CULTIVATION. Tissue cultures are of limited value in isolating the viruses. Types A9 and B1, 2, 3, 4, 5, and 6 grow well in monkey kidney monolayers and produce a cytopathic effect resembling that of the polioviruses. They produce a cytopathic effect in human amnion.

Apart from coxsackievirus A9, the other A viruses are isolated by the inoculation of suckling mice. Thereafter, some can be adapted to tissue culture. In monkeys, coxsackieviruses do not usually produce clinical diseases, but after inoculation a viraemia develops and later the virus is excreted for several weeks in the faeces. Types A7 and A14, however, possess the power to cause a mild paralysis in monkeys with lesions in the central nervous system resembling those

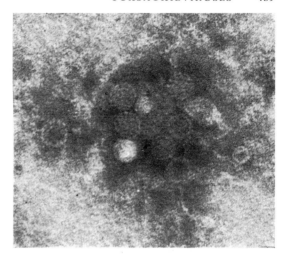

PLATE 45.2. Electron micrograph of a cluster of Coxsackie virus (A9) particles. (Phosphotungstic acid. × 152 000.) (From Swain and Dodds, 1967, *Clinical Virology*, Edinburgh: Churchill Livingstone.)

of poliomyelitis. Type A7, which has caused paralytic disease in man, is identical with the Russian Ab IV strain which was at first thought to constitute a fourth type of the poliomyelitis virus.

ANTIGENIC CHARACTERS. Thirty antigenic types have been defined by cross-neutralization tests in mice or tissue culture, and cross-complement-fixation reactions. Twenty-four have the pathogenicity of group A and six the characters of group B. Each of the six group-B types are subject to antigenic variation and sera from convalescent cases may show heterotypic responses. Coxsackievirus A9 is intermediate in some of its properties between the echo and coxsackie groups and has some antigenic relationship with A23 and echovirus 9.

CLINICAL FEATURES

Group A Viruses

These viruses give rise to a number of different illnesses. Aseptic meningitis, indistinguishable clinically from that caused by other enteroviruses is caused by a number of types, e.g. 2, 4, 7, 9, or 23. Type A7 has given rise to epidemics of aseptic meningitis with some cases of paralytic disease in Scotland, Russia and elsewhere. The paralysis is not as severe in its after-effects as that due to polioviruses. Herpangina is an acute feverish disease, characterized by lesions in the mouth consisting of papules on the anterior pillars of the fauces; these papules become vesicles and finally shallow ulcers with a greyish base and punched out edge. There are usually 5 to 10 lesions and the illness lasts about 4 days. Types 2, 4, 5, 6, 8, 10, and 23 have been isolated at various times from these infections. 'Hand, foot and mouth' disease presents as a painful stomatitis with a vesicular rash on the hands and feet. Typically, it lasts about a week; most of the cases are seen in the summer in children aged 1 to 10 years. The viruses usually implicated are types 5 and 16.

Coxsackievirus A21 (COE) has caused epidemics of colds in camps of military recruits and B strains have been associated with upper respiratory infections, bronchitis, and pneumonia in young children.

Group B Viruses

Epidemic myalgia or Bornholm disease, so-called because it was first described on the Danish island of Bornholm, is characterized by fever and the sudden onset of agonizing stitch-like pains in the muscles of the chest, epigastrium or hypochondrium. Although the disease is most frequently recognized in its epidemic form, many sporadic cases occur. Epidemic myalgia may be complicated by pleurisy and pericarditis.

In newborn infants, severe and often fatal mycocarditis has been reported and the causative virus has been found in high concentrations in the mycocardium at autopsy. Epidemics have occurred in nurseries and are found at a time when other evidences of group B virus activity are present in a community. The baby is presumably infected by its mother and is highly susceptible to the virus, like the infant mouse. Myocarditis and pericarditis can occur in children and adults and virus has been isolated from pericardial fluid.

Aseptic meningitis, sometimes with cases of paralysis is a common infection due to group B virus. Occasionally a rash is present.

It is important to note that when a group B coxsackievirus is active in a community a

Table 45.2.

Clinical syndrome	Poliovirus types	Coxsackievirus types		Echovirus types
		A	B	
Neuronal damage				
Paralysis, sustained	1, 2, 3	4, 7, 9, 23	—	2, 4, 9, 11, 13, 16
Paralysis, transient	1, 2, 3	2, 9	3, 4, 5	1, 9, 16
Encephalitis	1, 2, 3	—	3*	9, 19
Aseptic meningitis	1, 2, 3	2, 4, 7, 9, 23*	1, 2, 3, 4, 5*, 6	1, 2, 3, **4***, 5, **6***, 7, **9***, 11, 12, 13, 14, 15, 16, 18, 19, 20, 21, 22, 25
Enteritis	—	—	—	**6***, 8, 11, 14, 18, 19, 20, 22, 23, 24, 28
Herpangina	—	2, 3, 4, 5, 6, 8, 10	—	—
Epidemic pleurodynia (Bornholm disease)	—	—	1, 2*, 3*, 4*, 5*	—
Colds and respiratory illnesses	—	21* (COE)	1, 3	6, 8, 11, 20*, 22, 25, 28*
Myocarditis	1, 2, 3	—	2, 3, 4, 5	—
Pericarditis	—	—	2, 3, 4, 5	—
Rashes, maculopapular or vesicular	—	2, 4, 9	1, 3, 5	2, 4, 6, **9***, 14, **16***, 18
*Hand, foot and mouth disease	—	5, 16	—	—

The figures in heavy type indicate the commoner serotypes.
*An asterisk indicates strains known to have been associated with epidemics.

spectrum of illnesses may extend from a 'flu-like' illness to epidemic myalgia and aseptic meningitis.

PATHOGENESIS

Coxsackieviruses are widespread in alimentary tracts of children and young adults and are disseminated in the summer and autumn months to a considerable proportion of children, especially those living under unhygienic conditions. The viruses are present in the gut for short periods, sometimes no more than a week; they are excreted in the faeces and have been recovered from sewage and flies.

The table on page 470 shows the relationship of the enteroviruses discussed in this chapter and the clinical disease.

LABORATORY DIAGNOSIS

VIRUS ISOLATION. The virus can readily be isolated from throat swabs or faeces during the first two weeks of the infection and can also be recovered from the cerebrospinal fluid from cases of aseptic meningitis. Stools and throat swabs are treated with antibiotics clarified by slow centrifugation in the manner used in isolation of the polioviruses, and inoculated into monkey kidney tissue cultures and HeLa cells. Human amnion cells may also be used but the viruses may not grow readily in them on primary inoculation. Cytopathogenic agents growing in these cultures will include all the group B types and group A type 9. If this procedure yields no virus the specimens should be inoculated into mice no older than 48 hours by the combined intracerebral and intraperitoneal routes. The optimum age of mice for inoculation is 24 hours for group B and 48 hours for group A. Subsequently, viruses will be placed in their appropriate groups according to the histological appearances of the lesions they produce. The causal relationship of a newly isolated virus to the illness should be confirmed by demonstrating a rising titre of homologous antibodies in the patient's serum. The final identification of the numerical serotype is carried out by neutralization tests in tissue cultures or, if this is not possible, in infant mice. The procedures are burdensome, for there are 30 possible type-specific antisera to set against the unknown virus and, unless some information is available as to the prevalent infecting type, it may require much time to complete the task.

SEROLOGICAL TESTS. Neutralization and complement-fixation reactions may be of value provided that the first serum has been taken within three days of the onset of the disease. Again the large numbers of viruses in the group often make these tests impractical unless there is some clue as to the nature of the prevailing virus.

IMMUNITY. Type-specific antibodies develop quickly after infection with coxsackieviruses. They are usually estimated by neutralization tests, but haemagglutination-inhibition tests can be applied to the viruses that cause haemagglutination. Complement-fixation tests can be used but they detect group rather than type specific antibodies. There is some doubt about the duration of immunity to some of the coxsackievirus although there is a long-lasting immunity to many.

EPIDEMIOLOGY

As an enterovirus infection, spread is most likely to be by the faecal/oral route with a high incidence within families. In a much smaller number of cases the virus is disseminated from focal lesions in the oropharynx. Aseptic meningitis, epidemic myalgia and herpangina all occur characteristically as epidemics. The peak incidence is usually in the summer months and large epidemics may occur. In the summer of 1951 a widespread epidemic of Bornholm disease occurred in Great Britain and in 1959 a high incidence of aseptic meningitis due to coxsackieviruses was reported in Scotland. In 1965 there was an outbreak of coxsackievirus B5 which was found not only in Great Britain but also in Scandinavia. Usually half the persons involved in epidemics are under the age of ten years and three-quarters under twenty. Herpangina is seen in very young children under five years of age in day nurseries and kindergarten schools, where it spreads rapidly. Sporadic cases of all the clinical forms of infection occur and often the patients are young adults who have acquired the infection presumably from family contacts. For a review of the coxsackieviruses see Plager (1962) and Kibrick (1964).

RHINOVIRUSES

The viruses of this group are responsible for the most frequent of all human infections, the 'common cold'. Most people suffer from 2 to 4 colds every year and, although the primary infection is not a severe one, secondary bacterial infection often follows with temporary incapacity. These viruses cause the loss of many million man-hours of work.

DESCRIPTION

The viruses belong to the picornavirus group and are distinguished from the other members by being destroyed at pH 3 to 5. There are at least 55 serotypes of rhinoviruses.

CULTIVATION. The viruses are divided into three groups according to the tissues of optimal growth. 'M' (monkey) strains grow and produce a cytopathic effect in monkey kidney monolayers and also in continuous lines of malignant human cells such as HeLa and HEp2. 'H' (human) strains are most easily isolated in human embryonic kidney cultures and in diploid cells from human embryonic lung W138 (Hayflick and Moorehead, 1961). 'O' (organ) strains grow only in organ cultures of human embryo respiratory epithelium. Some of these 'O' strains can be adapted to human embryo respiratory fibroblasts and are designated 'O–H' strains.

Both M and H strains require for their growth a temperature of 33°C, a pH (7·0) lower than that commonly used, and the use of revolving drums to maintain the oxygen tension of the cell cultures by rotation. Infected cultures are maintained in a medium containing 0·03 per cent sodium bicarbonate, 0·25 per cent lactalbumin hydrolysate and 2·0 per cent calf serum in Hanks' saline with antibiotics.

VIABILITY. Rhinoviruses can be preserved at −70°C and survive freeze drying rather better than most picornaviruses. Drying in air at atmospheric temperature quickly inactivates the viruses. They are stable to heat treatment at 50°C for 30 minutes but sensitive to pH fluctuations and are quickly inactivated at pH 3 to 5. They survive overnight exposure to 20 per cent ether.

VIRUS MULTIPLICATION. The viruses replicate in the cytoplasm of infected cells and give a CPE which coincides with release of virus particles in the same way as other picornaviruses.

Clinical Features

After infection has occurred the patient develops a cough and sneezing is common. A clear watery nasal discharge appears followed by a mucoid or purulent discharge. Laryngitis with hoarseness of the voice occurs frequently in adults and the nasal sinuses usually become infected. Rhinoviruses have frequently been isolated during acute exacerbations of chronic bronchitis.

PATHOGENESIS

When rhinoviruses are instilled into the nose of human volunteers a mild sore throat and cough are the premonitory signs which precede the profuse nasal discharge of typical common cold. The incubation period is 48 to 96 hours. Chimpanzees are the only other creatures known to be susceptible to these viruses. The viruses can be recovered from the secretion of the nose and throat but only rarely from the faeces.

The mechanism of infection with rhinoviruses has been clarified by the organ culture technique of Hoorn and Tyrrell (1965) which was introduced for the study of respiratory viruses. The virus settles on the ciliated nasal epithelial cells, enters the cells and spreads from cell to cell in the epithelium. The cilia become immobilized and both cilia and cell degenerate as the virus replicates. Although it is often suggested that bacterial invasion of the damaged tissue occurs and is responsible for the purulent nasal discharge which is a feature, the engulfing of dead or virus damaged epithelial cells by phagocytes of various sorts may be the primary cause of this discharge.

The infection of the nasal sinuses is due to bacterial secondary infection superimposed on a primary virus infection.

IMMUNITY. Circulating antibodies mainly of the lgG type appear in response to a rhinovirus infection in both natural infections and those induced in volunteers. There is a good correlation in volunteers between circulating neutralizing antibody titres and resistance to challenge with small doses of homologous virus; those with high titres are not infected. A protective high titre can be obtained by injection of a formaldehyde-treated vaccine. It is important to note that this immunity is specific to the type of virus to which neutralizing antibodies are present. The person is not protected against a different serological type of the rhinovirus. The fact that there are 55 types of rhinovirus indicates the difficulties in attempting to produce an efficient composite vaccine. The nasal secretions contain antibodies of the secretory IgA type and presumably they play a role in the prevention of infection. Rhinoviruses cause interference in cell cultures and are susceptible to human interferon; whether interferon is important in recovery from the cold is not clear but it may play a part in the resistance of a person recovering from a cold from being reinfected for about four weeks.

Laboratory Diagnosis

Nasal washings are taken with saline and an equal quantity of bacteriological broth. Nasal swabs and throat swabs in transport medium are used also for isolation. The specimens after treatment with penicillin and streptomycin should be inoculated immediately or stored at $-70°C$ or lower. The cells used for culture are either W1—38 or human embryo kidney cells and the cultures after being set up are incubated at 33°C at pH 7·0 to 7·3 in a roller drum apparatus. If a rhinovirus is present a focal CPE develops. Final identification is made by neutralization tests.

A serological diagnosis can be made from paired sera, the first being taken during the acute stage of the illness, the second about three weeks later, but due to the large number of virus types this is rarely practicable.

Epidemiology

The incidence of colds is greatest in the winter months when outside temperatures are falling, but the reason for the seasonal variation has never been satisfactorily explained. Deliberate exposure of volunteers to wet and chilling does not increase their susceptibility to colds. Common colds are probably transmitted by the same mechanisms as those in influenza and other respiratory infections. About 10 per cent of colds compel their victims to absent themselves from work. Colds in the home are often introduced by pre-school and schoolchildren who contract the infection from their playmates. In general, adults under the age of 30 are more susceptible than those over 40 (Lidwell and Williams, 1961).

Prophylaxis

As has been mentioned above there is at present no suitable vaccine for prevention of the common cold, due to the difficulty of evolving a suitable composite vaccine.

The only available method for prevention of spread is for the infected person to eschew the company of his or her fellow human beings, a counsel of perfection not liable to be practised by many.

Reoviruses (respiratory enteric orphan viruses), one of which was classified as echovirus 10, have occasionally been recovered from mild fevers in children but have been more constantly associated with diarrhoea than with respiratory symptoms.

Para-influenza viruses, the respiratory syncytial virus, the adenoviruses, and *Mycoplasma pneumoniae* have all been found in association with cold-like illness.

REVIEWS AND REFERENCES

BUTLER, N. R., BENSON, P. F., WILSON, B. D. R., PERKINS, F. T., UNGAR & BEALE, A. J. (1962) Poliomyelitis and triple antigen efficiency given separately and together. *Lancet*, i, 834.

CLARKE, S. K. R., COOK, G. T.; EGGLESTONE, S. I., HALL, T. S., MILLER, D. L., REED, S. E., RUBENSTEIN, D., SMITH, A. J. & TYRRELL, D. A. J. (1972) A virus from epidemic vomiting disease. *British Medical Journal*, iii, 86.

DOLIN, R., BLACKLOW, N. R., DUPONT, H., BUSCHO, R. F., WYATT, R. G., KASEL, J. A., HORNICK, R. & CHANOCK, R. M. (1972) Biological properties of Norwalk agent of acute infectious non-bacterial gastroenteritis. *Proceedings of the Society of Experimental Biology and Medicine*, **140**, 578.

HALE, J. H., DORAISINGHAM, M., KANAGARATNAM, K., LEONG, J. W. & MONTEIRO, E. S. (1959) Large-scale use of Sabin-type 2 attenuated poliovirus vaccine in Singapore during a type 1 poliomyelitis epidemic. *British Medical Journal*, i, 1541.

HAMLIN, M. H., DAVIS, P. M. & MACRAE, A. D. (1963) The typing of enteroviruses in tissue culture by neutralization with composite antiserum pools. *Journal of Hygiene (Cambridge)*, **61**, 479.

HAYFLICK, L. & MOORHEAD, P. S. (1961) The serial cultivation of human diploid cell strains. *Experimental Cell Research*, **25**, 585.

HENDERSON, D. A., WITTE, J. J., MORRIS, L. & LANGMUIR, A. D. (1964) Paralytic disease associated with oral poliovaccines. *Journal of the American Medical Association,* **190**, 41.

HOORNE, B. & TYRRELL, D. A. J. (1965) On the growth of certain newer respiratory viruses in organ culture. *British Journal of Experimental Pathology*, **46**, 109.

HSIUNG, G. D. (1962) Further studies on characterization and grouping of echoviruses. *Annals of the New York Academy of Sciences*, **101**, 413.

KIBRICK, S. (1964) Current status of coxsackie and echovirus in human disease. *Progress in Medical Virology*, **6**, 27.

LIDWELL, O. M. & WILLIAMS, R. E. O. (1961) The epidemiology of the common cold. *Journal of Hygiene (Cambridge)*, **59**, 303, 109.

MINISTRY OF HEALTH (1963) *Reports on Public Health and Medical Subjects*, 107. London: H.M.S.O.

SABIN, A. B. (1959) Present position of immunization against poliomyelitis with live virus vaccines. *British Medical Journal*, i, 663.

STOTT, E. J. & KILLINGTON, R. A. (1972) Rhinoviruses. *Annual Review of Microbiology*, **26**, 503.

TYRRELL, D. A. J. (1968) Rhinoviruses. *Virology Monographs*, **2**, 68.

WEIR, I. B. L., JAMIESON, W. M. & GREEN, D. M. (1964) Poliomyelitis in Dundee, 1962. *British Medical Journal*, ii, 853.

WENNER, H. A. & BEHBEHANI, A. M. (1968) Echoviruses. *Virology Monographs*, **1**, 3.

WORLD HEALTH ORGANIZATION (1962) Requirements for poliomyelitis. *World Health Organization Technical Report Series*, **203**.

WORLD HEALTH ORGANIZATION (1962) Requirements for biological substances. Requirements for poliomyelitis vaccine (oral). *World Health Organization Technical Report Series*, **237**.

ZAHORSKY, J. (1929) Hypermesis hiemes or winter vomiting disease. *Archives of Pediatrics*, **46**, 391.

46. Hepatitis Viruses Infectious and Serum Hepatitis

Viral hepatitis in human beings is a syndrome caused by a variety of viruses of widely different taxons. In neonates and children, sporadic cases of hepatitis may be caused by rubella, adenovirus, some enteroviruses (e.g. Coxsackie B), cytomegalovirus and *Herpesvirus hominis*. Biochemical evidence of hepatitis, mostly symptomless, is frequent in infectious mononucleosis. In tropical and semi-tropical areas yellow fever virus is an important cause of hepatitis. In addition, cases of hepatitis may be due to various non-viral organisms such as leptospira, *Coxiella burnettii* or toxoplasma.

However, most cases of hepatitis, particularly in outbreaks in temperate climes, are caused by one or other of two distinct, but similar viruses (or families of viruses); respectively those of infectious hepatitis (synonyms: virus hepatitis A, AVH, IH) and serum hepatitis (virus hepatitis B, BVH, SH, etc.). In other words, the term 'virus hepatitis' usually means virus hepatitis A or B.

THE VIRUSES OF HEPATITIS A AND B

These viruses have been particularly difficult to cultivate in laboratory animals or in cell or organ culture although promising methods are now emerging. Consequently, much of our knowledge of the properties of the agents and the pathogenesis of the disease is derived from inoculation experiments with human volunteers in various countries during World War 2 and subsequently in the United States, particularly at the Willowbrook State School, New York. Despite the inevitable limitations of this information it is well established that virus A is distinct from virus B; the distinguishing attributes are listed in Table 46.1. Crucial differences are those in the incubation periods; case mortality; antigen composition (i.e. the viruses do

not cross-immunize); the age incidence and secondary attack rates; the predominant routes of transmission of infection and duration of viraemia; and finally, the recent discovery that patients and carriers of hepatitis B virus have in the blood and liver a distinctive lipoprotein known variously as Australia antigen, Hepatitis-Associated-Antigen, SH Antigen or Hepatitis B surface antigen (HB_SAg; in brief Hb ag). There are at present no antigens of practical diagnostic value for Hepatitis A virus. The epidemic hepatitis associated antigen ('Milan' antigen), once thought to be specific for Virus A, is now considered to be a host-specified lipoprotein increased in various liver diseases including hepatitis A; the antigen found in the faeces from hepatitis A patients by workers in Melbourne (Australia) is still being assessed, and is not yet accepted as specific for this infection.

The association of Hepatitis B antigen with virus B is most clearly demonstrated in the studies in Willowbrook State School in which it was found that over 95 per cent of those experimentally infected with MS2 (the prototype virus B strain) became HB ag positive whereas none of those induced with MS1 (the prototype virus A strain) did so. In addition, studies of 'point source' or 'common vehicle' outbreaks of virus A—i.e. outbreaks which can be characterized epidemiologically as virus A—have not revealed HB ag in a proportion higher than would be found by chance in the healthy population at large.

Apart from acute hepatitis, HB ag is found in a small proportion of ostensibly healthy persons (about 1/800 to 1/1 000 of blood donors in the United Kingdom, but the prevalence ranges from 5 to 10 per cent in tropical Africa, Southeast Asia and the Far East) some of whom are found to have a degree of liver disease detected by biochemical tests or liver biopsy. It has been suggested that a proclivity to chronic carriage is genetically determined and may even be related

Table 46.1. Differential Features of Infectious and Serum Hepatitis.

	Infectious Hepatitis (IH: Virus A)	Serum Hepatitis (SH: Virus B)
Prototype strains	MS1	MS2
Australia- or hepatitis-associated antigen (HB$_s$ Ag)	−	+
Incubation period		
to illness	30–40 days*	40–200 days
to seroconversion	−	(29–43 days (parenteral))
HB$_s$ Ag positive	−	(68–81 days (oral))
Clinico-pathological aspects		
onset	Acute	Slow
arthralgia, rash	−	+
fever	Common	Rare
main prevalence	6–20 years	20 years and over
mortality	0·1–1%	1–37%
raised SGOT	3–19 days	35–200 days
raised IgM	Common	Rare
thymol turb./flocc.	+++	±
Virus in body		
blood	°Mid-incubation period to onset and during acute illness	°87 days before onset, during and after illness
faeces	°16 days before to 8 days after onset Neg. 19–33 days	°Vol. tests negative
urine	°Present acute illness	Unknown (HB$_s$ Ag present)
liver	...	'Virus' (28 nm) in nucleus. HB$_s$ Ag in cytoplasm
nasopharynx	°Variable	°One positive observation
Chronic carriers		
blood	Rare	Up to 13 years (? lifelong)
faeces	Rare	...
Immunity		
homologous	Present, 1 year	Present, 1·5 years
heterologous (*in vivo* and *in vitro*)	Absent	Absent
'normal' immunoglobulin	Protects	Partial or no protection
Transmission		
parenteral route	+	+++
oral route	+++	+
respiratory route	?	
skin/conjunctiva	?	±
non-parenteral contact spread	+++	+
Virus size		
filtration	Seitz	Gradocol 52 nm
electron microscopy	...	20–45 nm
Heat		
56° × 30 minutes	Survived	Survived
60° × 4 hours	...	Survived
60° × 10 hours (albumin)	...	Inactivated
100° × 1 minute	Inactivated	Immunogenicity survived
85° × 60 minutes	...	HB$_s$ Ag inactivated

Key: * Dose dependent.
    ... No information.
    ° Limited observations with volunteers.

to possession of certain histocompatibility anti-gens. HB ag is also found in some cases of polyarteritis nodosa and glomerulonephritis, in a proportion of cases of chronic persistent or chronic aggressive hepatitis which varies markedly from country to country, in cirrhosis of the liver (10 to 30 per cent; including alcoholic cirrhosis, but not in primary biliary cirrhosis), in primary hepatoma (0 to 80 per cent in Africa) and systemic lupus erythematosis. It would be premature to assume a cause and effect relation-ship between Virus B and disease in all of these states; the relation may be indirect in that the disease predisposes to antigen carriage. Thus patients with immunological defects, particu-larly in the cell mediated component, e.g. in lepromatous leprosy, leukaemias, Down's syn-drome, chronic uraemia, aplastic anaemia, as well as those receiving corticosteroids or chemi-cal immunosuppressants, once infected, tend to carry HB ag for long periods and are also often, perhaps always, viraemic although the relation between the titre of antigen and the titre of virus is unknown at present. It should be noted that the prevalence in patients with leprosy and Down's syndrome may owe as much to being in an institution as to their immune defects.

DESCRIPTION OF VIRUSES A AND B AND DIAGNOSTIC ANTIGENS

Studies with volunteers have established that the infective agents pass filters which hold back bacteria; in the instance of Virus B, a membrane of average pore size 52 nm. These results, plus the resistance to inactivation by ether and phenolic disinfectants and a degree of heat resistance greater than that of most viruses (Table 46.1), recall the properties of an entero- or parvovirus. Acute-phase sera from hepatitis A patients, including those from volunteers inoculated with the Willowbrook MS1 strain, produce, some 4 to 6 weeks after inoculation, abnormal liver function tests in a small South American monkey, the marmoset (*Saguinus sp.*). With some isolates serial passage has been pos-sible and cross-challenge experiments suggest more than one type of hepatitis A virus. These results with non-human primates have not yet

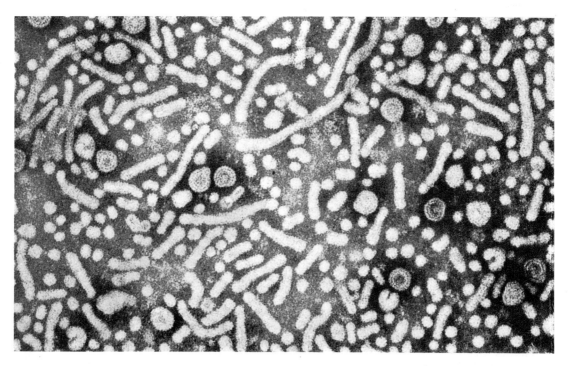

PLATE 46.1. Hepatitis B surface antigen and Dane particles. (× 130 000.) (By courtesy of Dr A. Keen, University of Capetown.)

been translated into an in vitro cell or organ culture technique for hepatitis A virus.

Chimpanzees, rhesus monkeys and possibly other non-human primates develop antigen after inoculation with HB ag positive blood associated with a clinically mild or inapparent infection. Expense, and the need to conserve large non-human primates, properly limit the practical exploitation of these observations in diagnosis and research. Other recent observations suggest that hepatitis B virus may multiply in organ cultures of human foetal liver with the production of large amounts of HB ag. HB ag can be purified from the serum of cases or carriers and may be seen by negative contrast staining in the electron microscope (Plate 46.1). Three morphological forms are present in varying proportions; small spherical particles 20 nm diameter, long tubular forms of the same diameter, and larger (42 nm diameter) forms with a complex internal structure, the 'Dane' particles. All three particles are agglutinated by antibody to HB ag made in hyperimmunized animals or human beings (multiply transfused haemophiliacs). This suggests they have similar surface antigens; recent research demonstrates a serologically distinct internal 'core' antigen in the 'Dane' particle and this antigen binds an antibody present in serum from convalescent hepatitis B patients. Current virological speculation supposes that the 20 nm forms of Australia antigen are the capsid proteins of the virus, self-assembled into the various morphological forms and generally without a nucleic acid core, whereas the larger 'Dane' particle may be the complete virion. Chemical studies indicate that hepatitis B antigen is an unusual lipoprotein which migrates with the α proteins of serum on electrophoresis, is resistant to digestion with proteolytic enzymes, and with antigenic determinants resisting heat up to 80°C (see Prophylaxis and Control). Attempts to find nucleic acid have had varying success; a low proportion (2 to 5 per cent) of ribonucleic acid and an RNA dependent DNA polymerase have been reported by some workers; recent reports describe a double stranded circular DNA, MW 1.6×10^6 daltons, and a DNA dependent DNA polymerase in the 'core' of the Dane particle (Robinson and Greenman, 1974). HB ag has been sub-typed by Le Bouvier and others; there is a common antigen 'a' and sub-types 'y' or 'd'. Class Y (i.e. type ay) predominates in certain epidemiological circumstances, e.g. dialysis associated hepatitis; intravenous drug addiction.

HB ag in serum or other body fluids, may be detected serologically with antisera from hyperimmunized human beings (haemophiliacs) or animals. Techniques range from simple double diffusion in agar or immunoelectroosmophoresis (IEOP) through complement fixation and immune adherence to radioimmunoassay with ^{125}I tagged antigen and double antibody or solid phase techniques (Chap. 2, Vol. II). Tanned or chromate-treated erythrocytes may also be coated with antigen and used to measure antibody by haemagglutination or antigen by inhibition. Radioimmunoassay is several thousand times more sensitive than IEOP in terms of the antigen titre attained. This does not mean, however, that it will detect several thousand times more carriers in, for example, blood donors; perhaps only twice as many; this is because the amount present is usually above the threshold of the least sensitive test. Antibody to HB ag is rarely detected by ID or IEOP in patients convalescent from virus B infection; it may be detected by haemagglutination or radioimmunoassay or evidence of past infection may be obtained by lymphocyte transformation on exposure to purified HB ag or by the macrophage migration inhibition technique.

CLINICAL ASPECTS AND PATHOGENESIS

Infections with virus A are often clinically indistinguishable from those of virus B; there is a prodrome of malaise, limb pain and headache, accompanied by low fever which diminishes as jaundice develops with dark urine and light stools. Symptomless, or minor, atypical infections are probably very common with either virus, particularly with virus A in young children. Specific symptoms and signs which favour a diagnosis of virus B infection are an insidious onset with arthralgia and urticaria and sometimes with polyarteritis nodosa—effects thought to be mediated by circulating antigen–antibody complexes with antigen in excess. With virus B hepatitis the amino-transferase values are often higher and abnormal for longer periods and the course generally more severe. Hepatic coma and death are commoner in virus B than in virus A infections but not all patients with hepatic coma of presumed viral origin have HB ag. Other points implicating virus B are a history of parenteral inoculation (e.g. dental operations, vaccine inoculation, tattooing, intravenous drug abuse or injection of blood or blood products) 1 to 4 months before onset. The age of the patient may be helpful—most hepatitis under 15 years is likely to be virus A except in certain institutions. A history of contact with another case of hepatitis in the family or institution, or of consumption of oysters or other shell food some 25 to 40 days before onset of illness are pointers to a virus A infection. Final differentiation of the two types of hepatitis depends on laboratory tests.

Hepatitis virus A is present in the faeces (and possibly in the urine) of clinical and subclinical cases in the late incubation period, during the period of acute hepatitis and during early convalescence. It is also present in the blood in the early stages of the disease. The site of viral multiplication is presumably the hepatocyte, but the mechanism of liver damage is unknown. Spread of virus to other individuals and the portal of entry is by the oropharynx and the intestinal tract; i.e. faecal–oral spread, a situation resembling that observed with poliovirus and other enteroviruses. As the virus is present in the blood, transmission and entry by parenteral routes is also possible and is postulated to explain, for example, cases of post-transfusion hepatitis with incubation periods under 40 days. As some of the latter patients have HB ag this view may well be incorrect, and parenteral transmission of virus A may be much less common than is supposed. The significance of the respiratory tract as a route of infection in virus A is uncertain; anicteric hepatitis developed only in a minority (< 10 per cent) of experiments in which nasopharyngeal washings from patients with hepatitis A were sprayed into the nose and throat of volunteers.

Hepatitis virus B is present in the blood of cases and carriers, and in all fractions of plasma from carriers except immunoglobulin prepared by the cold ethanol fractionation method. Indirect evidence suggests that it is present in synovial and other body fluids such as lymph,

pleural and peritoneal fluids and is associated with buffy coat cells. However, the freezing and washing procedures involved in the production of stored packed erythrocytes render these less icterogenic. Carriage of virus B in the blood may continue for many years, perhaps even lifelong. This viraemia is closely paralleled by the presence of HB ag but it cannot at present be assumed that virus is always present with or to the same titre as antigen. Antigen is regularly present in the hepatocytes of cases and carriers of hepatitis B. It has been reported (not always with confirmation) in the faeces, urine, bile and saliva.

Our ideas on the portal of entry of virus B and the route of transmission are undergoing change at present. It is still correct that an important mode of infection, particularly for the production of clinical disease, is tissue penetration—any manoeuvre which places the blood, body fluids or cells from a carrier through the skin of another person. In addition studies at Willowbrook School have shown that serum with MS2 strain of virus is infective when given by mouth and several accounts of dialysis-associated hepatitis indicate that the accidental aspiration of infected blood into the mouth while pipetting samples, or the splashing of blood onto the skin, oral mucosa or conjunctiva, can lead to infection. It is sometimes assumed that these observations equate to faecal–oral transmission as with virus A. However, faeces from cases of virus hepatitis B were not shown to be infective for volunteers and the age distribution and secondary attack rates in the households of persons with virus B are quite different from those with virus A.

The production of disease in hepatitis B, although not yet completely understood, promises to be of considerable interest immunologically. Infection of the hepatocyte by the virus does not necessarily lead to cell destruction; thus some chronic symptomless carriers have little biochemical or histological evidence of pathological changes in the liver although by immunofluorescence their hepatocytes contain HB ag, i.e. the infection is non-cytocidal. Because similar findings obtain in leukaemics and immunosuppressed persons whereas healthy persons with normal immunological competence may have a severe disease, it is supposed that disease results from the host's immunological response to a non-cytocidal viral infection of the hepatocyte. Other evidence suggests that the component of the immune response most probably involved in disease production is that of the thymus-dependent lymphocyte which, in general, plays an important part in the 'rejection' of virus infected cells as with tumour cells or homografts. Complexes of HB ag and antibody, in antigen excess, probably cause tissue damage by mechanisms discussed in detail under 'serum sickness' (see Chap. 11); besides arthralgia, periarteritis nodosa and urticaria as prodromal aspects of hepatitis B, complexes may also be small enough to enter the glomerular filter and cause glomerulonephritis. It is less clear whether these complexes also cause liver damage; the present balance of evidence is against the possibility.

LABORATORY DIAGNOSIS

The main differential diagnosis to be made is between virus A and virus B, so all patients with suspected viral hepatitis should be tested for HB ag. Other general laboratory tests are of limited value although IgM values may be raised and the thymol flocculation tests are positive in virus A infections and not in virus B. Sporadic or atypical cases may be due to infectious mononucleosis, or infections with cytomegalovirus (CMV), Q fever rickettsiae, leptospirae, or the enteroviruses and adenoviruses, depending on age group and epidemiological setting. Clinical and epidemiological information may point to the probable diagnosis and render extended laboratory testing unnecessary, but if exhaustive investigation seems required a specimen of faeces should be collected at the time when the patient is first seen (near to onset of illness) and should be tested for enteroviruses. Serial specimens of sera are also obtained and may be tested initially for complement-fixing antibody to adenovirus group, CMV and *Herpesvirus hominis* antigen, *C. burnetii* phase 2, toxoplasma and (broadly reactive) leptospiral antigens. Infectious mononucleosis can be excluded by total and differential leucocyte counts and the appropriate serological tests (Chap. 41).

Tests for HB ag will usually be by IEOP and with clinical cases of the disease, as distinct from carriers, this may be of low sensitivity as antigen is complexed with antibody. Serum specimens may be examined for antigen by electron-microscopy or radioimmunoassay in critical circumstances (e.g. a patient in a dialysis unit); they should also, when definitive information is required, be tested for the development of antibody to HB ag by radioimmunoassay (RIA) or haemagglutination. It has been observed, for example, that dialysis unit staff who contract hepatitis from their patients, may not develop antigen detectable by IEOP but may be antigen positive by RIA or develop antibody detectable by RIA or haemagglutination.

Treatment and Serotherapy

There is no specific therapy for viral hepatitis although the biochemical monitoring of the patient and the recognition of impending hepatitic coma is of the greatest importance. Attempts at serotherapy of hepatic coma with specific immune globulin from plasma with antibody to HB ag suggest that a controlled trial would be worthwhile but the treatment is still developmental.

EPIDEMIOLOGY

Hepatitis A

Virus hepatitis A is a major public health problem, is endemic in most parts of the world with superimposed minor, or occasional, major epidemics; along with measles and sexually transmitted disease, it is one of the major uncontrolled infectious diseases of our time. Spread is in the main by person-to-person contact with numerous subclinical cases which aid the process. A high proportion (30 to 50 per cent) of cases have a history of exposure to a previous case of hepatitis, most often in a child, and over 30 per cent of children and 10 per cent of adults at risk may be infected in family outbreaks. In Western nations the disease appears to be in the process of evolving from a near universal infection in early childhood to a sporadic infection of children and young adults; an age shift reminiscent of the changes observed with poliomyelitis and other enteroviruses. The main prevalence of the disease is in the autumn and early winter; this may represent a spread in summer, but given the lengthy incubation period, the peak of the prevalence is reached later than with the enteroviruses. Apart from this pattern of spread, viral contamination (probably faecal) of aliments sometimes gives rise to large outbreaks in which milk, water or food is the vehicle of infection. American or Scandinavian investigations have shown that oysters and certain types of clam, harvested from sewage-contaminated estuaries, are sometimes responsible for infective hepatitis A. One oyster may be enough to infect and it appears that measures adequate to clear these molluscs of enteric bacteria may not be adequate for enteroviruses and hepatitis viruses. It is generally considered that the person-to-person spread takes place by the faecal–oral sequence but the possibility cannot be excluded that spread also occurs from the oropharynx by contamination of fomites or expulsion of droplets—the epidemiological evidence is inconclusive and a few outbreaks attributed to airborne infection are recorded. This pattern is clearly different from that of recognized respiratory viruses such as influenza or measles.

Hepatitis B

A recent major change in epidemiological thinking has resulted from the finding that a substantial proportion of sporadic cases of hepatitis have HB ag and that antibody surveys of healthy populations reveal a widespread experience of virus B not simply limited to populations exposed to frequent parenteral therapy.

The epidemiology of hepatitis B is clear enough in relation to blood transfusion or use of blood products, tissue penetration with inadequate asepsis in, e.g. haematological clinics, diabetic, dental or venereal disease clinics (examples of 'syringe transmitted jaundice'), drug addiction with 'mainline' heroin, tattooing and so forth. Spectacular outbreaks have occurred in recent years in maintenance dialysis and kidney transplantation units where the factors of frequent blood or plasma transfusion, immunosuppression resulting in prolonged viraemia, and a need for frequent access to the extra-corporeal circulation combine to produce rapid lateral spread of virus B among patients and, by tissue penetrating accidents, from patients to staff.

The unresolved epidemiological questions in relation to virus B relate to spread of virus among young adults in the general population without obvious parenteral exposure. It has been noted in this general group that infection is commoner in the sexual partners of cases or carriers of hepatitis B virus. It is possible that oral or genital contact may be the occasion of infection particularly in the light of the finding that HB ag may be present in saliva; also a bloodborne virus might be excreted into the female genital tract at the menses or shed from minor lesions. The secondary attack ratio among the contacts of cases of parenterally acquired hepatitis B is low (around 2 per cent) in sharp contrast to the rates observed in family contacts of virus A. At present this argues against faecal–oral spread of virus B as observed with virus A.

CONTROL AND PROPHYLAXIS

It is now well established that unselected gamma-globulin (IgG) in doses of 0·02 to 0·12 ml per kg is an effective seroprophylactic for Virus A in institutions or 'high risk' groups such as the military, Peace Corps personnel and others working in endemic areas. IgG is much less effective in the prophylaxis of Virus B infection in post-transfusion hepatitis, in dialysis units and the like. This may be related to its generally low and variable content of antibody to HB ag. Recently, specific immunoglobulin (SIgG) has been prepared from plasma with substantial amounts of antibody to HB ag. Experience in the U.S.A., France and in the U.K. indicates that this may be of value when given prophylactically to staff involved in tissue penetration accidents in dialysis units, etc. Finally, preparations of HB ag have been heated for a short time at 99 to 100°C and used as 'vaccines' in subjects at Willowbrook State School who were subsequently challenged with the MS2 strain of virus B. Protection was achieved by these inoculations and it is clear that if the virus could be propagated consistently in culture the way would be open for control by active immunization as with other virus diseases.

REFERENCES AND FURTHER READING

KOFF, R. S. (1971) *Critical Reviews in Environmental Control*, **1**, 383.

MacCALLUM, F. O. (ed.) (1972) Viral hepatitis. *British Medical Bulletin*, **28**,

ROBINSON, W. S. & GREENMAN, R. L. (1974) DNA polymerase in the core of the human hepatitis B candidate. *Journal of Virology*, **13**, 1231–1236.

WORLD HEALTH ORGANIZATION (1973) Scientific group on viral hepatitis. *World Health Organization Technical Report Series*, No. 512.

47. Arboviruses

Encephalitis: Yellow Fever: Dengue

The term arbovirus is not derived from the Latin *arbor* a tree, though many of the viruses in this group are in fact associated with sylvatic environments, but is simply a contraction, introduced in 1963, of the term 'arthropod-borne'. Arboviruses are defined (W.H.O., 1967) as 'viruses which are maintained in nature principally, or to an important extent, through biological transmission between susceptible vertebrate hosts by haematophagous arthropods; they multiply and produce viraemia in vertebrates, multiply in the tissues of arthropods and are passed on to new vertebrates by the bite of an arthropod after a period of extrinsic incubation.' This definition excludes viruses which are conveyed by arthropods by 'mechanical' means, i.e. without a cycle of multiplication in the arthropod. Although arthropod transmission is a basic characteristic of the group, arboviruses can, sometimes, be transmitted by other means, such as by the respiratory or alimentary routes.

The evidence on which any given virus is allocated to the group varies widely. In a few cases the complete natural cycle of transmission has been demonstrated as, e.g. for yellow fever virus by the classic experiments of the Yellow Fever Commission of the U.S. Army led by Walter Reed. In Cuba in 1900 these workers showed from experiments on man that a mosquito (*Aedes aegypti*) transmitted the disease by its bite, and that an interval of some 12 days was necessary between the mosquito taking its infective meal and its being able to convey the infection to another person. Further, they showed that the disease could be transmitted by inoculation of blood from a sick to a well person during the first 1 or 2 days of the illness but that it could not be transmitted by contact with patients or their fomites; also, that elimination of *Aedes aegypti* prevented urban epidemics. More usually, the complete natural cycle has not been demonstrated and allocation of a virus to the group is made on partial evidence—epidemiological observations of field situations, such as the circumstances of isolation of the virus, reinforced by studies on its behaviour in the laboratory, such as on its transmission between vertebrate hosts by arthropod vectors; or evidence, from titration or serial passage, of multiplication of the virus in arthropod tissues.

Besides these characters, associated with the transmission cycle, certain other characteristics are accepted as indicating that an agent is an arbovirus: susceptibility to ether and to sodium desoxycholate; the presence of RNA in the virus; antigenic relationship with an established arbovirus.

Some 252 viruses were included in the group according to W.H.O. (1967). The total number included at present in the systematic catalogue of the arboviruses (Taylor, 1967; American Committee on Arthropod-borne Viruses, 1970, 1971) is 257. The names by which arboviruses are designated may indicate the diseases with which they are associated, such as yellow fever, chikungunya, Rift Valley fever and Kyasanur Forest disease. Often, however, isolations were not associated with any specific named disease ('orphan' viruses) and thus many virus names epitomize the localities, such as West Nile, Cache Valley, Ilheus, Bwamba, or the hosts, such as *Anopheles* B, *Wyeomyia*, *Trivittatus*, from which the viruses were isolated; or compound these two, such as Entebbe bat salivary gland, Dakar bat.

CLASSIFICATION AND DESCRIPTION

The table presents the main arboviruses known to cause disease in man, classified according to antigenic groups (W.H.O., 1967; Taylor, 1967) and also according to the disease syndromes they cause, and according to their vectors.

Significant groupings within the arboviruses were first noticed in relation to the susceptibility of certain mouse strains and to inactivation by a substance in milk. Two groups were indicated, groups A and B of the present classification, which is based mainly on haemagglutination inhibition (HI) or complement fixation (CF) reactions, sometimes on neutralization (N). Groups are antigenically distinct from one another and ungrouped viruses are not apparently related to other viruses; however, because of the large number of arboviruses, all possible comparisons are seldom performed. More detailed classifications of some groups are possible by absorption of antiserum with heterologous and homologous virus and differences may be found even within one arbovirus species; e.g. American and African strains of yellow fever virus may be distinguished.

The Catalogue (Taylor, 1967) recognizes 23 groups comprising 155 viruses and 49 ungrouped agents. As regards initial isolation, 97 were made from mammals (40 from man, 11 from domestic vertebrates and 28 from feral vertebrates) and 107 from arthropods (84 from mosquitoes, 19 from ticks and 3 from *Phlebotomus*). Some 45 arboviruses are associated with human disease, of which about 20 are important.

It is to be emphasized that the grouping of arboviruses is purely an ecological one and is heterogeneous in relation to systems of virus

Table 47.1. Main arboviruses associated with human disease.

Group A[1]
  Encephalitis—mosquito transmitted
    Eastern equine encephalitis (EEE)
    Venezuelan equine encephalitis (VEE)
    Western equine encephalitis (WEE)
  Pyrexia—mosquito transmitted
    Chikungunya
    Mayaro
    O'nyong-nyong
    Semliki Forest
    Sindbis
Group B[1]
  Encephalitis—mosquito transmitted
    Ilheus
    Japanese encephalitis (JE)
    Murray Valley encephalitis (MVE)
    St. Louis encephalitis (SLE)
  Encephalitis—tick transmitted
    Louping ill
    Powassan
    Tick-borne encephalitis
  Pyrexia—mosquito transmitted
    Dengue, types 1–4
    Spondweni
    West Nile (WN)
    Wesselsbron
    Yellow fever (YF)
    Zika
  Pyrexia—tick transmitted
    Kyasanur Forest disease (KFD)
    Omsk haemorrhagic fever (OHF)
Group C
  Pyrexia—mosquito transmitted
    Apeu
    Caraparu
    Itaqui
    Marituba
    Murutucu
    Oriboca

Bunyamwera group
  Pyrexia—mosquito transmitted
    Bunyamwera
    Germiston
    Guaroa
    Ilesha
Bwamba group
  Pyrexia—mosquito transmitted
    Bwamba
California group
  Encephalitis—mosquito transmitted
    California encephalitis
    Tahyna
Guama group
  Pyrexia—mosquito transmitted
    Catu
Simbu group
  Pyrexia—mosquito transmitted
    Oropouche
Tacaribe group[2]
  Pyrexia
    Junin
    Lassa fever
    Machupo
Phlebotomus fever group
  Pyrexia—*Phlebotomus* (sandfly) transmitted
    Neapolitan sandfly fever
    Sicilian sandfly fever
Ungrouped
  Pyrexia—mosquito transmitted
    Rift Valley fever
  Pyrexia—tick transmitted
    Colorado tick fever[3]
    Crimean haemorrhagic fever
Taxonomic groups:
  1. Togaviruses, mainly
  2. Arenaviruses
  3. Reovirus (diplornavirus)
  4. Rhabdoviruses

classification based on the characteristics of the virion. Information about these characteristics is still fragmentary for the arboviruses but at least four taxonomic groups are represented among them (Table 47.1)—the reoviruses (diplornaviruses), rhabdoviruses, arenaviruses and togaviruses. Most group-A and group-B arboviruses appear to be togaviruses. Togaviruses are single-stranded RNA viruses of icosahedral shape enclosed in a lipid envelope (this last character correlates with their sensitivity to ether and sodium deoxycholate). The virions are 20 to 60 nm in diameter. They multiply in the cytoplasm and mature by budding from cytoplasmic membranes. Of the non-arboviruses only rubella virus and lactic dehydrogenase virus of mice (LDH) fall into the togavirus group.

Other taxonomic groups are more sporadically represented (Table 47.1), the reoviruses by Colorado tick fever virus and some arboviruses of animals, e.g. blue-tongue and African horsesickness, the rhabdoviruses by bovine vesicular stomatitis virus, and the arenaviruses by the Tacaribe complex (Melnick, 1970; Fenner and White, 1970).

Classical reovirus (ECHO 10) is widespread in man and is therefore frequently isolated from patients with a variety of illnesses—fever, respiratory, gastro-intestinal or nervous diseases and so on, though its etiological relationship to the clinical condition is frequently dubious. The virus has been recovered from mosquitoes which may transmit it mechanically (Andrewes and Pereira, 1972). Some reoviruses of present interest are transmitted by ticks or biting diptera.

All arboviruses so far studied contain RNA.

ARBOVIRUS INFECTION OF THE VERTEBRATE HOST

Clinical Picture and Pathogenesis

Many arbovirus infections in man are inapparent or subclinical and their occurrence can be detected only by demonstration of a rise in specific antibody titre in the serum of the subject. A considerable number, however, cause significant clinical disease and some, e.g. yellow fever, may cause extensive and highly lethal epidemics. The clinical outcome depends on the extent of the virus multiplication in the body and its localization in particular tissues. Clinical pictures of the disease caused by any given virus may vary widely though in epidemics enough patients occur with typical clinical syndromes for a diagnosis to be indicated. Different viruses may produce closely similar clinical manifestations, e.g. the pyrexias caused by West Nile and by dengue viruses.

After infection, an incubation period of at least a few days intervenes before the appearance of clinical manifestations. These are characteristically abrupt in onset and coincide with or follow soon after the appearance of viraemia. The duration of the viraemia is typically short (only a few days). Sometimes the clinical manifestations are limited to this period of viraemia and the disease resolves directly to recovery. Sometimes there may be a remission of a few days and thereafter a recrudescence of pyrexia and new clinical manifestations which are determined by localization of virus in particular organs (e.g. jaundice, encephalitis, albuminuria). Such a process is referred to as diphasic and the associated temperature curve as 'saddle-back'. Sometimes the initial viraemic period is asymptomatic and clinical signs only appear with the second phase.

The clinical picture induced by any given arbovirus varies widely. For instance, dengue, traditionally regarded as an inconvenient but not major fever, has recently been shown to be associated sometimes with a severe haemorrhagic, and often lethal, illness. This outcome may not be a special characteristic of the strain but a sensitization phenomenon associated with sequential infection with several strains (Halstead, 1966; Smith, 1968; Downs, 1970). The clinical syndromes most characteristic of the various arboviruses are indicated in the Table and are:

PYREXIA. The febrile illness may be of an undifferentiated sort, with or without rashes, lymphadenopathy or arthralgia. Such a febrile illness may be the whole attack or it may be the precursor of more serious disease. The pyrexia may be associated with haemorrhages, mainly in the gastrointestinal tract and lungs rather than cutaneously; this syndrome is frequently lethal and yellow fever is the classical example of it.

ENCEPHALITIS. A typical clinical picture is of

fever with progressively more severe headache, nausea, stiff neck and back, progressing to more marked signs of CNS involvement—stupor, coma and paralysis in severe cases. Some encephalitogenic virus infections are frequently fatal, or are prone to cause severe motor and mental sequelae in patients who do recover.

The arboviruses are classified in Table 47.1 by these main clinical types but even in the case of the most lethal infections many of the cases may be of inapparent or of undifferentiated fever.

Isolation in Laboratory Animals; Cell Cultures

Arboviruses in nature occur in a wide variety of host species, both mammals and birds, but may be specific in their ability to infect particular animal species. For instance, early work with yellow fever virus was greatly impeded by the need to use monkeys as experimental animals. The rapid development of work on yellow fever, and indeed on arboviruses generally, owes much to the development of methods for propagating virus in hosts normally insusceptible, such as the intracerebral inoculation of mice, and to the exploitation of highly susceptible hosts such as suckling mice, embryonated eggs and tissue cultures. Arboviruses grow readily in suckling mouse brain and brain triturates provide potent virus suspensions. Chorioallantoic, yolk-sac and intraembryonic routes of inoculation are used with embryonated eggs. Some arboviruses produce pocks on the chorioallantoic membrane. The most commonly used cell culture systems are chick embryo, hamster kidney and HeLa cells. Primary hamster kidney cells are widely susceptible to arboviruses. Many arboviruses are cytopathic in cell culture.

Arbovirus Infection in the Invertebrate Host

Cyclical transmission by an arthropod depends on the ingested virus being able to penetrate the gut wall, and on its being able subsequently to multiply in tissue cells, including those of the salivary glands. The concentrations of virus required to penetrate the gut wall vary widely between mosquito species, some being completely refractory and others being able to be infected with as little as antilog 1·5 mouse LD50. After an 'eclipse phase', during which virus is not detectable in the arthropod, multiplication of virus takes place, to levels several thousand-fold those ingested, in suitable hosts. In contrast, in unsuitable hosts, virus levels fall off rapidly. Virus persists in infected arthropods for long periods, generally for their life span, and does not seem to have any pathological effect on the arthropod host. In ticks, infection is retained from stage to stage of their metamorphosis (trans-stadial transmission), and transovarial transmission occurs in some species. In contrast, in mosquitoes, transovarial transmission has not been demonstrated, but it may occur in *Phlebotomus* (sandflies).

These factors, determining the ease with which arthropod hosts may become infected, and how long infection persists in them, are of great importance for assessing epidemiological situations, indicating which species are likely to be concerned as vectors and, as the viraemia in the vertebrate host is ordinarily brief, how virus persists during interepidemic periods.

Recently arboviruses have been grown in cultures of the tissues of their vector arthropods —mosquitoes and ticks.

ISOLATION AND IDENTIFICATION OF ARBOVIRUSES

Isolation of arboviruses is most usually attempted by the inoculation of the sera, or of tissue suspensions, of suspected infected hosts, man or animal, or by the inoculation of suspensions of arthropod tissues, into susceptible animals, embryonated eggs or tissue cultures. Prompt processing and inoculation of materials are important for success; or in field situations, materials, as for example wild-caught arthropods, may be stored in solid CO_2 or in liquid N_2 for transport to a central laboratory for processing. Intracerebral inoculation of suckling mice is probably the most sensitive method but some viruses can be isolated equally well or more easily in cell cultures. Recognizable pathogenic effects in inoculated mice, or cultures, may not develop at first passage and several blind passages may be required before the virus is adapted to cause such effects, as for instance with dengue virus (W.H.O., 1967).

Identification of a virus isolate, after its preliminary categorization as an arbovirus isolate by filtration experiments and by study of its sensitivity to ether and to sodium desoxycholate, is by study of its antigenic characteristics in relation to a range of specific antisera. Ascription to a group is made with HI and CF techniques but final identification is usually by a neutralization test, as being most specific.

Laboratory Diagnosis

The most definitive method of diagnosis of arbovirus infection is, of course, the isolation and identification of virus. Isolation attempts are, however, often unsuccessful because the viraemia is characteristically short, hardly extending beyond the onset of clinical symptoms. Isolation may be attempted also from the cerebrospinal fluid, or in fatal cases from brain tissue. Serological identification of an illness with a particular arbovirus depends on the demonstration of a rise in antibody titre, particularly neutralization titre, temporally related to the illness. Diagnosis may be established also by finding characteristic histopathological lesions in the tissues of the host obtained by biopsy or necropsy, e.g. the mid-zonal necrosis of the liver lobule which is characteristic of yellow fever (Strode, 1951).

Details of the techniques involved in the isolation and recognition of arboviruses are given by Casals (1967), Work and Hammon (1964) and Work (1964).

TRANSMISSION AND EPIDEMIOLOGY

The possible patterns of transmission by which arboviruses may be maintained and transmitted to man in nature are summarized in Figure 47.1. Arbovirus (and other) infections are often zoonoses—infections of animals that may be transmitted to man—and this is a useful concept. However, it should not be forgotten that this is not a categorical definition for any particular agent but that cycles of transmission may alter from place to place and temporally. It is probably more profitable, rather than to categorize an infection as a zoonosis, to keep in mind all the various possible cycles of transmission and to realize that different parts of the total possible patterns of transmission may be accentuated, or suppressed, in different epidemiological situations (Fig. 47.1). For instance, introduction of virus into a human population may be a terminal event—variously called accidental, dead-end, sentinel or tangential infection—or it may be followed by intrahuman transmission as in an urban yellow fever epidemic.

What avenues of transmission are actually followed in the field are rarely susceptible of proof and epidemiological interpretations are usually based on a stochastic summary of available evidence—e.g. the incidences of antibody to the virus in different vertebrate species (indicating the extent of their involvement in transmission patterns), the frequency of isolation of virus from different arthropod species, the temporal and spatial distribution of possible vertebrate hosts in relation to the activity of arthropod vectors, with laboratory evidence as to the capability of different arthropod species to maintain and transmit the virus; and so on.

Long term survival of arboviruses often presents a problem. The large vertebrate host cannot, usually, act as a long term reservoir as viraemias are characteristically short and lead either to the death of the host or to its developing a long term solid immunity precluding further viraemic episodes. And, although the virus infection in the arthropod vector is non-pathogenic and is co-extensive with the life of the arthropod, many vectors, such as mosquitoes, are typically short lived. Many mechanisms have been invoked to account for long term interepidemic virus survival. Viruses persist for periods of many months, in poikilothermic or hibernating vertebrates and in overwintering mosquitoes, and viraemias may increase on exposure to warmth. Cycles in small vertebrates with rapid population turnover may provide a supply of non-immune juveniles adequate for continuous transmission. Transstadial and transovarial transmission in ticks extends to periods of years the survival in them of the viruses they carry. Virus may be periodically re-introduced into an area by migrating birds. In extensive tropical forest virus may persist as a wandering epidemic in forest animals only returning to any given locality when the prevalence of immune

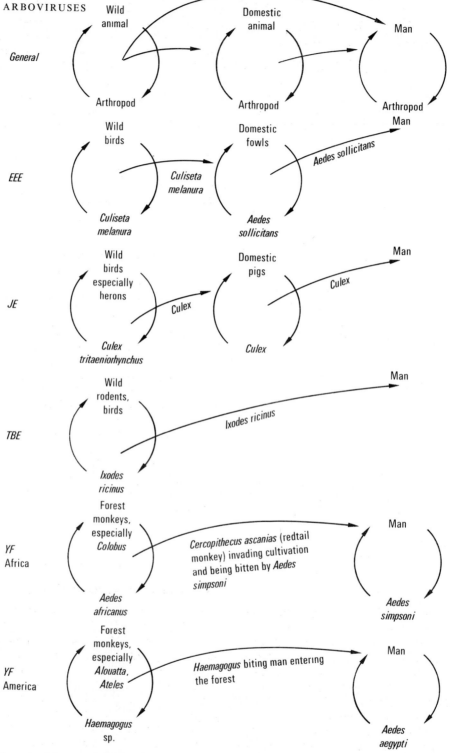

FIG. 47.1. The parts of the general diagram (indicating all possible cycles and routes of transmission) which occur in nature vary from place to place and temporally. Representative examples are given: viz. Eastern equine encephalitis (EEE), Japanese encephalitis (JE), tick-borne encephalitis (TBE) and yellow fever (YF) in Eastern Africa and America.

individuals in the population has been denuded by death and by replacement by juveniles.

Incrimination of an arthropod species as a vector usually involves the recovery of virus from unfed specimens of it in the wild, demonstration in, the laboratory of its capability to become infected and to transmit to new hosts, and on field evidence of its behaviour.

The majority of arboviruses are mosquito-transmitted and the main theatre of their occurrence the tropics, particularly forest areas. However, many may also invade temperate zones, particularly those that are tick-transmitted.

Generally, tick-borne viruses do not develop in mosquitoes; some mosquito-borne viruses will, however, develop in ticks. Although emphasis is placed on cyclical transmission non-cyclical transmission may sometimes be important as, e.g. under a dinner table, where a few mosquitoes, disturbed in their feeding, may successively bite the ankles of several guests.

PROPHYLAXIS AGAINST ARBOVIRUS INFECTIONS

Protection against arbovirus infection by means of vector control is practicable in some situations, such as that of urban yellow fever in which the breeding places of the vector mosquito are readily identified and an organization easily set up to deal with them. Vector control in sylvatic environments is more difficult, because of the multiplicity, and often inaccessibility, of the breeding places of the vector species, e.g. tree-holes, leaf axils. Control of tick populations related to domestic animal and human hosts is more promising. Besides efforts to reduce the vector population, protection from vectors by the use of protective clothing and bed nets, screening and repellents, are important.

Vaccines, either live attenuated or inactivated, are theoretically possible for any arbovirus infection. However, the development of an attenuated live vaccine for any given arbovirus is a major operation, necessitating large production staffs and extensive testing before use in a human population. In this situation, the only vaccine which has come into general use is that for yellow fever. Inactivated vaccines avoid some difficulties but protection is deemed to wane significantly in less than a year, which compares unfavourably with the 10 years or so protection afforded by live YF vaccine. The foregoing are very general comments. The multifariousness and complexity of the factors affecting the development, trial, and prophylactic application of arbovirus vaccines are fully discussed by Smith (1971) who concludes that lack of clear commercial interest, rather than technical difficulty, is the main barrier to the development of arbovirus vaccines.

No useful specific therapy is available against arbovirus infections.

ARBOVIRUS INFECTIONS AS CLINICAL SYNDROMES

In this section the viruses are grouped primarily under the heads of the leading clinical symptoms with which they are characteristically associated. Reference may be made to the tables for details of their antigenic grouping and mode of transmission. Attention will be paid particularly to epidemiology as it is this aspect which has attracted most attention and which is in any case the most important as regards the prevention of human infection. For more extended general treatments see van Rooyen and Rhodes (1968), Cohen (1969), Fenner and White (1970) and Smith (1968) and, for primarily epidemiological treatments, Andrewes (1967), Downs (1970) and Simpson (1971).

VIRUSES ASSOCIATED WITH ENCEPHALITIS

Western Equine Encephalitis (WEE)

WEE virus occurs in western states of the U.S.A. and of southern Canada and also extends into South America. Most human infections are inapparent, only some 1 in 1 000 showing clinical symptoms. Mild cases are characterized by fever with headache and vomiting, sometimes stiffness of the neck and back. More severe cases progress to stupor and coma; convulsions may occur, particularly in children. The case mortality is about 3 per cent. Recovery is usually complete without sequelae.

The pathological picture is of an aseptic meningitis. The meninges are congested and oedematous with mononuclear infiltration. Focal neuronal destruction, petechial haemorrhages, demyelination with mononuclear infiltration affect particularly the basal ganglia, pons and cerebellum.

Eastern Equine Encephalitis (EEE)

EEE virus occurs in the eastern U.S.A. and Canada and in Central and South America. Its distribution overlaps to some extent that of WEE. EEE is a much more severe disease than is WEE. Inapparent infection is rare and mortality may be high, as much as 60 to 75 per cent. Symptoms are similar to those of WEE but more severe, leading to a lethal outcome in as little as 5 days. Mental deficiency and paralyses are common sequelae. Pathological lesions are similar to those of WEE.

Venezuelan Equine Encephalitis (VEE)

VEE resembles WEE in usually being a mild infection. It occurs in the northern half of South America and around the Caribbean.

Epidemiology of Equine Encephalitides

As regards WEE and EEE, outbreaks of encephalitis in horses have been known in the U.S.A. for 80 years. They may be severe; in 1938 it is estimated that 184 000 horses were infected, with a 90 per cent case mortality (Andrewes, 1967). Incidence in man is usually lower than that in horses. Natural cycles of transmission of virus take place in birds by mosquitoes, particularly *Culex tarsalis* (WEE). Infections in birds are inapparent except in introduced birds such as pheasants. Infections in man are tangential from the main wild cycle though sometimes another cycle of transmission is thought to be interposed. For instance, in New Jersey in 1959 it is believed that *Culiseta melanura*, probably the main vector in wild bird cycles, was introduced by wind into a populated area and infected mainly chickens; *Aedes sollicitans* was then involved in transferring virus from infected chicks to man.

Less is known of the transmission cycles of VEE but it is presumed to be mosquito-transmitted from perhaps wild rodents to horses and to man but as virus has been isolated from the throat, perhaps droplet infection may also occur.

The mechanisms by which these viruses survive the winter in temperate climates when adult mosquitoes are virtually or completely absent, present a problem. Transovarial transmission is unlikely. Although the viruses have been isolated from northward migrating birds in Alabama, there are definite antigenic differences between EEE virus derived from South and from North America. Possibly virus persists unusually long in the blood of certain hosts, perhaps hibernating bats or even snakes (Andrewes, 1967); or in overwintering mosquitoes.

Japanese Encephalitis (JE)

JE virus occurs over a wide area of Asia, from eastern Siberia to Malaysia. It is particularly important in Japan and has been extensively studied there. Although most infections are inapparent or mild, some 1 in 500 infections develop encephalitis which is of a severe type similar to that caused by EEE virus, with a mortality as high as 90 per cent and mental impairment, personality changes and paralyses as sequelae. Although the incidence of encephalitis is low, the actual number of cases occurring in such densely populated areas such as in Tokyo, is considerable; in one epidemic there were about 8 000 (Andrewes, 1967).

EPIDEMIOLOGY. Birds, particularly herons, are the wild vertebrate hosts and the virus is transmitted among them by mosquitoes of the genera *Aedes* and *Culex*. The epidemiological picture has been worked out in detail especially in relation to Tokyo. Black crowned night herons and egrets breed in large heronries near the city and their breeding season coincides with the time of maximum prevalence of the main vector *Culex tritaeniorhynchus*. The nestling night herons are fed on by the mosquitoes and a high proportion of these become infected, so acting as 'amplifier' hosts and greatly increasing the amount of virus circulating in the mosquito population from late June to September. Pigs also are infected and undergo inapparent infections. Man is in closer contact with his pigs than he is with the wild bird hosts and so pigs can act importantly as 'link' hosts for the infection of man. Only in man, the 'dead-end' host, does clinical disease occur.

St Louis Encephalitis (SLE)

SLE virus occurs in the western and mid-western states of the U.S.A., around the Caribbean and in South America. Most infections are in-apparent and even when apparent tend to be clinically mild except in elderly patients.

EPIDEMIOLOGY. Considerable epidemics appear from time to time, the last in 1964. The vectors are *Culex* spp.—*C. tarsalis* in the western states, *C. quinquefasciatus* and *C. pipiens* in the mid-west. Cases occur mainly in the late summer perhaps because of an 'amplifier' effect in wild hosts similar to that reported for JE virus. Chickens and sparrows living in close association with man are likely 'link' hosts facilitating the transmission of the virus to man.

Murray Valley Encephalitis (MVE)

MVE virus occurs in eastern Australia and in New Guinea. The virus is closely related to JE virus and like it induces a severe disease with a high mortality and a high incidence of sequelae in recovered cases.

EPIDEMIOLOGY. *Culex annulirostris* is the main vector mosquito species and the main wild hosts are pied cormorants and other water birds. Studies of the incidence of specific antibody in birds have been made on the yolk of their eggs. Epidemics in man have been associated with seasons of heavy rainfall encouraging southward migration of bird hosts. There is a high incidence of antibody, some 80 to 90 per cent, in aborigines in north Australia, a situation which may serve as an immunological barrier to the introduction to Australia of JE virus. Epidemics of ence-phalitis in Australia occurring as far back as 1918 (Australian-X disease) are thought to have been caused by this virus.

Ilheus

Ilheus virus is the cause of mild encephalitic disease in Central and South America and in Trinidad.

California Encephalitis (CE)

CE virus was recognized first as a cause of encephalitis in man in the San Joaquin Valley of California in 1945. It was shown to be the cause of 285 cases of CNS disease in the U.S.A. between 1963 and 1968, mainly in the states of Ohio, Indiana, Wisconsin, Minnesota and Louisiana. The clinical disease varies from a mild undifferentiated febrile illness to acute CNS disease, even fatal.

Tahyna

Tahyna virus was found to be the cause of a mild illness mainly of a respiratory type in Czecho-slovakia since 1963.

EPIDEMIOLOGY OF CALIFORNIA ENCEPHA-LITIS AND TAHYNA. The vector mosquitoes are species of *Aedes*, *A. melanimon* for CE and *A. vexans* and *A. caspius* for Tahyna. Wild vertebrate hosts are believed to be mainly hares, rabbits and ground squirrels. Human infections occur mainly in the period July to September (Henderson and Coleman, 1971).

Tick-borne Encephalitis (TBE)

TBE virus occurs widely in the U.S.S.R. and in central Europe; the Russian and European viruses are closely related but antigenically dis-tinguishable. They are the cause of encephali-tides referred to in the past as Russian spring-summer encephalitis, Far-eastern Russian ence-phalitis and Central European tick-borne fever. The incubation period is 8 to 14 days. Onset is sudden, pyrexia with signs of cerebral involve-ment, photophobia, coma and paralyses. The bulbar centres and the cervical cord may be involved. Inapparent infections may occur. Mortality is highest in the Far-eastern form, reaching 30 per cent; paralyses may be perma-nent in recovered subjects. The Central European disease is often biphasic, the central nervous system involvement accompanying the second phase.

EPIDEMIOLOGY. The vectors of TBE are the hard-ticks *Ixodes ricinus* and *I. persulcatus*. Transovarial transmission of virus takes place in these species and infected individuals remain so for life. Thus the tick provides a long term reservoir for the survival of virus, though the full significance of transovarial transmission is not yet clear; being only about 10 per cent efficient, it is thought, considering the high mortality of tick larvae, unlikely to be sufficient in itself to ensure virus survival (Andrewes, 1967). The vertebrate hosts appear to be small rodents and ground-frequenting birds. The latter may, by their migrations, distribute infected ticks very widely and as virus persists in some species (such as ducks) for extended periods, they may be concerned also with the long term persistence of virus. Infection tends to be focal, perhaps because of ecological factors determining the presence of the complex of hosts and ticks necessary for virus survival. Infection of man is associated with contact with such foci, though it may also be acquired by the ingestion of goat milk.

Louping Ill

Louping (= leaping) ill is an encephalomyelitis of sheep occurring in hill pastures on both sides of the England–Scotland border, in northern Ireland and in south-west England. It is normally a disease of sheep though cattle are sometimes affected. The disease, typically, shows two phases, one of viraemia accompanied by high pyrexia and a second, some days later, of neurological incoordination, paralysis, even death. The second phase may be absent and, in sheep, the infection may be inapparent. Human cases derive from contact with infected sheep, or from laboratory infection; serous meningitis with some encephalitis is the presenting syndrome, but the illness is less severe than is associated with TBE encephalitis (Andrewes and Pereira, 1972).

Small rodents, *Cervus* (red deer) and *Lagopus* (grouse) have been shown to be naturally infected, apparently subclinically. *Ixodes ricinus* (a 'hard' tick) is the arthropod vector which may act as a long-term reservoir of infection. Concurrent infection of sheep with tick-borne fever (a rickettsial infection) may predispose to CNS invasion by louping-ill virus (Andrewes and Pereira, 1972).

Powassan

Powassan virus, first isolated from a child with encephalitis, occurs in northern U.S.A. and in eastern Canada. It has been isolated from the ticks *Dermacentor* and *Ixodes*.

VIRUSES ASSOCIATED WITH PYREXIA

Yellow Fever (YF)

Yellow fever was first recognized as a disease entity in the seventeenth century. For over two hundred years the disease was the cause of devastating epidemics in towns of the West Indies, Central America and the southern U.S.A. As recently as 1905 an epidemic in New Orleans caused 5 000 cases and 1 000 deaths (Strode, 1951). The discovery by Walter Reed and his colleagues in Cuba in 1900–1901 that the disease was due to a filtrable virus transmitted by *Aedes aegypti* opened up the possibility of the control of urban yellow fever by anti-mosquito measures. By the early 1930s these measures were thought to have eliminated yellow fever completely from the American continent. About that time, however, the appearance of cases of yellow fever away from cities and in localities in which *Aedes aegypti* did not occur, drew attention to the possibility of cycles of transmission not involving man—jungle yellow fever. From investigations of that situation in South America has stemmed much of the subsequent work on the epidemiology of yellow fever in America and in Africa, and indeed much of the work on arboviruses generally. Most of the work on yellow fever was supported by the Rockefeller Foundation and during these investigations six investigators died of yellow fever; vaccines did not become available until the 1930s.

Clinical Features and Pathology

As is typical of arboviruses generally, the severity of the clinical attack of yellow fever is very variable, ranging, even among the members of a single family, from inapparent infection, through mild fever to fulminant fatal attacks (Strode, 1951). The incubation period is some 3 to 6 days. The disease, when fully developed, consists of three clinical periods: of infection (coincident with viraemia); of remission; of intoxication. The dangerous aspects of the disease, intestinal haemorrhage (black vomit-blood altered by the gastric juices), albuminuria, liver damage, etc. are associated with this stage of the disease. The fatality rate is probably about 5 per cent of all cases. At necropsy the stomach and intestine show petechial mucosal haemorrhages and may contain partially digested blood. The liver shows mid zonal necrosis of the lobules and acidophilic masses formed from necrotic cells are also characteristic.

Laboratory Diagnosis

Attempts to isolate virus (by the intracerebral inoculation of the patient's serum into suckling mice) are likely to be successful only in the first day or two of the clinical disease. Otherwise, the YF virus antibody titre of acute and convalescent sera should be compared. *Post mortem* the liver lesion is characteristic and this was the basis of the programme carried on in the 1930s in South America—to procure samples of liver tissue from fatal fevers of less than 10 days duration by a special instrument (viscerotome) —to recognize the areas in which yellow fever was occurring.

Epidemiology

The basic sylvatic cycles of YF virus transmission in both Africa and America involve monkeys and forest mosquitoes and so the endemic yellow fever area is essentially that of the tropical forests of the two continents. Monkey species differ in their habits, e.g. in the extent to which they stay in the forest canopy or to which they may leave the canopy and invade ground-level or extra-forest environments. Similarly, forest mosquitoes are stratified as regards their biting habits, some species attacking at canopy level will seldom do so at ground level, and *vice versa*. The probable patterns followed by YF virus in its maintenance in sylvatic cycles and in its transmission to man are deduced from information of this sort—on the habits of possible wild animal hosts (together with information as to the prevalence of YF antibody in them in nature and on their capability to circulate virus in the laboratory) and on the habits of possible vectors (together with information on their capability to transmit virus in the laboratory).

In America many monkey species are involved but probably particularly *Alouatta* (howler monkey) and *Ateles* (spider monkey). The vectors transmitting virus among the canopy monkey population are mainly mosquitoes of the genus *Haemagogus*. These mosquitoes were once believed to be rather rare, but were noticed, once by chance, to be abundant, and biting man, in the vicinity of the crowns of newly felled forest trees. This episode drew attention to the importance of the forest canopy mosquito fauna in the epidemiology of yellow fever. It is believed that it is by the bite of *Haemagogus* mosquitoes, infected from wild animals and brought into contact with man by such operations as tree-felling, that most jungle-derived human infections in South America occur. Intra-human epidemics ensue only if the forester infected in this way returns to his village and the domestic mosquito *Aedes aegypti* is present there.

In Africa, again, many monkey species are involved but the high incidence of antibodies in the practically exclusively arboreal *Colobus* monkeys indicates the importance of the forest canopy cycles of transmission. The vector in the African forest canopy is principally *Aedes (S.) africanus*. The link between the forest canopy cycle and man is probably provided by monkey species, such as *Cercopithecus ascanias* (red-tail monkey), which raid into the plantations of the local inhabitants for bananas and other cultivated fruit. These plantations contain plants whose leaf axils contain water, e.g. banana trees, colocasias, in which *Aedes (S.) simpsoni* breeds. An infected monkey, viraemic but clinically undisturbed, entering the plantation may be fed upon by this mosquito species, which will transmit the infection in turn to its normal host, man. Intra-human epidemics may then ensue. This train of events, considering that African monkeys are clinically unaffected by the yellow fever viraemia, seems a very likely one. South American monkeys on the other hand are clinically affected and the presence of a yellow fever epidemic among them is often signalled by the presence of dead monkeys on the forest floor. This difference between African and

American monkeys in their clinical response to the disease is paralleled between African and South American Indian human populations and has been taken to indicate that yellow fever virus was comparatively recently introduced into America, perhaps at the time of the slave trade, and that American hosts, both monkey and human, have not yet adapted to its presence.

The long term survival of YF virus in forest cycles may seem precarious, as an epidemic in the wild monkey population leaves few non-immune individuals. Probably virus survival depends on continuous progression of the epidemic over such large areas of forest that it only returns to its previous track after a period long enough for a new susceptible primate population to grow up. Or cycles in other hosts, such as bats or bush babies (*Galago*) may be involved.

Control Measures

Control by anti-mosquito measures is straightforward in urban conditions but impracticable against jungle cycles of virus maintenance. Two live attenuated vaccines are available, both extremely effective. French neurotropic (FN) virus vaccine was developed at the Institut Pasteur, Dakar, Senegal and is produced in mouse brain. It is thermostable and is administered by scarification. Thus it is very convenient for use in the field in tropical conditions. It should not, however, be used for children under 14 years old among whom there have occurred cases of post-vaccinal encephalitis. The 17D vaccine developed by Theiler in New York in 1937 was attenuated by growth in tissue culture and is prepared in embryonated eggs. It is administered by subcutaneous inoculation by syringe or by jet injector. The vaccine is much less stable than the FN vaccine. Long period storage requires temperatures below $-20°C$ and vaccine life at $4°C$ is only about 3 months. The vaccine requires to be reconstituted immediately before use and, kept on ice, is potent for only about 1 hour. Post-vaccinal encephalitis is very rare with 17D vaccine, and occurs in children under 1 year of age. A booster dose is required 10 years after primary vaccination. Vaccination is a highly effective way of preventing yellow fever and may be used for the protection of individuals, for the establishment

of herd immunity to prevent epidemics or to form a barrier of an immune population against geographical spread of the disease (W.H.O., 1971).

Dengue

Dengue virus is widely distributed in the tropics and subtropics in both Old and New Worlds. In most cases the infection is inapparent or clinically mild but it may be a severe fever, diphasic in character, the first stage being marked by severe muscle and joint pains, photophobia and conjunctivitis, the second by a morbilliform rash, sometimes lymphadenopathy. A much more severe haemorrhagic type of the disease has appeared, mainly in children, in the Philippines, Malaysia, Vietnam, Thailand and India. The haemorrhagic fever occurred only in orientals, not in Caucasian people (Andrewes, 1967).

Haemorrhagic fever in indigenous people tends to be associated with areas where multiple dengue viruses cause disease—the classical dengue syndrome—in short-term residents. This, together with the accelerated, secondary, type of antibody response which takes place in haemorrhagic fever patients has led to the suggestion that the fever is a hyperimmune response in persons previously sensitized by another type of dengue virus. It is difficult to distinguish which type of virus is most responsible for the haemorrhagic outcome. However, type 2 was most frequently, though not exclusively, recovered from severe and fatal infections (Halstead, 1966; Smith, 1968).

EPIDEMIOLOGY. Dengue is transmitted by day-biting mosquitoes of the genus *Aedes*. In urban situations the cycles of transmission are intra-human and the vector *Aedes aegypti*. Andrewes (1967) has drawn attention to a difference in the characteristics of dengue epidemics according to whether they occur within the equatorial belt, where the mean monthly temperature exceeds 18°C throughout the year, or outside that zone. Within the zone where *Aedes aegypti* exists throughout the year transmission is continuous, outbreaks are localized. Outside that zone, transmission is intermittent, occurring only in the summer months and dengue outbreaks tend to be large, involving whole populations and millions of cases. There is evidence that species of monkeys, lemuroids and squirrels may be involved in sylvan cycles of transmission—jungle dengue.

Chikungunya

Chikungunya virus occurs in East, Central and South Africa and in India and south-east Asia. It is the cause of an acute dengue-like pyrexia of sudden onset, associated with intense joint and muscle pains and a rash. In African epidemics case fatality was minimal but the virus has since been found in Thailand associated with a severe haemorrhagic fever, in which dengue viruses also were involved (Andrewes, 1967). The name of the virus derives from an African language word meaning 'the thing causing bending up', from the contorted position of patients induced by the joint pains.

O'nyong-nyong

O'nyong-nyong virus is closely related to chikungunya and produces a practically identical clinical syndrome except that lymphadenopathy also occurs. The name of the virus has the same meaning as chikungunya.

EPIDEMIOLOGY OF CHIKUNGUNYA AND O'NYONG-NYONG. Chikungunya virus was first reported from an epidemic occurring in a rural African population living on a sandstone plateau in South Tanzania; some 180 000 cases occurred among a population of 200 000. Because of the porous nature of the plateau, water was at a premium and was stored in large clay jars dug into the floor of the huts. These provided large populations of *Aedes aegypti* within the houses and this species was considered to be the vector. Wild vertebrate hosts have not been identified but serological evidence suggests a cycle in nature involving non-human primates (Downs, 1970).

O'nyong-nyong appeared as an epidemic in north-west Uganda in 1959 and progressed across the north of Uganda along a course of some 500 miles, disappearing in western Kenya; about 5 million people are estimated to have been infected. Unusually for mosquito-borne arboviruses, which are mainly transmitted by culicine mosquitoes particularly the genera *Culex* and *Aedes*, o'nyong-nyong virus appears to have been transmitted by anophelines; it was isolated from both *Anopheles gambiae* and *Anopheles funestus*. Extra-human vertebrate hosts are not known; interpretation of studies on the sera of African animals is complicated by the serological overlap between this virus and related ones.

West Nile (WN)

West Nile virus occurs throughout eastern Africa from South Africa to Egypt and occurs also in France and southern Asia from Israel to the Philippines. Most infections occur in children and are inapparent or clinically mild; epidemics affecting all ages have occurred in Israel. Affected people showed fever, sore throat, lymphadenopathy and sometimes a morbilliform rash.

EPIDEMIOLOGY. Infection of man is tangential from cycles involving wild birds, probably mainly crows, house sparrows, pigeons and herons. The vectors are mosquitoes *Culex univittatus* and *C. pipiens*, the latter species perhaps important in ensuring virus survival, as it overwinters as an adult.

Rift Valley Fever (RVF)

RVF virus is endemic in sheep and cattle in East and South Africa. Mosquitoes of the genera *Aedes*, *Eretmapodites* and *Culex* are likely vectors. Primary vertebrate hosts probably include sheep, cattle, wild bovines and wild rodents. Man is most commonly infected by handling sick or dead animals but sometimes by mosquito bite.

Besides those viruses discussed individually, above, there are many agents which have been identified as the cause of mild fevers in man, or are known to infect man from serological evidence, and which are presumed to be mosquito-transmitted on such evidence as virus isolation from mosquitoes or from sentinel susceptible animals. Examples of these, classified according to the region of the world from which they come, are:

Africa: Bunyamwera, Bwamba, Germiston, Ilesha, Semliki Forest, Sindbis, Spondweni, Wesselsbron, Zika.

South America: Guaroa, Apeu, Carapara, Itaqui, Mayaro, Marituba, Murutucu, Oriboca, Catu, Oropouche.

Kyasanur Forest Disease (KFD)

KFD virus appeared as a new disease in the Kyasanur Forest in Mysore Province, South India, in 1957. It may be extending its range at present. The clinical infection is often mild, characterized mainly by fever, headache, conjunctivitis, vomiting and diarrhoea. However, severe haemorrhagic cases occur, with alimentary tract haemorrhage and epistaxis. Recovery from an attack may be slow. The case fatality may be as much as 10 per cent.

EPIDEMIOLOGY. At the same time as the occurrence of the human cases in villages near the Kyasanur Forest, dead monkeys, mainly langurs (*Presbytis*) and bonnet-macaques (*Macaca radiata*) were found in the forest. The vector arthropod among the monkeys was a tick, *Haemaphysalis spinigera*. The basic cycle of transmission appears to be by *Haemaphysalis* ticks among jungle fowl in which antibodies to KFD were found. Antibodies occurred also in some small mammals but these mainly carried *Ixodes* ticks not *Haemaphysalis*. It seems likely that both human and monkey infections are tangential episodes from this forest-bird-tick cycle. Transovarial transmission occurs in *Haemaphysalis*.

Omsk Haemorrhagic Fever (OHF)

OHF virus occurs in the U.S.S.R. and in Roumania. Clinically the disease resembles KFD. The virus is transmitted in cycles involving rodents and ticks of the genus *Dermacentor*. Musk-rats, rodents occurring in the area but not indigenous to it, suffer from fatal infections; and men have been infected by handling the musk-rats.

Colorado Tick Fever

Colorado tick fever occurs in the moister parts of the north-west U.S.A. and in Alberta, Canada. Often it is an inapparent or mild infection but it may be a severe diphasic fever with haemorrhagic and encephalitic complications in children. Basic cycles of transmission involve ground squirrels and chipmunks, transmission being by the wood-tick *Dermacentor andersoni*. Man is infected tangentially.

Sandfly Fever (SF)

SF virus occurs from the Mediterranean basin eastwards through the central U.S.S.R. to India. The infection in man may be inapparent or it may be a fairly severe fever characterized by myalgia, conjunctivitis and retro-orbital pain. The incubation period is 7 to 10 days. Two serological types of the virus are known, the Naples and Sicily strains, respectively. They are transmitted by sandflies (*Phlebotomus papatasii*) which resemble mosquitoes but are much smaller and breed not in water but in sand, dust and soil. There is evidence, though not conclusive, that transovarial transmission takes place from one generation of *Phlebotomus* to another. As regards vertebrate hosts, so far only man has been shown to be infected but the possibility of other vertebrates being concerned is indicated by the occurrence of some similar viruses in rodents and in a sloth in Brazil.

Argentinian and Bolivian Haemorrhagic Fevers; Lassa Fever

The South American haemorrhagic fevers are caused, respectively, by Junin and Machupo viruses of the Tacaribe group. Their main clinical pictures are pyrexia, nasal, intestinal and uterine haemorrhage, petechiae and purpura, with a fatality rate as high as 20 per cent. Although these viruses have been isolated from rodents and from mites, attempts to isolate Machupo virus from arthropods during the course of an epidemic, failed. From this and from the demonstration of the presence of Machupo virus in the urine of chronically-infected rats, it is doubtful if these viruses are in fact arthropod-borne (Casals, 1971).

Lassa fever, characterized by severe muscle pains, a haemorrhagic rash and a high case fatality appeared in 1969 among Americans living at Lassa, Nigeria. Lassa fever virus also belongs to the Tacaribe group (Casals, 1971).

REFERENCES

AMERICAN COMMITTEE ON ARTHROPOD-BORNE VIRUSES (1970) Catalogue of arthropod-borne viruses of the world. *American Journal of Tropical Medicine and Hygiene*, **19**, 1082–1160.

AMERICAN COMMITTEE ON ARTHROPOD-BORNE VIRUSES (1971) Catalogue of arthropod-borne and selected viruses of the world. *American Journal of Tropical Medicine and Hygiene*, **20**, 1018–1050.

ANDREWES, C. H. (1967) *The Natural History of Viruses.* London: Weidenfeld and Nicolson.

ANDREWES, C. H. & PEREIRA, H. G. (1972) *Viruses of Vertebrates.* 3rd edn. London: Ballière, Tindall.

CASALS, J. (1967) Immunological techniques for animal viruses. In *Methods in Virology.* Edited by K. Maramoroschk and H. Koprowski. New York: Academic Press.

CASALS, J. (1971) Arboviruses: Incorporation in a general system of virus classification. In *Comparative virology.* Edited by K. Maramoroschk and E. Kurstak. New York: Academic Press.

COHEN, A. (1969) *Textbook of Medical Virology.* Oxford: Blackwell Scientific Publications.

DOWNS, W. G. (1970) Arboviruses: epidemiological considerations. In *Infectious Agents and Host Reactions.* Edited by S. Mudd. Philadelphia: W. B. Saunders Co.

FENNER, F. O. & WHITE, D. O. (1970) *Medical Virology.* New York: Academic Press.

HALSTEAD, S. B. (1966) Mosquito-borne haemorrhagic fevers of south and south-east Asia. *Bulletin of the World Health Organization*, **35**, 3–15.

HENDERSON, B. E. & COLEMAN, P. H. (1971) The growing importance of California arboviruses in the etiology of human disease. *Progress in Medical Virology*, **13**, 404–461.

MELNICK, J. L. (1971) Classification and nomenclature of animal viruses, 1971. *Progress in Medical Virology*, **13**, 462–484.

RHODES, A. J. & VAN ROOYEN, C. E. (1968) *Textbook of Virology.* 5th edn. Baltimore: Williams and Wilkins.

SIMPSON, D. I. H. (1971) Arbovirus diseases. *British Medical Bulletin*, **28**, 10–15.

SMITH, C. E. G. (1968) Recent advances in arbovirus research. *Abstracts in Hygiene*, **43**, 1397–1436.

SMITH, C. E. G. (1971) Arbovirus vaccines other than yellow fever: achievements, problems, needs. *Proceedings of International Conference on the Application of Vaccines against Viral, Rickettsial and Bacterial Diseases of Man.* Scientific Publication No. 226. Washington: Pan American Health Office.

STRODE, G. K. (Ed.) (1951) *Yellow Fever.* New York: McGraw-Hill Book Co. Inc.

TAYLOR, R. M. (1967) Catalogue of the arthropod-borne viruses of the world. *U.S. Department of Health, Education and Welfare, Public Health Service*: Publication No. 1760.

WORLD HEALTH ORGANIZATION (1971) W.H.O. expert committee on yellow fever. Third report. *World Health Organization Technical Report Series* No. 479.

WORLD HEALTH ORGANIZATION (1967) Arboviruses and human disease. *World Health Organization Technical Report Series* No. 369.

WORK, T. H. (1964) Isolation and identification of arthropod-borne viruses. In *Diagnostic Procedures for Viral and Rickettsial Diseases.* Edited by E. H. Lennette and W. J. Schmidt. New York: American Public Health Association.

WORK, T. H. & HAMMON, W. McD. (1964) Arbovirus infection in man. In *Diagnostic Procedures for Viral and Rickettsial Diseases.* Edited by E. H. Lennette and W. J. Schmidt. New York: American Public Health Association.

48. Rhabdoviruses   Rabies

Rabies, one of the zoonoses, is primarily a disease of warm-blooded animals, particularly carnivores, and including vampire, fruit and insect-eating bats. The dog amongst domestic animals is the commonest source of infection for man: the virus is excreted in the saliva and any person bitten by a rabid (mad) dog is liable to develop rabies, sometimes called hydrophobia because of the difficulty and fear in swallowing water. The disease in man and in most clinically infected animals is rapidly fatal but more prolonged infections occur in vampire bats. Rabies is not endemic in the domestic or wild animal life in Britain, but may be imported by animal pets (particularly dogs and cats) or rarely by exotic animals intended for zoos and the like. The system of 6 months quarantine for imported canines and felines from 1886 accompanied in the early years by the muzzling of dogs, was successful in eradicating rabies from animal life in Britain from 1902 until it was re-introduced in 1918 by an illegally imported dog. The infection persisted among dogs for 4 years and 144 persons bitten by rabid dogs had courses of rabies vaccine but there were no human cases of the disease. From 1922 to 1970, close on 100 000 imported animals have been quarantined; of these 27 developed rabies including two dogs retained for more than 6 months for special reasons.

In 1969, a dog imported from Germany developed rabies about a week after release from 6 months quarantine. Although only the owner was bitten by the dog, 41 contacts were given full courses of rabies vaccine: there were no cases of infection. In addition, the almost total destruction of all wild life in an area of 3 000 acres where the dog was thought to have been at large for a short time was carried out, and this drastic action may have helped to prevent further spread. Another episode occurred in the same year when a dog admitted from Pakistan developed rabies 3 months after release from quarantine; there were no human or animal cases of infection. These incidents led to an extension of the quarantine period, initially for 8 and then for 12 months, and the inclusion in the quarantine regulations of a list of exotic animals that might be imported. These stringent measures were deemed necessary, particularly at a time when rabies was spreading among the wild life of Western Europe with special involvement of foxes; for example, rabies was diagnosed in 675 animals in Europe in 1969 so that the risk to animal life in Britain was obvious. In 1972, the quarantine was reduced to 6 months, but with the requirement that all quarantined animals be given a dose of an acceptable rabies vaccine on entry and a second dose one month later.

DESCRIPTION

The properties of the rhabdoviruses have not yet been well defined; they consist of several viruses from different sources with structural resemblances. Rabies virus closely resembles the well-studied animal virus of vesicular stomatitis: it is bullet-shaped, 75 to 80 nm wide and up to 180 nm long. Haemagglutinating spikes project from the lipoprotein envelope. The single-stranded RNA is enclosed in an internal nucleocapsid with helical symmetry. There is only one serotype and specific antibody is demonstrable by neutralization and complement fixation tests. The virus can be grown in a variety of tissue culture cells, e.g. baby hamster kidney (BHK) and characteristic acidophilic inclusions develop in the cytoplasm. Virions are found in the cytoplasmic matrices and also bud from the cytoplasmic membrane, but little new virus is released and most cells survive. The virus grows well in the tissues of 7-day old chick embryos and this source has been used for the preparation of vaccines.

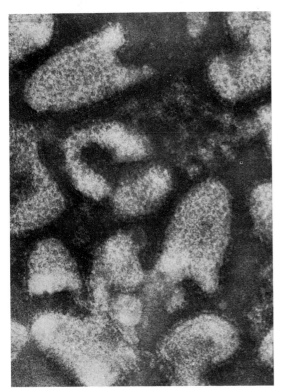

PLATE 48.1. Rabies virus grown in BHK cells; note bullet-shaped particles: stained PTA. 150 × 100 nm. (Courtesy of Dr C. R. Madeley. Institute of Virology, Glasgow.)

Animal Pathogenicity

Rabies virus naturally infects a wide range of mammals from domesticated dogs, cats and cattle to foxes, wolves, coyotes, jackals, skunks, racoons, mongooses, squirrels and bats. The virus invades the blood and the central nervous system of the host and is excreted in the saliva, milk and urine. These materials can be used to transmit the infection to laboratory animals, including rabbits, mice and guinea-pigs. Freshly isolated strains of the virus are known as 'street virus' and will kill laboratory animals with a severe encephalitis after an incubation period which varies from 1 to 12 weeks according to the species inoculated. Multiple eosinophilic inclusions known as Negri bodies are found in the nerve cells especially in the hippocampus, and measure $0.5\ \mu m$ to $20\ \mu m$ in diameter. Negri bodies are specific to rabies infection and their detection in nerve tissue enables a diagnosis of

rabies to be made. Serial brain-to-brain passages of the virus in rabbits yields an attenuated or 'fixed' strain of the virus which is no longer able to multiply in extraneural situations. Negri bodies are scanty in the brains of animals inoculated with the fixed virus.

PATHOGENESIS

The usual portal of entry is the bite and rabies virus from the infected saliva is introduced into the depths of the wound. Occasionally the virus may gain access through a pre-existing scratch or abrasion if this has been contaminated with saliva. The virus multiplies locally in the tissues, invades adjacent nerve fibres, and spreads centrally to infect the neurones in the brain and spinal cord. The virus is thought to enter and travel along the neurones of peripheral nerves. Although bite wounds are the usual mode of entry, rare instances have been reported of infection by inhalation in bat-infested caves where there was bat-rabies or by ingestion through eating rabid cattle. The highly susceptible fox and coyote (but not the more resistant dog and cat) have been experimentally infected by inhalation from exposure in caves.

The incubation period varies from ten days to two years after the bite of a rabid animal; its duration may depend on the distance the virus has to move from the point of entry to reach the brain. Average figures are: for bites on the leg 60 days, on the arm 40 days and on the head 30 days. The incubation period is shorter in children than in adults. Occasionally, when severely lacerated wounds of the head and shoulders have been heavily infected, the virus may be carried to the brain via the bloodstream; in such cases the incubation period is short.

From the neurones which show little or no cytopathic effect, the virus may spread to other tissues including the salivary glands where it multiplies in the acinar cells, the adrenals, kidneys, pancreas and myocardium. It may also infect the conjunctiva or cornea so that examination of exudate or corneal impression smears by immunofluorescence may be useful as a diagnostic procedure (Cifuentes et al., 1971).

The first symptoms of the disease are headache, fever, a profound sense of apprehension, and a feeling of irritation at the site of the bite. The patients complain of a dry throat and thirst, but they will not drink. High fever, difficulty in swallowing and the consequent fear of water become the dominant symptoms, and the patient passes into delirium with generalized convulsions. The outcome is invariably fatal.

Histopathological examination of the brain shows, in addition to the Negri inclusion bodies in the neurones of cerebellum and hippocampus, a polio-encephalitis affecting usually the brain stem and spinal cord and characterized by perivascular cuffing with lymphocytes and plasma cells, parenchymal microgleal response, and sometimes neuronophagia. The inflammatory reaction appears early whereas the Negri bodies are more commonly found in cases with a long illness (Dupont and Earle, 1965).

LABORATORY DIAGNOSIS

In man the history and clinical findings are usually so characteristic that laboratory confirmation is not always necessary. The virus, however, is present in the saliva and may also be isolated from specimens of the brain and spinal cord and salivary glands obtained at necropsy. The material, if thought to be contaminated, is treated with antibiotics and then inoculated intracerebrally in mice; the animals develop a flaccid paralysis of the limbs and die within 10 to 14 days.

If there is the slightest reason to suspect a dog of rabies, the animal should be kept in strict isolation and observed for a period of ten days; if it survives for this period, rabies may safely be excluded. If unmistakable symptoms of rabies are observed, the animal is killed (preferably with chloroform) and the diagnosis is confirmed by laboratory examination. If the laboratory is at some distance, the head is removed, wrapped in a cloth soaked in 50 per cent glycerol saline, and forwarded in crushed ice. Diagnosis depends on the demonstration of the virus in brain tissue and salivary glands by immunofluorescence which gives a specific diagnosis within a few hours and at an early stage of the infection: later, inclusion Negri bodies are demonstrable in the cytoplasm of the nerve cells in the hippocampus. If need be, confirmation is obtained by intra-cerebral inoculation of mice with the infective tissue.

EPIDEMIOLOGY

The epidemiology of rabies is determined by the animal sources of infection. Dog and cat rabies constitute the most important source because 95 per cent of human infections are derived from these animals. In the dog the incubation period is as a rule 2 to 8 weeks, but it may be as long as eight months. The disease is characterized by two clinical forms. In 'furious' rabies the animals become aggressive, vicious and excited; they snap and bite at the approach of any other creatures. In 'dumb' rabies paralysis of the muscles of the head and neck occurs and the dog cannot chew its food; its owner, believing it has some object in its throat, may attempt to remove the obstruction and contaminate his hands with infected saliva. About 50 per cent of rabid dogs excrete the virus in their saliva. They are infectious for only about ten days before their death.

Many species of wild animals suffer from rabies. One of the most important carriers is the fox, which may transmit the infection to domestic animals. The spread of rabies among wild life from central into western Europe has involved the fox particularly. In Canada many cases of cattle rabies have been attributed to this source of infection. In eastern Europe, and the Middle East, wolves and jackals have transmitted the infection, and in India, South Africa and some West Indian countries, the mongoose is an endemic reservoir. Other species which are able to transmit rabies are rats, badgers, opossums, musk-rats, racoons, skunks (a common reservoir in the U.S.A.), chipmunks, squirrels and possibly other small mammals.

Rabies may infect all the usual domestic animals, including the horse, cow, sheep, goat or pig. Often the animals are infected by the bite of rabid foxes, or other wild animals.

In Trinidad and South America rabies is transmitted by the vampire bat *Desmodus rotundus murinus*. The bat is the only species so far recognized which suffers a prolonged and mainly inapparent infection with rabies virus. In North America fruit- and insect-eating bats are also known to harbour the virus, and when rabid are able to transmit the infection to other bats, animals and man. Isolated instances of rabies among bats have been reported from a few European countries so there may be a remote possibility of the introduction of the infection to Britain from Northern France.

CONTROL MEASURES

Control of rabies which has a world-wide distribution would be possible only by the eradication of the infection among the many species of wild life as well as the domestic animals that are susceptible. Eradication of the infection from the wild life of a country in which rabies is endemic is virtually impossible, but more active measures against certain species, e.g. foxes in European countries, would greatly lessen the risks of infection among domestic animals, e.g. dogs and cats.

Since in endemic areas dogs are the main source for human infection, an active or compulsory vaccination programme for all domesticated dogs and cats and the rounding up of strays can greatly reduce the human hazard. In this way, human rabies has virtually disappeared from the U.S.A. although annually, there are over 4 000 reported cases of animal rabies, mainly in wild life. In Britain, Australia, New Zealand and numerous other smaller islands, the application of quarantine regulations have been remarkably effective in controlling the introduction of rabies.

Specific Prophylaxis

Between 1946 and 1969, 8 fatal cases of rabies have been confirmed in Britain; in each case the infection was acquired abroad and in 6 was due to the bite of a rabid dog (Macrae, 1969). But every year 25 to 35 persons have been given prophylactic courses of vaccine after suspected exposure abroad; in special incidents at home, e.g. at Edinburgh Zoological Gardens in 1965 (Sharp and McDonald, 1967) and at Camberley in 1969 (see above), a considerable number of possible contacts of rabid animals have been vaccinated. The rationale of prophylactic vaccination after infection may have occurred is that with a long incubation period, the vaccine may stimulate the production of antibody early enough and in sufficient amount to neutralize the virus before it gains access to the CNS neurones. The principle is somewhat analogous to the vaccination of smallpox contacts.

If the risk of rabies is great, as happens when there is a high probability that the animal concerned is rabid, and there are multiple bites on the head, face, neck or arms, immediate action is necessary and passive protection should be given by injecting hyperimmune horse serum or concentrated immunoglobulin preferably around the injured tissues and within 12 to 24 hours after the incident. The dose of the serum is 0·5 ml per kg body weight and that of the immunoglobulin is at least 40 International Units (1 iu = 1 mg) per kg body weight. The administration of antibody must be followed by a minimum of 10, and preferably 14, injections of vaccine to stimulate active immunity and 2 booster injections thereafter; this is necessary because passively injected antibodies have a suppressive effect on the early development of antibodies by the patient himself.

Various vaccines are used to confer active immunity. One type in general use in many countries is the Semple vaccine which contains a 4 per cent suspension of the brain of rabbits infected with the 'fixed' rabies virus inactivated by 0·5 per cent phenol. A number of similar vaccines prepared from infected rabbit or sheep brain are also used and inactivation is achieved by ultra-violet light, formalin or other agents. Vaccines of this type suffer from the serious disadvantage that the nervous tissue they contain may sensitize a small proportion (1 in 4 000 to 1 in 10 000) of persons being immunized who later may develop an allergic type of encephalitis. In order to avoid such 'neuroparalytic accidents' other types of vaccines containing no nervous tissue have been developed. Of these, the inactivated duck embryo vaccine, first introduced in the U.S.A., is now the vaccine mainly used in Britain although it is apparently less effective in producing virus-neutralizing antibody than brain tissue or tissue culture vaccines (Crick and Brown, 1970).

A possible disadvantage of daily injections of a weakly potent antigen is that the antibody response is predominantly IgM which does not easily reach the tissues where antibody is most needed. This difficulty could be overcome by the use of more potent rabies vaccines produced for example in tissue culture (not yet licensed for human inoculation) and the injection of the vaccine at longer intervals to encourage the early appearance of IgG antibody (Rubin *et al.*, 1971).

Attenuated strains of the living virus have also been developed. Of these the Flury low egg passage (LEP) strain, which has been carried through 40 to 60 egg passages, has been extensively used in a vaccine for the immunization of dogs. An inactivated tissue culture vaccine is also available for dogs. A high passage strain (HEP) carried through more than 180 egg passages is recommended for the vaccination of cats and cattle.

For the protection of staff who may be at some risk of exposure to rabies, e.g. veterinary surgeons, attendants in quarantine kennels and zoos, a schedule of two doses of duck embryo vaccine at an interval of 6 weeks followed by a booster 6 months later, is recommended, and this course may be followed by further booster doses if the risk of continued exposure exists.

REFERENCES AND FURTHER READING

CIFUENTES, E., CALDERON, E. & BIJENGA, G. (1971) Rabies in a child diagnosed by a new intra-vitam method: the cornea test. *Journal of Tropical Medicine and Hygiene*, **74**, 23.

CRICK, J. & BROWN, F. (1970) Efficacy of rabies vaccine prepared from virus grown in duck embryo. *Lancet*, i, 1106.

DUPONT, J. R. & EARLE, K. M. (1965) Human rabies encephalitis: a study of 49 fatal cases with a review of the literature. *Neurology*, **15**, 1023.

MACRAE, A. D. (1969) Rabies in England. *Lancet*, ii, 1415.

RUBIN, R. H., DIERKS, R. E., GOUGH, P., GREGG, M. B., GERLACH, E. H. & SIKES, R. K. (1971) Immunoglobulin response to rabies vaccine in man. *Lancet*, ii, 625.

SHARP, J. C. M. & McDONALD, S. (1967) Effects of rabies vaccine in man. *British Medical Journal*, iii, 20.

WORLD HEALTH ORGANIZATION (1966) Fifth report of expert committee on rabies. *World Health Organization Technical Report Series*, no. 321.

49. Slow and Oncogenic Viruses

Scrapie: Kuru: Animal Virus Tumours

It is appropriate to consider slow and oncogenic viruses together. Much of the interest in both subjects stems from a renewed appreciation of the value of comparative virology and pathology.

The central feature which slow and oncogenic viruses have in common is the long continued association of all or part of the virus with the host; host genetic factors are also of crucial importance and with the age, immunological and hormonal state of the host may, in large measure, determine the outcome of any particular host-virus combination. In general, the associated, as distinct from infectious, diseases occur sporadically and only exceptionally do they assume epidemic features. There are two main patterns of pathogenesis. Some slow viruses (the spongeiform encephalopathies) are due to unusual agents, perhaps not viruses in the classical sense; others are conventional viruses which evade or modify the immune response of the host. The oncogenic viruses overlap with the latter group and in addition have developed special integrative arrangements with the host cell genome.

SLOW VIRUS INFECTIONS

These may be divided into two principal groups.

1. Those in which the nature and morphology of the causative agents has not yet been established and in which there is no demonstrable immune response; the spongeiform encephalopathies.

2. Those in which 'typical' viruses are involved and in which an immune response, although present, cannot apparently halt the disease process and indeed may contribute to the development of lesions.

THE SPONGEIFORM ENCEPHALOPATHIES

This group comprises scrapie disease of sheep, Kuru and Creutzfeld-Jakob disease of man, and mink encephalopathy; all four are essentially degenerative diseases of the CNS without inflammatory response.

Scrapie

The prototype disease is scrapie in sheep. It gets its name from the presenting clinical sign of pruritus but locomotor ataxia is also a prominent feature. The familial pattern of the disease in nature initially led to the conclusion that the disease was inherited and governed by a single recessive autosomal gene. Further observations revealed that although the disease is not highly infectious, lateral transmission occurs. Experimentally the disease was first transmitted to sheep and later to goats. Later, transmission to mice enabled quantitative methods to be applied to the characterization of the agent. Even studies with mice are difficult because of the long incubation periods involved—rarely less than 4 months even with the largest doses. The length of incubation period and the rate of proliferation of the agent in the mouse spleen and brain depends on the 'sinc' gene. The histopathological type and anatomical distribution of the resulting brain lesions also depend on the genotype of the mice and the origin of the agent; with certain genotypes of mice, strains of scrapie agent with differing incubation periods and lesion profile can be distinguished. This is important because the agent cannot be assayed in cell culture. Cultures of glial cells have been established from infected mouse brain. These show more vigorous cell growth than comparable cultures from uninfected brain and there is an increase in the titre of scrapie agent in step with the increase in cell numbers.

In experimental animals the disease can be transmitted by a number of different routes with a wide variety of tissues; the smallest doses are required intracerebrally and the greatest concentration of agent is found in brain. In such systems it has been shown that the agent is filterable and transmissible in series, thus resembling a virus. However, the agent is remarkably resistant to physical and chemical inactivation; for example, it resists boiling, treatment with formaldehyde and β propiolactone, and digestion by nucleases and proteases. It is not inactivated by large doses of X and ultraviolet radiation; findings difficult to reconcile with the presence of a nucleic acid genome. Moreover, it is partially sensitive to the action of 0·1 M periodate, urea, and 90 per cent phenol and also to strong alkali and acid solutions. These properties, together with the heat resistance and insensitivity to nucleases and proteases, have led to the suggestion that the 'information' of the agent is carried in a carbohydrate rather than a nucleic acid template, perhaps as altered polysaccharide constituents of cell membrane. If substantiated, this would be of great biological interest. Other workers have concluded that the findings, particularly the small target size, might be explained by the presence of very small amounts of nucleic acid. They point to the virus of potato spindle tube disease which has an RNA genome of about 500 000 MW and which is capable of functioning in the absence of helper virus.

TRANSMISSIBLE MINK ENCEPHALOPATHY is a disease of mink which has occurred in minor epizootics perhaps after consumption of bovine or ovine tissues. It does not spread readily by contact and once the epizootic is over the disease does not tend to recur in the herd even though progeny of affected mink may still be present. The agent of mink encephalopathy can be distinguished from that of scrapie only by its host range; the former can, it is claimed, be transmitted to rhesus monkeys unlike scrapie which will, however, infect mink.

Kuru

Kuru is a slowly progressive neurological disease in human beings and is confined to the Fore people of the Eastern Highlands of New Guinea, among whom the incidence has been high. Other tribes or outsiders living in the region have not been affected. Originally, it was a disease of women and children of both sexes but the disease has now largely disappeared from children. Epidemiological data suggests an incubation period of from 4 to 20 years. Transmission is probably by the oral route because the gradual disappearance of the disease in the young may be related to the discontinuation of the practice by women and children of eating the organs, particularly brain, of deceased relatives (as a mark of respect).

As the pathology of this disease resembled that of scrapie transmission experiments were attempted with a wide selection of experimental animals. The disease was reproduced by injection of chimpanzees with CNS tissues from Kuru patients. The incubation period was initially up to 3 years but on serial passage diminished to about 1 year. Kuru has also been reproduced with typical features in spider, capuchin, squirrel and rhesus monkeys, the last of which with an incubation period of more than 8 years.

Creutzfeld-Jakob disease is an uncommon form of human pre-senile dementia. Histopathological and ultrastructural changes resemble those seen in experimental Kuru and the disease has also been transmitted to chimpanzees.

SLOW VIRUS DISEASES ASSOCIATED WITH CLASSICAL VIRUSES

Visna and Maedi

Visna is a meningo-leukoencephalomyelitis and maedi a slowly progressive pneumonia. They are confined to sheep and were first recognized in Iceland and transmitted to normal sheep by filtrates of tissues of infected animals with an incubation period often of several years. A typical syncytial cytopathic effect occurred in cells cultured from diseased organs and in cell cultures (e.g. sheep choroid plexus) prepared *de novo* and then inoculated. The pathogenesis of the disease was studied by cell culture and virus was demonstrated in whole blood, CSF and saliva of infected sheep during the (incubation) period. Similarly the virus can be recovered from brain, lung and spleen of experimentally inoculated sheep long before the development of clinical signs. The animals develop complement-fixing and later neutralizing antibodies but these do not appear to limit the spread of the disease.

The isolates from visna and maedi are closely similar and are enveloped viruses, lipid solvent sensitive, of 85 nm diameter with an internal ribonucleoprotein component characteristic in common with the leukoviruses. Their replication is dependent on host DNA synthesis and is inhibited by base analogues and the transcription inhibitor actinomycin D (Chap. 13) as with leukoviruses. The virions include a reverse transcriptase. Visna is not oncogenic in animals although it transforms cell cultures. The ability to produce syncytia is associated with the virions and its demyelinating ability in the CNS may be linked with this capacity.

Sub-acute Sclerosing Panencephalitis (SSPE)

This is a rare disease of children and young adults. There is progressive failure of intellectual function with, sometimes much later, neurological signs including ataxia. Remissions are rare and the disease progresses to dementia and death. The CSF has no pleocytosis but there is an elevated IgG content in the fluid and also in extracts of brain tissue. Perivascular lymphocytic hyperplasia and diffuse microglial infiltrations are found in both grey and white matter and some degree of demyelination is usually present. Eosinophilic intranuclear cytoplasmic inclusion bodies may be seen in neurones and glial cells. The degenerative changes are thought to be secondary to the inflammatory changes. Electromicrographs reveal myxovirus-like tubular structures and immunofluorescence the presence of measles antigen. Further, such patients had high levels of measles antibody in their serum and CSF. Finally, measles virus was isolated by co-cultivation and cell fusion techniques with standard cell lines and cells from the CNS and found to be antigenically similar to measles virus from other sources, although one study concluded that they resembled vaccine, rather than wild strains. There is also some evidence that SSPE strains may be more neurotopic in hamsters.

SSPE material inoculated into ferrets produces a diffuse encephalomyelitis after several months. The animals neither developed measles antibody nor was measles virus isolated from their brains. In other studies particles resembling a papovavirus have been seen in cells from a culture of SSPE brain; as a similar virus has been isolated from a renal patient on long term immunosuppression, it may be that this anomalous finding represents both an unusual immunological response to measles virus and infection with another virus in circumstances of viral immunosuppression. Despite these equivocal results the bulk of the evidence suggests measles virus as the aetiological agent of SSPE.

Aleutian Disease of Mink

The disease is named after the condition found in a certain type of mink with the 'Aleutian' genes which gives a commercially valuable colour of pelt; its pathological features are plasmacytosis and a positive Coombs' test, amyloidosis, hyaline glomerulonephritis, polyarteritis nodosa and hypergammaglobulinaemia, which simulate autoimmunity; it is therefore noteworthy that this disease is infectious in mink farms and is transmissible with cell-free filtrates to the susceptible genotype of mink. Once infected, the mink carries the virus in the tissues, serum and urine for the remainder of its life and often dies of glomerulonephritis. The glomerular lesions are of the 'immune complex' variety (Chap. 14) and infectious virus can be isolated from them.

Other persistent virus infections of animals characterized by immune complex disease are lymphocytic choriomeningitis and lactic dehydrogenase viruses of mice and a leukaemia virus infection of New Zealand Black mice; in the latter a variety of 'autoimmune' antibodies (e.g. antinuclear factor) are formed in addition to leukovirus-antibody complexes. A speculative interpretation of the findings with this general category of slow virus infection suggests a virally induced defect of cell mediated immunity—with a consequential failure to eliminate the clones of infected cells—and with a sustained formation of viral and antitissue antibodies by unaffected B lymphocytes freed from 'feedback' control.

ONCOGENIC VIRUSES

Four (pox; adenovirus; herpes; papova) of the seven groups of DNA animal viruses and one (leukovirus) of the groups of the RNA animal viruses are oncogenic in nature or under special experimental circumstances. Historically, the RNA tumour viruses (oncorna viruses) were the first to be recognized when Peyton Rous and other pioneers described the avian sarcoma of the leukosis complex of fowls in the early 1900s; in the 1970s the leukovirus again appear to be the important oncogenic viruses in nature.

Although a DNA oncogenic virus such as polyoma causes few tumours in mice under natural conditions, studies of its oncogenicity and that of SV40 and certain adenoviruses in new-born mice, hamsters and other rodents, have been most fruitful in elucidating the mechanisms of tumour production. Similarly, much of the published work on in vitro transformation of cells also relates to one or other of these three viruses; these studies are central to our understanding of events at a cellular and molecular level (see reference to review articles below). Transformation refers to a stable, heritable change in cells exposed to high multiplicities of such oncogenic viruses. While some cells undergo a lytic or cytocidal infection, others acquire a range of new properties including loss of contact inhibition of movement and macromolecular synthesis, membrane changes evidenced by lectin agglutinability and new transplantation antigens, increased plating efficiency *in vitro*, and ability to form tumours in the hamster cheek pouch. Infectious virus and structural protein is rarely detected in transformed cells although it may sometimes be induced with radiation or chemicals; virus-specified early proteins, detected as tumour or T antigens or unusual enzyme, may be found. Other evidence of the presence of a virus genome in the cell is provided by detection of viral mRNA, molecular hybridization experiments with cell and virion DNA, and genetic experiments to 'rescue' virus markers by superinfection with mutant strains of virus.

Attention here will be concentrated on those viruses associated with naturally occurring tumours.

ONCOGENIC DNA VIRUSES

1. PAPILLOMA viruses are members of the Papovaviridae. The virion, 52 to 54 nm in diameter, contains double-stranded DNA and has an icosahedral capsid with 72 capsomeres. They are ether stable and heat resistant.

Infectious warts of man are caused by a papovavirus and occur in various morphological forms on the hands, feet, larynx or genitalia. Antibodies to virus purified from wart tissue may be detected by gel diffusion, complement fixation and passive haemagglutination in many cases. The lesions may persist for variable periods, but often regress spontaneously. Experimental transmission to man has been reported with incubation periods of 2 to 8 months. Spread may be indirect or direct, including sexual contact. As yet, the viruses have not been grown in cell culture or experimental animals.

Papillomata in other species. The Shope papilloma causes a benign wart in the cottontail rabbit; when adapted to the domestic rabbit the papillomata may become malignant and metastisize. Cells from the tumour may contain infectious DNA and novel enzymes (arginase) but no infectious virus. The Shope virus is apparently distinct from the virus of naturally occurring oral papillomatosis in domestic rabbits. Other papovaviruses cause papillomata in cattle, dogs and horses.

2. ADENOVIRUSES. Attempts have been made to link adenovirus with human tumours by examining tumours for virus or virus-coded products such as viral mRNA or by serological surveys of cancer patients and controls for the presence of antibodies to the T antigens of adenoviruses. Although virus has on occasion been isolated, in general the molecular biological tests and serological surveys have failed to implicate adenoviruses.

3. HERPESVIRUSES. The association of the Epstein Barr virus (EBV) with infectious mononucleosis and with the Burkitt lymphoma and the suspected association of *Herpesvirus hominis*, serotype 2, with human cervical carcinoma are dealt with in Chapter 41.

The well known tendency of herpesviruses to persist as latent infections complicates the evaluation of their significance when they are demonstrated in tumours.

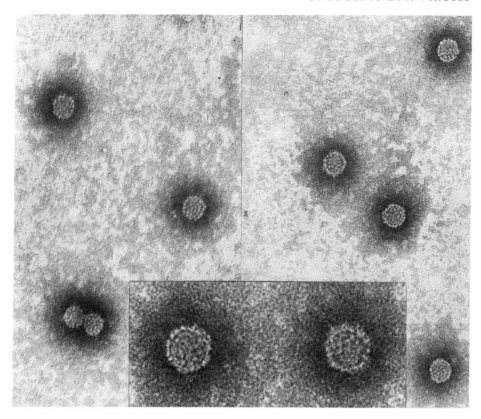

PLATE 49.1. An electronmicrograph of a partially purified suspension of the tissue of a plantar wart. The hexagonal shape of the wart virus particles and the surface capsomeres are clearly defined by negative staining with phosphotungstic acid. × 100 000 (inset × 200 000). (From Swain and Dodds, 1967, *Clinical Virology*. Edinburgh: Churchill Livingstone.)

Oncogenic non-human primate herpesviruses. *Herpes saimiri* and *Herpesvirus steles* were both isolated from spontaneously degenerating monkey kidney cells in tissue culture. Both cause lymphomata when injected into primates of species other than those from whose kidney cell cultures they originated.

Marek's disease of chickens. A herpesvirus has been isolated from fowls with the natural disease and transmission experiments indicate that it is the causative agent. The virus can be grown in chicken kidney cells with characteristic cytopathic effect and is cell associated. The fine structure of the virion is that of typical herpesvirus but there is no antigenic relation with other herpesviruses. The lesions in the fowl usually involve the nerves which become heavily infiltrated with round cells—(hence neurolymphomatosis) with resultant paralysis of wings or legs. Lymphoid tumours are also seen. An acute form of the disease also occurs with lymphoid infiltration of the liver and other viscera. Virus is present in the oral secretions and feather follicles and spread takes place by contact. The dust in poultry houses may remain infectious for several weeks. Live attenuated viruses have been used as vaccines and their prophylactic effect has provided further evidence of the causative role of the virus in the tumour.

The Lucké Frog Carcinoma. The cells of this adenocarcinoma of the kidney contain intranuclear inclusions which are particularly evident when the tumour-bearing frogs are held in the cold. Electronmicroscopy of such inclusions reveal the presence of typical herpes virions. However, there is evidence from cell culture studies that more than one kind of herpesvirus may be present and that these may occur in association with a papovavirus; definitive evidence on the etiological role of the herpesvirus is therefore still lacking.

Cottontail Rabbit Lymphoma. The virus (*Herpes sylvilagus*) gives rise to lymphomata when injected into young cottontail rabbits. It was originally isolated from a spontaneously degenerating kidney cell culture from young cottontail rabbits. Thus it is of special interest because of its ability to induce tumours in the same species from which it was originally isolated.

4. POXVIRUSES. Yaba virus causes a subcutaneous histiocytoma in rhesus monkeys. The disease occurred spontaneously in, and can be readily transmitted to, monkeys. Tumours appear on the head and limbs after a short incubation period and often ulcerate. They regress within a month or two. There are reports of an accidental laboratory infection in man and in inoculated cancer patients; the virus produced local skin lesions which regressed within a few weeks. The morphology of its virion and certain other characteristics closely resemble those of vaccinia, but there is no antigenic relationship.

The virus grows on the chick embryo chorio-allantoic membrane and also in cell cultures of human and simian origin.

ONCOGENIC RNA VIRUSES

LEUKOVIRUSES. This is the only genus of RNA viruses that causes tumours in nature. They are pleomorphic but usually spherical particles of 90 to 120 nm in diameter (see Plate 49.2). A, B and C type particles are described. The nucleoid of A type particles is less dense and these are thought to be immature forms often seen in association with the Golgi apparatus. The RNA-containing nucleoid in B and C type particles is electron dense, some 55 nm in diameter and central in position in C type particles and eccentric in B type particles. The nucleoid is separated by a clear 'halo' from the electron-dense surface membrane which may be single or double.

The genome, a single strand of RNA, is divisible into four segments and has a molecular weight of $10/13 \times 10^6$ daltons; about 20 per

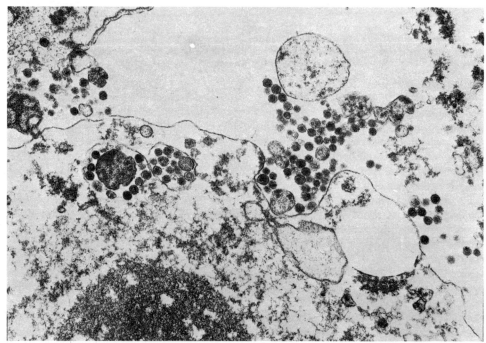

PLATE 49.2. Feline leukaemia virus particles in vesicles and at cell membrane. × 20 000. (By courtesy of Dr Helen Laird, Department of Veterinary Pathology, Glasgow University.)

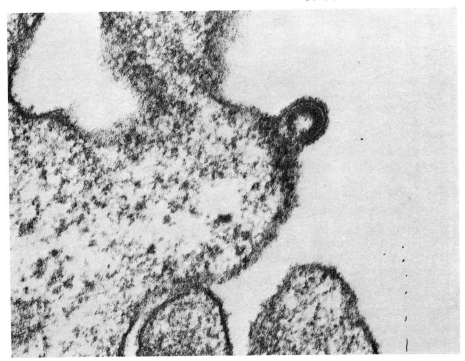

PLATE 49.3. Maturing feline leukaemia virus at cell membrane. ×80 000. (By courtesy of Dr Helen Laird, Department of Veterinary Pathology, Glasgow University.)

cent of the virion. The outer envelope may have a spiked appearance in negative contrast preparations in the electron microscope and contains lipoprotein soluble in lipid solvents and disaggregated by detergents. In all cases, assembly of the replicated viral components takes place at the cell membrane; first the nucleoid is located under the membrane which then thickens and buds off a particle (Plate 49.3).

It has been recognized for some years that the replication of these viruses required synthesis of host cell DNA—one cell division being enough —and that nucleic acid base analogues and inhibitors of enzymes in the synthetic pathway for DNA would inhibit multiplication; also that actinomycin D (a transcription inhibitor) blocked replication. All of this suggested that a DNA template was required for virus multiplication. Recently a series of enzymes has been discovered which copy the viral strand of RNA (an RNA dependent DNA polymerase or 'reverse transcriptase') in DNA giving an RNA/DNA hybrid. This is then copied by another polymerase to make a double-stranded

DNA which is often, perhaps invariably, integrated into the chromosome DNA of the host cell (see lysogeny, Chap. 13). In this situation it may be replicated with the host DNA and under the control of the host regulator genes; or the viral gene may be expressed and transcribed (the step inhibited by actinomycin D) with formation of viral nucleoprotein and envelope proteins and the liberation of mature, infective, virions (Plate 49.3). The outcome of the cell-virus encounter depends very much on the genetic composition of the host and with the mouse leukoviruses the genes determining resistance or susceptibility have been identified in some instances. The internal or 'gs' antigens, probably nucleoproteins or internal virion proteins, have specificity for the group and may even cross-react with leukoviruses of another species (see Interspec antigen: Table 49.1) while the envelope proteins are type specific and determine the range of cells (genetically determined) which can be infected. Cells replicating leukoviruses are not killed and continue to divide while shedding virus. New antigens, some depressed host coded and some virus

Table 49.1. Cross-reactivity of some leukoviruses.

GS antigens	Mouse	Rat	Hamster	Cat	Bovine	Avian
1	+	−	−	−	−	−
2	+	−	−	−	−	−
3*	+	+	+	+	[+] ?	−

*Note interspecies antigen (interspec.).

coded, are found on the cell membrane; the murine, avian and other sarcoma viruses will transform cells *in vitro* and this effect is accompanied by a variable degree of expression of the viral genes, e.g. some sarcomas do not shed infective virus or form morphological virions.

THE AVIAN LEUKOSES AND SARCOMAS

Lymphoid leukosis, erythromyeloblastic leukosis and various forms of sarcomata in fowls are caused by leukoviruses with similar physical and morphological properties but with different biological effects. These viruses will multiply in chick embryo cells in culture without cytopathic effect. Some members of the group can act as helper virus for Rous sarcoma virus and for other members of the group and some of the features of this association have been described in Chapter 13. Others are detectable by their ability to interfere with the growth of Rous sarcoma virus. The term RIF (Resistance Inducing Factor) is used for viruses showing this property. Lymphoid leukosis is the most common naturally occurring disease and its presence can be demonstrated by the RIF test. Although many isolates of virus have been tested, it has been difficult to reproduce the neoplastic disease experimentally, related perhaps, to the finding that transmission under natural conditions may take place both horizontally and vertically. A proportion of birds infected vertically are immunologically 'tolerant' and may continue to excrete virus over long periods, without signs of disease. Leukosis-free flocks have been reared from embryos from immune hens and by rigid quarantine of the newly hatched chicks and the flock.

Avian Sarcomata occur sporadically and in variable incidence from flock to flock; very few are transmissible with cell-free filtrates or even with cells. Most information about the state of

the viral genome in sarcomas has come from the study of a few laboratory passaged tumours such as the Rous sarcoma.

AVIAN ERYTHROBLASTOSIS AND MYELOBLASTOSIS. Clinical signs are of anaemia and weakness which lead to death. It seems that many cells support virus multiplication but only certain 'target' cells are transformed and give rise to the leukosis. The presence of myeloblastosis virus may be manifested by high levels of adenosine triphosphatase in the plasma of the infected birds. This enzyme is associated with the virion and can be used quantitatively to estimate the titre of virus. It seems that, as an enzyme associated with the cell membrane, it is inadvertently included in the virion when it buds from the cells. Virions from cells without adenosine triphosphatase do not contain the enzymes.

THE MURINE LEUKAEMIAS AND LYMPHOMAS

Much of the earlier work with these viruses was concerned with the development of inbred strains of mice which showed a high incidence of spontaneous viral tumours; as with the avian leukoses the genotype of the host is of primary importance. From such mice Gross transmitted leukaemia by injecting new-born mice of low leukaemia strains with cell-free tumour filtrates.

The murine leukoviruses have been subdivided into the thymic group which include Gross, Moloney and Graffi's chloroleukaemic strains and the splenic group which includes the Friend and Rauscher strains and the virus of murine erythroblastosis. Many of the strains described produce leukaemias experimentally but it is uncertain whether this happens in nature. The murine leukoviruses have the general attributes described earlier and contain group specific internal complement fixing antigen. Serological analysis of the envelope antigens suggests that Friend, Moloney and Rauscher viruses are closely related but Gross virus is distinct. Analysis of virus induced membrane antigens in cells infected with these viruses supports these distinctions. Most of the group multiply in embryonic mouse cell cultures without producing cytopathic effect.

MOUSE SARCOMA VIRUSES (MSV). Two mouse sarcoma viruses have been described which are morphologically similar and serologically related to the viruses of the Friend-Moloney-Rauscher subgroup. The situation is reminiscent of that with the avian viruses in that 'helper viruses' of the murine leukaemia group are required.

MAMMARY TUMOUR VIRUS OF MICE. The Bittner agent or mammary tumour virus (MTV) closely resembles the other leukoviruses with B type particles having regularly arranged spikes on their outer membranes. The virus is usually latent, only producing mammary adenocarcinomata in mice of suitable genotype and under the influence of oestrogens.

FELINE LYMPHOSARCOMA. Leukoviruses also cause lymphosarcomas in cats and are transmitted vertically from one generation of animal to the next: it is also spread horizontally from animal to animal, as shown by well documented instances of contagious spread of lymphosarcoma through small colonies of cats. Feline lymphosarcoma virus multiplies in cultures of feline embryonic cells without a cytocidal effect; it also grows in human cells. There are several internal (gs) antigens, one of which cross-reacts with murine leukaemia viruses (Table 49.1). Apart from defined leukoviruses of birds, mice and cats, there is morphological evidence of leukoviruses in a wide variety of normal and tumour tissue of animal species including guinea-pigs, hamsters and cattle.

A human rhabdomyosarcoma cell line has been established which produced tumours in kittens. A cell line (RD114B) from one of these kitten tumours, having a human karyotype, has been shown to release C type particles. Antigenic studies of the virus indicate that it is distinct from other known mammalian leukoviruses.

Viruses of this type have been recovered from naturally occurring tumours including mammary tumours, of non-human primates and this finding strengthens the possibility that such viruses will be isolated from naturally occurring tumours of man. Progress with human cancer viruses is, however, still hampered by the lack of a leukovirus of indisputable human origin. Particles resembling mouse mammary tumour virus have been seen in the milk of women of 'high cancer' families and in the women of the Parsee sect in India, an inbred group with a high incidence of breast cancer. It is claimed that the particles contain the reverse transcriptase but recent evidence has blurred these initially encouraging findings. The discovery of the reverse transcriptase has provided a very valuable tool for the investigation and detection of suspected leukoviruses, particularly in human tumours where the conventional approach of inoculation of new-born members of the species is not possible. The matter of enzyme specificity is highly important. Most of the earlier published work used synthetic RNA templates to demonstrate the reverse transcriptase; with such methods activity is found in certain normal, as well as in tumour, cells. When specific RNA templates from purified leukovirus virions are used, differences can be shown between the enzymes present in normal cells and those in leukoviruses. Hybridization experiments with the synthetized DNA and viral RNA together with immunological data confirm that the activity in normal cells is distinct from that in leukoviruses.

One of the many current theories of cancer causation—the oncogene hypothesis—infers the ubiquitous distribution of a DNA copy (the virogene) of all, or part, of a leukovirus integrated in the host chromosome of most species. These virogenes are normally repressed and only become activated in whole or in part when induced by carcinogenic stimuli (radiation, chemicals, hormones, etc.). Recent immunological research has underlined the importance of immunological responses, particularly the cell mediated response, in the development of or resistance to virus-induced tumours. A variety of immunosuppressive techniques, including neonatal thymectomy, chemicals, X-irradiation and antilymphocytic serum, alter the susceptibility of strains of mice normally genetically resistant to the oncogenic effects of polyoma virus. With the leukoviruses there is evidence that immunological reactions which lead to proliferation of white cell precursors or to the transformation of lymphocytes (as for example during graft versus host reaction) may induce virogenes carried by the cells with production of infective virions and subsequently the onset of leukaemia or lymphosarcoma.

REFERENCES

ANDREWES, C. H. & PEREIRA, H. G. (1972) *Viruses of Vertebrates*. 3rd edn. London: Ballière, Tindall.

BLACK, P. H. (1968) The oncogenic DNA viruses: A review of *in vitro* studies. *Annual Review of Microbiology*, **22**, 391.

DULBECCO, R. (1970) Topoinhibition and serum requirement of transformed and untransformed cells. *Nature, London*, **227**, 802.

GREEN, M. (1970) Oncogenic viruses. *Annual Review of Biochemistry*, **39**, 701.

HEUBNER, R. J. & TODARO, C. J. (1969) Oncogenes of RNA tumour viruses and determinants of cancer. *Proceedings of the National Academy of Sciences*, **64**, 1087.

MCALLISTER, R. N., GILDEN, R. V. & GREEN, M. (1972) Adenoviruses in human cancer. *Lancet*, **i**, 831.

ROYAL COLLEGE OF PHYSICIANS (1972) *Symposium on Host-Virus Reaction with Special Reference to Persistent Agents.* London: Royal College of Physicians.

TEMIN, H. M. (1970) Malignant transformation by viruses. *Perspectives in biology and medicine*, **14**, 11.

TEMIN, H. M. (1971) Mechanism of cell transformation by RNA tumour viruses. *Annual Review of Microbiology*, **25**, 609.

VIGIER, P. (1971) RNA oncogenic viruses, structure, replication and oncogenicity. *Progress in Medical Virology*, **12**, 240.

WORLD HEALTH ORGANIZATION (1972) *Oncogenesis and Herpesvirus. W.H.O. International Agency for Research on Cancer, Lyon.* Publication 2. London: H.M.S.O.

Volume I: Part 4
Other Pathogenic Microorganisms and Associated Diseases

The genus *Chlamydia* includes organisms previously called the psittacosis-lymphogranuloma venereum-trachoma group (PLT organisms) or the TRIC group (*trachoma-inclusion conjunctivitis* organisms). The generic name *Bedsonia* has also been used in recognition of the pioneering work of Sir Samuel Bedson and his colleagues who isolated and characterized the agent of psittacosis during its prevalence in the early 1930s; however, by the rules of nomenclature, *Chlamydia* has priority.

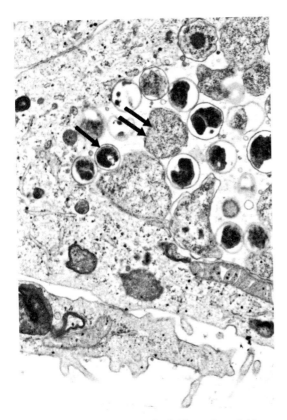

PLATE 50.1. Electronmicrograph of thin section of chlamydial inclusion; (a) ↑, small elementary body; (b) ↑↑, 'initial' body. × 15 000. (By courtesy of Dr Douglas R. Anderson, Miami.)

Bedson and his colleagues correctly concluded that the psittacosis organisms multiplied by binary fission like bacteria but other workers confused them with viruses because they are filterable and obligate intracellular parasites. It is now clear that the chlamydiae are small prokaryotes that have evolved to a highly parasitic existence in the cytoplasm of cells; they do not constitute a 'missing link' between the bacteria and the viruses (Moulder, 1966).

Chlamydiae are widely distributed in birds and mammals and are responsible not only for considerable human disability (trachoma is the commonest world-wide cause of blindness) but also for economically important diseases of livestock (e.g. enzootic abortion of ewes).

BIOLOGICAL PROPERTIES AND CLASSIFICATION OF CHLAMYDIAE

The organisms are small, non-motile, Gram-negative obligate intracellular parasites which have two forms of cell. There is a small, 300 nm diameter form (Plate 50.1(a)), which has a compact electron-dense nucleoid; this is the highly infectious, stable, extracellular, transport form, or elementary body, of the organism. Then there is a larger form, 800–1200 nm in diameter, without a dense nucleoid (Plate 50.1(b)), the 'initial body' of the light microscopists of the early 1900s, which is intracellular and constitutes the replicating form of the organism. Reaction with the Gram stain is negative and weak, but both forms stain well with the Macchiavello, Castenada or Gimenez stains and also by Giemsa. The organisms grow in the cytoplasm of their host cells forming characteristic micro-colonies or inclusion bodies which are made up of a mixture of the larger and smaller cells. Some organisms, viz., trachoma-inclusion conjunctivitis, lymphogranuloma venereum and murine and hamster pneumonitis.

have compact inclusions with a glycogen matrix and constitute subgroup A of the chlamydiae. Others do not have a glycogen matrix and are categorized as subgroup B. The two groups also differ in susceptibility to sulphadiazine and D-cycloserine (Table 50.1). Apart from these differences all the organisms are similar in morphology and share a common antigen or antigens, usually detected by complement fixation with boiled suspensions of the organism. The group CF antigens are resistant to nucleases and proteases, but are inactivated by lecithinase A and by sodium periodate. They can be extracted from the organism with deoxycholate or chloroform-methanol by the Folch technique; in sum these properties suggest a complex of lipid and carbohydrate. A soluble haemagglutinin (i.e. one separable from the cell particle) is formed by some chlamydiae and has properties resembling those of the group antigen; it agglutinates murine and vaccinia-sensitive fowl erythrocytes. Individual strains or species can be characterized by heat-labile, type-specific antigens which are left in the cell after extraction with deoxycholate. Viable suspensions of chlamydial elementary bodies are toxic when inoculated intravenously in mice. The toxins can be neutralized with specific antisera and the reaction is used to subdivide strains within groups. Immunofluorescence with dots of antigen on slides can be used to subdivide strains into types A to I and to measure type specific antibody (Treharne et al., 1972; Wang et al., 1973).

Electron micrographs of thin sections of the small cell show a thin cell wall and a limiting cytoplasmic membrane; cholesterol is not demonstrable in cell extracts (cf. Mycoplasma). Inside the cytoplasmic membrane there are ribosomes of the 70S type found in bacterial cells; protein synthesis on these is inhibited by broad spectrum antibiotics such as tetracyclines, erythromycin, chloramphenicol; aspects of clinical importance. The DNA is concentrated in the central nucleoid and is double-stranded, with a G plus C ratio in the range of 39–41 per cent, according to the organism, and a genome size about 950×10^6 daltons, which approximates to that of Mycoplasma hominis; the latter is, however, capable of multiplication in cell-free media. So a small genome size is not the simple explanation for the parasitism of the chlamydiae. N-acetylmuramic acid has been demonstrated in several species and isolated cell walls are sensitive to lysozyme. Lysine and D-alanine, but not diaminopimelic acid, appear to be components of the cross-linking peptide chains. Further evidence of a cell wall resembling that of bacteria is provided by the action of penicillin and D-cycloserine (an analogue of D-alanine) in inhibiting cell-wall formation and giving rise in infected cells to large, irregularly shaped bodies essentially analogous to bacterial spheroplasts. Despite this sensitivity to penicillin in experimental systems, the antibiotic is not of great clinical value in treating infections. Subgroup A chlamydiae are more susceptible to D-cycloserine and the effect is less easily reversed by D-alanine

Table 50.1. Illustration of the division of some strains of Chlamydia into subgroups A and B (after Moulder, 1966).

Agent	Inclusion Morphology	Glycogen	Sulphadiazine sensitivity	D-cycloserine sensitivity
Subgroup A				
Lymphogranuloma venereum	Compact	+	+	+++
Inclusion conjunctivitis	Compact	+	+	+++
Mouse pneumonitis	Compact	+	+	+++
Subgroup B				
Psittacosis	Diffuse	−	− or +	+
Ornithosis	Diffuse	−	−	+
Meningopneumonitis	Diffuse	−	−	+
Feline pneumonitis	Diffuse	−	−	+
Guinea-pig conjunctivitis	Diffuse	−	−	+
Bovine encephalomyelitis	Diffuse	−	−	++

than with group B; a differentiating feature (Table 50.1).

GROWTH OF CHLAMYDIAE IN LABORATORY HOSTS

The first members to be propagated in the laboratory were the psittacosis organisms (subgroup B) which are pathogenic for mice by the intraperitoneal route and can be seen as cytoplasmic microcolonies in the cells in impression smears from the spleen or liver of infected mice. Organisms could also be propagated in the mouse lung, after intranasal inoculation; a procedure carrying the double hazard of infection for the operator during the inoculation of the mice and also that of contamination with the mouse pneumonitis agent (Nigg's 'virus'). Strains of lymphogranuloma venereum can be adapted to intracerebral growth in mice. Avian strains can also be propagated in birds, if a chlamydia-free stock is available, and some mammalian strains produce fever and emaciation in guinea pigs with an antibody response in convalescence. The next major advance was the use of the yolk sac of 7–8 day-old chick embryos after the method devised by Cox for the growth of rickettsiae. This enabled large amounts of various members of subgroups A and B to be grown for serological, morphological and biochemical studies.

Even with these new techniques, the organisms from trachoma and inclusion conjunctivitis continued to elude cultivation although their relation to the group had been recognized for many years; indeed, Lindner, Halberstaedter, von Prowazek and others had seen, as early as 1910, the characteristic inclusion bodies in conjunctival epithelial cells, and in cells from the cervix of mothers with children suffering from inclusion blennorrhoea or from the urethra of men with 'non-specific' urethritis. Finally T'ang, in 1957, cultured the trachoma agent in the yolk sac; a lower temperature of incubation and antibiotics (e.g. streptomycin) which suppressed the accompanying conjunctival bacteria and allowed survival of the chick embryos were crucial factors. Shortly afterwards, Collier, Jones and their colleagues propagated an inclusion conjunctivitis agent in the yolk sac. The sensitivity of yolk sac inoculation for the isolation of strains is low and serial 'blind' passage is sometimes required which is time-consuming, expensive, and open to the danger of cross-contamination. Recently, it has been established that chlamydiae will grow in cell culture, particularly if their penetration into cells is aided by centrifugation of the inoculum on to the cells or if adsorption is increased with DEAE-dextran. The introduction of irradiated or IUDR treated cells (McCoy, Hela or BHK cells) for the primary isolation of TRIC agents has provided a much more sensitive alternative to yolk sac culture and has substantially changed our view of the ecology and natural history of TRIC infections.

The growth of chlamydiae in experimentally inoculated rodents or birds, or in yolk sacs or cell cultures can be detected by staining impression smears by Giemsa (Colour Plate 13), Macchiavello, Gimenez stain or by acridine orange fluorescence which reveals characteristic inclusions with green (mature, DNA-rich) forms and red (intermediate, RNA-rich) forms. The inclusions may also be stained by immunofluorescence with an antiserum directed against the group antigen and the appropriate fluorescein-antiglobulin conjugate (Colour Plate 15). The inclusions of subgroup A chlamydiae have, for many years, been detected by staining the glycogen with iodine (Colour Plate 14); in tissue sections (e.g. mouse lung with mouse pneumonitis agent), the periodic-acid-Schiff method gives striking results. Antibody response in experimental animals may also be used as an index of infection but latent infection of laboratory animals (e.g. guinea-pig inclusion conjunctivitis) may complicate interpretation of serological results.

Developmental Cycle of Chlamydia in Cells

The small, 300 nm, rigid, highly infective, extracellular elementary bodies (EB) of the chlamydiae are taken into the cell by phagocytosis. Unlike the rickettsiae there is no active mechanism of cell penetration dependent on ATP. After phagocytosis the EB lies in a membrane-bounded phagosome but is evidently resistant to digestion by hydrolytic lysosomal enzymes. Recent studies of trachoma elementary bodies show that they contain, in addition to ribosomal and t-RNA, a DNA-dependent-RNA polymerase bound to the chromosome of the organism; in the presence of the four nucleoside triphosphates, m-RNA is synthesized by this enzyme on the DNA chromosome. This process continues throughout the developmental cycle and is irreversibly inhibited by the semi-synthetic antibiotic rifampicin; this may have therapeutic implications for the future. The increased RNA synthesis is accompanied by rearrangement of the cell to form the larger, 800–1200 nm, reticulate or initial body. Its increased RNA content is well shown in the acridine orange stain and its DNA is dispersed through the cell in contrast to that in the EB. The reticulate body is of lower infectivity than the small EB and more easily disrupted by sonic treatment. There is evidence that the peptidoglycans of its cell wall are, unlike those of EB, not cross-linked by peptide chains. This 'loosening of the stays' may increase permeability of the cell for the energy-rich ATP and other compounds that the organism cannot synthesize and must derive from the host cell; hence its role as an 'energy parasite'. The use of the inhibitor, cycloheximide, that inhibits protein synthesis on eukaryotic but not on prokaryotic ribosomes reveals that the chlamydiae synthesize their own DNA and protein and do not use the translation apparatus of the host cell, unlike viruses. Certain members of the group have been grown in enucleated cells and indeed, host cell DNA synthesis is depressed in chlamydial-infected cells; probably thereby reducing competition for nucleotides and other precursors which might be used in common by parasite and cell. It is likely that the facilitating effect of X-irradiation of cell cultures on the growth of chlamydiae is connected with inhibition of host cell DNA synthesis and of metabolic competition.

The larger reticulate forms divide a number of times by binary fission and then condense to the smaller EB, with division of the larger form by cross septa resembling mesosomes and cross-linking of the amino sugar chains of the cell wall. The cycle takes about 24 to 48 hours. The glycogen synthesis by subgroup A agents to form an inclusion matrix is due to the presence of a unique glycogen synthetase with a different substrate specificity to that in uninfected cells and therefore presumably genetically determined by the chlamydiae. Studies of the metabolism of reticulate bodies are difficult, but the activities of isolated EB's have been investigated. This has revealed that chlamydiae possess limited enzymic equipment that can, for example, utilize substrates such as glucose-6-phosphate with the evolution of CO_2, or incorporate carbon from it into fatty acids. Electron transport systems and cytochrome are lacking and there is no evidence that these 'vestigial' enzymes participate in energy-yielding reactions. Their presence, however, is another link with bacteria and further differentiates them from viruses. The subgroup A strains that are sensitive to sulphonamides synthesize their own folic acid whereas the resistant strains, subgroup B, convert host cell folic acid to their own specific form of the vitamin.

CHLAMYDIAL INFECTIONS IN ANIMALS AND MAN

Infections in Birds and Animals

The clinical and laboratory aspects of infection with *Chlamydia* in birds and domestic and other mammals are described by Meyer, Eddie and Schachter (1969) and by Storz (1971), with a useful series of references. The special supplement to the American Journal of Ophthalmology (Conference, 1967) may also be consulted. The most important avian infection is psittacosis occurring in, and named after, psittacine birds such as parrots, parakeets and cockatoos. Ducks, pigeons, chickens, turkeys, fulmars and certain gulls may also be infected and the condition in these hosts is called ornithosis. The acute avian disease is characterized by diarrhoea, emaciation and wasting of the pectoral muscles, rash and purulent nasal discharge. The lungs are rarely involved but there may be a seropurulent exudate in the air sacs, an enlarged spleen and liver with necrosis and inflammation of serous membranes. Birds are infected as fledglings and may remain latently infected thereafter; during the initial infection, or during relapses under stress (e.g. overcrowding in cages, underfeeding during transfer as stock or holding in pet shops), organisms may be shed in large amounts in their droppings or exudates. After drying this contaminated material may be dispersed as a dust by the flapping of wings and may be inhaled and infect other birds, animals or human beings in contact.

The organism may be isolated from the spleen of latently infected birds, or antibody to the group CF antigen can be demonstrated by the direct or indirect CF reactions in those birds whose sera do not fix complement.

Other members of subgroup B cause infection of sheep, cattle, goats and pigs. In sheep, there is an economically important disease, enzootic abortion of ewes (EAE), characterized by abortion or premature lambing in the last three weeks of gestation. The gross appearance of the aborted placenta resembles that found in *Brucella abortus* infection; examination of impression smears made from the cotyledons and stained by Macchiavello, or the modified Ziehl-Neelsen stain used by veterinarians, reveals large numbers of elementary bodies and the agent can be isolated in chick embryo yolk sac, mouse lung or in cell culture. Sheep may be infected by exposure to contaminated pastures and lambs born of infected ewes may harbour infection into maturity and abort during pregnancy. A formolized vaccine from infected yolk sacs is of value in prophylaxis. Subgroup B agents infecting cattle, sheep, goats and pigs may cause enteritis, encephalomyelitis, pneumonitis, arthritis or conjunctivitis; findings of comparative interest for such conditions as Reiter's syndrome in man. Human exposure to these mammalian agents rarely results in overt disease, but antibody may be provoked. Feline pneumonitis and keratoconjunctivitis and infections of many small wild mammals are also caused by chlamydiae. Mouse pneumonitis, caused by a subgroup A organism, is latent in some mouse stocks and may be activated to a fatal pneumonia by serial 'blind' passage, by the intranasal route, of lung suspensions from ostensibly healthy mice; it may also contaminate viruses or other agents being passaged by this method. Sulphadiazine is sometimes added to the diet of the mice to control the infection.

Infections in Man: Clinical and Laboratory Aspects

Chlamydial infection of man takes two main clinical forms, a febrile, predominantly respiratory illness with the organisms of psittacosis-ornithosis and, rarely, other members of subgroup B, and the clinically quite dissimilar ocular or genital infections with the trachoma-inclusion conjunctivitis-lymphogranuloma venereum (LGV) organisms of subgroup A.

1. PSITTACOSIS or ORNITHOSIS is acquired by inhalation of infected aerosol or dust from birds during handling as pets, or with chickens, pigeons, geese and turkeys, while killing, plucking and cleaning for the table. It is therefore an occupational hazard for bird fanciers, pet shop and poultry farm workers, butchers, fishmongers, and those in certain animal feed and fertilizer plants. The incubation period is about ten days and the illness ranges from an 'influenza-like' syndrome with general malaise, fever, anorexia, rigors, sore throat and headache and photophobia, to a severe illness, with typhoidal state, delirium and pneumonia with numerous well demarcated areas of consolidation; these may resemble bronchopneumonia, but the bronchi and larger bronchi are involved as a secondary event and sputum is scanty.

Organisms from psittacines and turkeys tend to be more virulent than those from chickens and pigeons and fatality rates up to 20 per cent may be seen in untreated cases, particularly in the elderly. For this reason the importation of exotic birds is regulated even though it is recognized that ornithosis is present in native birds; for example, in the numerous pigeons that nest on civic buildings. Although the pneumonic form of the illness may focus clinical attention, the organism is blood borne through the body, and there may be a meningoencephalitis, arthritis, pericarditis or mycocarditis, or a predominantly typhoidal state with enlarged liver and spleen and even a rash resembling that of enteric fever. A subacute endocarditis resembling that complicating Q fever has also been described.

The organism may be found in the sputum during the pneumonic illness, but person to person spread is exceptional; however, with certain highly virulent strains physicians and nurses have been infected from patients.

Clinically, the condition has to be differentiated from bacterial pneumonia and from atypical pneumonias caused by influenza and parainfluenza virus, adenovirus, *Mycoplasma pneumoniae* and *Coxiella burnetii*; also from generalized septicaemias such as typhoid. A history of exposure to birds is useful and blood counts and routine sputum examination help to exclude bacterial pneumonia. A specific diagnosis depends on the culture of the organism from sputum or heparinized blood during the acute illness, or from the lung, liver or spleen of fatal cases; also by the demonstration of high or changing titres of CF antibody to the chlamydial group antigen during convalescence. Sputum, blood or tissue suspensions, treated with streptomycin, neomycin or polymyxin if bacteria are present, are inoculated intraperitoneally and intracerebrally into mice. Yolk sac or cell culture may also be used, but bacterial contamination may be a problem. The organisms are detected and identified in these hosts by staining and serological reactions by methods described in Vol. II. The paired sera are examined not only for CF antibody to chlamydial group antigen, but also for antibody to myxo- and paramyxoviruses, Q fever, *M. pneumoniae*, adenovirus, respiratory syncytial virus. A four-fold or greater rise (or fall in late convalescence) of CF antibody to the group antigen gives a more secure diagnosis; moderate, unchanging levels of CF antibody should be interpreted with caution as these are not infrequently observed in the population at large, perhaps in relation to the prevalence of subgroup A organisms. Account has also to be taken of the fact that intensive antibiotic therapy may delay the development of antibody. Chlamydiae are sensitive to tetracycline, erythromycin and chloramphenicol. Tetracycline is widely used and is effective in reducing the case fatality from psittacosis; successful clinical response can occur with failure to eliminate the organism and subsequent chronic carriage.

2. TRIC-LGV, SUBGROUP A CHLAMYDIAE, comprise a group of infections transmitted by contact, mainly sexual, in developed countries but also eye to eye in undeveloped countries where trachoma is endemic. LGV is the more invasive; it starts as a small painless papule or ulcer (lymphogranulomatous chancre) on the external genitalia or internally, some five to ten days after exposure. Infection then spreads to the regional lymph nodes (inguinal, perirectal or paraaortic), with suppuration in many cases, and sometimes a generalized infection with fever, and, variably, rash, arthritis, conjunctivitis and meningoencephalitis. In the late stages of the disease chronic inflammation around lymphatics in the genital and rectal area leads to fibrosis with elephantiasis of the genitalia. Rectal strictures are common in women and male homosexuals. Isolation of the organism, in mice intracerebrally or in yolk sac, is difficult although LGV strains are more pathogenic for these hosts than the TRIC strains. In practice CF reactions are used with patients' sera and LGV group antigen from yolk sac. A skin test for delayed hypersensitivity to heat inactivated LGV antigen (Frei test) is also available. The Frei test antigen is the heat-stable one shared with other chlamydiae and the reaction remains positive long after the acute infection; consequently a positive result indicates only that infection with a member of the group has occurred at some time.

Trachoma, on the one hand, and on the other hand, *inclusion blennorrhoea* in neonates and *inclusion conjunctivitis* in adults, are caused by essentially similar organisms. The clinical syndromes are now recognized to overlap although there are epidemiological differences with trachoma. Three ocular syndromes are recognized; (a) *trachoma*: a follicular eye disease progressing to scarring and pannus; (b) TRICagent-*punctate keratitis*: a syndrome with subepithelial infiltration of the cornea, and (c) *inclusion conjunctivitis*: a follicular conjunctivitis resolving without sequelae and without corneal involvement (Jones *et al.*, 1966).

Inclusion blennorrhoea is a significant problem in the newborn; about 2–5 per cent of babies in a maternity hospital have eye sepsis and of these some 18 per cent have TRIC infections. Probably the figure would be higher with the more sensitive culture methods now available. The reservoir of infection for neonatal inclusion blennorrhoea is the adult urogenital tract and the baby is infected as it passes down the birth canal. As long ago as 1911 Lindner recognized inclusion blennorrhoea as a clinical entity not caused by ordinary bacteria and noted the similarity of the inclusion body in the conjunctival epithelial cells to the Halberstaedter-Prowazek body seen in cells from trachoma. This was further related to the findings of similar inclusion-bearing cells in cervical smears from the mothers of infants with inclusion blennorrhoea and in smears from the urethra of men with 'non-specific', i.e. non-gonococcal, urethritis. Subsequently, the adult condition, inclusion conjunctivitis, was recognized as 'swimming pool conjunctivitis', acquired by swimming in unchlorinated pools (presumably) contaminated by infected genital secretions.

These early cytological and clinico-epidemiological observations have, in recent years, been substantiated by the isolation of subgroup A organisms from children with inclusion blennorrhoea, from their mothers with inclusion cervicitis, and from their fathers with 'non-specific' urethritis. The organisms have also been isolated during general surveys of men presenting with non-specific urethritis and from their sexual consorts, some of whom had vaginal discharge, cervical follicles and proctitis. Yolk sac culture was used for these studies but is insensitive, readily invalidated by contaminating bacteria in the clinical specimen, and open to laboratory cross-contamination during the time consuming 'blind' passages of yolk sac material required to establish an isolate or confirm a negative result. Recently, Darougar, Kinnison and Jones (1971) have developed a simplified and sensitive, 'one passage', technique for isolation of TRIC agents in irradiated McCoy cells (probably mouse cells); this system is also more resistant to bacterial contamination than the yolk sac. Dunlop *et al.* (1971) applied this technique to the study of 41 men with non-specific urethritis and 21 of their sexual contacts. Chlamydiae were grown in 18/41 (44 per cent) of the men sampled by urethral swab and scraping and from the cervix or rectum of 5/21 (24 per cent) of the consorts. Clinically, a proportion of these women were suffering from salpingitis, cervicitis with purulent discharge, or vaginal discharge; the pattern of isolations of chlamydiae was broadly related to these abnormal clinical findings. However, there were sometimes infections with trichomonads and candida as well. Simultaneous infection of the genital tract with a variety of organisms not infrequently complicates clinical interpretations. Weak CF reactions with the patient's sera and a group CF antigen from LGV were commoner among the men and women from whom chlamydia had been isolated. Other investigations have shown that chlamydial punctate kerato-conjunctivitis or inclusion conjunctivitis presenting for treatment at ophthalmic clinics is accompanied, in a high proportion of cases, by chlamydial genital infection. Treatment of these genital infections is by a 21-day course of tetracycline, 250 mg, 4 times a day.

In the years since 1951 the prevalence of both gonococcal and non-gonococcal or non-specific urethritis has climbed steadily in the United Kingdom and at present the number of non-gonococcal cases is at least equal to, and probably many times greater than, those caused by gonococci. It is thus probable that chlamydial genital infections are widely distributed. In view of the tendency of chlamydiae to persist in the tissues a reappraisal of their possible role in acute and chronic non-bacterial salpingitis and deep pelvic inflammation, and in acute and chronic prostatitis and inflammation of the para-urethral glands is now required; also further investigations of such conditions as the urethral syndrome and 'non-bacterial' cystitis. Reiter's syndrome (non-gonococcal urethritis, conjunctivitis, arthritis) has also to be assessed in relation to these new findings. Subgroup A agents have been isolated from the urethra or conjunctiva of patients with Reiter's syndrome, but rarely from the joints. Schachter (1967) isolated chlamydia with subgroup B properties from the joints. Clearly further work is required.

The clinical aspects of trachoma and the environmental and epidemiological circumstances which account for the greater severity of the disease, compared with other chlamydial infection of the eye, are summarized by Thygeson and Hanna (1969) and by Nichols *et al.* (1971).

Laboratory Diagnosis

From the section on chlamydial infection in man it will be clear, in broad terms, that the organisms may be demonstrated in cells from the site of the lesion by light microscopy with material stained by Giemsa, Macchiavello or Gimenez stains, or by fluorescence microscopy with acridine orange stain, or by immunofluorescence with antibody against the group antigen. The organisms may be isolated by mouse or guinea-pig inoculation, or by culture in the chick embryo yolk sac or irradiated cell culture; the range of laboratory hosts chosen depends very much on the species to be isolated. Finally, sera from the infected man, mammal or bird may be examined for antibody but different clinical syndromes vary in the degree to which antibody is provoked. Generalizations are not possible and there is a wealth of technical detail to be observed for optimal results; the procedures are well described by Meyer and his colleagues (1969) and by Thygeson and Hanna (1969). Clinical differentiation of psittacosis from pneumonia due to viruses, rickettsiae or mycoplasmas may be effective but should be assisted by a broad approach in serological testing in the laboratory. Similarly, the expert will distinguish trachoma and inclusion conjunctivitis from other forms of kerato-conjunctivitis or follicular conjunctivitis; the laboratory may also look for the *Herpes simplex* virus, adenovirus and molluscum contagiosum in cases of diagnostic uncertainty.

Control

This depends on hygienic measures, e.g. ban on importation of psittacine birds, testing and culling of infected stock, protection of workers in high risk circumstances with gloves, safety glasses and dust masks. Trachoma has been treated by improvements in environmental hygiene and social circumstances coupled with topical or systemic use of sulphonamides or broad spectrum antibiotics, e.g. tetracycline. Chronic trachoma of low intensity has been difficult to treat on a mass scale. Vaccines prepared from killed chlamydiae have produced a protective effect in various experimental systems and in field trials (e.g. with trachoma), but are not yet well enough established for routine mass vaccination.

REFERENCES AND FURTHER READING

CONFERENCE (1967) On Trachoma and allied diseases. San Francisco, August 25–31, 1966. *American Journal of Ophthalmology*, **63**, Suppl. 1027/1.

DAROUGAR, S., KINNISON, J. R. & JONES, B. R. (1971) Simplified irradiated McCoy cell culture for isolation of Chlamydiae. In *Trachoma and Related Disorders Caused by Chlamydial Agents*, pp. 63–70. Edited by R. L. Nichols. Amsterdam: Excerpta Medica.

DUNLOP, E. M. C., HARE, M. J., DAROUGAR, S. & JONES, B. R. (1971) Chlamydial infection of the urethra in men presenting because of 'non-specific' urethritis', *ibid*, pp. 494–500.

JONES, B. R., AL-HUSSAINI, M. K., DUNLOP, E. M. C., EMARAH, M. H. M., FREEDMAN, A., GARLAND, J. A., HARPER, I. A., RACE, J. W., DU TOIT, M. S. & TREHARNE, J. D. (1966) Infection by TRIC agents and other members of the Bedsonia group; with a note on Reiter's Disease I Ocular Disease in adults. *Transactions of the Ophthalmological Society of U.K.*, **86**, 291.

MEYER, K. F., EDDIE, B. & SCHACHTER, J. (1969) Psittacosis—Lymphogranuloma verereum agents. In *Diagnostic Procedures for Viral and Rickettsial Infections*, pp. 869–903. Edited by E. H. Lennette and N. J. Schmidt, New York. American Public Health Association Incorporated.

MOULDER, J. W. (1966) The relation of the psittacosis group (Chlamydiae) to bacteria and viruses. *Annual Review of Microbiology*, **20**, 107–130.

NICHOLS, R. L., MURRAY, E. S., SCOTT, P. P. & McCOMB, D. E. (1971) Trachoma isolation studies in Saudi Arabia from 1957 through 1969. In *Trachoma and Related Disorders Caused by Chlamydial Agents*, pp. 517–528. Edited by R. L. Nichols. Amsterdam: Excerpta Medica.

REEVE, P. (1970) Trachoma and inclusion conjunctivitis agents in the British Isles. In *Modern Trends in Medical Virology*, pp. 186–203. Edited by R. B. Heath and A. P. Waterson. London: Butterworth.

SCHACHTER, J. (1967) Isolation of Bedsoniae from human arthritis and abortion tissues. *American Journal of Ophthalmology*, **63**, Suppl. 1082–1086.

STORZ, J. (1971) *Chlamydia and chlamydia-induced Disease*. Springfield, Illinois: Thomas.

TREHARNE, J. D., DAVEY, S. J., GRAY, S. J. & JONES, B. R. (1972) Immunological classification of TRIC agents and of some recently isolated LGV agents by the micro-immunofluorescence test. *British Journal of Venereal Diseases*, **48**, 18–25.

THYGESON, P. & HANNA, L. (1969) TRIC Agents. In *Diagnostic Procedures in Viral and Rickettsial infections*, pp. 904–930. Edited by Lennette and Schmidt. American Public Health Assoc. Inc., New York.

WANG, S. P., KUO, C. C. & GRAYSTON, J. T. (1973) A simplified method for immunological typing of trachoma—inclusion conjunctivitis—lymphogranuloma venereum organisms. *Infection and Immunity*, **7**, 356–360.

WENTWORTH, B. B., BONIN, P., HOLMES, K. K., GUTMAN, L., WIESNER, P. & ALEXANDER, E. R. (1973) Isolation of viruses, bacteria and other organisms from venereal disease clinic patients; methodology and problems associated with multiple isolations. *Health Laboratory Science*, **10**, 75–81.

51. The Rickettsiae Typhus: Q Fever

The family Rickettsiaceae includes the causative organisms of the two forms of typhus, and those of the spotted fevers and trench fever, together comprising the genus *Rickettsia*; also that of Q fever, now placed in a separate genus: *Coxiella*.

Rickettsiae have a very wide host range in nature and have been found in lice, fleas, ticks, mites, birds and in many species of mammals (Wisseman, 1968; Brezina, 1969). With the exception of epidemic typhus, maintenance of the organisms is enzootic and man is infected by accidental intrusion into cycles of transmission between arthropod and vertebrate hosts, or those between vertebrate hosts.

In past times epidemic typhus has been one of the great, lethal, infective scourges of man accompanying war, revolution and poverty. No doubt it remains in the wings to return in any period of social disruption; its last appearance in Europe was during the Second World War in the eastern theatre, in and subsequently around the Nazi concentration camps and in North Africa and Italy (Naples). Zinsser (1935) has chronicled the earlier social and political effects of typhus in *Rats, Lice and History*. Although foci of rickettsial disease remain in various areas of the world (Table 51.1), at present in developed western nations, given stable social circumstances, rickettsial diseases are uncommon. Only infrequent sporadic, imported, murine typhus, Brill-Zinsser disease, and sporadic cases or small outbreaks of Q fever are likely to be encountered in Europe with Boutonneuse fever in the Mediterranean littoral.

CLASSIFICATION AND BIOLOGICAL PROPERTIES OF RICKETTSIAE

Rickettsiae are small prokaryotic cells that, with one exception, have an obligate intracellular existence. The exception is *R. quintana*, which grows extracellularly in the louse gut and has been cultivated on modified blood agar. The rickettsial cells are pleomorphic and, on light microscopy, are rod-shaped, coccal, or occasionally filamentous organisms some 200 to 500 nm in diameter and 800 nm to 2·0 μm or more in length. They are Gram-negative in the main but *Coxiella burnetii* is Gram-positive with alcoholic iodine as a mordant.

The established rickettsiae making up the typhus, spotted fever, scrub typhus, trench fever and Q fever groups are given in Table 51.1. Some other rickettsiae— *R. sennetsu*, *R. montana*, *R. parkeri* and *R. canada*— of uncertain significance for man, have been described recently. On the basis of cross-protection and serological tests the spotted fever group have been arranged in 4 subgroups—(A) *R. rickettsii* and *R. sibirica*; (B) *R. conori* and *R. parkeri*; (C) *R. australis* and *R. akari* and (D) *R. montana*. *R. canada* appears to be related to the typhus group and may be maintained in a bird-tick cycle.

The genus *Rickettsia* differs in a number of ways from that of *Coxiella*. All species of pathogenic rickettsia release a 'soluble' CF antigen when shaken with ether; this is probably derived from a capsule. Similar material is not extractable from *C. burnetii* with ether. *C. burnetii* exists in two antigenic forms as detected with CF reaction: phase 1 in arthropod and vertebrate hosts and phase 2 on passage in the chick embryo yolk sac. This is a host-controlled variation resembling smooth-rough variation in bacteria. Phase 1 antigen can be removed by treatment with trichloracetic acid revealing phase 2. The phase 1 antigen of *C. burnetii*, a lipopolysaccharide, is heat-stable (resisting autoclaving at 121°C for 15 min) and the organism itself is more resistant to drying, to storage for long periods at room temperature, to heating at temperatures up to 60°C, and to exposure to phenolic disinfectants than most vegetative bacteria. Rickettsiae, on the other hand, are easily inactivated by these treatments. Studies of the nucleic acid base composition of *C. burnetii* and *R. prowazekii* indicate that the G + C percentage of the two organisms are quite different thus substantiating the separation of the former into a separate genus. Ormsbee (1969) lists further differences between *C. burnetii* and other rickettsiae and concludes that the two genera may be of very different origins with similarities resulting from convergent evolution in the selective circumstances of arthropod and animal cells. Studies of the fine structure of the rickettsial cell show that it is rod-shaped, 300 to 700 nm in diameter, and 0·8 to 2·0 μm or more in length. There is a thin multi-layered cell wall, about 7–10 nm thick, and an underlying cytoplasmic membrane, 6–8 nm, with the characteristic 'unit' membrane structure found in bacterial cells. Some rickettsiae, such as *R. prowazekii*, display the ether-soluble capsule. Internally there are ribosomes, 7–20 nm in diameter and presumably of the bacterial type. The nuclear material may be organized in a central body with radiating fibres (*C. burnetii*) or dispersed as a network of fibrils; a double-stranded DNA has been extracted from *C. burnetii*.

Cell walls of rickettsiae contain two amino sugars, glucosamine and muramic acid, and are sensitive to lysozyme. Diaminopimelic acid, an amino acid found in the cross-linking peptide chains of the cell walls of Gram-negative bacteria, is also found in rickettsiae including *C. burnetii*. These features, together with the general amino acid composition and the absence of techoic acid, a characteristic component of the cell walls of Gram-positive bacteria, all underline the resemblance between rickettsiae and Gram-negative bacteria. This lends some credence to the notion that rickettsiae evolved from the intestinal flora of arthropods (see Moulder, 1962).

Rickettsiae, other than *C. burnetii*, are unstable outside of host cells and their cytoplasmic membranes readily leak macromolecules such as RNA and intracellular ions into aqueous media. Consequently, special suspending media with sucrose, glutamate, bovine serum albumin and K^+, Mg^{2+} are used; this may be further supplemented with ATP, coenzyme I and coenzyme A, perhaps mimicking the intracellular environment found to be favourable by an organism with an especially permeable cell membrane. Significantly, *R. quintana* does not have a requirement for the intracellular ion, K^+.

With the exception of *R. quintana* the rickettsiae multiply intracellularly and by binary fission. Most form colonies of organisms in the cytoplasm, but *R. rickettsii* and *R. canada* may also be found in the nuclei of infected cells. *C. burnetii* probably also multiplies by binary fission although Kordova and associates have suggested a mode of division involving smaller, filterable forms (see Ormsbee, 1969, for discussion).

Rickettsial suspensions outside of cells have a variety of enzymes connected with metabolic pathways for the breakdown of carbohydrate or for the generation of energy (ATP) from some steps in the Krebs cycle; enzymic equipment varies from species to species, *C. burnetii* being the more active. Pathways for the synthesis of lipid and protein are also present. Moulder (1962) provides a useful discussion of the metabolic basis for the intracellular parasitism of rickettsia, chlamydia and malaria.

Ormsbee (1969) suggests that the host cell contribution may include primary substrates such as glutamate and pyruvate, factors such as ATP, NAD and coenzyme A; perhaps also nucleoside triphosphate precursors (see Chlamydia) and other cell pool components such as amino acids.

Rickettsiae have been propagated in mouse fibroblasts, Detroit 6 cells, HEp2, HeLa and other continuous cell lines. Multiplication is slow and growth of rickettsia in the cell causes little obvious damage until numbers increase to a point at which the cell bursts; there is no nuclear 'switch off' or rearrangement of cell metabolism as observed with viruses.

At the level of the whole animal concentrated suspensions of typhus rickettsiae, some spotted fever rickettsiae and scrub typhus rickettsiae will kill mice within a few hours of intravenous injection; *C. burnetii* does not do this. This toxic effect is neutralized by specific antiserum and the reaction is of value in subdividing rickettsial groups and measuring the potency and antigenicity of rickettsial vaccines.

RICKETTSIAL INFECTIONS IN MAN AND ANIMALS

Pathogenesis and Clinical Aspects of Human Infection

Human rickettsial infection results mainly from exposure to the various species of infected arthropod involved in the maintenance of the organisms in nature. Q fever differs in that although a few instances of human infection from tick-bite have been described, man is infected from the cycle of maintenance in domestic animals by inhalation of aerosols of *C. burnetii* from the products of conception of infected cattle, sheep or goats, or from the consumption of their milk or milk products. These modes of infection resemble those of brucellosis.

The tick-borne and mite-borne rickettsiae (spotted fever group and scrub typhus; Table 51.1) are inoculated into the skin through the mouth parts of the arthropod after a period of feeding; a lesion (eschar) may form at the site and is of clinical diagnostic import in scrub typhus, rickettsial pox and some other members of the spotted fever group. With the louse-borne and flea-borne rickettsioses, i.e. epidemic and murine typhus and trench fever, infection follows when the infected insect faeces is rubbed or scratched into abraded skin at the site of the bite or, conceivably, contaminates the conjunctiva or respiratory mucosa.

The rickettsiae probably multiply at the site of inoculation and from there are disseminated throughout the body. However, events during the 10–20 day incubation periods of the rickettsioses and of Q fever are unclear except that there is a rickettsiaemia during the latter part of the incubation period and early febrile phase of the illness. The typhus and spotted fever groups of organisms parasitize the endothelial cells of the small blood vessels. Experiments with non-human primates show that *R. rickettsii* will also multiply in the alveolar cells of the lung and in organs such as the spleen. The clinical aspects of the diseases, particularly the various forms of rash, may be understood in terms of the vascular involvement. In Q fever there is less clear-cut involvement of the vascular endothelium although peripheral thrombosis is one of the sequelae of the disease. There is a

Table 51.1. Summary of causative organisms in various rickettsioses, their distribution, hosts and vectors.

Category		Organism	Disease	Geographical distribution	Arthropod vector	Vertebrate host
Typhus group		*R. prowazekii*	Epidemic typhus and Brill-Zinsser disease (recrudescent typhus)	Worldwide	Body louse —	Man Man
		R. mooseri (*typhi*)	Murine or endemic typhus	Worldwide	Rat flea	Rats
Spotted fever group	A*	*R. rickettsii*	Rocky Mountain spotted fever	Western hemisphere	Tick	Small wild mammals, dogs, birds
		R. sibirica	Siberian tick typhus	Siberia, Mongolia	Tick	Wild animals and birds
	B	*R. conori* (*R. parkeri*)	Boutonneuse Fever —	Mediterranean littoral	Tick	Small wild mammals, dogs
	C	*R. akari*	Rickettsial pox, vesicular rickettsiosis	North-east U.S.A., U.S.S.R.	Gamasid mite	House mouse
		R. australis	Queensland tick typhus	Australia	Tick	Bush rodents
Scrub typhus		*R. tsutsugamushi*	Scrub typhus	Oceania	Trombiculid mite	Small wild rodents and birds
Trench fever		*R. quintana*	Trench fever	Europe, North Africa, Middle East, Mexico	Body louse	Man
Q fever		*Cox. burnetii*	Q fever	Worldwide	Two cycles: (1) Tick and small wild mammals (2) Cattle, sheep and goats by aerosol and milk without arthropod vector	

* Subgroup of spotted fever; group D not shown.

rickettsiaemia in Q fever and, as with the other rickettsioses, infection may involve any organ system. A substantial proportion (up to 50 per cent) of Q fever patients have pneumonia, often of a lobar type. There may be hepatitis with small foci of necrosis. These modes of presentation often dominate the clinical picture. Pneumonia also occurs in the other rickettsioses but is overshadowed by the other signs and symptoms.

This variation aside, the general features of the rickettsial infections are broadly similar. Onset of illness is often abrupt and may be recorded to the hour. Headache—frontal or retroorbital—is often very severe and resistant to analgesics. Fever (100–104°F), rigors and sweating, myalgia and arthralgia, anorexia, nausea and vomiting are all found, as in many other acute infections. 'Sore eyes' or photophobia with severe headache is a memorable feature of many Q fever cases and a useful differential point in history-taking. The rash of the typhus-spotted fever groups of infections appears four to seven days after onset of illness, first as macules or papules, that progress in severe cases (e.g. spotted fever) to petechial or haemorrhagic lesions, or in rickettsial pox, to vesicular lesions that simulate chickenpox. A small proportion of patients with epidemic or murine typhus do not have a rash, and a rash is very uncommon in Q fever.

The course and case fatality of the various rickettsioses, without chemotherapy, differs from group to group. Epidemic typhus, scrub typhus and the Rocky Mountain spotted fever group display an overall case fatality of 10–20 per cent or more with substantially higher rates in the over 50 age group. These rates are effectively reduced by treatment with tetracycline or chloramphenicol. Murine typhus, and trench fever have a negligible case fatality; likewise, although Q fever may be severe and very debilitating on occasion, it is rarely fatal. The duration of disease varies from 2–5 weeks with stupor, delirium or coma and uraemia as complications of severe typhus or spotted fever. Although the heart, kidneys and brain bear the brunt of acute typhus, sequelae are uncommon.

This composite account of the clinical features of the rickettsioses is necessarily superficial; admirable detailed accounts of the diseases are given by Snyder (1965) on epidemic and murine typhus; by Woodward and Jackson (1965) on the spotted fever group; by Smadel and Elisberg (1965) on scrub typhus; by Derrick (1937), Clark *et al.* (1951) and Powell (1960, 1961) on Q fever.

In Q fever a small proportion of clinical or subclinical infections, particularly in persons with pre-existing rheumatic heart disease, may lead to a chronic, subacute endocarditis with features resembling those of subacute bacterial endocarditis. The mitral or aortic valve may be involved with small compact vegetations containing microcolonies of *C. burnetii* (Andrews and Marmion, 1959; Marmion, 1962). A substantial number of cases of Q fever endocarditis have now been described in the United Kingdom and recently chronic liver disease has been recognized as a complication in some of the patients. Treatment is by prolonged antibiotic therapy (tetracycline and lincomycin) with valve replacement to correct mechanical defect or extension of the lesion. Q fever may also present as a pericarditis, meningoencephalitis, uveitis and optic neuritis. The organism has also been isolated from the human placenta but, as with cattle, sheep and goats, is not a significant cause of abortion.

It might be expected that other rickettsiae would give rise to chronic endocarditis; French workers have produced some interesting but not entirely conclusive evidence. Chronic infection with rickettsiae does, however, occur elsewhere, probably in the reticulo-endothelial system, and is exemplified by Brill-Zinsser disease or recrudescent typhus; a condition of considerable epidemiological importance and immunological interest. In the early 1900s Brill described a form of typhus in migrants to New York who had come from areas of eastern Europe where there had been outbreaks of epidemic typhus. Zinsser (1934) showed that *R. prowazekii* was present in the blood of these cases and that the condition was a relapse of an infection acquired many years previously. These cases have now been described in most parts of the world that have received migrants from eastern Europe or other endemic areas and substantial numbers have also been recognized in the residents of countries (e.g. Yugoslavia) that had epidemic typhus in the Second World War (Murray *et al.*, 1951).

Details of rickettsial infection in animals and of the veterinary aspects of Q fever are outside of the scope of this text (see Babudieri, 1959; Stoker and Marmion, 1955a). The general point may be made that rickettsial infections in animals are rickettsiaemic but usually trivial and that the vector arthropod mainly suffers no ill effects while transmitting infection transovarially or interstadially. Head and body lice, however, are killed as a result of infection with *R. prowazekii*.

LABORATORY DIAGNOSIS OF RICKETTSIAL INFECTIONS

The approach in laboratory diagnosis is the same, in principle, as with many viral and bacterial infections, viz. the organism may be isolated or the serological response to infection may be measured with antigens prepared from prototype strains of the organisms.

Isolation of rickettsiae in laboratory animals should not be attempted except in laboratories equipped with safety cabinets and other facilities, segregated animal accommodation and with staff who have been vaccinated against the rickettsiae to be handled; the processing of infected yolk sac material is a particular hazard for laboratory workers. Epidemic and murine typhus rickettsiae, and the majority of the spotted fever rickettsiae can be isolated in guinea-pigs; cotton rats are highly susceptible to *R. prowazekii*. White mice are used for scrub typhus and the vesicular rickettsioses such as rickettsialpox.

C. burnetii readily infects guinea-pigs and hamsters. The larger animals are bled before inoculation, their temperatures are taken for 3 weeks after inoculation and they are bled again 4–6 weeks after inoculation. The pre- and post-inoculation sera are tested with known antigens to ascertain the type of infecting organism and to detect a non-febrile infection. The inoculum, given intraperitoneally, is usually the clot from a blood specimen collected during the rickettsiaemia, and ground in sterile skimmed milk or in a special suspending medium without antibiotics. Febrile animals are bled, or killed and the brain, spleen or liver used for passage material for fresh animals or, after a few passages, to establish the rickettsiae in the yolk sac. A good account of the practical details is given by Elisberg and Bozeman (1969).

With Q fever it is considered that the demonstration that a guinea-pig has seroconverted to CF antibody positive after inoculation constitutes an 'isolation' of *C. burnetii*; visualization of the organism in impression smears of liver or spleen or adaptation of the strain to the yolk sac is not required for routine diagnosis and is a hazardous procedure.

Examination of patients' sera is based on specific CF reactions with purified rickettsial antigens extracted from infected chick embryo yolk sacs, and on the Weil-Felix reaction. The latter depends on fortuitous similarity of serological specificities of carbohydrate haptens found in certain rickettsiae and in non-motile, 'O' variants of *Proteus vulgaris* and *Proteus mirabilis*. Patients infected with *R. prowazekii*,

Table 51.2. Patterns of Weil-Felix reaction obtained with suspensions of *Proteus vulgaris* OX19 and OX2 and *Proteus mirabilis* OXK in various rickettsioses.

Disease category	Degree of reaction with *Proteus* strain		
	OX19	OX2	OXK
Epidemic typhus (other than Brill-Zinsser disease)	+ + + +	+	−
Murine typhus	+ + + +	+	−
Rocky Mountain spotted fever and other tick-borne rickettsioses	+ + + + or +	+ or + + +	−
Rickettsialpox	−	−	−
Scrub typhus	−	−	+ + + + (variable)
Q fever	−	−	−
Trench fever	−	−	−

R. mooseri, some of the spotted fever group and scrub typhus rickettsiae may develop agglutinins to the various proteus strains (Table 51.2); those with Brill-Zinsser disease, rickettsial pox and Q fever generally do not. The antibodies concerned are in the IgM class, heat-labile at 56°C, and develop rapidly. It is important to demonstrate a changing titre; false positive reactions in liver disease and other conditions are characterized by lower, unchanging levels.

The CF tests commonly utilize the group-specific, ether-soluble heat-stable antigens for, respectively, epidemic and murine typhus and for the spotted fever group. A positive reaction does not distinguish between infection with various members of the group; for this purpose washed rickettsial suspensions for CF or agglutination tests are required; now difficult to obtain. Antibody may also be measured by immunofluorescence with slide preparations of the appropriate rickettsia, also microagglutination (Fiset *et al.*, 1969).

In suspected Q fever, patients' sera are tested with suspensions of *C. burnetii* in phase 2 and if positive also with a phase-1 antigen. Patients with the acute, self-limiting form of Q fever show rising antibody levels to phase 2, usually over a titre of 80, and no or only low antibody levels to phase-1 antigen. In Q fever endocarditis the phase 1 CF antibody titres are of the same order or higher than those for phase 2 and are mostly over 1 000. Attempts should be made to isolate *C. burnetii* in suspected cases of sub-acute endocarditis that have only low titres of phase 2 antibody as the serological result alone is inadequate to sustain the diagnosis. Patients with Q fever endocarditis have raised IgM levels and this may differentiate them from subacute *bacterial* endocarditis. All cases of subacute endocarditis, with or without bacteria in blood culture, should be tested for Q fever CF antibody as double infections with bacteria and rickettsiae have been observed and *C. burnetii* does not respond clinically to penicillin.

Previous exposure to *C. burnetii* may be detected by skin tests with purified, inactivated vaccine; reactions give a typical delayed type hypersensitivity response. Antibody may also be detected by double antibody radio immunoassay with suspensions of *C. burnetii* tagged with ^{131}I or [125]I. The results of skin testing and radio immunoassay reveal a much wider experience of subclinical infection with *C. burnetii* than is found in surveys with the CF test.

The differential diagnosis of typhus, spotted fever and Q fever is clearly a complex matter. Early smallpox, enteric fever, meningococcal septicaemia, chickenpox (with the vesicular rickettsioses), leptospirosis, brucellosis and other medium term fevers may be confused with the condition and can be resolved by systematic testing along the lines described in other chapters.

EPIDEMIOLOGY OF THE RICKETTSIOSES

The ecosystems responsible for the maintenance of the various groups of rickettsiae in nature are summarized in Fig. 51.1. The interaction of these with human social patterns determines the prevalence of disease in man.

The geographical distribution of the rickett-sioses is outlined in Table 51.1. In general terms, it was noted that Q fever had virtually a world-wide prevalence corresponding to the distribution and movement of infected domestic animals. The wide distribution of rats and their ecto-parasites, particularly rat fleas, determines the prevalence of murine typhus. Scrub typhus is more sharply limited to the S.E. Asian sub-continent, Oceania and Australasia and similarly the location of the various members of the spotted fever group is determined by the distribution of the arthropod hosts, small wild animals. Epidemic typhus (*R. prowazekii*) is dependent on man for survival and is transmitted by head and body lice in circumstances of poverty and social disintegration that favour louse infestation—crowding, cold climate, lack of fuel and water for washing, no change of clothing. Lice are infected by feeding on a person with rickettsiaemia; consequently the patient with recrudescent typhus, Brill-Zinsser disease, plays a central role in initiating an epidemic. Although there have been claims to have demonstrated antibodies to *R. prowazekii* in domestic animals and to have isolated the rickettsia from them, experimental inoculations have not supported the concept of an alternative vertebrate host.

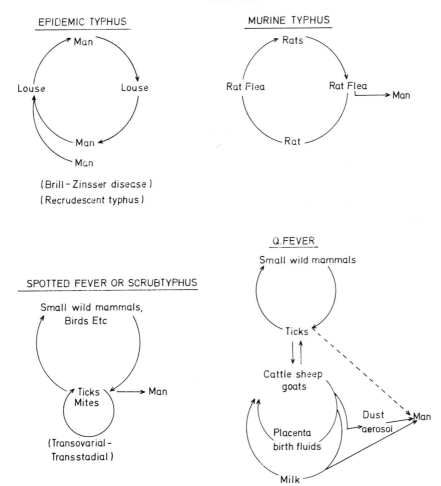

FIG. 51.1. Diagram of ecosystems for maintenance of rickettsiae.

Discussion of the ecology of vertebrate hosts and arthropods, vectors for murine typhus, spotted fever rickettsiae and scrub typhus are given by Snyder, 1965; Woodward and Jackson, 1965; Smadel and Elisberg, 1965, and Audy, 1961.

In the United Kingdom Q fever is the only significant rickettsial infection; in the period since 1940 there have been rare episodes of murine typhus on visiting ships and some indigenous cases of Brill-Zinsser disease; vesicular rickettsioses have not been observed. Cattle and sheep in many parts of the U.K. are infected with *C. burnetii* and the prevalence of infection in these animals and in man is greater in areas where both are present (summary by Marmion and Stoker, 1958). Limited surveys of chickens and other birds and small wild animals did not reveal infection. The organism has been isolated from one species of native tick (*Dermacentor punctata*) (Stoker and Marmion, 1955b). Serological surveys of rural populations in England showed that infection is widespread and Q fever is a significant cause of illness in the farming community and persons associated with it. Prevalence in urban communities is generally small. Exposure to cattle or sheep at parturition, or consumption of infected raw milk was a satisfactory explanation for many of the cases observed. Puzzling outbreaks occur as a result, no doubt, of the prolonged survival of *C. burnetii* on fomites.

Treatment and Control

Chemotherapy with tetracycline or chloramphenicol has radically improved the treatment and prognosis of all the rickettsial infections. Treatment of Q fever endocarditis is less satisfactory although the use of tetracycline combined with lincomycin or trimethoprim-sulphonamide (cotrimoxazole) is reported to be effective, greater experience is required.

Effective vaccines are available for epidemic and murine typhus, spotted fever and Q fever (P.A.H.O. conference, 1967), but the indications for their use are now limited. General hygienic control measures are described in detail by the American Public Health Association, 1960.

REFERENCES AND FURTHER READING

ANDREWS, P. S. & MARMION, B. P. (1959) Chronic Q fever 2 morbid anatomical and bacteriological findings in a patient with endocarditis. *British Medical Journal*, **ii**, 983–990.

AMERICAN PUBLIC HEALTH ASSOCIATION (1960) *The Control of Communicable Diseases in Man*. A.P.H.A., New York.

AUDY, J. R. (1961) The ecology of scrub typhus. In *Studies in Disease Ecology*, pp. 389–432. Edited by J. M. May, New York: Hafner.

BABUDIERI, B. (1959) *Advances in Veterinary Science*, **5**, 81–182.

BREZINA, R. (1969) *Current Topics in Microbiology*, **47**, 20–39. Springer, Berlin.

CLARK, W. H., LENNETTE, E. H., RAILSBACK, O. C. & ROMER, M. S. (1951) Q fever in California, VII. clinical features in one hundred and eighty cases. *Archives of Internal Medicine*, **88**, 155–167.

DERRICK, E. H. (1937) Q fever, new fever entity: clinical features, diagnosis and laboratory investigation. *Medical Journal of Australia*, **2**, 281–299.

ELISBERG, B. L. & BOZEMAN, F. M. (1969) Rickettsiae. In *Diagnostic Procedures for Viral and Rickettsial Infections*,

4th edn. Edited by E. H. Lennette and N. J. Schmidt, American Public Health Association Inc.

FISET, P., ORMSBEE, R. A., SILBERMAN, R., PEACOCK, M. & SPIELMAN, S. H. (1969) A microagglutination technique for detection and measurement of rickettsial antibodies. *Acta virologica*, **13**, 60–66.

MARMION, B. P. (1962) Subacute rickettsial endocarditis, an unusual complication of Q fever. *Journal of Hygiene and Epidemiology*, **6**, 79–84.

MARMION, B. P. & STOKER, M. G. P. (1958) The epidemiology of Q fever in Great Britain: An analysis of the findings and some conclusions. *British Medical Journal*, **ii**, 809.

MOULDER, J. W. (1962) *The Biochemistry of Intracellular Parasitism*, pp. 43–83. Edited by P. P. H. De Bruyn, Chicago Univ. Press.

MURRAY, E. S., PSORN, T., DJAKOVIC, P., SIELSKI, S., BROZ, V., LJUPSA, F., GAON, J., PAVLEVIC, R. & SNYDER, J. C. (1951) Brill's disease IV study of 26 cases in Yugoslavia. *American Journal of Public Health*, **41**, 1359–1369.

ORMSBEE, R. A. (1969) Rickettsiae (as organisms). *Annual Review of Microbiology*, **23**, 275–292.

P.A.H.O. CONFERENCE (1967) First international conference on vaccines against viral and rickettsial diseases of man. *Pan American Health Organisation/World Health Organisation*. Scientific Publication No. 147.

POWELL, O. (1960) Q fever: clinical features in 72 cases. *Australasian Annals of Medicine*, **9**, 214–223.

POWELL, O. (1961) Liver involvement in Q fever. *Australasian Annals of Medicine*, **10**, 52–58.

SMADEL, J. E. & ELISBERG, B. L. (1965) Scrub typhus rickettsiae. In *Viral and Rickettsial Infections of Man*, pp. 1130–1143. Edited by F. Horsfall and I. Tamm, Pitman.

SNYDER, J. C. (1965) Typhus fever rickettsiae. In *Viral and Rickettsial Infections of Man*, pp. 1059–1094. Edited by F. Horsfall and I. Tamm, Pitman.

STOKER, M. G. P. & MARMION, B. P. (1955a) The spread of Q fever from animals to man: natural history of a rickettsial disease. *Bulletin of the World Health Organization*, **13**, 781–806.

STOKER, M. G. P. & MARMION, B. P. (1955b) Q fever in Britain. Isolation of *Rickettsia burneti* from the tick *Haemaphysalis punctata*. *Journal of Hygiene (Cambridge)*, **53**, 322.

WISSEMAN, C. L. JNR. (1968) *Zentr. Bakteriol. Parasitenk Abt. I Orig.*, **206**, 299–313.

WOODWARD, T. E. & JACKSON, E. B. (1965) Spotted fever rickettsiae. In *Viral and Rickettsial Infections of Man*, pp. 1095–1129. Edited by F. Horsfall and I. Tamm, Pitman.

ZINSSER, H. (1934) Varieties of typhus virus and the epidemiology of the American form of European typhus fever (Brill's disease). *American Journal of Hygiene*, **20**, 513–522.

ZINSSER, H. (1935) *Rats, Lice and History*. Boston: Little.

52. Mycoplasma* Respiratory and Urogenital Infections

Mycoplasmas are small procaryotic cells, probably the smallest able to grow in cell-free culture media. The first member of the group, *Mycoplasma mycoides*, was isolated in 1898 from bovine pleuropneumonia. As other pathogenic or saprophytic isolates accumulated from veterinary or human sources they were known by a wide variety of names, the most popular of which was the pleuropneumonia group of organisms or pleuropneumonia-like organisms (PPLO): a term now superseded by *Mycoplasma* at genus level with *Mycoplasmataceae*, *Mycoplasmatales* and *Mollicutes* at the level of, respectively, Family, Order and Class. 'Mycoplasma' refers to the branching, pleomorphic nature of the cells of some species and *Mollicutes* ('soft skins') refers to the lack of a cell wall. A distinctive feature of most mycoplasmas is a requirement for sterol as a growth factor. One group of organisms, represented by *Mycoplasma laidlawii* will incorporate cholesterol but some can synthesize a carotenoid which they can use instead of cholesterol; these have been segregated in a separate genus, *Acholeplasma*. Finally, there are the T strain mycoplasmas (T for tiny colonies) which require cholesterol, split urea, and have a lower pH optimum for growth than 'classical' mycoplasmas.

Mycoplasmas are widely distributed in nature and have been detected in man, animals, plants and sources such as soil and sewage. They are of particular importance to veterinary microbiologists as various species cause economically important infections in the respiratory tracts, mammary glands and genital tracts, or synovia of cattle, sheep, goats, cats, mice and rats, swine and birds. The plant 'mycoplasmas', although, as yet, not well characterized, are associated with various insect transmitted diseases (e.g. aster yellows), previously thought to be viral. For detailed information on all these aspects reference should be made to the comprehensive text edited by Hayflick (1969) and the review by Davis and Whitcombe (1971). The present discussion will be limited to the general properties of the organisms, the human flora and human mycoplasmal disease.

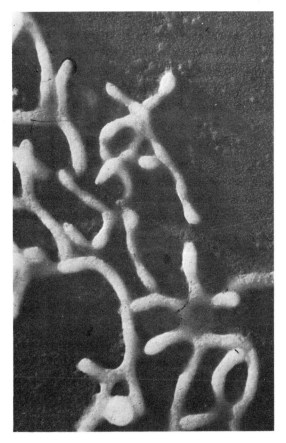

PLATE 52.1. *Mycoplasma mycoides*, gold shadowed electron micrograph, to show branching nature of a filamentous strain. × 28 800. (From Rodwell and Abbot, 1961, *Journal of General Microbiology*, 25, 201.)

* The abbreviation *M* for Mycoplasma is used throughout this chapter. In certain circumstances the abbreviation *Mycopl.* might be used to avoid confusion with other genera, e.g. Mycobacterium.

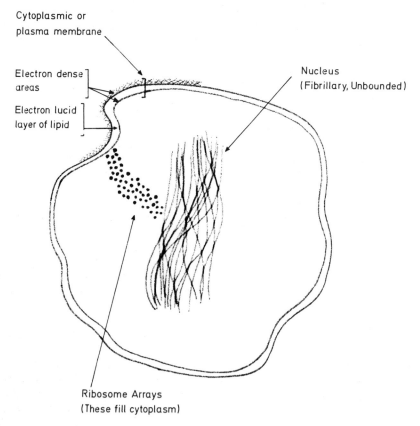

Fig. 52.1. Diagrammatic representation of a mycoplasma cell.

THE MYCOPLASMA CELL: MORPHOLOGY AND FINE STRUCTURE

Mycoplasma cultures, according to species, show short or long branching filaments with spherical coccal bodies in variable numbers in the filaments (Plate 52.1). Other species are predominantly cocco-bacillary. The morphology of the cells is also dependent on the tonicity and nutritive properties of the growth medium, particularly the ratio of saturated to unsaturated fatty acids which influences the membrane structure of the organisms. The minimal reproductive unit is a roughly spherical cell about 200 to 250 nm in diameter and the diagrammatic representation in Fig. 52.1 is based on this shape. It is from cells of this order of size, whatever the shape, that growth is initiated in cell-free media; such cells also make up, with larger forms (0·5 to 1·0 μm diameter) and cholesterol droplets, the substance of the characteristic agar-embedded colonies.

The cell is limited by a plasma membrane, 8 to 15 nm thick, with two electron-dense layers separated by a translucent layer (Fig. 52.1) as with the cell membrane of a bacterial or animal cell. Some species (*M. pulmonis, M. gallisepticum*) have surface spikes and may resemble *Myxoviruses*. The electron-lucent part of the membrane represents lipids with the long chains of the fatty acids inwards and polar groups to the external and internal parts of the cell; the electron dense part represents protein and carbohydrate. Chemical analysis of membranes shows substantial amounts of lipid and, unlike bacterial membranes, cholesterol or carotenol. The lipid is mainly phospholipid but glycolipids are found in some sugar-fermenting species and the sugar moieties of these are important serologic-ally as antigenic determinants in complement-fixing and neutralizing antibody reactions; in certain instances, they are also important in provoking a serological cross-reaction against fortuitously similar structural groupings in brain tissue or on erythrocytes of the host. The membrane polypeptide chain which may be external to the membrane, or perhaps interwoven with it, also contributes to cell antigens. The cholesterol (or carotenoid/carotenol) is interspersed between the phospholipid molecules and is thought to play an important part in maintaining membrane integrity in the face of varying external osmotic pressures and in the absence of a rigid cell wall as found in bacteria. The presence of the cholesterol renders the cell membrane suscep-tible to damage with agents that complex with sterols; i.e. saponin, digitonin and some polyene antibiotics (filipin, amphotericin B); the latter action is not of therapeutic importance but may be of significance in efforts to treat fungal con-tamination of mycoplasma cultures. The failure to see a cell wall in electron micrographs of thin sections of mycoplasmas is substantiated by the results of chemical analysis which have not detected either N-acetylmuramic acid, one of the characteristic amino-sugar units of the giant macromolecule *mucopeptide* or *murein* compris-ing the bacterial cell wall, or diaminopimelic acid, an unusual amino acid found in the cross-linking peptide chains of some mucopeptides. As would be anticipated mycoplasmas are com-pletely resistant to penicillin and cycloserine which act on various stages of bacterial cell wall synthesis and also to the enzyme lysozyme (muramidase) which acts on linkages between the mucopeptide units, N-acetyl glucosamine and N-acetyl muramic acid.

The mycoplasma membrane is also the site of many metabolic reactions involving membrane-bound enzymes and transport mechanisms. In *M. pneumoniae* there appears to be a specialized area (the 'foot') which attaches to neuraminic acid receptors on the animal cell surface; a needle-like aspirating tube is inserted into the cell which may enable the mycoplasma to inject nucleases and other enzymes and to take from the cell the products of enzyme action (e.g. nucleotides). This specific adsorption site is presumably related to the ability of colonies of some mycoplasma species to adsorb erythro-cytes (haemadsorption), tissue culture cells or sperm which have the appropriate neuramini-dase-sensitive receptors.

The cytoplasm of the mycoplasma does not contain an internal membrane (endoplasmic reticulum) or a defined mesosome as with bac-teria. In *M. gallisepticum* membrane-bounded vesicles ('blebs') have been observed. The cyto-plasm is packed with ribosomes and there is nuclear material (unbounded, no nucleoli) in fibrillary form (3 nm thickness), centrally placed or dispersed. The ribosomes are of the 70S variety and, as with bacteria, protein synthesis is inhibited, or modified, on these ribosomes by antibiotics such as puromycin, tetracycline, tylosin, kanamycin, streptomycin, erythromycin, chloramphenicol, etc.—an aspect of consider-able therapeutic importance; inhibitors of pro-tein synthesis on 80S ribosomes, such as cycloheximide, have no effect on mycoplasma ribosomes.

The content of DNA in mycoplasma cells ranges from 1·5 to 4 per cent of the dry weight of the cells; circular double-stranded genomes have been extracted from six or more species studied. The molecular weight of the genomes range from 444×10^6 to $1\,200 \times 10^6$ daltons; the lowest value, from *M. arthritidis*, is of interest by comparison with that of a large animal virus of the pox group (160 to 200×10^6) as an indication of the smallest amount of genetic information needed for the free-living existence. The guanine-cytosine ratios (G + C per cent) of the DNA cover a very wide range, 24 to 41 per cent, with *M. pneumoniae* and *M. gallisepticum* at the upper end of the range. The various species are arranged in clusters over this range and G + C per cent determinations are of substantial taxonomic value. Further details of chemical structure and metabolism of myco-plasmas may be found in Hayflick (1969) and in the review by Marmion (1967).

COLONY FORM AND CULTIVATION OF MYCOPLASMAS

Mycoplasmas are commonly grown in fluid, semi-solid ('sloppy agar') or soft solid media with a rich meat digest base and a high supplement (10 to 30 per cent) of animal protein—human serum or ascitic fluid, horse or swine serum—and yeast extract. Semi-defined media have been developed with a few highly investigated strains, e.g. *M. mycoides*. The T strain mycoplasmas have a specific requirement for urea which is obtained from the serum or from urea added as such. Most species of mycoplasmas are aerobes or facultative anaerobes, but some require microaerophilic conditions and CO_2. Most species grow best at 35 to 36°C but the *Acholeplasmas* have a lower temperature optimum (22 to 30°C).

Probably the best known character of mycoplasma is the 'fried egg' colony formed in solid media (Plate 52.2). According to Ruys, Razin and Oliver and others, the mycoplasma cell is drawn into the spaces of the agar gel and a colony forms as a ball-like structure (the embedded centre) which then grows up to the surface and along it in the superficial layer of liquid thus giving the peripheral zone of growth; credence is lent to this view by the observation of agar-embedded centres alone in suboptimal culture medium, and of colonies entirely on the surface of 'stiff' agar or on unusual media such as coagulated serum. The high concentrations of protein in serum in the media are not utilized as such. Serum rather serves as a source of cholesterol and fatty acids and other lipid precursors, and as a regulator (by binding) of their input; some fatty acids in greater than trace amounts are highly toxic for mycoplasmas. Combinations of fluid and solid media—'sloppy' agar, diphasic media with a slope of agar in a bottle of broth—are particularly valuable in adapting mycoplasmas to grow in artificial media.

Many species of mycoplasmas also grow readily in cell and organ cultures, in the lung and yolk sac of chick embryos and a few may be cultivated in laboratory animals such as hamsters. These methods all carry the hazard of contamination with extraneous mycoplasmas from the cell culture or animal, but may support growth of fastidious mycoplasmas more readily than cell-free media. Indeed, it is certain that there are organisms with the ultramicroscopic structure of mycoplasmas and with appropriate sensitivity to broad spectrum antibiotics, organic gold salts and arsenicals, which have not been cultured in cell-free media; grey lung 'virus' of mice and the plant pathogens are two examples.

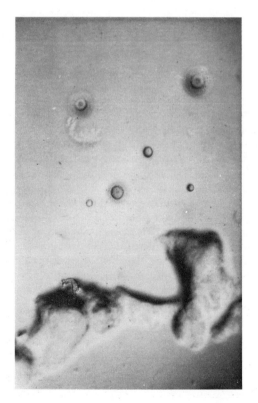

PLATE 52.2. Colonies of *M. hominis* on agar, showing 'fried egg' appearance.

CLASSIFICATION: BIOLOGICAL AND BIOCHEMICAL PROPERTIES OF MYCOPLASMAS

Mycoplasmas fall into three general physiological groups: (1) carbohydrate-fermenting non-sterol-requiring (represented by *Acholeplasma laidlawii*), (2) carbohydrate-fermenting, sterol-requiring and (3) non-carbohydrate-fermenting and sterol-requiring. The range of sugars fermented by groups (1) and (2) is limited; acid is produced from glucose, fructose, mannose, maltose, starch and glycogen and, with some avian species also from sucrose and galactose. A mycoplasma that ferments glucose usually ferments most of the other sugars so that fermentation patterns are of limited value in differentiating species. Studies with fermenting species such as *M. mycoides* suggest that the respiratory pathway terminates at the flavoprotein level and there are no haem-containing cytochromes or associated enzymes; most are catalase-negative. Terminal electron transfer to substances such as triphenyl tetrazolium produces a red formazan; the ability of some species (e.g. *M. pneumoniae*) to produce this under aerobic conditions is a useful identifying characteristic. Some fermenting species, such as *M. pneumoniae* or *M. fermentans*, are particularly vigorous producers of hydrogen peroxide and when their colonies are overlayed with guinea-pig erythrocytes in agar, areas of haemolysis, resembling β-haemolysis of *Strept. pyogenes* are produced. Weaker, α-haemolysis, is produced under similar conditions by some non-fermenting species in group (3).

The non-fermenting species utilize amino acids and fatty acids as carbon and energy sources. It appears some non-fermenting mycoplasma species, e.g. *M. arthritidis*, have cytochromes and cytochrome oxidase in their respiratory pathways and catalase, which is easily lost from the cells during washing, is also demonstrable. The arginine dihydrolase pathway, in which arginine is broken down to ammonia and CO_2 with generation of ATP, is important in many, but not all, of the non-fermentative mycoplasmas.

Practical use is made of the acid produced by fermentative mycoplasmas and of the ammonia produced by non-fermentative mycoplasmas in measuring growth by the change of the medium to acid or alkaline pH; inhibition of growth by antibody, the effect of which is enhanced by the presence of complement, inhibits the pH change and constitutes a valuable, sensitive method of antibody titration ('metabolic inhibition test'). Active proteases and lipases are not common in mycoplasmas, but *M. mycoides* will liquefy coagulated serum and lipolytic activity is the basis of the 'film and spots' phenomenon observed in the plate cultures of some species.

The replication of mycoplasmas has been the subject of much study and controversy. The predominantly cocco-bacillary species seem to follow a pattern of binary fission. With the filamentous species the division of the nucleus may not be synchronous with that of the filamentous cell so that several nuclei or 'elementary bodies' may be found in one filament and are eventually liberated by breakdown of the filament; the subject is critically reviewed by Freundt in Hayflick (1969).

ANTIGENIC ANALYSIS

The identification and species classification of mycoplasmas has, until recently, presented a problem in view of the limited range of colonial morphology and biochemical reactions. Systematic serological studies supplemented by techniques from molecular biology have brought order to the field in recent years. Serological studies with mycoplasmas have utilized most of the standard reactions. Given stable suspensions, agglutination has been used for antigenic classification and for measuring antibody in naturally and experimentally infected hosts; it is expensive in terms of antigen. Complement fixation has been widely employed for both purposes and reveals the most antigenic inter-relationships between species. Metabolic inhibition tests,

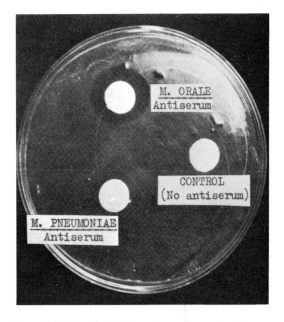

PLATE 52.3. Growth inhibition of mycoplasma by antiserum.

agglutination of latex particles or of tanned erythrocytes coated with fragmented myco-plasmas, are sensitive methods of measuring post-infection antibody. Mycoplasmas differ from the great majority of bacterial species in that their growth on solid media is inhibited by potent antisera in the *absence* of complement (Plate 52.3). The phenomenon is more species-specific than complement fixation and con-stitutes a simple, valuable, widely used, method of identifying strains and isolates of myco-plasmas; its sensitivity for measurement of antibody is, however, low. Immunofluorescence on colonies of mycoplasmas (Colour Plates 7a and b) yields similar species-specific results and is particularly useful in detecting mixtures of mycoplasma species. Double diffusion of anti-gens and antisera in agar or other gels has yielded useful information about the number and inter-relationship of antigens in mycoplasma species. Serological studies with mycoplasmas are some-times complicated by the tendency of these organisms to absorb and tenaciously hold de-natured globulin or other constituents from the serum-rich medium in which they are grown. This may result in misleading serological results in several ways. For example, human sera may contain rheumatoid factor or other antibodies that will react with the denatured serum pro-teins giving a false-positive result. Again, when rabbits or other animals are hyperimmunized with suspensions of mycoplasmas, the forma-tion of antibodies against these absorbed serum components will lead later to non-specific cross-reactions in tests with such antisera and other species of mycoplasma. Such problems may be offset to some extent, by growing the organisms in media containing only protein from the species of animal to be hyperimmunized or by suitable absorption of the antiserum with the medium components, e.g. horse serum or yeast cell products, likely to lead to the unwanted cross-reactions.

These serological methods are easily applic-able at a routine diagnostic level. A variety of more elaborate techniques are available to establish the species of an unknown mycoplasma or to substantiate a new species. These include comparison of the G + C ratios of established and unknown species, and nucleic acid hybridi-zation experiments with DNA extracted from the species under comparison, or between the DNA from one species and the mRNA trans-cribed from that of the other. Such studies have been particularly important in excluding the postulated (genetic) relationships between myco-plasmas and *Corynebacteria*, *Haemophilus sp* and streptococci arising from the hypothesis that mycoplasmas are stable L-phase variants of bacteria (see below). Comparison of gene products—the proteins of mycoplasma mem-branes or of the whole cell—by polyacrylamide gel electrophoresis gives characteristic patterns for each species; classification by this method correlates well with the result from nucleic acid hybridization and antigenic analysis.

Mycoplasmas and L-phase Organisms

Treatment of multiplying bacteria with sub-stances that interfere with various stages of cell wall synthesis, such as penicillin, D-cycloserine, bacitracin, vancomycin, glycine, or ones that attack linkages in the mucopeptide molecule, such as lysozyme or 'phage-associated murami-dase', in media of suitable osmotic composition results in the formation of spheroplasts or proto-plasts with, respectively, modified or no cell wall. If these structures can multiply as variants of the parent bacterium, they constitute L-phase organisms. They may be *stable* (i.e. do not revert to the normal bacterial form on removal of the inducer) or *unstable* (i.e. do revert).

The colonies of L-phase variants in solid media may bear a striking resemblance to those of mycoplasmas, probably a reflection of the lack of cell wall in both types of organism. The differences between the groups may be sum-marized as follows. The minimal reproductive unit of L-phase organisms is on the whole larger (*circa* 600 nm) than that of mycoplasmas, and filamentous forms are rare; L-phase variants usually retain the ability to synthesize muramic acid and diaminopimelic acid and the enzyme alanine racemase—parts of the machinery of cell wall synthesis—and may also retain surface antigens of the parent bacterium; mycoplasmas have a requirement for cholesterol as a growth factor whereas L-phase organisms will incor-porate exogenous sterol to save endogenous synthesis; some mycoplasmas are pathogenic whereas L-phase organisms are non-pathogenic until they revert to the parent bacterium *in vivo* or unless they produce potent endo- or exotoxins. Finally, L-phase organisms have the nucleic acid base ratios of, and show homology with, the nucleic acid of the parent bacterium, whereas mycoplasmas have not shown nucleic acid homology with any of the bacteria from which they were supposed to have been derived.

A detailed account of the biology of L-phase organisms and their relation to disease is given in various chapters of Hayflick (1969) and in Guze (1968).

MYCOPLASMAS OF HUMAN ORIGIN

The human mycoplasma flora consists of some 8 or 9 species which are listed in Table 52.1. Of these *M. pneumoniae* is the only unequivocal pathogen although *M. hominis* may act as a low-grade pathogen in certain circumstances. The T-strains comprise a large group of separate antigenic subtypes whereas the other species are single antigenic types although there is a substantial degree of antigenic overlap in the *M. salivarium-M. orale* complex.

CLINICAL ASPECTS AND EPIDEMIOLOGY OF HUMAN MYCOPLASMA INFECTIONS

1. Infection with Mycoplasma Pneumoniae

In the late 1930s the syndrome of primary atypical pneumonia (PAP) was described (atypical in the sense that it was not attributable to any of the bacteria that commonly cause pneumonia). Experiments by the Commission on Acute Respiratory Diseases in the 1940s established that the condition was due to a filtrable agent and Eaton and colleagues isolated an agent in cotton rats and hamsters and subsequently in chick embryos which was related then, and in later studies using immunofluorescence, to cases of PAP developing cold haemagglutinins and *Streptococcus MG* agglutinins. The agent was subsequently identified as a mycoplasma—*M. pneumoniae*—by Marmion and Goodburn (1961) and Chanock, Hayflick and Barile (1962).

Clinically, *M. pneumoniae* infections take the form of a febrile bronchitis or pneumonia with an insidious onset of generalized symptoms—malaise (which may overshadow respiratory symptoms), myalgia, sore throat or headache. Cough, which starts around the third day, is characteristically non-productive, troublesome and sometimes paroxysmal. Coryza is unusual but nausea and vomiting may be a feature. About a third of the patients have earache and some may have myringitis; although *M. pneumoniae* has been isolated from otitis media, surveys do not suggest that it is an important cause of otitis. Radiographic examination of the chest may show partial or complete consolidation of a dependent segment of lower or middle lobes of greater extent than the paucity of physical signs would suggest. Complications include rashes—urticaria, maculo-papular rash, erythema multiforme or nodosum and the Stevens-Johnson syndrome (erythema multiforme, vesicular and bullous lesions on mucocutaneous junctions) and also meningitis and encephalitis. Haemolytic anaemia is sometimes observed in patients with high titres of cold haemagglutinins.

Infection with *M. pneumoniae* is probably worldwide although most reports have been from northern temperate zones and from Australasia. PAP was prevalent in military camps during World War II and subsequently. It tends to spread slowly in institutional groups and as family outbreaks in the general population. Probably the infection is endemic in the population but tends to peak prevalences at 3 to 5 year intervals without any pronounced seasonal incidence. The highest prevalence is in the age group 5 to 15 years and the sexes are equally affected. In these age groups *M. pneumoniae* may be the major cause (20 to 40 per cent) of all non-bacterial pneumonias. The school age child is the most important 'vector' of infection and frequently constitutes the index case in a family; more than 70 per cent of family contacts may be infected, the proportions being higher in the younger members. Of those infected about three-quarters have clinical manifestations. The case-to-case interval is about 3 weeks. The organism may be carried in the throat for periods up to 2 months or longer after natural clinical recovery or successful antibiotic treatment.

LABORATORY DIAGNOSIS OF
M. PNEUMONIAE INFECTIONS

Routine Laboratory Findings

The white blood cell count is usually within normal limits or only slightly raised in contrast to bacterial pneumonia. The erythrocyte sedimentation rate is often markedly elevated. Cold haemagglutinins or *Streptococcus MG* agglutinins occur in about 30 to 60 per cent and 10 to 20 per cent of cases respectively. These two reactions depend on fortuitously shared haptens (saccharides) between the mycoplasma, the streptococcus and the I antigen of red cells. A positive Coombs test and reticulocytosis may be observed in conjunction with the cold haemagglutinins.

Specific Laboratory Diagnosis

A throat swab with transport medium or a specimen of sputum is taken for culture and inoculated onto plates and into diphasic medium (Chap. 5, Vol. II). Serum is collected as soon after onset of illness as possible and again after 3 weeks. Sera are tested by complement fixation and by metabolic inhibition tests. The complement-fixing reactions may be done with suspensions of the whole organism, heated or unheated, or with organisms grown on glass to avoid anti-complementary effects (see Vol. II). Alternatively, the glycolipid haptens may be extracted from the organism with chloroform-methanol and make an excellent concentrated CF antigen free from anti-complementary activity. The organism is not easy to isolate from clinical material and prolonged incubation of diphasic medium with periodic subculture may be required. Isolates are identified by glucose fermentation, β-haemolysis, haemadsorption and growth inhibition with specific antiserum. In one series the organism was isolated from 65 per cent of patients showing a fourfold rise of CF antibody; conversely of those from whom the organism was isolated only 4 per cent had very low or no CF antibody titre.

2. Infection with M. Hominis and T Strains

In contrast with the substantial body of evidence relating *M. pneumoniae* to human respiratory infection the role of *M. hominis* and T strains in genito-urinary infections is much less certain. There are good reasons for supposing that some cases of ovarian abscess, salpingitis, puerperal sepsis, haemorrhagic cystitis are caused by *M. hominis*. The relation of this mycoplasma to vaginitis, cervicitis, and urethritis in women and non-gonococcal urethritis in men is uncertain as both *M. hominis* and T strains are found in a substantial number of persons without symptoms and, basically, are probably related to the carrier's degree of sexual promiscuity; the incidence of T strains is, however, higher in patients with non-gonococcal urethritis and the question remains unresolved. It should be noted that some cases of non-gonococcal urethritis are caused by organisms of the *Chlamydia* group. No firm evidence has been adduced relating mycoplasma infection to Reiter's syndrome, rheumatoid arthritis, leukaemia or malignant disease.

Treatment and Prophylaxis of Mycoplasma Infections

Infection with *M. pneumoniae* may be treated with tetracycline (1 g/day) for 2 to 3 weeks or similarly with erythromycin. *M. hominis* is less sensitive to erythromycin so that tetracycline is the best all round choice. Chloramphenicol, streptomycin and other antibiotics to which mycoplasmas are sensitive *in vitro* are rarely used clinically. It has been shown that recruits with antibody to *M. pneumoniae* develop pneumonia less frequently when exposed in training camps than do those without such antibody; hence vaccination could, theoretically, be of value in controlling the infection. However, conventional inactivated *M. pneumoniae* vaccines produced 'vaccine enhanced' disease. Efforts to produce live attenuated vaccines with temperature-sensitive mutants are reported.

MYCOPLASMAS AND CELL CULTURES

The extensive use of cell cultures during the last two decades has revealed substantial problems and errors arising from the unsuspected contamination of cell cultures with mycoplasmas. There may be as many as 10^7 mycoplasmas/ml of culture without any gross cytopathic effects.

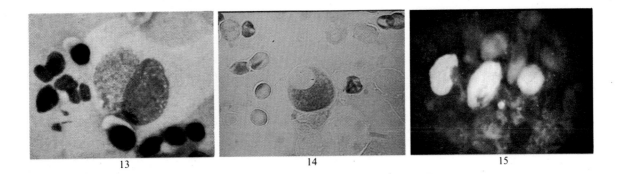

13   14   15

Plate 13   TRIC agent inclusion. Conjunctival scraping. Stained with Giemsa and examined by bright-field illumination. (By courtesy of Dr J. Treharne, Institute of Ophthalmology, London WC1.)

Plate 14   TRIC agent inclusion in conjunctival scraping. Stained with iodine. Bright-field illumination. (By courtesy of Dr J. Treharne.)

Plate 15   TRIC agent inclusions in conjunctival scraping. Stained by direct immunofluorescence with RBA counterstain. (By courtesy of Dr J. Treharne.)

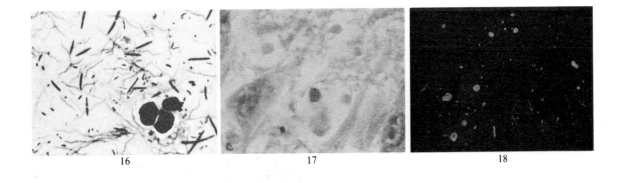

16   17   18

Plate 16   Film from a case of gingivo-stomatitis after staining for 10 min with dilute (1 in 10) carbol fuchsin. Large numbers of *Borr. vincentii* and fusiform bacilli (*Fusiformis fusiformis*) are seen. (From Gillies and Dodds *Bacteriology Illustrated*, 3rd edn. Churchill Livingstone, 1973.)

Plate 17   Section of hippocampus of brain of dog suffering from rabies. The large round or oval eosinophilic inclusion bodies (Negri bodies) in the cytoplasm of the nerve cells are diagnostic of the conditions. (Haemalum and alcoholic eosin. × 1000.) (By courtesy of Dr L. N. Markson, Central Veterinary Laboratory, Weybridge.)

Plate 18   Rabies virus in brain tissue. Immunofluorescent staining. (By courtesy of Dr L. M. Markson, Central Veterinary Laboratory, Weybridge.)

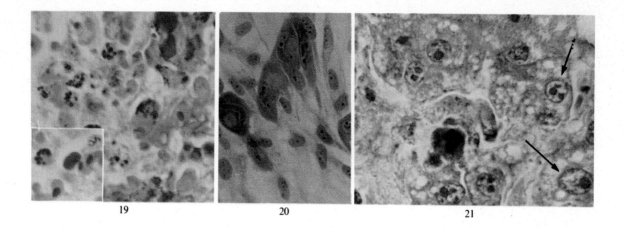

Plate 19   A section through a pock produced by the cowpox virus on the chorio-allantoic membrane of a chick embryo. The eosinophilic intracytoplasmic inclusions are obvious; they are often multiple and vary in size from small dots to large irregular masses. × 1000. Mann's stain. (From Swain and Dodds *Clinical Virology*, Churchill Livingstone, 1967.)

Plate 20   Intranuclear inclusions of cytomegalovirus in culture of human fibro-blasts. (Haematoxylin and eosin.)

Plate 21   A section of liver from a fatal case of yellow fever. The arrows point towards the sharply defined eosinophilic intranuclear inclusions, *Torres bodies*. Mann's stain. × 800. (From Swain and Dodds *Clinical Virology*, Churchill Livingstone, 1967.)

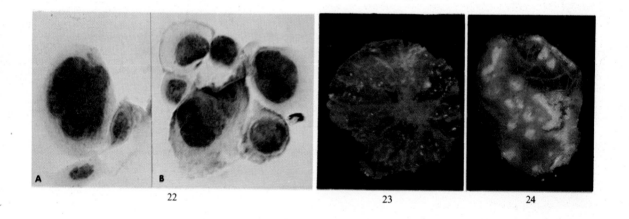

Plate 22   Scrapings from the base of a vesicle from a case of herpes varicella. (*a*) A large multinucleate giant cell. (*b*) A syncytial mass of cytoplasm containing several nuclei. Similar appearances would be seen in scrapings from chicken pox lesions. (Giemsa stain). × 550. (From Swain and Dodds *Clinical Virology*, Churchill Livingstone, 1967.)

Plate 23   *Herpes hominis* virus type 1 on chorio-allantoic membrane.

Plate 24   *Herpes hominis* virus type 2 on chorio-allantoic membrane.

Table 52.1. Biological properties of various species of mycoplasma of human origin.

Species	Degree of growth		Hydrolysis of		Fermentation of sugars		Aerobic reduction of Tetrazolium	Haemolysis	Haemadsorption	Yeast extract	Growth in thallium acetate (0.01%)	Growth in Methylene Blue (0.001%)	Animal pathogenicity
	aerobic	anaerobic or micro-aerophilic	Arginine	Urea	glucose	mannose							
M. hominis	++	+	+	–	NC	NC	NC	±	Neg	NR	++	–	None (Mice)
M. salivarium	–	++	+	–	NC	NC	NC	–	Neg	NR	++	–	..
M. orale Type 1	±	++	+	–	NC	NC	NC	–	Pos**	R	++	–	..
M. orale Type 2	±	++	+	–	NC	NC	NC	–	Neg	NR	++	–	..
M. orale Type 3	–	++	+	–	NC	NC	NC	–	Pos**	R	++	–	..
M. fermentans	±	++	+	–	A	NC	NC	–	Neg	NR	++	–	Subcut. abscesses in mice
M. pneumoniae	++	+	–	–	A	A	F	β (sheep, guinea-pig rbc)	Pos*	R	++	++	Pneumonia in hamster, some sp. of mice and cotton rats
*M. primatum**	±	++	+	–	NC	NC	NC	–	Neg	..	++	–	None (mice)
T-strains	–	++	–	+	NC	NC	NC	± (guinea-pig rbc)	Pos	R	–	..	

Key: ± to +++ = increasing degree of growth or size of colony.
A = acid produced; NC = no change; F = formazan produced.
± or – = no or green change in erythrocyte overlay.
* Mainly simian; one human isolate (Navel). Some workers include *M. Lipophilia* in the human flora (see Purcell and Chanock, 1969).

** with chicken erythrocytes; variable, but see Purcell and Chanock, 1969.
* with rat, guinea pig, monkey and chicken erythrocytes.

β = change resembling β haemolysis
NR/R = not required/required.
.. = information not available.

The depletion of arginine in the cultures interferes with the replication of viruses such as adenovirus and herpes virus. The mycoplasma nucleases alter the nuclear material of the cell and nucleic acid metabolism (e.g. thymidine incorporation) and there is substantial interference with cell membrane function as a consequence of the mycoplasmas lined up on its surface.

Many of the properties of mycoplasmas, e.g. filterability, sensitivity of infectivity to lipid solvents, viral interference by arginine depletion, haemadsorption, resemble those of a myxo- or leuko-virus and have been mistaken for them. The mycoplasma cells on the surface of cells in cultures have been misidentified as rubella virions. Misleading serological results arise from the same species of mycoplasma in different species of cell or virus.

The mycoplasma species commonly found are *M. hominis, M. orale I, M. hyorhinis* (a swine species probably from trypsin). Sporadic isolations include *M. pulmonis* (mice), *M. gallisepticum* (chickens), *A. laidlawii* and *M. arginini*. These contaminants probably came originally from the oropharynx of the operators or the ingredients of the cell culture media. They are now spread and maintained by cross-infection among different lines of cell during handling, either as the result of aerosol formation or of contamination of bulk media used for successive sets of cultures.

Contamination is best detected by anaerobic culture of a cell suspension on plates and in sloppy mycoplasma agar. Immunofluorescence with antisera to the common contaminating mycoplasma species and 'flying coverslip' of cells is also effective.

Eradication of the mycoplasmas is difficult as testified by the large number of methods described. Treatment with the antibiotic Tylosin and sodium aurothiomalate as described by Cross, Goodman and Shaw (1967), probably offers the best chances of success. In addition, treatment with antiserum against the mycoplasma may also be of value.

REFERENCES AND FURTHER READING

CHANOCK, R. M., HAYFLICK, L. & BARILE, M. F. (1962) Growth on artificial medium of an agent associated with atypical pneumonia and its identification as a PPLO. *Proceedings of the National Academy of Sciences, U.S.A.,* **48**, 41.

CROSS, G. F., GOODMAN, M. R. & SHAW, E. J. (1967) Detection and treatment of contaminating mycoplasmas in cell culture. *Australian Journal of Experimental Biology and Medical Science,* **45**, 201–212.

DAVIS, R. E. & WHITCOMBE, R. F. (1971) Mycoplasmas, Rickettsiae, and Chlamydiae; possible relation to yellow diseases and other disorders of plants and insects. *Annual Review of Phytopathology,* **9**, 119–154.

GUZE, L. B. (1968) (ed.) *Microbial Protoplasts, Spheroplasts and L forms.* Baltimore: Williams and Wilkins.

HAYFLICK, L. (1965) Cell cultures and mycoplasmas. *Texas Reports on Biology and Medicine,* **23** (suppl. 1), 285–303.

HAYFLICK, L. (1967) (ed.) Biology of the mycoplasma. *Annals of the New York Academy of Sciences,* **143**, 1–824.

HAYFLICK, L. (1969) (ed.) *The Mycoplasmatales and the L-phase of Bacteria.* Amsterdam: North Holland.

MACPHERSON, I. (1968) Mycoplasmas in tissue culture. *Journal of Cell Science,* **1**, 145–168.

MARMION, B. P. & GOODBURN, G. M. (1961) Effect of gold salts on Eaton's primary atypical pneumonia agent and other observations. *Nature,* **189**, 247.

MARMION, B. P. (1967) The mycoplasmas; new information on their properties and their pathogenicity for man. In *Recent Advances in Medical Microbiology,* edited by A. P. Waterson. London: Churchill.

PURCELL, R. H. & CHANOCK, R. M. (1969) Mycoplasmas of human origin. In *Diagnostic Procedures for Viral and Rickettsial Infections,* 4th edition, pp. 786–825. Edited by Lennette and Schimdt. American Public Health Association Inc.

53. Pathogenic Fungi

Fungi and yeasts constitute the *Eumycetes*. They are eukaryotes with a differentiated nucleus and rigid chitinous cell walls and were formerly regarded as plants without chlorophyl or differentiation of root, stem and leaves. They are now regarded as neither plants nor animals and are grouped with protozoa, slime moulds and most algae as Higher Protista. Bacteria, including all the actinomycetes, are prokaryotes and belong to the Lower Protista.

Role in Nature and Human Life

The yeasts and fungi are heterotrophs, needing organic compounds as nutrients, and their role in nature is as scavengers, breaking down the complex carbohydrates and proteins of the dead bodies of other organisms. Only a few of them are pathogens and most of those affecting man are facultative, rather than obligate, parasites. Unlike most microorganisms, fungi have mainly been of service to man, as in the making of bread, fermented drinks, cheese and, more recently, useful organic chemicals including antibiotics. They have caused only a small proportion of infectious disease in the past, but with the increasing control of those due to bacteria and viruses through sanitation, education, immunization and chemotherapy, they are becoming more important. Nowadays there are as many reported deaths from mycoses (fungus infections) in the U.S.A. as there are from whooping cough, diphtheria, scarlet fever, typhoid, dysentery and malaria put together (Emmons, Binford and Utz, 1970). Furthermore, the superficial fungus infections, such as athlete's foot, though not dangerous, are extremely common. Britain is fortunate in that the potentially fatal mycoses that may affect otherwise healthy people are rare but, as in any technologically developed country, our ability to prolong the life of those dying from other diseases and to control most bacterial infections,

has led to an increase in infections due to 'opportunist' organisms, including many common fungi, which can establish themselves in debilitated people and are resistant to the commonly used antibiotics.

CLASSIFICATION

The *Eumycetes* can be divided into four morphological groups, each of which includes some pathogenic varieties.

1. The *moulds* (filamentous, mycelial fungi) grow as long filaments or hyphae which branch and interlace to form a meshwork or mycelium, and reproduce by the formation of various kinds of spores. The major part of the mycelium, the *vegetative mycelium*, grows on and penetrates into the substrate, absorbing nutrients for growth. Other hyphae constitute the *aerial mycelium* and protrude from the vegetative mycelium into the air; they form, and disseminate into the air, various kinds of spores. When grown to a large size on artificial medium, the mycelium is seen as a filamentous mould colony; this may become powdery on its surface due to the abundant formation of spores. The ringworm fungi are examples.

2. The *yeasts* are unicellular fungi which occur mainly as single spherical or ellipsoidal cells and reproduce by budding. On artificial media they form compact colonies with a creamy, mucoid or pasty consistence (e.g. like those of staphylococcus). *Cryptococcus neoformans* is the only important pathogen.

3. The *yeast-like fungi* grow partly as yeasts and partly as long filamentous cells joined end to end, forming a 'pseudo-mycelium', e.g. *Candida albicans*.

4. The *dimorphic fungi* grow either as filaments or as yeasts, according to the cultural conditions. Growth usually takes place in the mycelial form on culture media at 22°C and in the soil,

but in the yeast form on media at 37°C and in the animal body. *Histoplasma capsulatum* is the most important of them.

The systematic classification of the fungi, which is unfortunately not a convenient basis for the description of fungi of medical interest, is made on different lines from the simple morphological classification given above. Four classes are distinguished, mainly according to the nature of their sexual spores.

1. The *Phycomycetes* form usually non-septate hyphae and asexual 'sporangiospores' contained within a swollen spore case, or 'sporangium', borne at the ends of aerial hyphae (Fig. 53.1). Sexual spores are also found and are of two varieties ('oospore' and 'zygospore').

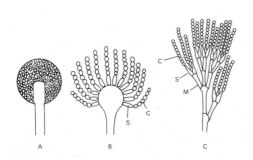

FIG. 53.1. (a) *Mucor* sp: sporangium containing sporangiospores. (b) *Aspergillus fumigatus:* conidiophore bearing sterigmata and conidia. (c) *Penicillium* sp: conidiophore bearing metulae, stergmata and conidia. (All × 160.)

2. The *Ascomycetes* form septate hyphae and various kinds of asexual spores including 'conidia' which are abstricted successively from the ends of specialized (often aerial) hyphae called 'conidiophores' (Fig. 53.1). Sexual 'ascospores' are formed, usually eight together, within a sac or 'ascus'.

3. The *Basidiomycetes* form septate hyphae and sexual 'basidiospores', usually four in number, from the ends of club-shaped structures called 'basidia'.

4. The *Fungi imperfecti* comprise all those of which the sexual or 'perfect' state has not yet been described and which therefore cannot be placed with certainty in one of the other three classes. Many imperfect fungi form septate hyphae and asexual conidia resembling those of *Ascomycetes*,

and their closest affinities lie with this class. A majority of the pathogenic moulds, yeasts, yeast-like fungi and dimorphic fungi belong to the group *Fungi imperfecti*. Various asexual spores are shown in Figs. 53.1 to 53.4.

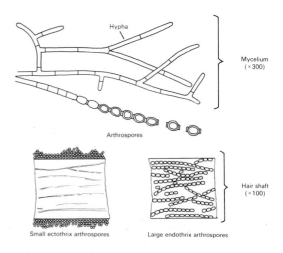

FIG. 53.2.

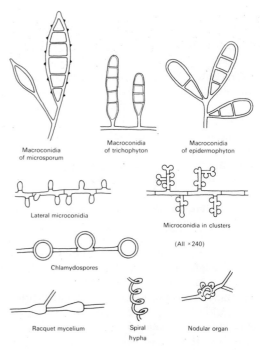

FIG. 53.3.

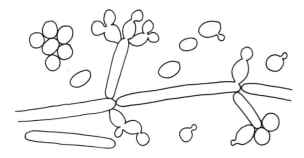

FIG. 53.4. *Candida albicans*: hyphae forming a pseudo-mycelium and giving rise to budding yeast-like cells (blastospores). (× 400.)

DESCRIPTION

It is difficult to generalize about the *Eumycetes,* but the medically relevant members have a number of common features. The basic elements of the morphology have been mentioned. The form of the spores is used in classification but their function in nature is reproduction and dissemination, usually by air. To display the microscopic features of fungi without disturbing the colony, cultures may be made in hanging drops of fluid medium or on the side of small agar blocks on a slide. The growth requirements of these heterotrophs are simple but for optimal growth and the development of yeast forms in the dimorphic fungi richer media may be required. Some fungi also need specific nutrients and can be used to assay these substances. Special media may be necessary for optimal sporulation. The fungi are all aerobes so that culture tubes need loose caps or cotton wool plugs. Growth occurs over a wide temperature range generally with an optimum about 28°C; a few grow poorly if the temperature is as high as 37°C. Fungal colonies grow more slowly than bacteria, taking several days or even weeks to appear. The features observed for identification are the rate of growth, the texture of the surface and the production of pigment. The appearances of fungal colonies are much more variable than those of bacterial colonies.

Susceptibility to physical and chemical agents varies but even the resistant spores are destroyed by the sterilization procedures used for bacteria. Heavy metal ions and non-ionic detergents such as Tego are convenient and effective chemical fungicides. In general, the fungi and yeasts are not as sensitive to acid as are bacteria and tolerate a pH below 6. Therapeutic antifungal agents are still few; two polyenes, nystatin and amphotericin B, are well established and others such as pimaricin and saramycetin are coming into use; griseofulvin inhibits dermatophytes and 5-fluorocytosine and clotrimazole are effective against yeasts. Antibacterial antibiotics usually have no effect either *in vivo* or *in vitro.* Cycloheximide inhibits many fungi but not the dermatophytes; it is too toxic for therapy, but can be used in selective media for the culture of dermatophytes.

The practical application of these growth requirements and susceptibilities to the isolation of fungi from clinical specimens, which are often contaminated with quicker growing bacteria, is the general use of a glucose peptone agar of acid pH containing either chloramphenicol or penicillin plus streptomycin. This is usually called Sabouraud's medium though it is very different from what he used. Incubation is carried out in air for three weeks, ideally in a 28°C incubator but often in practice at both room temperature and 37°C instead.

Metabolic activities are little used either for classification or laboratory diagnosis, except among the yeasts, nor is antigenic analysis much used, except in trying to develop useful serological tests. Animal pathogenicity varies, but the mouse is susceptible to most human pathogenic fungi. Animal inoculation is useful for isolating fungi from the environment but is usually no better than culture for clinical specimens.

The diseases caused by fungi have, like their agents, some features in common. An oversimplified grouping is into superficial infections acquired by contact (e.g. tinea, candidosis); subepidermal infections acquired by trauma (e.g. mycetoma); and systemic infection acquired by inhalation, e.g. histoplasmosis. The source of the first is usually man or animals and that of the other two is spores in the soil. The basis of pathogenicity is not known. The yeast, *Cryptococcus neoformans* has a capsule but no aggressins or toxins have been shown to be relevant to fungal disease in man. The infections run a slow course; the tissue reaction is often granulomatous but may be negligible; diagnosis is usually based on direct microscopy (often of biopsies) and the naked eye and microscopical features of the organism in culture; treatment is slow even when successful and prevention is by avoidance (if possible) rather than by immunization. The systemic infections share these features and also have others in which they resemble pulmonary tuberculosis. They are acquired by inhalation; the initial focus in the lung is commonly asymptomatic and the infected person develops a positive delayed-type hypersensitivity reaction demonstrable in a tuberculin-type skin test with fungal antigen. There may be calcification or cavitation of the focus and possibly subsequent reactivation of the disease; and finally, if it disseminates, the infection carries a serious prognosis.

Laboratory diagnosis of the mycoses requires particularly careful collection of specimens as they are often contaminated with faster growing organisms, fungal as well as bacterial. For microscopy, the associated tissue cells need to be 'cleared', i.e. rendered transparent, with KOH or dimethyl sulphoxide, and, except for yeasts, wet unstained preparations are more revealing than dry, stained smears. Sections of biopsies stained by the periodic-acid-Schiff or methenamine-silver techniques may be extremely valuable. Culture is essential for identification of most fungi and proves useful in guiding treatment. Serological and skin tests may help but need experienced interpretation.

YEASTS AND YEAST-LIKE FUNGI

Yeasts are unicellular fungi. The cells are spherical, oval or elongated and reproduce by budding from one or more points. The buds usually separate, but one or two generations of buds may remain attached to each other. In such cases, when the cells are elongated and the terminal buds the longest, yeasts may appear filamentous (Fig. 53.4). This form is called a pseudomycelium. The yeasts producing a pseudomycelium are usually called yeast-like fungi, but the term, though established, is unsatisfactory and the distinction is not important medically; all yeasts will therefore be treated together. They stain Gram-positively.

The genera of yeasts of medical significance are *Candida, Torulopsis, Cryptococcus* and *Pityrosporum*. It has always been a problem to decide which species within these genera are pathogenic and which are not and, as the strains isolated from man become more fully identified and our understanding of opportunism grows, it is more and more difficult to draw a sharp dividing line.

CANDIDA

This is a genus of 'yeast-like fungi', several species of which occur naturally and can cause disease in man; about 90 per cent of the infections are due to *C. albicans*.

C. albicans is normally present in the mouth, intestine and vagina. It is responsible for infections in these sites and elsewhere when there is a disturbance of local conditions or impairment of the defence mechanisms.

Description

C. albicans grows normally as a thin-walled, non-capsulated oval yeast, 2·5 to 4·0 μm in diameter, but can give rise to pseudomycelium in the body and when aeration is poor also in culture. At temperatures below 26°C in nutritionally poor media such as cornmeal agar it characteristically produces thick-walled resting cells 7 to 17 μm in diameter, called chlamydospores. No sexual forms are known.

Characteristic also of *C. albicans* is the production of curved, elongated germ tubes within three hours when the yeast is transferred from a peptone-containing medium to mammalian serum at 37°C. The yeast and pseudomycelial forms stain readily with the Gram stain (Gram-positive) as well as with mycological stains.

Growth requirements are simple and on blood agar or Sabouraud's medium, colonies usually reach 0·5 mm in diameter after 18 hours and develop into high convex, off-white colonies 1·5 mm in diameter after two days. The behaviour of *C. albicans* in other media, its capacity to assimilate and ferment carbohydrates and its failure to split urea are used in differentiating it from other yeasts (torulopsis, cryptococcus) and from other candida species.

Candida is tolerant of acid and not sensitive to any of the antibacterial antibiotics; it thrives in its normal sites in the body when broad-spectrum antibiotics restrain the growth there of the normal bacterial flora. It is uniformly sensitive to the polyene antibiotics and clotrimazole and usually sensitive to 5-fluorocytosine.

Candida species are closely related antigenically to one another and none of their antigenic components has been found of practical value either in recognizing species or in understanding their pathogenicity.

C. albicans is pathogenic for rabbits, guinea-pigs and mice. When it is given intravenously to rabbits or mice, abscesses develop in the kidney. Other species are not pathogenic for animals except C. tropicalis and C. stellatoidea when given in large doses to mice. The basis of the pathogenicity either for animals or man is not known.

INFECTIONS DUE TO C. ALBICANS

C. albicans is part of the normal flora of the mouth, intestine and vagina and it may also be isolated in health from adjacent skin, though other yeasts normally predominate. It is also an opportunistic pathogen giving rise to local inflammation under a wide variety of circumstances. Infection is usually endogenous though cross-infection may occur, as between infants in a nursery. The inflammatory reaction is normally mild and superficial with a polymorphonuclear exudate but systemic invasion may occur in drug addicts and patients on immunosuppressive or cytotoxic therapy.

The sites affected are principally mucosae where candida is normally present in health and on moist areas of the skin. Infection of the mucosa is known as 'thrush'. Less common manifestations are secondary infections in the lower respiratory tract and urinary infections. Septicaemia with localization in meninges, endocardium, bone-marrow or kidney may occur in patients seriously ill with other conditions. The opportunistic candida infections may occur in pregnancy, neonatal debility, senility, minor trauma, continued exposure of the skin to moisture or when the patient is debilitated by diabetes or alcoholism. Addiction

to drugs and the medical profession's increasingly active disturbance of the normal body flora with antibiotics and of the natural defensive reactions of the body with immunosuppressive drugs and cytotoxic agents have led to pulmonary and systemic infections with candida among other opportunistic invaders becoming a significant problem in the hospital medicine of today.

The commonest candida infection is vaginitis, or *vaginal thrush*. Pregnant women are particularly susceptible. There is a whitish discharge with a pH below 5·2 and, microscopically, some pus cells and many yeasts, including pseudomycelial forms, can be seen. In infections due to trichomonas and bacteria, the discharge is more purulent and less acid.

Oral thrush occurs in debilitated or bottle fed infants. Creamy white patches are found covering red, raw areas of mucous membrane and tongue. It also occurs in adults in angular cheilitis, in 'sore mouth' caused by ill-fitting dentures and, all too frequently after prolonged courses of oral antibacterial therapy.

Infections of the *skin* are common in diabetes, especially where the skin is frequently moist or mildly traumatized. Lesions are characterized by erythema, exudation and desquamation and occur commonly in the axilla and groin, on the vulva and glans penis, in the inframammary folds and around the umbilicus. It may involve the whole napkin area in infants. In those whose hands or feet are frequently in water, it affects the interdigital clefts, the skin folds round the nail and sometimes the nail itself.

Infections of the *intestine* occur in infants, the aged and those on long courses of oral antibiotics. There may be pruritis ani or diarrhoea, and a great increase in the proportion of yeasts in the faecal flora but little cellular exudate.

Bronchial and *pulmonary candidosis* also occur but are not common. When yeasts are persistently present in sputum it is usually because they have colonized pockets of secretion in a bronchial tree damaged by bronchiectasis, tuberculosis or carcinoma. The sputum then contains many yeasts but is often mucoid and gelatinous rather than purulent.

Systemic infections may occur when the organism is inoculated directly into the tissues as in drug addicts, after heart valve operations, in severe generalized disease such as leukaemia especially when treated with cytotoxic drugs, steroids and antibiotics, and occasionally in small children with no clear predisposing condition. There is often no obvious local site of preceding candida infection.

Laboratory Diagnosis

The organism survives well in exudate collected on swabs and may even multiply if there is delay in transmission to the laboratory. It may be demonstrated microscopically in wet preparations or Gram-stained smears and grows readily on blood agar or Sabouraud's medium. The growth of competing bacteria may be restrained by incorporating antibacterial antibiotics. Usually it is unnecessary to identify the species of a yeast from clinical material, but *C. albicans* may often be quickly identified by its colonial appearance and by obtaining a positive result in the germ-tube test. More formal identification requires in addition, the demonstration of pseudomycelium production, which separates it from other genera of yeasts, and a characteristic pattern of assimilation of sugars, which differentiates it from other species of *Candida*.

The interpretation of a finding of *C. albicans* depends on a comparison of the numbers of the organism, both absolute and in relation to other organisms, with the numbers normally expected in the specimen and also on knowing whether previous specimens in the series have shown similar results.

The significance of small numbers of yeasts in a single specimen of vaginal discharge cannot always be assessed even with experience and judgment. A single isolation from blood may or may not be significant. It must therefore neither be dismissed as a contaminant nor be considered as evidence of septicaemia. Further attempts must be made to demonstrate its presence. Even if further cultures are negative, the first isolation may have been a signal that casual breaches in the normal defences of the body are occurring.

Serology and skin testing are not yet of established value in diagnosis. Patients with chronic candida infections and healthy members of the general population may have similar levels of agglutinins and precipitins in their sera.

Treatment and Prevention

It is important before treating a candida infection to try to identify the underlying circumstances that have allowed it to establish itself. If the underlying disturbance such as poor hygiene or diabetes can be corrected, the body will usually deal with the yeast. Treatment will, however, shorten the process. When the underlying condition cannot be altered quickly as in pregnancy, debility or serious disease, the usual treatment is to give the polyene nystatin locally. Nystatin is very poorly absorbed from the gut so that systemic infections must be treated with amphotericin B, another polyene (which unfortunately has to be given intravenously), with 5-fluorocytosine or with clotrimazole. Superficial infections can also be treated with other polyenes and one of them, trichomycin, is often used in vaginitis as it is effective against trichomonas as well as against candida. However, if this is done to avoid making an aetiological diagnosis, the underlying reasons for the infection will not be clear and appropriate further action to prevent recurrence cannot be taken.

Endogenous infections cannot be prevented by immunization, but can be made less likely by good medical practice and avoiding injudicious use of antibacterial antibiotics and immunosuppressive and cytotoxic agents. Cross-infection in nurseries can be controlled and prevented by the general measures that apply to infections transmitted by contact, fomites or infected dust.

Other Species of Candida

Several species of *Candida* other than *C. albicans* occur naturally in man—*C. tropicalis*, *C. pseudotropicalis*, *C. krusei*, *C. parapsilosis*, *C. stellatoidea* and *C. guilliermondii*. The sites are similar to those where *C. albicans* is found, but the frequency with which each species is found differs with the site. *C. albicans* predominates in the mouth, *C. parapsilosis* on the skin and *C. stellatoidea* and *C. albicans* may be present in equal numbers in the vagina. Like *C. albicans*, all the other species can cause disease, *C. tropicalis* most commonly, but together they are not responsible for more than 10 per cent of human cases of candidosis.

The tests used to differentiate the species of

Candida include the ability to produce germ tubes in mammalian serum; the type of growth on Sabouraud agar, in Sabouraud broth and on blood agar; the pattern of growth and production of chlamydospores in nutritionally poor media; the fermentation and assimilation of sugars; and pathogenicity in experimental animals.

TORULOPSIS

This genus is very similar to *Candida* but produces no pseudomycelium. One species, *T. glabrata*, is found in the same body sites as *C. albicans* and has been shown to be an opportunistic pathogen capable of establishing itself in the blood, lungs and urinary tract of debilitated patients (Langston and Eickhoff, 1970). The colonies on sheep's blood agar are much smaller than those of *Candida* and, of the commonly used sugars, only glucose and trehalose are assimilated or fermented. It is differentiated from *Cryptococcus* by its lack of a capsule and failure to hydrolyse urea.

CRYPTOCOCCUS

This genus of yeasts produces no pseudomycelium and differs from both *Candida* and *Torulopsis* in possessing a urease. There is one pathogenic species, *C. neoformans*, which is widespread in nature and present in particularly large numbers in pigeon faeces. It has been isolated from human faeces and skin. It causes sporadic, chronic and often fatal disease in man and in a variety of domestic animals.

Description

C. neoformans is a spherical yeast with a capsule of variable thickness. Cells measure from 5 to 20 μm in diameter and the capsule can be well seen in wet India ink preparations. The yeast is stained by Gram's method (positive) and by PAS, and its capsule by mucicarmine. It has simple growth requirements and grows more quickly at 37°C than at 22°C (at which temperature growth may not be apparent for two weeks). Cultures are cream to brownish in colour and may be so mucoid as to flow down an agar slope. No germ tubes develop in mammalian serum at 37°C. The only metabolic activity of note is the splitting of urea which differentiates *Cryptococcus* from other yeasts found in human material. The perfect state of *C. neoformans* is a basidiomycete, *Leucosporidum neoformans* (Shadomy, 1970).

C. neoformans is pathogenic for mice and intraperitoneal injection of a culture or exudate produces enlarged mesenteric glands and spleen and gelatinous masses in abdomen and brain after three to four weeks. It does not induce new growths but was named *neoformans* because the local lesion following subcutaneous inoculation looked to early workers like a myxoma.

Pathogenesis

The route of infection and pathogenesis of cryptococcosis in man are not yet well understood, but appear to be similar to those in tuberculosis. The commonest mode of infection is probably by the inhalation of dust contaminated with pigeon faeces. Birds are not susceptible to infection with *C. neoformans*, possibly because of their high body temperature, but their faeces provide a very rich and apparently selective medium for the growth of the yeast. The initial lesion in man is a small granuloma in the lung which heals with fibrosis but without calcification. Blood-borne dissemination may occur to lymph nodes, skin, bones or meninges. In any site the yeasts may be few and the reaction slight or there may be many yeast cells with a relatively acellular granulomatous reaction. Large lesions produce their effects mainly by their size. Skin lesions may ulcerate. Meningeal infection normally leads to a slow and irregularly progressive meningoencephalitis, which is fatal if untreated. The disease is unfortunately often only recognized at necropsy and even then may be mistaken for tuberculosis. Histologically the gelatinous exudate is found to consist almost entirely of encapsulated yeasts with very few inflammatory cells.

Laboratory Diagnosis

Specimens submitted include cerebrospinal fluid, biopsy material, sputum and exudate from skin lesions. In the cerebrospinal fluid the cellular reaction and chemical changes resemble those in tuberculous meningitis and if the capsules are small and the diagnosis not considered, the organisms may be mistaken for lymphocytes or red blood cells. Wet films should be made and mixed with India ink to show up the capsule by contrast. Cultures from cerebrospinal fluid are made on Sabouraud and blood agar and kept for at least two weeks. The small, off-white colonies, if they are scanty and not examined microscopically, may be mistaken for micrococci and the diagnosis may be missed. Identification is based on the presence of capsules, growth at 37°C, the failure to produce any pseudomycelium, the presence of urease and the results of intraperitoneal injections into mice.

Serological tests may provide epidemiologically valuable evidence of subclinical infection. For example, antibodies are much commoner in pigeon fanciers than in the general population. They are not yet of any diagnostic help in the individual patient. Skin tests are not of any value even epidemiologically.

TREATMENT AND PREVENTION. The organism is sensitive to amphotericin B, 5-fluorocytosine and clotrimazole. Whilst our knowledge of the natural course of the disease is limited and dissemination remains a possibility, treatment is usually indicated even though a lesion may appear localized and not progressive. Prevention and control are not yet practicable.

PITYROSPORUM

This is a genus of yeasts which reproduce by budding from a wide base and appear to have an absolute nutritional requirement for lipid. Two species are found in man, *P. ovale* and *P. orbicularis*.

P. ovale is oval or bottle-shaped, 2 to 3 μm × 4 to 5 μm. It is Gram-positive and a normal inhabitant of the skin. It is particularly evident in scales from dandruff and though some consider it may play a part in the aetiology of pityriasis capitis and seborrhoeic dermatitis, it is generally regarded as being only a harmless saprophyte. Growth occurs in 3 to 5 days at 37°C on Sabouraud or malt

extract agar smeared with oleic acid, olive oil or butter fat.

P. orbicularis, previously called *Malassezia furfur*, is thick-walled and more variable in size and shape than *P. ovale*, but may be cultured in the same way. It is regarded as the cause of pityriasis versicolor, a chronic asymptomatic infection of the skin of the trunk which is not uncommon in tropical countries. The lesions are brownish, desquamating macules which fluoresce bright yellow in Wood's light. Gram-stained smears of skin scrapings or sellotape strippings will show yeasts and short lengths of pseudomycelium. Culture is rarely carried out. Treatment is soap and water followed by applications of sodium thiosulphate solution or salicylic acid ointment.

FILAMENTOUS FUNGI

Most of the 100 000 species of fungi are filamentous, i.e. they are *moulds* and their classification is complex. Most are harmless saprophytes but about 100 species are true or opportunistic pathogens of man; these are widely scattered among the taxonomic groups.

COMMON SAPROPHYTIC MOULDS

Most moulds occur in the soil and their airborne spores often contaminate foodstuffs, media and laboratory specimens. Some can also occur as secondary invaders, e.g. in the external ear or lung. It is important to note, however, that *their presence in diagnostic cultures must not be taken as denoting an aetiological relationship*. Varieties commonly encountered include *Rhizopus*, *Mucor*, *Aspergillus* and *Penicillium*. *Rhizopus* and *Mucor* are phycomycetes with non-septate hyphae, asexual sporangiospores, and sexual zygospores which are formed by conjugation of two hyphae at their tips (Fig. 53.1). *Aspergillus* and *Penicillium* species are either ascomycetes or fungi imperfecti, having septate hyphae, asexual conidia and in some cases sexual ascospores. Their colonies are commonly pigmented yellow, green or black. The conidial chains of *Aspergillus* arise from finger-like 'sterigmata' which radiate without branching from the expanded bulbous tip of the conidiophore. Those of *Penicillium* arise, brush-like, from sterigmata borne on the tips of several terminal branches of the conidiophore (Fig. 53.1). The important antibiotic substance, penicillin, is derived from *Penicillium notatum* and *P. chrysogenum*.

DISEASES CAUSED BY FILAMENTOUS FUNGI

A clinically recognizable disease, such as ringworm or mycetoma, may be caused by a number of different fungi (and sometimes by other types of microorganism) but one fungus does not often give rise to quite different diseases. It is therefore convenient and economical to describe the filamentous fungi in relation to the kinds of disturbance caused in man.

1. Infections of keratinized tissue: dermatophyte infections, (ringworm), other infections of hair and skin.

2. Infections of other exposed surfaces: bronchopulmonary infections, infections of the nose and sinuses and gastrointestinal tract, otomycosis, ophthalmic infections.

3. Infections of deeper tissues: mycetoma, chromoblastomycosis, subcutaneous phycomycosis.

4. Sensitization.

5. Poisoning.

The importance of fungal infections lies in their being often disfiguring or disabling and thus interfering with the patient's wellbeing or working capacity; they are themselves rarely a cause of death. The prevalence and geographical distribution of the conditions and the fungi responsible are very variable. The ringworms are very common and world wide, but some of their causative agents have limited distributions. The other conditions are not common; mycetoma affects the unshod in warm climates, and opportunistic infections spreading on exposed surfaces in seriously ill patients are becoming an increasing problem in the specialist hospital practice of the technologically advanced societies. The source of an infecting fungus may be other people, animals, dust or the soil and it is acquired by contact, through the air or by accidental inoculation. Sensitization may accompany clinical infection, but also occurs without it. Poisoning is by the ingestion of fungi that are themselves toxic or of food material rendered toxic by the growth of fungi in it.

DERMATOPHYTE INFECTIONS: RINGWORM OR TINEA

These very common infections of skin, hair and nails are caused by members of a group of some 30 to 40 related filamentous fungi that can digest keratin. The saprophytic members of this group, which normally live in the soil and from which the human and animal pathogens have probably been derived, play an important role in nature, breaking down the keratinized tissues of dead animals and scurf and hair spread from live ones. From 1843 when the first member of the group was described until quite recently, only the asexual forms of any of these fungi were known. They were therefore placed in the Fungi Imperfecti in three genera, *Epidermophyton*, *Microsporum* and *Trichophyton* distinguished by the morphology of their large asexual spores, or 'macroconidia' (Fig. 53.3). Recently, however, the sexual forms of 'perfect states' of about half the *Microsporum* and *Trichophyton* species have been identified. They belong to two genera of the Ascomycetes, *Nannizzia* and *Arthroderma* respectively. The species whose perfect states have been identified are mostly soil organisms but include some common pathogens, both zoophilic and anthropophilic. No free-living or perfect states have yet been found for the highly adapted human dermatophytes *Epidermophyton floccosum*, *Microsporum audouinii* or *Trichophyton rubrum* and they may have disappeared in the course of evolution.

About half the species of these keratinophilic fungi so far recognized have been isolated from disease in man or animals and in this chapter they will all be referred to as dermatophytes and by their old generic names, because they will undoubtedly be so called by doctors long after their perfect states have been recognized. Because fungi are no longer classified as plants, the soil species may sometimes now be referred to as saprobes rather than saprophytes.

Although separated into different genera, the dermatophytes have many features in common and can conveniently be described together. Mycological and dermatological texts may be consulted for fuller details of the differences between the species, their geographical distribution and their manifestations.

The following six species are responsible for 90 per cent of the dermatophyte infections of man in Britain: *Microsporum audouinii*, *M. canis*, *Trichophyton rubrum*, *T. mentagrophytes*, *T. verrucosum*, and *Epidermophyton floccosum*.

DESCRIPTION

The dermatophytes causing infection in man live normally on the keratinized surfaces of man or domestic animals and only occasionally in the soil. They do not invade non-keratinized tissues.

Their *morphology* in the host is simple, consisting only of hyphae and arthrospores formed by segmentation of a hypha into a row of separate thick-walled cells (Fig. 53.2). In artificial culture, two kinds of asexual spores, microconidia and macroconidia are also formed (Fig. 53.3). The microconidia are unicellular, small (2 to 5 μm), round or pear-shaped, borne laterally or terminally, singly or in clusters. The macroconidia are multicellular and their size, shape and surface are used to differentiate the genera (Fig. 53.3). In *Microsporum* they are usually numerous, spindle-shaped, with a rough surface and 5 to 15 segments and measure from 40 to 150 μm in length. In *Epidermophyton*, they are pear-shaped with a smooth surface and 2 to 4 segments, and measure 30–40 μm. Two or three often arise from the same hypha. In *Trichophyton* they are generally scanty and often irregular in shape; characteristic ones are smooth, cylindrical, with 2 to 6 segments and 10 to 50 μm long. In some species the hyphae may show identifying features such as spirals, expansions just proximal to the septa ('racquet' hyphae) or irregular terminal protrusions looking like antlers. The production of sexual spores is not necessary for diagnosis but it can however be observed in some species grown on soil 'baited' with hair or on special media. Two different strains of a fungus may be required for 'mating'.

The basic growth requirements of the dermatophytes are those of any heterotroph, but some species require, in addition, specific nutrients such as thiamine, histidine or inositol. Many require richer media for optimum growth and special media for optimum sporulation. All grow at room temperature, but 26 to 28°C is the optimum for growth of most dermatophytes.

Sabouraud's medium is suitable for isolation and is improved by adding cycloheximide which inhibits many common contaminants but does not affect dermatophytes. A further modification is Dermatophyte Test Medium (Taplin *et al.*, 1969) on which all dermatophytes produce enough alkali to turn the medium red.

Colonial appearances may be characteristic of species but often vary considerably within species and even in the same strain and on different makes of the same medium, so considerable experience is required for recognition. The relevant features are the rate of growth and the folding and zoning of the colony, its surface texture and the pigmentation of the colony and of the medium.

The sensitivity of dermatophytes to physical and chemical agents is similar to that of other fungi. Spores are not killed by the mild wet heat of laundering so their destruction in clothes may require boiling or formaldehyde vapour. The benzoic and salicylic acids of Whitfield's ointment are fungicidal. Griseofulvin is fungistatic to all dermatophytes *in vitro* but not all infections respond to treatment with it.

Metabolic activities are only rarely used in the identification of the dermatophytes though their common ability to utilize keratin is the basis of their role in nature and in disease. Their antigenic structure is not used in either identification or classification.

PATHOGENICITY

The basis of pathogenicity of the dermatophytes is not understood. The fungus grows in the keratinized layers of the skin, throughout the thickness of nails and on and inside hair shafts, the keratin being attacked by extracellular enzymes. Except in very rare circumstances the hyphae do not penetrate into living tissue and the mechanisms by which these superficial infections stimulate an inflammatory reaction are not clear. It could be a reaction to products of fungal metabolism (though no such substances have been demonstrated) or to fungal constituents. The sensitization of distant uninfected areas of skin, as in cheiropompholyx implies that fungus antigens must diffuse out of the keratinized layers.

Different species have predilections for different hosts. Man is the main or only source of the *anthropophilic* species and another animal that of the *zoophilic* species. The most important anthropophilic species are *M. audouinii*, *T. rubrum*, *T. mentagrophytes* (*var. interdigitale*), *E. floccosum*, *T. sulphureum* (*T. tonsurans*), *T. schoenleinii* and *T. violaceum*. Infections due to them are often mild and may persist throughout life, flaring up only occasionally. Those due to *M. audouinii* usually disappear at puberty.

Of the zoophilic species, *T. verrucosum* from cattle and *T. mentagrophytes* (*var. granulare*) and *M. canis* from dogs and cats are the commonest agents of infection in man. They often cause a more severe reaction but are more readily cured than infections with anthrophilic species. Human infection with species normally present in the soil, e.g. *M. gypseum*, does occur but is rare.

As well as a variable pathogenicity for different hosts, the dermatophytes vary in their ability to attack particular structures or areas of the body. *M. audouinii* usually confines its attacks to the hair of children under the age of puberty and no *Microsporum* species attacks nails. *T. rubrum* is a common cause of skin and nail infections but does not attack hair. *E. floccosum* usually attacks the skin of groins or feet, rarely attacks the upper half of the body and never the hair.

Mycologists classify the dermatophytes on the basis of the morphology of their perfect states where known, but for the purposes of medical microbiology identification is based on colonial appearances and on the morphology of the macroconidia, the microconidia and the hyphae *in vitro*. Recognition is aided in practice by a knowledge of the source of the specimen and in the case of hair infections by the relationship of the spores to the hair shaft.

DISEASES DUE TO DERMATOPHYTES

The usual name given to these infections is ringworm or tinea, and this name is qualified by the name of the site affected, e.g. tinea capitis or tinea pedis, but special names are also used in dermatology for particular manifestations, e.g. kerion, cheiropompholyx, favus.

When skin is infected the fungus spreads radially in the dead keratinized layer in the form of branching hyphae with occasional arthrospores. The inflammatory reaction from living tissue below may be very mild and only a little dry scaling or hyperkeratosis is seen. More commonly there is irritation, erythema, oedema and some vesiculation especially at the spreading edge and this irregular pink periphery gave rise to the name ringworm. Animal strains of dermatophyte, secondary infection or vigorous treatment may give rise to an exaggerated reaction with weeping vesicles, pustules and ulceration. Clinically characteristic appearances may be associated with particular species, e.g. tinea imbricata with *T. concentricum*. The species that commonly attack the skin are *Trichophyton* spp., *E. floccosum* (groins and feet) and *M. canis*.

Infection of the nails renders them irregular, discoloured and friable. The fungus grows deep into the substance of the nail. The species usually responsible are *T. rubrum* and both human and animal strains of *T. mentagrophytes*.

When the scalp is infected the fungus grows in the horny layer of the epidermis and down into the hair follicles. The hyphae surround and invade the hair shaft and once within it, they grow towards the area of new keratin production. The hair continues to grow and the hyphae break up into long chains of arthrospores, in some species only within the shaft (endothrix infections) but more commonly mainly on the outside (ectothrix infections) (Fig. 53.2). After two to three weeks' growth the weakened hair breaks off, leaving either a black dot at the follicle mouth as in endothrix infections or a 2 to 3 mm grey, spore-covered stump in the ectothrix varieties.

The species that produce ectothrix infections are *Microsporum spp.* and *T. mentagrophytes* (all with small spores of 2 to 3 μm) and *T. verrucosum* (with large spores of 4 to 6 μm). The endothrix infections are caused by *T. tonsurans, T. violaceum, T. soudanense* and *T. schoenleinii*. The last is the normal cause of favus.

In chronic infections of skin and nail, the patient becomes sensitized to fungal antigens and irritating vesicular lesions (cheiropompholyx) develop from time to time, most often between the fingers. They contain no fungus, but skin tests demonstrate a delayed hypersensitivity reaction to fungal antigen.

LABORATORY DIAGNOSIS

The laboratory diagnosis of ringworm is based on direct demonstration of fungal hyphae and arthrospores in the keratinized tissue by microscopy and on colonial appearances and hyphal and conidial morphology in culture. Genera are distinguished according to the morphology of the macroconidia and species by a combination of microscopic and colonial features. Metabolic activities are rarely relevant and skin tests, serology and animal inoculation are not used.

It is particularly important to collect appropriate material with as little contamination as possible. Cleansing of the area should be followed with 70 per cent ethanol, especially for nails. From skin lesions, scales, preferably 2 to 3 mm in diameter, should be scraped outwards with a blunt scalpel from the active periphery of the lesion and the domes of any vesicles snipped off.

Good material from nails is not easy to obtain. It is best to take scrapings from the nail with a scalpel but discard the most superficial samples. Some of the friable material from under the nail may be taken but ordinary nail clippings are not satisfactory: they often fail to yield any fungus.

For good results from hairs careful selection is important. The dusty stumps of ectothrix infections and the black dots of some endothrix infections can be recognized by the naked eye and if suspicious hairs are scanty, a Wood's lamp may show the fluorescence of hairs infected by *Microsporum spp.* and *T. schoenleinii*. The hairs when located should be plucked from the follicles with fine forceps. Specimens should be folded up in black paper, which makes it easier not to lose the material.

In surveys of tinea capitis, it is quick and convenient to collect spores by brushing the child's hair with a sterilizable and reusable, massage brush (Midgley and Clayton, 1972). Samples from the environment can be taken with convenient pieces of sterilized carpet with a short, stiff nap.

In the laboratory, the specimen is 'cleared' (i.e. the keratinized cells are rendered transparent so that the fungal filaments and spores are easier to see) usually with 20 per cent KOH or 40 per cent dimethylsulphoxide. The hyphae appear as slightly greenish, branching threads running across the outlines of the colourless cells of skin or nail. In hairs, the arthrospores are easier to see than the hyphae and their size (2 to 3 μm or 3 to 5 μm) and their position within or outside the hair shaft may allow a presumptive diagnosis of the species.

Culture is carried out by implanting fragments of specimen on Sabouraud's medium (preferably with added cycloheximide) or on Dermatophyte Test Medium. Contamination can be reduced by brief immersion of the specimen in 70 per cent ethanol. The best temperature is about 28°C; room temperature is slower but adequate. Colonies of dermatophytes may be visible in two or three days but some *Trichophyton* species may take two weeks. Cultures are not usually reported as negative until after three weeks.

Identification is based on the rate of growth, surface texture and pigment production of the colony, combined with the microscopical morphology of hyphae and spores, which is most clearly seen in young cultures.

Treatment and Prevention

Oral griseofulvin is the treatment of choice for hair infections and those due to *T. rubrum*. It may be less effective for infections of the skin and nails, particularly those of the feet and those due to the human strains of *T. mentagrophytes*, for which the older remedies, such as Whitfield's ointment, which contains salicylic and benzoic acids, should be tried first. Treatment with griseofulvin acts by preventing infection of the newly formed keratin and needs to be continued until previously infected keratin has been replaced. Ten days may be sufficient for a skin lesion and three weeks for hair, but months may be required for thick, horny skin and a year or more for nails, though nail infections often defeat all measures. Skin infections appear to respond well to a new local agent, tolnaftate.

Dermatophyte infections are not easy to prevent. They are carried by arthrospores, which are very resistant to environmental conditions and may be transmitted by direct contact, by indirect contact (e.g. brushes, clothes, duckboards) or through the air. Rising standards of hygiene in the home, at school and in hairdressing establishments have made dermatophyte infections less common: keeping feet clean and dry, hair well cared for, and avoiding the sharing or exchanging of caps, socks and underclothes, all reduce the likelihood of acquiring anthropophilic dermatophytes, such as *M. audouinii*. Communal baths and changing rooms, however, continue to be a source of infection and ordinary washing and laundering do not kill spores.

Knowledge of the transmissibility of animal ringworm from domestic pets infected with *M. canis*, from cattle and laboratory animals and from slow-moving wild animals like the hedgehog may reduce but does not prevent infections being acquired by children and occupationally exposed workers. It is usual to get rid of infected domestic pets as their treatment is difficult.

Other Infections of Hair and Skin

Three organisms infect hair and produce palpable nodules. The filamentous fungi, *Piedraia hortae* and *Trichosporon beigelii*, cause black and white piedra respectively. The bacterium *Corynebacterium* (*Nocardia*) *tenuis*, in combination with various micrococci, causes trichonocardiosis axillaris. *Cladosporum wernickii*, a fungus, causes tinea nigra and *Cornebacterium* (*Nocardia*) *minutissimum* causes erythrasma.

INFECTIONS OF OTHER EXPOSED SURFACES

Airborne fungal spores may reach any part of the respiratory tract, its associated sinuses, the conjunctivae or the ear canal, or may be ingested. Under normal circumstances they are eliminated but if the defences are impaired some organisms that are generally non-pathogenic may establish themselves and are then described as opportunistic pathogens. Impairment of the defences may be local or general, due to such natural causes as trauma, previous infection, diabetes or malignant disease or to medical intervention. Antibiotic therapy disturbs the normal ecology; cytotoxic drugs damage normal as well as abnormal cells; and steroids and other immunosuppressive drugs, used for moderating the body's natural (but not always beneficial) reactions to unfamiliar cells or antigens, often moderate them to the point where the body can no longer eliminate opportunistic fungi.

Bronchopulmonary Infections

Though fungal spores are being inhaled all the time, infection is rare. It is commonest in agricultural workers, who either have preexisting pulmonary disease or are on steroids and the organism is most frequently a species of *Aspergillus*. This genus is very widespread, common in decaying vegetation and the commonest contaminant in the laboratory. The most important species causing disease in man are *A. fumigatus*, which also causes pulmonary infection in birds and mycotic abortion in cattle, and *A. niger*.

Description of Aspergillus

The genus has septate hyphae and reproduces by asexual conidia (Fig. 53.1) produced in chains from elongated cells called *sterigmata*, which are themselves borne on the expanded end or vesicle of a specialized aerial hypha, the conidiophore. The morphology of these asexual sporing structures is used in species identification. Some species form sexual ascospores.

The growth requirements are simple and some species, such as *A. fumigatus*, are tolerant of temperatures up to 50°C. Colonies grow rapidly and are white and velvety at first but soon become green, yellowish or black and powdery as the conidia are formed.

Endotoxins are produced by *A. fumigatus* and though they may play a role in animal diseases, their relevance to disease in man has not been demonstrated.

Several types of bronchopulmonary disease occur and they may be mixed. The simplest is the 'saprophytic' colonization of a pre-existing cavity in which the fungus grows as a mycelial mass ('fungus ball' or aspergilloma). It slowly expands the cavity but there is no tissue invasion and there may be no symptoms or only a slightly productive cough. Various species may be responsible. Sometimes a true infection may occur in seriously ill patients on steroids. There is invasion of the lung with tissue destruction and a purulent granulomatous reaction. The fungus invades blood vessels causing thrombosis, and septic emboli may lodge in brain, heart and kidneys. The sputum contains blood and pus as well as fungal elements and the prognosis is poor. *A. fumigatus* is the commonest agent. Thirdly, the fungus may produce sensitization of the patient who then reacts to the inhalation of spores with asthmatic symptoms and production of mucofibrinous sputum containing eosinophils, i.e. an extrinsic allergic alveolitis.

Laboratory Diagnosis

Fresh sputum should be examined as a wet preparation for hyphae and sporing heads, pus cells and erythrocytes. The fungi causing bronchopulmonary disease grow easily and rapidly on Sabouraud's medium provided that cycloheximide has not been incorporated. The genus and the common species are readily identified by colonial appearances and the characters of the sporing structures.

Because of their frequency as contaminants, demonstration of an aspergillus species in a single specimen is of little significance except perhaps when it is *A. fumigatus* which is not a common contaminant. Repeated isolations or a demonstration of sporing heads in fresh sputum indicate that a particular species is established in the pulmonary tract.

Immunological reactions have been extensively studied but agreement has not yet been reached on the value either of serological tests or skin tests in bronchopulmonary infections due to aspergillus species. Animal inoculation is not used.

Treatment of these infections is not yet satisfactory. The pre-existing condition is usually serious or difficult to remedy. Vaccines and iodides have been used and more recently polyene antibiotics, both by their ordinary routes and by inhalation. Surgical resection may sometimes be employed with success.

INFECTIONS OF OTHER MUCOUS MEMBRANES

Fungus infections of the nose and adjacent sinuses and of the gastro-intestinal tract sometimes occur in patients with severe acidosis due to uncontrolled diabetes or in the late stages of terminal disease. The organisms are normally saprophytic members of the class *Phycomycetes*, usually belonging to the genera *Absidia*, *Rhizopus* or *Mucor*. The infection develops into a cellulitis with the organism showing a predilection for blood vessels as an aspergillus does when invading the lungs. Sinus infections spread rapidly to the orbit and brain and most cases have been fatal. The gastro-intestinal lesions are usually ulcers and if they are terminal, it may be very difficult to decide whether tissue invasion occurred before or after death, unless there is a cellular reaction, blood vessel invasion or septic infarcts.

The phycomycetes are common free-living fungi with non-septate hyphae and reproduce asexually by the production of large numbers of spores within a sporangium which develops at the end of an aerial hypha (Fig. 53.1). They grow and sporulate rapidly.

Wounds very rarely become infected with filamentous fungi.

Otomycosis

Chronic infections of the ear canal are usually bacterial but in 10 to 20 per cent of cases the predominant organism is a fungus belonging to one of the genera *Aspergillus*, *Rhizopus*, *Mucor* or *Penicillium*; most commonly it is *A. niger*. These opportunists are apparently able to colonize the area only after bacterial infection has damaged the surface. Relapses after treatment are common, local susceptibility may remain and it may be very difficult to re-establish the normal flora.

Ophthalmic Infections

After injury, bacterial infection and treatment with antibacterials and steroids, the cornea may be infected by opportunistic saprophytes, belonging to a number of genera including *Aspergillus*, *Fusarium*, *Cephalosporium*, *Curvularia* and *Penicillium*. These infections are still rare but important because they are destructive and early treatment is effective. Material for culture must be taken by curetting deep into the base or at the edge of the ulcer as ordinary swabs usually yield no fungus (Wilson and Sexton, 1968). *Fusarium* infections may be resistant to amphotericin B and require pimaricin, another polyene antibiotic.

INFECTIONS OF DEEPER TISSUES

These infections are a group occurring mainly in warm climates in people whose bare skin is exposed to soil, dust and recurrent minor trauma. The commonest and most widespread syndrome is *mycetoma* which may be due either to filamentous fungi or to higher bacteria belonging to the aerobic actinomycetes (see Chap. 24). Two other syndromes are *chromoblastomycosis* and *subcutaneous phycomycosis*; each may be caused by more than one fungus.

The infections are chronic and usually remain localized and are believed to be acquired by the traumatic inoculation of opportunistic organisms normally present in the soil or on thorns.

MYCETOMA

The condition most commonly affects the foot ('madura foot'). It presents as a swelling often with several sinuses discharging pus which may contain granules varying in size (0·5 to 2 mm) and in colour (black, red or buff), according to the organism responsible. Fungal agents include *Madurella mycetomi*, *M. grisea*, *Allescheria boydii* (of which the asexual conidial state is *Monosporium apiospermum*), *Cephalosporium falciforme*, *Phialophora jeanselmei* and *Leptosphaeria senegalensis*, but the list is still increasing. The chief actinomycetes responsible are *Nocardia brasiliensis*, *N. asteroides*, *Streptomyces somaliensis*, *S. madurae* and *S. pelletieri*. The disease is locally destructive to soft tissue, bone, tendon and nerve, but rarely spreads, even to lymph nodes.

Laboratory Diagnosis

The best specimen is an unfixed deep biopsy but pus or granules may be collected. Discharges and sinus swabs are always contaminated. Grains may be collected by allowing the sinuses to discharge into surgical gauze. The size and colour of the grains, which are colonies of the organism, may suggest the species responsible.

Wet preparations and Gram-stained smears should be made after crushing the granules if necessary. The size of the hyphae will show whether the organism is a fungus (more than 2 μm in width) or an actinomycete (usually less than 1 μm). In sections, the pattern and staining reaction of the granules often allow a tentative diagnosis of the species responsible.

Culture for the fungi should be carried out at 26°C on Sabouraud's medium (without cycloheximide); and for the actinomycetes at 37°C on blood agar or Loewenstein-Jensen medium. The fungi are all filamentous and septate but their colonial and microscopic appearances differ widely. Their identification is for experts. Some are sensitive to antibiotics *in vitro* but none is sensitive *in vivo*. The actinomycetes grow readily as dry, waxy or crumby colonies often reaching 2 to 3 mm in 3 to 5 days and showing buff or reddish pigment. The organisms appear as irregular Gram-positive filaments which branch but readily break up into short bacilli and cocci. *Nocardia spp.* may be semi-acid-fast and are sensitive to many antibacterial antibiotics, sulphones and sulphonamide-trimethoprim mixtures both *in vitro* and *in vivo*.

Streptomyces spp. have aerial filaments which terminally break up into coccoid forms in chains and look like conidia on a simple conidiophore. The species of *Streptomyces* causing mycetoma are less responsive to anti-bacterial therapy than those of *Nocardia*.

Serum antibodies and skin tests may be used to distinguish fungal from actinomycotic myce-toma but not to distinguish one fungal or actinomycetic cause from another.

The only effective treatment used to be surgery and still is for fungal mycetoma. Nocardial and some streptomyces infections respond to long courses of dapsone and to cotrimoxazole.

Prevention is not at present possible but the conditions are likely to disappear with better standards of living.

CHROMOMYCOSIS

This disease, formerly called chromoblasto-mycosis, is a chronic warty dermatitis, usually of legs and feet, caused by traumatic inoculation of one of five closely related pigmented fungi which normally grow on wood. Several of them were formerly called Hormodendrum but they are now called *Phialophora pedrosoi*, *P. com-pactum*, *P. verrucosa*, *P. dermatitidis* and *Clado-sporium carrionii*.

Laboratory diagnosis is based on finding typical pigmented cells in crusts or biopsies. All five species have brown, thick-walled rounded cells, 5 to 10 μm in diameter, splitting up by septation into small clusters. Culture yields slow growing, dark brown or greenish black colonies. Microscopically, the hyphae are brown and several types of spores are produced. Specific identification within this closely related group is usually left to a reference laboratory.

Treatment is not satisfactory. Early lesions may be excised but neither surgery nor medical treatment has been successful with late lesions.

SUBCUTANEOUS PHYCOMYCOCIS

Phycomycetes such as *Absidia* spp. and *Rhizopus* spp. can infect and penetrate the mucous membranes of the nose, sinuses and stomach when patients are *in extremis* but two others,

Basidiobolus haptosporus and *Entomophthora coronata* can establish themselves and spread in the subcutaneous tissue of healthy subjects. *Basidiobolus* infections occur over a wide area between Indonesia and West Africa and affect the trunk and proximal parts of the limbs in children; *Entomophthora* infections involve the perinasal area of the face in adults and occur in parts of the Caribbean, Africa and Asia. How they reach the subcutaneous tissues is uncertain. The reaction is an eosinophilic granuloma which forms an easily palpable, well defined, firm subcutaneous lump but does not normally penetrate either skin or deeper tissue. There is no ulceration or discharge and laboratory diagnosis is usually made from histological examination of a biopsy. The responsible fungus can easily be grown from pieces of fresh biopsy. The col-onies grow rapidly and soon cover the whole Petri dish. The hyphae are wide (5 to 10 μm) with occasional septa; characteristic sexual zygospores are produced within a week. Treat-ment with iodide is usually satisfactory and since most cases are in young people and complications and sequelae are rarely seen it is probable that the disease often resolves naturally.

FUNGI CAUSING SENSITIZATION

Many fungi grow readily in decaying vegetation and poorly stored agricultural produce. If their spores are repeatedly inhaled by agricultural workers, lasting sensitization may result, even when no infection is established. Recently described examples are in maple bark strippers (Emanuel, Wenzel and Lawton, 1966) and in malt workers (Riddle *et al.*, 1968) who may become sensitized to spores of *Cryptostroma corticale* and *Aspergillus clavatus* respectively.

Similar but much more widespread is the condition known as farmer's lung (Pepys *et al.*, 1963) in which the principal organism is *Micromonospora faeni*, a thermophilic actino-mycete, previously known as *Thermopolyspora polyspora*. It grows abundantly in wet hay that has heated up to 50°C. Normal persons may become sensitized and subsequent exposure to such hay or to an artificial aerosol of spores causes acute allergic alvec1itis and respiratory distress within 4 to 5 hours. Repeated exposure may lead to a chronic insidious disease with permanent lung damage due to an interstitial granulomatous reaction and subsequent fibrosis. Gel diffusion and other serological tests show specific antibodies in most patients. Antibodies are also demonstrable in a proportion of asymptomatic fellow workers but not in unexposed persons.

FUNGI CAUSING POISONING

There are two kinds of poisoning by fungi, mycetism and mycotoxicosis. In mycetism, the toxic substances are constituents of a fungus large enough to be eaten for itself. In mycotoxicosis, the fungus is a contaminant of, and has produced toxic products in, some other food.

Quite a number of fungi contain substances that are pharmacologically active when taken by mouth. They are usually well known to, and sometimes used by, the local population. The effects of mycetism include diarrhoea, jaundice, haemoglobinuria and hallucinations, but death is rare.

An example of mycotoxicosis was the poisoning by aflatoxin of turkeys that had fed on ground nuts infected with *Aspergillus flavus*. It was subsequently discovered that aflatoxin increases the incidence of hepatoma in certain experimental animals, but only when given in amounts not likely to be taken naturally.

Ergot poisoning is a mixture of mycotoxicosis and mycetism. The rye is not only contaminated with *Claviceps purpurea*, but the grain is virtually replaced by the alkaloid-containing tissue of the fungus.

DIMORPHIC FUNGI

The majority of fungi are filamentous, some exist only as yeasts and others change from one form to the other depending on the conditions of growth. These last are called dimorphic fungi and include a number of pathogens, *Sporothrix schenckii*, *Blastomyces dermatitidis*, *Paracoccidioides brasiliensis*, *Histoplasma capsulatum* and *H. duboisii*. As saprophytes in the soil and in culture at 22°C, they are filamentous but in culture at 37°C and as parasites in the body, they

grow as yeasts. Another pathogen, *Coccidiodes immitis*, is dimorphic in a different way; in culture it is mycelial, both at 22°C and at 37°C, but in the body it forms thick-walled spherules in which asexual sporulation occurs.

The dimorphic fungi have a number of features in common. Most of them live in the soil and the infections they cause are not communicable from man to man. *Sporothrix schenckii* differs from the others and resembles the opportunistic organisms of mycetoma in requiring traumatic implantation to establish itself and in producing a chronic local pyogenic infection with little tendency to disseminate. All the other infections due to dimorphic fungi are acquired by inhalation and their natural histories have many points in common with tuberculosis. The process is slow, the cellular reaction granulomatous and the infection is accompanied by a tuberculin-like sensitivity. The primary infection is often asymptomatic and only a small proportion of the infections progress, but if dissemination does occur the prognosis is not good. Microscopic recognition of the agent is important in diagnosis, growth in culture is slow, serology of uncertain assistance and treatment difficult.

SPOROTHRIX SCHENCKII

This dimorphic fungus lives in the soil and has been found on wood and plants but is not a plant pathogen. After traumatic inoculation into the subcutaneous tissue it causes a chronic pyogenic granulomatous infection which ulcerates and spreads some way along the draining lymphatics. General dissemination is rare.

In the body or in culture at 37°C, the form is a yeast, spherical or cigar shaped and up to $3 \times 10 \, \mu m$ in size. At 22°C it is filamentous and septate with many asexual conidia borne mainly at the ends of lateral hyphae. Its sexual or perfect state has not been recognized but may belong to the genus *Ceratocystis* as their asexual conidial states are indistinguishable.

Culture at 37°C on cysteine glucose blood agar yields soft greyish yellow bacterial type colonies in 2 days. On Sabouraud's medium at 22°C a wrinkled colony with no aerial mycelium develops nearly as quickly and slowly darkens almost to black.

Infection with *S. schenckii* usually follows injury to the hands with contaminated splinters or thorns but may be acquired from infected animals. A local 'chancre' forms and small subcutaneous abscesses develop along the line of the inflamed draining lymphatics.

Laboratory Diagnosis

The best specimen is pus, aspirated from a sub-cutaneous abscess, both because incisions heal poorly and to avoid contamination. The organisms are scanty and rarely recognized in smears either when stained by Gram's method or even using fluorescent antibody techniques. For culture, heavy inocula should be made on cysteine glucose blood agar and Sabouraud's medium. Intraperitonal inoculation of specimens into mice may fail if organisms are few but if infection is established (as by inoculation of cultures) much larger numbers of organisms are seen in the exudates than in any human pus.

Biopsies show a typical purulent granuloma and occasional diagnostic 'asteroid bodies' may be seen. These are yeasts surrounded by a stellate cuff of eosinophilic debris, consisting of a mixture of yeast antigen and host antibody together with other material from the exudate and are similar to the clubs of actinomycosis, the outer layers of the grains in mycetoma and the eosinophilic granular debris which surrounds the large hyphae in subcutaneous phycomycosis.

Serum antibodies are usually present, most frequently agglutinins to the yeast phase. Skin tests with yeast-phase antigen show a tuberculin-like response which (unlike the tests for histoplasmosis, blastomycosis and coccidioidomycosis) appears to be specific.

Treatment systemically with iodides is extremely effective so other antifungal chemotherapy is rarely necessary. Local treatment is usually ineffective, but it is interesting that raising the ambient temperature reduces the severity of experimental infections in animals and local hot dressings or rubifacients have cured localized lesions in man.

Prevention of this largely occupational infection is difficult but the outbreak in the Transvaal mines due to contamination of wood used in them was brought to an end by treating the wood.

BLASTOMYCES DERMATITIDIS

This fungus has been found in the soil and its perfect state is an ascomycete, *Ajellomyces dermatitidis*. Man is probably infected by inhalation but the main manifestations are chronic, pyogenic, granulomatous lesions of the skin. The disease used to be called North American blastomycosis but it also occurs widely in Africa and most mycologists agree that the fungus does not properly belong to the genus *Blastomyces*. In the absence of agreed new names however, the organism will be referred to here as *Blastomyces dermatitidis* and the disease as blastomycosis.

In the mammalian host and in the moist creamy colonies that grow on culture at 37°C, the fungus takes the form of a thick-walled, almost spherical yeast, 8 to 15 μm or more in diameter. It is multinucleate and produces a thin-walled, broad based bud which remains attached until it is as large as the parent cell.

In cultures below 30°C, the fungus grows as a white mould, waxy at first but cottony and brownish later. It may exceed 5 cm in diameter in 2 weeks, becoming granular and sporing freely or it may remain small and develop few spores. Microscopically the hyphae are broad, thick-walled and closely septate. Microconidia of very variable size are produced on lateral branches. Old cultures show terminal chlamydospores.

Natural infection occurs in man and the dog but the sources, occasions and contributing factors have not been defined. The primary infection is normally respiratory and slowly progressive, leading first to general dissemination with the skin being principally affected, and then subsequently to death with lesions in bone, kidneys and central nervous system. The liver, spleen and gastrointestinal tract are usually spared. Mice can be infected experimentally.

Laboratory Diagnosis

Sputum, scrapings from the skin or droplets of pus from the microabscesses at the edge of skin lesions should be examined microscopically for typical thick-walled budding yeasts. Biopsies may also provide a presumptive diagnosis. Cultures should be set up on Sabouraud's medium (without chloramphenical or cyclo-heximide) below 30°C and on blood agar at 37°C and incubated for at least four weeks for conclusive diagnosis.

Inoculation into mice protected with anti-biotics against concomitant bacteria may be helpful. Serological and skin tests are available but their interpretation is difficult.

Treatment with iodides, hydroxystilbamidine and amphotericin B may be effective but natural resistance is poor and a hypersensitivity reaction following treatment may lead to deterioration.

PARACOCCIDIOIDES BRASILIENSIS

The natural habitat of this fungus is not known and it appears to infect only man. It causes 'South American blastomycosis', which is a chronic, progressive, pyogenic, granulomatous disease with a predilection for lymphatic tissue. Its main lesions are in mucous membranes, lymph nodes, skin, spleen and intestine. It is eventually fatal if not treated and common enough in Brazil to be a health problem.

The fungus in the body and in the creamy colonies formed in culture at 37°C is a large spherical or oval yeast, up to 30 μm or more in diameter. Buds may be single but some larger cells are often covered all over with numerous regularly arranged buds, 1 to 5 μm in diameter, attached by narrow necks.

At temperatures below 30°C, the whitish colonies grow slowly taking perhaps 3 weeks to reach 1 cm and vary in form. The hyphae are septate and freely branching with terminal chlamydospores but no typical conidia.

The infection in man is believed to be ac-quired by inhalation but the first manifestations are usually ulceration of the mucous membrane of the mouth or nose with extension to local lymph nodes. Lymphatic and haematogenous spread occurs later and involves the lungs (if it does not actually start there), the spleen, the liver and the lymphatic tissue of the intestine. The skin may be involved by spread from mucous membranes, by blood-borne dissemina-tion or by direct auto-inoculation.

Laboratory Diagnosis

Skin crusts, ulcer scrapings and pus contain abundant yeasts. Cultures should be set up on blood agar at 37°C and on neutral or alkaline Sabouraud's medium below 30°C. Animal inoculation leads to infection but has no advantage over culture. Serological tests are available but are more useful as guides to progress than in diagnosis. Skin tests are not helpful.

Treatment is not yet very satisfactory. Sul-phonamides may halt the progress of the earlier stages of the disease but are not usually curative. Amphotericin B appears to be curative but some cases relapse and a long follow-up will be necessary to be sure.

HISTOPLASMA

Histoplasma capsulatum is a dimorphic fungus found in many parts of the world in soil enriched with the droppings of certain birds and mammals. When its spores are inhaled by a mammalian host they develop into yeasts which set up an intracellular infection of the histiocytes. The clinical manifestations in man vary from an asymptomatic pulmonary infection to fatal generalized disease. There are many parallels with tuberculosis.

In soil or after 2 weeks in culture at 28°C, *Histoplasma capsulatum* grows as a white or brownish slightly woolly mould. The septate mycelium bears 2 to 5 μm microconidia on lateral branches and diagnostic, spherical 8 to 14 μm macroconidia which have thick walls covered with blunt projections and are often described as 'tuberculate chlamydospores' (Fig. 53.5). In the mammalian body or in culture at 37°C, *H. capsulatum* grows as an oval yeast no bigger than 3 to 4 μm in size and forms moist, buff, yeast-like colonies. Growth does not occur much above 37°C and perhaps for this reason the organism does not apparently infect birds though it flourishes in soil enriched with their droppings.

Infection occurs naturally in rodents, dogs, cats and bats as well as in man. Most human infections are acquired by inhalation and the

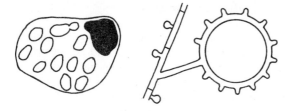

FIG. 53.5 *Histoplasma capsulatum*: left, yeast-like cells in macrophage; right, mycelium from culture bearing microconidia and a tuberculate chlamydospore. (× 400.)

usual outcome is a small calcified peripheral focus in the lung and a tuberculin-type sensitivity to histoplasmin. In some areas of the United States, 90 per cent of the population appear to have had inapparent infections. A larger dose of spores, as from cleaning out old hen houses or exploring bat-infested caves, leads to an acute though usually benign pneumonitis. Primary infections may progress to chronic cavitating disease or may take that form when reactivated later in life. Progressive disseminated disease, with an enlarged liver and spleen, anaemia and foci in adrenals, meninges and brain, is rare but more likely to occur at the end of life and in patients who also have Hodgkin's disease, leukaemia or lymphoma.

Histologically the reaction to the yeasts is primarily a diffuse histiocytic granuloma with large numbers of yeasts in some cells. Clinically, radiologically, in biopsies and even at necropsy the disease has been mistaken for tuberculosis.

Laboratory Diagnosis

This is as often made from histological examination of biopsies of skin or mucous membranes as from microbiological examinations. Smears of suspected material should be stained with Giemsa to demonstrate the intracellular yeasts forms and cultures set up at 26°C on Sabouraud's medium and at 37°C on cysteine glucose blood agar and incubated for 3 weeks. Serological tests are useful and the complement-fixation test the most reliable, though positive reactions may be found after a histoplasmin skin test and also in blastomycosis and cryptococcosis. Skin tests have the same significance in histoplasmosis as in tuberculosis, i.e. a positive result

indicates current or previous infection, most often asymptomatic.

Treatment is not required for most infections but for symptomatic disease amphotericin B may be given and local lesions, even in the lung, may sometimes be excised. Disseminated disease has a poor prognosis and amphotericin B or the newer polyene, saramycetin, which can be given subcutaneously, should be tried.

Prevention is not practised except by the avoidance of known sites of exposure.

Histoplasma duboisii is the name given to the organism found in a large proportion of African cases. The yeasts both in the body and in culture are much larger than in *H. capsulatum* infections (which also occur in Africa) and may measure $7 \mu m \times 15 \mu m$. In culture at 26°C *H. duboisii* and *H. capsulatum* are indistinguishable.

The clinical manifestations in 'African histoplasmosis' also differ from the classical ones. The usual tissues involved are the skin, subcutaneous tissue and bones, especially of the cranium. The lungs are not commonly involved and disseminated lesions do not carry a poor prognosis. Laboratory diagnosis is made in the same way as for *H. capsulatum* but the large yeasts must be distinguished from *Blastomyces* and the skin test is often negative even when the patient is not at all ill. Treatment is on the same principles. The source and route of infection and the proportion of infections that remain asymptomatic are unknown.

COCCIDIOIDES IMMITIS

This fungus lives in hot, dry soil and causes natural infections in wild rodents, man and many of his domestic animals. It is dimorphic, but the two forms depend not on the temperature at which the organism is growing, but on whether growth is *in vivo* or *in vitro*. Infection is acquired by inhalation and is normally asymptomatic. It has many parallels with tuberculosis and histoplasmosis. Most of the recognized cases have occurred in the south-western United States.

The organism grows as a fungus both at room temperature and at 37°C, producing a white cottony colony in a few days. The hyphae are septate and lateral branches break up into highly infectious arthrospores which easily become airborne and are a serious hazard in the laboratory (Fig. 53.6). No sexual reproduction is known.

In the host, the arthrospores germinate to form a small cell 2 to 5 μm in diameter which then grows steadily while its nucleus undergoes repeated division and the cell wall both expands and thickens. This body is known as a spherule. Individual spores form round each nucleus and, when the mature spherule reaches 60 μm or so, they are released into the tissue to repeat the cycle.

This process of asexual reproduction occurs in the phycomycetes and suggests that *Coccidioides immitis* is probably phycomycete and the spherule a sporangium. No perfect state has yet been described.

Infections with coccidioides are normally asymptomatic or mild (though erythema nodosum and pneumonia may occur) and the patient is left with a delayed type of hypersensitivity to coccidioidin and perhaps a calcified focus or dry, thin-walled cavity in the lung. More severe disease may occur in migrant workers and military personnel first exposed to infected dust as adults. Progressive disease occurs only rarely, but dissemination may then be miliary or to skin, bones and central nervous system and the mortality is 50 per cent. For this reason, very strict precautions are necessary against the risk of laboratory infection from cultures or infected animals.

Laboratory Diagnosis

Wet preparations of sputum or other material are examined for sporangia and biopsies may be taken. Culture should be set up on blood agar or Sabouraud's medium; the temperature is not important but medium should be in tubes or bottles as cultures in Petri dishes produce many airborne infective spores. Colonies grow in a few days. Animal inoculation is slower than culture but may be used for confirmation.

Serological tests are more useful for prognosis than diagnosis. Precipitins are found early on but do not persist. Complement-fixing antibodies may not develop, or only slowly, but then persist till recovery or death.

Treatment is needed only for progressive cases; amphotericin B should be used. Prevention of fungus diseases is rarely attempted and then is usually based on avoiding exposure rather than on increasing host resistance but in the case of coccidiomycosis both live attenuated and dead vaccines have been tried in animals with some success.

RHINOSPORIDIUM SEEBERI

This organism has not been grown in culture nor has infection been established experimentally in animals. It stains like a fungus in tissues and resembles some species of *Synchytrium* which are obligate plant parasites. Natural infections occur in man, horses, mules and cows and in most parts of the world, though most reports have come from India and Ceylon. Affected persons usually give a history of repeated immersion in rivers or ponds.

The infection causes the development of polyps in the submucosa of the nose, mouth and other areas, in the conjunctiva and occasionally in the skin. There is no tendency to disseminate. The organism is present in the form of globular cysts, 10 to 350 μm in diameter, which have thick walls with outer chitinous and inner cellulose layers and a thin pore area through which the very large numbers of contained spores escape. At maturity spores are 6 to 7 μm in diameter and have a thick chitinous wall.

LABORATORY DIAGNOSIS. A polyp may be examined histologically or a portion may be crushed in water between slide and coverslip. Some large cysts and many small spores should be seen. Treatment is surgical.

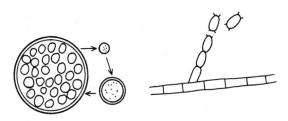

FIG. 53.6 *Coccidioides immitis*: left, mature spherule containing endospores and immature spherules as found in tissues; right, mycelium segmenting to form arthrospores in culture. (× 200.)

REFERENCES

BARLOW, A. J. E. (1968) The cutaneous mycoses. *British Journal of Hospital Medicine*, **1**, 115.

BENEKE, E. S. (1968) *Medical Mycology Laboratory Manual*, 3rd Edn. Minneapolis: Burgess Publishing Co.

BENHAM, R. W. (1957) Species of candida most frequently isolated from man: methods and criteria for their identification. *Journal of Chronic Diseases*, **5**, 460.

BORKER, E., INSALATA, N. F., LEVI, C. & WITZEMAN, J. S. (1966) Mycotoxins in feeds and foods. *Advances in Applied Microbiology*, **8**, 315.

BOYCOTT, J. A. (1961) The nature of vaginal discharge. *Lancet*, **1**, 1071.

CONANT, N. F., SMITH, D. T., BAKER, R. D. & CALLAWAY, J. L. (1971) *Manual of Clinical Mycology*, 3rd Edn. Philadelphia: Saunders.

EMANUEL, D. A., WENZEL, F. J. & LAWTON, B. R. (1966) Pneumonitis due to *Cryptostroma corticale* (Maple bark disease). *New England Journal of Medicine*, **274**, 1413.

EMMONS, C. W., BINFORD, C. H. & UTZ, J. P. (1971) *Medical Mycology*, 2nd Edn. London: Henry Kimpton.

MACKENZIE, D. W. (1964) Serum tube identification of *Candida albicans, Journal of Clinical Pathology*, 15, 563.

MARKS, M. I., LANGSTON, C. & EICKHOFF, T. C. (1970) *Torulopsis glabrata*—an opportunistic pathogen in man. *New England Journal of Medicine*, **283**, 1131.

MIDGLEY, G. & CLAYTON, Y. M. (1972) Distribution of dermatophytes and Candida spores in the environment. *British Journal of Dermatology* **86** (Suppl. 8), 69.

MOSS, E. S. & McQUOWN, A. L. (1969) *Atlas of Medical Mycology*, 3rd Edn. Baltimore: Williams and Wilkins Co.

REBELL, G. & TAPLIN, D. (1970) *The Dermatophytes—their Recognition and Identification*, Revised Edn. Miami, Fa.: University of Miami Press.

REPORT (1970) Mycoses in Great Britain and Ireland 1967–70. *British Medical Journal*. **ii**, 185.

RIDDELL, R. W. (1951) Laboratory diagnosis of common fungus infections. In *Recent Advances in Clinical Pathology*, p. 77, 2nd Edn. S. C. Dyke. London: Churchill.

RIDDLE, H. F. V., CHANNELL, S., BLYTH, W., WEIR, D. M., LLOYD, M., AMOS, W. M. G. & GRANT, I. W. B. (1968) Allergic alveolitis in a malt worker. *Thorax*, **23**, 271.

SARGEANT, K., SHERIDAN, A., O'KELLY, J. & CARNAGHAN, R. B. A. (1961) Toxicity associated with certain samples of groundnuts. *Nature*, **192**, 1096.

SMITH, H. (1968) Biochemical challenge of microbial pathogenicity, *Bacteriological Reviews*, **32**, 164.

SYMMERS, W. ST. C. (1966) Deep mycoses in the U.K. *American Journal of Clinical Pathology*, **46**, 514.

TAPLIN, D., ZAIAS, N., REBELL, G. & BLANK, H. (1969) Isolation and recognition of dermatophytes on a new medium. *Archives of Dermatology*, **99**, 203.

TASCHDJIAN, C. L. (1957) Routine identification of *Candida albicans*: current methods and a new medium. *Mycologia*, **49**, 332.

THOM, C. & RAPER, K. B. (1945) *A manual of the Aspergilli*. Baltimore: Williams and Wilkins Co.

WILSON, L. A. & SEXTON, R. R. (1968) Laboratory diagnosis in fungal keratitis. *American Journal of Ophthalmology*, **66**, 646.

WINNER, H. I. & HURLEY, R. (Eds) (1966) *Symposium on Candida Infections*, Edinburgh: Livingstone.

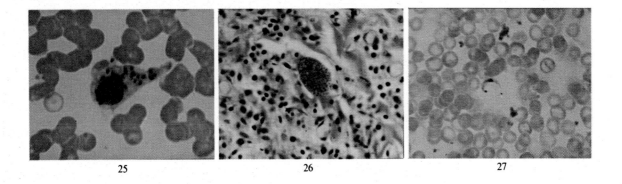

Plate 25   *Leishmania donovani*, amastigotes in macrophage in bone-marrow smear; Giemsa's stain.

Plate 26   *Trypanosoma (S) cruzi*, amastigotes in pseudocyst in heart muscle; haematoxylin and eosin stain.

Plate 27   *Trypanosoma (S) cruzi*, trypomastigote in peripheral blood; Giemsa's stain.

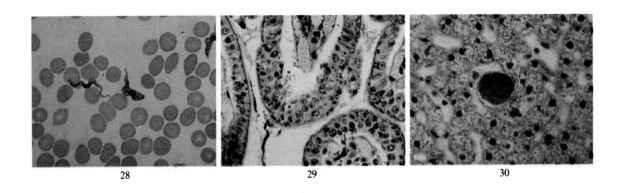

Plate 28   *Trypanosoma (T) brucei rhodesiense*, trypomastigotes in peripheral blood; Giemsa's stain.

Plate 29   *Toxoplasma gondii*, schizonts in epithelium of gut of cat; silver stain; courtesy of Dr W. M. Hutchison.

Plate 30   *Plasmodium cynomolgi* of *Macaca* sp. (monkey), primary exo-erythrocytic schizont in liver parenchyma cell; resembles *P. vivax* of man; Giemsa-colophonium stain.

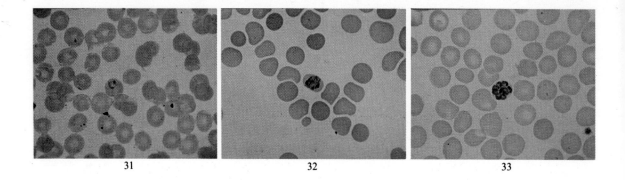

31 32 33

Plate 31   *Plasmodium vivax*, trophozoite—signet ring form; Giemsa's stain.

Plate 32   *Plasmodium malariae*, trophozoite—band form; Giemsa's stain.

Plate 33   *Plasmodium malariae*, mature erythrocytic schizont ('daisy head'); Giemsa's stain.

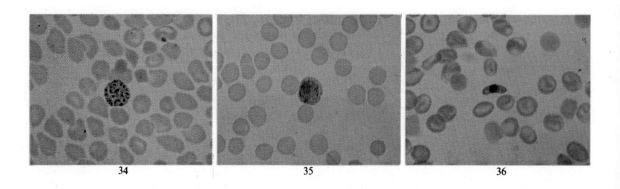

34 35 36

Plate 34   *Plasmodium vivax*, mature erythrocytic schizont; Giemsa's stain.

Plate 35   *Plasmodium vivax*, gametocyte; Giemsa's stain.

Plate 36   *Plasmodium falciparum*, gametocyte; Giemsa's stain.

54. Protozoa

Leishmaniasis: Trypanosomiasis: Amoebiasis: Malaria: Toxoplasmosis

Introduction

Some protozoal diseases, especially malaria and sleeping sickness, are household words as important causes of human morbidity and mortality in the tropics, and the discoveries of their etiology and of their mechanisms of transmission are classical contributions to the history of human medicine. Nevertheless, partly because of the general limitation of protozoal diseases to the tropics, and so to 'tropical medicine', and partly because of an illogical separation of protozoology and helminthology, under a restricted designation of 'parasitology', from other groups of pathogenic organisms such as the bacteria and the viruses, protozoal diseases have recently had little prominence in temperate climate medicine. Their importance is at present enlarging, as modern communications increase the contacts of the indigenous United Kingdom population with tropical environments and as the proportion of immigrants from tropical countries in the United Kingdom population rises. Examples of the dangers of protozoal diseases in these contexts are the fatalities in returning tourists due to unrecognized *Plasmodium falciparum* malaria and the transmission by transfusion, of malaria, Chagas' disease and other protozoal infections of the blood when immigrant donors are concerned. A working knowledge of protozoal diseases of man is therefore no more a requirement only for the tropical practitioner but more and more essential for the temperate climate doctor also.

Some of the diseases of man of protozoal causation are of minor importance for such reasons as being of low pathogenicity, or of only limited distribution, or of rare occurrence. Examples are vaginitis due to infection with *Trichomonas vaginalis*, dysentery due to *Balantidium coli*, or meningo-encephalitis due to *Naegleria* sp. In such cases as these, awareness of the possibility of protozoal causation is important as diagnosis may easily be missed if only bacterial or viral detection procedures are applied. However, the main importance of the protozoa lies in their providing several of the 'grandes endémies' which are such potent factors in delaying the development of the warm countries of the world. These are:

Leishmaniasis, caused by infection with *Leishmania* spp., may be visceral, involving especially the spleen, liver and bone marrow, and characteristically lethal (kala-azar), or cutaneous or mucocutaneous involving skin or skin and mucous membranes (tropical sore, espundia and allied conditions), not characteristically lethal but often seriously disfiguring.

Trypanosomiasis is caused by infection with *Trypanosoma brucei* ssp. *gambiense* and *rhodesiense* (African sleeping sickness) or with *Trypanosoma cruzi* (Chagas' disease of Central and South America). These diseases are characteristically lethal either early, in an acute stage, or later as a result of chronic involvement of, mainly, the central nervous system or of the heart musculature. *Trypanosoma* spp. in Africa exert, also, an important indirect effect on human affairs; they cause a disease, called nagana, in domestic stock, to the extent that cattle and horses are virtually excluded from many regions, with consequent limitation of the availability of protein for human diet, and of animal transport. Regions so affected have been estimated to amount in total area nearly to that of the United States of America.

Amoebiasis, infection with *Entamoeba histolytica*, is an important cause of dysentery, with ulceration of the gut mucosa, as well as of metastatic lesions such as liver and brain abscess.

Malaria, infection with one or other of four species of *Plasmodium*, has probably influenced human affairs more than any other single disease and remains a major cause of morbidity and mortality affecting some 360 million people.

The mechanisms of transmission of all these infections are now well known and effective specific chemotherapy is usually available so that there is seldom difficulty in protecting or treating small populations under good administrative conditions, such as incoming technical personnel. Great progress has been made with the more difficult problem of the reduction of infection in indigenous populations, but control or eradication schemes usually require continuous surveillance to guard against recrudescence, and vast areas and populations still remain infected.

CLASSIFICATION AND DESCRIPTION

The taxonomy and nomenclature of the protozoa are complicated (Honigberg *et al.*, 1964) and are greatly simplified in this chapter. Essentially the protozoal parasites of man (most important pathogenic genera in brackets) fall into four groups:

Flagellates (Superclass Mastigophora) comprising organisms moving by means of flagella, reproducing asexually by binary fission; parasites of the lumen of the intestine or of the genito-urinary tract (*Giardia, Trichomonas*) and of tissues (*Leishmania, Trypanosoma*).

Amoebae (Superclass Sarcodina) comprising organisms moving by means of pseudopodia, reproducing asexually by binary fission; parasites of the gut lumen, or free-living, also invading tissues (*Entamoeba, Naegleria*).

Malaria and allied parasites (Subphylum Sporozoa) comprising organisms of restricted motility, with multiple asexual reproduction (schizogony) but also with a sexual cycle of development and subsequent multiplication (sporogony); parasites of tissues (*Plasmodium, Toxoplasma*).

Ciliates (Subphylum Ciliophora) comprising organisms moving by means of cilia, reproducing asexually and sexually; parasites of the gut lumen but also invading tissues (*Balantidium*).

Protozoa are single-celled (or acellular) animals in which one cell is capable of performing all necessary functions. Generally protozoal cells are of the order of 5 to 50 μm in dimension and consist of a nucleated mass of cytoplasm enclosed in an external cell wall of single unit membrane. Depending on species and on stages in life-histories, there is great variety of cell shape and nuclear arrangement (Figs. 54.1 to 54.7 and Colour Plates 25–36). There may be one, several or many similar nuclei within one cytoplasmic body, and in one group, the Ciliophora, organisms possess two dissimilar nuclei—a macronucleus concerned with the vegetative function of the organism and a micronucleus concerned with sexual reproduction.

Organelles, parts of the cell modified and developed to fulfil special functions, add to the elaboration and the resulting variety has perhaps been an important factor in leading study of the subject more into morphological and observational channels than towards experimental and inferential ones, in contrast to trends in the fields of bacteriology and virology. The most conspicuous organelles are those concerned with cell shape (e.g. axostyles, internal skeletal structures; pellicles, superficial stiffened coats), with locomotion (e.g. pseudopodia, ephemeral expansions of the cytoplasm; flagella, long lashing filaments; cilia, short beating filaments) or with nutrition (e.g. cytostomes, invaginations of the cell wall adapted to ingest solid particles; cytopyges, similarly adapted for the extrusion of solid waste). Some morphological characters may be seen in the living organism, particularly with phase-contrast microscopy, but many details require staining or electron microscopy for their demonstration. Stains most employed are the Romanowsky stains (polychromed methylene blue and eosin—Giemsa's stain; Leishman's stain) for blood films or tissue smears, iodine for gut lumen parasites and haematoxylin and eosin and Giemsa-colophonium for tissue sections.

Locomotion is mainly by means of pseudopodia (amoeboid) or by means of flagella or cilia. Amoeboid movement implies the temporary expansion of the body in a given direction as a pseudopodium, the drawing up of the body into that extension, with progressive repetition. Pseudopodia in parasitic protozoa are generally broad and blunt (lobopodia). Although amoeboid movement is not confined to the amoebae (occurring, e.g. in the intracellular trophozoite of the Sporozoa) it is in this group that it is most conspicuous. Flagella and cilia are of essentially similar structure, both being cylindrical, contractile, filamentous, extensions of the cytoplasm, showing, in ultramicroscopic section, a circle of nine double microtubules placed around a central pair of single microtubules. Flagella and cilia can be distinguished, broadly, by being, respectively, few in number, say up to eight per organism, long and whip-like, lashing individually, and short, many in number, forming a brush-like coating on the organism, and beating in a co-ordinated manner—metachronal rhythm; but an absolute distinction is not possible and integradations exist. Besides these methods of locomotion some organisms, e.g. certain stages of Sporozoa, move in a slugwise way, called gregarine movement.

Biological Activities

The *physiology* of the parasitic protozoal cell, delimited from a liquid, or nearly liquid, ambient, by the unit membrane cell boundary, is clearly closely bound up with the transport of materials across that boundary. Tissue-inhabiting protozoa are likely to be maintained at osmotic pressure and pH levels close to those of the blood plasma. Nevertheless some tissue protozoa, such as trypanosomes, can survive large alterations in the tonicity of the ambient, e.g. reductions sufficient to lyse erythrocytes. Gut-lumen protozoa may be expected to be even more accommodating. Tissue-inhabiting protozoa tend to be aerobic in their respiration in the same way as metazoan cells, degrading glucose to carbon dioxide and water, but the blood stream forms of *Trypanosoma brucei* are an exception; glucose is degraded only as far as pyruvic acid. As a rule gut-lumen protozoa subsist only at low oxygen tension, a point to be remembered when attempting their isolation in culture. Both gut-lumen and tissue-infecting organisms are, in their vertebrate host, protected from large changes of environmental temperature. In the case of tissue-inhabiting protozoa, temperature reduction may reproduce the conditions in their invertebrate vectors and so induce the morphological changes associated therewith (see below). Gut-lumen parasites are typically adversely affected by lower temperatures, often forming resistant cysts to survive these, and other, adverse conditions.

Nutrition in the parasitic protozoa is holozoic, the ingestion of already formed molecules of proteins, carbohydrates and so on and their refabrication for the organism's own purposes. Ingestion may be phagotrophic, in which large particles are actively and evidently ingested as, e.g. by being engulfed by the pseudopodial action of an amoeba, or saprozoic, in which simpler materials, the products of digestion of organic material by bacterial or host or other enzymes, are ingested without evident phagotrophy. How far this process is simply by diffusion through the cell wall and how much by pinocytosis (a process of phagotrophy on an ultramicroscopic scale, in which vacuoles of the ambient fluid of the parasite are pinched off by invagination of the limiting membrane of the cell) doubtless varies from one parasite and one situation to another.

Excretion of soluble waste products appears to be mainly by diffusion through the cell wall. Solid residues and food vacuoles may be extruded through the cell wall either adventitiously as in amoebae or through a special cytopyge, as in the Ciliophora. Or solid waste material may simply be relinquished at cell division as is the haemozoin (malaria pigment) by *Plasmodium* spp. at schizogony in the erythrocytic cycle.

Asexual reproduction of parasitic protozoa is most commonly by binary fission. The nucleus divides first, by a simplified form of mitosis, and later the cytoplasm divides to form two pieces, each containing one daughter nucleus, by the deepening of a constriction round the organism. Some organelles may divide nearly coincidentally with the time of cell division as, e.g. the kinetoplast of the trypanosomes, others may be formed again by one of the daughter cells, e.g. the cytostome of Ciliophora. Another form of asexual reproduction is schizogony. In this process, the parent cell (schizont) produces, by successive nuclear divisions followed by the allocation of portions of cytoplasm to each daughter nucleus, a number of individual organisms, varying from 4 to say 40 000, called merozoites. This process is characteristic of the Sporozoa.

Sexual reproduction takes place in the Sporozoa and Ciliophora. In the Sporozoa certain special individuals (gametocytes) give rise to gametes, often unequal—aniso-gametes, e.g. small flagellate male gametes and larger non-flagellate female gametes. The zygote formed by the fusion of the gametes produces large numbers of uninucleate sporozoites by a process called sporogony, essentially similar to schizogony (see above). In the Ciliophora two organisms conjugate. Their vegetative macronuclei disintegrate and the micronuclei produce, after various divisions, a pair of gametic nuclei. One of each pair then migrates to the opposite organism where it fuses with the remaining nucleus forming the zygotic nucleus. The organisms then separate and the zygotic nucleus gives rise to both the macronucleus and the micronucleus of the new individual organism.

MODES OF SPREAD

Transmission mechanisms of parasitic protozoa from host to host vary from very simple to highly complicated. With some of the gut-lumen parasites, such as *Entamoeba gingivalis* of the mouth and *Trichomonas vaginalis* of the male and female genital tracts, direct host to host transfer is frequently possible and no special transmission forms are developed. With others, such as *Entamoeba histolytica* and *Ent. coli* of the colon, transfer depends on faecal contamination of food of the host and a resistant cyst is developed to survive the intervening period outside the host. Parasites that are essentially parasites of the deep tissues, e.g. *Leishmania*, *Trypanosoma* and *Plasmodium*, mainly depend on some blood-sucking arthropod for their transmission between hosts. Sometimes transmission is thought to be by direct transfer of organisms from one host to another on the mouthparts of the arthropod by the interruption of its blood meal on one host and its resumption on another. But more usually the parasite goes through a defined cycle of development in the arthropod, leading through stages in which the organisms are non-infective to the mammal host, to the appearance of infective forms (sometimes called metacyclic) in either the mouth parts or the salivary glands of the

arthropod, or in its rectum. Such development is designated as cyclical transmission and changes in the environments in which the organisms subsist during its process are correlated with changes, often complicated, in their form and function.

Many of the protozoal infections of man are not exclusive to him. Many of them occur also in wild or domestic mammals, sometimes called reservoir hosts. This is the concept of the zoonosis—an infection of animals transferable to man. This term, useful though it has been in emphasizing the importance of infections in animals in the epidemiology of human disease, should be used with some circumspection as the transmission patterns of any given pathological agent are not fixed and immutable but may vary from one ecological situation to another. It is perhaps more useful to think flexibly of the transmission patterns of agents as possibly involving wild and domestic animals and man, with variable possibilities of maintaining transmission within any one of these categories and of transfer between them in any direction. In some ways the cycles of transmission resemble those followed by the arboviruses (q.v.).

FLAGELLATES

FLAGELLATE INFECTIONS OF HOLLOW VISCERA

Three species, *Retortamonas intestinalis*, *Enteromonas hominis* and *Chilomastix mesnili* (Fig. 54.1, a, b, c) may be quickly dismissed, as not being clearly pathogenic. Although they are often detected in diarrhoeic stools there is little evidence that they are causally involved and their occurrence could as well be due to their being carried along by diarrhoea induced by other agents. They are cosmopolitan in their distribution and are transmitted by cysts. Their prevalence is indicative of the degree of faecal contamination of food.

The three flagellate species discussed above are characteristically located in the caecum. *Giardia lamblia*, on the other hand, occurs mainly in the glandular crypts of the duodenal-jejunal mucosa. It is a pear-shaped organism,

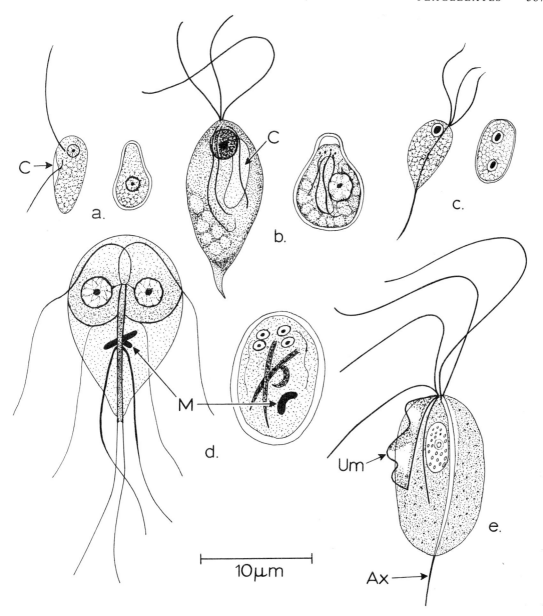

FIG. 54.1. Flagellates of hollow viscera. (a) *Retortamonas intestinalis*, trophozoite and cyst. (b) *Chilomastix mesnili*, trophozoite and cyst. (c) *Enteromonas hominis*, trophozoite and cyst. (d) *Giardia lamblia*, trophozoite and cyst. (e) *Trichomonas vaginalis*, trophozoite. Ax—axostyle; C—cytostome; Um—undulating membrane; M—median body.

binucleate, with 8 flagella arranged in a complicated bilaterally symmetrical pattern (Fig. 54.1d). The 'ventral' surface of the organism is concave and is used as a sucking disc to attach the organism to the mucosa. Transmission is by means of cysts and infection is commonest in young children though epidemics among adults have been reported. Generally infection is commensal and silent but is fairly frequently associated with duodenal irritation, excess mucus secretion and dehydration with chronic steatorr-hoeic diarrhoea. The steatorrhoea has been attributed to the coating of the mucosal surface of the small bowel with organisms, causing interference with fat absorption. Occasionally the gall bladder may be invaded, with associated colic and jaundice. Diagnosis is by recognition of the trophozoites or cysts in the faeces. Quinacrine and metronidazole are usually effective chemotherapeutic agents.

Three species of *Trichomonas* occur in man —*T. tenax* in the mouth, *T. hominis* in the caecum and *T. vaginalis* in the male and female genito-urinary system. All these species are morphologically very similar but are considered separate species because, experimentally, they are not able to be transferred from one to another of these sites of infection, because they show antigenic differences. No cysts are known for any of the three species and transmission is presumably by transfer, respectively by saliva, faecal contamination of food and coitus. All three species are cosmopolitan, and their prevalence is dependent on standards of hygiene. *T. tenax* may affect 25 per cent or more of persons in European populations, *T. hominis* less. Both species feed mainly on ingested bacteria, necrotic mucosal cells and such like, and seem usually to be non-pathogenic. Cases of respiratory tract infection have, however, been reported. *Trichomonas vaginalis*, also, is cosmopolitan in its distribution and frequently infects both sexes. Overall prevalence in women of child-bearing age has been estimated at 25 per cent. Probably the prevalence in males is similar but diagnosis of the parasite in the male genito-urinary tract is more difficult. Usually infection is a silent one, but it is sometimes associated with an acute vaginitis—desquamation and erosion of the vaginal epithelium with leucocyte infiltration and copious frothy greenish or yellowish exudate, containing large numbers of organisms. A chronic state may ensue with long term presence of organisms. Infections in the male are generally symptomless or associated with mild urethritis. Diagnosis is mainly by recognition of the organism in secretions, centrifugate of urine, or vaginal or urethral scrapings, by direct examination or by culture. Transmission is mainly by coitus but direct female to female transmission also occurs in poor sanitary con-texts. Metronidazole is an effective specific chemotherapeutic agent although infections resistant to it have been noted.

FLAGELLATE INFECTIONS OF THE TISSUES

These are caused by two closely related genera, *Leishmania* and *Trypanosoma*, which are remarkable in having, besides the nucleus, another structure containing a quantity of deoxyribonucleic acid (DNA)—the kinetoplast (Fig. 54.2). In stained preparations the general form of the body of the organism, the nucleus, the kinetoplast, and the flagellum (sometimes with an attached undulating membrane) are conspicuous and provide characters for the differentiation of species. They are important, also, in relation to the developmental changes undergone by the parasites in their various hosts; certain characteristic forms are named (Fig. 54.2). Broadly: the amastigote form is that adopted by organisms in intracellular phases of their development; promastigote and epimastigote forms occur mostly in the gut lumen of insect vectors; the trypomastigote form is characteristic of *Trypanosoma* spp. in the vertebrate host while they are living in blood and tissue fluids, and of the infective forms arising after the cycle of development in the insect host. But cycles of development are often complicated and exceptions exist to this general pattern.

LEISHMANIASIS

Leishmania spp. are essentially parasites of the cells of the reticulo-endothelial system of their vertebrate hosts, in which (Colour Plate 25) they exist as amastigotes. They are widely distributed in mammal and reptile hosts as well as in man. There is negligible morphological difference among the named species of the genus and the specific names are rather convenient labels to designate particular complexes of geographical distribution, clinical appearance, biological behaviour, etc. All *Leishmania* spp. are readily cultured, as promastigote forms, on

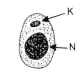

Amastigote (leishmania form or
Leishman-Donovan body)

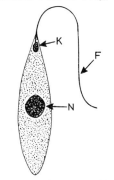

Promastigote (leptomonad form)

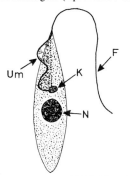

Epimastigote (crithidial form)

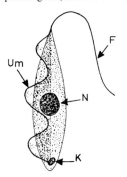

Trypomastigote (trypanosome form)

FIG. 54.2. Forms which may be adopted by *Leishmania* and *Trypanosoma* spp. In brackets are given the terms for the forms under the old nomenclature now being superseded. F—flagellum; K—kinetoplast; N—nucleus; Um—undulating membrane.

blood agar media. *Cricetulus griseus* (hamster) is a highly susceptible host much used experimentally. *Leishmania* spp. are transmitted by psychodid flies of the genera *Phlebotomus* and *Lutzomyia* (sand-flies) in whose gut lumen they develop as promastigotes.

Two general types of leishmaniasis are distinguished—visceral, and cutaneous or muco-cutaneous.

Leishmania donovani, Visceral Leishmaniasis

Visceral leishmaniasis is widely distributed, though focally, in tropical and subtropical Asia and Africa, in the Mediterranean area and in tropical South America. Kala-azar is the vernacular name of the disease in which Leishman first demonstrated the parasite in 1903. A wide range of *Phlebotomus* spp. have been shown or suggested to be vectors.

The incubation period varies between 10 days and more than a year and onset may be sudden or insidious. Irregular malaise, headache and fever with progressive enlargement of the spleen and, less markedly, of the liver, progressing with dysentery and bleeding from mucous membranes to a cachectic state, are classical clinical signs. Untreated, the disease is generally fatal either in the acute stage or, by intercurrent infection, after some 2 to 3 years of chronic illness. Diagnosis depends mainly on the demonstration of amastigotes in macrophages in smears of sternal bone marrow, lymph node, spleen or liver biopsies or in the peripheral blood, or on culture of these materials.

In the insect vector, ingested amastigotes transform to promastigotes and multiply in the midgut and pharynx, to such an extent that the gut lumen may become 'blocked'. When the insect attempts to feed again, the blood flow is obstructed, and at the relinquishment of the attempt, infective promastigotes are regurgitated into the bite. Epidemiological patterns vary. In India, transmission cycles appear to be purely intra-human. In other areas, however, other vertebrate hosts are suspected to act as reservoirs. In central and southwestern Asia, in Mediterranean areas, and in Brazil, where the disease mainly affects children under six years of age, dogs, domestic or wild, are found infected and may be infected experimentally with *Leishmania* from human patients. In Kenya and the Sudan wild rodents, *Tatera*, *Xerus*, *Rattus* and *Acomys* spp., have yielded isolations of *Leishmania* and are suspected as reservoirs.

Treatment is by pentavalent antimonial drugs (e.g. sodium stibogluconate) or by diamidines. Prevention is mainly by disrupting the cycles of transmission by such measures as protection from bite by sandflies, control of sandflies by clearing their breeding sites, or by insecticides, and by the reduction of extrahuman reservoirs such as dogs. Post-kala-azar dermal leishmanoid, a condition observed most frequently in India, develops after incomplete treatment with antimony; depigmented areas and nodules develop in the skin. Such lesions contain *L. donovani* and may be of importance epidemiologically as sources of infection for the vector *Phlebotomus*.

Leishmania tropica and L. brasiliensis
Cutaneous and Mucocutaneous Leishmaniasis

Cutaneous or mucocutaneous leishmaniasis occurs widely in tropical and subtropical areas of Southwest Asia, North Africa, West Africa and Central and South America. Although not based on any clear morphological or other general difference, it is convenient to discuss the Old World cutaneous leishmaniasis, as caused by *Leishmania tropica*, separately from the cutaneous and mucocutaneous leishmaniases of the New World as caused by *Leishmania brasiliensis*.

L. tropica infection occurs in the Mediterranean littoral of Europe, in much of southwest and central Asia, and in the northern half of Africa. It is convenient to refer to it generically as tropical sore although it receives many local names—Aleppo boil, Delhi boil, Biskra button, etc., in different parts of its range. The sores occur mainly on skin surfaces exposed to bite by *Phlebotomus*—the extensor surfaces of the forearms, and on the legs and face—and may be single or multiple. Incubation periods vary from a few days to several months. The sores are initially reddish papules which then develop a crust of brownish scales which breaks down to leave shallow ulcers with sharp raised edges. Sores usually heal spontaneously leaving a depressed depigmented scar. The subject be-

comes, after some eight months, immune to further infection.

Diagnosis is by direct recognition of amastigotes by microscopy in smears of tissues aspirated from marginal areas of the sore, in macrophages or neutrophils or free in tissue fluids; or by culture of such materials. Parasites may be scarce in later stage lesions.

Different types of lesion, correlated with different epidemiological situations are recognized. For instance, in Turkestan, 'dry' (*L. tropica minor*) and 'wet' types (*L. tropica major*) occur. *L. tropica minor* infections are slow of onset (with incubation periods of 2 to 8 months), and of development (lasting a year or more), and ulceration tends to be delayed. *L. t. major* lesions are more rapidly progressive (of some 2 to 6 weeks incubation and 3 to 6 months development) and they tend to ulcerate earlier. Epidemiologically, *L. t. minor* infection is an urban disease, transmitted all the year round; dogs are suspected as reservoirs. *L. t. major* infection is a rural disease, transmitted mainly in the summer and the autumn; *Rhombomys* and *Meriones* spp. (gerbils, burrowing desert rodents) show leishmanial sores on the nose and ears and are suspected as natural reservoirs of infection.

Treatment is, generally, superfluous as the sores heal spontaneously, the parasites are restricted to the lesion and do not metastasize, and healing is followed by resistance to reinfection. However, where lesions are likely to be disfiguring, sodium stibogluconate may be used. Artificial immunization has been accomplished by the inoculation of material from sores or of culture organisms. Protection against bites of *Phlebotomus* can be afforded by repellents or by screens or fine-mesh nets.

Leishmania brasiliensis is essentially similar in its morphology, general pathology, and transmission and epidemiology, to *L. tropica* of the Old World. There is, however, a series of fairly distinct clinical conditions associated with it in different parts of its range in the New World and these are conveniently separated under different subspecific names.

L. b. mexicana, the cause of chiclero ulcer, or Bay Sore, occurs in Mexico, British Honduras and Guatemala. The disease is a rural one, occurring mainly in people entering virgin forest, such as gum latex collectors (*chicleros*).

The incubation period is 2 to 6 weeks and the lesions affect mainly the ear. Ulceration leads slowly to extensive necrosis and cicatrization. The condition is chronic, painless, with alternate phases of ulceration and healing. There is little or no tendency to metastasize.

L. b. peruviana, the agent of Uta and similar conditions, occurs in Costa Rica, Panama, French Guiana, Peru, Ecuador and Venezuela, sometimes to altitudes over 1 000 m. The lesion of Uta is similar to that of *L. tropica* with an incubation period of 2 to 6 weeks and lasting 6 to 48 months. Most lesions heal in 12 to 15 months leaving a depigmented scar. Metastasis is rare.

L. b. brasiliensis and *L. b. guyanensis* are agents of Espundia, cutaneous leishmaniasis with a tendency to metastasize to muco-cutaneous junctions and mucous membrane. *L. b. brasiliensis*, showing a high incidence of naso-oropharyngeal metastasis, occurs in Venezuela, Brazil, Paraguay and North Argentina, and is associated with humid forests at altitudes below 1 000 m. The incubation period of the disease is 2 to 12 months. A primary lesion like that of *L. b. peruviana* may heal and then later break down to flat weeping ulcers. Secondary metastatic involvement affects mainly the nose and pharynx but also the larynx and face and limbs. These lesions may follow, or accompany, the primary lesion. Hyperplasia of the mucosa leads to polyp formation, ulceration and extensive necrosis. Great deformity, e.g. loss of the nose, or of the voice may occur. Spontaneous recovery is rare and septicaemia or broncho-pneumonia are common terminal episodes.

L. b. guyanensis is similar but shows only a low incidence of oropharyngeal metastasis, and is more mild clinically; it occurs in the Guianas, Costa Rica and Panama; metastasis takes place in only some 5 per cent of cases.

L. b. pifanoi, associated with a disease known as *leishmaniasis tegumentaria diffusa*, occurs in Bolivia and Venezuela. The initial localized nodular lesion ulcerates and disseminates to satellite cutaneous lesions, macules, plaques or papules, involving nearly the whole dermis but not tending to involve viscera.

All these infections are associated with forest or rural environments and the organisms transmitted by the infecting sandflies are derived, most probably, from wild animal hosts. These natural hosts are still little known but *Dasypus* (armadillo), *Proechimys* (spiny rat), *Ototylomys*, *Nyctomys*, *Heteromys* (rodents), *Potos* (kinkajou), among many other wild mammals, have been found naturally infected with *Leishmania* spp. Treatment is, as for kala-azar, with anti-monial drugs, but metronidazole has also been reported effective.

TRYPANOSOMIASIS

The organisms of the genus *Trypanosoma* fall into two main groups (Hoare, 1966):

Stercoraria—Trypanosoma spp. that, after multiplication in the midgut of the insect vector, typically pass posteriorly, and produce the forms infective to the vertebrate host (metacyclic forms) in the rectum; transmission, therefore, is by the 'posterior station', 'contaminative', by the introduction of infective forms in bug faeces to new hosts *via* skin abrasions or mucous membranes.

This group includes two trypanosome species infecting man in America—*Trypanosoma (Schizotrypanum) cruzi*, the agent of Chagas' disease, and *Trypanosoma (Herpetomonas) rangeli*, a non-pathogenic species.

Salivaria—Trypanosoma spp. that, after multiplication in the midgut of the insect vector, typically pass anteriorly, producing the forms infective to the vertebrate host (metacyclic forms) in the mouth parts or salivary glands; transmission is, therefore, by the 'anterior station', 'inoculative', by the introduction of metacyclic forms by the bite of the vector.

This group includes *Trypanosoma (Trypanozoon) brucei*, subspecies *gambiense* and *rhodesiense*, the agents of African sleeping sickness, and also the trypanosomes indirectly important to man as causes of nagana in cattle—*T. (Duttonella) vivax*, *T. (Nannomonas) congolense* and *T. (T.) brucei brucei*.

American Trypanosomiasis: Chagas' Disease

Chagas' disease occurs mainly in Central America, in Mexico and Costa Rica, and in South America, in all the states south as far as northern Argentina. Some 30 million people are estimated to be at risk and some 7 million infected at the present time. The agent, *T. (S.) cruzi*, is transmitted by the faeces of blood-sucking bugs of the family Reduviidae, the kissing, barber or assassin bugs, species of *Panstrongylus*, *Rhodnius* and *Triatoma*.

The incubation period is some 7 to 14 days. There is frequently a lesion at the site of infection, the chagoma, an indurated swelling of the skin, or unilateral conjunctivitis with palpebral oedema, Romaña's sign. When recognized, the acute stage of the disease is characterized by pyrexia, headache, local or generalized oedema, and signs of heart involvement. The acute stage is seen most in children and is believed to involve a mortality of about 5 per cent, mainly due to meningo-encephalitis. Recovery may appear to be complete but after some decades disturbance of the physiology of hollow organs may supervene — myocardial insufficiency, interference with bundle conduction, heart block; 'mega' conditions of the oesophagus, colon and other viscera in which there is interference with peristaltic function and distension of the organ. These late effects appear mainly in the third to fifth decades of life, when the economic productivity and family responsibility of the individual are at their greatest. Sudden death under exertion is commonly the terminal event in chronic Chagas' disease. It appears to be due, mainly, to cardiac arrest, rather than to embolus of the thrombi which form in the heart, or to rupture of the apical aneurysm which is characteristic of the Chagas heart.

Infection is by the introduction of trypomastigotes from the faeces of the vector bug into the host. These invade many types of cell, but mainly macrophages and muscle cells, transforming to amastigotes. Repeated binary fission of the amastigotes in the host cell transform it into a cyst-like cavity packed with amastigotes—the pseudocyst (Colour Plate 26). A proportion of the amastigotes in the cyst transform to trypomastigotes and leave the cyst, circulating in the body and infecting further cells. Not all the amastigotes released from the pseudocyst transform; some degenerate and induce local inflammatory lesions and Köberle (1968) believes these are responsible for the diminution in the number of the ganglion cells of the autonomic nervous system which results, later, in disturbance of heart and gut function. Trypomastigotes circulating in the blood are 15 to 20 μm long, often C-shaped, with an acutely-pointed posterior end and a large kinetoplast (Colour Plate 27). Besides invading and infecting further cells of the vertebrate host these trypanosomes are able to multiply in the gut of the vector bug. They do not divide in the blood. They may be numerous in the blood during the acute phase and may persist in the blood during the chronic phase, but at such low concentrations that they are difficult to demonstrate.

Laboratory Diagnosis

Diagnosis by demonstration of the parasite in the peripheral blood by microscopy is sometimes easy in the acute stage. The extremely low concentrations of trypanosomes in the peripheral blood in the chronic stage makes microscopical diagnosis always difficult. The amount of blood examined can be increased, e.g. by the use of thick films. But multiplicative methods, blood culture, the inoculation of animals, and xenodiagnosis, are more likely to be successful and, particularly the last, are much used. Xenodiagnosis consists of allowing laboratory-bred clean bugs to feed on suspect hosts, maintaining the bugs in the laboratory long enough for any ingested organisms to multiply, and then examining the gut contents of the bugs for their presence. Although certainly a highly sensitive way of recognizing infection, xenodiagnosis is laborious, and slow to yield answers —it may be necessary to keep the bugs for some 60 to 90 days to detect all infections. And, as it involves extensive handling of bugs containing infective forms, it is dangerous. The complement fixation (CF) test is widely used for screening of populations for *T. cruzi* infection and for diagnosis, though variability in antigen preparations has caused difficulties. Haemagglutination and immunofluorescence tests have been developed and are in process of evaluation.

The transmission cycle of *T. (S.) cruzi* is shown in Figure 54.3. Several species of reduviid bugs are involved in different parts of central and south America, most importantly, *Rhodnius prolixus*, *Triatoma infestans* and *Panstrongylus megistus*. Mostly these insects feed at night so transmission is mainly in the dark, in low quality

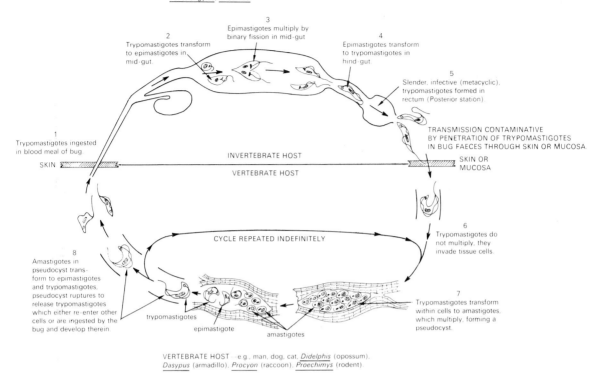

FIG. 54.3. Life cycle of *Trypanosoma* (*Schizotrypanum*) *cruzi* in vertebrate and invertebrate hosts.

housing, in rural or peri-urban areas. Probably the most important transmission cycles are intra-human or between domestic animals such as dogs and cats and the human population. There are occasional records of transmission, transplacentally, by milk and by laboratory accident. Transmission by blood transfusion is important: it may be guarded against by CF testing of donor bloods.

Epidemiology

T. (*S.*) *cruzi*-like organisms occur in a wide variety of wild mammals—*Dasypus* (armadillo), *Didelphis* (opossum), *Neotoma* (wood-rat), *Procyon* (raccoon), as examples. These animals seem likely to act as reservoirs of human infection and possibly man may be infected directly from sylvatic cycles involving these animals by forest bugs entering houses; but the respective importances of the various possible channels of infection are difficult to assess.

Control and prevention of Chagas' disease is by protection against the bite of infected bugs by the improvement of housing structure so as to deny them harbourage, and by insecticides. Although some drugs, nitrofurans, have some efficacy against the parasite, a really effective chemotherapeutic agent of low toxicity to man has not yet been discovered.

T. (*H.*) *rangeli*, although non-pathogenic to man, requires to be mentioned at this stage. It occurs in man in Guatemala and El Salvador of Central America and in the South American states of Colombia, Venezuela, and Chile. It is readily distinguished in the peripheral blood from *T.* (*S.*) *cruzi*, being 26 to 36 μm in length and having a kinetoplast only 1 to 2 μm in diameter, very much smaller than that of *T. cruzi*. It infects also domestic dogs and cats and wild *Cebus* (capuchin monkey) and *Didelphis* (opossum). It, also, is transmitted by reduviid bugs, *Rhodnius* and *Triatoma* spp., apparently by both inoculative and contaminative routes. As well as the *T. cruzi*-like development in the lumen of the gut, the haemacoele is invaded and infective trypanosomes eventually appear in the salivary glands.

The infection appears to be non-pathogenic in the vertebrate host; it may, however, kill the vector bug.

AFRICAN TRYPANOSOMIASIS—SLEEPING SICKNESS

Two broadly different clinical patterns of sleeping sickness may be distinguished, associated with two named species of the infective agent, now perhaps more conveniently regarded as 'subspecies' of *Trypanosoma* (*Trypanozoon*) *brucei*. And there is a third 'subspecies', which is a morphologically identical organism occurring in wild and domestic artiodactyls (two-toed ungulates) and in insect vectors, but not capable of infecting man. As below:

T. brucei brucei—a parasite mainly of wild and domestic artiodactyls, not infecting man.
T. brucei gambiense—a parasite of the insidious, slow onset, sleeping sickness in man, with an incubation period extending to several years, Gambian or *T. gambiense* sleeping sickness.
T. brucei rhodesiense—parasite of the acute rapid onset, rapidly progressing, sleeping sickness whose incubation period is typically a matter of weeks, Rhodesian or *T. rhodesiense* sleeping sickness.

All are transmitted by the bite of dipterous flies of the genus *Glossina* (tsetse flies).

Sleeping sickness is widely distributed, but focally, in sub-Saharan Africa as far south as latitude 20°S. It is essentially a village or rural disease. Despite the extensive slave trade out of Africa the disease did not become established elsewhere in the world. Broadly, though there are exceptions, the slow onset *T. b. gambiense* disease occurs in West Africa and the more acute *T. b. rhodesiense* disease is distributed in East and Southeast Africa.

As in Chagas' disease there is often a lesion at the site of infection—the so-called trypanosome *chancre*. This is an indurated swelling (which later becomes an area of dry shining desquamation) in which trypanosomes inoculated by the bite of the infecting *Glossina*

multiply, mainly in the subcutaneous fat immediately deep to the dermis. This initial lesion is variably noticed as related to the systemic disease, perhaps more in the *T. rhodesiense*, because of its shorter incubation period, than in the *T. gambiense* disease. Thereafter, there is a stage of dissemination in blood and lymph of the host. Although this is the main obvious development, it is to be realized that the organisms are by no means confined to these tissues but invade widely. This stage is characterized by an irregularly remitting pyrexia, headache and, particularly, lymphadenopathy. The lymph nodes of the posterior cervical triangle are particularly affected; this, known as Winterbottom's sign, is reported to have been well known to slavers. The later stage of the disease is that of invasion of the central nervous system—slow speech, tremors of hands and tongue, unsteady gait progressing to coma and death, usually from intercurrent infection. The outcome of the untreated infection was until recently presumed always to be death but recent serological evidence indicates that there may be considerable numbers of 'healthy carriers' in an endemic situation (e.g. Bentz and Macario, 1963).

During the period of lymphatic and blood stream involvement, when trypanosomes are numerous in these fluids, there is increased fragility of erythrocytes, rise in serum potassium, a fall in serum albumin and a rise in globulin. The rise in globulin is particularly in the IgM, and is probably related to the repetitive appearance of a new antigenic variant of the infecting organism with each parasitaemic wave. The increase in IgM is dramatically large and is of diagnostic significance (see below). Lymph nodes are enlarged and haemorrhagic and contain many trypanosomes. Myocarditis occurs, even bundle branch block, but less conspicuously than in Chagas' disease. There is damage to the endothelium of capillaries with leakage of plasma into the surrounding tissues and disturbance of the circulation in small vessels. The later stage of the disease is that of a chronic meningo-encephalitis. The cerebrospinal fluid pressure is raised and there is an increase in its protein content and of its cells (mainly lymphocytes); both these changes are of diagnostic importance. The brain substance is infiltrated, mainly perivascularly, by lymphocytes, plasma cells and macrophages; demyelinization of fibres takes place, particularly near cellular infiltrates. Characteristic of the infection is the occurrence of morula cells, cells containing a large eosinophilic morula (perhaps composed of IgM), considered to be degenerate plasma cells. The pathological process is essentially similar in both types of the disease except for modifications related to the different rates of development; for instance, brain lesions are less marked in the more acute *T. rhodesiense* disease than they are in the more chronic *T. gambiense* one.

The organisms in the vertebrate host are trypomastigotes, with a blunt posterior end and small subterminal kinetoplast (Colour Plate 28) no intracellular amastigote phase as occurs in *T. (S.) cruzi* has been described. The trypomastigotes are pleomorphic, varying widely in length and usually categorized into long slender forms, as long as 35 μm, and with a considerable free flagellum, and short stumpy forms, as short as 15 μm, often without any free flagellum. Intermediate forms occur. The representation of these two forms in the blood varies with the stage of the infection. It is believed that the infection consists of a series of parasitaemic waves each of which, in its crescendo stage is composed mainly by long forms, in its diminuendo stage mainly by short forms; and that these waves are associated with antigenic change on the part of the organism, each wave being antigenically different from preceding and succeeding waves; and that, in preparation for establishment in the vector *Glossina*, the short forms are adapted for transfer from the blood environment to that of the lumen of the insect gut.

Laboratory Diagnosis

The diagnosis of sleeping sickness in its chronic stage is broadly comparable to that of Chagas' disease: it is the detection of organisms at extremely low concentrations. However, there are differences of emphasis. Salivarian trypanosomes are less easily cultured than are stercorarian and so blood culture is little used. Also, because even under optimum conditions only small proportions of *Glossina* become infected, xenodiagnosis is not useful. Animal inoculation is valuable in *T. rhodesiense* situations as most strains of this type readily infect laboratory rats or mice; it is less useful in *T. gambiense* situations as strains of this type characteristically only occasionally infect laboratory mice or rats and require to be established in more susceptible but less easily available hosts, young *Cercopithecus* (monkeys) or in *Cricetomys* (giant rat). It has recently been shown (Lanham, 1968) that there is a difference in surface charge between trypanosomes and the blood cells with which they are intermixed which allows them to be separated on anion-exchange columns. A large volume (e.g. 10 ml) of the blood of a suspect host may be passed through the column; blood corpuscles are preferentially retained on the material of the column (DEAE cellulose) while trypanosomes pass through and may be concentrated by centrifugation from the eluate which is otherwise free of cells. This method is extremely sensitive, allowing the recognition of the presence of trypanosomes at concentrations as low as 4 per ml.

The cell and protein content of the cerebrospinal fluid is of diagnostic and prognostic significance. Protein concentrations of over 30 mg per 100 ml and cell concentrations of over 5 per mm^3 are regarded as indicative of central nervous system involvement and therefore of requirement for treatment with arsenicals (see below). Centrifugation of cerebrospinal fluid and examination of the deposit for trypanosomes, or its inoculation to susceptible animals, are additional procedures.

Immunological diagnosis of African trypanosomiasis in man is complicated by the multiplicity of different antigenic types of the organisms which are produced during the course of the infection. Thus tests to recognize these variant antigens are only significant if positive; negative results may simply be due to the non-inclusion of the appropriate antigen in the test. Such tests are those based on agglutination, lysis, and neutralization of infectivity. Tests based on the stable antigens of trypanosomes—complement fixation, immunofluorescence—are more likely to be useful at a generic level but they miss a considerable proportion of cases which can be shown to be infected by 'parasitological'

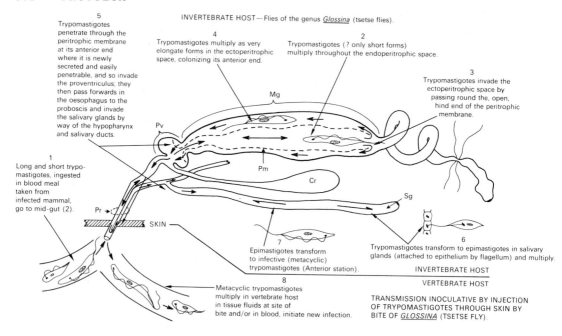

INVERTEBRATE HOST—Flies of the genus *Glossina* (tsetse flies).

5
Trypomastigotes penetrate through the peritrophic membrane at its anterior end where it is newly secreted and easily penetrable, and so invade the proventriculus; they then pass forwards in the oesophagus to the proboscis and invade the salivary glands by way of the hypopharynx and salivary ducts.

4
Trypomastigotes multiply as very elongate forms in the ectoperitrophic space, colonizing its anterior end.

2
Trypomastigotes (? only short forms) multiply throughout the endoperitrophic space.

3
Trypomastigotes invade the ectoperitrophic space by passing round the, open, hind end of the peritrophic membrane.

1
Long and short trypo-mastigotes, ingested in blood meal taken from infected mammal, go to mid-gut (2).

Mg
Pv
Pm
Cr
Sg
Pr
SKIN

7
Epimastigotes transform to infective (metacyclic) trypomastigotes (Anterior station).

6
Trypomastigotes transform to epimastigotes in salivary glands (attached to epithelium by flagellum) and multiply.

INVERTEBRATE HOST
VERTEBRATE HOST

8
Metacyclic trypomastigotes multiply in vertebrate host in tissue fluids at site of bite and/or in blood, initiate new infection.

TRANSMISSION INOCULATIVE BY INJECTION OF TRYPOMASTIGOTES THROUGH SKIN BY BITE OF *GLOSSINA* (TSETSE FLY).

VERTEBRATE HOST—e.g., man, bovids, equids.

FIG. 54.4. Life cycle of *Trypanosoma* (*Trypanozoon*) *brucei* sspp. in invertebrate hosts (*Glossina*). Pm—peritrophic membrane; P—proventriculus; Mg—midgut; Sg—salivary gland; Cr—crop; Pr—proboscis.

means. In this situation much attention has been attracted by a non-specific approach—the estimation of the level of IgM in the serum and CSF. This, as was pointed out by Mattern (1968) is of such an order that there is little danger of confusion with other diseases, especially if the CSF IgM content is taken into account. Estimation of serum IgM, easily and rapidly performed by several methods, especially by radial immunodiffusion in agar gel containing antiserum specific for IgM, is thus a useful screening procedure. It is this method, together with immunofluorescence techniques, which have indicated that there exists in African populations exposed to infection a significant proportion of persons with silent infections who may act as healthy carriers (Bentz and Macario, 1963).

The process of development of *T. brucei* in *Glossina* is detailed in Fig. 54.4, and hardly requires further comment. Non-cyclical transmission, by miscellaneous species of biting flies, often canvassed in the veterinary context, seems

not to be regarded as important in the human one.

Epidemiology

Patterns of transmission and epidemiology are difficult to prove but some are plausibly proposed and may be accepted as probable for each of the two main epidemiological situations. Transmission of the *T. gambiense* type disease seems to be mainly by intra-human cycles. The slow onset of the disease predisposes to the long term presence of infected persons to act as sources for the infection of *Glossina*. Transmission is mainly associated with the repetitive attack of restricted populations of *Glossina* on the human population. An example of this kind of situation is the village in the savannah zone sited close to a watercourse fringed with woodland infested with *Glossina palpalis*. The people visit the stream bed for water and for washing and are then exposed to attack by a *Glossina* population restricted to the riverain woodland by the aridity of the general countryside surrounding. In such a situation the fly population feeds repetitively on the humans and so transmission occurs without other animal hosts being necessarily involved; all categories of the population, men, women and children, may be involved, but mainly the women, as especially concerned with water collection and washing. In contrast, transmission of the *T. rhodesiense* disease seems to be much more a zoonosis. Because the disease is typically acute, infected persons are rapidly removed from the epidemiological picture, either by death or by treatment. The disease is mainly associated with visits by honey-hunters, fishermen, game-watchers, and such like, to areas sparsely inhabited by man but with abundant antelope populations. Incidence tends to be higher in males than in other members of the population.

Treatment

Efficient therapeutic and prophylactic drugs are available for African trypanosomiasis. Suramin is the drug of choice for cases without central nervous system involvement, melarsoprol (an arsenical drug) for later stage cases when the central nervous system has been invaded. Pentamidine can be used as a prophylactic. Policies differ depending on local situations; for instance prophylactic drugs are used in *T. gambiense* areas in which incubation periods are prolonged and detection of infection difficult, discouraged in *T. rhodesiense* areas in which infections may be expected to declare themselves at an early date and so be able to be specifically treated. Similarly, anti-*Glossina* measures such as insecticiding or destruction of the vegetation of the *Glossina* habitat may be economically feasible in *gambiense* contexts but less so in *rhodesiense* situations which may involve huge areas of sparsely inhabited bush.

AMOEBAE

Eight species of amoebae infect man. Seven of these are essentially primary parasites of the gut lumen, one, of the tissues of the central nervous system.

Amoebic Infection Primarily of the Gut Lumen

The seven species concerned are:
Entamoeba gingivalis, Ent. coli, Ent. hartmanni, Ent. histolytica; Endolimax nana; Iodamoeba bütschlii; Dientamoeba fragilis.

These organisms vary in size, with species or stage of development, from some 5 to 50 μm in diameter; most are between 7 and 35 μm. Differentiation of species both as trophozoites and as cysts tends to be difficult, depending on size and on details of nuclear structure and of cytoplasmic inclusions, difficult to observe. Only one species, *Entamoeba histolytica*, is regarded as an important pathogen.

ENTAMOEBA HISTOLYTICA: AMOEBIC DYSENTERY AND SEQUELAE

E. histolytica is a cosmopolitan parasite of man but clinical manifestations of infection are more common in tropical and subtropical regions than in temperate climates. Recorded prevalences vary widely, from say 5 to 20 per cent of individuals in temperate climate communities to 20 to 50 per cent in tropical ones. Such figures are heavily influenced by the methods used; for instance, a single stool examination without concentration will discover only about one-third of infected individuals. And *Ent. hartmanni* (see below) may not be differentiated, in which case the figures are likely to be about twice those for *Ent. histolytica* alone.

Ent. histolytica infection of the intestine may be asymptomatic or cause clinical symptoms of varying degrees of intensity up to that of acute dysentery. Symptoms tend to develop gradually, intermittent diarrhoea and constipation, abdominal discomfort, nausea, vomiting and loss of appetite.

Infection is acquired by the ingestion of cysts in contaminated food or water. Amoebae establish themselves first in the mucosal crypts of the intestine and then penetrate into the submucosa where they multiply, forming abscesses. These rupture to the gut lumen and develop into ulcers with raised undermined edges and necrotic centres. The amoebae extend the ulcer laterally below the epithelium and muscularis layers so that an ulcer with over-hanging shaggy edges is formed, the 'flask' ulcer. The region most involved initially is that of the appendix, caecum and ascending colon. Spread from the initial region, by amoebae carried along the gut, produce further lesions, particularly in the sigmoid colon and rectum. The ulcers are, of course, invaded also by bacteria. They may perforate into the peritoneal cavity.

Extra-intestinal Amoebiasis

From the intestinal lesions amoebae and bacteria may spread by lymphatic and blood vessels more widely in the body. Hepatitis occurs and it is controversial how far this condition is caused by actual metastases of amoebae and how far by simple increase in the exposure of the liver to bacterial and toxic influences from the gut lesions. Doubtless both factors are operative in

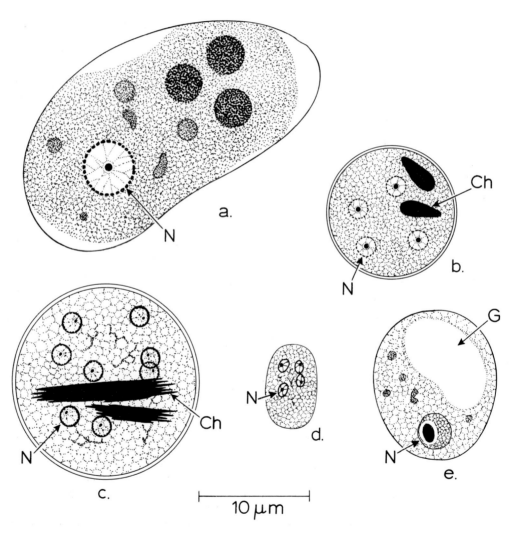

FIG. 54.5. (a) *Entamoeba histolytica*, trophozoite with ingested erythrocytes. (b) *Entamoeba histolytica*, mature cyst. (c) *Entamoeba coli*, mature cyst. (d) *Endolimax nana*, cyst. (e) *Iodamoeba bütschlii*, cyst. N—nucleus; Ch—chromatoid bodies; G—glycogen vacuole.

varying degrees. Amoebic abscess occurs most commonly in the liver and in its right lobe, because of the usual initiation of gut lesions in the caecal region. Clinical symptoms are mainly intermittent fever, night sweats, and pain in the upper right abdominal quadrant.

Liver abscesses may attain a large size and be palpable. Typically they show a central liquid core, composed of necrotic liver and blood cells, fat, etc., with connective tissue strands, surrounded by a layer of normal liver tissue being invaded by amoebae. They are usually bacteriologically sterile. They may rupture in several directions—to the surface, to the peritoneum, colon, pleural cavity or lung. Amoebic abscesses are rare in other sites. Amoebic brain abscesses may occur concurrently with or subsequent to liver abscess. They are small, perivascular, occurring mainly in the cerebrum and are usually rapidly fatal.

Cutaneous amoebiasis is secondary to intestinal amoebiasis, the skin being invaded, particularly in the perianal and perineal regions, as extensions from rectal infections. Other sites sometimes affected are those at the rupture of a liver abscess or at a colostomy or on the penis as a result of unnatural sexual practices.

Laboratory Diagnosis

The parasitological diagnosis of amoebiasis depends on the demonstration of the parasite in the stool, in scrapes of ulcers obtained by sigmoidoscopy, or in the aspirate of an abscess. For stools, a direct microscopical examination is made of small samples, including any mucus observed, emulsified, respectively, in physiological salt solution and in a solution of iodine in potassium iodide. Trophozoites, and the nuclear and chromatoid characteristics of cysts may be observed in the unstained film; cyst nuclei may be further observed in the iodine. Emulsification of a sample in 1 per cent eosin may be useful, showing up trophozoites and cysts unstained against a stained background. Repetitive examination may be necessary as cyst production may be intermittent. Concentration techniques are available, flotation in 33 per cent zinc sulphate solution, and emulsification

in formalin with ether and centrifugation; Sargeaunt's stain (malachite green) is used to demonstrate chromatoid bodies (see below) in cysts after concentration. Cultivation, also, is useful, on an egg-slant medium with horse serum and rice starch. Faecal material may be preserved and stained by the 'MIF' technique (with sodium merthiolate, iodine and formalin) so that it may be satisfactorily examined for cysts for at least a year afterwards.

The main morphological characteristics of *Ent. histolytica* are:

Trophozoite (Fig. 54.5a) 10 to 60 μm in diameter; cytoplasm clearly differentiated into ectoplasm and endoplasm, sometimes with ingested erythrocytes; nucleus vesicular with small central karyosome and fine peripheral granules of chromatin.

Cyst (Fig. 54.5b) 10 to 20 μm in diameter, spherical, with 4 nuclei when mature; chromatoid bodies (ribonucleoprotein reserve) blunt-ended rods.

Mainly, *E. histolytica* requires to be distinguished from *E. hartmanni* and *E. coli* which are closely similar but non-pathogenic:

Ent. hartmanni (trophozoites 5 to 14 μm; cysts 4 to 10 μm) corresponds to what used to be designated the small, non-pathogenic, race of *E. histolytica*. It is distinguished from *E. histolytica* by its smaller cysts ($< 10 \mu$m in diameter), by the diffuse type of vacuolation in the cyst, and by immunofluorescence.

Ent. coli trophozoites are similar to those of *E. histolytica* but their nuclear structure is more coarsely granular and they do not ingest erythrocytes. The cysts (Fig. 54.5b) tend to be larger (10 to 33 μm) than those of *E. histolytica* and typically show 8 nuclei when mature; chromatoid bodies in the cyst are splinter-like.

As regards the serological diagnosis of *E. histolytica* infection, complement fixation, agglutination and immunofluorescence tests are available and are mostly useful for indicating extra-intestinal involvement.

The four other, non-pathogenic, amoebae infecting the human gut lumen may be quickly dismissed:

Ent. gingivalis occurs in the mouth and upper pharynx. It is essentially similar in structure to *E. histolytica* (Fig. 54.5a). It ingests bacteria, host leucocytes, epithelial cell debris and occasionally erythrocytes. No cyst has been described and transmission is presumably direct.

Endolimax nana occurs mainly in the caecum. Its nucleus has a large eccentric karyosome and little peripheral chromatin. Mature cysts (5 to 14 μm) contain 4 nuclei.

Iodamoeba bütschlii occurs mainly in the caecum. The nucleus has a large central or eccentric karyosome. Cysts (5 to 18 μm) are usually uninucleate and show a conspicuous vacuole, packed with glycogen, which stains brown with iodine, hence the name of the genus (Fig. 54.5e).

Dientamoeba fragilis is a small amoeba which occurs mainly in the glandular crypts of the colon. Commonly, individual organisms have two nuclei whose karyosomes are made up of several granules. No cyst is known.

EPIDEMIOLOGY

Transmission of *Ent. histolytica* is by the ingestion of cysts, which typically occur in formed rather than in dysenteric stools; the latter usually contain only trophozoites. Cysts will remain viable under moist cool conditions for some 30 days but are killed by desiccation and heat (50°C). They are resistant to antiseptics such as mercuric chloride, formalin and chlorine. The contamination of food by cysts is associated with: contaminated water supplies; low standards of hygiene in food handling; transport by flies and cockroaches, in which cysts can survive 48 hours; the use of human faeces as manure; low standards of personal hygiene, such as in mental institutions. Large water-borne epidemics have been reported; 1409 infections occurred in two hotels in Chicago in 1933, due to leakage of sewage into the water supply.

As regards hosts of *E. histolytica* other than man, dogs, kittens and guinea pigs may be infected, often pathogenically, with strains from symptomless humans. Dogs and monkeys have been found naturally infected but are considered of little significance in the epidemiology of the human disease.

The measures for the control of amoebiasis are obvious, the detection and treatment of cyst-passers, the improvement of diagnostic surveillance, of hygiene in relation to water supply, of food handling, toilet customs, and so on; although these matters are not always easily susceptible of improvement in primitive communities.

Treatment

Emetine hydrochloride with chloroquine, or metronidazole are drugs of choice when the liver is involved. Emetine may be contra-indicated by its cardiotoxicity. Abscesses regress on treatment but if evacuation is necessary, aspiration is to be preferred to surgical drainage. For the intestinal infection emetine hydrochloride is ineffective and metronidazole, emetine bismuth iodide and diloxanide furoate are recommended. 'Cyst passers', without clinical symptoms, may be treated where their incidence in the population is low as in the U.K. and the U.S.A.

Primary Amoebic Meningo-encephalitis

Since 1964 there have been some 40 records of primary meningo-encephalitis ascribed to infection with amoebae of the genera *Hartmanella* and *Naegleria*, previously thought to be free living organisms occurring in damp soil. Although prodromal symptoms of upper respiratory tract infection may occur, the onset is typically sudden, with headache and fever, progressing to vomiting, neck and back rigidity and mental confusion, coma and death in some 4 to 7 days. Organisms occur in pockets, packed with amoebae, around capillaries, mainly in the cerebral grey matter. Symptoms resemble meningococcal meningitis but the turbid cerebrospinal fluid contains erythrocytes and amoebae instead of neutrophils and diplococci. Cases have been reported from Australia, Czechoslovakia, U.S.A. and U.K. Infection is associated with swimming in freshwater lakes or pools or playing in muddy water; infection directly through the nasal mucosa and cribriform plate is presumed. Amphotericin B may be effective in treatment; early institution of treatment is important.

Symptomless infection of the throat with *Hartmanella* sp. has been found in infants, and amoebae from such cases will, in mice, invade the central nervous system via the nasal mucosa.

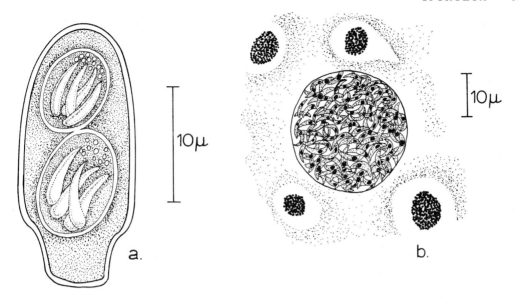

Fɪɢ. 54.6. (a) *Isospora belli* sporulated oocyst from faeces. (b) *Toxoplasma gondii*, cyst in mouse brain.

SPOROZOA

The distinction made for the flagellates and for the amoebae between parasites which are primarily of the gut lumen or of tissues, is less clear in the Sporozoa as these are all essentially parasites of cells. However, a general distinction still holds true, between those which are parasites of the margins of the gut lumen, the gut epithelium (*Isospora*, *Toxoplasma*) and those which are parasites of deeper tissues (*Plasmodium*, *Sarcocystis*, *Pneumocystis*, *Babesia*).

Iꜱᴏꜱᴘᴏʀᴀ, Tᴏxᴏᴘʟᴀꜱᴍᴀ: Sᴘᴏʀᴏᴢᴏᴀɴ Iɴꜰᴇᴄᴛɪᴏɴꜱ ᴏꜰ ᴛʜᴇ Gᴜᴛ Eᴘɪᴛʜᴇʟɪᴜᴍ

Human infection with *Isospora belli* and *I. hominis*, regarded previously as hardly more than curiosities, have taken on a new significance with the demonstration by Hutchison and his colleagues (see below) that *Toxoplasma gondii* passes through a similar cycle of development and is therefore likely to be closely-related. Information on the *Isospora* spp. infecting man is scanty but by analogy with *Isospora* infections in other animals the course of infection is probably as follows. Sporozoites ingested in food initiate one or several schizogony cycles in the epithelial cells of the lower ileum or caecum. Later, male and female gametocytes are produced in the same situation and from a resulting zygote, formed in the gut lumen, is derived an oocyst which on 'sporulation', outside the body, develops two sporocysts each enclosing 4 sporozoites (Fig. 54.6a). Clinical manifestation of infection is limited to mild, brief, self-terminating diarrhoea.

Toxoplasma gondii occurs in a wide range of mammalian and avian hosts as crescentic organisms some 6 μm long (zoites) which invade cells, mainly macrophages, multiplying in them till the cell is packed with organisms, the pseudocyst. Rupture of the cell releases the organisms to infect other cells. Proliferation occurs widely in the body but particularly in the central nervous system, muscles and lungs. In this longer term, chronic, stage, infected cells may be up to 60 μm in diameter and contain thousands of parasites enclosed in a tough membrane—the cyst (Fig. 54.6b).

Only some 200 clinical cases of toxoplasmosis are reported annually in the U.K. but serological tests indicate that some 30 per cent of the population have undergone infection. Symptomatology in post-partum infection is mild, lymphadenitis with or without fever, but infection persists for long periods in a latent phase. Prenatal infection is more serious, the fetal nervous system being vulnerable; cerebral calcification, chorio-retinitis, hydrocephalus or microcephalus and psychomotor disturbances are common after pregnancies proceeding to term; or stillbirth may be the outcome.

Although toxoplasma infection has been known to be widespread in the U.K. population since serological tests for its recognition were introduced about 1948, the transmission of the disease has been a puzzle. Transmission by ingestion or handling of infected meat was known but this could not explain the high incidence in the general population nor the common occurrence of the disease in herbivorous animals. The work of Hutchison, Dunachie, Siim and Work (1970) showed that *Toxoplasma gondii* went through a cycle of development in the epithelial cells of the gut of cats similar to that known for *Isospora* spp. Perhaps *Toxoplasma* should now be included in the genus *Isospora* and perhaps cats are importantly involved in the epidemiology of the human disease.

Laboratory Diagnosis

Organisms may be recognized in smears of biopsy or necropsy tissues or in deposits from centrifuged CSF, stained with Romanowsky stains. But identification of organisms may be difficult. Intracerebral and intraperitoneal inoculation of mice is preferable; peritoneal exudates and brain smears Romanowsky-stained are examined for organisms after 6 to 10 days, or in animals dying.

The Sabin-Feldman dye test, complement fixation and the fluorescent antibody test are the most useful serological tests. The dye test depends on the fact that living *T. gondii* lose their affinity for methylene blue when treated with homologous antiserum; normal human serum also is necessary in the test, as an 'activator'.

MALARIA: SPOROZOAN INFECTIONS OF THE DEEP TISSUES

The trenchant effects of malaria on human affairs up until about the time of World War 2 are discussed by Hackett (1937). Malaria appears most dramatically as the prime disease of military importance, capable of incapacitating such large numbers of troops that military operations may be endangered. But the disease has a less noticeable, more insidious impact in endemic situations; freedom from clinical disease in the adult population is purchased by a high infant mortality, and standards of living and cultural levels are depressed.

Malaria is widely distributed in the world, not only in the tropics and the subtropics but as far north as the Arctic circle. There are few countries where some species of anopheline mosquito capable of transmitting under suitable conditions of temperature, do not exist. Of the tropics, only some Pacific islands are free from *Anopheles* and so have never been malarious. Recent schemes of malaria eradication, under the aegis of the World Health Organization, have greatly contracted the distribution of malaria and many areas, e.g. south Europe, which were malarious before World War 2, are now free; however, many areas, in particular sub-Saharan Africa, remain virtually unchanged and some 360 million people still live in malarious areas. Also, setbacks have been numerous and the present consensus of opinion (Bruce-Chwatt, 1969) is that the outcome of malaria eradication schemes may be compromised by lack of administrative organization and basic health services.

Malaria in man is caused by infection with one or other of four species of *Plasmodia—Plasmodium vivax*, *P. malariae* or *P. ovale* and *P. (Laverania) falciparum*, *P. falciparum* is by far the most important.

The life cycles and transmission patterns of all four species are fundamentally similar (Fig. 54.7), though there are differences which are important in relation to pathogenicity and treatment. Closely related parasites occur in non-human primates in both the Old and New Worlds and some infections have been exchanged between man and other primates in both directions. However, it is considered (W.H.O., 1969) that infections of non-human primates present little danger to the health of man and so, in general, consideration here may be limited to intra-human transmission cycles, i.e. from patient to patient.

IN MAN

IN ANOPHELINE
MOSQUITO

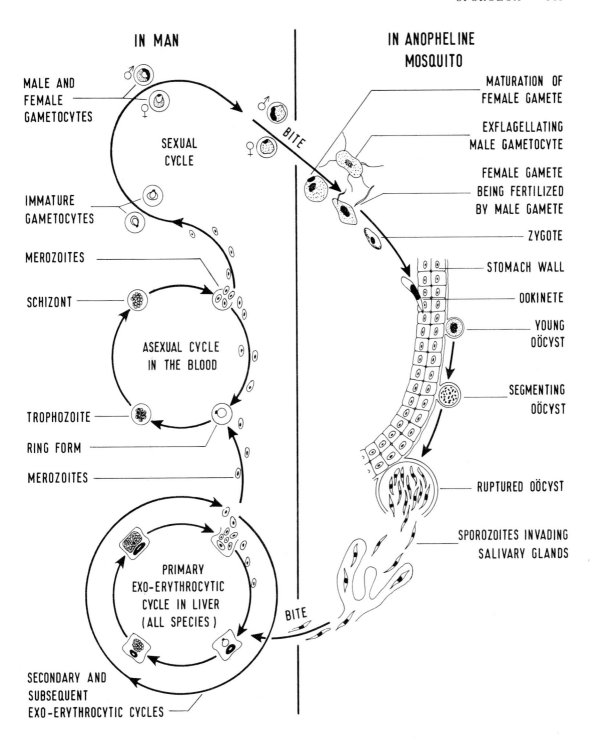

MALE AND
FEMALE
GAMETOCYTES

SEXUAL
CYCLE

BITE

MATURATION OF
FEMALE GAMETE

EXFLAGELLATING
MALE GAMETOCYTE

FEMALE GAMETE
BEING FERTILIZED
BY MALE GAMETE

IMMATURE
GAMETOCYTES

ZYGOTE

STOMACH WALL

MEROZOITES

SCHIZONT

OOKINETE

YOUNG
OÖCYST

ASEXUAL CYCLE
IN THE BLOOD

SEGMENTING
OÖCYST

TROPHOZOITE

RING FORM

MEROZOITES

RUPTURED OÖCYST

SPOROZOITES INVADING
SALIVARY GLANDS

PRIMARY
EXO-ERYTHROCYTIC
CYCLE IN LIVER
(ALL SPECIES)

BITE

SECONDARY AND
SUBSEQUENT
EXO-ERYTHROCYTIC CYCLES

FIG. 54.7. Life cycle of *Plasmodium vivax* in man and in the female anopheline mosquito.

Life Cycle

The basic cycles of development in human and invertebrate hosts (always a female *Anopheles* mosquito) are shown in Figure 54.7. Infection of the human host is by sporozoites inoculated by the bite of the mosquito. Sporozoites are spindle-shaped organisms some 12 μm in length. They pass to the liver where they invade parenchyma cells, grow and become schizonts—the primary exo-erythrocytic schizonts. The curious nomenclature of these forms arises from the fact that they are of comparatively recent discovery, long after the erythrocytic cycles of schizogony (see below) were well known. These schizonts, in the liver parenchyma cells, take some 5 to 15 days to develop. Fully developed, they are up to 60 μm in diameter and each produces some tens of thousands of merozoites (Colour Plate 30). These merozoites, released on rupture of the host cell, have two destinations. They may invade further liver parenchyma cells and initiate secondary, and continuing (apparently for periods of many years) cycles of exo-erythrocytic schizogony in these cells; or they may enter erythrocytes, initiating the erythrocytic schizogony cycle. Secondary and subsequent cycles of exo-erythrocytic schizogony in the liver cells occur only in *P. (Plasmodium)* spp.—*P. vivax*, *P. malariae* and *P. ovale*. In *P. (Laverania) falciparum* only a single primary exo-erythrocytic schizogony cycle takes place, a point of importance with regard to relapse and treatment (see below).

The growth of the merozoites that enter erythrocytes is fundamentally the same for all four species. The organism first becomes vacuolated so that in stained preparations it presents a 'signet ring' appearance—a ring of blue cytoplasm round a vacuole, interrupted at one point by the red-staining nucleus (Colour Plate 31). The parasites continue to enlarge (trophozoites, Colour Plate 32) to form the erythrocytic schizont. When this stage is reached, the nuclear material divides up into some 5 to 32 portions (Colour Plate 33) about which the cytoplasm condenses to form a corresponding number of merozoites, that are released into the plasma on the rupture of the containing erythrocyte. These merozoites invade other erythrocytes, initiating further cycles of erythrocytic

schizogony. Also, some merozoites give rise to sexual forms, gametocytes (Colour Plates 35 and 36), which develop further only if they are ingested by a suitable vector *Anopheles*. In that vector, female gametocytes round up and become female gametes, while male gametocytes 'exflagellate'—produce some 8 flagellate male gametes (Fig. 54.7), which fertilize the female gametes. The resulting zygotes are motile organisms, called oökinetes, which penetrate the wall of the midgut of the mosquito, settling on its haemocoelic aspect and developing to oöcysts (Fig. 54.7). A fully developed oöcyst, some 60 μm in diameter, contains large numbers of sporozoites. On its rupture into the haemocoele of the mosquito the sporozoites pass to the salivary glands whence they may be inoculated into a new vertebrate host.

SYMPTOMATOLOGY AND PATHOLOGY

Clinical and pathological effects in malaria are exclusively related to the erythrocytic cycle, the exo-erythrocytic phase in the liver is pathologically silent. The paroxysm is due to the rupture of the infected erythrocytes and the release into the blood plasma of the merozoites, the remains of the red cell cytoplasm and the excretory products of the schizont (including malaria pigment). Thus the incubation period of the disease will be at least the duration of the primary exo-erythrocytic cycle plus the duration of one erythrocytic cycle. Typically it is 8 to 30 days but may be extended to weeks, months or even years. Onset is usually sudden and the periodical paroxysms of pyrexia and sweating—the malaria rigor—related to the periodicity of erythrocytic schizogony, are well known. However, symptoms may be variable, particularly with *P. falciparum* infections. The disease may present first with gastrointestinal, cerebral or other symptoms, and periodic rigors may be absent.

There are certain differences between the species which have important clinical implications:

1. The numbers of merozoites produced by the primary exo-erythrocytic schizont is 10 000 to 15 000 in *P. vivax*, *P. malariae* and *P. ovale*, 30 000 to 40 000 in *P. falciparum*. Also the rate of development of the primary exo-erythrocytic

schizont is faster in *P. falciparum*, taking 5 to 6 days, as compared with 7 to 8 days for *P. vivax*, about 9 for *P. ovale* and 13 to 16 for *P. malariae*.

Thus *P. falciparum* is the parasite most likely to produce the largest numbers of merozoites invading the blood, at the earliest time after infection.

2. The periodicity of erythrocytic schizogony in *P. vivax*, *P. ovale* and *P. falciparum* is 48 hours and so, as the pyrexia induced by the infection tends to be similarly periodic, they give rise to 'tertian' malaria, the peaks of pyrexia being on the 'third' day. In *P. malariae* the periodicity of the erythrocytic cycle is 72 hours and the pyrexia 'quartan'.

3. The numbers of merozoites produced by each erythrocytic schizont varies with the species, being higher (up to 24 per schizont) in *P. vivax* and *P. falciparum*, and lower in *P. ovale* and *P. malariae* (5 to 12 per schizont).

Taking all these factors into account *P. falciparum* emerges as the parasite with the highest potential for multiplication in the human host. Its pre-erythrocytic schizogony produces the largest numbers of merozoites and is short; its erythrocytic cycle is short and the number of merozoites produced tends to be large. At the other extreme, *P. ovale* and *P. malariae* have exo-erythrocytic schizonts yielding comparatively small numbers of merozoites; their erythrocytic cycles of schizogony are longer, and the numbers of merozoites they produce tend to be small.

Besides being pre-eminent as regards reproductive potential, *P. falciparum* also tends to localize, except for early trophozoites (ring-forms) and gametocytes, in the capillaries of internal organs. These capillaries may become blocked with masses of infected cells, free parasites, pigment and phagocytic cells. The effect appears to be related to increased adherence of infected cells to the endothelium and increase in blood viscosity associated with parasitized cells being less easily deformed than uninfected cells. Petechial, 'ring', haemorrhages surround affected capillaries. Neuroglial cells invade necrotic foci, the malarial granuloma. Many tissues are affected, brain, spleen, liver, bone marrow, intestines, etc., and the clinical picture is largely dependent on the distribution and intensity of the lesions. Particularly serious

is involvement of the brain which is the cause of most of the deaths from *P. falciparum* infection. This picture is a simplified one and it has been suggested that stickiness and sludging are later events and that malaria pathogenesis is mainly related to disturbance of the oxygen metabolism of the tissue cells, not because of defects in oxygen transport but rather because of pathological changes in the metabolizing cells. In chronic malaria there is typically anaemia, enlargement and hardening of the spleen, hepatomegaly and pigmentation of tissues.

Although *P. falciparum* is the most immediately pathogenic of the four species, it is not liable to relapse as it undergoes only a single, primary, cycle of exo-erythrocytic schizogony in the liver cells. In the other species, blood schizogony may be re-initiated for periods of many (up to 40) years from continuing secondary and subsequent cycles of exo-erythrocytic schizogony in the liver. Reappearances of *P. falciparum* infection, derived from the erythrocytic cycle and termed 'recrudescences', are more limited, to a year or so.

Laboratory Diagnosis

From diagnostic and prognostic points of view two steps are important. (1) the distinction of malaria parasites from other structures which may resemble them and; (2) the differentiation of *P. falciparum*, as the main lethal parasite, requiring urgent treatment, from the other species. To be accepted as malaria parasites the structures should show, in Romanowsky-stained films, definite blue cytoplasm and red nuclear material and be intracellular in the erythrocyte. The various stages of the four parasite species differ in many characters, such as size, morphology, arrangement of the merozoites, the alterations which they cause in the host erythrocyte and so on. These differences will be detailed in Volume 2 but some representative forms are shown in colour in the Plates (29 to 34). One important point with relation to *P. falciparum* should be emphasized. In this species the larger trophozoites and the schizonts are confined to the deeper capillaries so that, typically, only early trophozoites (ring forms) and gametocytes (crescents, Plate 34) occur in the peripheral circulation.

Transmission and Epidemiology

The cycle of development in the female anopheline mosquito (Fig. 54.7) takes, at 20°C, some 16 days for *P. vivax*, 30 for *P. malariae* and 22 for *P. falciparum*. Epidemiological patterns are exceedingly complex, being affected by many factors; the intensity of anopheline breeding and its relation to human communities, the susceptibility of local *Anopheles* spp. to infection, their predilection to enter houses and to feed on the human host, the effect of meteorological conditions on the speed of development of the parasite and the vector, or the longevity of the vector; and so on. Attempts have been made to produce mathematical models of epidemiological situations.

Treatment and Prevention

The efficacy of the natural drug quinine against malaria is well known. Although not discarded it is nowadays largely replaced by synthetic chemotherapeutic agents, which vary in their efficacy and application to different stages of the development of the parasite:

Primary exo-erythrocytic schizonticides. Drugs acting in this way (and on sporozoites) are designated 'causal prophylactics' as they prevent any clinical infection. Proguanil (biguanide); pyrimethamine (diaminopyrimidine).

Erythrocytic schizonticides. These drugs are mainly applicable in the treatment of the developed disease or for its suppression. Chloroquine and amodiaquine (4-aminoquinolines); mepacrine (9-amino-acridine).

Secondary exo-erythrocytic schizonticides are used for 'radical treatment', the prevention of relapse. Pamaquine, primaquine (8-aminoquinolines).

Gametocytocides affect gametocytes so that they cannot develop subsequently in the anopheline vector. Pamaquine, primaquine (8-aminoquinolines).

With the widespread use of synthetic drugs *Plasmodium* spp. may develop resistance to them. Most important has been the appearance of *P. falciparum* strains resistant to 4-aminoquinolines widely in the tropics—Brazil, Thailand, Vietnam, etc.

Antimalarial drugs fall into three main groups (Hunsicker, 1969):

(a) Drugs inhibiting the synthesis of new DNA and read-out of RNA so interfering with the synthesis of many enzymes—quinoline derivatives.

(b) Aminobenzoic acid antagonists—sulphonamides and sulphones.

(c) Folic acid reductase inhibitors; pyrimethamine, proguanil, which interfere, respectively, with the formation and metabolism of folic acid.

Drugs of groups (b) and (c) affect primarily the dividing parasite and so are generally slower in action than are the quinolines. Also, since they affect only one metabolic pathway, resistance to them is more likely to occur. In practice, sulphonamides and sulphones are used, not as primary drugs but as synergists to folic acid reductase inhibitors to improve rapidity of action and reduce the chance of resistance.

Anti-malarial control measures are manifold, comprising: reduction of the vector populations by control of their breeding places (in swamps, lakes, streams, etc.) and increasingly, nowadays, by residual insecticidal attack on adult mosquitoes; recognition and treatment of infected persons; protection against bites by screening or by insect repellents; chemoprophylaxis; etc. The measures adopted depend on local situations and whether an attempt is being made to eradicate the infection or simply to limit its transmission.

Immunity to malaria is associated mainly with IgG immunoglobulins and with the erythrocytic cycle of schizogony. As judged by parasite rates in infected communities, immunity is high in the neonate, from maternal antibody, low from 4 months to 3 years (when the child is acquiring immunity from repeated infection and at which period the main mortality occurs), increasing from then onwards to adult life. Immunofluorescence techniques are available for the recognition of antiplasmodial antibody. Some genetic factors affect susceptibility to malaria, e.g. sickle cell gene; *P. falciparum* trophozoites appear to have difficulty in metabolizing the abnormal haemoglobin associated with this gene.

Other Pathogenic Sporozoa

There remain a few sporozoan parasites of man, hardly more than curiosities, about which a few words should be said:

Sarcocystis lindemanni. Trophozoites, crescentic bodies about 12 μm long, very similar to those of *Toxoplasma*, occur in sarcocysts 1 to 2 mm long, divided up into compartments by trabeculae, in muscle, mainly of the larynx, oesophagus and diaphragm.

Sarcocystis occurs commonly in other animals, e.g. sheep and cattle. Infection probably occurs by ingestion.

Babesia spp. are common parasites of the erythrocytes of rodents and cattle, and are transmitted by ixodid ticks. Four human cases are recorded, all but one in persons who had been splenectomized; two were fatal.

Pneumocystis carinii. Not indisputably a protozoon, *P. carinii* occurs in the lung as spherical organisms about 10 μm in diameter, uninucleate, or about 12 μm in diameter containing 8 nuclei ('cyst'). It is associated, in man, with an interstitial plasma cell pneumonia in babies premature or with immunoglobulin deficiencies, or with immunosuppression in geriatric patients. It has been recorded in dogs, and rodents in the Old and New Worlds. Its transmission mechanism is unknown.

CILIOPHORA

Balantidium coli; Balantidial dysentery

Balantidium coli occurs in the colon of man, other primates, pigs and a variety of other mammals, in many parts of the world. The trophozoites feed on bacteria as parasites of the lumen but also on cells of the gut epithelium, and invade the tissues.

Clinically the disease resembles amoebiasis with diarrhoea or dysentery, abdominal colic, nausea and vomiting. The stools may contain blood and mucus. Balantidial ulcers of the mucosa resemble those of *E. histolytica*, but further extensions appear to be rare though the intestinal lymphatics and the mesenteric lymph nodes may be invaded; and balantidial peritonitis and vaginitis have been reported.

Diagnosis depends on the demonstration of *B. coli* either as trophozoites or as cysts in the faeces. Infection in man tends to be related to contact with pigs, in farm-workers, or in the tropics with people who keep pigs in close association with their living quarters. Diodohydroxyquin and tetracycline appear to be effective drugs.

Conclusion

Protozoology is at present in a state of transition. For long mainly observational and descriptive, the subject is now being increasingly influenced by other fields of microbiology and is extending rapidly its experimental aspects, particularly in immunology (Lumsden, 1967) and in biochemistry. Particularly influential in this development has been the introduction of methods for the viable preservation of organisms at low temperatures—cryopreservation (Polge and Soltys, 1957; Cunningham, Lumsden and Webber, 1963). Cryopreservation avoids the continuous selection, and so modification, of organismal populations which takes place when they are maintained by serial passage in laboratory animals or in cultures; it allows the setting up of reference collections of organism materials which remain stable over periods of at least several years, thus greatly facilitating reproducible experimentation.

The foregoing summary of medical protozoology attempts only to pick out essential principles and points of interest. For systematic treatments *in extenso* the reader is referred to Baker (1970), Belding (1965), Faust, Russell and Jung (1970), Garnham (1966), Hoare (1949), Kudo (1966), Levine (1941), Lumsden (1967), Weinman and Ristic (1968) and Wenyon (1926).

REFERENCES

BAKER, J. R. (1970) *Parasitic Protozoa*. London: Hutchinson University Library.

BELDING, D. L. (1965) *Textbook of Parasitology*. 3rd Edn. New York: Appleton-Century-Crofts.

BRUCE-CHWATT, L. J. (1969) Malaria eradication at the crossroads. *Bulletin of the New York Academy of Medicine*, **45**, 999–1012.

BENTZ, M. & MACARIO, C. (1963) Le traitement systematique des individus porteurs d'hyper-beta-2-macroglobulinémies en zone d'endemie trypanique. *Bulletin de la Société de*

588 PROTOZOA

CUNNINGHAM, M. P., LUMSDEN, W. H. R. & WEBBER, W. A. F. (1963) Preservation of viable trypanosomes in lymph tubes at low temperature. *Experimental Parasitology*, **14**, 280–284.

FAUST, E. C., RUSSELL, P. F. & JUNG, R. C. (1970) *Clinical Parasitology*. Philadelphia: Lea and Febiger.

GARNHAM, P. C. C. (1966) *Malaria Parasites and other Haemosporidia*. Oxford: Blackwell Scientific Publications.

HACKETT, L. W. (1937) *Malaria in Europe*. London: Humphrey Milford.

HOARE, C. A. (1949) *Handbook of Medical Protozoology*. London: Ballière, Tindall and Cox.

HOARE, C. A. (1966) The classification of the mammalian trypanosomes. *Ergebnisse der Mikrobiologie, Immunitätsforschung und Experimentelle Therapie*, **39**, 43–57.

HONIGBERG, B. M., BALAMUTH, W., BOVEE, E. C., CORLISS, J. O., GOJDICS, M., HALL, R. P., KUDO, R. R., LEVINE, N. D., LOEBLICH, A. R., WEISER, J. & WENRICH, D. H. (1964) A revised classification of the Protozoa. *Journal of Protozoology*, **11**, 7–20.

HUNSICKER, L. G. (1969) The pharmacology of the antimalarials. *Archives of Internal Medicine*, **123**, 645–649.

HUTCHISON, W. M., DUNACHIE, J. F., SIIM, J. C. & WORK, K. (1970) Coccidia-like nature of *Toxoplasma gondii*. *British Medical Journal*, **i**, 142–144.

KÖBERLE, F. (1968) Chagas' disease and Chagas' syndromes: the pathology of American trypanosomiasis. *Advances in Parasitology*, **6**, 63–116.

KUDO, R. R. (1966) *Protozoology*. 5th Edn. Springfield: Charles C. Thomas.

LANHAM, S. M. (1968) Separation of trypanosomes from blood of infected rats and mice by anion-exchangers. *Nature, London*, **218**, 1273–1274.

LEVINE, N. D. (1961) *Protozoan Parasites of Domestic Animals and Man*. Minneapolis, Burgess Publishing Co.

LUMSDEN, W. H. R. (1967) The demonstration of antibodies to protozoa. In *Handbook of Experimental Immunology* edited by D. M. Weir, Edinburgh: Blackwell Scientific Publications.

MATTERN, P. (1968) Etat actuel et resultats de techniques immunologique utilisées a l'Institut Pasteur de Dakar pour le diagnostic et l'étude de la trypanosomiase humaine africaine. *Bulletin of the World Health Organization*, **38**, 1–8.

POLGE, C. & SOLTYS, M. A. (1957) Preservation of trypanosomes in the frozen state. *Transactions of the Royal Society of Tropical Medicine and Hygiene*, **51**, 519–526.

WEINMAN, D. & RISTIC, M. (Eds) (1968) *Infectious Blood Diseases of Man and Animals*. New York: Academic Press.

WORLD HEALTH ORGANIZATION (1969) Amoebiasis. *World Health Organization Technical Report Series*, 421. Geneva: World Health Organization.

WORLD HEALTH ORGANIZATION (1969) Parasitology of malaria. *World Health Organization Technical Report Series*, 433. Geneva: World Health Organization.

Volume 1 : Part 5
Diagnosis, Treatment and Control of Infections

55. Infective Syndromes and Diagnostic Procedures

The practice of good clinical medicine requires the intelligent use of laboratory services. The aid of the bacteriology department is necessary for the accurate diagnosis of many common infections and the selection of a suitable antimicrobial agent for the treatment of the patient may be impossible without knowledge of the *in vitro* sensitivity of the causal microorganism. The bacteriological results, however, should always be interpreted in relation to clinical findings and the results of other investigations.

Sterile containers and swabs of various types are provided by the laboratory, but unless the clinician accepts responsibility for the careful collection and prompt submission of suitable specimens, laboratory examinations may be useless. Delay in transit can result in the death of some delicate bacteria and viruses whereas other clinically insignificant bacteria may be able to multiply in the material sent for examination. The effects of delay can sometimes be overcome by the use of special transport media. Specimens *must be* clearly labelled and accompanied by a completed laboratory request form giving relevant clinical details. This information is often essential in deciding how a particular specimen will be treated in the laboratory. The laboratory diagnosis of an infection can be accomplished in two different ways: either the microorganisms responsible for the infection can be isolated and identified, or serological evidence of the host's reaction to the pathogen can be obtained.

I. Isolation of the Causal Microorganisms

Bacteria

Isolation of the causal bacterium is the most satisfactory method of laboratory diagnosis. It may be relatively easy to do, but sometimes it is difficult or even impossible. The evaluation of cultures inoculated with samples taken from sites which have a normal bacterial flora requires experience; potentially pathogenic bacteria have to be distinguished from commensal organisms and isolation of a potential pathogen is not necessarily significant.

The way in which a specimen is treated in the laboratory largely depends on its source and nature although the routine method may be modified if there are special circumstances noted in the patient's history. The laboratory examination of bacteriological specimens, however, follows a standard pattern.

1. DIRECT FILMS. Films made from the material submitted are usually examined after they have been stained, but some direct films, e.g. those made from faeces and urine, may yield additional information if they are examined unstained ('wet films'). Gram's method is the staining technique universally used and, if tuberculous infection is suspected, Ziehl-Neelsen-stained films are also prepared. In addition films stained by Leishman's or another Romanowsky stain may be necessary to study the nature of the cells in an exudate.

2. CULTURE. The specimen is inoculated on to solid and into fluid culture media.

   (a) *Solid media.* Blood agar is the most widely used medium in diagnostic bacteriology and plates of this medium, seeded with the material sent for examination, are often incubated in a variety of different atmospheric conditions. These range from air (aerobic conditions) through varying degrees of reduced oxygen tension to completely anaerobic conditions; the addition of carbon dioxide may be necessary for the growth of certain bacteria. On blood agar, colonies of many of the common pathogens can be recognized after overnight incubation. Other types of media in routine use include *specially enriched media* which promote the growth of exacting pathogens, e.g. heated blood agar for isolation of the gonococcus and haemophilus, and *selective media* which inhibit some organisms but allow others to grow. Many selective media have been devised to facilitate the isolation of a particular pathogen from a mixture of commensal organisms, e.g. desoxycholate-citrate agar for the isolation of intestinal pathogens. The solid medium allows the estimation of the relative numbers of bacteria of different species present in the specimen.

(b) *Fluid media.* Bacteria may not grow on solid media if only a few viable organisms are present in the specimen, or if the material submitted contains substances that inhibit bacterial growth (e.g. antibiotics). Inoculation of a suitable fluid medium, however, not only ensures the rapid multiplication of small numbers of organisms but also dilutes the concentration of inhibitory substances sometimes allowing growth to take place. Note, however, that such cultures yield no information about the relative number of pathogenic organisms actually present in the original specimen. Growth in fluid media is investigated by making films from the broth and subculturing on to solid (usually selective) media. The most important fluid medium for general use is Robertson's cooked-meat broth which allows the growth of both aerobic and anaerobic organisms.

3. ANTIBIOTIC SENSITIVITY TESTS. By determining the sensitivity of pathogenic bacteria to the various antibiotics the laboratory can aid the practitioner in the treatment of bacterial diseases. In general there is good agreement between the in-vitro sensitivity of the infecting organism to a given antibiotic and the clinical response observed when that drug is given to the patient (see Chap. 56).

The simplest way to carry out these tests is by the disk diffusion method. Here a number of paper disks or tablets containing different antibiotics are placed on the surface of an agar plate that has been uniformly spread with the isolated pathogen. After overnight incubation the plate is examined for zones of inhibition of growth around the various disks. A zone of inhibition indicates that the organism is sensitive to the antibiotic contained in the disk: growth right up to the disk margin indicates resistance. It is sometimes possible to use the specimen submitted, e.g. pus, urine, as the inoculum instead of the isolated pathogen to speed laboratory reporting. This method is called primary sensitivity testing.

Viruses

The isolation of viruses is time-consuming, expensive and requires special laboratory resources. Attempts to isolate viruses are often futile unless the specimens are properly preserved, and sent to the laboratory by a rapid method. The isolation of viruses is attempted usually in the investigation of outbreaks and rarely in the case of individual patients except in diseases of importance for which some well recognized prophylactic measure can be applied, e.g. smallpox and poliomyelitis. Swabs on wooden applicator sticks are the most suitable for taking materials from the throat, mouth, skin lesions, rectum, vagina, etc. Immediately after use the stick is broken to a short length and the swab is inserted into a screw cap container to which has been added about 2 ml of a suitable transport medium (e.g. medium 199 or 1 per cent skim milk containing 50 units penicillin and 50 μg streptomycin per ml) or CVTM (charcoal virus transport medium). Samples of faeces may also be placed in a transport medium.

Specimens for virus isolation should be collected and transmitted at temperatures laid down by the virus laboratory which must be consulted beforehand. It is often convenient in hospital practice to store the specimen in the ice trays of a domestic refrigerator. For transport to the laboratory the specimens in their containers may be surrounded with ice, or preferably an ice-salt mixture, in a suitable jar or tin. *Do not send such specimens by post.* The best way of transmitting frozen specimens to a laboratory at some distance is to pack them in special insulated box or thermos flask surrounded by 'dry ice' (i.e. solid carbon dioxide). Such containers are sometimes available on demand at the laboratory. See Appendix 1.

II. SEROLOGICAL DIAGNOSIS

Serological tests to detect antibodies against the infecting microorganism provide a useful means of indirect diagnosis. These tests are of especial value in virology where isolation of the virus responsible for the infection may be difficult or impossible. In diagnosing bacterial infections, however, serological methods are less often used but there are two particular instances where such tests are routine, viz. the examination of the patient's serum for agglutinating antibodies against the salmonellae responsible for enteric fever (Widal Reaction) and *Brucella abortus* when investigating the cause of an unknown fever, and the examination of the patient's serum for complement-fixing or flocculating antibodies in the diagnosis of syphilis.

Serological Diagnosis of Virus Infections

Serological tests for complement-fixing, neutralizing and haemagglutination inhibiting antibodies, often give valuable diagnostic information; they form the usual routine means of laboratory investigation in some virus infections. Since small traces of antibody may persist long after recovery and are frequently demonstrable in normal healthy individuals the examination of a single sample of serum seldom yields information of any value. Exceptions are seen in cases of infections with the chlamydiae where the single observation of a high antibody titre may be significant. In most other infections the results of serological tests are of diagnostic significance only if there has been at least a fourfold rise of antibody titre during the period between the onset of the illness and convalescence.

It is therefore essential to send at least two samples of serum to the laboratory; the first taken as soon as possible after the onset of the disease and the second after about 2 to 3 weeks.

For the tests, 1 to 2 ml of clear serum showing no trace of haemolysis is required. The serum should be removed from the clot within 24 hours of collection and then kept at 4°C or lower. When both acute and convalescent samples have been collected they may be sent to the laboratory by post. Whole blood is unsuitable for transmission by post.

RESPIRATORY TRACT INFECTIONS

Infections of the Upper Respiratory Tract

The upper respiratory tract is frequently the site of general and localized infections involving the mouth, or pharynx, nose, nasopharynx, larynx and trachea.

The primary infection is often viral in origin and secondary bacterial infection is most often due to the potential pathogens resident in the upper respiratory tract, e.g. pneumococci, streptococci, *H. influenzae* and staphylococci. The area affected is usually obvious and examination will be directed to the site affected. The most useful procedure is to take a swab direct from the surface; if exudate, membrane or pus is present some of this should be sampled. Films may be prepared from the swabs after cultures have been inoculated, or smears may be prepared directly from the membranes, exudate or surface by means of a swab or loop and stained by suitable stains.

Acute mouth infections, such as *stomatitis*, are most common in young babies, children and older persons, especially when the patient is debilitated as the result of intercurrent disease, or when the mouth has not been given proper hygiene. The more common organisms involved are aerobic and anaerobic streptococci, Vincent's organisms, and Candida species; viruses involved may be those of herpes simplex, Coxsackie group A, and measles.

SORE THROAT. This syndrome, characterized by acute inflammation of the tonsillar and faucial areas (acute tonsillitis, acute pharyngitis) with or without exudate, which may be loose or adherent, is most commonly due to *Strept. pyogenes*. But many cases of acute sore throat, and especially the milder cases, are virus infections (e.g. adenoviruses), and it is important to distinguish between streptococcal and non-streptococcal infections since the former respond to penicillin therapy which is also effective in preventing septic and non-septic complications, including acute rheumatic fever. Virus infections, on the other hand, do not respond to antibiotics and should not be treated with these substances unless there is evidence of a secondary bacterial infection. Other causes of sore throat with exudate are diphtheria and Vincent's angina; exudate is also frequently present in certain forms of mononucleosis (glandular fever), in granulocytopoenia and in the leukaemias. An important contributing factor in the last three of these diseases is the diminution or inefficiency of the granular white cells which normally act as scavengers in keeping the mucous membranes clean.

Acute adenitis, sinusitis, otitis media, rhinitis, laryngitis, tracheitis or peritonsillar abscess (quinsy), may accompany or follow the acute throat infection. Chronic lesions may be due to leprosy, syphilis and tuberculosis. Actinomycosis with involvement of deeper tissues and the formation of abscesses is a rare cause of infection in the cervico-facial region.

Infections of the Lower Respiratory Tract

In the lower respiratory tract (trachea, bronchi, bronchioles and lung tissue) there is often a primary infection by a virus, e.g. adenoviruses, myxoviruses, respiratory syncytial virus, herpesvirus, picornavirus and thereafter there is a secondary infection by pathogenic microorganisms from the upper respiratory tract and by spread through the blood and lymph channels; more rarely there is direct extension of infection from other affected tissues, such as the liver. The mucous membrane of this part of the respiratory tract is probably sterile in health, but direct examination involves bronchoscopy or lung biopsy, neither of which is indicated in the normal course of the diagnosis of infection.

Sputum from patients with acute bronchitis, acute exacerbations of chronic bronchitis, bronchiolitis and pneumonia, should be examined bacteriologically. In most cases the sputum will consist of a mixture of exudate from the affected mucous membrane or lung tissue and saliva. The more purulent material is likely to contain specific pathogens and therefore examination should be directed to this part by spreading the sputum in a dish so that the purulent material may be picked directly with a loop. Alternatively, the sputum may be homogenized by adding saponin and incubating for half an hour, or by shaking the sputum with glass beads, or by digestion with pancreatin; in this way random sampling of the sputum specimen will include any pathogens present.

DIRECT FILM. Films made from the sputum and stained by Gram's method are of limited value and give no indication of the number of viable organisms present: further the presence of commensal organisms in saliva may confuse the picture. Direct films may be of value in the diagnosis of pneumococcal and staphylococcal infections of the lung. If tuberculosis is suspected, a direct film stained by Ziehl-Neelsen's method is examined for acid- and alcohol-fast bacilli.

CULTURE. Sputum is plated on blood agar for aerobic, anaerobic and carbon dioxide incubation and on heated blood agar incubated in carbon dioxide with diagnostic antimicrobial disks. An optochin disk may be placed on the plates for the differentiation of pneumococci from *Strept. viridans*. In specific infections the significant organisms such as pneumococci, *Haemophilus influenzae* and *Staphylococcus aureus* are usually isolated in large numbers. If tuberculosis is suspected the sputum is homogenized and concentrated prior to culture; sometimes guinea-pig inoculation is also performed. The methods are described in Chapter 22, and given in detail in Vol. II.

ACUTE INTESTINAL INFECTIONS

Acute diarrhoea with or without vomiting is a very common complaint that may be due to a variety of causes. Infection with known or unknown bacteria, viruses or protozoa is a major contributor but specific bacterial pathogens can be recovered from not more than around 20 per cent of the 'infective diarrhoeas'. The most common identifiable intestinal pathogen in Britain is *Shigella sonnei*; the salmonella species, and the food poisoning enterotoxic strains of *Staph. aureus* and *Cl. welchii* are less commonly incriminated. The aid of the laboratory is essential in arriving at a diagnosis and specimens of faeces should be sent for bacteriological examination. A specific infection must never be excluded on the basis of one negative report and a series of specimens may have to be submitted for investigation.

Specimen Collection

A sample of faeces is a much better specimen than a rectal swab. However, if many contacts of a patient with an infective diarrhoea have to be investigated it is often more convenient to take rectal swabs. It is necessary to ensure that these swabs sample the contents of the *rectum* and that they are not merely placed in the anal orifice. Faeces should be passed into a clean pot which does not contain any antiseptic and the specimen should be collected free from urine. A sample of the specimen is transferred with the spoon provided to a sterile glass universal container and this should be sent to the laboratory as soon as possible. Alternatively, an adequate sample of the faeces in the pot may be sent on a swab. If delay is inevitable, the specimen should be transported in glycerol saline because this prevents the intestinal commensal organisms overgrowing any enteric pathogens that may be present (see Appendix I).

If amoebic dysentery is suspected the specimen must be available for examination *within a few minutes* of being passed if the motile vegetative form of *Entamoeba histolytica* is to be recognized. The record of the history sent with the specimen should include information about recent foreign travel as patients who have been abroad are more likely to be infested with intestinal protozoa, worms, and infected with salmonellae.

URINARY TRACT INFECTIONS

The diagnosis of urinary tract infection cannot be made without bacteriological examination of the urine. Patients with classic symptoms of urinary infection may have a sterile urine and asymptomatic patients may have infected urine. The chemotherapy of proven infection may be controlled by in-vitro sensitivity tests and the outcome assessed by examination of the urine at the conclusion of treatment. Follow-up of patients who have had a urinary infection is essential because relapse may be clinically silent (see Chap. 29).

Specimen Collection

Specimens are usually collected in universal containers, but for the collection of mid-stream specimens from females it is an advantage to provide a wide-mouthed container such as a 12-oz honey-pot. Alternatively, disposable plastic pots with tight-fitting lids may be used for urine specimens.

From male patients a mid-stream specimen

of urine (MSU) should be submitted, the middle of the urinary flow being collected. Formerly, for bacteriological examination, a catheter specimen of urine (CSU) was always collected from female patients so that contamination of the specimen with organisms from the ano-genital region was avoided. This practice, however, is no longer regarded as justifiable because catheterization may introduce infection—a risk, under ideal conditions, estimated at between 2 and 6 per cent. As a result voided specimens are now submitted from women and these compare satisfactorily with catheter specimens. It is now considered unnecessary to clean the ano-genital region before taking the specimen and there is evidence that in infants such cleaning increases the bacterial count. The patient passes urine with the labia separated and the middle of the stream is collected for examination.

Once collected, the specimen must be transported to the laboratory *without delay* because urine is an excellent culture medium supporting the rapid growth of many bacteria. If delay of more than 1 to 2 hours is unavoidable the multiplication of bacteria in the urine should be prevented by storage in a refrigerator, or the specimen may be transported in some form of special container that maintains low temperature. A simple container which utilizes a standard one pint vacuum flask has been devised for this purpose (Elliott and Sleigh, 1963). Urine may also be preserved by adding boric acid to a final concentration of 1·8 per cent (Porter and Brodie, 1969).

If tuberculosis of the urinary tract is suspected the first urine passed in the day is the most suitable specimen (early morning urine). Three complete early morning urines should be sent to the laboratory where microscopical, cultural and animal tests will be carried out on the centrifuged deposit.

Bacterial Counts

The results of culture are not always clear-cut, and in recent years studies of the actual number of bacteria present in otherwise normal but contaminated and infected urines have been made. Viable counts may be performed either by a pour-plate method or by inoculating the surface of media with known volumes of urine (Miles and Misra method). Colony counts are made after incubation for 24 to 48 hours.

SEMI-QUANTITATIVE CULTURE OF URINE. Although quantitative urine culture yields extra information it is time-consuming and also requires considerable amounts of laboratory materials. Consequently, a number of semi-quantitative methods have been introduced and the results of these simplified techniques compare well with quantitative examinations carried out on the same specimen. There are two basic semi-quantitative methods, the first in which a loop of standard diameter is used and the second, the dip slide, in which a thin layer of suitable agar either as a coating on a slide or in a metal or plastic spoon is dipped into a fresh specimen of urine.

In the loop method, the loop is charged with the uncentrifuged urine and plated out on solid media in a standard way (McGeachie and Kennedy, 1963). After overnight incubation the plate culture is inspected for colonies and the results evaluated in accordance with a pre-arranged scheme.

In the dip slide method, the slide coated with agar or the spoon containing agar is dipped into a fresh specimen of urine, the excess urine is drained off and the specimen or spoon sent in a suitable container to the laboratory. Incubation is carried out at 37°C and the number of organisms per ml estimated by comparing the slide with a chart showing bacterial counts. Culture at 15 to 18°C gives comparable results.

When properly taken urine specimens are examined, contamination never produces more than 10^4 organisms per ml and usually accounts for less than 10^3 organisms per ml. These counts, inconstant and varying from specimen to specimen taken from the same patient, represent bacteria from the urethra and external genitalia which have entered the urine during collection of the specimen. Infected urines contain more than 10^4 organisms per ml, usually more than 10^5 organisms per ml and often up to 10^8 organisms per ml. These high counts, fairly constant in serial specimens taken from the same patient, are the result of bacterial multiplication in the urine within the urinary tract.

Significant bacteriuria (counts greater than 10^5 organisms per ml) may sometimes be found, in the absence of symptoms or pyuria, in patients who subsequently develop symptoms of urinary infection. There is good evidence of a frequent association between asymptomatic bacteriuria and pyelonephritis.

MENINGEAL INFECTIONS

The clinical signs of meningeal irritation always suggest infection of the meninges but they may occur in association with certain other acute infections not involving the meninges (meningismus) and they may also be seen in patients with non-infective conditions such as subarachnoid haemorrhage. Infants, however, may have meningitis without the usual localizing signs. Patients suspected of having meningitis should always have a specimen of cerebrospinal fluid (CSF) examined in the laboratory as soon as possible. Prompt identification of the causal organism is important because until an exact bacteriological diagnosis has been made the proper antimicrobial therapy cannot be prescribed.

Specimen Collection

When cerebrospinal fluid is obtained by lumbar puncture it is essential to take rigorous precautions to prevent the introduction of infection. (It is safe to remove 5–10 ml of CSF *as long as intracranial pressure is not increased*.) The sample is best collected in one or two sterile screw-capped containers. Test-tubes with cotton-wool plugs should not be used because if they are shaken or fall over, the CSF may be absorbed by the plug. The specimen must be dispatched to the laboratory at once; delay may result in the death of delicate pathogens such as meningococci, the disintegration of leucocytes and the reduction in the concentration of sugar in the CSF. Specimens should not be kept in the refrigerator, which kills *H. influenzae*.

Examination for Cells

In acute bacterial meningitis there is a great increase in the number of leucocytes in the CSF, which, as a result, generally becomes turbid. Up to several thousand cells per mm^3 is a common finding and early in the disease almost all of them are polymorphs. In tuberculous meningitis there are fewer cells in the CSF (200–500 per mm^3) and lymphocytes predominate, but some polymorphs are usually present. Virus infections of the meninges result in an 'aseptic' type of meningitis; between 50 and 1 000 cells per mm^3 are found and they are virtually all lymphocytes.

Biochemical Examination

Part of the specimen should be submitted for quantitative biochemical estimation of the protein, sugar (glucose) and chloride content of the fluid. The Lange colloidal gold test depends on the relationship between gammaglobulins and other protein fractions in the CSF. Three abnormal types of curve are recognized, the paretic, the leutic and the meningitic.

Examination for Microorganisms

ACUTE PURULENT MENINGITIS. The CSF is turbid. The three bacterial species most commonly responsible are *Neisseria meningitidis*, *Diplococcus pneumoniae* and *Haemophilus influenzae*. These organisms usually reach the meninges via the bloodstream and can sometimes be isolated simultaneously by blood culture. Meningitis can also result from direct spread to the meninges from infections in neighbouring structures, e.g. middle ear, paranasal or frontal sinuses. Bacteria may also gain access to the meninges after careless lumbar puncture or from infected neurosurgical wounds. Thus a wide variety of organisms including *Staphylococcus aureus*, *Streptococcus pyogenes*, *Pseudomonas pyocyanea*, *Escherichia coli* and anaerobes such as *Bacteroides* species and anaerobic streptococci can also cause meningitis.

In the laboratory the CSF is centrifuged and films stained by Gram's stain are examined. A diagnosis can often be made at this stage. Cultures are made on blood and heated blood agar and incubated at 37°C aerobically, anaerobically, and in 5–10 per cent CO_2. A primary sensitivity test is carried out if a large number of organisms is seen in the stained film.

ACUTE NON-PURULENT BACTERIAL MENINGITIS. The CSF is usually not turbid. Such meningitis may be due to *Mycobacterium tuberculosis* or *Leptospira*. In tuberculous meningitis a veil clot appears in the CSF on standing, and on microscopy by Ziehl-Neelsen stain, acid- and alcohol-fast bacilli may be found in it along with lymphocytes. Cultures are made with the deposit on Löwenstein-Jensen medium and guinea-pigs are inoculated. Diagnosis of leptospiral meningitis is made by serological tests.

VIRAL (ASEPTIC) MENINGITIS. The CSF is not turbid. The commonest viruses responsible for this disease are members of the picornaviruses group, echoviruses, coxsackieviruses and, least frequently, polioviruses. Aseptic meningitis may also occur as a complication of other virus diseases such as mumps (sometimes unassociated with parotitis), chickenpox, measles, infectious hepatitis and herpes zoster.

Echoviruses and coxsackieviruses can usually be isolated directly from the CSF. They may also be present in the faeces. A sample of CSF should be sent as early as possible and faeces may also be submitted. Second samples of both specimens should be sent two or three days later. If faeces are not available, a rectal swab is a reasonably satisfactory alternative. These viruses may also be recovered from throat swabs or oropharyngeal washings but, in the case of the polioviruses, with considerably less frequency. Cerebrospinal fluid from cases of aseptic meningitis seldom, if ever, contains polioviruses. These materials may be held for up to 24 h at 0°–4°C, in a domestic refrigerator, but for longer periods they should be preserved frozen at −30°C or in 50 per cent glycerol saline.

Paired sera should also be sent for serological diagnosis. Table 55.1 shows the findings in the CSF in different types of meningitis.

WOUND INFECTIONS

Wound infections may be *endogenous* or *exogenous*. Endogenous infections (*auto-infections*) are caused by organisms that were leading a commensal existence elsewhere in the host's body; for example abdominal surgical wounds may become infected with organisms from the large bowel after an operation that has involved incision of the colon. In exogenous infections

Table 55.1. Findings in the cerebrospinal fluid in different types of meningitis.

Test	Normal	Acute bacterial meningitis	Tuberculous meningitis	Aseptic meningitis
Appearance	clear and colourless	turbid	clear or opalescent	usually clear
Total protein	15–40 mg/100 ml	greatly increased	moderately increased	slightly increased
Sugar	50–70 mg/100 ml	greatly reduced	reduced	normal
Chloride	700–740 mg/100 ml	reduced	reduced	normal
Cell count	0–3 lymphocytes per mm³	greatly increased—all polymorphs	increased—mainly lymphocytes, some polymorphs	increased—lymphocytes predominate
Culture on artificial media	sterile	causal bacterium isolated	*M. tuberculosis* isolated	negative

the source of the infecting organism is outwith the host who becomes infected; *cross-infection* is a particular example of exogenous infection where the causal organism is spread from person to person. Infection may occur after accidental or intentional trauma of the skin or other tissues; the latter type is often called 'post-operative sepsis'.

Specimen Collection

Pus or exudate from infected wounds is usually sampled by means of a swab which must be well soaked in the exudate. A specimen of the pus itself is always preferable and may often be obtained by using a syringe or pipette to transfer the material to a sterile tube or screw-capped bottle. If only a small amount of exudate is available it should be allowed to run into a capillary tube; after sealing both ends the tube can be sent to the laboratory inside a glass tube or bottle. Pieces of tissue removed at operation, or curettings from infected sinuses and other tissues are sometimes sent for bacteriological examination: these specimens are homogenized in a tissue grinder with a little broth and subsequently treated in the same way as exudates. Delay in the transit of specimens to the laboratory must be avoided, especially in the case of swabs where the exudate may dry into the cotton-wool.

REPRODUCTIVE SYSTEM INFECTIONS

In the nursing mother, breast abscesses may occur and are due to *Staphylococcus aureus*.

Cellulitis of the breast is due to *Streptococcus pyogenes*.

Infection of the upper part of the female genital tract (salpingitis and oophoritis) may be part of a generalized infection or it may be localized, but in either case bacteriological diagnosis by examination of specimens obtained from the accessible lower tract is rarely possible. The commonest organisms found are coliforms followed by streptococci. *Mycobacterium tuberculosis* and *Neisseria gonorrhoeae* are important pathogens although not so common.

Acute infections in the female are fairly common after delivery, e.g. puerperal sepsis or septic abortions. *Streptococcus pyogenes*, *Clostridium welchii*, *Bacteroides* species and coliform bacteria are the principal organisms found. Acute cervicitis also occurs in non-pregnant women, and some cases are venereal and some due to herpesvirus. Cervical swabs should be taken with the aid of a speculum under direct vision. The swab should be put into Stuart's transport medium if a bacterial infection is suspected.

Acute and chronic vaginitis and vulvo-vaginitis may be due to a variety of causes and many organisms may be responsible. Acute vaginitis due to *Trichomonas vaginalis* and vaginal thrush due to *Candida* species (particularly in pregnant women) are the most important infections. Exudate can be readily obtained by swabbing and direct smears on slides for microscopic examination: or exudate may be collected by pipette or spoon for wet films.

In the male, acute urethritis and prostatitis are fairly common; many cases have a venereal origin, due to *Neisseria gonorrhoeae*, chlamydiae or *Mycoplasma* species.

CONJUNCTIVAL INFECTIONS

A variety of bacteria may produce acute conjunctivitis. The gonococcus produces severe ophthalmia neonatorum and *Staph. aureus* is a common cause of 'sticky eye' in newborn babies in maternity hospitals. *Diplococcus pneumoniae*, *Haemophilus influenzae* (Koch-Weeks bacillus) and *Moraxella lacunata* are other common infecting species. Certain adenoviruses and other viruses produce conjunctivitis together with an upper respiratory infection, and the TRIC agents cause acute and chronic infections, e.g. inclusion blennorrhoea and trachoma. Severe infections with *Ps. pyocyanea* have followed the use of contaminated eyedrops.

Purulent exudate from an inflamed conjunctiva should be treated as pus. Direct microscopy frequently shows microorganisms and a presumptive diagnosis can often be made: this is particularly important in the early detection of gonococcal ophthalmia. Small numbers of Gram-positive cocci, small Gram-negative bacilli or Gram-positive bacilli may indicate no more than the normal commensal flora but the pneumococcus, gonococcus, *Haemophilus* spp., *Staph. aureus* and coliform bacilli may be seen in numbers sufficient to suggest a diagnosis. The cultures must always be incubated in the presence of carbon dioxide.

In many cases there is a minimum of exudate and diagnosis is facilitated by the inoculation of media and the preparation of smears for direct microscopy at the bedside. For this purpose a platinum loop (diameter 1 mm) and slopes of heated blood agar in 1-oz screw-capped bottles are useful. Swabs coated with exudate are best sent to the laboratory in Stuart's transport medium.

Many cases of conjunctival inflammation are not bacterial in origin. In infections with adenoviruses or herpesviruses scrapings from the conjunctiva, put in a fluid virus transport medium, are used for isolation in tissue cultures. For the demonstration of TRIC agents scrapings taken from the conjunctiva are spread on slides, stained with Giemsa's stain and examined for basophilic inclusion bodies, or stained by a fluorescent conjugated antiserum and examined by fluorescent microscopy.

PYREXIA OF UNKNOWN OR UNCERTAIN ORIGIN

Patients who have a significant and persistent fever (greater than 100°F), the cause of which cannot be readily diagnosed on clinical examination, are classified as having a 'pyrexia of uncertain origin' (PUO). Many such cases are due to infection and their diagnosis will depend upon the employment of any methods to demonstrate the presence of a specific pathogen in the blood or tissues; thus while every effort must be made to recover the causative organism, recourse to indirect methods of diagnosis must also be made, particularly serological methods to demonstrate specific antibody. The patient should be asked if he has been abroad recently, so that the possibility of an exotic infection may be considered.

The procedure to be followed is usually along the following lines:

1. Examination of the Blood

(a) BLOOD FILMS. Direct films of the patient's blood should be prepared and examined to exclude the presence of circulating parasites such as plasmodia; this examination will also indicate the white cell picture of the peripheral blood and such information may be a help in diagnosis.

(b) BLOOD CULTURE. This should be carried out on several occasions each day or on successive days. In cases of bacteraemia such as occurs in subacute bacterial endocarditis the number of organisms in the blood may be very small; to increase the chance of their recovery a series of cultures over a period of several hours should be taken. The presence of antibacterial agents increases the difficulty of recovering the causative organism and, with the exceptions of benzylpenicillin and sulphonamides, their inhibitory effects can best be countered by dilution of the blood. Antibody and leucocytes may also inhibit growth of bacteria in the specimen and their effect may be counteracted by diluting the blood 1 in 10 in broth. Special media are required for isolation of *Brucella* and an atmosphere containing 10 per cent CO_2 is necessary for the isolation of *Brucella abortus*.

(c) ANIMAL INOCULATION. In some infections, e.g. leptospirosis, brucellosis and rickettsial diseases, animal inoculation carried out with freshly drawn blood may be more successful than attempts at culture in artificial media.

(d) EXAMINATION OF THE SERUM. Part of the blood drawn for blood culture may be set aside, allowed to clot and the serum used for antibody studies. Serological studies should be done at an interval of 5 to 10 days during the acute phase of the disease and later during the convalescent stages. This allows demonstration of any rise or fall in the amount of antibody; the unequivocal interpretation of a single result is often impossible. Examinations of paired specimens should always be made for antibodies to the enteric group of salmonellae (Widal test) and the brucella species.

It may be necessary to carry out as many tests as the laboratory is able to perform, in which case fairly large quantities of serum will be required (5 to 10 ml). If possible, indication of the most likely causes of the infection is helpful as this will direct attention to a more limited number of tests.

2. Examination of the Urine

Routine examination should be carried out to exclude infection of the urinary tract and it should be remembered that urinary tract pathogens such as *Esch. coli* may be present only on intermittent occasions in chronic pyelonephritis. Occasionally *Salmonella* spp. can be isolated from the urine. Repeated examinations may be necessary.

If genito-urinary tuberculosis is suspected, three entire early morning specimens or a 24-hour specimen of urine should be submitted; pyuria is usually present and *Myco. tuberculosis* may be seen after centrifugation and staining of the urine deposit; in leptospirosis, leptospires may be demonstrated by dark field examinations of the fresh alkalized urine.

3. Examination of Faeces

This should be carried out particularly for organisms of the enteric and dysentery groups and for other causes of intestinal disease, in-

cluding protozoa and the ova of helminths. In suspected virus infections it is advisable to match isolation of a virus with rise in the homologous antibody titre of the serum.

4. Examination of Tissues

Biopsy of tissue such as a lymph node may be carried out. The tissue is best cultured, e.g. for *M. tuberculosis*, after grinding it in a homogenizer or tissue blender. It is essential to avoid contamination, especially when fluid cultures are used for the cultivation of the pathogens.

5. Examination of Other Body Fluids

Other body fluids should be examined microscopically and by culture if clinical signs or symptoms indicate this. Aspiration of secretions such as bile may be advisable to confirm suspected infection of the gall-bladder, liver or biliary passages, cerebrospinal fluid in meningitis and bone marrow in enteric fever.

6. Skin Tests

In a number of subacute and chronic infections, hypersensitivity to the constituents of the causative organism develops. The inoculation of small quantities of suitable preparations of the bacterial products, e.g. tuberculin, brucellin, the Frei antigen, results in a localized delayed-type hypersensitivity reaction at the site of inoculation in patients with present or past infection. The results of such tests may be helpful in making a diagnosis.

REFERENCES

ELLIOT, W. A. & SLEIGH, J. D. (1963) Container for transport of urine samples at low temperature. *British Medical Journal*, i, 1142.

McGEACHIE, J. & KENNEDY, A. C. (1963) Simplified quantitative methods for bacteriuria and pyuria. *Journal of Clinical Pathology*, **16**, 32.

PORTER, I. A. & BRODIE, J. (1969) Boric acid preservation of urine samples. *British Medical Journal*, i, 353.

GENERAL READING

LENNETTE, E. H. & SCHMIDT, N. (1969) *Diagnostic Procedures for Viral and Rickettsial Infections*, 4th edn. New York: American Public Health Association, Inc.

MAY, J. R. (1972) *Chemotherapy of Chronic Bronchitis*, 2nd edn. London: The English Universities Press Ltd.

O'GRADY, F. & BRUMFITT, W. (1968) *Urinary Tract Infection*. London: Oxford University Press.

STOKES, E. J. (1968) *Clinical Bacteriology*, 3rd edn. London: Arnold.

56. Strategy of Antimicrobial Therapy

The ideal bacteriological management of patients with infection in whom it is intended to use antibacterial agents is: (a) to establish a clinical diagnosis; (b) to confirm the nature of this infection by isolation of the causative organism in the laboratory; (c) to prescribe the antibiotic or chemotherapeutic agent as indicated by sensitivity tests carried out on the organism; (d) to conduct laboratory examinations during and after treatment to ensure that therapy has been effective, and that superinfection with resistant organisms has not occurred; (e) where necessary to measure tissue or body fluid levels of the antibacterial agent, either to make certain that adequate dosage is being given or to avoid a situation that might lead to toxic sequelae; (f) to carry out follow-up examinations on the patient so that clinical and bacteriological cures can be checked.

It must at once be said that it is only possible and practical to follow such a strategic plan in a minority of cases in hospital, and even fewer in general practice. Most patients who are diagnosed as suffering from infections are treated with antimicrobial drugs on an empirical basis. Generally the results of such treatment are good, in large part because the natural defences of the body are adequate to overcome the infection in the majority of patients and the antibacterial agent merely assists these mechanisms. Thus the activity of the antimicrobial agent does not require to be highly specific nor of the highest order to bring about a successful result. Many infective syndromes such as acute respiratory bacterial infections, superficial boils or acute diarrhoeas do not require the assistance of chemotherapy for satisfactory resolution, although it may be a difficult clinical decision to withhold such therapy in many patients.

More serious infections such as lobar pneumonia, pyelonephritis and osteomyelitis do require chemotherapy, and this is more effective when specific antibacterial agents against the causative organism are used. Frequently however, the microorganism cannot be isolated from such patients either because material for examination is not available, and this is particularly so in children, or circumstances do not allow the organism to grow on culture in the laboratory. In such cases a judicious choice of an antimicrobial agent known to be active against the most likely infecting agent must be made.

In very serious infections, such as bacterial endocarditis, purulent meningitis or bacteriaemic shock, the patient will require chemotherapy urgently as a life-saving measure. Although every effort must be made to isolate the causative organism and examine its specific sensitivity to antimicrobial agents, therapy must be commenced at the earliest possible moment on the basis of experience in the treatment of such infections. Whenever possible, however, a specimen for laboratory examination should be collected from the patient *before the start of therapy*.

An infection may be suspected from the results of clinical examination but the primary causative organism may be viral and not bacterial as frequently happens with acute respiratory tract infections; as yet no chemotherapeutic agents available have any direct effect upon these organisms. Many clinicians believe, however, that chemotherapy is helpful in such cases since it controls secondary invasion by bacterial pathogens and thus shortens the clinical course of influenzal-like infections and the common cold.

A further reason for commencing treatment with antimicrobial agents before full laboratory information is available, is that the delay can be inconvenient for both patient and doctor. In such cases the results of laboratory examination may lead to modification or withdrawal of chemotherapy at a later stage.

There are thus many reasons why patients are treated with antimicrobial drugs without laboratory examinations having been made, or before the results of such examinations are made available. If material for examination in the laboratory cannot be obtained from the patient before therapy is begun, the isolation of microorganisms from tissues and circulating body fluids after antimicrobial therapy has commenced is very much more difficult. The microbiologist finds this situation frequently in patients with meningitis who are admitted to hospital with signs of the disease but who have had chemotherapy before admission. In such cases even one dose of penicillin or tetracycline before examination of the cerebrospinal fluid will so suppress organisms such as *Neisseria meningitidis* that they are both difficult to see in smears and to isolate on culture. It is wrong to argue that such empirical therapy is incorrect since early administration of a suitable antibiotic likely to be effective against the most

common pathogens can be life saving. The diagnosis of meningitis or isolation of the causative agent may be more difficult but this is a relatively small price to pay for the very low case fatality which now pertains in this infection. The decision to proceed with chemotherapy in these infections must be made on clinical grounds and the probability of the nature of the infecting organism.

PREDICTABLE SENSITIVITY TO ANTIBACTERIAL SUBSTANCES

Because most infections are treated on an empirical basis chemotherapy may be guided by

Table 56.1. Predictable sensitivities (fixed antibiograms) for commonly occurring bacterial pathogens.

Group of organisms	Strains usually sensitive to	Frequently sensitive to
Strept. pyogenes	P E L A Ceph	T
Diplococcus pneumoniae	P E L Ceph A	T
Strept. faecalis	A Ceph C E L	
Anaerobic streptococci	A P E L	T
Strept. viridans	P E L Ceph	
Haemophilus influenzae	A T Cot C	E L Ceph
Other Haemophilus spp.	A T Cot	E L Ceph
Proteus mirabilis	A K Su Cot C	
Other Proteus spp.	K Cot C	
Pseudomonas pyocyanea	Poly Genta	Carb
N. gonorrhoeae	K Cot	P
N. meningitidis	Su P A C	
S. typhi and *S. paratyphi*	C A	Cot
Brucella	T Su Cot K	A
Bacteroides	T E C	L
Pasteurella	P S K	A

Groups of bacteria whose strains are more variable in sensitivity:
Staphylococcus aureus

1. 'Penicillin-sensitive'	P T E C A Ceph	
2. 'Antibiotic-sensitive'	T E C A Ceph	
3. 'Antibiotic-resistant'	C Flu L Fus	
Escherichia		
1. Antibiotic-sensitive	A Su T Cot Ceph K Nal Fur	
2. Antibiotic-resistant	K Cot	
Shigella	should always be tested if chemotherapy is contemplated	
Salmonella (other than *S. typhi* and *S. paratyphi*)	should always be tested if chemotherapy is contemplated	

N.B. This table is intended as a guide and is not exhaustive. Local conditions or changes in bacterial ecology may modify individual entries.

P = penicillin	Carb = carbenicillin	Genta = gentamicin
E = erythromycin	T = tetracycline	Flu = flucloxacillin
A = ampicillin	Su = sulphonamide	Fus = fusidic acid
Ceph = cephalosporins	Cot = cotrimoxazole	Nal = nalidixic acid
L = lincomycin	C = chloramphenicol	Fur = nitrofurantoins
K = kanamycin	Poly = polymyxin	

a knowledge of the probable causative organisms although it may not be possible to isolate and identify them (Table 56.1). In other patients the organism may have been isolated but it is unnecessary to carry out sensitivity tests since the sensitivity of the organism can be predicted with a high degree of accuracy. This knowledge can save time, allow treatment to be begun, and reduce the amount of unnecessary work carried out in the laboratory.

Thus strains of many of the common pathogens (Table 56.1) are similar in their sensitivity to most of the antibacterial agents being either 'resistant' or 'sensitive'. The description of 'resistance' and 'sensitivity' is a *clinical* one; it is usual to select a concentration of the drug which is known to be the average attained in the serum or more occasionally in certain body fluids or tissues after normal dosage. Organisms susceptible to concentrations less than this are usually regarded as 'sensitive'; those growing in higher concentration are 'resistant'. The correlation between this interpretation and the clinical results of treatment is generally good but not complete. Discrepancies may in part be due to the failure to attain adequate concentrations in the tissues resulting in clinical failure; similarly, higher than expected concentrations may be attained so that organisms designated as 'resistant' are susceptible to the prescribed dosage. However, there are many other factors involved in the outcome of the host–parasite relationship in infection and it would be surprising if there was a complete correlation between *in vitro* sensitivity tests and the results of chemotherapy in the patient. Therefore meticulous accuracy in carrying out sensitivity tests may be pointless since the range of variables including drug levels in the patient's tissues is large. Sometimes, however, when a patient is seriously ill with an infection, it may be necessary to carry out detailed laboratory sensitivity tests of the isolated organism to assist in choice of the most effective antibacterial agent for treatment, e.g. in cases of subacute bacterial endocarditis.

Organisms with Predictable Sensitivity

Groups of organisms such as *Haemophilus influenzae* and *H. parainfluenzae* are almost always sensitive to chloramphenicol, tetra-cyclines, ampicillin and cotrimoxazole; they are relatively resistant to penicillin (Table 56.1). Thus, the clinician who knows or suspects that infection is due to *H. influenzae* has a choice of drugs for treatment, and his choice will be influenced by his own personal experience, by possible toxicity of the drug and the chance of hypersensitivity reactions. Other drugs such as erythromycin, lincomycin and the cephalosporins are active against only some strains of *H. influenzae* so that treatment of infections due to this group of organisms with these antibiotics may not be clinically effective.

Regular patterns of sensitivity to many antimicrobial drugs can be shown for streptococci, pneumococci, *Pasteurella, Salmonella, Clostridium, Proteus mirabilis*, etc. (Table 56.1). These patterns may be used as a guide to chemotherapy and the choice of drug. The use of the predictable antibiogram must be qualified by possible differences in the occurrence of resistant strains in certain geographical areas, e.g. the frequency of tetracycline-resistant streptococci or pneumococci; such information may be obtained from local microbiological laboratories.

Organisms with Variable Sensitivity

Other groups of pathogenic bacteria such as staphylococci, escherichiae and some other Gram-negative bacilli, contain a proportion of strains which vary in their sensitivity to antimicrobial drugs. There is therefore greater need to carry out individual sensitivity tests against strains of these organisms when they are isolated; if this is not possible because the causative organism cannot be isolated, it is useful to know the most likely active agents suitable for chemotherapy.

Staphylococcus aureus (syn. *pyogenes*) may be divided into three groups for this purpose:

1. Strains that are penicillin-sensitive (i.e. do not produce penicillinase). These strains are almost invariably sensitive to all the other antistaphylococcal antibiotics, which include chloramphenicol, tetracyclines, cotrimoxazole, ampicillin, the cephalosporins, cloxacillin, flucloxacillin, erythromycin, lincomycin and fusidic acid. The amino-sugar drugs are also effective, particularly gentamicin.

Penicillin-sensitive strains are frequently found in general practice but their incidence is much smaller in hospital infections.

2. Strains that are antibiotic-sensitive but penicillin-resistant because they produce penicillinase. Such strains are sensitive to all the anti-staphylococcal antibiotics except penicillin.

The majority of strains of *Staphylococcus aureus* isolated from patients in hospital and a fair proportion in the general population belong to this group.

3. Antibiotic-resistant strains, all of which produce penicillinase and in addition are resistant to one or more of the other anti-staphylococcal antibiotics, most frequently streptomycin, tetracycline or erythromycin, more rarely lincomycin, fusidic acid or cloxacillin and almost never chloramphenicol. Resistant strains of this type are usually found in patients with infections contracted in hospital.

In general it is reasonable to recommend a choice of cloxacillin, flucloxacillin, lincomycin, clindamycin, fusidic acid, gentamicin or chloramphenicol for the treatment of staphylococcal infections in hospital and the final choice must depend upon the clinician.

Escherichia includes many strains of variable sensitivity but most strains of *Esch. coli* in infections among the general population are sensitive to the anti-escherichia drugs, agents which include ampicillin, cephalosporin, sulphonamide, cotrimoxazole, tetracyclines, kanamycin, nalidixic acid and the nitrofurantoins. The drugs are suitable for *Esch. coli* infections of the urinary tract, but when there is any doubt about the sensitivity of the strain or the response of the patient, individual sensitivity tests must be carried out, particularly in hospital where resistant strains are more likely to occur.

ANTIBIOTIC POLICY

An 'individual' antibiotic policy is the manner in which the individual practitioner or consultant wishes to use antimicrobial drugs. The plan may follow the lines of strategy laid down in this chapter, but to a considerable extent it must be influenced by the usage of antibiotics by other medical colleagues in the area. A number of factors suggest that a more ordered and systematic use of antimicrobial drugs might be of benefit in the general strategy of chemotherapy.

Probably the most important of these is the factor of acquired resistance among some strains of bacteria to antibacterial agents that are commonly used. Whatever the ultimate mechanism of such acquired resistance, it is well established that the prevalence of antibiotic resistant strains is generally proportional to the extent of use of any particular antibiotic in the area. The antibiotic acts as a powerful selective factor in the spread of resistant bacteria and restriction of its use should have the opposite effect of reducing the proportion of resistant strains. The acceptance of this thesis has encouraged 'restrictive' policies such as a temporary ban on the use of penicillin to reduce the incidence of penicillin-resistant staphylococci, or of erythromycin to prevent the appearance of erythromycin-resistant strains, e.g. in infant nurseries. Some local success in hospital practice has been obtained by these policies.

Another advantage of an antibiotic policy is that of clinical convenience. If only a restricted range of antibiotics is available for treatment the dilemma of choice is reduced and only outstanding clinical or bacteriological reasons justify the use of antibiotics outwith the defined group. In extreme instances the use of a single antibiotic over a period has been suggested; such a policy could reduce the chances of error in prescription and also the financial cost of antibiotic therapy.

Periodic changes of antibiotics used for the treatment of infection in the general community might help to avoid the emergence of resistance among pathogenic bacteria and also prevent the increase in the environment of opportunistic pathogens such as *Pseudomonas* and *Achromobacter* which can give rise to troublesome infections. In addition the therapeutic value of antibiotics may be retained over longer periods by such a rotational policy.

The development of a large range of antibacterial substances suitable for clinical application (Table 56.2) makes the serious consideration of such antibiotic policies on a wider scale more practicable and the slowing down in the rate of discovery of new antimicrobial drugs makes them more pertinent.

Table 56.2. Major antimicrobial drugs: uses and modes of administration.

Antibiotic	Route of administration	General antibacterial spectrum	Particular indications
PENICILLINS			
benzyl penicillin ('penicillin')	parenteral oral	Gram-positive organism	Streptococcal and pneumococcal infections
phenoxymethyl penicillin	oral		
benzathine penicillin	parenteral		Long acting for venereal infections
ampicillin	oral and parenteral	Gram-positive and Gram-negative	Respiratory and urinary tract infections. Gall-bladder and bowel infections
carbenicillin	parenteral and oral	Gram-negative	Pseudomonas infections
cloxacillin		Gram-positive cocci	Staphylococcal infections
flucloxacillin			
AMINO-GLYCOSIDES			
streptomycin	parenteral	Gram-negative bacilli	Tuberculosis
kanamycin	parenteral	Gram-negative organisms	Infections due to Gram-negative coliform bacilli
gentamicin	parental	Gram-negative organisms	Pseudomonas infections
framycetin	topical	Gram-negative organisms	Bowel preparation
neomycin	topical	Staphylococci	Wound dressing
TETRACYCLINES			
tetracycline	oral	wide range	Respiratory infections: Coxiella, mycoplasma and rickettsial infections
oxytetracycline	oral	wide range	Respiratory infections: *Bacteroides*
chlortetracycline	oral	wide range	
demethylchlortetracycline	oral	wide range	Respiratory infections: *Bacteroides*
doxycycline	oral low dosage	wide range	
CEPHALOSPORINS			
cephaloridine	parenteral	wide range	
cephalothin	parenteral	wide range	
cephalexin	oral	wide range	
PEPTIDES			
bacitracin	topical oral	Gram-positive organisms	Wound dressing Bowel preparation
Polypeptide			
polymyxin E	parenteral	restricted	Pseudomonas infection
colistin	parenteral	restricted	Pseudomonas infection
OTHERS			
erythromycin	oral and parenteral	Gram-positive organisms	Streptococcal infection *Chlamydia, Coxiella, Bacteroides*
lincomycin	oral	Gram-positive organisms	Streptococcal and pneumococcal infections
clindamycin	oral	Gram-positive organisms	Staphylococcal infections
fusidic acid	oral	Gram-positive organisms	Staphylococcal infections
chloramphenicol	oral and parenteral	wide range	Salmonella, rickettsial, haemophilus and bacterial infections
novobiocin	parenteral	Gram-positive organisms	Streptococcal infections
cycloserine	oral	Gram-negative bacilli	Chronic urinary infections Tuberculosis

Table 56.2 (continued)

Antibiotic	Route of administration	General antibacterial spectrum	Particular indications
I.N.A.H.	oral	Mycobacteria	Tuberculosis
P.A.S.	oral	Mycobacteria	Tuberculosis
ethambutol		Mycobacteria	Resistant and atypical
rifampicin	oral	wide range	Urinary infections: Tuberculosis
sulphadimidine	oral	some Gram-positive and Gram-negative bacteria	Urinary tract infections
sulphathiazole, many other sulpha compounds	oral and parenteral		Meningococcal meningitis
cotrimoxazole (mixture of trimethoprim and sulphamethoxazole)		wide range	Respiratory infections. Urinary tract infections
nalidixic acid	oral	Gram-negative bacilli	Urinary tract infections
nitrofurantoins	oral	Gram-negative bacilli (not proteus)	Urinary tract infections

CHEMOTHERAPY OF SYSTEMIC INFECTIONS

Serious Generalized Infection

Patients with serious and often overwhelming generalized infection are not infrequently seen in hospital practice. They include patients with 'bacteriaemic shock' (better described as 'bacterial shock syndrome', since the presence of organisms in the blood stream is not necessary for the toxaemic collapse) and others with the symptomatology of acute infection without localizing signs. These syndromes may be related to post-operative infection, to instrumentation such as catheterization, or to the aggravation of a previously mild infection, e.g. extension of infection from the middle ear to the brain, or infection superimposed upon disease where there is reduction in the natural resistance of the patient. Such a situation may arise in renal failure, in immune deficiency states, in blood dyscrasias and in many forms of neoplastic disease. Many of the specific measures used in the treatment of these diseases further reduce resistance to infection, e.g. inhibition of antibody production in transplantation surgery or the use of cytotoxic drugs in leukaemia. Often, the clinical features characteristic of infection will be muted or absent in these patients so that

the seriousness of their situation will be masked.

Wherever possible blood, urine and other body fluids and exudates should be submitted to the laboratory before treatment is begun in an effort to isolate the causative organisms. However these patients may require immediate treatment with antibacterial drugs and often there will be little indication of the nature of the infecting organism: further, more than one infecting species may be involved, especially when the source of the infection is within the abdomen. Chemotherapy must therefore cover as wide a range of organisms as possible, e.g. the Gram-positive cocci, the Gram-negative coliform bacilli, and anaerobes such as bacteroides and anaerobic streptococci. In such cases a combination of kanamycin or gentamicin with ampicillin should be prescribed, to which may be added, if thought desirable, tetracycline or lincomycin. When the causative organism(s) are isolated, therapy may be changed or restricted as indicated by the predictable sensitivity of the organism, to be confirmed by subsequent laboratory tests. If the patient's infection fails to respond after three days' treatment, a change may be indicated, e.g. the use of alternative active antibiotics or a purely empirical choice to cover organisms which may as yet be unidentified. It must always be remembered that such patients are suffering from toxaemia and toxins already formed are unaffected by antibacterial therapy. Unfortunately the few specific antitoxic sera available are rarely indicated, e.g. anti-gas gangrene or anti-tetanus serum, but large doses, e.g. 100 ml or more per day of human pooled immunoglobulin may be helpful. Supportive treatment will include correction of fluid and electrolyte imbalance and appropriate treatment of any coexisting renal, cardiac, respiratory or hepatic failure.

Urinary Tract Infections

Urinary infections presenting with symptoms for the first time and cases of asymptomatic bacteriuria are most often uncomplicated when they occur in adolescent and adult females, as seen in general practice and in maternity clinics. More than 90 per cent are due to infection with *Esch. coli* and most strains are sensitive to a wide range of antimicrobial drugs. The treatment of these patients is therefore the prescription of the drug of choice (Table 56.2) from the group of drugs known to be active against *Esch. coli*. In about three-quarters of the cases eradication of the organism is achieved after a course of therapy lasting ten days: the remainder will respond to a second course of the same or a different antibacterial agent, but if the bacteriuria still persists, fuller investigation of the genito-urinary tract is required. Failure to eradicate the infecting organism is usually unrelated to *in vitro* resistance of the organism but rather to abnormality in the urinary system. Recurrence of bacteriuria is unfortunately quite common within weeks or months after a short course of treatment, and it is most important that all patients have their urine bacteriologically examined 3 to 7 days after the cessation of any antibacterial treatment and again after one month. Sensitivity tests of any organisms isolated may reveal a change in antibiotic sensitivity and such change is usually an indication of a fresh infection with an organism which may be resistant to the antibiotic already used (see Chap. 29). This information will indicate the need for further therapy with different antibacterial agents.

Infection of the urinary tract sometimes occurs after instrumentation such as catheterization or cystoscopy; it is almost unavoidable if in-dwelling catheters are used and may also occur after operations such as prostatectomy. Sometimes the infection is endogenous but more often the strains causing these infections are derived from the hospital environment and are resistant to one or more of the commonly used antibacterial agents. In some patients several bacterial species are present, which makes effective treatment more difficult. Sensitivity tests are carried out on these isolates to help in the choice of antibiotics and a combination of drugs is sometimes required. The most useful antibacterial agents are ampicillin, cotrimoxazole and gentamicin; combinations of ampicillin and sulphonamide, or of cotrimoxazole and carbenicillin; gentamicin or a polymyxin may be used if serious pseudomonas infection is present.

In chronic pyelonephritis it may be important to control the bacteriuria and progression of the disease by using long-term or continuous treatment with antibiotics such as ampicillin, tetracycline, cotrimoxazole and sulphonamides. Unfortunately some patients may become reinfected with different species which are resistant to the drug in use and the bacteriuria will not be controlled even during treatment, so that alternative drugs must be used. Thus long-term therapy may require periodic bacteriological re-assessment and sensitivity tests on the flora isolated to indicate when changes in therapy are required. Combinations of antibacterial agents (see below) may reduce the chances of the appearance of reinfection with resistant bacteria and may be advised. The components of such mixtures may be selected on the basis of the results of sensitivity tests of the infecting strains or selected at random from the list of 'commonly used urinary tract antibacterial agents' (Table 56.2). A large series of combinations can thus be permutated from the oral drugs available and each combination given for a period of a few weeks before starting the series once again. This form of therapy can be effective in maintaining low bacterial counts.

Respiratory Infection

Respiratory tract infections are extremely common and although many are primary virus infections, those that are more severe and prolonged usually indicate secondary bacterial infection: successful treatment of the bacterial infection can make the patient more comfortable, shorten the period of illness and reduce the chances of serious complications. Some infections are often related to specific bacterial pathogens such as sore throat due to *Streptococcus pyogenes*, lobar pneumonia due to the pneumococcus and atypical pneumonia due to *Mycoplasma pneumoniae*. Laboratory diagnosis of these conditions is important since the most effective treatment depends upon the use of antibiotics specifically active against the causative organisms. Acute exacerbations of chronic bronchitis are almost invariably associated with either pneumococcus or haemophilus and treatment may be carried out with a wide range of antimicrobial drugs effective against this flora, such as ampicillin, tetracycline, cotrimoxazole and cephalosporins. The results are equally good with any of these different agents and the need for detailed laboratory diagnosis is reduced.

Sore Throat, Pharyngitis and Sinusitis

A number of bacteria may be associated with these infections including *Streptococcus pyogenes*, pneumococcus, *Haemophilus influenzae* and other haemophilus species, and Vincent's organisms. The most important infections from the point of view of the development of sequelae are those due to *Strept. pyogenes* and therefore the treatment of choice is penicillin, which should be given for at least seven days to ensure eradication of the organism. All the other important bacterial pathogens will also respond to this treatment with the exception of some haemophilus infections. If haemophili are regarded as significant, treatment should be with tetracycline, cotrimoxazole or possibly a cephalosporin.

If for some reason penicillin cannot be prescribed, the antibiotic of choice would be erythromycin or lincomycin because these two drugs are active against virtually all strains of *Strept. pyogenes*. Ampicillin should be avoided if there is any likelihood of mononucleosis because it tends to cause a rash and prolong the disease. The increased proportion of strains of *Strept. pyogenes* resistant to tetracycline may make the use of this group of antibiotics inadvisable in streptococcal sore throat. Vincent's angina will usually respond to treatment with metronidazole.

Lower Respiratory Tract Infections

Lobar pneumonia is most frequently due to the pneumococcus and penicillin is the drug of choice; erythromycin, lincomycin or cephalexin are good alternatives. Infection due to klebsiellae or other organisms isolated by culture will require treatment with antibiotics indicated from the results of sensitivity tests. Chloramphenicol is usually effective in such cases if this information is not available. Coliform bacilli, rarely involved in pulmonary infections but frequently isolated from sputum cultures, rarely require specific treatment.

Mycoplasma infections respond best to tetracycline or possibly erythromycin.

Bronchopneumonia is most frequently associated with pneumococcal, streptococcal or haemophilus infection so that ampicillin, cephalexin, tetracycline or cotrimoxazole should be effective. More rarely bronchopneumonia is due to *Staphylococcus aureus* and effective antistaphylococcal antibiotics are urgently required for treatment. Normally the choice would be made from cloxacillin, flucloxacillin, fusidic acid, lincomycin or clindamycin.

In chronic infection such as bronchiectasis, lung abscess or fibrocystic disease, antimicrobial treatment should be prescribed after the detailed examination of laboratory cultures and subsequent sensitivity tests. Combinations of active antibiotics may be more effective in some of these patients. Acute exacerbations of chronic bronchitis are best treated with ampicillin, tetracycline or cotrimoxazole prescribed for not less than ten days, or until the exacerbation abates.

In general the effectiveness of treatment is greater the earlier in the disease that chemotherapy is begun.

Infective Endocarditis

Whenever possible treatment of cases of endocarditis should be related to the results of sensitivity tests made on the organism isolated from the blood. The variety of organisms causing infective (bacterial) endocarditis is greater than it was 30 years ago, partly because of the development of various forms of medical and surgical treatment in other diseases which carry with them a risk of infection of the endocardium. *Strept. viridans* is now isolated from only about one half of patients, and the organisms from the remainder are usually relatively resistant to penicillin. In a proportion of cases believed to be infective on clinical evidence (approximately 25 per cent) no organism can be isolated and treatment must be empirical. There has therefore been an increasing tendency to use combinations of antibiotics such as penicillin and streptomycin for the treatment of bacterial endocarditis.

It seems to be important to kill all the organisms growing in the heart valve tissue since the normal defence mechanisms of the body find it difficult to penetrate this site to assist the antibacterial effect of the antibiotic. It is therefore necessary in such patients to carry out bactericidal tests with antibiotics against the causative organisms and it may also be helpful to monitor the progress of the patient by means of assays of the bactericidal effect of his serum against the causative organism.

Post-operative infections may involve a heart valve and endocardium, particularly after operations for replacement of the heart valves with prostheses. Frequently it is difficult to isolate the causative organism from these patients and there may be doubt as to whether or not infection has become superimposed. The risk of withholding treatment, however, may be considered so great that empirical treatment must commence, and as staphylococcal infection may occur in such circumstances it is best to include an anti-staphylococcal antibiotic.

Rare causes of infective endocarditis in which blood cultures are negative include infections with *Coxiella burnetii* or certain chlamydiae. The diagnosis of these conditions depends largely upon indirect methods such as measuring serological titres, as it is difficult to isolate the organisms. An etiological diagnosis is most important as treatment with an appropriate antibiotic such as tetracycline, erythromycin or lincomycin may be life saving.

Meningitis

The degree and quality of pleocytosis is usually sufficient to differentiate viral from bacterial meningitis, even if the bacteria cannot be seen, in which case initial treatment is best carried out with a combination of penicillin or ampicillin with chloramphenicol and sulphonamide: this combination ensures adequate treatment of infections with Gram-negative coliform bacilli, most common in neonates, and of infections with *N. meningitidis*, *Haemophilus influenzae* and pneumococci which are the most common causes of meningitis in young children. It is also effective against most other bacteria which may cause meningitis, e.g. *Strept. pyogenes* and other streptococci, and more rarely staphylococci, leptospires, etc.

When a definite diagnosis is established treatment may be continued as indicated, but generally chloramphenicol is the drug of choice for haemophilus infections, sulphonamides (with penicillin) for meningococcal infections, and penicillin for pneumococcal infections. Kanamycin or gentamicin is the drug of choice for coliform infections. *Pseudomonas pyocyanea* meningitis may occasionally occur as a nosocomial infection and should be treated with full doses of gentamicin or colistin plus sulphonamide. At all times consideration must be given to the possible need for intrathecal administration of antibiotics to supplement the oral or parental therapy being given.

Intestinal Infections

The consensus of current medical opinion is that cases of Sonne dysentery, salmonella food-poisoning and infection with type-specific *Esch. coli* do not require chemotherapy. Such therapy usually does not lead to more rapid eradication of the causative organism; instead it may make intestinal carriage more likely and increase the risk of the selection of antibiotic resistant strains. The most important treatment is symptomatic, e.g. a kaolin mixture with correction of any upset in fluid balance in the patient. More seriously affected patients such as those with typhoid and paratyphoid fever and *Shigella flexneri* infections may warrant treatment with the appropriate antibiotic, e.g. chloramphenicol or ampicillin for salmonellae and neomycin or colistin for shigellae.

Spread of infection from the bowel to the liver or the blood stream may occur, or may be more local, e.g. abdominal abscess and peritonitis. These are usually serious infections and associated with severe toxaemia. The causative organisms are likely to be varied and frequently include anaerobes such as bacteroides and clostridia. Subphrenic, retrocolic or pelvic abscesses may form and it may not be immediately possible to carry out laboratory examinations to identify the causative organisms. Drainage is a most important aspect of treatment but antibiotics can assist recovery of the patient; cephalosporins or an amino-glycoside plus ampicillin are useful in empirical treatment and tetracycline, erythromycin or lincomycin should be added if bacteroides is likely to be present.

Acute peritonitis after non-specific inflammation of the bowel such as appendicitis is usually effectively controlled with ampicillin or a cephalosporin.

Liver Infections

Specific bacterial infections of the liver and portal pyaemia are best treated with large doses of penicillin or the antibiotic most effective against the organism isolated. Abscesses occur most frequently in the liver due to spread via the portal tract by Gram-negative bacilli from the intestines, or to retrograde spread in the biliary passages by streptococci and clostridia from the gall-bladder. Ampicillin is selectively concentrated in the bile and is frequently useful in treatment of cholecystitis. Amoebic abscess requires prompt and specific treatment and its possibility should always be kept in mind, particularly in any patient who has been abroad.

In all cases of liver infection function of the organ is impaired and if severe may lead to secondary effects on other organs such as the heart and kidneys. Treatment must involve correction of these effects.

Bone and Joint Infections

Most infections of bones and joints are due to *Staph. aureus*. Large doses of penicillin and a cloxacillin should be given to cases of acute osteomyelitis contracted outside hospital (probably due to a penicillin-sensitive strain) and a combination of a cloxacillin with either fusidic acid or lincomycin to neonatal and other cases contracted in hospital (probably due to a penicillin-resistant hospital strain). In subacute or chronic cases of osteomyelitis when long-term treatment is needed, the high concentration of lincomycin in bone makes it the drug of choice.

Streptococcus strains are responsible for many cases of septic arthritis, and penicillin is the drug of choice, given in high dosage for 4 to 12 weeks. Where other organisms are involved, either as primary agents or as secondary invaders in chronic disease, specifically directed therapy is required.

Host Factors

The ultimate choice of the most appropriate antimicrobial drug for treatment may be determined by the history and responses of the patient. If he is hypersensitive to a drug such as penicillin then obviously neither this antibiotic nor those closely related can be prescribed and alternatives must be used. Side-effects may be produced by the antibacterial agents such as nausea and vomiting, diarrhoea or pruritis, and be severe enough to warrant changing treatment. The treatment of intercurrent disease in the patient may contraindicate certain antibiotics either because there is specific organ deficiency, e.g. the failure of the liver to detoxicate in hepatitis or because of therapy with other drugs which can make the antibiotic more toxic, e.g. the administration of the diuretic frusamide and cephaloridine. Frank toxicity, such as ototoxicity from the use of the amino-glycosides must always be borne in mind and particularly in patients who are expected to have poor excretion of the drug, e.g. anyone over the age of 40 or anyone known to have poor renal function.

The absorption of oral antibiotics varies from patient to patient and if poor may be a cause of failure of treatment. Infection may be localized and circumscribed so that penetration of the antibiotic is difficult and the only alternative is surgical drainage. Obstruction to the flow of body fluids may also militate against success and this is important in urinary tract infections, biliary infections and some cases of respiratory infection so that more radical interference is indicated to relieve the obstruction.

When antibiotics are given intravenously they should be administered directly into the vein and not added to other infusion fluids; the reasons for this are that adequate blood levels of the drug may not otherwise be obtained owing to excretion outpacing administration of the antibiotic and also possible incompatibility between the antibiotic and the contents of the fluid. In all cases the manufacturer's instructions and recommendations about the administration of the drug should be closely followed.

ANTIBIOTIC PROPHYLAXIS

There may be some confusion about the term chemoprophylaxis and its application to clinical medicine. Some authorities advise that the prophylaxis of infection should not be attempted with antibacterial drugs since this may result in the selection of resistant organisms which subsequently cause infection and possible spread to other individuals; or that there may be superinfection with highly resistant organisms such as yeasts or staphylococci. The evidence for this is equivocal as indeed is much of the evidence for the efficacy of chemoprophylaxis.

Probably the most widely accepted use of antibiotics for prophylaxis of infection is in patients who have suffered an attack of rheumatic fever or are known to have had rheumatic carditis when long-term penicillin prophylaxis has been justified for the prevention of further streptococcal infection and rheumatic relapse (Chap. 16).

Generally the use of antibiotics as blanket cover to prevent the development of infection is deprecated since it masks the clinical development of infection and makes bacteriological diagnosis very difficult. However, clinicians are reluctant to deny some patients antibiotic cover after prolonged and extensive operations where the exposure of tissue has been great. In such circumstances antibacterial substances may be used topically, e.g. sprays of antibiotic mixtures or antibiotic powder may be spread over the wound; antibiotics, particularly anti-staphylococcal antibiotics, may also be given parenterally before and after operations such as those for the insertion of prostheses, and the administration of penicillin *immediately* before, and for some days after, dental extraction is common.

The use of antibiotics on a large scale for the treatment of undetermined acute upper respiratory tract infection is perhaps not strictly speaking prophylaxis as infection of some sort already exists. However, more serious bacterial infection may be aborted by such therapy and it may be argued that the reduction in its incidence is a justification for the use of antibiotics in this way.

A further controversial use of antibiotics is to modify or reduce the flora of the intestinal tract. This form of prophylaxis is used by some surgeons to supplement bowel toilet before large bowel surgery, thereby reducing the likelihood of post-operative infection. The popularity of this procedure is waning for the lack of unequivocal evidence of its efficacy but there is little argument that some form of bowel toilet whether it be physical or chemical, benefits the post-operative course of these patients. It is certain that the technique of such antibiotic prophylaxis requires more study.

The long-term treatment of chronic infection should not be confused with prophylaxis and may be of great value in the continuous management of chronic urinary tract infection as described above, and the treatment of some cases of chronic bronchitis and chronic lung disease.

COMBINATIONS OF ANTIBIOTICS

'The resistance of certain parasites is a purely chemical question which can be solved only by chemical means: the road leading to its solution which provides the best results is that of combined therapy. . . . Combined therapy is best carried out with therapeutic agents which attack entirely different chemoreceptors in the parasite . . . a simultaneous and varied attack on the parasite in accordance with the military maxim, march apart but fight combined' (Ehrlich, 1913).

The strategical approach to chemotherapy cannot ignore the case for combinations of antibacterial agents, but their therapeutic use is as yet relatively limited. The combination of two or more antibacterial agents is accepted as the method of choice for the treatment of tuberculosis since by this means the selection and possible spread of strains resistant to individual components of the combination are greatly reduced. It is known that if only one drug is used there is a very high chance of resistance developing within a few weeks with persistence or relapse of the infection.

The potentiation of the antibacterial effect of some drugs can result from a combination with others. Sometimes this is referred to as synergism and is exemplified by cotrimoxazole ('septrin', 'bactrim') which is a combination of sulphamethoxazole and trimethoprim; each of these drugs has a low level of antibacterial activity but acts against different pathways in the bacterial metabolism. Together they are active against a wide range of bacterial pathogens and this is reflected in the increasing use of the compound in clinical practice. Resistance is a relatively rare phenomenon.

Other mixtures of antibiotics which are used include combinations of sulphonamide and colistin as this mixture has a synergistic effect *in vitro* upon *Ps. pyocyanea*, and the clinical results of treatment may be better than with colistin alone. Cloxacillin and methicillin have a certain effect in reducing the production of penicillinase in bacteria and can therefore be used in combination with other penicillins of higher specific activity such as benzyl penicillin or ampicillin ('Ampiclox'); such combinations have some use in pediatrics and may also be more effective in coliform and pseudomonas infections.

A further and more subtle effect of a combination may be an increase in the bactericidal action compared with that of the individual components alone. Thus in *Strept. faecalis* endocarditis the bactericidal effect of penicillin may be low although the organism is inhibited by a concentration lower than that obtained in the patient's serum. The addition of streptomycin may dramatically increase the cidal effect of the mixture which is much more likely to effect cure.

ASSAY OF ANTIBIOTICS

It is possible to determine by biological and sometimes chemical tests the amount of antibiotic in the serum of patients undergoing antibiotic therapy. As the concentration in the serum is usually accepted as the significant level for determining whether or not an organism is 'sensitive' or 'resistant', such assays may be used to monitor the effectiveness of treatment. In practice, however, it is rarely necessary to do this and the marked variations in levels in the same patient from time to time make the results of limited value. The most satisfactory measure of the efficacy of therapy is the assessment of the clinical and if possible bacteriological response.

More important may be the monitoring of the levels of antibiotics such as the amino-glycosides which are known to be toxic. It is generally agreed that the serum levels of kanamycin should not exceed 15 μg/ml so as to avoid nerve deafness and it may be desirable to carry out assays in certain patients receiving this and similar antibiotics, particularly when there is known impairment of renal function. Regular assays are very necessary in patients undergoing renal dialysis or transplantation to assist in the management of the dosage of antibiotics. A disadvantage of most techniques is the delay in the result of the bacterial assay since it may be too late to know 24 hours later that the serum level was above the toxic limit. More rapid methods are available for certain antibiotics, but are not in common use. Chemical techniques are generally not sufficiently sensitive but they are available for cycloserine and chloramphenicol assay. It is probable that as much useful information on the accumulation of antibiotic in blood can be obtained by measuring the blood urea or creatinine clearance and reliable results of such tests can be made available much more quickly.

The interpretation of the results of antibiotic assays in the serum may be difficult, if the patient is having or has recently received other antibiotics. With the exception of penicillin it is not possible to selectively remove one antibiotic in order to assay the other component of the mixture. The usual technique is to run parallel biological assays with organisms resistant to one but sensitive to another, but errors in such estimations easily arise and their routine use is not recommended. Further, it is important to know the relationship of the sample being examined to the time of dosage: the maximum levels are obtained by measuring the serum between half and one hour after the previous dose. Cumulative effects are shown by sequential tests carried out on samples taken at the same time each day.

In patients with chronic infections such as bacterial endocarditis it may be thought important to monitor the bactericidal effect of the serum against the causative organism. In such patients the serum should kill at a dilution of not less than 1 in 4, i.e. it should contain at least four times the minimum inhibitory concentration for the infecting organism.

Thus the indications for the routine assay of antibiotics are relatively few: they should always be carried out in close consultation with the microbiologist to ensure the correct timing of samples and to avoid errors due to multiple therapy. The results must be interpreted in the full context of the patient's condition.

Antiviral Chemotherapy

As yet there are few antiviral agents that can be used in treatment. One of the few which is clinically effective is iodo-de-oxyuridine (IUdR) which has been used in the treatment of herpetic keratitis and also in herpetic encephalitis (see Chap. 13).

Other drugs such as the isoquinolines, amantadines and moroxyuridine are under investigation and the thiosemicarbazones (Marboran) have been used for the prophylaxis of smallpox.

FURTHER READING

GARROD, L. P., editor (1960) Antibiotics in medicine. *British Medical Bulletin*, **16**, no. 1.

GARROD, L. P., LAMBERT, H. P. & O'GRADY, F. (1973) *Antibiotic and Chemotherapy*. Edinburgh: Churchill-Livingstone.

GEDDES, A. M. & WILLIAMS, J. D. (1973) *Current Antibiotic Therapy*. Edinburgh: Churchill-Livingstone.

SMITH, HILLAS (1969) *Antibiotics in Clinical Practice*. London: Pitman Medical.

Proceedings from the International Conference on Nosocomial Infections (1971) Chicago: American Hospital Association.

57. Epidemiology and Control of Community Infections

Epidemiology may be literally interpreted as the study of phenomena among the people, the unit of observation being a group of people in the general community or in closed or semi-closed communities (e.g. hospitals and other institutions). A commonly used definition of epidemiology is the science concerned with the distribution and determinants of disease or disability in a community. There is no suggestion in such a definition that epidemiology is solely concerned with the study of epidemics of infectious diseases although this restricted use of the term was in the past widely adopted, mainly because infectious diseases were responsible for a large proportion of the morbidity and mortality in the community and at times spread as great pestilences through many countries. However, the broader concept of epidemiology as defined was accepted, at least in the U.K., more than a century ago. For example, the Epidemiological Society of London defined epidemics in 1862 as 'including the diseases classified as zymotic or miasmatic; many local and constitutional diseases which at times assume an epidemic character; and certain endemic and indigenous diseases such as goitre, pellagra and beri-beri which are peculiar to regions and countries'. In more recent years, epidemiological studies have greatly advanced our knowledge of the aetiological factors and pointed the way to control measures in a wide range of non-communicable diseases including organic heart disease, hypertension, peptic ulcer, cancers, chronic respiratory diseases, accidents and suicides.

In this chapter, our main concern is with the part which the microbiologist plays in conjunction with other members of the epidemiological team in the study of endemic-epidemic infections as they are manifested in different communities. As in police and detective investigations of crime, skill, thoroughness and persistence in the collection of relevant data are essential to success. To quote Frost, 'Epidemiology is something more than the total of its established facts. It includes their orderly arrangement into chains of inference which extend more or less beyond the bounds of direct observation. Such of these chains as are well and truly laid guide investigation to the facts of the future; those that are ill made fetter progress'.

In comparison with the physician who is concerned with the diagnosis, prognosis and treatment of a disease syndrome in an individual patient, the epidemiologist or the epidemiological team, mainly concerned with communicable diseases, studies the sources and modes of spread of an infection occurring endemically or erupting as an epidemic in the community together with all the social and environmental factors that may be involved, with the objective of predicting future trends and recommending control or preventive measures. Just as the physician tackles his individual problem in a methodical fashion—history, physical examination, laboratory aids and clinical course—so the epidemiologist measures incidence rates and relates them to *time*, *place* and *persons*; this involves incubation period, the epidemic curve among affected persons, attack rates by age, sex and race, possible sources and vehicles or vectors of infection, and many other relevant (or irrelevant) factors. Although much of his information may be inaccurate or incomplete, he eventually pieces the data together to form an epidemiological syndrome. These stages in the study of endemic or epidemic infections are often referred to as respectively the *descriptive* and *analytical* phases, which lead to certain deductions or hypotheses, to be further tested by control measures, just as the physician may confirm or refute a presumptive diagnosis by the patient's response to a specific treatment.

It must at once be stated that numerous illuminating studies into the epidemiology of specific infectious diseases were made in the pre-bacteriological era. An outstanding example was the work of John Snow, a London physician and anaesthetist, whose studies on cholera more than a century ago (and 40 years before the cholera vibrio was identified) proved that the materies morbi was excreted from the intestines of infected patients and that sewage-polluted water was the main vehicle for spread of the infection. By painstaking 'shoe leather' epidemiological investigation he showed that in central London during an epidemic period, deaths from cholera were at a rate of 71 per 10 000 houses receiving their water through one company (Southwark and Vauxhall) which collected and distributed water from the lower, grossly polluted, reaches of the Thames whereas in the same area the rate was only 5 per 10 000 houses which used the water supplied by the Lambeth company with a relatively clean intake from the higher reaches of the river. Epidemiological studies of similar merit were contributed by Budd, a West Country doctor, on typhoid fever, Villemin, a Frenchman, on tuberculosis, and Panum, a Dane, on measles in the Faroe Islands, and all before the aetiological agents of these diseases were discovered. A modern analogy in a non-infectious disease is the incrimination of cigarette smoking in the aetiology of lung cancer although the carcinogenic agent has not yet been identified.

THE ROLE OF THE LABORATORY

With the steady increase in the availability and quality of laboratory services, particularly in the past 50 years, clinical diagnosis of infective syndromes can be checked and much useful epidemiological evidence obtained. Among the early epidemiological benefits of the laboratory diagnosis of infectious diseases was the recognition that healthy carriers of various kinds—contact, convalescent, chronic—could be essential links in the chain of infection in a community. The importance of water, milk and foods as vehicles of infection was also confirmed. Later, intensive bacteriological studies of outbreaks or endemic infections rectified data collected from notifications of diseases. For example, the trend in recent years of Sonne bacillary dysentery to have a higher incidence among primary school children than among pre-school nursery children was confirmed by intensive bacteriological examination of cases of diarrhoeal disease in general practice (Gillies, 1965). The realization that in endemic areas typhoid fever and cholera have their highest incidence among young children was only made possible by similar intensive laboratory studies, as was the evidence that more than half of the acute sore throats seen in general practice are caused by pathogens, mostly viruses, other than *Strept. pyogenes* (Ross *et al.*, 1971). Thus, in the field of public health and preventive medicine, the microbiologist is an essential partner with health administrators and clinical colleagues in the collection of precise epidemiological data on communicable diseases as they occur either endemically or in epidemics in the general community and in institutions such as schools, day and residential nurseries and in residential institutions of various kinds.

Although the epidemiological methods to be used in the investigation of infections are similar, irrespective of the nature and composition of the community, special attention will be focused here on (1) infections in the general community and (2) hospital (or nosocomial) infections. In the first category, large populations of all ages are living under very variable conditions and under different health authorities but vulnerable to the same infectious diseases which know no administrative boundaries. In such circumstances, the microbiological services are likely to be most effective if relevant microbiological data collected in peripheral and regional public health laboratories are submitted weekly to a central unit where they are analysed and quickly re-distributed for information to the collaborating microbiologists and health officers. In the collection and analysis of laboratory data on nosocomial infections, the hospital laboratory concerned with both the curative and preventive aspects of infection, plays an important role in assessing the shape and size of the problem and in instituting and monitoring control measures, particularly in areas of high risk such as maternity nurseries, paediatric wards, intensive care units, organ transplantation and renal dialysis units.

COMMUNITY INFECTIONS

Collection of Data

For the epidemiological study of communicable diseases in a general community, the collection and analysis of reliable morbidity and mortality data is essential. At first emphasis and reliance were placed on mortality data and from 1837 the official registration of all births, deaths and marriages to the local Board of Guardians (instead of voluntary records in the parish church registers) and the further assembly of these area records in the General Register Office was quickly utilized by the first Government Medical Statistician, William Farr, to illustrate many of the public health hazards of the time, e.g., the relationship of bad housing and poor sanitation to the high mortality rates in the large towns. The lessons to be learned from the mortality data were expounded by men like Edwin Chadwick and John Simon and led to the Great Sanitary Awakening in the latter half of the nineteenth century. However, *mortality data* could give only a very limited and often lopsided picture of the causes and prevalence of sickness in a community and, increasingly, efforts have been made to obtain reliable *morbidity data* from various sources. For communicable diseases, the Infectious Diseases Notification Act (1889) with later Acts and Regulations has made compulsory the notification by doctors of a wide range of infectious diseases. Unfortunately, this source of information may be misleading in that some infections, e.g. diphtheria, may be over-notified on clinical diagnosis and, more commonly, others are grossly under-notified, e.g. whooping-cough, even when diagnosed clinically. Even so, notifications act as indicators of seasonal and secular changes in the incidence of various infectious diseases as well as supplying valuable information on sex, age, geographic distribution, etc., of individual infections. It is important to note that notifications give a measure of the *incidence* of diseases, that is, the number of new cases occurring in a population of given size within a period of time, usually one year, and expressed as the *incidence rate* per 100 000 population or, where children are predominantly affected, the rate per 100 000 children in specified age-groups. Incidence must not be confused with *prevalence* which measures the number and the rates of cases suffering from a disease at one point of time—sometimes called point-prevalence. As examples, the incidence rate of measles which is a disease of short duration will, particularly in an epidemic year, greatly exceed the prevalence rate, whereas in tuberculosis, a chronic infection, prevalence rates are likely to exceed incidence rates.

In order to calculate incidence and prevalence rates in a country or community, a regular census, usually every 10 years, must be taken so that the age and sex structure of the whole population is known. If the census is taken at regular intervals, an estimation can be made of the population at any point of time between two censuses.

Laboratory Investigations

Since clinical notifications are often incomplete and inaccurate, laboratory examinations are needed to confirm or refute a diagnosis, particularly when the clinical syndrome, e.g. acute diarrhoea, sore throat with exudate, meningitis, may be caused by a number of different pathogens. Facilities for the collection and transmission to the laboratory of specimens from patients with infective conditions are offered by most Health Authorities but are often not fully utilized by general practitioners (Thomson, 1971).

Immunological surveys on random samples or special groups of the population can yield useful information about the prevalence of specific infections in a community. Skin tests as in diphtheria and tuberculosis and serological assays for antibodies as in poliomyelitis have been used extensively as epidemiological evidence on the proportion of susceptible or immune children in different age-groups and therefore as pointers for immunization programmes. Thus, in school outbreaks of diphtheria (which still happen) Schick testing of the contacts will indicate which children are susceptible and in need of immediate protection by passive-active immunization. Tuberculin tests among children in different age groups and in successive years gives a measure of the prevalence of tuberculosis in a community and is used in school children to separate the susceptibles who may be offered BCG vaccination from those already infected; among the latter those with large reactions need close surveillance for some years to detect the onset of clinical disease. Serological tests for polio antibodies have shown that in crowded areas, and particularly in communities with low standards of environmental sanitation, a large proportion of the children have been latently infected before five years of age.

Sources and Spread

In the search for sources and modes of infection, occurring either endemically or in explosive outbreaks, the active cooperation of the microbiologist is usually essential. The part which carriers may play as sources of infection, e.g. the chronic gall-bladder carrier in typhoid fever, the nasal carrier in streptococcal infections and the many contact carriers in outbreaks of Sonne dysentery, can be brought to light only by thorough bacteriological examinations. Similarly, the incrimination of water, milk or specific articles of food as vehicles, or the importance of utensils like slicing knives and mixing bowls in disseminating infection in butchers' and bakers' establishments, depends on the work of the laboratory detective.

Improvements in microbiological methods both for the isolation of pathogens and for their precise identification have helped to sharpen the laboratory tools for solving the mysteries that sometimes enshroud outbreaks of infection. There are many fascinating episodes of this kind that have been soberly recounted in official reports (see *Some Notable Epidemics* by H. H. Scott and the *Collected Papers* of Wade Hampton Frost) or have been more dramatically told by Geddes Smith in *Plague on Us* and by Roueche in *Eleven Blue Men* and other stories.

The microbiologist may not always be the central figure in such dramas but he plays an essential role in collecting the evidence and helping to fit together the pieces in the jig-saw puzzle. The introduction and use of new detective devices such as serotyping, phage-typing and bacteriocine-typing have helped greatly in identifying sources and modes of spread. As examples, the sudden appearance of new salmonella serotypes as causes of bacterial food-poisoning in Britain during the second world war was shown to be associated with the finding of those same serotypes in dried egg consignments imported from North America: later, outbreaks of paratyphoid fever were probably related to infected frozen egg imported from China and other sources. Outbreaks of typhoid fever due to a particular, sometimes unusual, phage type may be traced to a human carrier or a vehicle (e.g. canned corn beef) of the same phage type. *Staphylococcus aureus* type 80/81 became known to be a particularly pathogenic type which spread readily through hospital wards and maternity nurseries, and pyocine typing has proved useful in tracing sources and spread of *Ps. pyocyanea* in skin and urinary tract infections in institutions.

Experimental Epidemiology

Studies using laboratory animals as experimental models have also extended our knowledge of the factors that may contribute to the endemic-epidemic spread of infection in a community. Outstanding examples are the long-term studies by Greenwood, Topley and their colleagues on salmonella infections in colonies of mice; of Webster, Lurie and others on the influence of selective breeding of mice and rabbits in raising or lowering resistance to infection; of Dubos and others in assessing the significance of nutritional factors in relation to susceptibility and severity of infections; and in a more natural setting, the work of Fenner on the effects of partial immunity in the host and lowered virulence in the parasite on the evolution of myxomatosis in rabbits.

CONTROL OF COMMUNITY INFECTIONS

The more precise our knowledge about the links in the chain of infection from the source to the susceptible host in each specific infectious disease the more prepared we are to attack and break the weaker link (or links). Sources and modes of spread of infection were discussed in Chapter 8, to which reference should be made for the broad outlines. Obviously if a pathogen can be eliminated from its source or breeding ground, it cannot be transmitted to a new host. Examples of infectious diseases in which this form of attack is the most practicable are the treponematoses (syphilis, yaws, etc.) and gonorrhoea, since these diseases are mostly spread by clinically ill patients and the other links in the chain are less amenable to attack. Mycobacterial infections also yield to direct attack on the source as has been proven by the dramatic response of tuberculosis, and in some degree leprosy, to mass chemotherapy.

The intestinal infections represent a group of diseases (typhoid, dysentery, cholera, food poisoning) in which the vehicles for transmission are most susceptible to attack by securing clean water, clean milk, clean food, clean hands and the control of flies. The availability of potable water within the household is one of the most effective measures for countering the ravages of intestinal infections and also in dealing with other infections that are susceptible to attack by good standards of personal and household hygiene, e.g. skin infections and infestations—impetigo, pediculosis, scabies, etc. Water and mud may also harbour pathogens like leptospires and the eggs and larvae of various parasites, but in infections associated with these species, direct attack on the animal or intermediate host may be most effective. In the prevention of water and food-borne infections close liaison between the health officer, the public health inspector and the microbiologist must be ensured in order to monitor and maintain satisfactory standards of cleanliness and safety in water, milk and food supplies and in the establishments concerned with their distribution. Although methods of sewage disposal are nowadays satisfactory in most sophisticated countries, environmental sanitation is still a major problem in developing areas, particularly in warm climate countries where parasitic infections are prevalent. Many simple and inexpensive methods for sewage disposal have been devised but local customs and poor education hamper progress and the short-term answer may be to concentrate attention on the host by prophylactic vaccination as in typhoid fever, and hopefully, in bacillary dysentery or by early and adequate treatment as in cholera and infantile gastroenteritis.

Among insect-borne infections, many suc-cesses have been achieved in the control of malaria, yellow fever, dengue, louse-borne typhus, etc., by direct attack on the vector with insecticides often aided by measures to reduce the reservoir of infection or protect the host by insect-repellant methods or chemoprophylaxis. Sometimes there may be a bonus from the widespread use of insecticides as for example, a marked reduction in the incidence of plague following the campaigns against malaria.

In the protection of the host, the two most effective measures are prophylactic vaccination where it has been shown to be needed (see Chapter 58) and improved standards of nutrition, particularly in young children. The implementation of these measures is often very difficult and needs public cooperation through health education by the methods that are likely to be most appropriate and effective in countries and communities with widely different cultural beliefs, socio-economic status and educational standards.

SURVEILLANCE

The term surveillance has recently become popular in international epidemiological parlance. It may be broadly interpreted as epidemiological research into the natural history of disease associated with the continuous observation of its occurrence. Surveillance of communicable disease connotes the active follow-up of specific infections in terms of morbidity and mortality in time and place, keeping track of the sources and spread of the infecting agent, and the study of conditions that may favour or inhibit the spread of infection in the community. Again, it requires team work with the obvious involvement of the microbiologist; it permits prognostic forecasts about future trends and allows objective assessment of deliberate control measures.

Specific examples may best illustrate some of the uses of surveillance in the control of infectious diseases: (a) When typhoid fever with its annual autumnal waves ceased to be a major epidemic disease in Britain following the country-wide use of piped water supplies and the proper disposal of sewage, attention became increasingly focused on chronic carriers as the ultimate source of infection. Intensive field investigations of individual outbreaks allied to improved laboratory methods, e.g. tests for Vi antibodies and phage typing, often led to the detection of the chronic carrier as the culprit. A national register of typhoid carriers was established and known carriers were either persuaded to undergo cholecystectomy or, later, prolonged treatment with ampicillin, or were barred from serving food in restaurants, shops and the like. As a result, outbreaks of typhoid fever traceable to an indigenous source are now rare in Britain and most cases can be related to the acquisition or importation of infection from abroad. Sometimes the lessons learnt from good epidemiological surveillance are forgotten or not acted upon as happened when, despite well documented outbreaks of typhoid fever signalling the dangers of imported canned meat from suspected factories, a large epidemic of some 500 cases occurred in Aberdeen due to the contamination of canned meat from a South American factory that used polluted river water for cooling the imperfectly sealed cans after sterilization. (b) In Britain a large series of controlled prophylactic trials in the 1950s had shown that pertussis vaccine satisfying certain criteria could give a high degree of protection against whooping-cough among young susceptible children. Yet, ten years later, it became evident from a wide clinical and laboratory survey sponsored by the Public Health Laboratory Service, that the currently used pertussis vaccines were not giving a significant degree of protection. This disturbing finding led to a careful overhaul of the antigenic properties and the required standards for pertussis vaccine and to the evidence (as judged by laboratory tests) that the protective efficacy of vaccines made by different manufacturers could vary considerably. (c) The national campaign against poliomyelitis, first with killed and later with live vaccine, which resulted in the virtual disappearance of paralytic polio, has been followed by an intense epidemiological surveillance at both clinical and laboratory levels in order to monitor the continued effectiveness and safety of the vaccine and to detect viruses other than the polio virus which may cause infantile paralysis. (d) Since influenza frequently spreads in pandemics affecting many countries, the need for

international surveillance was obvious. Under W.H.O. sponsorship a network of 80 national influenza reference centres has been set up and established in 55 countries with two international centres in London and Atlanta, U.S.A., respectively. In this way, early identification of new influenza virus types is facilitated and vaccines against a new antigenic type may be prepared in time to protect the more susceptible members of the community as well as doctors and nurses who have to deal with sudden upsurges of cases. At the national level, besides the early warnings from sudden increases in hospital admissions, sickness payments and deaths from respiratory infection, the collaboration between laboratory services and spotter physicians who send specimens from cases of influenza for virus identification has given most useful information.

Increasing collaboration between the medical and veterinary laboratory services in the surveillance of some of the zoonoses, e.g. salmonella infections, brucellosis, leptospirosis, has shed new light on the extent, sources and geographical distribution of these animal to man diseases.

HOSPITAL INFECTIONS

Historically, hospitals have a notorious reputation for infection. The hazards of puerperal sepsis and the horrors of septic infection in the pre-Listerian era have been well documented; yet the dictum of Florence Nightingale, made over a century ago, that 'the very first requirement in a hospital is that it should do the sick no harm' is still not being met. Fever hospitals allowed the segregation of patients with the more contagious fevers but as these have been largely controlled there is now only a limited need for such hospitals: it is often more convenient to have isolation units attached to general hospitals. Many infections that occur in the community are amenable to treatment in the patient's home and specific chemotherapy achieves rapid cure; thus relatively few patients are admitted to hospital specifically for the treatment of their infections, although many may and do have infections incidental to the condition which necessitates their admission to hospital. Infection acquired in hospital (noso-comial infection) is common and resists strenuous efforts to eliminate it. Many factors are involved in its spread; these are reflected in the great difficulties experienced in its control.

Hospital infections when they occur include cross infections, i.e. infections spread from person to person, and post-operative surgical wound infections, but these terms must not be regarded as synonymous. To appreciate the full problem of infections in hospital the following categories must be taken into account:

1. Infections contracted and developing outside hospital which require admission of the patient, e.g. pneumonia.

2. Infections contracted outside hospital which become clinically apparent when the patient is in hospital, e.g. measles.

3. Infections contracted and developing within hospital, e.g. wound infections.

4. Infections contracted in hospital but not becoming clinically apparent until after the patient has been discharged, e.g. some infections in babies.

If all these infections are taken into consideration their number is considerable and may amount to over 30 per cent of the total admissions in a general hospital. The pattern of infection differs between hospitals and sometimes from one geographical area to another. Certain types of hospital will have characteristic patterns of infection, e.g. intestinal infections are common in mental hospitals associated with overcrowding and the difficulty in maintaining good personal hygiene; surgical hospitals have a higher proportion of wound infections whilst units specializing in purely elective surgery such as orthopaedics, have a lower infection rate than those carrying out emergency work where the patients are more likely to have infected tissue *ab initio*.

Endogenous Infections

A high proportion of infections that are clinically apparent in hospital are endogenous, the infecting organism being derived from the patient; such are urinary tract and pulmonary infections developing in recumbent patients and precipitated by lack of normal movement and function and sometimes the lowering of resist-ance from intercurrent disease or treatment. These infections are difficult to prevent because it is almost impossible to control the commensal flora and potential pathogens on the skin and mucous membranes. Bacteriological monitoring of patients on admission to detect such potential hazards is not feasible on a wide scale though it may be considered for certain individuals; e.g. in patients going for major cardiac surgery or transplantation, it may be considered advisable to suppress *Staphylococcus aureus* or clostridia by intense local antisepsis. Abnormal flora may be detected in debilitated patients, e.g. overgrowth of candida in the mouth, so that special care is goven to oral hygiene to prevent thrush.

Exogenous Infections

Exogenous infections acquired from other patients or from staff carriers are specially dangerous because the causal organisms are often strains that have been selected in the hospital community for high infectivity and drug-resistance. They are, however, potentially preventable by the practice of hygienic precautions based on knowledge of their sources and modes of spread. The concentration of patients, with and without infection, ensures dissemination of large numbers of micro-organisms, e.g. in airborne dust, bed-linen and fomites, so that most individuals in hospital become contaminated with this institutional flora as is shown by the rapid changes in the surface flora of both patients and staff soon after their entry into hospital. The situation has been aggravated in recent years by the steady increase in the number of elderly patients who often have to stay in hospital for longer periods than is usually the case with younger patients and who are less resistant to exogenous or endogenous infection.

The mechanisms of transmission of exogenous infections in hospital include those dependent on *contact* with the hands and clothing of attendants and with contaminated instruments, equipment, bed-linen and other fomites; on *airborne dust*, contaminated *food* and *eating utensils*, and *airborne secretion droplets*, probably in that order of importance. Under-staffing with nurses and overcrowding with patients greatly increase the risks of infection by making it difficult for the nurses to adhere to hygienic and aseptic procedures and by enhancing contamination of the air with infected dust.

EMERGENCE OF DRUG-RESISTANT BACTERIA

The use of antiseptics, chemotherapy and aseptic techniques produces strongly selective pressures so that sensitive species of microorganisms are not allowed to survive and those that are more resistant are encouraged. Sometimes this leads to the local multiplication of opportunist bacteria such as pseudomonads and klebsiella in disinfectant solutions, water supplies or wet bathroom equipment, and these potential pathogens may contaminate patients and give rise to infection. The widespread use of antibiotics, which tends to be more concentrated within the hospital environment, produces similar selective pressures so that antibiotic-resistant variants of the common bacteria such as staphylococcus, streptococcus and coliform bacilli come to predominate among the bacteria present in patients, staff and the environment. The mechanism may be either the emergence, multiplication and subsequent spread of spontaneous mutants present in the original microbial population, or the preferential spread of strains originally resistant, but another important mechanism is the spread of heritable drug-resistance factors among the bacteria themselves. Resistance transfer factors (RTF) are known to confer resistance in Gram-negative bacilli to one, two or several antibiotics and it is possible that the transfer of similar factors, such as phage transmission of plasmids between different strains of staphylococci, may affect resistance in other species. The epidemic spread of intestinal infections may be more common in hospital because the close proximity of patients and staff may allow the transfer of resistance factors to sensitive coliform bacilli in a newly admitted patient from a patient already colonized with resistant organisms.

It has even been shown that the consumption of food contaminated with drug-resistant organisms such as escherichia, pseudomonas and klebsiella can give rise to colonization of the gut. In hospital, therefore, there is (a) a higher proportion of antibiotic-resistant strains of the common pathogens such as *Staph. aureus* and *Esch. coli*, and (b) a greater number of strains of resistant opportunistic organisms such as pseudomonas, klebsiella and proteus. Many cross-infections are caused by these organisms and endogenous infection may also result after prior colonization of the hospital patient with such antibiotic-resistant and opportunist organisms, thereby prejudicing the effective treatment of these patients.

Table 57.1. Commonly occurring microorganisms in hospital infections.

Respiratory infections	Urinary tract infections	Superficial infections	Wounds
Respiratory viruses	Esch. coli (antibiotic-sensitive)	Staph. aureus	Staph. aureus
Mycoplasma H. influenzae	Esch. coli (antibiotic-resistant)	Micrococci Coryne-bacteria	Streptococci
Pneumococcus		Coliform bacilli	Esch. coli
Strept. pyogenes	Strept. faecalis Proteus mirabilis	Bacteroides	Proteus
			Pseudomonas
	Klebsiella		Bacteroides Fusiformis
Candida Pseudomonas Klebsiella	Pseudomonas		Coryne-bacteria Staph. albus Clostridia

Gastro-intestinal infections
Enteropathogenic Esch. coli Shigella sonnei Salmonella species Viruses

Surgical Wound Infection

Surgical wound infection costs the health services millions of pounds annually. The reported incidence varies widely, depending on the nature of the surgery undertaken and on the clinical criteria used to define infection; it is lowest (less than 1 per cent) in elective orthopaedic surgery and highest (10 to 15 per cent or more) after operations on the lower bowel. Infection may be *endogenous*, due to transfer into the wound of staphylococci (or occasionally streptococci) carried by the patient in his nose and distributed over his skin or of coliform bacilli released from his bowel during operation. Alternatively, it may be *exogenous*, due to staphylococci or coliform bacilli derived from other patients or healthy staff carriers; the organisms may be transferred into the wound *during operation*, e.g. through the surgeon's punctured gloves or moistened gown, on imperfectly sterilized surgical instruments and materials, or by airborne theatre dust, or *post-operatively*, in the ward, from contaminated bed linen, by airborne ward dust or in consequence of a faulty wound dressing technique. The site and extent of infection and the time it is first recognized after the date of operation often help to establish whether exogenous infection was acquired during operation or post-operatively in the ward; a clustering of cases according to their surgical attendants, ward nurse or location in the ward may suggest a common source.

The high rate of wound infections following bowel operations has led to a widespread use of pre-operative medication with unabsorbable broad-spectrum antibiotics, e.g. neomycin, given in an attempt to 'sterilize' the bowel lumen. Although such treatment will suppress many of the species present in the normal bowel flora, there is no evidence that it is more effective in preventing post-operative infection than physical methods such as washing out the large bowel. There is, however, considerable evidence that the routine systemic administration of prophylactic antibiotics may not only fail to control wound infection but may make it more likely. In the same way, the widely practised treatment of operation wounds in theatre by irrigation, spraying or dusting with antibiotic solutions, aerosols or powders often fails to prevent infection. The elements of surgical practice that are important for the prevention of wound infection are careful cleansing and disinfection of the skin of the operation site, careful use of sterilized instruments and materials, and gentle handling of tissues to avoid damage which may reduce their resistance to bacteria.

Exogenous surgical wound infection is preventable and recognition of its existence is the first step in prevention. It is part of good surgical practice, therefore, to record in a special register brief details of the nature of each operation along with details of the staff involved, the state of the wound each time it is dressed, and the site, nature and extent of any infection which arises. A properly kept 'wound book' of this kind, examined daily, will rapidly reveal any undue rate of wound infection, and the details entered in it will often give a clue to the point at which preventive measures have broken down.

METHODS OF PREVENTION AND CONTROL

The continuing change in medical and surgical techniques and the changing composition of patients being treated in hospital are altering the problems of hospital infection and of its prevention and control. A study of the epidemiology of hospital infection must begin with information about the number and nature of the cases as they occur and the relevant data are obtained from both clinical and laboratory sources. Not all cases of infection have material sent to the laboratory for examination so it is important that a proper record be kept in the ward of the clinical infections as they occur, detailing their nature and treatment and any peculiar circumstances. The microbiologist should also keep a record of the organisms isolated in each unit with appropriate information about antibiotic sensitivity, phage or serotype or other identifying markers. All this may be termed surveillance.

Probably the best way to carry out surveillance is to appoint one person, the Control of Infection Officer, to correlate all the information; he or she will work in association with a group of the hospital staff including a surgeon, physician, administrative and nursing officers and a microbiologist, who constitute a Control of Infection Committee. Some hospitals appoint a senior nurse as the Control of Infection Officer and this can be very successful if such a person can work freely between the wards and the laboratory in cooperation with the microbiologist and the clinician. The epidemiological information collected should enable steps to be taken to prevent the spread and recurrence of infection in individual units.

Table 57.2. Hospital infection: sources, spread and control

Sources	Routes of spread	Prevention	
Cases and carriers among patients and staff	Contact	Washing of hands 'No touch' technique	No admittance of staff with infection
	Droplets	Bed spacing Barrier nursing	
	Airborne dust	Room isolation Air filtration Unidirectional airflow	Reduce activity of personnel Measures to reduce dust
Ancillary and domestic staff			
Visitors	Food Milk	Sterilization and disinfection	Certified supplies
Other sources	Apparatus		

The actual procedures to control nosocomial infections and their spread within the hospital depend upon the nature of the infection but in general follow the principles already outlined. They include:

1. *Asepsis.* Aseptic techniques play an important part in reducing the hazard of infection in surgery and numerous diagnostic and therapeutic procedures. Sterilization procedures must be regularly monitored and are perhaps best supervised by the microbiologist. Much progress has been made in recent years in reducing the danger of infection from instruments, needles, and syringes, by the provision of pre-sterilized packs, including the use of disposable items, and more recently this sterile supply service has been extended to the sterile theatre tray service. The use of sterile apparatus will not avoid the spread of infection if there is carelessness in its use and whenever possible strict 'no touch' techniques must be used coupled with strict personal hygiene on the part of the operator. These routines are rigidly laid down in theatre practice but are less well implemented at ward level, e.g. in the performance of dressings. Many hospitals have instruction sheets on the procedures for wound dressings which should preferably be carried out in a separate dressing station.

2. *Antisepsis and disinfection.* Chemical disinfectants have a limited part to play in preventing infection and there is widespread waste of these substances because of a lack of appreciation of their limitations. The use of disinfectants in floor and wall washing is virtually useless because of the short time of contact and the inactivation of the disinfectant properties by dirt and organic matter. Adequate concentrations of disinfectant can be effective at localized sites in certain circumstances, e.g. the disinfection of hard surfaces such as trolley tops and the chemical sterilization of milk feeding bottles or thermometers, providing that there has been initial physical cleansing and adequate time for the disinfection process. Great care must be taken to use only fresh reagents in clean containers and to check that no opportunist organisms have colonized the reagents (see P.H.L.S. Monograph Series, No. 2, 1972).

3. *Isolation.* Patients may be at risk of infection, particularly if they have a decreased resistance, and patients may also be a source of infection to others. Therefore all hospitals should be provided with adequate isolation facilities of approximately 2 single-bedded cubicles per 100 beds so that patients at risk or a hazard to others can be completely separated and nursed in isolation. In this way all routes for the spread of infection can be severed in both directions.

'Barrier nursing' is a term used to describe the attempts to 'isolate' a patient when strict physical segregation is not possible. The patient is nursed in the same multi-bedded ward as other patients and is exposed to an interchange of airborne microorganisms with them, but is protected by the practice of strict aseptic precautions against the transmission of infection by contact with the hands or clothing of attendant staff or with contaminated equipment. Such a regime is difficult to carry out in a busy hospital ward and may do more harm than good by producing a false impression of isolation. It is commonly employed in cases of suspected dysentery or other intestinal infections. All attendants, wearing clean gowns, must wash their hands before and after visiting the patient. All articles, including eating utensils, are kept strictly for the sole use of the patient and his excreta are disinfected. After discharge all disposable material should be destroyed and the clothing, bedding, etc., used by the patient, disinfected by a special wash.

'Cubicle' or 'single-bedded room' isolation, by which the patient is nursed by himself in a room separated by a door and corridor from other patients' rooms, confers a substantial measure of protection against air-borne cross-infection. The protection is greatest if a system of unidirectional exhaust ventilation with clean or filtered air is used. Cubicle isolation should be practised in conjunction with aseptic nursing precautions against infection by contact. Comparative studies of cross-infection with heterologous types of *Streptococcus pyogenes* and *Corynebacterium diphtheriae* in scarlet fever and diphtheria wards have shown that the adoption of strict barrier nursing techniques in multi-bedded wards has brought about only slight or moderate reductions in the cross-infection rate, whilst cubicle isolation plus aseptic nursing has virtually eliminated cross-infection (e.g., Allison and Brown, 1937; Wright, Shone and Tucker, 1941).

4. *Instrumental Procedures.* The procedures used in the treatment and diagnosis of patients are important factors in hospital infection: they may debilitate the patient and thereby reduce his resistance, or introduce organisms directly into the tissues as in surgery, cannulation or catheterization. Anaesthetic machines and respirators may facilitate the spread of organisms from patient to patient and incubators can be a fruitful source of opportunist organisms to contaminate premature infants. The greatest care must be taken to ensure that any diagnostic or treatment procedures are carried out as carefully as possible and with a minimum of disturbance to the patient, and that all apparatus is free from pathogenic organisms. Instruments used to penetrate the body surfaces must be sterile and apparatus used on the surfaces should be free from pathogens.

5. *Personnel.* Hospital staff are the major reservoirs of organisms in the hospital environment and therefore potential sources of infection. Apart from this it has been clearly shown that infection rates are higher among people in a semi-closed community as there are increased contacts and chances of contamination. All staff in attendance on patients should be free from obvious infection; this may be very difficult to regulate and various surface infections such as boils and respiratory infections may pass unnoticed. All staff should be encouraged to report such incidents and alternative duties not involving the exposure of patients should be available. Under certain circumstances, particularly in units that have high risk patients, bacteriological monitoring of staff may be undertaken.

6. *Ward Design.* The movement of personnel and apparatus within wards or special units is known to affect the rate of infection. Good design which reduces unnecessary movement and helps to maintain the rest and quiet of the patient will therefore contribute to a reduction in infection. Adequate space will reduce the concentration of organisms in the environment and enable proper spacing of beds, thereby reducing the hazard of cross infection, e.g. by droplets or dust from bed to bed.

The flow of material from the 'clean' to the 'dirty' sides of a unit, with a minimum crossing of paths, is also important. There should be adequate air flow with a required number of air changes (e.g. ten) per hour to reduce the intake of organisms and to dilute out pathogens. The separation of patients in small rooms may do little to reduce the risk of cross infection unless to-and-fro air flows are prevented and rigorous aseptic nursing procedures are also adopted. The full isolation of a patient requires a well designed unit to ensure the physical isolation of the patient and include the provision of air pressure barriers. Outpatient departments including dressing stations must also be so designed as to facilitate unidirectional traffic.

7. *Administration.* The administrative officer(s) of the hospital should take an intimate

interest in the problem of infection and should be on the Control of Infection Committee. A Medical Superintendent, when there is one, may be well suited to act as chairman of such a committee. The monitoring of ancillary staff, including kitchen and domestic staff, to check on their illnesses is important since such persons may be an important source of respiratory and intestinal infections. High standards of portering must be maintained and steps taken to ensure that the transfer of materials within the hospital does not carry an infection hazard. Laboratory specimens, particularly from areas of high risk of infection such as hepatitis, e.g. dialysis units and transplant wards, must be properly sealed in impervious bags and suitably labelled to indicate their nature so as to reduce the chance of contamination, not only of laboratory staff, who should be aware of the risks, but of other persons who may come into contact with the specimens in transit.

8. *Antibiotic Policy*. It has been emphasized that antibiotics act as selective agents in the hospital environment by encouraging the emergence and spread of antibiotic-resistant and opportunistic bacteria (Chap. 56). At present the only reasonable possibility of controlling this hazard is to operate an antibiotic policy which releases the ecological pressure. A restrictive policy involving the complete withdrawal of one or more antibiotics from clinical use may reduce the appearance of bacterial strains resistant to these drugs, and has been tried successfully with penicillin and ampicillin. In one neurosurgical hospital a serious epidemic of meningeal, pulmonary and urinary infections with antibiotic-resistant klebsiellae was brought rapidly to an end by the complete cessation of the use of antibiotics for prophylaxis and therapy (Price and Sleigh, 1970). Another policy that may be helpful is the rotational use of different sets of antibiotics for successive periods; this procedure should achieve the same ends as restriction and be more convenient in clinical practice.

Antibiotics, if spilt into the hospital environment and inhaled, may lead to staff becoming carriers of resistant organisms.

It may be concluded that the judicial use of antimicrobial drugs in acute infections plus isolation, the blocking of channels of spread, and protection of the susceptible host allows the epidemiologist, the microbiologist, the health officer and physician to reduce the load of infection and control its spread, whether locally within the family, within a hospital or within the general community. Success will depend upon full cooperation between all of these persons and the fullest utilization of the information that is available. This team effort requires to be expeditiously carried out at all times and maintained with enthusiasm.

REFERENCES AND FURTHER READING

ALLISON, V. D. & BROWN, W. A. (1937) Reinfection as a cause of complications and relapses in scarlet fever wards. *Journal of Hygiene, Cambridge*, **37**, 153.

CONTROL OF COMMUNICABLE DISEASES IN MAN (1970) 11th Edn. New York: American Public Health Association.

FENNER, F. & RATCLIFFE, F. N. (1965) *Myxomatosis*. Cambridge University Press.

FROST, W. H. (1941) *Collected Papers*. A Contribution to Epidemiological Method. Edited by K. F. Maxcy, London.

GEDDES SMITH (1941) *Plague on us*. London.

GILLIES, R. R. (1965) Longitudinal Family Studies in Scotland. In *Comparability in International Epidemiology*. New York: Milbank Memorial Fund.

PICKLES, W. N. (1939) *Epidemiology in Country Practice*. Bristol: Wright & Son.

PRICE, D. J. E. & SLEIGH, J. D. (1970) Control of infection due to *Klebsiella aerogenes* in a neurosurgical unit by withdrawal of all antibiotics, *Lancet*, **ii**, 1213.

PROCEEDINGS OF INTERNATIONAL CONFERENCE ON NOSOCOMIAL INFECTIONS (1970) Chicago: American Hospital Association.

ROSS, P. W., CHRISTY, S. M. K. & KNOX, J. D. E. (1971) Sore Throat in Children: its Causation and Incidence. *British Medical Journal*, **ii**, 624.

SCOTT, H. H. (1934) *Some Notable Epidemics*. London.

TAYLOR, I. & KNOWELDEN, J. (1964) *Principles of Epidemiology*. 2nd Edn. London: Churchill.

THOMSON, W. A. R. (1971) *Calling the Laboratory*. 3rd Edn. Edinburgh: Churchill-Livingstone.

WILLIAMS, R. E. O., BLOWERS, R., GARROD, L. P. & SHOOTER, R. A. (1966) *Hospital Infection*. 2nd Edn. London: Lloyd-Luke.

WRIGHT, H. D., SHONE, H. R. & TUCKER, J. R. (1941) Cross-infection in diphtheria wards. *Journal of Pathology and Bacteriology*, **52**, 111.

58. Prophylactic Immunization

The principles of artificial immunization, both active and passive, have been discussed in Chapter 10. Here, the applications of these principles in immunization programmes and schedules for the prevention or control of certain microbial infections are considered. It must be emphasized that prophylactic immunization is only one of several measures that may be used for the control of infectious diseases and that its cost and efficacy must be assessed against other forms of attack such as chemotherapy and chemoprophylaxis, environmental sanitation, insect vector control and improved nutrition. Sometimes it is profitable to use two or more of these measures simultaneously, e.g. environmental sanitation and immunization against typhoid fever, and chemotherapy and BCG vaccination against tuberculosis. Again, a large proportion of the morbidity and mortality from infection is not preventable by immunization or presents great difficulties to its application; for example, the complex of diarrhoeal diseases and respiratory infections that takes a heavy toll of life and health among young children in poor and overcrowded communities is not amenable to control by specific vaccines; nor are the common bacterial infections associated with haemolytic streptococci, pneumococci and coliform bacilli, nor many virus infections, although encouraging efforts are being made in this direction.

RATIONALE OF IMMUNIZATION

The objective of immunization is to produce, without harm to the recipient, a degree of resistance as great as, or greater than, that which follows a clinical attack of the natural infection. With this objective in mind, those communicable or infectious diseases amenable to control by vaccination may be considered in four main groups; toxic, acute bacterial, chronic bacterial, viral and rickettsial infections. In the first group, e.g. diphtheria and tetanus, the brunt of the infection is due to a specific poison or toxin which can be purified artificially, rendered harmless by treatment with formaldehyde (i.e. conversion to toxoid) and used as an effective antigen or prophylactic, particularly if it is absorbed on to a mineral carrier, e.g. aluminium hydroxide or aluminium phosphate. (These alum salts are tissue irritants and therefore should be used in the lowest concentration required for an adjuvant action.) The potency of toxoid antigens can be measured and standardized with great accuracy, and the antitoxin level produced in the blood of the inoculated person gives a reliable indication of the degree of his resistance to a particular infection, e.g. diphtheria.

Among the acute bacterial infections there are two categories as far as immunization procedures are concerned; (a) pyogenic infections (staphylococcal, streptococcal, pneumococcal and coliform) against which vaccines are largely ineffective, since there are many different antigenic types within the species, e.g. some 80 types of pneumococcus, so that an infection or artificial immunization with one type does not protect against infection with other types; (b) infections like whooping-cough, cholera, plague and anthrax, where there is only one or two main antigenic types of organism, so that a vaccine prepared with the prevalent infecting organism might be expected to give a reasonable degree of protection. Pathogenic organisms contain many different antigenic components of which probably only one or two are particularly concerned with the virulence of the organism. It is important to try to identify and certainly to preserve these 'protective antigens' in vaccine preparations.

Another difficulty is that in bacterial infections like whooping-cough and cholera, the disease affects predominantly the epithelial surfaces so that humoral antibodies produced as a result of parenteral vaccination may not gain easy access to the site where the pathogen is producing the infection. For this and other reasons it is essential to test vaccines against whooping-cough and cholera in properly controlled field trials so that objective assessment of their value may be obtained.

So far, the assumption has been implicit that the production of a specific protective antibody is the main requirement for effective immunization. When the chronic bacterial infections are considered (e.g. typhoid, brucellosis, tuberculosis), it must be concluded from knowledge of their natural behaviour that the specific humoral antibodies that can at present be identified play little part in overcoming the infection. Thus, antibodies to the specific antigens of the typhoid and brucella bacilli are demonstrable in the blood of the patient within a week of onset of the clinical illness, but the fever may go on for many weeks before clinical recovery. In addition, relapses in these *continued fevers* are not uncommon despite the presence of high concentrations of specific antibodies. In contrast to the acute bacterial infections, the infecting organisms in chronic infections are for the most part intracellular parasites, and it seems likely that what is called cellular or cell-mediated immunity may be more important in overcoming the infection than the presence of humoral antibodies. The development of tissue hypersensitivity probably plays a part in raising resistance to infection or re-infection in these and some other infections. It may be noted that in tuberculosis and brucellosis a live attenuated vaccine is needed to produce immunity.

In the viral infections humoral antibodies may be protective but, again, cellular immunity seems to be important in some diseases. Thus, children with hypo-gammaglobulinaemia can recover from virus infections like measles, chickenpox and mumps with an apparently good immunity but without detectable humoral antibody, whereas they rapidly succumb to acute bacterial or toxic infections. Such children can also be successfully vaccinated with small-pox and BCG vaccines. These findings indicate that specific humoral antibodies do not play a major role in recovery from some virus diseases. On the other hand, immunity to certain infections seems to be related to the presence of antibody; human immunoglobulin has been used effectively to prevent or ameliorate measles and infectious hepatitis; killed viral vaccines, which probably act mainly in virtue of the production of humoral antibody, protect against diseases like poliomyelitis and influenza.

IMMUNE RESPONSE AND DURATION OF IMMUNITY

The newborn baby may contain in its blood antibodies to the agents of certain toxic, bacterial and viral infections according as the corresponding antibodies are present in the mother's blood. This passive immunity gives protection to the infant at a time when it is poorly equipped to produce specific antibodies, but it interferes to a varying extent with the infant's capacity to respond to the stimulus of injected or ingested toxoids or vaccines in the early months of life. For example, measles vaccines elicit little or no antibody response in most children under 9 months of age because of the presence of maternal antibody; polio antibodies in breast-milk may interfere with oral vaccination in the early months of life. The capacity of the infant's tissues to produce specific antibody to injected antigens is poorly developed in the first few months of life although some response is obtained to powerful antigens such as alum-adsorbed toxoids. However, the tissues of the newborn infant will usually respond to BCG and smallpox vaccines with resultant immunity, probably because the protection is cell-mediated.

When a good specific antibody response is being sought to a toxoid or killed antigen, the usual procedure is to give three doses of the antigen at spaced intervals. The first dose of antigen evokes a low level of antibody after a latent period of approximately two weeks, but after the second dose the amount of antibody produced has multiplied tenfold that of the original response and after a third dose may be increased a hundredfold. The first or 'priming' dose of toxoid will be more effective the larger it is; or if it is released slowly as from a mineral carrier; or if it is mixed with certain bacterial vaccines, e.g. tetanus toxoid plus typhoid vaccine, diphtheria toxoid plus pertussis vaccine. The mineral carrier and the bacterial vaccine act as adjuvants (see below) for the toxoid. The second and subsequent doses are effective in much smaller amounts than the first, and without the help of adjuvants. With most antigens the response is much better if the two doses are spaced out at an interval of six to eight weeks, and, provided the priming dose is adequate, the response to the second dose will still be maximal even if given six months after the first. A third or booster dose is recommended at a varying interval after the second dose but administratively is most conveniently given after 4 to 6 months (see schedule *a*). Where there is reason to believe that a community has acquired a basic immunity from the widespread occurrence of clinical or inapparent infection, as in influenza and, in some countries, typhoid fever, one dose of antigen may be enough to act as the secondary stimulus.

The *duration* of immunity after the basic course can be measured precisely in the case of toxic infections in accordance with the level of specific antitoxin in the blood or, less precisely, in diphtheria, by the Schick test. Recent studies have shown that a protective concentration of diphtheria antitoxin may persist in the blood of children for several years after primary immunization in early infancy; after a primary course of three doses of tetanus toxoid, a satisfactory antitoxin titre may persist for as long as ten years.

The duration of immunity after injections of killed bacterial vaccines cannot be equated with the presence of demonstrable antibody; for example, after a course of three doses of pertussis vaccine given to children (average age one year) there was no change in the degree of protection in successive six months during a follow-up period of two-and-a-half years, although antibodies were no longer demonstrable in a considerable proportion of the children within a year after immunization. Again, in the continued fevers, e.g. typhoid and brucellosis, antibody titres give no measurement of the degree of protection. In certain viral infections, e.g. influenza, systemic antibody titres are related to the degree of protection, but in other diseases, e.g. measles and respiratory syncytial infection, antibodies to killed vaccine may be causally associated with severe reactions on exposure to natural infection, possibly due to tissue hypersensitivity.

Adjuvants

Antigens may be incorporated in or mixed with an adjuvant in order to increase the antibody response. Adjuvants are most effective in enhancing the response to the less particulate protein antigens, such as toxoids and virus vaccines. Three main types of adjuvant have been used in human and veterinary medicine—a gel of aluminium hydroxide or aluminium phosphate, a water-in-mineral oil emulsion or a suspension of Gram-negative bacilli. All three adjuvants act in varying degree by creating a depot from which the antigen is slowly and continuously released over a period of days or weeks. The alum adjuvants and probably the oily emulsion also help to make the antigen more particulate, which again enhances the antibody response. Thus, the response to two doses of an alum-adsorbed diphtheria toxoid may be five times greater than that to three doses of plain toxoid, and the antibody titre after 0·2 ml of influenza virus vaccine in a water-in-oil emulsion will considerably exceed that following 1·0 ml of a saline virus vaccine. With these two antigen adjuvants, antibody titres also persist at a higher level for a much longer period of time. Gram-negative bacterial suspensions seem to act in virtue of their content of lipopolysaccharide (endotoxin) which, by disrupting host cells with the release of DNA derivatives, leads to increased antibody production, but the enhancing effect may not be as great or as predictable as with the other two types of adjuvant.

Because of the tissue reaction to the alum and oily adjuvants, with the consequent tendency to form a local granuloma and sometimes a sterile cyst, injections should be given either deep subcutaneously (in the case of alum adjuvants) or intramuscularly (for oily adjuvants).

Age of Commencement of Immunization

There is good evidence that the newborn child responds poorly and in a different fashion to a variety of antigens, as compared with an infant a few months old. However, with powerful antigens like tetanus toxoid, good antibody responses may be obtained even in premature infants. A complicating factor that frequently inhibits or restricts the infant's response to some of the commonly used antigens when given parenterally is the acquisition of maternal antibodies via the placenta. Antibodies to polio virus may be present in mother's milk and may interfere with the activity of poliovirus vaccine given orally in early infancy.

These passively acquired antibodies in the infant, e.g. diphtheria antitoxin and polio and measles viral antibodies, gradually disappear in the course of a few months, so that diphtheria toxoid will usually elicit a good antibody response when given after three months and killed polio vaccine when given after six months of age; in the case of measles, traces of specific antibody may restrict the response to live vaccine if given before nine to twelve months of age. On the other hand, there seems to be little or no transfer of protective antibodies against pertussis, so that infections occur, and are most severe, in the first six months of life and artificial immunization may be started as early as three months of age. Primary vaccination against smallpox is necessary early in infancy in communities where the infection is endemic but may not be effective if done in the first month of life. BCG vaccination may be successfully performed at birth, since there is no transfer of immunity to tuberculosis, but the age of commencement of vaccination programmes against tuberculosis and other preventable infections must be adjusted to the known epidemiology of these diseases in the community (Table 58.2).

Dosage and Spacing of Vaccines

The primary antibody response is directly related to the dose of antigen and the practice, now largely discarded, of giving a smaller primary dose followed by a larger second dose is immunologically wrong. With prophylactic reagents that produce little reaction, such as the toxoids, there is no difficulty in ensuring an adequate 'priming' dose, whereas large doses of some bacterial vaccines, e.g. pertussis or typhoid vaccines, may cause both local and systemic reactions, so that the vaccinator is tempted to reduce the recommended dosage. With inactivated virus vaccines, it may be economically or technically difficult to give an adequate primary dose; on the other hand the use of live bacterial or virus vaccines, which multiply in the host's tissues, should ensure adequate stimulation of the antibody-producing mechanism.

After an adequate primary dose of antigen, there is multiplication of clones of antibody-producing cells, which, with their descendants, will quickly respond to further stimulation by the same antigen, even when given in a smaller dose. In the past, the mistake was frequently made of giving the second dose too soon (seven to ten days) after the first. Now it is known that the minimal interval for a maximal response to the second dose is 40 days and that thereafter the degree of response does not vary much for the next six months. As an example, Brown *et al.* (1964) found that the antibody titres to the three common antigens, diphtheria and tetanus toxoids and pertussis vaccine, were uniformly higher when two doses of this triple vaccine were given at a *two-month* rather than at a one-month interval. If, however, the antibody response to the primary dose is very weak, because of poor or insufficient antigen (as was the case with the early inactivated polio vaccines), the interval between the first and second doses should not be too great.

Once a clone of antibody-producing cells has 'memorized' the capacity to respond to a particular antigenic stimulus, a booster dose, given perhaps years later, will evoke a rapid outpouring of antibody. This phenomenon has been particularly well demonstrated in such infections as tetanus, yellow fever and rabies, where an injection of the antigen has elicited excellent antibody responses at intervals of 10 to 25 years after the basic immunization.

CONTROLLED STUDIES OF PROPHYLACTIC VACCINES

Evaluation of prophylactic vaccines and toxoids by means of carefully designed and controlled field trials has resulted in a revolutionary change in the accuracy with which the degree of protection afforded to the inoculated can be assessed. Public health programmes for the use of vaccines so tested can now be planned with the assurance that a known degree of effectiveness will be obtained. Vaccines submitted to controlled field trials include those against whooping-cough, tuberculosis, typhoid fever, influenza, poliomyelitis and measles. It may be noted that although BCG and typhoid vaccines had been available and in use for many years prior to the time the new methods of field testing were generally applied, they had ultimately to be submitted to controlled trials before a true assessment of their value could be made. It is only by statistically acceptable studies which give unbiased information that controversy is settled and confident use can be made of the vaccines on a large scale. Well-planned studies, though costly, save money, time and misplaced effort in the long run and give information not otherwise obtainable on dosage, combined antigens, duration of immunity and the like.

Combined field and laboratory studies of vaccines aim at providing confidence in the efficacy of future vaccination programmes, which can only rarely be attained if the studies do not observe two basic principles, which may be called (1) the principle of comparability and (2) the principle of reproducibility.

(1) *The Principle of Comparability* ensures confidence that an observed degree of protection apparently conferred upon a population group by vaccination was due to the vaccination and not to other chance influences. It requires comparison of the incidence of the disease in two or more groups, and precautions to ensure that these groups can be regarded as identical in all respects except for the factor of vaccination.

The most convincing evidence will be obtained if one of the groups in a field trial ('the control group') remains unvaccinated, or is vaccinated with an unrelated vaccine. If it is not feasible to have a control group, comparisons may be made between groups inoculated with vaccines that are prepared in different ways, or sometimes between groups treated with the same vaccine but a different dosage schedule.

(2) *The Principle of Reproducibility* ensures confidence in obtaining, in future vaccination programmes, the same degree of protection as was observed in the initial field trial. It requires precautions to ensure that the vaccine which was proved to be of value in the field trial can be prepared again at the same level of safety and potency and can, if possible, be validly tested for these properties in a laboratory assay.

A field trial can show only whether or not the actual preparation of vaccine used in the trial was successful. What is then needed is confidence in the ability to reproduce this particular preparation or of preparing an equally or more efficient vaccine. The method of preparation must therefore be meticulously described and the laboratory studies must include assays of different vaccines in experimental animals, in order to develop, if possible, a laboratory method yielding results that parallel those obtained in the field; this procedure permits the assessment of the protective value of future vaccine preparations by laboratory assay alone.

If the essential protective antigen of a microorganism could be isolated, identified and quantitatively assessed with chemical exactitude and if the mechanism of the production of immunity by the host were understood, there would clearly be no need to do more than to measure the amount of protective antigen in the first successful vaccines tested. It could then be ensured that all subsequent vaccines contained similar or greater amounts of the essential constituent. Such measurement can be made with some approach to accuracy with toxoids such as the diphtheria or tetanus prophylactics, but with many bacterial and virus vaccines, killed or living, this is not possible, and the principle of reproducibility must therefore be carefully observed. In these circumstances, it is necessary to compare a series of vaccines in field studies and at the same time to submit them to as many laboratory studies as possible in the hope that variations of protective power in the field will occur, which will be reflected in one or more laboratory tests. The laboratory test which gives results most closely corresponding to the protective value in the field trials may then be adopted as the test for standardizing future batches of vaccine.

Whether or not a laboratory test for the protectiveness of a particular antigen is found to correlate with its efficacy in field trials, manufacturers of vaccines for commercial use are required in Britain and in many other countries to satisfy certain standards pertaining to the purity, safety, potency and stability of their products. In addition, the World Health Organization has established certain internationally agreed requirements for a number of microbial vaccines in common use; antigens used in immunization programmes sponsored in any way by W.H.O. must conform with these requirements. At national level, some system for continuing surveillance of the efficacy of prophylactic vaccines and periodic checks on the occurrence of local or systemic reactions or sequelae should be instituted.

Controlled Trials of Pertussis Vaccines

The series of controlled vaccine trials against whooping-cough carried out in Britain during a 10-year period afford good examples of the application of the principles of comparability and reproducibility of immunization programmes. Pertussis vaccines had been used both in the prevention and treatment of whooping-cough for many years; a high degree of protection was apparently obtained in the Danish use of pertussis vaccines to control epidemics of the infection in the Faroe Islands and later in American studies on the control of endemic whooping-cough. But these reported successes did not conform to the tenets of a properly controlled trial and, under the sponsorship of the Medical Research Council, a series of pertussis vaccine studies was begun in Britain in 1946; a total of some 50 000 children mostly in the age range 6 to 24 months and 25 different vaccines were involved during the next 10 years. Data from the first trial are given here (Report, 1951). Children in the age range 6 to 18 months (average 12·2 months) recruited with parental consent from five different urban areas in England were divided by random sampling into two groups, one group to be given pertussis vaccine (3 doses at monthly intervals) and the other group an anticatarrhal vaccine. Code numbers were used for each batch of vaccine and neither the staff concerned with administering the vaccine nor the recipients or their parents knew which child received which vaccine (double-blind trial). The two groups were remarkably similar in all respects (Table 58.1)

Table 58.1. Similarity of vaccinated and unvaccinated groups in pertussis vaccine trials.

	Vaccinated			Unvaccinated			Grand Total
	Male	Female	Total	Male	Female	Total	
Total No. of children given 3 inoculations	1,823	1,978	3,801	1,932	1,825	3,757	7,558
Average age (months)	12.1	12.3	12.2	12.2	12.2	12.2	12.2
Average duration of observation per child (months)	26.9	27.2	27.1	27.2	27.2	27.2	27.1
Average No. of children under 14 years per household	1.8	1.8	1.8	1.8	1.8	1.8	1.8
Breast-feeding:							
No. breast-fed	1,457	1,575	3,032	1,540	1,471	3,011	6,043
Average duration of breast-feeding (months)	5.4	5.3	5.3	5.3	5.4	5.4	5.4
No. not breast-fed	321	350	671	344	308	652	1,323
No. where history not known	45	53	98	48	46	94	192
No. of cases of certain other infectious diseases in children during the trial:							
Measles	440	480	920	471	420	891	1,811
Chicken-pox	138	151	289	139	141	280	569
Bronchopneumonia	50	45	95	53	41	94	189
Diphtheria	0	1	1	1	0	1	2
TOTAL	628	677	1,305	664	602	1,266	2,571
No. known to be:							
Immunized against diphtheria	1,592	1,736	3,328	1,716	1,609	3,325	6,653
Vaccinated against smallpox	1,151	1,240	2,391	1,205	1,141	2,346	4,737

so that if the incidence of whooping-cough in the follow-up period was significantly lower in the pertussis vaccine group, the difference would be due only to the vaccine. After vaccination was completed, each child was visited regularly for 27 months or more by a nurse investigator who reported on the incidence of any suspicious symptoms and further clinical and laboratory observations were made on suspect cases. The incidence of whooping-cough among the 3 801 vaccinated and 3 757 control infants was respectively 149 and 687, giving attack rates of 1·45 and 6·72 per 1 000 child months, i.e. a protection rate of 78 per cent in the vaccinated group. Among young children exposed in the home to an infected sibling the attack rates were 18·2 per cent in the vaccinated and 87·3 per cent in the control group; and when whooping-cough did occur in a vaccinated child, the infection was on average much less severe and of shorter duration than in unprotected children (Fig. 58.1). During this and later trials with different pertussis vaccines, different laboratory tests were carried out to discover, if possible, a method of assay that would correlate with the results of the field trials. A test involving the intracerebral injection of a challenge strain of *Bord. pertussis* into

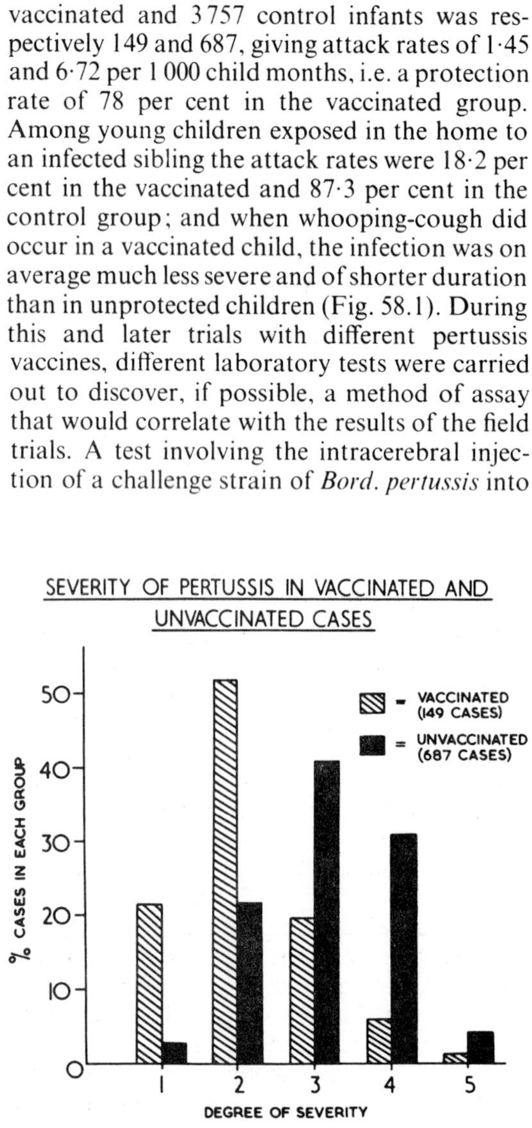

batches of previously vaccinated mice was found to give reasonably good correlation (Fig. 58.2) and this mouse-brain test was adopted for the assay of future pertussis vaccines although later events suggest that the standard British requirements were, perhaps, set too low (see Pittman, 1970).

HAZARDS OF IMMUNIZATION

It is axiomatic that prophylactic agents, before they are issued for use, should have been shown to be safe as well as effective, and the Therapeutics Substances Act regulations require certain tests for sterility and toxicity to be carried out on these prophylactics. Nonetheless, there are certain incidental hazards associated with the injection of immunizing agents. The first of these relates to the syringe and needle to be used for the injection. The best way to ensure that a syringe and needle are sterile is to heat the assembled outfit in a hot air oven at a temperature of 160°C for one hour. The next best is the use of high pressure steam in an autoclave or pressure cooker which, with the syringe dismantled, can again ensure absolute sterility, i.e. the destruction of both sporing and non-sporing microorganisms. Although boiling does not kill the more resistant sporing organisms, this procedure is accepted as reasonably safe for the re-sterilization of syringes that have already been properly sterilized in a hot air oven or autoclave. In other words, where many injections are being given, as at a baby clinic, repeated boiling of the syringe and needle for ten minutes may be accepted as adequate protection against the risk of transference of infection. A sterile syringe and needle must be used for each injection to avoid the risk of transferring the agent of serum hepatitis, for a syringe, if used for repeated injections even with a fresh sterile needle each time, may carry over minimal amounts of tissue fluid. The skin should, of course, be cleansed and preferably treated with a quick acting antiseptic such as 2 per cent iodine in 70 per cent alcohol immediately before the injection. For smallpox vaccination, the skin should simply be cleansed with soap or methylated ether and then allowed to dry. It is unwise to give an injection to a

SEVERITY OF PERTUSSIS IN VACCINATED AND UNVACCINATED CASES

FIG. 58.1. Severity of pertussis in vaccinated and unvaccinated cases.

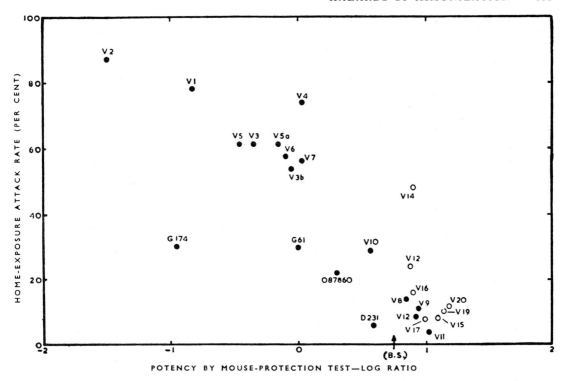

FIG. 58.2. Chart showing the relationship, with 25 pertussis vaccines, between home-exposure attack rate in the field and potency as estimated by the mouse-potency test. The log potency of the British Standard Vaccine is shown by the arrow.

child who is obviously suffering from skin sepsis; and smallpox vaccination should be avoided in a child with eczema, because of the risk of generalized vaccinia (Chap. 40).

In regard to reactions, there is as a rule little or no local or systemic reaction after the injection of plain toxoids, but when an alum salt is added to the toxoid there is usually some local reaction because of the irritant effect of the alum. For this reason the injection should be given deep subcutaneously so that any fibrous nodule at the site of injection is not easily felt. A hazard that has recently emerged is the occurrence of local or generalized hypersensitivity reactions to tetanus toxoid that has been administered too frequently. With killed bacterial vaccines, the amount of local or systemic reaction is usually greater than with toxoids and with both TAB and pertussis vaccines there may be local swelling associated with some febrile reaction within the first

24 to 72 hours after inoculation. After injections of pertussis vaccine, rare cases of encephalopathy, manifested by convulsions and coma and followed sometimes by mental deterioration, have been reported. It is impossible to estimate the risk of this hazard, but it occurs in probably less than one in 1 million injections and has been noted particularly in the U.S.A. and Sweden. Other disturbing reactions to pertussis vaccine are a state of shock (the child becomes very pale and may lose consciousness) and persistent screaming, usually manifested within 1 to 6 hours after an injection. The incidence is apparently more common among infants under 6 months of age and may vary with different vaccines. Efforts are being made to reduce the risk of these toxic effects but meanwhile it is advisable to avoid giving pertussis vaccine to children with a history of repeated convulsions and to children who are convalescent from some other illness.

The disastrous accidents that may happen due to errors in the production, distribution and use of vaccines have been reviewed by Wilson (1967).

IMMUNIZATION PROGRAMMES

When the comparative efficacy and safety of a particular vaccine have been ensured, the health authority has to consider very carefully the indications for its large-scale use and the priority it should be given in relation to other measures designed to maintain or improve the health of the community or to control specific preventable diseases.

To plan rationally, the health authority needs reliable epidemiological information on morbidity and mortality rates for diseases in general and for preventable infections in particular. It must be emphasized that priorities among infections preventable by vaccination in economically advanced countries with temperate climates may not be, and often are not, the priorities of developing countries with tropical or subtropical climates. Each country must determine the age, sex, secular, and socio-economic distribution of each specific infection and the geographical localization of the main reservoirs, since the plan of campaign for immunization programmes will often depend on this kind of information. If certain infections are most prevalent among young children in poor, overcrowded urban communities—diphtheria, whooping-cough and tuberculosis are examples—the primary attack in the immunization campaign should be directed at these endemic reservoirs: or clinical infection may first manifest itself in more well-to-do urban areas, as may happen with poliomyelitis; or it may be more common in rural areas, as with tetanus.

Another factor that needs careful thought is the interdependence between infection and nutrition. Malnutrition may not affect the incidence of infectious diseases, but it often contributes to the severity of the infection. Would it then be more profitable, in terms of community health, to hasten inprovements in nutritional standards so as to lessen the toll of morbidity and mortality from the generality of infections than to give priority to specific immunization programmes against, say, measles and whooping-cough?

The aim of immunization programmes is the control of infection in the community rather than individual protection. A lower level of herd immunity than is necessary for solid individual protection can effectively reduce the incidence of most preventable diseases if a high proportion of the susceptible community is immunized. Thus, in diphtheria, there is a rapid reduction in both morbidity and mortality rates when 60 to 70 per cent of pre-school and school children are effectively immunized. It is stated that smallpox may be controlled when 80 to 90 per cent of the whole community has been successfully vaccinated. Tetanus is an exception to this general rule in that protection of a proportion of the population does not reduce the risk to the non-immunized individual.

For countries with well-developed systems for the collection of morbidity and mortality data relating to communicable diseases plus good medical services, it should be relatively easy to decide what vaccinations should be carried out and how best the programme can be effected. Nonetheless, delays and lack of coordination in the application of knowledge frequently occur even when a good organization is available. There is also the risk that the incidence and importance of a disease may be underestimated or miscalculated if notification is poor, or mortality rates are falling, e.g. in tuberculosis and whooping-cough, or deaths are attributed to secondary causes, e.g. bronchopneumonia after measles or whooping-cough. In countries with limited medical services it is essential that strenuous efforts be made to provide satisfactory vital statistics and, by sample surveys or other means, to obtain a reasonably accurate assessment of the main causes of morbidity and mortality.

In the United' Kingdom most of the immunization work is done either at child welfare clinics or by the family doctor or pediatrician. Whilst there are obvious advantages in having the immunizations carried out by the family doctor, it is essential that there should be a well-organized system for ensuring that the child receives the vaccines at the appropriate age and time intervals, that there is an efficient system of recording the immunizations and of any reactions and complications after administration of the vaccines, and that a continuing surveillance be maintained to assess the efficacy and safety of the vaccination programme.

An immunization campaign carried out without provision for its continuation as a routine procedure will not give satisfactory results—except where complete eradication is achieved. Therefore, in planning immunization schedules, provision must be made to ensure receptivity by the public and, particularly, to secure the cooperation of parents who have to bring their children to the doctor or clinic for repeated inoculations. These measures are essential for the successful execution of the programme.

In the planning and execution of immunization programmes, immunological points that merit special emphasis are: (1) the use of combined antigens and the simultaneous administration of killed and live vaccines; (2) the incorporation of adjuvants in killed vaccines; (3) the age of commencement; and (4) the dosage and spacing of the antigens.

VACCINATION SCHEDULES

In the consideration of vaccination schedules for his community, the Health Officer must keep in mind four main precepts: the need, efficacy, safety and ease of administration of each prophylactic vaccine. In Britain it is generally agreed that protection of the susceptible population against diphtheria, whooping-cough, poliomyelitis and tetanus is to be recommended and can best be achieved by immunization. Other communicable diseases against which prophylactic vaccination is highly effective, but the need for nation-wide use less generally accepted, are tuberculosis, measles and rubella. Vaccination against virus influenza may be recommended for groups at special risk whilst immunization against typhoid fever,

Table 58.2. (a) Schedule of immunization in countries with adequate public health services.

Age	Vaccine	Interval	Notes
During the first year of life	Diph/Tet/Pert.* and oral polio vaccine (first dose)		The earliest age at which the first dose should be given is 3 months, but a better general immunological response can be expected if the first dose is delayed to 6 months of age
	Diph/Tet/Pert. and oral polio vaccine (second dose)	Preferably after an interval of 6 to 8 weeks	
	Diph/Tet/Pert. and oral polio vaccine (third dose)	Preferably after an interval of 4 to 6 months	
During the second year of life	Measles vaccine		
At 5 years of age or school entry	Diph/Tet and oral polio vaccine or Diph/Tet/Polio vaccine		These may be given, if desired, at 3 years of age to children entering nursery schools, attending day nurseries or living in children's homes
Between 10 and 13 years of age	BCG vaccine		For tuberculin-negative children
All girls aged 11 to 13 years	Rubella vaccine	There should be an interval of not less than 3 weeks between BCG and rubella vaccination	All girls of this age should be offered rubella vaccine whether or not there is a past history of an attack of rubella (see note 8)

*Diph/Tet/Pert.   Diphtheria formol toxoid, tetanus formol toxoid and killed pertussis bacilli.

cholera and yellow fever should be restricted to those going abroad either as visitors or as immigrants to areas where these infections are still endemic. Fortunately, the vaccines for the four diseases in the first mandatory group are, besides being effective and safe with minor qualifications for pertussis vaccine, easily administered in that all four prophylactics can be given at the same time—diphtheria and tetanus toxoids plus pertussis vaccine as combined killed antigens (DPT) injected parenterally and live polio vaccine given orally; all four are best given in the first year of life from 3 months of age onwards. Various other combinations are recommended to suit the needs of other countries, but the combination of two or more live vaccines, e.g. smallpox and yellow fever vaccines, measles, mumps and rubella vaccines is not presently advised for use in Britain.

It will be noted that in the first schedule (Table 58.2), smallpox vaccination has been omitted. This is because the W.H.O. global programme for the eradication of smallpox has been so successful that the risk of smallpox being imported to Britain has been markedly reduced and vaccination against smallpox is no longer recommended as a routine procedure. It is essential, however, that health service staff, including doctors and nurses, ambulance staff and public health workers, who may come in contact with suspected cases and laboratory staff who may have to handle infective material should be adequately vaccinated. Travellers going abroad will be advised by the travel agencies which countries require a valid certificate of vaccination against smallpox and against other diseases, e.g. cholera and yellow fever, before entry.

Two vaccination schedules are given here as flexible models (a) for areas with well-developed medical services, and (b) for areas with limited medical services. Schedule (a) is modified from that recommended in a recent memorandum on Immunization against Infectious Diseases (1972). It is envisaged that schedule (b) will be used in countries with endemic smallpox and typhoid fever but a low incidence of clinical poliomyelitis. In such areas poliomyelitis vaccine should not be employed routinely, but should be available to those at special risk of clinical disease, e.g. in urban areas, particularly those with reasonably good environmental sanitation and household hygiene.

Table 58.2 (b) Schedule of immunization in countries with limited public health services.

Visit	Age	Prophylactic
1	0–1 month	[1] BCG vaccination
2	3–5 months	Diph/Tet/Pert. vaccine (alum adsorbed) [2] Oral polio vaccine [3] Smallpox vaccination
3	6–8 months	Diph/Tet/Pert. and oral polio vaccine (2 months after first dose) BCG vaccination if omitted at 0–1 month
4	1–2 years	[4] Typhoid and oral polio vaccine [5] Measles vaccine
5	5–6 years (school entry)	Tetanus + [4] typhoid vaccine
6	11–12 years	Tetanus vaccine

Note: This schedule aims to give basic protection in the minimum number of visits.

[1] BCG vaccination should be done in the neonatal period if the baby is born in an institution.

[2] Oral polio vaccine should be given if there is evidence of cases of paralytic poliomyelitis among young children.

[3] Primary smallpox vaccination in infancy is recommended in countries where the infection is still endemic or where there is a fair risk of importation. The result (successful or not) is checked at the next visit.

[4] If typhoid fever is endemic in the area, one dose may act as a booster at school entry; in hyperendemic areas, 1 to 2 doses may be given in the second year of life.

[5] Measles vaccine may be given in countries where the infection and its complications cause high morbidity and mortality; but it is expensive.

REFERENCES AND REVIEWS

BROWN, G. C., VOLK, V. K., GOTTSHALL, P. Y., KENDRICK, P. L. & ANDERSON, H. D. (1964) Responses of infants to DTP-P vaccine used in nine injection schedules. *Public Health Reports*, **79**, 585.

IMMUNIZATION AGAINST INFECTIOUS DISEASE (1972) London: HMSO.

PITTMAN, M. (1970) *Bordella Pertussis*. In *Infectious Agents and Host Reactions*, Edited by Stuart Mudd. Philadelphia: Saunders.

REPORT (1951) The prevention of whooping-cough by vaccination. Medical Research Council Investigation. *British Medical Journal*, **i**, 1464.

WILSON, G. S. (1967) *The Hazards of Immunization*. London: Athlone Press.

WORLD HEALTH ORGANIZATION (1971) *International Conference on the Application of Vaccines against Viral, Rickettsial and Bacterial Diseases of Man*. Pan-American Health Organization/World Health Organization.

Appendices

Appendix 1

CONTAINERS AND SWABS FOR THE COLLECTION OF SPECIMENS

Specimens for bacteriological investigation should be forwarded as soon as possible to the laboratory in robust, leak-proof, sterile containers. It is essential that each container should bear the name of the patient from whom the specimen is submitted and the accompanying form should be accurately completed. Relevant clinical data must indicate the probable clinical diagnosis, information regarding recent or current chemotherapy and, especially if a serological investigation is required, relevant details of previous immunization should be given.

GLASS TUBES AND UNIVERSAL CONTAINERS. These are suitable for submission of specimens of exudate, pus, blood, cerebrospinal fluid, urine and faeces. Strong glass test-tubes, $4 \times \frac{3}{8}$ in, with rubber bungs or bark corks, may be used. They should be sterilized in the autoclave with the bungs or corks loosely fitted and thereafter pressed in. Tubes with bark corks may be sterilized in the hot-air oven.

The screw-capped bottle known as a universal container is recommended; it consists of a strong moulded glass bottle, $3\frac{1}{4}$ in high $\times$ $1\frac{1}{8}$ in diameter, capacity 1 oz (28 ml), with a flat base and wide mouth. These bottles are supplied already cleaned and capped in 1-gross boxes. They are sterilized by autoclaving with the caps loosely screwed on; after sterilization the caps are tightened. They cannot be sterilized in the hot-air oven, as the rubber washers will not withstand the temperature.

The screw-capped universal container has many advantages over the glass tube. It is stronger, and the screw cap keeps the mouth of the container sterile whereas dust collects at the rim of a stoppered tube. The contents of a universal container cannot leak or become contaminated and, as it is quite stable on its base, it is particularly convenient when specimens are taken at the bedside.

For the collection of serous fluids, e.g. pleural fluid, the universal container is suitable. The addition of 0·3 ml of a 20 per cent solution of sodium citrate to the container prior to autoclaving (with the cap fitted) is recommended for the collection of fluids that may coagulate on standing. This avoids difficulty in performing cell counts or centrifuging procedures with such fluids.

Blood may be submitted in a universal container but a small quantity for serological investigation is more conveniently sent in a sterile glass tube fitted with a rubber bung. The blood clot may be cultured in a selective medium, e.g. for enteric organisms. Blood intended primarily for blood culture should be submitted in a special blood culture bottle.

For the collection of *faeces*, a small squat bottle of about 2 oz capacity, or a glass specimen tube 2 in $\times$ 1 in, fitted with a bark cork in which a small metal spoon is fixed, is sometimes used: but containers having a cap or top fitted with an *attached spoon* may be troublesome; on removal of the cap, some of the specimen is withdrawn on the spoon resulting in contamination of the cap or the working surface. Such containers also have the disadvantage that any fermentation of the faeces tends to blow out the cork and cause leakage of the contents. The corks have to be discarded after use. The shoulder on the bottle makes cleaning difficult.

For small quantities of faeces the universal container is recommended. A small spoon made of tin plate $3\frac{3}{8} \times \frac{3}{8}$ in may be included in the container prior to sterilization. A portion of faeces is taken up in the spoon and the whole dropped into the container and the cap screwed on. Alternatively, a wide-mouth 2-oz screw-capped jar, known as a 'pomade pot', is used and the faeces taken up in small cardboard spoons (such as are used for ice-cream cartons). These containers may be transmitted to the laboratory by post, the package labelled 'Pathological Specimen'.

When there is likely to be a delay of some hours before laboratory cultivation can be carried out, neutral glycerol-saline should be added to the faeces.

For small quantities of *urine*, e.g. for the diagnosis of most cases of urinary tract infection, the universal container is used (see Chap. 29). For larger quantities, e.g. complete early morning specimens, 20-oz screw-capped bottles are convenient.

DISPOSABLE SPECIMEN CONTAINERS. Screw-capped waxed cardboard cartons of 2-oz capacity (such as are used for cream and ice-cream) are suitable for the collection of sputum and faeces. A similar carton with a sealable top is available for urine specimens. Because of postal regulations these waxed cartons *cannot* be sent through the post.

1. Aluminium containers (2 in in diameter by 1 in deep) suitable for the collection of faeces or sputum can be despatched through the post.

2. Plastic containers—made of polystyrene and/or polypropylene—are available, already sterilized, with or without spoons, anticoagulants, labels, from a number of manufacturers (Sterilin, Stayne (Bydand), Searle). These containers are made in a variety of sizes and are suitable for urine, faeces, pus, blood, etc. It should be noted that not all of these containers have been authorized for sending by post as some have push-on caps rather than screw-caps; some types have been known to leak during transmission. In the British Standards Institution Publication BS 4851 (1972) specifications for Medical Specimen Containers for Haematology and Biochemistry are laid out including details of a leakage test. A separate standard covering specimen containers for microbiology is being prepared. Attention is drawn to the work of Cash (1971) on a special type of double plastic envelope suitable for the transport of 'high risk' specimens such as blood for examination for hepatitis virus B.

3. Recently, disposable glass specimen containers have become available from various suppliers (Stayne (Bydand), Labco).

All disposable containers should be destroyed in a furnace after use.

SWABS. A swab usually consists of a piece of aluminium or tinned iron wire, 15 gauge and 6 in long. One end is made rough for about $\frac{1}{2}$ in by squeezing it in a small metal vice or the cutting edge of pliers. Around this end a thin pledget of absorbent cotton-wool is tightly wrapped for about $\frac{3}{4}$ in. The wire is placed in a narrow thick-walled test-tube, 5 in $\times \frac{1}{2}$ in, and the top of the tube is plugged with cotton-wool. Alternatively, and where swabs have to be sent by post, the wire should be $4\frac{1}{2}$ in long and the top inserted into a bark cork which stoppers the tube. The tube with swab should be sterilized in the autoclave and not in the hot-air oven, as in the latter the wool may char and give rise to tar-like products which may be inimical to bacteria on the swab. It is important to autoclave cork-stoppered tubes with the cork loose and to press in the cork after sterilization. Tubes plugged with cotton-wool should be dried after autoclaving.

Instead of wire, swabs may be prepared from thin wooden sticks $6\frac{1}{2}$ in long that are specially made for the purpose, and are known as 'Peerless' wooden applicators. A cotton-wool pledget is wrapped round one end as above, and the tube is plugged with cotton-wool. They cannot be used conveniently with a bark cork, but have the advantage that the stick can be broken off short when the swab has to be placed in transport medium in a screw-capped container.

DISPOSABLE SWABS. A variety of types of swab, e.g. plain, serum coated, charcoal coated, are available (Exogen, A. R. Horwell). These come in cardboard or clear plastic tubes, or plastic envelopes already sterilized. The swab in its tube or envelope is destroyed in a furnace after use.

The swabs may also be purchased loose and unsterile, for assembly and sterilization in tubes. This type of swab is also useful in the laboratory for other purposes, e.g. seeding of media for disk sensitivity tests.

When taking specimens from babies and young children it is often necessary to employ a very fine swab so that small orifices, such as the aural meatus, may be negotiated without gross contamination from the external surfaces. These are made in the same way as the swabs described above but with fine rigid wire such as that supplied as ENT probes by George Stone and Son, 35 High Park Street, Liverpool 8. To avoid damage to the tissues, the end of the wire should be fused in a Bunsen flame before fixing a tiny pledget of cotton-wool to it.

Swabs are very useful for taking specimens from:

(a) Throat: in cases of suspected diphtheria, tonsillitis, etc.

(b) Wounds, discharging ears, or surgical conditions, e.g. fistula, sinus, etc. Some of the purulent material is taken up on the cotton-wool.

(c) Post-nasal or naso-pharyngeal space: for this purpose the terminal $\frac{3}{4}$ in is bent through an angle of 45 degrees, and in use is inserted behind the soft palate. This procedure is useful for obtaining specimens from suspected meningococcal carriers and for the early diagnosis of whooping-cough.

For the diagnosis of whooping-cough a 'pernasal' swab is preferable to the post-nasal swab: this is made from 7 in of flexible copper wire or nichrome SWG 25 (0·51 mm diameter), the terminal $\frac{1}{4}$ in being bent back to take the pledget of cotton-wool, a very thin layer of which is wound firmly round it. Ready-made pernasal swabs with a finger loop may be purchased from McQuilken & Co., 15 Sauchiehall Street, Glasgow. The swab is contained in a $6 \times \frac{1}{2}$ in test-tube plugged with cotton-wool. The swab is passed gently back from one nostril, along the floor of the nasal cavity until it reaches the posterior wall of the naso-pharynx, rotated gently and it is then withdrawn.

(d) Rectum: rectal swabs are very useful in bacillary dysentery cases or contacts, especially in young children.

(e) Cervix uteri: in gonorrhoea and puerperal infections. A longer wire, 9 in, is preferable for these specimens.

Where some time may elapse before the swab is examined and especially where delicate pathogens are concerned, e.g. meningococcus or *Bord. pertussis*, it is advantageous to place the swab in transport medium. A bark cork is used as a stopper and the wire pushed through the cork so that the cotton-wool is clear of the agar. After the specimen has been taken, the swab is inserted into the tube and the wire pushed down until the cotton-wool pledget is in contact with the transport medium.

A special method for preserving the viability of the gonococcus in swabs is described in Vol. II, Chapter 28. The problem of bacterial survival is not confined to the Neisseriae, since slow-drying is known to be lethal to most bacterial species. Transport media for various species are described in Vol. II, Chapter 6. Rubbo and Benjamin (1951), as a result of their comparative findings with many different pathogens, recommend the use of a serum-coated cotton-wool swab to prolong viability. The swabs are prepared by dipping the cotton-wool on a wooden applicator into undiluted ox serum for 10–30 s, spreading them out on sheets of blotting-paper, drying in an incubator at 37°C for about half an hour, and finally sterilizing in the autoclave at 121°C for 20 min. The finished product is a compact honey-coloured pledget, 3–5 mm in diameter, in which the cotton-wool fibres are firmly bound to each other and to the applicator. Clinicians may need to be warned about the unusual appearance of these swabs so that they will not think they have already been used. For a more detailed account of swabs and swabbing methods see Cruickshank (1953).

Appendix 2

POSTAL REGULATIONS

The Postmaster-General has laid down the following instructions for sending pathological material through the post and these should be rigorously observed:

'ARTICLES SENT FOR MEDICAL EXAMINATION OR ANALYSIS. Deleterious liquids or substances, though otherwise prohibited from transmission by post, may be sent for medical examination or analysis to a recognized Medical Laboratory or Institute, whether or not belonging to a Public Health Authority or to a qualified Medical Practitioner or Veterinary Surgeon within the United Kingdom, by *letter post, and on no account by parcel post*, under the following condition:

'Any such liquid or substance must be enclosed in a receptacle, hermetically sealed or otherwise securely closed, which receptacle must itself be placed in a strong wooden, leather or metal case in such a way that it cannot shift about, and with a sufficient quantity of some absorbent material (such as sawdust or cotton-wool) so packed about the receptacle as absolutely to prevent any possible leakage from the package in the event of damage to the receptacle. The packet so made up must be conspicuously marked "Fragile with care" and bear the words "Pathological Specimen".

'Any packet of the kind found in the parcel post, or found in the letter post not packed and marked as directed, will be at once stopped and destroyed with all its wrappings and enclosures. Further, any person who sends by post a deleterious liquid or substance for medical examination or analysis otherwise than as provided by these regulations is liable to prosecution.

'If receptacles are supplied by a Laboratory or Institute, they should be submitted to the Secretary, General Post Office, in order to ascertain whether they are regarded as complying with the regulations.'

The following receptacles have been approved by the Postmaster-General:

For universal containers, media bottles and 2-oz pots, a leatherboard box, internal size $4\frac{3}{8}$ in $\times$ $2\frac{1}{8}$ in $\times$ $1\frac{7}{8}$ in deep with metal-bound edges and full-depth lid, is used. The glass container is wrapped in a piece of cellulose tissue, 19 in $\times$ $4\frac{1}{2}$ in, and then fits securely in the box which is placed in a shaped gummed envelope having a tag for the postage stamps.

Swabs or cultures in tubes are wrapped in cellulose tissue and placed in hinged metal boxes having rounded corners, size $6\frac{1}{4}$ in long, $2\frac{1}{2}$ in wide and 1 in deep. Leatherboard boxes with metal-bound edges of the same size are also permitted. These are placed in stout manilla envelopes which have a tag at the end for the postage stamps.

For the 8-oz pots and the 1-lb jars, a larger piece of cellulose tissue is required, while the leatherboard box is similar in construction to the one mentioned above and large enough to take these receptacles.

Gummed labels printed with the name and address of the laboratory and the information required by the Post Office Regulations are often issued by laboratories when sending out the postal materials.

Appendix 3

THE LABORATORY DIAGNOSIS OF BACTERIAL INFECTIONS OF MAN

Nature of infection	Specimens to be submitted for examination	Media for primary inoculation	Atmosphere for incubation	Techniques and selective agents for separation	Further steps for identification of the causal organism	Indirect methods of diagnosis	Antibiograms Fixed — Sensitive	Fixed — Resistant	Variable
Actinomycosis and related infections	Exudates Tissue	Blood agar Shake culture in glucose agar	Aerobic Micro-aerophilic Anaerobic	Prolonged culture Washing of granules			P.K.C*.T.		
Anthrax	Exudate Blood culture (Sputum, Faeces)	Nutrient agar Blood agar	Aerobic		Animal pathogenicity		P.C.T.K.		
Brucellosis	Blood culture Serum	Liver infusion agar and broth Blood agar	Aerobic Air + CO_2		Dye sensitivity tests Animal pathogenicity Specific antisera	Agglutination tests CFT	K.C.T.E.Su.		
Cholera	Faeces	Alkaline selective medium	Aerobic	Surface growth on alkaline peptone water	Haemolysis Biochemical tests Specific antisera		C		T
Clostridial	Exudate Tissue Blood culture	Blood agar Cooked-meat broth	Anaerobic	Neomycin Differential heating	Biochemical tests Toxin neutralization tests Animal pathogenicity		C.T.P.A.	K	Su.H.serotherapy
Diphtheria	Exudate (membrane) Throat swab	Blood agar Loeffler's medium Blood tellurite media	Aerobic		Biochemical tests Toxin neutralization tests Animal pathogenicity		P.E.L.		
Gonococcal	Exudate from urethra, cervix, rectum, conjunctiva Serum	Blood agar Heated blood agar Thayer-Martin medium	Air + CO_2 (high humidity)		Oxidase tests Biochemical tests	Complement fixation test	C.T.K.		P.H.A.
Haemophilus	Sputum Exudate from eye CSF Blood culture	Blood agar Heated blood agar Levinthal or Fildes agar	Aerobic Air + CO_2	Penicillin	Growth requirement Specific antisera*		K.C.T.M.	P	E.L.H.
Leptospiral	Blood culture Serum Urine	Serum broth enrichment media	Aerobic Micro-aerophilic	Animal inoculation	Dark ground microscopy Specific antisera	Agglutination tests	P.K.T.		
Meningococcal	CSF Blood culture Post nasal swabs (carriers)	Blood agar Heated blood agar	Air + CO_2 (high humidity) Anaerobic		Oxidase test Biochemical tests Specific antisera*		P.C.A.H.		Su.M.
Pasteurella	Exudate Aspirate (bubo) Blood culture Sputum Serum	Blood agar Nutrient agar	Aerobic		Biochemical tests Animal pathogenicity	Agglutination tests*	K.C.T.M.		T.P.
Pneumococcal	Sputum CSF Blood culture Exudate (ear, eye, etc.) Throat swab	Blood agar	Air + CO_2 Anaerobic	Optochin	Biochemical tests Specific antisera* Animal pathogenicity		P.C.E.M.H.	K.	Su.

The Laboratory Diagnosis of Bacterial Infections of Man —*continued*

Nature of infection	Specimens to be submitted for examination	Media for primary inoculation	Atmosphere for incubation	Techniques and selective agents for separation	Further steps for identification of the causal organism	Indirect methods of diagnosis	Antibiograms Fixed Sensitive	Antibiograms Fixed Resistant	Antibiograms Variable
Proteus	Urine Exudate	MacConkey's agar 4% agar	Aerobic	Inhibition of swarming	Biochemical tests		K.C.M.	T.	Su.A.H.
Pseudomonas	Urine Exudate CSF	Blood agar Nutrient agar MacConkey's agar	Aerobic	Chloroxylenol or Cetrimide	Pigment production Oxidase test Phage typing* Pyocine typing*		Poly.		Su.C.T.K.B.
Salmonella — Enteric Fever	Blood culture Faeces Urine Serum	MacConkey's agar. DCA Wilson & Blair's medium	Aerobic	Enrichment broth media	Biochemical tests Specific antisera Phage typing*	Agglutination tests (Widal reaction)	C.A.		T.M.H.
Salmonella — Food poisoning	Faeces Vomit Food Blood culture	MacConkey's agar. DCA Wilson & Blair's medium	Aerobic	Enrichment broth media	Biochemical tests Specific antisera Phage typing*		C.A.		T.M.H.
Shigella	Faeces	MacConkey's medium DCA	Aerobic	Enrichment broth media	Biochemical tests Specific antisera Colicine typing*				Su.C.T.K.Poly.
Staphylococcal	Exudates Anterior nares Flexures } Carriers Tissue Blood culture Serum	Blood agar milk agar	Aerobic	7–10% NaCl (faeces, food)	Coagulase test (Phosphatase test) Phage typing*	Anti α-staphylolysin*	Ox.		P.K.C.T.E.A.M.F.
Streptococcal — caused by *Strept. pyogenes*	Exudates Throat swab High vaginal swab Blood culture Serum	Blood agar	Aerobic Anaerobic	Crystal violet	(Lancefield grouping) Bacitracin sensitivity — Lancefield Group A Griffith typing*	Antistreptolysin O.* Anti-DNAase anti-hyaluronidase*	P.C.E.‡L.M.	K.	T.
Streptococcal — caused by other α & β haemolytic streptococci	Exudate Blood culture	Blood agar	Aerobic Anaerobic	Crystal violet	Bacitracin resistance — other Lancefield Groups		E.L.M.	K.	P.C.T.A.
Treponemal	Exudate Serum				Dark ground microscopy	Complement fixation tests Flocculation tests (VDRL) Immobilization and fluorescent antibody tests* *Trep. pallidium* haemagglutination inhibition	P.C.T.		
Tuberculosis Mycobacteria	Sputum Exudate Urine CSF	Egg media, e.g. Löwenstein-Jensen	Aerobic (6–8 weeks)	Concentration and preparation of specimen	Differentiation from *atypical* forms by various tests	Tuberculin skin test			S.I.Pas.T.R.
Whooping cough	Pharyngeal/laryngeal swab Cough plate Throat washings	Special blood media, e.g. Bordet-Gengou	Aerobic	Penicillin	Specific antisera.		C.T.H.M.		

Antibiograms
Fixed, (sensitive/resistant) = invariable or very frequently obtained results of *in vitro* tests.
Variable   = strains vary significantly in their sensitivity to the antibiotics listed.

B = Carbenicillin	A = Ampicillin	K = amino-sugars	P = Penicillin
F = Fusidic acid	C = Chloramphenicol	M = Cotrimoxazole	Poly = Polymyxins
H = Cephalosporins	E = Erythromycin	Ox = Cloxacillin, Flucloxacillin	S = Streptomycin
L = Lincomycin, clindamycin	I = Isonicotinic acid hydrazide	Pas = Para-amino-salicylic acid	Su = Sulphonamides
		R = Rifampicin	T = Tetracyclines

* Although many pathogenic bacteria are sensitive to chloramphenicol the use of this drug should be restricted to typhoid fever, *H. influenzae* meningitis and serious infections when its administration may be strongly indicated.

* Tests requiring special laboratory facilities.

‡ A few reports of resistance have appeared in isolated areas.

Appendix 4

THE LABORATORY DIAGNOSIS OF VIRAL, CHLAMYDIAL, RICKETTSIAL AND MYCOPLASMAL INFECTIONS OF MAN

Disease	Detection of virus			Detection of serum antibodies	
	Material required	Transport to laboratory	Tests used	Dates for collection of sera	Tests used
Variola	1. Serum in pre-eruptive phase	By hand or by post	Virus cultivation Microscopy for elementary bodies Electron-microscopy Cultures on allantoic membrane Agar gel precipitation, immune electro-phoresis for viral antigen	Before 5th and after 15th day	Comp. fixation; Neutralization
Vaccinia Cowpox	2. 6 films on slides made from scrapings of macules and papules	,,			
	3. Vesicle fluid in capillary tubes	,,			
	4. Crusts in screw-capped bottles	,,			
Varicella Herpes zoster	Vesicle fluid	By hand or by post	Microscopy for elementary bodies and giant cells Electron-microscopy Complement fixation for viral antigen Tissue culture	Before 5th and after 15th day	Comp. fixation
Herpes simplex	1. Vesicle fluid	Frozen	Electron-microscopy Egg, animal, or tissue culture inoculation	Before 5th and after 15th day	Comp. fixation; Neutralization
	2. Crusts or scrapings from bases of lesions on slides	Frozen			
	3. Skin or brain from autopsy	In glycerol saline and frozen			
Cytomegalic virus infection	Respiratory secretions, urine, venous blood	By hand or frozen	Microscopy for inclusions, immuno-fluorescence, virus isolation	At any time	Comp. fixation
Infectious mononucleosis	Venous blood	By hand or by post	Not practicable	Before 3rd and after 15th day	Paul Bunnell, immunofluorescence
Influenza	1. Throat washings in first 48 hours	Frozen	Egg, ferret or tissue culture inoculation	Before 3rd and after 15th day	Comp. fixation; Haemagglutination-inhibition Indirect immuno-fluorescence
	2. Throat swab (children)	Frozen			
	3. Lung tissue at autopsy	Frozen			
Acute Respiratory Disease due to: (a) Parainfluenza viruses, RSV, etc.	Throat washings or throat swabs	Frozen	Tissue culture inoculation	Before 3rd and after 15th day	Neutralization; Comp. fixation Haemagglutination-inhibition (group) Indirect immuno-fluorescence

The Laboratory Diagnosis of Viral, Chlamydial, Rickettsial and Mycoplasmal Infections of Man—*continued*

Disease	Detection of virus			Detection of serum antibodies	
	Material required	Transport to laboratory	Tests used	Dates for collection of sera	Tests used
(b) Adenoviruses	1. Throat washings or throat swab	By hand or by post	Tissue or organ culture inoculation	Before 3rd and after 15th day	Comp. fixation (group); Neutralization (type)
	2. Conjunctival swab	,,	,,		
	3. Sputum	,,	,,		
(c) Rhinoviruses and coronaviruses	4. Nasal secretions	,,	,,		Plaque reduction
Measles	Throat and oral swab	Immediate	Tissue culture inoculation	Before 3rd and after 15th day	Neutralization; Comp. fixation
Mumps	1. Saliva during first 3 days	Frozen	Egg inoculation, monkey kidney or human epithelial cells	During first 6 days and after 21st day	Comp. fixation; Haemagglutination-inhibition
	2. Cerebrospinal fluid in first 3 days of encephalitis				
Rubella (German measles)	1. Throat secretions	Immediate	Culture in primary monkey or human embryonic cells or cell cultures, e.g. GRK or BHK	From onset of disease or at any necessary time	Haemagglutination-inhibition Comp. fixation
	2. Tissues from mother or embryo				
Encephalitis (Herpes; Louping ill, and Arthropod borne virus infections)	1. CSF in first 4 days	Frozen	Animal inoculation	Before 5th and after 14th day	Haemagglutination inhibition; Neutralization; Comp. fixation
	2. Brain from autopsy in glycerol saline	Frozen			
Lymphocytic choriomeningitis	1. CSF ⎫ in first 2. Citrated blood ⎬ 4 days	Frozen	Animal inoculation	Before 10th day, after 21st day and again after 50 days	Comp. fixation
Poliomyelitis	1. Whole blood during prodromal period	By hand or frozen	Inoculation of animal or tissue cultures	Before 3rd and after 14th day	Neutralization; Comp. fixation
	2. Pharyngeal swab during first week	By hand or frozen			Metabolic inhibition tests
	3. Faeces	By hand or by post			
	4. Brain or spinal cord from autopsy	In glycerol saline by hand or by post	Inoculation of animal or tissue cultures		
ECHO Virus infections; Coxsackie virus infections; Bornholm disease; Herpangina; Aseptic meningitis	1. Faeces or rectal swabs ⎫ during 2. Swabs from ⎬ first oral lesions ⎭ 3 days 3. CSF	By hand or frozen	Suckling mouse inoculation Tissue culture inoculation	Before 5th and after 21st day	Neutralization; Comp. fixation haemagglutination inhibition in some
Hepatitis A & B	Venous blood	By hand or by post	Immune electrophoresis: radio-immune assay, electron-microscopy, comp. fixation, haemagglutination-inhibition	At any time	Immune electrophoresis, comp. fixation, haemagglutination-inhibition
Rabies	1. Saliva	Frozen	Animal inoculation		
	2. Animal brain One half in glycerol saline One half in Zenker's solution	By hand or by post	Indirect immuno-fluorescence Animal inoculation Examination for Negri bodies		Neutralization

The Laboratory Diagnosis of Viral, Chlamydial, Rickettsial and Mycoplasmal Infections of Man—*continued*

| Disease | Detection of virus | | | Detection of serum antibodies | |
	Material required	Transport to laboratory	Tests used	Dates for collection of sera	Tests used
Psittacosis	1. Sputum ⎱ in 2. Citrated ⎰ acute blood ⎰ phase	Frozen	Egg or animal inoculation, or Infection of McCoy irradiated cells	If possible before 6th day and after 21st day	Comp. fixation
	3. Lung and spleen from autopsy	Frozen	Egg or animal inoculation		
Lymphogranuloma venereum	1. Pus from bubo	Frozen	Animal or egg inoculation	After 21st day, and if possible before 10th day	Comp. fixation
	2. Biopsy material	One portion of biopsy material to be frozen, another fixed in Zenker's fluid	Histological picture. Frei's test positive after 2 weeks		
Primary atypical pneumonia	Sputum in first 4 days	Frozen	Animal, egg or tissue culture inoculation Special medium for PPLO	Before 7th and after 14th day	Comp. fixation for Q. fever, psittacosis, influenza; Myco-plasma, Strep M.G. agglut.; Cold. agglutinins
Trachoma; Inclusion conjunctivitis	Smears of scrapings from tarsal conjunctiva	By hand or by post	Microscopy for elementary bodies and inclusions Egg or tissue culture inoculation		Comp. fixation
Rickettsial infections	Whole blood	Immediate	Animal or egg inoculation	Before 6th day After 21st day	Weil-Felix, agglu-tination and Comp. fixation

Note.—Routine tests for all the virus infections listed may not be available. In special emergencies the laboratory should always be consulted. This table has been considerably modified from that in *Virus and Rickettsial Diseases*. Edward Arnold and Company, London (1961).

Appendix 5

DOCUMENTATION OF SPECIMENS IN THE LABORATORY

Specimens should be dealt with as expeditiously as possible after arrival at the laboratory, and efforts to deliver the material rapidly from the patient must not be vitiated by unnecessary delays consequent upon specimens lying about unattended. Great care must be taken to identify specimens and request forms on arrival at the laboratory so that when their future separation occurs no mistake will arise: this is best carried out by having a responsible person label all specimens and corresponding forms with a duplicate serial number. For this purpose serial numbers printed on gummed paper, in duplicate, triplicate, etc., may be purchased; these are also useful for identifying tubes and culture plates that are used for the examination of the specimen. Different colours and prefixes may be usefully employed to distinguish different types of specimen or series of examinations and this facilitates record keeping and identification, e.g. T for tuberculosis, U for urine examination. These serial numbers can be used for chronological clerking of specimens which serves as a cross reference system to an alphabetical filing system.

In most cases it is valuable to examine and report on each specimen in the light of previous knowledge of the patient. The information given by practitioners on bacteriological request forms is not usually sufficient for this and it is preferable to have the results of previous bacteriological examination(s) available in each case. This can be done by filing the results of all examinations on a card for each patient; it is more informative and less time-consuming if all laboratory findings are recorded on the reverse side of each request form and to file this in a small envelope or folder for each patient along with a copy of the report issued. This occupies less filing space. The colour of the folders may be changed at six month intervals and one year's work is kept readily available. At the end of each six month period files more than one year old are removed for storage and later destroyed.

As each specimen arrives at the laboratory, the file for the patient is withdrawn and it accompanies the specimen throughout its examination; in this way the bacteriologist may direct his examination and interpret his findings in the light of all the previous reports.

REFERENCES

CASH, J. D. (1971) An envelope designed to facilitate safer transport and rapid identification of 'high risk' specimens in hospital laboratories. *Journal of Clinical Pathology*, **24**, 367.

CRUICKSHANK, R. (1953) Clinical pathology in general practice—taking swabs. *British Medical Journal*, **ii**, 1095.

ELLIOT, W. A. & SLEIGH, J. D. (1963) Container for transport of urine specimens at low temperature. *British Medical Journal*, **i**, 1142.

HOUGHTON, B. J. & PEARS, M. A. (1957) Cell excretion in normal urine. *British Medical Journal*, **i**, 622.

MCGEACHIE, J. & KENNEDY, A. C. (1963) Simplified quantitative methods for bacteriuria and pyuria. *Journal of Clinical Pathology*, **16**, 32.

STRAKER, EDITH, HILL, A. B. & LOVELL, R. (1939) A study of the nasopharyngeal bacterial flora of different groups of persons observed in London and South-East England during the years 1930 to 1937. London: H.M.S.O.

RUBBO, S. D. & BENJAMIN, M. (1951) Some observations on survival of pathogenic bacteria on cotton-wool swabs. Development of a new type of swab. *British Medical Journal*, **i**, 983.

GENERAL READING

BEDSON, S. P., DOWNIE, A. W., MACCALLUM, F. O. & STEWART-HARRIS, C. H. (1967) *Virus and Rickettsial Diseases of Man*, 4th edn. London: Arnold.

STOKES, E. JOAN (1960) *Clinical Bacteriology*, 2nd edn. London: Arnold.

THOMSON, W. A. R. (ed.) (1971) *Calling the Laboratory*, 3rd edn. Edinburgh: Livingstone.

Appendix 6

ABBREVIATIONS AND CONVERSION FACTORS

Mass

g   = gram
kg = kilogram (1 kg = 1000 g)
mg = milligram (1 mg = 0·001 g)
μg = microgram (1 μg = 0·001 mg)
lb = pound weight avoirdupois
      (1 lb = 453·6 g)

Length

m   = metre
cm = centimetre (1 cm = 0·01 m)
mm = millimetre (1 mm = 0·001 m)
μm = micrometre (10^{-6} metre)
nm = nanometre (1 nm = 10^{-9} m)
in = inch (1 inch = 2·54 cm)
ft = foot (1 ft = 12 in)

Area

in^2 = square inch (1 in^2 = 6·45 cm^2)

Volume

l   = litre (1 l = 1·76 pints)
ml = millilitre (1 ml = 0·001 l)
μl = microlitre (1 μl = 0·001 ml)
oz = fluid ounce (1 oz = 28·41 ml)
ft^3 = cubic foot (1 ft^3 = 28·3 l)

Temperature

X°C = X degrees Centigrade
Conversion of X° Centigrade to X° Fahrenheit:
$$X°F = 1·8X°C + 32$$

Time

h = hour   min = minute   s = second

Other Abbreviations

N   = normal (e.g. 2 N HCl)
M   = molar (e.g. 0·1 M Na_2CO_3)
rev/min = revolutions per minute
mV   = millivolt
parts/10^6 = parts per million
LD50   = average lethal dose
MLD   = minimum lethal dose
MHD   = minimum haemolytic dose
per cent   The percentage concentration of solution is stated as g of solute per 100 ml of solution, i.e. as per cent (w/v). Unless otherwise indicated the solvent is *water*. Per cent (v/v) = ml of substance per 100 ml of mixture, as in gas mixtures.
g   = force of gravity

See *Units, Symbols and Abbreviations* for further details. Obtainable from Editorial Office, Royal Society of Medicine, 1 Wimpole St., London, W1M 8AE.

Index

Index

Filmset in 'Monophoto' by Technical Filmsetters Europe Ltd,
and
Printed by T. & A. Constable Ltd, Edinburgh, Scotland